FRONTIERS IN PERITONEAL DIALYSIS

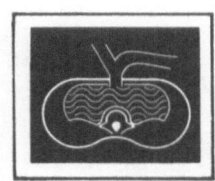

FRONTIERS IN PERITONEAL DIALYSIS

EDITED BY JOHN F. MAHER, M.D.
PROFESSOR OF MEDICINE
UNIFORMED SERVICES UNIVERSITY OF THE HEALTH SCIENCES
BETHESDA, MARYLAND, U.S.A.

JAMES F. WINCHESTER, M.D.
ASSOCIATE PROFESSOR OF MEDICINE
GEORGETOWN UNIVERSITY MEDICAL CENTER
WASHINGTON, D.C., U.S.A.

Springer-Verlag Berlin Heidelberg GmbH

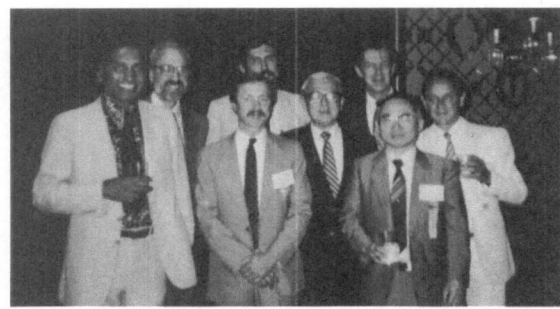

Officers and Councillors of the International Society for
Peritoneal Dialysis; from left to right, R. Gokal (U.K.),
K. Nolph (U.S.A.), J. Winchester (U.S.A.), A. Treviño-
Becerra (Mexico), F. Boen (Netherlands), J. Maher
(U.S.A.), K. Ota (Japan), J. Bergström (Sweden); not
shown N. Thomson (Australia).

THIS PUBLICATION IS SUPPORTED IN PART
BY A GRANT FROM THE NATIONAL KIDNEY FOUNDATION, INC.

SUPPORTERS OF THE III INTERNATIONAL SYMPOSIUM ON
PERITONEAL DIALYSIS

Abbott Laboratories
American Kidney Fund
AMP/DELMED Dialysis Group
Amuchina
E.I. Dupont De Nemours & Co., Inc.
Fresenius Foundation
Fogarty International Center, NIH
Gambro Lundia AB
W.L. Gore and Associates, Inc.

Merck, Sharpe and Dohme
National Institute of Arthritis, Diabetes and
    Digestive and Kidney Diseases
National Kidney Foundation of the National Capital
    Area
Pfizer Pharmaceuticals
Stuart Pharmaceuticals Division of ICI Americas,
    Inc.
Travenol Laboratories

ISBN 978-3-662-11786-6   ISBN 978-3-662-11784-2 (eBook)
DOI 10.1007/978-3-662-11784-2
Library of Congress Catalog Card Number: 85-80199

Contents

SECTION II. TECHNOLOGY, ACCESS, SOLUTIONS

SECTION V: COMPLICATIONS, PERITONITIS, AND RESPONSE TO INFECTION

Preface

The III International Symposium on Peritoneal Dialysis was held in Washington, DC, June 17 to 20, 1984. The 980 attendees came from all continents, 30 countries, and more than half were from the United States of America. The diversity of attendance was reflected by a similar dispersion of geography and scientific interests found in the 295 abstracts submitted for presentation. These *Proceedings* encompass 125 manuscripts of papers presented at the Symposium as standard slide presentations, posters or components of panel discussions.

This Symposium was considerably larger than its two successful predecessors, in Chapala, Mexico, 1978, and in W. Berlin, FRG, 1981. Indeed, the organization of the Symposium has become sufficiently formidable that we are pleased that the newly founded International Society for Peritoneal Dialysis now represents a resource to facilitate future Symposia. The President of the new Society is Dr. John F. Maher. The reader should note that the IV International Symposium on Peritoneal Dialysis will be held in Venice, Italy, June 9 to 13, 1987, and also that information about joining the Society can be obtained from the Secretary-Treasurer, Dr. J. F. Winchester, Georgetown University Hospital, Washington, DC, 20007, USA.

Without the timely contributions of the authors, these *Proceedings* would not have been possible. Moreover, in their role as organizers of the Symposium, the Editors appreciate the help of the Executive, Scientific, and Local Organizing Committee of the Symposium.

The success of the Symposium also reflects the generous support of numerous organizations and foundations listed. Without their assistance the expenses of the Symposium would have been overwhelming.

These *Proceedings* have been generously supported by a grant from Abbott Laboratories, by the National Kidney Foundation and by contributions from Gambro AB, Travenol Laboratories, and The National Institute of Health.

The International Society for Peritoneal Dialysis was established to promote knowledge about peritoneal dialysis. The *Peritoneal Dialysis Bulletin*, the official publication of the Society, has already promoted such knowledge commendably. The Editors earnestly hope that these *Proceedings* will foster increased knowledge and enlighten and update the reader about the current techniques, results and problems associated with peritoneal dialysis.

JOHN F. MAHER, M.D.
JAMES F. WINCHESTER, M.D.
EDITORS

SECTION I

Morphology, Physiology, Kinetics, Drugs

J.W. Dobbie and M.A. Zaki

1

The Ultrastructure of the Parietal Peritoneum in Normal and Uremic Man and in Patients on CAPD

SUMMARY

The peritoneum was examined by electron microscopy using biopsy specimens of normal tissue of uremic patients commencing CAPD and of patients after three days to 28 mo of CAPD. The normal and uremic peritoneum demonstrate a cobblestone or waved ridge pattern of mesothelial cells with abundant microvilli. Definite ultrastructural changes in the mesothelial and submesothelial tissues occur after exposure to dialysis fluid, which are more pronounced after multiple attacks of peritonitis.

INTRODUCTION

In 1730, James Douglas gave the first modern description of the structure of the human peritoneum. He observed that it was "everywhere smooth and even and lubricated by a fluid in order to preserve it from those inconveniences which otherwise have followed from its continual attrition with other viscera."[1] As Douglas observed, the peritoneum is designed to reduce friction as internal organs move one over the other. With the advent of continuous peritoneal dialysis, it should be appreciated that the use of the peritoneum as a dialysing membrane may frustrate the natural functions of this most delicate of tissues.

From the University Department of Medicine and Renal Unit, Glasgow Royal Infirmary, Glasgow, Scotland.

Hitherto, scant interest has been shown in the morphology of the peritoneum, and what little information is available, has been derived from studies on the experimental animal.[2-6] Increasing clinical concern over the long-term effects on the peritoneum of continued exposure to dialysis fluid, and to repeated attacks of chemical or bacterial peritonitis, has recently stimulated an interest in its ultrastructure.[7-9] Thus the use of an increasingly popular form of life support system has called to account our lack of basic knowledge on the morphology of the peritoneum.

MATERIAL AND METHODS

Ten peritoneal biopsies were obtained at routine surgical operations from 10 patients whose peritoneum was normal on microscopic inspection and who had no history either of previous peritonitis, abdominal operations, or serious pathology of the abdominal viscera. Twenty peritoneal biopsies were obtained from 20 patients with end-stage renal failure at the time of insertion of their first peritoneal catheter. Twenty biopsies were obtained from 20 patients who had been treated with continuous ambulatory peritoneal dialysis (CAPD) for periods ranging between 3 days and 28 months. The biopsies were carefully removed from the parietal peritoneum of the anterior abdominal wall, immediately on opening the abdominal cavity. The tissue was not touched, rubbed, or stretched either manually or with swabs or instruments, but was immediately immersed in cold, buffered, isotonic fixative (2% glutaraldehyde in Sorensen's phosphate buffer). The tissue for light and transmission electron microscopy (TEM) was postfixed in 1% osmic acid and embedded in Epon. The tissue for scanning electron microscopy (SEM) was subjected to critical-point drying and sputter-coated with gold. Both random and serial sections were cut from the prepared blocks. Tracings made from the serial sections were used to make three-dimensional reconstructions of the mesothelial cells and their organelles. Sections mounted on formvar-coated, carbon-reinforced slit grids were used to construct montages of strips of mesothelium in order to study the spatial relation-ships between cellular components of the mesothelium and the underlying structures.

RESULTS

No significant qualitative differences were observed in the ultrastructure of biopsies obtained from normal controls or uremic patients.

Normal Peritoneum

At low magnification, SEM of normal human peritoneum shows a pavementation pattern. The ap-

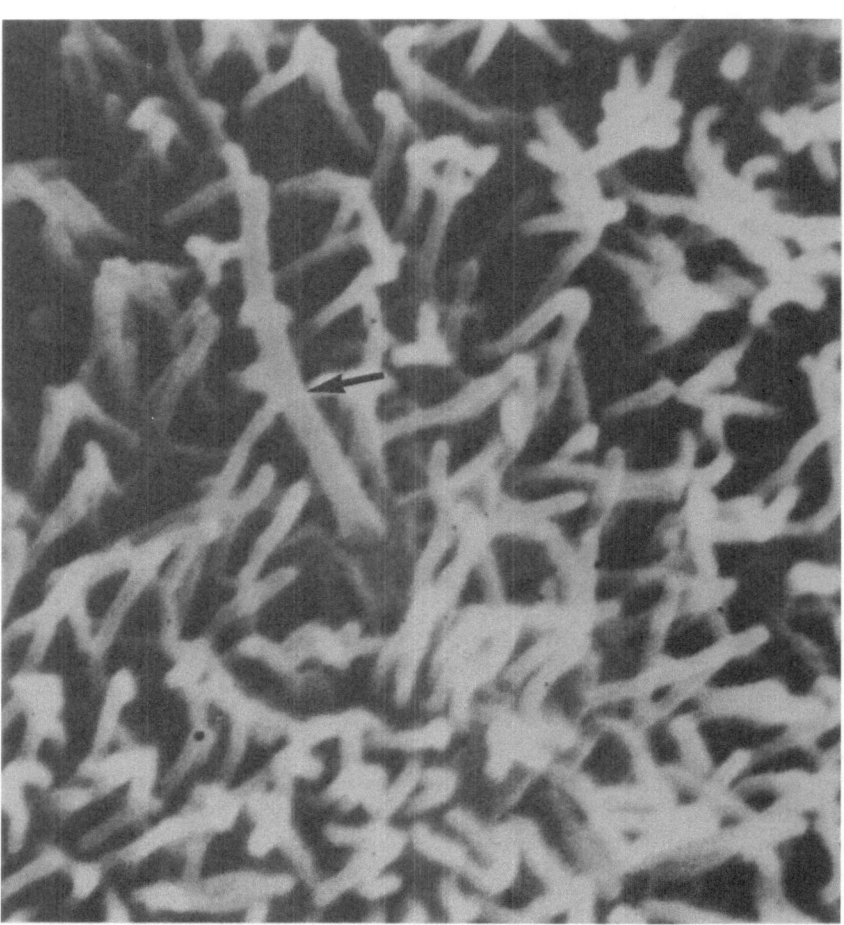

Fig. 1. SEM of normal human parietal mesothelium (anterior abdominal wall), showing a thick carpet of profuse microvilli. A cilium is arrowed. Magnification × 37,500.

pearance and interpretation of scanning electron micrographs of mesothelium, however, are complicated by the presence of underlying structures that may undergo differential changes in shape and size during fixation and dehydration. Thus a cobblestone pattern may be seen in areas of the peritoneum that have been fixed in a relaxed state, and a waved ridge pattern may be seen in other areas that have undergone stretching.

Normal human parietal mesothelium is covered by a thick carpet of profuse microvilli, whose features are best demonstrated by SEM (Fig. 1). Examination at high magnification with SEM reveals the other characteristic feature of mesothelial cells, the surface pits representing the openings of the micropinocytotic vesicles. In addition to the microvilli, other small rounded surface projections, known as blebs, may be seen. In normal mesothelium these are few in number, but in damaged peritoneum, their numbers are markedly increased.

TEM of normal human mesothelium demonstrates a nucleus that is oval or cigar-shaped in profile. In contracted cells it may also assume a highly convoluted form with cytoplasmic invaginations. The relative abundance of nuclear pores, two prominent nucleoli, and the preponderance of euchromatin over heterochromatin, point to a cell of active synthetic ability. In some nuclei, between the inner nuclear membrane and the outer margin of the heterochromatin, there may be found a homoge-

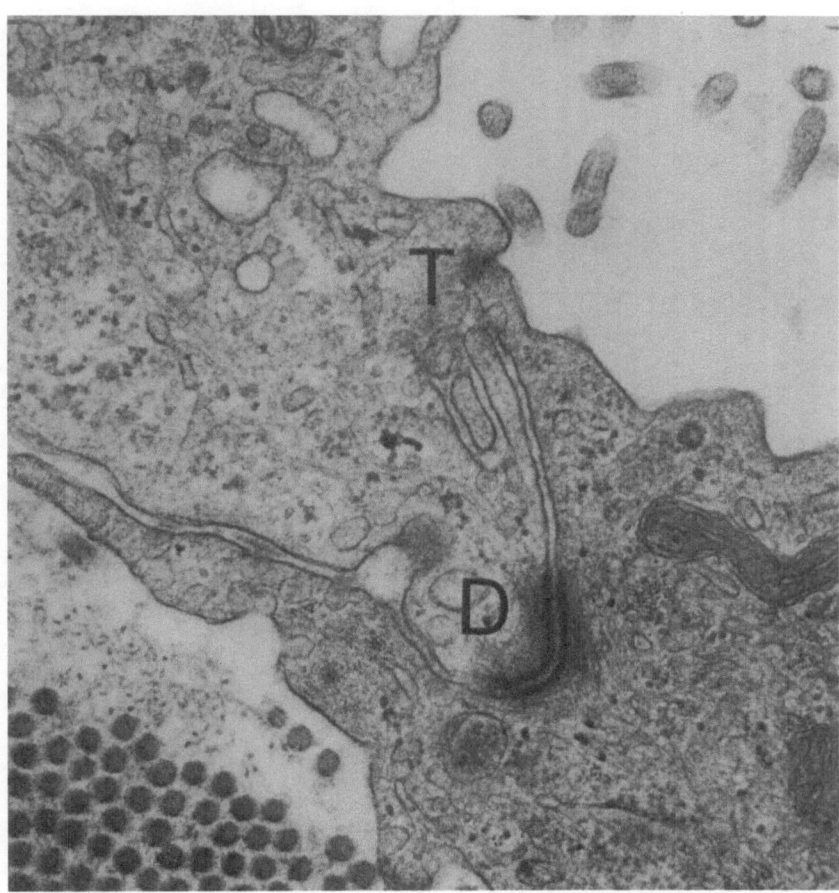

Fig. 2. TEM of normal human mesothelium showing a junctional complex. The tight junction (T) is nearest to the surface. Desmosome (D). Magnification × 61,900.

neous band of moderate electron density, which constitutes the fibrous lamina. Serial electron micrographs demonstrate the relative abundance of mitochondria, which are significantly greater in number than that encountered in endothelial cells. Short lengths of rough endoplasmic reticulum (RER) and free ribosomes are scattered throughout the cytoplasm. A Golgi apparatus of moderate development is present in all cells. Micropinocytotic vesicles are found along both inner and outer margins of the cell

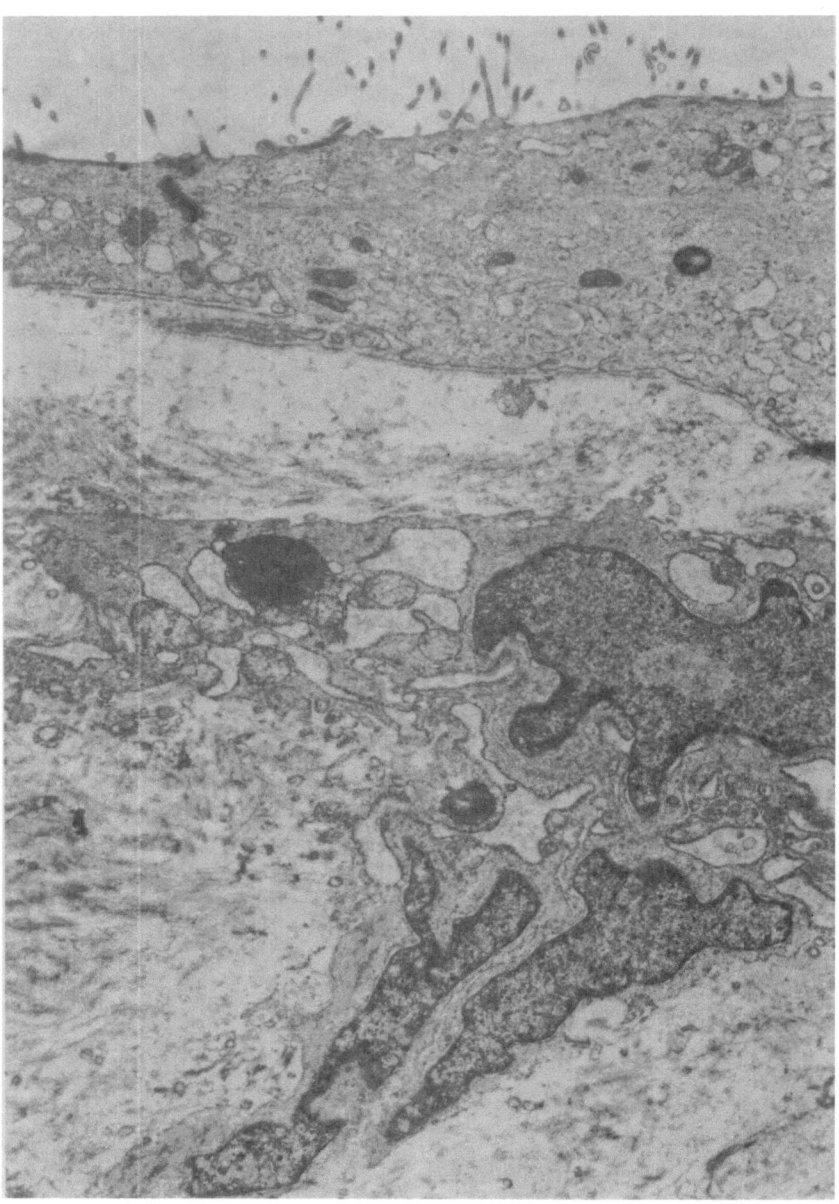

Fig. 3. TEM of peritoneum from patient who had been on CAPD for 28 months, demonstrating submesothelial edema and an active fibroblast close to the basement membrane. Magnification × 9,900.

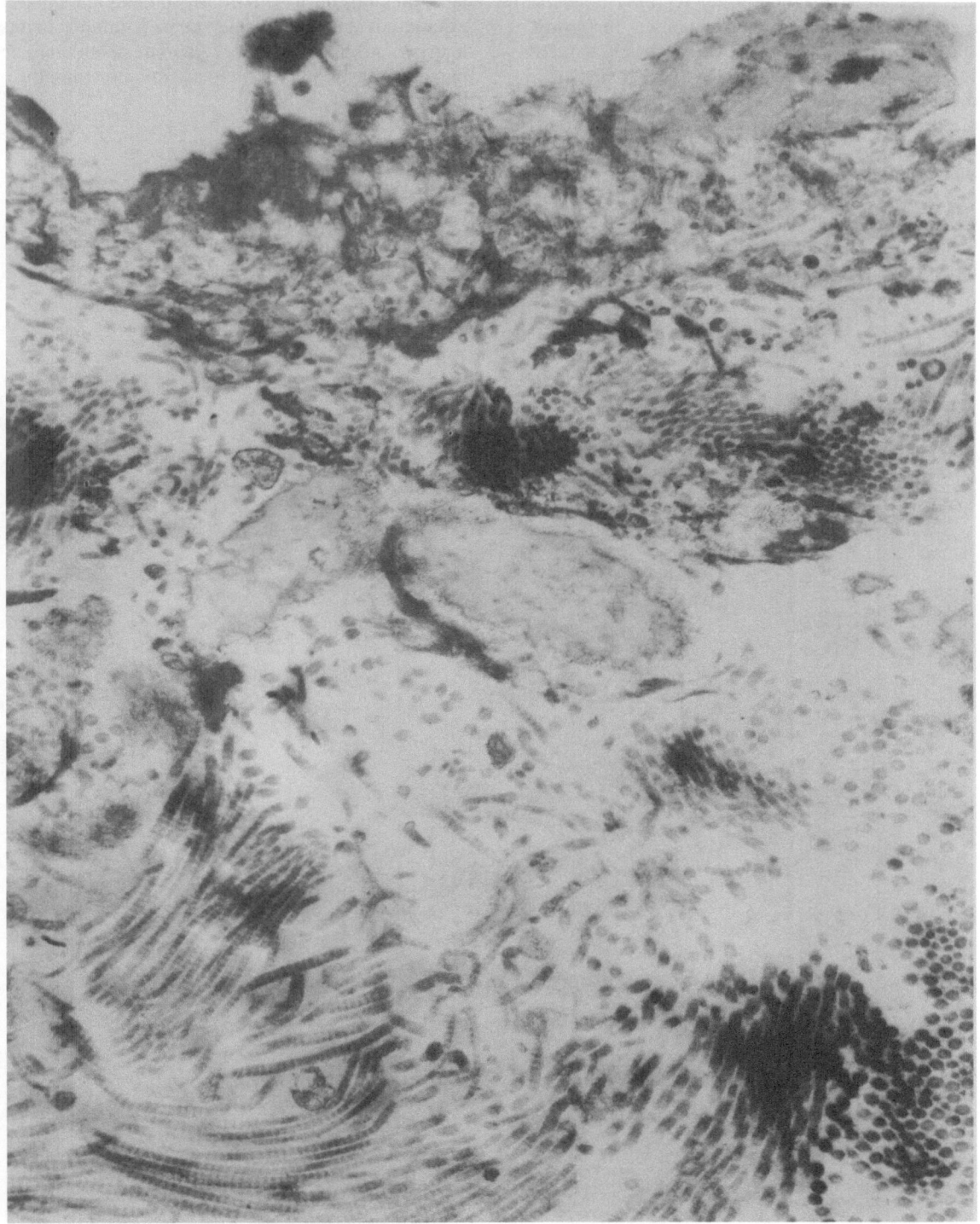

Fig. 4. TEM of peritoneal biopsy obtained from a patient during an episode of fungal peritonitis, showing mesothelial cell denudation, the surface being covered with a fibrin web. The underlying stroma is edematous and the collagen fibers disorganized. Magnification × 20,930.

and also along the junctional regions, along with areas of specialized cell attachment. Phagosomes and lipid vacuoles are only occasionally encountered.

Normal mesothelial cells overlap one on the other in the manner of roof tiles. The apical portion of the mesothelial junctional complex contains a tight or occludens junction, which is macular rather than zonular in type (Fig. 2). Beneath this there are one or two well-developed desmosomes. The basal portion of the cells form a complex series of interlocking processes. The cells rest on a thin basement membrane. The tissue immediately underlying the mesothelium consists of orderly bundles of regularly orientated collagen fibers, set in a homogeneous matrix of ground substance. At some depth there lie bands of elastic fibers, the occasional resting fibroblast, and mast cells.

Peritoneum Exposed to Dialysate

In biopsies obtained from patients after only a few days exposure to dialysate, SEM shows patchy open intercellular clefts. The overall appearances in

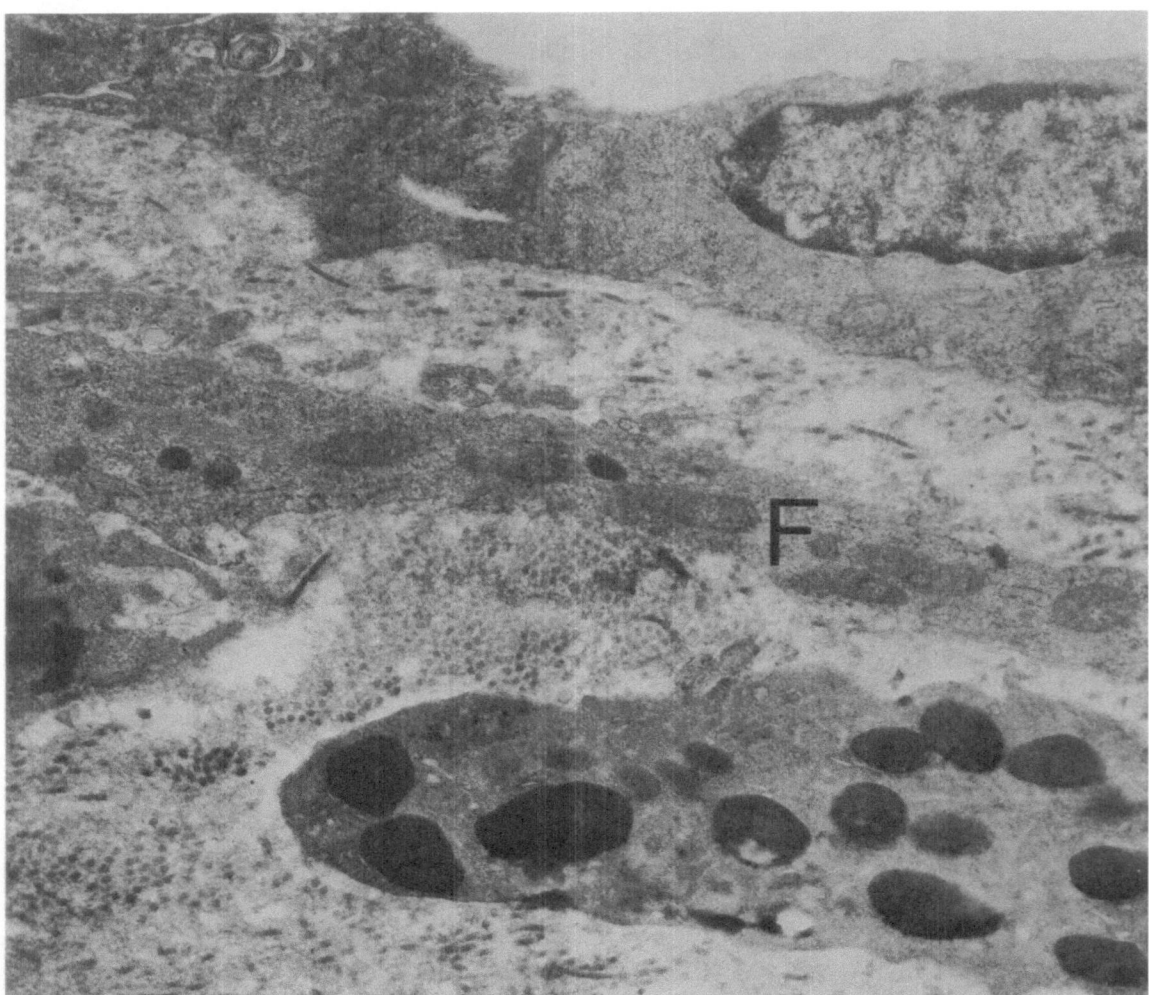

Fig. 5. TEM of peritoneum following a recent episode of bacterial peritonitis. The mesothelial cell cytoplasm is more dense than normal. There is loss of microvilli and micropinocytotic vesicles. The stroma is edematous. Active fibroblasts (F) and mast cells lie close to the mesothelium. Magnification × 20,930.

such specimens suggest that the cause of cell separation is cell shrinkage. TEM of such biopsies show increased density of the cell cytoplasm and a striking development of the RER. Micropinocytotic vesicles, though larger, are less numerous. Minimal edema of the submesothelial tissues may be evident.

With increased periods of exposure to dialysate, active fibroblasts begin to appear immediately under the mesothelium. In biopsies obtained from patients with a history of one or more episodes of peritonitis, the submesothelial stroma shows increased disorganization of the collagen fibers, increased numbers of active fibroblasts, and mast cells (Fig. 3).

Biopsies obtained during an episode of peritonitis frequently show denudation of mesothelial cells. The surface is covered with a layer of fibrin of variable thickness, a continuous cordon of elongated fibroblasts lie immediately beneath the surface, while the edematous stroma is infiltrated with macrophages and acute inflammatory cells and mast cells (Figs. 4 & 5). SEM of nondenuded areas usually show grossly damaged mesothelial cells whose surfaces, devoid of microvilli, are covered in blisters and blebs. Biopsies examined by SEM 2–3 weeks after recovery from peritonitis, still show a grossly irregular, warty, mesothelial surface (Figs. 6 & 7).

Peritoneal biopsies obtained 6–12 weeks after cessation of dialysis, continue to exhibit distinctly irregular pavement patterns of the mesothelium, with accentuation of the intercellular clefts.

DISCUSSION

Peritoneum is a delicate tissue, and if not handled with care, is easily damaged. Collection, fixation, and processing for SEM or TEM must be carried out with maximum regard for the integrity of the fragile monolayer of cells in order to minimize the creation of artifact.

Analysis of the fine structure of the mesothelium in comparison with its sister tissue, the endothelium, is of relevance in understanding its function as a lining membrane and its reaction to injury. Observations on the mesothelial cell with respect to its nuclear composition; its relative abundance of RER, free ribosomes, and mitochondria; and the development of the Golgi apparatus, all suggest a cell possessing synthetic capability significantly greater than that of endothelium. The interest and preoccupation of physiologists and nephrologists in the possible role of the large population of micropinocytotic vesicles in the permeability of the peritoneum is perhaps misplaced. The structural features of the

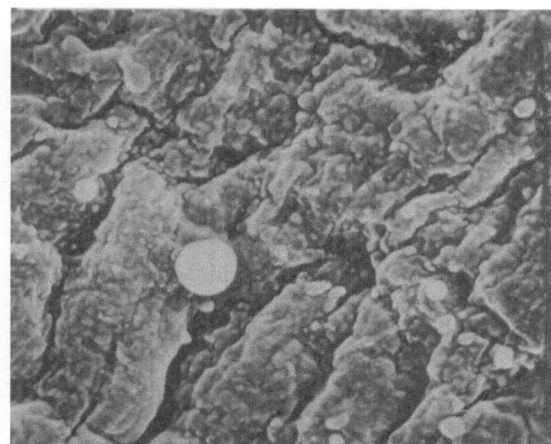

Fig. 6. SEM of specimen shown in Figure 5, showing an irregular warty mesothelial surface, devoid of microvilli. Magnification × 1,650.

cell suggest that the role of the mesothelium is more that of a secretory tissue, whereby lubricant (serous) fluid is liberally delivered by the vesicles into, and entrapped by, the thick web of microvilli. Thus, the signs of possible increased synthetic activity of the mesothelial cells on first exposure to dialysate may be a compensatory response by the cell to the elution of its surface lubricant film by constant washing with dialysate. Therefore, any ultrastructural deviations

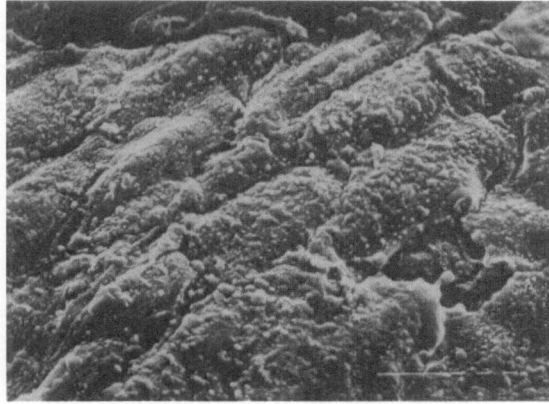

Fig. 7. SEM of biopsy of peritoneum obtained from a patient who had been on CAPD for 11 months and had suffered three episodes of bacterial peritonitis. The biopsy was taken 2 weeks after recovery from the last episode of peritonitis. There is evidence of cell separation and the mesothelial surface is covered with blebs. Magnification × 1,620.

from normality encountered in mesothelium exposed to dialysate may not in fact denote damage.

Our observations indicate that exposure to dialysate results in a variable degree of cell shrinkage and subsequent cell separation. This phenomenon, when extensive, may be of relevance to the problem of loss of ultrafiltration in some patients on CAPD.

Perhaps the most significant observations in this investigation with respect to the effects of peritoneal dialysis are the changes in the submesothelial tissues following episodes of peritonitis. The migration of active fibroblasts underneath the mesothelium, the disorganized and occasionally edematous stoma, together with the increased numbers of mast cells, indicate reactive fibroplasia.

In conclusion, there are definite ultrastructural changes in the mesothelium and submesothelial tissues associated with exposure to dialysis fluid. These changes, which may be minimal in patients who have had no recorded episodes of peritonitis, become more pronounced where there is a history of multiple attacks of peritonitis.

ACKNOWLEDGMENT

This study was generously supported by Travenol Laboratories.

REFERENCES

1. Douglas J: A description of the peritoneum. London: J Roberts, Warwick Lane, 1730

2. Odor DL: Observations of the rat mesothelium with the electron and phase microscopes. J Anat 95: 433, 1954

3. Felix MD, and Dalton AJ: A comparison of mesothelial cells and macrophages in mice after the intraperitoneal innoculation of melanin granules. J Biophys Biochem Cytol 2(Suppl): 109, 1956

4. Baradi AF, and Hope J: Observations on ultrastructure of rabbit mesothelium. Exp Cell Res 34: 33, 1964

5. Andrews PM, and Porter KR: The ultrastructural morphology and possible functional significance of mesothelial microvilli. Anat Rec 177: 409, 1973

6. Gotloib I, Robinovich S, Rodella H, Medline A, and Oreopoulos DG: Ultrastructure of the rabbit mesentery. In Gahl GM, Kessel M, and Nolph KD (Eds), Advances in peritoneal dialysis: Proceedings of the 2nd international symposium on peritoneal dialysis. Amsterdam: Excerpta Medica, 1981, p 27

7. Dobbie JW, Zaki MA, and Wilson L: Ultrastructural studies on the peritoneum with special reference to chronic ambulatory peritoneal dialysis. Scott Med J 26: 213, 1981

8. Dobbie JW, Zaki MA, and Wilson L: The morphology of the peritoneum with special reference to peritoneal dialysis. In Parsons FM, and Ogg CS (Eds), Renal failure—who cares? Lancaster: MTP Press, 1982, p 179

9. Verger C, Brunschvicg O, LeCharpentier Y, Lavergne A, and Vantelon J: Peritoneal structure alterations on CAPD. In Gahl GM, Kessel M, and Nolph KD (Eds), Advances in peritoneal dialysis: Proceedings of the 2nd international symposium on peritoneal dialysis. Amsterdam: Excerpta Medica, 1981, p 10

N. DiPaolo, G. Sacchi, U. Buoncristiani, P. Rossi, E. Gaggiotti,
C. Alessandrini, L. Ibba, and A.M. Pucci

2

The Morphology of the Peritoneum in CAPD Patients

SUMMARY

The structure of the peritoneum has been studied by scanning and transmission electron microscopy and by light microscopy in 38 biopsies of 22 patients undergoing CAPD. Before CAPD the mesothelium was characterized by flattened cells with protruding nuclei, numerous microvilli and many pinocytotic vesicles. After prolonged CAPD there is a reduction and subsequent disappearance of microvilli and a vacuolar separation of cells from the basement membrane, accompanied by widening of intercellular junctions. Neither ultrafiltration rate nor small solute clearance change with these structural alterations. During peritonitis there is extensive cellular necrosis with denuding of the basement membrane. After recovery the mesothelium is replaced by thick fibrous connective tissue.

INTRODUCTION

Much more research has been carried out by light microscopy (LM), transmission electron microscopy (TEM) and scanning electron microscopy (SEM) on the morphology of the peritoneal membrane in animals than in human beings.[1-3] The introduction of CAPD has given an additional impetus to this study in man. The human peritoneal membrane, very similar to that of animals, is made up of a monocellular layer of mesothelium which rests on a continuous basement membrane (BM) overlying several strata of collagen fibers, fibroblasts, blood vessels, and lymphatics, which make up the connective tissue. The mesothelium is substantially the same in all peritoneal areas, with flat cells having an oval nucleus. Several cytoplasmatic organules are present. Microvilli and vesicles are the most important characteristic elements.[1] Careful study (TEM and SEM) of the peritoneal mesothelium shows numerous microvilli on the free surface of the cells, with the quantity varying according to the organ.

The microvilli are not uniformly distributed and are absent in some areas, not due to artifact.[4] The mesothelial cells, which play an important role in peritoneal transport, have oval vesicles grouped mainly on the luminal and basal borders, which at times are arranged in single file cutting across the cells.

The mesothelial cells have tight junctions, zonulae adherens, desmosomes, and intercellular channels in the basal border with a continuous and homogenous BM.[5,6] The submesothelial area consists of interstitial and connective tissue, fibers, collagen bundles, fibroblasts, macrophages, lymphatics and blood vessels, as well as granular material, microfibrillar structures and areas of sparse structure.

If it is true that only the mesothelium situated above the capillaries (2.6% of the total mesothelial surface) is involved in the active solute exchange,[7] and if 80% of the capillaries cannot be perfused,[8] then the active surface is only 0.52% of the mesothelium, which is very close to the theoretical 0.6% of the "pore" theory.[9]

From the Nephrology and Dialysis Departments of Siena and Perugia, and the Anatomy and Histology Institutes, University of Siena, Italy.

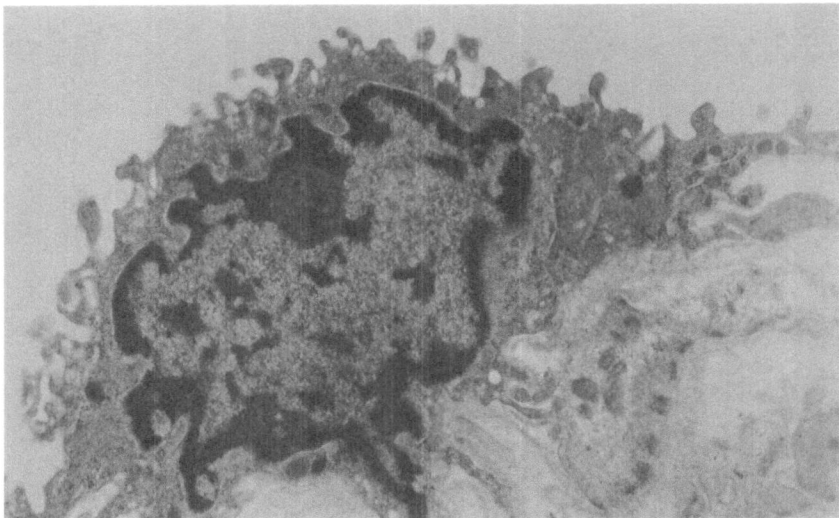

Fig. 1. Mesothelial cell of the parietal peritoneum with many small microvilli near the nucleus. (TEM 10,000 ×).

The presence and wide distribution of the lymph vessels (4% of the surface) suggest their importance in transport. Furthermore, the absence of a continuous BM in the lymphatic wall could indicate a lesser resistance to filtration than the blood vessels; even the fibroblasts of the interstitium might play an active part in solute transport.[10]

The mesothelium in rats on peritoneal dialysis does not reveal morphological alterations in the absence of peritonitis.[11] During these episodes, LM reveals an increase in the wall thickness of the mesothelium, made up of one or more layers of oval cells, hypervascularization, and the presence of a fibrous submesothelial layer. The TEM also shows interstitial edema with many fibroblasts and mast cells, and in some areas the mesothelium has disappeared. With the SEM, we noted intercellular zones between the mesothelial cells that are crossed by cytoplasmic interdigitation, where oval cells are present. A study of peritoneal regeneration in animals after mechanical damage demonstrates that new mesothelial cells originate in the subperitoneal

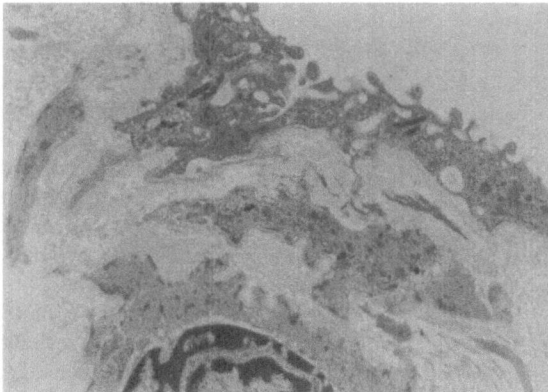

Fig. 2. The borders of this mesothelial cell of the parietal peritoneum are almost completely covered by long microvilli. (TEM 7,700 ×).

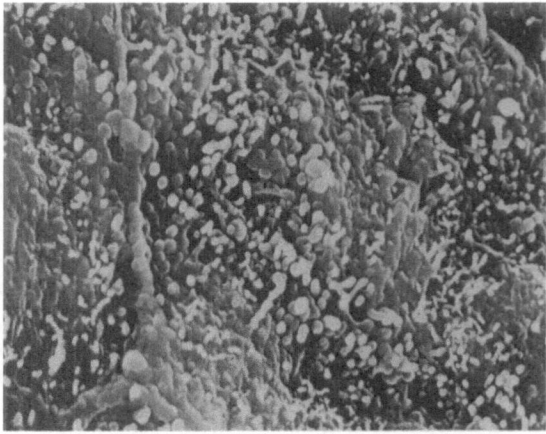

Fig. 3. The parietal peritoneum appears full of microvilli. (SEM 3,100 ×).

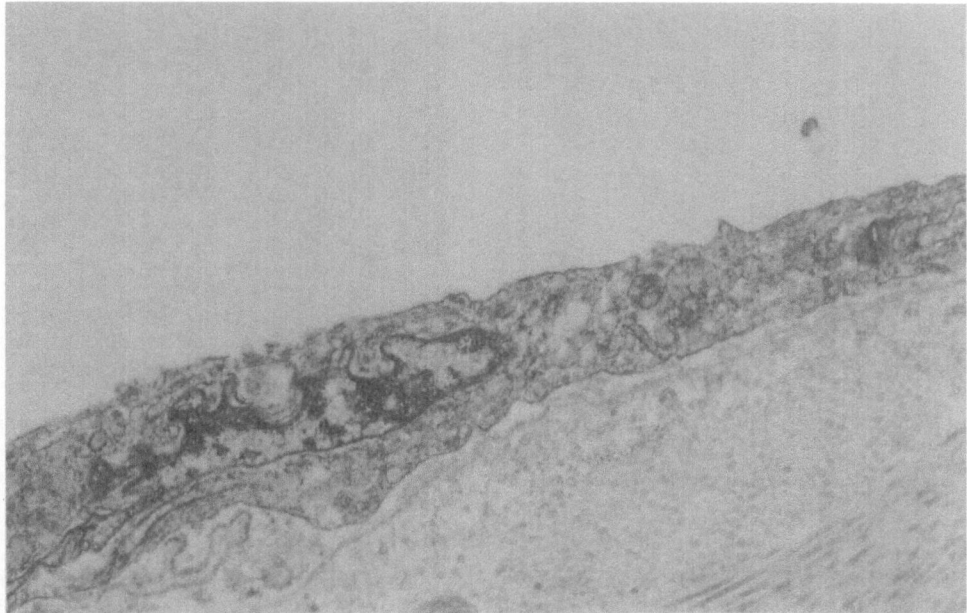

Fig. 4. After 12 mo CAPD with one episode of peritonitis, this patient presents more or less complete absence of microvilli. (TEM 13,500 ×).

connective tissue, while the contribution of the surrounding integral mesothelium is negligible.[12]

The peritoneal membrane in patients on CAPD for one year shows a partial or total disappearance of the mesothelium in most patients, with variation from patient to patient and from sample to sample. When mesothelial cells are present, they may appear to be either thin or cubical with intercellular spaces of varying dimensions and a normal BM. The submesothelial tissue appears fibrous and thicker, and there is often hypervascularization, with changes in the capillary wall.

The fibrous thickening of the submesothelial layer could very well represent a defense against the

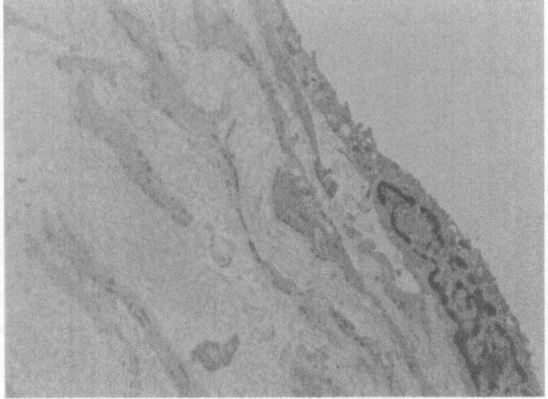

Fig. 5. After 15 mo CAPD with two episodes of peritonitis, the luminal cellular membrane is badly damaged, while the connective tissue seems normal. (TEM 3,500 ×).

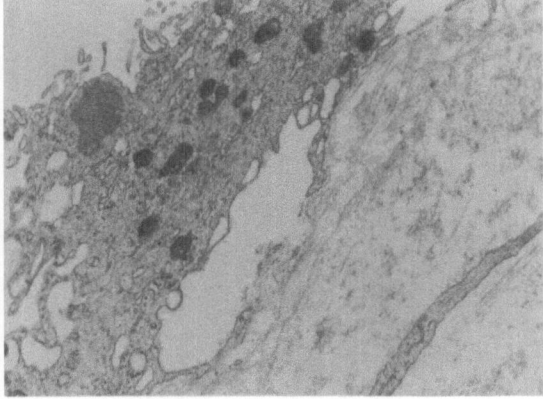

Fig. 6. After 24 mo CAPD with four episodes of peritonitis vacuoles begin to appear in the base of the mesothelial cell and the connective tissue is edematous. (TEM 7,700 ×).

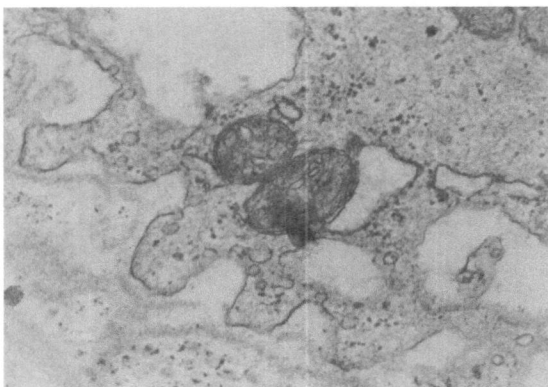

Fig. 7. Using higher magnification for the same case as in Figure 6 we note progressive detachment of the mesothelial cells from the basement membrane. (TEM 35,500 ×).

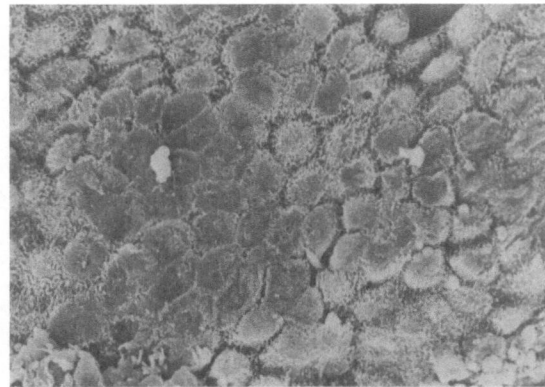

Fig. 9. After 36 mo CAPD with four episodes of peritonitis, extended areas of peritoneum are covered by cells distinctly separate from one another. (SEM 655 ×).

hyperpermeability of glucose and the consequent loss of ultrafiltration capacity.[13, 14] In CAPD patients with previous episodes of peritonitis, there is a sclerotic thickening of the peritoneum with hypervascularization and infiltration of mononuclear cells, but with no signs of birefringent material or giant cells.[15, 16] Some CAPD patients have also been reported to have intestinal occlusion caused by fibrous material, structurally different from the postsurgery and drug-induced fibrosis.[17, 18]

MATERIALS AND METHODS

As there are insufficient data on peritoneal morphology, it is impossible to interpret correctly any variations in peritoneal transport observed over a period of time. Since we also use surgery in our departments for the insertion, removal, and replacement of the peritoneal catheter, we were able to perform 38 peritoneal biopsies on 22 subjects with no discomfort whatsoever for these patients. The specimens were obtained only from the parietal peritoneum, and not from the intestinal or mesenteric peritoneum, to avoid trauma in the patients and also because specific literature does not mention any substantial structural differences between the various peritoneal areas.[4]

Eight patients had peritoneal biopsies before starting CAPD, and 19 patients after from 8 to 40 months. Six patients had biopsies during episodes of peritonitis, and five underwent repeat biopsy after from 1 to 4 months. Bouin's fixative was used for

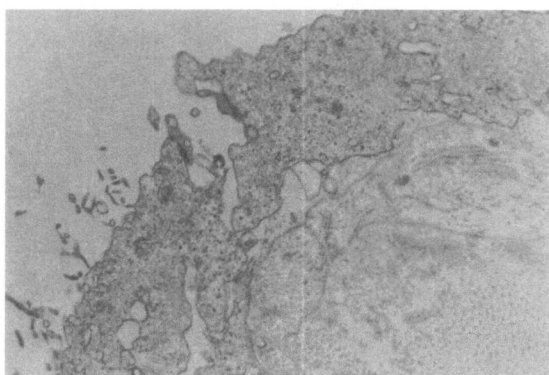

Fig. 8. After 19 mo of CAPD with two peritonitis episodes we note the opening of the intercellular junction. (TEM 10,000 ×).

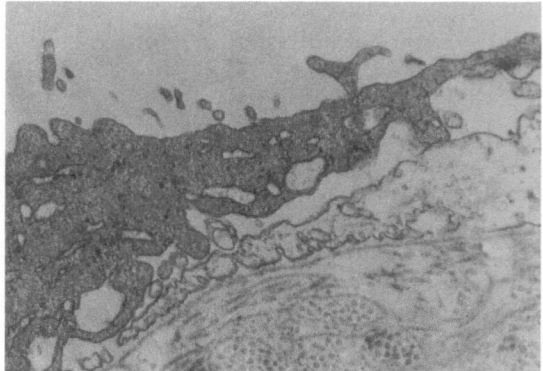

Fig. 10. During peritonitis the intercellular junctions widen and this may also occur between normal and damaged cells. (TEM 12,500 ×).

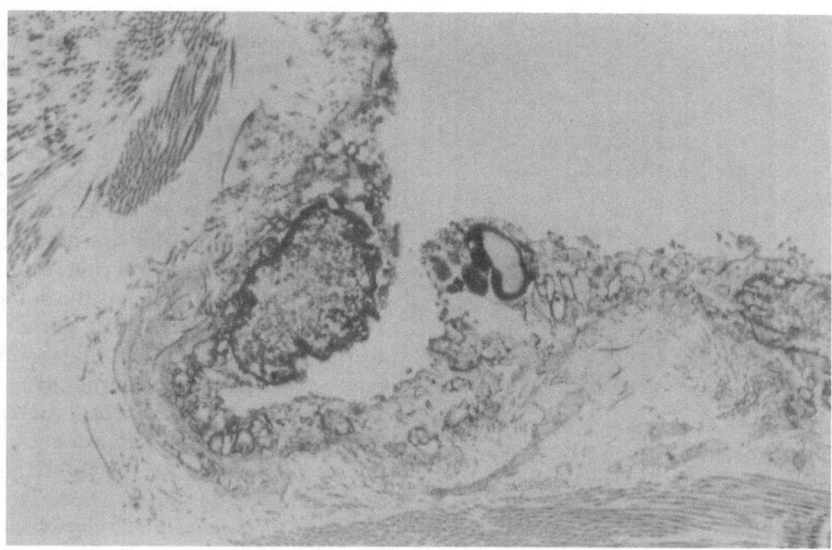

Fig. 11. During peritonitis the mesothelial cell is badly damaged and cyto-plasmatic borders become detached from the cells. (TEM 4,600 ×).

LM, and gluteraldehyde fixative for TEM and SEM. The samples were examined by LM, TEM, and SEM.

In all the patients, before or just after the peritoneal biopsy, we calculated creatinine and urea clearances and measured drainage volumes. Creatinine and urea clearances were calculated using the formula $D/P \times Vd/t$ where Vd is the peritoneal drainage volume (ml), t is the duration of dialysis exchange (min), D is the dialysate concentration,

and P is the plasma concentration. Drainage volume was calculated following three 2L exchanges containing 1.5% dextrose. Paired data were analyzed statistically.

RESULTS AND DISCUSSION

Before CAPD, the mesothelium appeared to be made up of flattened cells with protruding nuclei and numerous microvilli of varying lengths on the

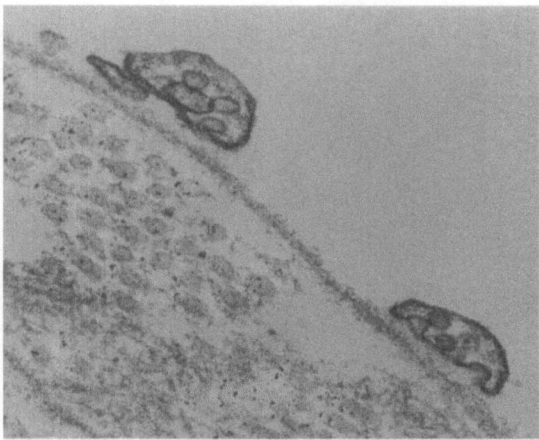

Fig. 12. During peritonitis only fragments of the cytoplasm are adhering to the peritoneal basement membrane (BM). (TEM 35,500 ×).

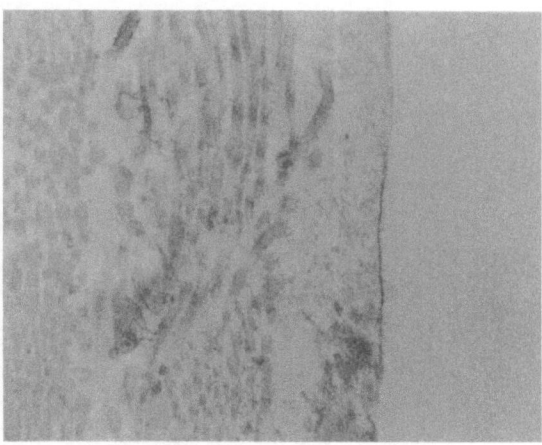

Fig. 13. During peritonitis the mesothelium is no longer visible and only the BM is in contact with the dialysis solution (TEM 31,500 ×).

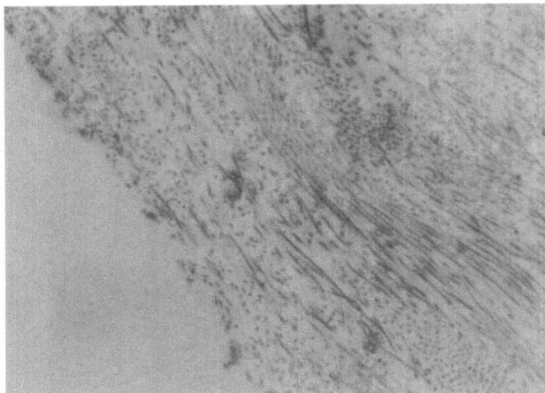

Fig. 14. Bare bundles of collagen fibers, without the protective mesothelial layer. (TEM 10,000 ×).

luminal side of both the nuclei and the cytoplasmic borders (Fig. 1). Others have reported differences in both number and length of cells and microvilli in animals according to the organs examined.[2] In the human parietal peritoneum, the cell number was constant, but microvilli length varied (Fig. 2). With SEM (Fig. 3) the peritoneum appeared so full of microvilli the individual cells could not be seen. According to some authors,[3] these microvilli have

specific transport functions, increasing the exchange surface, while other authors[2] maintain that the function of the microvilli is principally mechanical protection against friction between organs. On TEM (Fig. 4) we noted many pinocytotic vesicles in the mesothelium cells and a very irregular surface border resting on a continuous BM. The importance of these vesicles in peritoneal transport has already been emphasized. Biopsies performed after 10–40 months of CAPD give varying results, but nevertheless are all characterized by the notable frequency of structural alterations, which seem to be related not to the length of the dialysis treatment, but to the number of episodes of peritonitis.

The modifications are progressive and start with a reduction and subsequent disappearance of the microvilli (Fig. 5), the absence of which is evident both with SEM and TEM. The cell membrane begins to show signs of damage following the disappearance of the microvilli (Fig. 6), and at this point, large vacuoles appear at the basement of the mesothelial cells (Fig. 7). These vacuoles produce progressive separation of the cell membrane from the BM. With high magnification (Fig. 8), these vacuoles, responsible for detachment of the mesothelium from the BM, are clearly seen as they merge, creating even larger zones, which increase the separa-

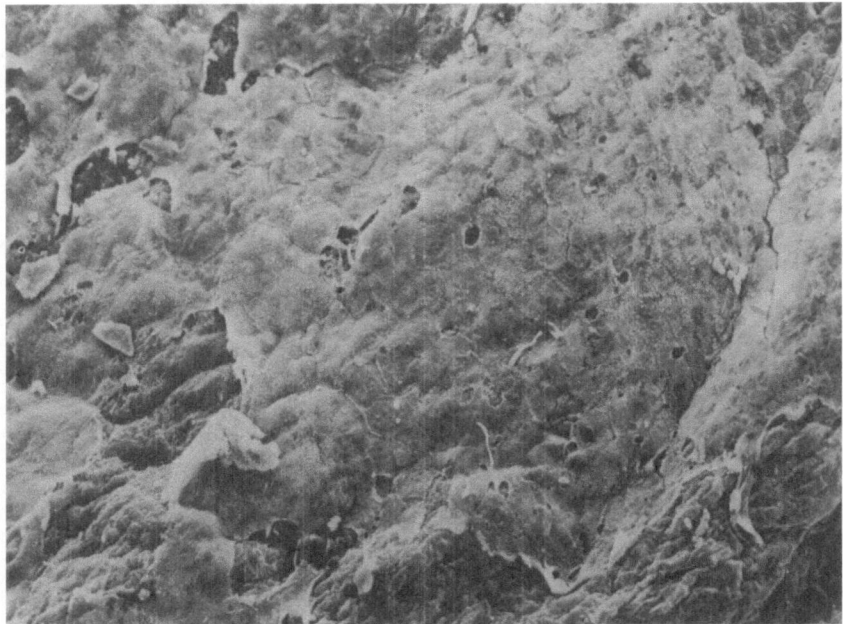

Fig. 15. During peritonitis, the mesothelium is seen flaking away from the underlying connective tissue. (SEM 178 ×).

tion of the mesothelium from the connective tissue (Fig. 9).

We also noted widening of the intercellular junctions (Fig. 10). This phenomenon is also clearly seen with the SEM, where extended areas of peritoneum are covered by cells distinctly separate from one another and microvilli are no longer present (Fig. 11). In patients with no episodes of peritonitis, the underlying connective tissue appears quite sound, with no alterations in the blood and lymph capillaries.

During peritonitis extensive cellular necrosis is noted, and the remaining mesothelial cells show large vacuoles and a progressive disappearance of cytoplasmatic borders. The most important and dramatic aspect can be observed with SEM (Fig. 12), where with low magnification we see that the mesothelium is flaking away from the underlying connective tissue, leaving behind the bare BM. In the remaining cells, there are no normal cytoplasmic organelles, while there are a few pinocytotic vesicles and the cytoplasm appears clear and full of fine fibrillar material (Fig. 13). Occasionally, cellular fragments may be found sticking to the apparently sound BM (Fig. 14), but in large areas only the connective tissue is exposed for contact within the abdominal cavity (Fig. 15).

One to four months after peritonitis, near areas of mesothelium, apparently sound but often without microvilli, there are zones where the mesothelium is

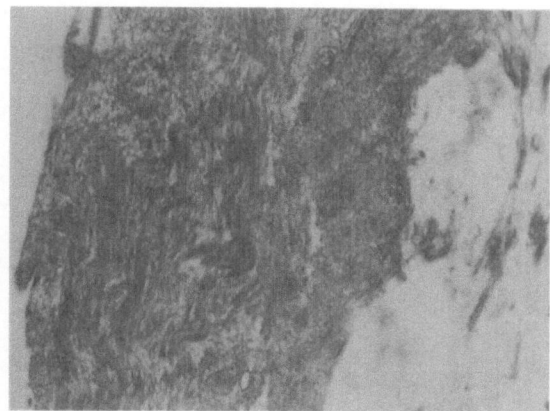

Fig. 16. Submesothelial fibrosis; the mesothelium has completely disappeared. (TEM 16,500 ×).

absent and the underlying connective tissue has thickened and produced extended areas of fibrosis. The position of, and distance between, the peritoneal vascular system and the other connective structures also appears altered. TEM confirms observations with the LM, that there is no mesothelium (Fig. 16), but only thick fibrous tissue. The SEM often shows a surface that can be evaluated only with difficulty due to the presence of fibrin (Fig. 17). Some authors[13] have observed foreign birefringent material, probably plastic, in the peritoneal connective tissue.[13] We have only seen this once,

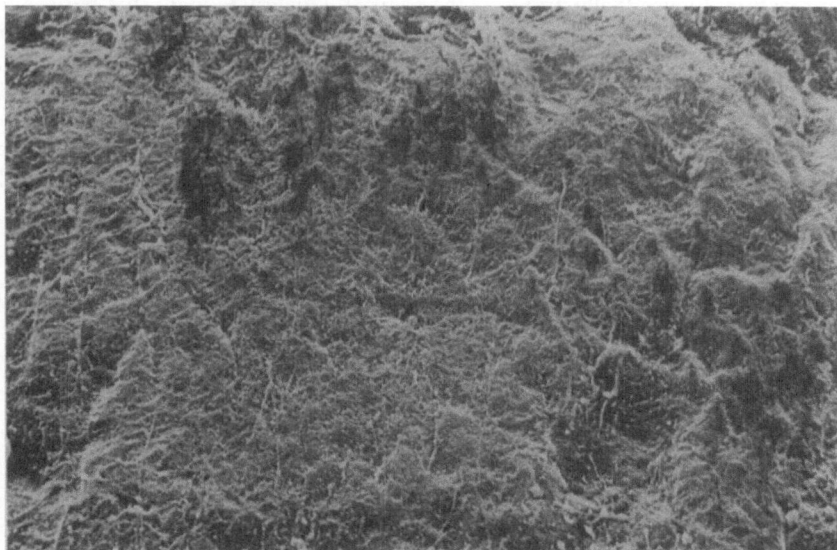

Fig. 17. 3 mo after peritonitis, the peritoneal surface can be evaluated only with difficulty due the presence of fibrin. (SEM 1,150 ×).

MORPHOLOGY OF PERITONEUM DURING CAPD
(study of 38 peritoneal biopsies)

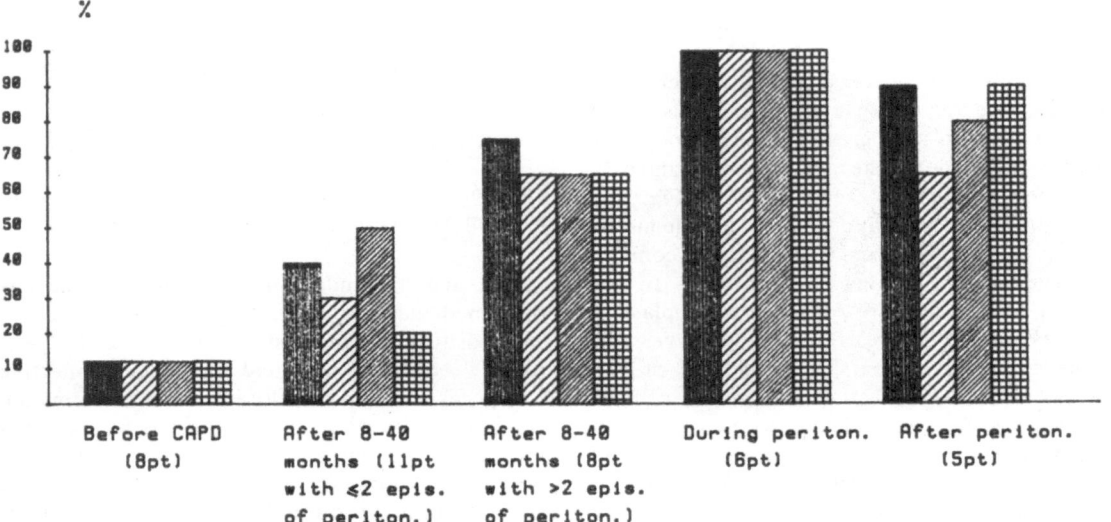

Fig. 18. Composite of morphological alterations observed during this study.

where the presence of many foreign bodies pro-voked a cellular reaction. Figure 18 illustrates all the alterations observed during this study. To facilitate comprehension we have divided the 19 cases examined from 9 to 40 months after CAPD into two groups, one of which includes 11 patients with two or less episodes.

With the cases so divided it was not possible for us to evaluate statistically due to the sparse data, but is still clearly evident that peritonitis plays a major role in provoking permanent anatomical damage to the peritoneal membrane. However, we did not observe significant modifications in the clearance of creatinine and urea, while with regard to the drainage volume, there was only the expected decrease observed during peritonitis (Table 1).

Table 1. Creatinine (CCr) and Urea (Cu) Clearances (ml/min) and Drainage Volume (V, ml) in CAPD (Mean ± SD).

	BC (8)	AC (11)	ACP (8)	DP (6)	AP (5)
CCr	13.8 ± 0.7	12.1 ± 1.4	11.6 ± 1.1	14.2 ± 2.4	13.3 ± 1.9
Cu	16.9 ± 1.2	15.4 ± 2.2	14.2 ± 0.8	15.8 ± 1.5	14.9 ± 0.7
V	2214 ± 46	2178 ± 56	2126 ± 62	1926 ± 28*	2127 ± 43

* $P < 0.05$ versus all the others. The number of patients studied shown in ( ).
BC = before CAPD.
AC = after 8–40 months CAPD with ≤2 peritonitis episodes.
ACP = after 8–40 months CAPD with >2 peritonitis episodes.
DP = during peritonitis.
AP = after peritonitis.

CONCLUSION

In morphological studies of the peritoneum, peritoneal biopsies of patients undergoing peritoneal dialysis have shown various alterations, which, according to other investigations, were caused not only by peritoneal infections, but also by chronic osmotic damage due to the use of commercial solutions. Our study shows that, evaluation of the alterations observed 8 to 40 months after CAPD would indicate that part of the damage is permanent, but it is not associated with clinical signs of decrease in peritoneal clearances or drainage volumes (Table 1).

REFERENCES

1. Gotloib L: Anatomy of the peritoneal membrane. In LaGreca G (Ed), Proceedings of the 1st international course on peritoneal dialysis. Milan: Wichtig Editore, 1982, p 17
2. Andrews PM, and Porter KR: The ultrastructural morphology and possible significance of mesothelial-microvilli. Anat Rec 177: 409, 1981
3. Odor R: Observation of the rat mesothelium with the electron and phase microscopes. Am J Anat 95: 433, 1954
4. Baradi AF, and Rao SN: A scanning electron microscope study of mouse peritoneal mesothelium. Tissue Cell 8: 159, 1976
5. Gotloib L, Rabinovich S, Rodella H, Medline A, and Oreopoulos DG: Ultrastructure of the rabbit mesentery. In Gahl GM, Kessel M, and Nolph KD (Eds), Advances in peritoneal dialysis: Proceedings of the 2nd international symposium on peritoneal dialysis. Amsterdam: Excerpta Medica, 1981, p 10
6. Gotloib L, Digenis GE, Rabinovich S, Medline A, and Oreopoulos DG: Ultrastructure of normal rabbit mesentery. Nephron 34: 248, 1983
7. Henderson LW: The problem of peritoneal membrane area and permeability. Kidney Int 3: 409, 1973
8. Nolph KD: The peritoneal dialysis system. Contrib Nephrol 17: 44, 1979
9. Nolph KD, Popovich RP, Ghods AJ, and Twardowski Z: Determinants of low clearance of small solutes during peritoneal dialysis. Kidney Int 13: 117, 1978
10. Lawrent TC: The ultrastructure and physical-chemical properties of interstitial connective tissue. Pfluegers Arch 336: 21, 1972
11. Verger C, Luger A, Moore HL, and Nolph KD: Acute changes in peritoneal morphology and transport properties with infectious peritonitis and mechanical injury. Kidney Int 23: 823, 1982
12. Rafferty AT: Regeneration of parieta and visceral peritoneum in electron microscopical study. J Anat 115: 375, 1973
13. Verger C, Brunschivic O, LeCharpentier Y, Lavergne A, and Vantelon J: Peritoneal structure alterations on CAPD. In Gahl GM, Kessel M, and Nolph KD (Eds), Advances in peritoneal dialysis: Proceedings of the 2nd international symposium on peritoneal dialysis. Amsterdam: Excerpta Medica, 1981, p 576
14. Verger C, Brunshvicg O, LeCharpentier Y, Lavergne A, and Vantelon J: Structural and ultrastructural peritoneal membrane changes and permeability alterations during CAPD. Proc Eur Dial Transplant Assoc 18: 199, 1981
15. Gandhi VC, Humayun HM, Ing TS, Daugirdas JT, Jablokow VR, Iwatsuki S, Geis WP, and Hand JE: Sclerotic thickening of the peritoneal membrane in maintenance peritoneal dialysis patients. Arch Intern Med 140: 1201, 1980
16. Schmidt RW, and Blumenkrantz M: Peritoneal sclerosis: A sword of Damocles for peritoneal dialysis? Arch Intern Med 141: 1264, 1981
17. Bradley JA, McWhinnie DL, Hamilton DNH, Starnes F, MacPherson SG, Seywright M, Briggs JD, and Junor BJ: Sclerosing obstructive peritonitis after CAPD. Lancet 19: 113, 1983
18. Parsoo I, Haffeie AA, and Naicker S: Intestinal obstruction due to adhesions complicating CAPD. Peritoneal Dial Bull 3: 43, 1983

L. Gotloib, A. Shustak, P. Bar-Sella, and V. Eiali

3

Fenestrated Capillaries in the Human Parietal Peritoneum and Rabbit Diaphragmatic Peritoneum

SUMMARY

Fenestrated capillaries account for 1.7% microvessels examined under electron microscopy in only one of 20 human peritoneal samples examined. The fenestrae were closed by diaphragms 70 Å thick. In New Zealand white rabbits fenestrae were seen in 3.2% of observed capillaries, with diaphragms 60 Å to 90 Å thick. The glycocalix covering the fenestrae diaphragms may limit the passage of anionic blood components, particularly proteins, as has been demonstrated in other studies.

INTRODUCTION

Microvessels in human and rodent parietal[1,2] and visceral peritoneum[2-4] have been classically described as being of the continuous type, according to the classification of Majno.[5] In this study, the existence of fenestrated capillaries in human parietal peritoneum and diaphragmatic peritoneum of the rabbit is demonstrated. The heterogeneity of the peritoneal microcirculation may well imply that the mechanisms of water and solute transfer across the peritoneum during peritoneal dialysis are much more complicated than suggested by *in vivo* kinetic whole organ studies.

From the Department of Nephrology and the Kornach Laboratory for Experimental Nephrology, and the Laboratory of Electron Microscopy, Department of Pathology, Central Emek Hospital, Afula, Israel.

MATERIAL AND METHODS

Samples of parietal peritoneum taken from 20 patients were examined under electron microscopy. This population included six chronic uremic nondiabetic, nondialyzed patients; five chronic uremics (one of them diabetic) on intermittent peritoneal dialysis; and nine nonuremic, nondiabetic patients. In uremics, biopsies were taken at the time of implantation or removal of a subcutaneous intraperitoneal prosthesis.[6] In nonuremics, samples were taken at the time of elective abdominal surgery. All procedures were carried out with the patient under general anesthesia. Biopsies were taken from macroscopically apparent normal areas of parietal peritoneum immediately after laparotomy was completed. Pieces of tissue of approximately 0.5 cm² were fixed by means of 2.5% glutaraldehyde in 0.1 M sodium cacodylate buffer at pH 7.2 and temperature of 4°C, overnight. After rinsing in the same buffer, tissues were postfixed in 2% osmium tetroxide for one hour, then dehydrated in ethanol and imbedded in Epon 812. Semi-thin sections were stained with 1% toluidine blue and examined by light microscopy. Thin sections were stained with uranyl acetate and lead citrate.

The number of blocks per biopsy ranged between eight and ten, whereas the number of examined grids was four to five per block. In total, 176 vascular profiles were observed.

Mesenteric, diaphragmatic and parietal peritoneal (from the ventral abdominal wall) samples were taken from five apparently normal New Zealand female rabbits, weighing between 2.90 and 3.45 Kg (mean ± 1 SD = 3,18 = 0,19 Kg). Under general anesthesia (halothane 0.5–1.5% and oxygen 4 L/min) and aseptic conditions, 150 ml of 2.5% glutaraldehyde solution buffered with 0.1 M sodium cacodylate at pH 7,2 was infused into the abdominal cavity through a 14-gauge needle. Approximately 20 minutes after the infusion was completed, the fluid was drained and macroscopically avascular areas of mesentery, diaphragmatic peritoneum, and the peritoneum of the ventral abdominal wall were excised through aseptic laparotomy.[3] Damage by handling the mesothelial surfaces was carefully avoided. At the end of the experiment, the animals were sacrificed by withdrawing the oxygen supply.

Pieces of tissue of approximately 0.5 cm² were processed for electron microscopy by the same technique used for human parietal peritoneum. All sections were finally examined using a Philips 300 electron microscope.

Five blocks from each peritoneal segment of each animal were prepared (total number: 75 blocks). Generally, five grids from each block were examined under electron microscopy (mesentery, 121 grids; diaphragmatic peritoneum, 123 grids; parietal peritoneum, 119 grids). A total of 284 vascular profiles was examined.

RESULTS

In humans, three fenestrated capillaries were found in only one of the 20 cases, a nonuremic, nondialyzed 42-year-old woman. Since the total number of observed microvascular profiles was 176, the contribution of fenestrated capillaries to the analyzed microvascular population was 1.7%. Endothelial cells, which showed an average thickness of 60 nμ, were remarkably thinner than those of continuous capillaries (average thickness approximately 650 nμ). Pinocytotic vesicles were observed, but showed a lower density distribution than that observed in endothelial cells of continuous capillaries of human parietal peritoneum (L. Gotloib, unpublished observations) and of other human organs.[5] Fenestrae were apparently closed by diaphragms, showing an average thickness of 70 Å (Fig. 1).

In rabbits, 284 vascular profiles were studied (202 from mesentery, 51 from diaphragmatic peritoneum, and 31 from the parietal peritoneum). Assuming that microvascular density of mesentery represents maximal peritoneal vascularization, it appears that diaphragmatic and parietal peritoneum

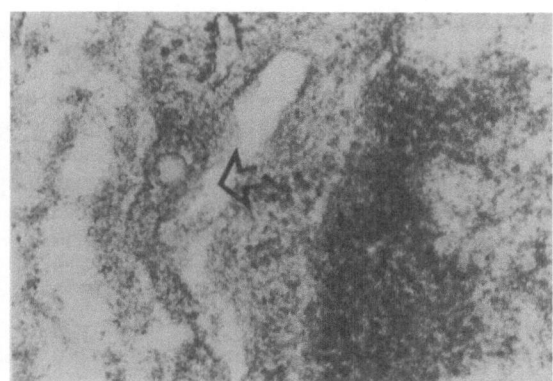

Fig. 1. Fenestrated capillary in human parietal peritoneum. One fenestra apparently closed by a diaphragm (bottom) can be observed on the mesothelial aspect of the capillary. The thin endothelial layer shows occasional pinocytotic vesicles. Arrow: capillary lumen. (× 65,000).

were respectively four and seven times less perfused than mesentery.

Nine fenestrated capillaries were observed in tissue samples of diaphragmatic peritoneum obtained from three of five rabbits. They represented 3.2% of the total number of observed capillaries. Here again, fenestrae were apparently closed by diaphragms, whose thickness ranged between 60–90 Å (Fig. 2).

In both human and rabbit fenestrated capillaries, fenestrae occupied approximately two-thirds of the endothelial cell border, whereas the remaining part of the cell showed a continuous thin layer of endothelium (Fig. 1).

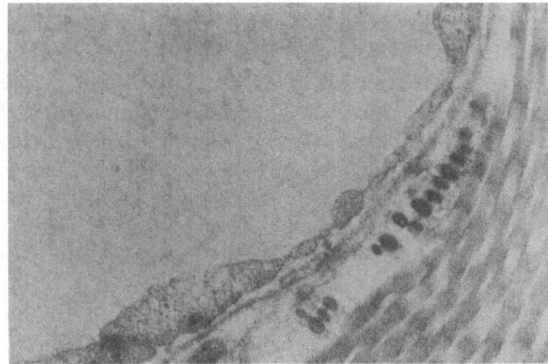

Fig. 2. Fenestrated capillary in rabbit diaphragmatic peritoneum. The thin endothelial layer lies on a continuous basement membrane. Pinocytotic vesicles are present. (× 47,000).

DISCUSSION

The mechanisms for water and solute transfer across capillary walls still remains one of the prime unsolved problems of modern physiology.[7] Identification of pathways and mechanisms governing the transfer of substances across the peritoneum during peritoneal dialysis is an even more formidable challenge, in part due to the fact that the role of mesothelial cells should be added to that ascribed to the peritoneal microvascular wall, and to the heterogeneous density and ultrastructure of peritoneal microcirculation.

Morphological studies have described human and rabbit peritoneal microvessels as being of the continuous type.[1-3] However, frog mesentery has a very low proportion of fenestrae only in venous capillaries and venules.[8] Even though most of the capillaries observed in this study were of the continuous type, the existence of fenestrated capillaries in both human parietal and rabbit diaphragmatic peritoneum is demonstrably a small fraction of the total number of observed vascular profiles.

Diaphragmatic fenestrated capillaries represented 3.2% of the total number of observed microvessels in the rabbit peritoneum. This figure is well within the range of 1–10% of the fractional area of large pores estimated by Simionescu et al.[9] for the continuous and fenestrated intestinal capillary circulation.

Fenestrated capillaries have been observed in endocrine glands, in rete mirabile, in tissues in which the main function is the production and/or secretion of fluids, and in rat prostate and omentum.[9-15] On the other side, several tissues have mixed populations of both continuous and fenestrated capillaries in quite different proportions.[4-16]

Endothelial cells of fenestrated capillaries are pierced by fenestrae (200–1200 Å diameter), which may be either open or closed by a diaphragm[4,9,10] that has a diameter between 50–70 nm.[10] High concentrations of negatively charged groups (heparin and heparan sulphate) on the blood front of fenestral diaphragms have been demonstrated in pancreatic and intestinal capillaries,[11,12,16] in peritubular capillaries of the mouse kidney cortex,[17] and in the fenestrated capillary bed of the rat optic choriocapillaries.[14,15] It has been suggested that the electric charge of the glycocalix covering the fenestral diaphragms may play a role in restricting the transmural passage of anionic blood components,[16] essentially plasma proteins. This prediction was demonstrated by Pino,[14] who showed a clear restriction of the passage of albumin (Stokes-Einstein effective radius = 35 Å) and of IgG (Stokes-Einstein effective radius = 55 Å) by a fenestrated endothelium. The fact that different microvascular beds can show different proportions of anionic sites could imply that they may also have different permeability to anionic proteins.[18,19] The possible existence of anionic sites in the fenestral diaphragms described in this study remains to be demonstrated, as well as the presence of fenestrated capillaries in other portions of the peritoneum.

The heterogeneity of the peritoneal microcirculation distribution and density, and the presence of fenestrated capillaries in parietal peritoneum and of transendothelial channels in mesenteric capillaries,[2] suggest that, *in vivo*, whole organ peritoneal permeability studies may eventually represent a rough average of several unknown individual values which, with an unknown statistical distribution, come from different segments of the peritoneum.

REFERENCES

1. Odor DL: Observations of the rat mesothelium with electron and phase microscopes. Am J Anat 95: 433, 1954
2. Gotloib L: Anatomy of the peritoneal membrane. In LaGreca G, Biasoli B, and Ronco C (Eds), Peritoneal dialysis. Milan: Wichtig Editore, 1982, p 17
3. Gotloib L, Digenis GE, Rabinovich S, Medline A, and Oreopoulos DG: Ultrastructure of normal rabbit mesentery. Nephron 34: 248, 1983
4. Wolff JR: Ultrastructure of the terminal vascular bed as related to function. In Kaley G, and Altura BM (Eds), Microcirculation. Baltimore: University Park Press, 1977, p 95
5. Majno G: Ultrastructure of the vascular membrane. In Handbook of physiology, Section II, Circulation, Vol III. Washington, D.C.: American Physiology Society, 1965, p 2293
6. Gotloib L, Nisencorn I, Garmizo AL, Galili N, Servadio C, and Sudarsky M. Subcutaneous intraperitoneal prosthesis for maintenance peritoneal dialysis. Lancet 1: 1318, 1975
7. Renkin EM: Multiple pathways of capillary permeability. Circ Res 41: 735, 1977
8. Bundgaard M, and Frokjae-Jensen R. Functional aspects of the ultrastructure of terminal blood vessels: A quantitative study on consecutive segments of the frog mesenteric microvasculature. Microvasc Res 23: 1, 1982
9. Simionescu N, Simionescu M, and Palade GE: Permeability of intestinal capillaries: Pathway followed by dextrans and glycogens. J Cell Biol 53: 365, 1972
10. Casley-Smith JR: Endothelial fenestrae in intestinal villi: Difference between the arterial and venous end of the capillaries. Microvasc Res 3: 49, 1971

11. Charonis AS, and Wissig SL: Anionic sites in basement membranes. Differences in their electrostatic properties in continuous and fenestrated capillaries. Microvasc Res 25: 265, 1983

12. Katsuyama T, Poon KC, and Spicer SS: The ultrastructural biochemistry of the basement membranes of the exocrine pancreas. Anat Rec 188: 373, 1977

13. Peters KR, and Milici AJ: High resolution scanning electron microscopy of the luminal surface of a fenestrated capillary endothelium. J Cell Biol 97: 336a, 1983

14. Pino RM: Restriction to endogenous albumin and IgG by the rat choriocapillary endothelium. J Cell Biol 95: 99a, 1982

15. Pino RM: Anionic sites on the choriocapillary endothelium. J Cell Biol 97: 337a, 1983

16. Simionescu M, Simionescu N, Silbert J, and Palade G: Differentiated microdomains on the luminal surface of the capillary endothelium. II. Partial characterization of their anionic sites. J Cell Biol 90: 614, 1981

17. Kanwar YS, and Farquhar MG: Anionic sites in the glomerular basement membrane. J Cell Biol 81: 137, 1979

18. Bankston PW, and Milici AJ: A survey of the binding of polycationic ferritin in several fenestrated capillary beds: Indication of heterogeneity in the luminal glycocalyx of fenestral diaphragms. Microvasc Res 26: 36, 1983

19. Clementi F, and Palade GE: Intestinal capillaries. I. Permeability to peroxidase and ferritin. J Cell Biol 41: 33, 1969

B. Rippe, G. Stelin, and J. Ahlmén

4

Lymph Flow from the Peritoneal Cavity in CAPD Patients

SUMMARY

In order to study lymph flow from the peritoneal cavity during continuous ambulatory peritoneal dialysis (CAPD), plasma uptake of IP radio-iodinated serum albumin (RISA) (^{125}I-HSA) was monitored over 6 to 8 hours in CAPD patients. The mean ($\pm$SEM) fractional plasma appearance rate of RISA was constant over 6 to 8 hours, and amounted to 0.44 $\pm$ 0.14%/h. This corresponded to a lymph flow of 11.1 $\pm$ 1.4 ml/h, but to only about 20% of the measured fractional peritoneal disappearance rate of tracer (2.50 $\pm$ 0.79%/h). Thus, tracer was likely to be trapped in the tissues surrounding the peritoneal cavity during non-steady state conditions.

The peritoneal lymph flow is thus relatively high, and should be taken into account in evaluation of fluid exchange between plasma and peritoneal cavity. Furthermore, if colloid tracers are to be used as intraperitoneal volume indicators, corrections have to be made for their relatively rapid disappearance from the peritoneal cavity.

INTRODUCTION

CAPD is now a common therapy for end-stage renal disease patients.[1] Absorption of colloids and particles from the peritoneal cavity into blood appears to occur almost exclusively via the subdiaphragmatic lymphatics.[2-4] Thus, particles up to the size of erythrocytes seem to be able to enter the

"lymphatic lacunae" in the diaphragm through gaps between the mesothelial cells overlying them, and to be further transported to the blood via retrosternal lymphatics and the right lymphatic duct.[5] The rates of peritoneal fluid and colloid absorption have been monitored in various animal models by numerous investigators,[2, 5-7] and it is generally agreed that the protein clearance between peritoneum and blood is a good measure of the lymph flow from the peritoneal cavity.[8]

Peritoneal lymph flow estimations have mostly been performed in patients with disturbed peritoneal fluid dynamics, such as ascitic patients.[8] In view of the important role that lymph flow plays in the fluid balance across the peritoneal membrane, we decided to measure the clearance of RISA (^{125}I-albumin) from the peritoneal cavity in patients undergoing CAPD. None of these patients had a history of liver disease.

Several studies have suggested that the peritoneal to plasma clearance of a macromolecule closely reflects the lymph flow from the peritoneal cavity.[2-8] After IP administration of a macromolecular tracer, it will saturate the plasma compartment very slowly, and tracer accumulation in plasma will therefore become almost linear with time.[2, 8] Furthermore, during the first few hours of tracer accumulation in the vascular space, tracer transport to the extravascular space (including back transport to the peritoneal cavity) will be negligible.[8] The local diffusive back-flux of a macromolecular tracer from the peritoneal cavity to plasma is probably also very small,[3, 8] because macromolecule transport from blood to the interstitial space (including the peritoneum) is essentially unidirectional and takes place

From the Department of Nephrology, Sahlgrenska Hospital, University of Gothenburg, Sweden.

almost solely by convection along a blood–tissue hydrostatic pressure gradient.[9-12] This largely unidirectional flux is then drained into the lymphatics. Thus, Henriksen et al.[8] showed that the plasma appearance of IP IgG and albumin occurred simultaneously after a certain delay. This was then followed by an almost identical fractional plasma absorption rate of the two different sized proteins. This is in line with studies in the rat showing that peritoneal to plasma absorption of erythrocytes and fibrinogen occurred at the same rate after an identical delay.[2] Both these studies indicate that large molecules and particles are absorbed from the peritoneal cavity via nonrestrictive water-conductive pathways such as lymph vessels, and not to a significant extent by local diffusion across the interstitium.

PATIENTS AND METHODS

Ten CAPD patients (7 men and 3 women) with a mean age of 56 years (range 36–71 years) and with end-stage renal disease of diverse causes participated in the study. They all used four daily 2 L exchanges of dialysis fluid (Dianeal®, Travenol, Deerfield, IL). The patients had been on CAPD for an average of 13.7 months (1–29 months) when the studies were performed. None of them showed any clinical signs of liver pathology.

The patients were given 5–10 μCi ^{125}I-albumin (^{125}I human albumin, Amersham Int, UK) in the first of their four daily exchanges of dialysis fluid. The tracer was carefully mixed with the dialysis fluid before its instillation. Blood samples were drawn at 0, 40, and 60 minutes after instillation, and then every hour for a total of 7–8 hours. Samples from the dialysate were taken at 0, 20, 40, 60, and 90 minutes, and then every hour up to 8 hours, when dialysis solution exchange was performed. Sampling from the dialysate was performed by draining 400 ml into the bag over 2–3 minutes and aspirating 1–2 ml into a sterile syringe. Radioactivity was measured with a gamma scintillation spectrometer (Selektronik Automatic System, Model 45). A minimum of 10,000 counts was measured. The fraction of unbound activity (free ^{125}I) was determined from the radioactivity in the supernatant after precipitation of the dialysate with 10% trichloroacetic acid. It amounted on average to 1.5% of total activity. No correction was made for this small fraction, however, as it was assumed to be rapidly distributed in the whole extracellular compartment, and hence considered not to contribute significantly to the plasma tracer activity.[8]

The intraperitoneal fluid volume (V) was determined as a function of time (V(t)) in separate experiments before or after the tracer experiments but under otherwise identical conditions. To check these measurements, however, two V(t)-values (in addition to the initial and final dialysate volumes) were obtained during the tracer experiments. To determine V(t) during dialysis the dialysate was rapidly drained into the CAPD bag and weighed, and this was done at 20, 50, and 90 minutes, and then every 2 hours during the dwell. The drained volume (V_D) was determined from the total bag weight corrected for the weight of the empty CAPD bag and of the connecting tubings and also for the density of the dialysate. The V_D versus time curves were almost identical from one dwell to another in the same patient for dialysis solutions containing identical dextrose concentrations. The drained volume plus the residual IP volume (V_R) gave the total intraperitoneal fluid volume, i.e. $V = V_D + V_R$. The peritoneal residual volume was determined at the end of the tracer experiments from the concentration of tracer remaining in the peritoneal fluid (after mixing) following the shift to the subsequent tracer-free bag. It amounted to between 7–16% (mean 10.5%) of the total intraperitoneal fluid volume.

CALCULATIONS AND DEFINITIONS

The peritoneal to plasma clearance of tracer (Cl, ml/h; equivalent to peritoneal lymph flow) was assessed by dividing the plasma absorption rate of tracer (M, CPM/h) by the mean intraperitoneal tracer concentration ($\overline{C}$, CPM/ml) during the time period studied (T, h). The plasma absorption rate of tracer was linear with time and was defined as; M = ($C_p(T) \times V_p$)/T, where V_p is the plasma volume in ml and $C_p(T)$(CMP/ml) was the plasma concentration of tracer at time T(h). The peritoneal tracer concentration varied as a function of time, (C(t)), and the average tracer concentration from time zero to time T is then:

$$\overline{C} = \int_{t=0}^{t=T} C(t)\,dt/T.$$

Furthermore, the peritoneal to plasma clearance of tracer (Cl) is:

$$Cl = \frac{(C_p(T) \times V_p)/T)}{\int_{t=0}^{t=T} C(t)\,dt/T} \qquad (1)$$

To obtain $\overline{C}$, the peritoneal tracer concentration over time was fitted to a power function of the type $C(t) = A \cdot t^{-b}$, where A and b were arbitrary values chosen to get the best least squares fit of the experimental data. This function was then integrated between time 0 and T (usually 6.5 h). $C_p(T)/T$ was obtained by linear regression analysis of the plasma concentration of tracer versus time (t) h. Plasma volume (V_p) was calculated from the formula BV = $(100 \times V_p)/(100 - Ht)$, where "BV" stands for blood volume and "Ht" for whole body hematocrit as calculated from venous Ht. Blood volume was obtained from a nomogram (Scientific Tables, Ciba Geigy AG) for relating blood volume to age, sex, and body weight. Body surface area (BSA) was calculated using the DuBois formula.

The fractional plasma absorption rate (FPAR) of tracer was defined as the amount of tracer appearing in plasma per hour (M, CPM/h, see above) divided by the mean intraperitoneal dose of tracer during the experiment. The latter was on an average 8% lower than the given dose (see below).

The fractional peritoneal disappearance rate of tracer (FPDR) was defined as the fractional fall in the peritoneal tracer content per hour expressed in percent of given dose. FPDR was determined from the intraperitoneal tracer dose versus time curve, which was linear (r > 0.95) when plotted on a semilogarithmic scale. The intraperitoneal tracer content at any time (D(t), CPM) was obtained from the product of IP tracer concentration C(t) and peritoneal fluid volume, i.e., D(t) = C(t) × V(t).

RESULTS

Figure 1 shows the plasma RISA concentration (C_p) plotted against time after IP tracer administration in a typical patient (GK). After a delay varying from 10–40 minutes, the plasma accumulation of RISA was linear with time, the linear regression coefficients (r) exceeding 0.95 in all patients. This pattern was identical to that observed earlier in the rat[2] and in cirrhotic patients.[8] In Figure 2 the intraperitoneal RISA dose (upper panel), the peritoneal RISA concentration (middle panel) and the total peritoneal fluid volume for Dianeal (13.6 g/l anhydrous dextrose) (lower panel) were plotted against time for the same patient as in Figure 1. The RISA time-dose curve was plotted on a semilogarithmic scale. The concentration versus time data for RISA were fitted to a power function using power regression analysis (hatched line), and the mean intraperi-

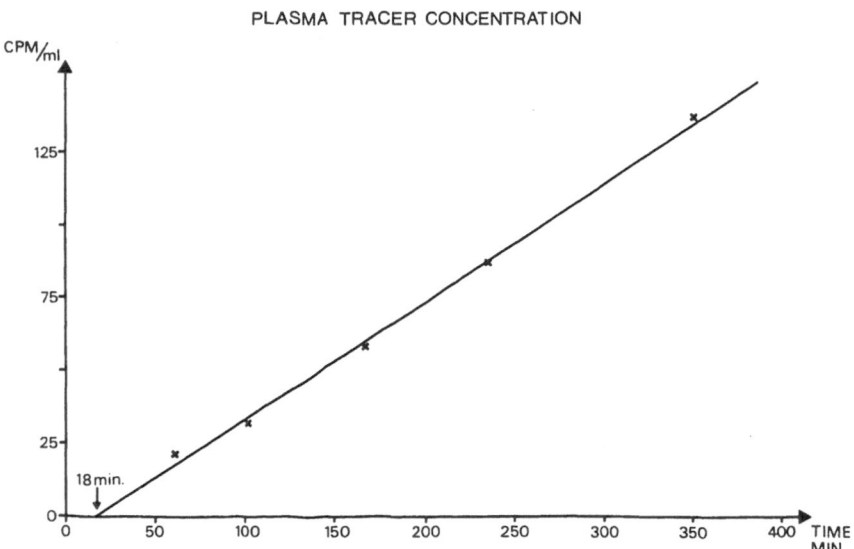

PLASMA TRACER CONCENTRATION

Fig. 1. The linear plasma accumulation of RISA in one of the patients investigated (G.K.) is shown. The equation for the linear regression of plasma RISA concentration (Cp, CPM/ml) versus time (t, min) was here Cp = −7.49 + 0.41t (r = 0.998). In this patient, tracer appearance time was 18.3 min, obtained from the intersection of the regression line with the abscissa.

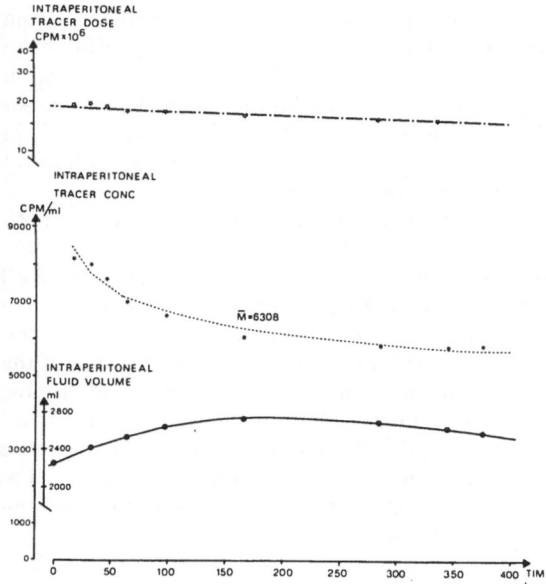

Fig. 2. The IP dose and concentration of RISA (upper and middle panels), together with the total IP fluid volume (lower panel), plotted against time in patient G.K. The IP RISA dose decreased exponentially with time, as evident from the linear time–dose relationship (r = −0.936) shown in the semilogarithmic plot (upper panel). The IP RISA concentration varied due to both alterations in total IP fluid volume with time and to disappearance of RISA from the dialysis fluid (3.02%/h). The peritoneal RISA disappearance rate could only be determined from *independent* measurements of dialysate volume and of tracer concentration in the dialysate.

toneal RISA concentration (C) was obtained from the average value of this function over the interval 0–400 minutes. Only part of the variation in peritoneal tracer concentration with time could be explained by the IP volume shifts. The remaining variation was apparently due to loss of RISA from the peritoneal fluid, as evident from the upper panel. The amount of RISA in the dialysate (obtained from concentration multiplied by volume) showed an exponential decrease with time, amounting to 3.02%/h in this patient.

Data for all the patients investigated are summarized in Table 1. The fractional plasma absorption rate represented only about 20% of the peritoneal tracer disappearance rate. This is in excellent agreement with a recent study in the rat.[2] Furthermore, the peritoneal to plasma clearance of tracer (Cl)

Table 1. Compiled Patient Data.

Pat	BSA (m²)	PV (L)	FPAR %/h	FPDR %/h	Cl ml/min/ 1.73 m²	FPAR/ FPDR
GJ	1.43	2.480	0.57	2.02	16.6	28.4
MM	2.05	4.259	0.59	2.82	14.9	20.8
BA	1.68	3.623	0.46	2.06	10.9	22.3
GK	1.64	2.903	0.44	3.02	11.8	14.6
LB	1.78	3.016	0.60	3.88	14.5	15.5
HB	1.68	2.943	0.28	1.00	6.9	28.2
GA	1.99	3.907	0.31	2.94	7.0	10.6
HK	1.75	3.748	0.58	2.74	15.7	21.3
IB	1.96	3.717	0.32	2.59	7.6	12.4
SI	1.96	4.347	0.23	1.91	4.8	11.8
	Mean		0.44	2.50	11.1	18.6
	SEM		0.05	0.25	1.1	2.1

FPAR: Fractional plasma absorption rate.
PV: Plasma volume.
FPDR: Fractional peritoneal disappearance rate.
BSA: Body surface area.
Cl: Peritoneal to plasma clearance of tracer.
Pat: Patient.

varied considerably from patient to patient. Patient SI, with the lowest Cl value, had an appendiceal abscess over 20 years earlier and was more extensively studied using γ-scintigraphy with ^{99}Tc-labeled sulphur colloid added to the dialysis solution as the macromolecular tracer. After a shift to "cold" dialysate, tracer was observed in the diaphragm, the parasternal lymphatics, and lymph glands, and also in the retroperitoneum of the right lower quadrant (the site of the former abscess) for up to 15 hours after the shift.

DISCUSSION

This study represents the first attempt to measure peritoneal lymph flow in patients with virtually normal peritoneal membranes and portal vein pressures. Henriksen et al.[8] investigated the peritoneal to plasma clearance of RISA and IgG in eight patients with ascites due to hepatic cirrhosis and in one with carcinomatous ascites. The calculated fluid absorption via the lymphatics was on average 61 ml/h in the cirrhotic patients and only 4 ml/h in the patient with peritoneal carcinosis.[8] These values probably reflect the markedly increased protein turnover between plasma and peritoneum in hepatic cirrhosis[13] and the decreased lymphatic absorption of proteins in carcinomatous ascites.[14] Estimations of lymph flow under more physiological conditions should fall somewhere in between, in agreement with the present data.

Our peritoneal lymph flow estimate is probably too low, however, as no corrections were made for tracer spillover from plasma to interstitium during the course of the experiment. Henriksen et al.[8] found that under similar conditions, as in the present study, such a correction would increase the estimated lymph flow by 7–20% (mean 14%) in cirrhotic patients with a somewhat elevated plasma disappearance rate of proteins. Correcting the present values by 14% increased the average lymph flow estimate from 11.1 to 12.6 ml/h (0.21 ml/min), and both these values are in close agreement with the value of 10.3 ml/h recently obtained in the rat and converted to 70 kg man, using (body weight)$^{0.7}$ as the scaling factor.[2]

The significance of these results lies in the fact that lymph flow is an important determinant of the Starling equilibrium governing fluid balance over the peritoneal membrane. When the dialysate crystalloids have attained osmotic equilibrium with plasma, usually after 4–6 hours of peritoneal dialysis,[15] absorption of peritoneal fluid will occur solely due to the classical Starling forces and by lymphatic drainage. Thus,

$$J_v = LpA (\Delta P - \delta \Delta \pi) - L \quad (2)$$

where J_v represents fluid flow from plasma to peritoneum (negative values stand for absorption), LpA represents the peritoneal membrane filtration coefficient, ΔP represents the effective hydrostatic pressure gradient between plasma and the peritoneal cavity, γ is the total protein osmotic reflection coefficient, $\Delta \pi$ is the oncotic gradient over the peritoneal membrane, and L is the lymph flow from the peritoneal cavity. γ is a function of the selectivity of the peritoneal membrane for plasma proteins. A value of unity characterizes a completely protein-impermeable membrane, whereas $\gamma = 0$ characterizes a membrane that does not discriminate between proteins and water. Rippe et al.[16, 17] reported a γ of 0.9 for cat peritoneal membrane, in agreement with estimates for continuous capillary beds.[18]

After 4–6 hours of peritoneal dialysis, when there are no major crystalloid osmotic forces acting across the peritoneal membrane,[15] J_v has been determined to be −0.9 to −1.1 (ml/min) by Pyle et al.[19, 20] Inserting $J_v = -1.0$, $\delta = 0.9$, $\Delta P = 10$ mm Hg,[21] $\Delta \pi$

= 20 mm Hg (from a calculated average plasma oncotic pressure of 20.1 ± 1.1 mm Hg (±SEM) in the present patients) and L = 0.2 (ml/min) into Equation 2, gives LpA = 0.1 (ml/min/mm Hg). This value for the peritoneal membrane filtration coefficient is in good agreement with that obtained by Rippe et al.[16, 17] in the cat (scale to 70 kg man).

The increment in initial volume flow to the peritoneal cavity (ΔJ_v) for a shift in dialysis fluid dextrose (anhydrous) concentration from, e.g., 13.6 g/l (76 mmol/L) to 38.6 g/l (214 mmol/L) can be used to assess the peritoneal osmotic conductance for glucose.[16, 17] The latter is defined as the product of the peritoneal filtration coefficient (LpA) and the osmotic reflection coefficient for glucose (δg). If we assume that the effective exchange area (A) and the hydraulic conductivity (Lp) remain essentially constant when shifting between the two dextrose concentrations, we have:

$$\frac{\Delta J_v}{RT (214 - 76)} = LpA\delta g \quad (3)$$

according to van't Hoff's law as corrected using the osmotic reflection coefficient (δ) for solute-permeable membranes. Here, RT stands for the product of the gas constant and the temperature in degrees Kelvin. Using the value of ΔJ_v of 5–11 (ml/min) from Pyle et al.,[19, 20] and 0.1 (ml/min/mm Hg) for LpA from the present study, gives a δg of 0.02–0.04, which again agrees well with the study of Rippe et al.[16, 17] on cat peritoneal membrane.

Both the calculated peritoneal filtration coefficient and the estimated osmotic reflection coefficient for glucose derived using a peritoneal to plasma lymph flow of 0.2 ml/min are at variance with the values obtained by Pyle et al.[19, 20] The reason for this discrepancy is not known. Our data, however, agree with modern hydrodynamic theories,[22] and with the estimate of the effective "small pore" radius in the peritoneal membrane based on transperitoneal clearances of various endogenous substances.[23] They are also in line with estimates of mesenteric capillary permeability in various animal models.[22] An osmotic reflection coefficient for glucose of 0.02 thus fits a peritoneal small pore radius of approximately 6 nm.[24]

The obtained discrepancy between the fractional plasma absorption rate and the peritoneal disappearance rate of tracer is remarkable. It has, however, recently been thoroughly investigated in rats and found to be due to local trapping of tracer under non-steady-state conditions in tissues surrounding the peritoneal cavity.[2] Thus, Flessner et al.[2] found that about 30% of the given tracer dose was trapped in the anterior muscle wall of the abdomen, while some 17% was found in the intestine and liver.[2] Only 18% of the peritoneal disappearance rate could be ascribed to plasma absorption of tracer,[2] in line with the present results. The reason for this loss of tracer to compartments outside the rapidly exchanging lymphatic compartment and the plasma compartment is not known. Local trapping in the interstitium (in, e.g., macrophages) may be responsible for this tracer "loss."

The fractional disappearance of RISA from the peritoneal cavity was surprisingly high (2.5%/h). Thus, if colloid tracers are to be used as intraperitoneal volume indicators, corrections have to be made for their rapid disappearance from the dialysate. Failure to correct for the RISA-disappearance in this experiment would, for example, have given an overestimation of the total IP volume by some 50 ml/h based on tracer-dilution calculations. It is also erroneous just to compensate the intraperitoneal dose of tracer for plasma tracer uptake, as this only represents a fraction of the total tracer loss from the peritoneal fluid. The possibility then exists that the volume versus time curves presented in many earlier studies[19,20] using tracer-dilution to assess IP volume and correcting the IP tracer amount for plasma tracer uptake are incorrect. These studies are likely to have overestimated the IP volume and to have underestimated the fluid absorption from the peritoneal cavity to the blood.

ACKNOWLEDGMENTS

We are indebted to Travenol Laboratories, Inc., and ACO Läkemedel, AB, for financial support.

REFERENCES

1. Popovich RP, Moncrief JW, Nolph KD, Ghods AJ, Twardowski ZJ, and Pyle WK: Continuous ambulatory peritoneal dialysis. Ann Intern Med 88: 449, 1978
2. Flessner MF, Parker RJ, and Sieber SM: Peritoneal lymphatic uptake of fibronogen and erythrocytes in the rat. Am J Physiol 244: H89, 1983
3. Yoffrey JM, and Courtice FC: Lympatics, lymph and the lymphomyeloid complex. London: Academic Press, 1979, p 295
4. Bettendorf U: Lymph flow mechanism of the subperitoneal diaphragmatic lymphatics. Lymphology 2: 3, 1978
5. French JE, Florey HW, and Morris B. The absorption of particles by the lymphatics of the diaphragm. Q J Exp Physiol 45: 88, 1960
6. Courtice FC, and Steinbeck AW: Absorption of protein from the peritoneal cavity. J Physiol London 114: 336, 1951
7. McKay T, Zink J, and Greenway CV: Relative rates of absorption of fluid and protein from the peritoneal cavity in cats. Lymphology 11: 106, 1978
8. Henriksen JH, Lassen NA, Parving HH, and Winkler K. Filtration as the main transport mechanism of protein exchange between plasma and the peritoneal cavity in hepatic cirrhosis. Scand J Clin Lab 40: 503, 1980
9. Lassen NA, Parving HH, and Rossing I: Filtration as the main mechanism of overall transcapillary protein escape from the plasma (editorial). Microvasc Res 7: 1, 1974
10. Rippe B, Kamiya A, and Folkow B: Transcapillary passage of albumin, effects of tissue cooling and increases in filtration and plasma colloid osmotic pressure. Acta Physiol Scand 105: 171, 1979
11. Rutili G, Granger DN, Parker JC, Mortillaro NA, and Taylor AE: Analysis of lymphatic protein data IV. Comparison of the different methods used to estimate reflection coefficients and permeability surface area products. Microvasc Res 23: 347, 1982
12. Taylor AE, and Granger DN. Exchange of macromolecules across the circulation. Handbook of Physiology 1984 (in press)
13. Henriksen JH, Ring-Larsen H, Lassen NA, Parving HH, and Winkler K: Plasma-to-ascitic fluid transport rate of albumin in patients with decompensated cirrhosis. Relation to intraperitoneal albumin. Clin Physiol 3: 423, 1983
14. Feldman GB: Lymphatic obstruction in carcinomatous ascites. Cancer Res 35: 325, 1975
15. Nolph KD, Popovich RP, Ghods AJ, and Twardowski Z: Determinants of low clearance of small solutes during peritoneal dialysis. Kidney Int 13: 117, 1978
16. Rippe B, Perry MA, and Granger DN: Permselectivity of the peritoneal membrane. Microvasc Res 25: 253, 1983
17. Rippe B, Perry MA, and Granger DN: Permselectivity of the peritoneal membrane. Microvasc Res (in press)
18. Rippe B, and Haraldsson B: Capillary permeability in rat hindquarters as estimated by measurements of osmotic reflection coefficients. Acta Physiol Scand (Suppl) 508: 60, 1982
19. Pyle WK, Popovich RP, and Moncrief JW. Mass transfer in peritoneal dialysis. In Gahl GM, Kessel M, and Nolph KD (Eds), Advances in peritoneal dialysis: Proceedings of the 2nd international symposium on peritoneal dialysis. Amsterdam: Excerpta Medica, 1981, p 41
20. Pyle WK, Moncrief JW, and Popovich RP. Peritoneal transport evaluation in CAPD. In Moncrief JW, and

Popovich RP (Eds), CAPD update. New York: Masson Publishing, 1980, p 35

21. Henriksen JH, Stage JG, Schlichting P, and Winkler K: Intraperitoneal pressure: Ascites fluid and splanchnic vascular pressues, and their role in prevention and formation of ascites. Scand J Clin Lab Invest 40: 493, 1980

22. Crone C, and Christensen O: Transcapillary transport of small solutes and water. Int Rev Physiol 18: 149, 1979

23. Rippe B, Stelin G, and Ahlmén J. Basal permeability of the peritoneal membrane during continuous ambulatory peritoneal dialysis (CAPD). In Gahl GM, Kessel M, and Nolph KD (Eds), Advances in peritoneal dialysis: Proceedings of the 2nd international symposium on peritoneal dialysis. Amsterdam: Excerpta Medica, 1981, p 5

24. Drake R, and Davis E: A corrected equation for the calculation of reflection coefficients. Microvasc Res 15: 259, 1978

R.L. Dedrick, M.F. Flessner, J.M.Collins, and J.S. Schultz

5

A Distributed Model of Peritoneal Transport

SUMMARY

A simplified distributed model of peritoneal solute transport is described, and found to agree with several observations in mammalian species. The model enables prediction of peritoneal transport from measurements of diffusivity in tissue, capillary permeability and capillary surface area.

INTRODUCTION

We were motivated to examine the physiology of peritoneal transport in connection with intraperitoneal drug administration for the treatment of abdominal cancer.[1] Important issues concern the depth of drug penetration into tumor and sensitive normal tissue, the scaling up of preclinical studies in rodents to humans, and the rate of drug absorption into the systemic circulation. We have developed a spatially distributed mathematical model to examine these issues,[2-4] and it appears to provide a useful way of looking at peritoneal dialysis in attempting to elucidate mechanisms and improve clinical practice.

THEORY

The concept of a spatially distributed model and a comparison of this approach with a lumped mem-

brane model is illustrated in Figure 1. Detailed mathematical descriptions are available elsewhere.[1-5] The kinetics of peritoneal dialysis have been described generally on the basis of a peritoneal membrane separating peritoneal fluid from blood (Fig. 1a),[6] and this description has led to some rather sophisticated and robust lumped mathematical models of the transport process.[7-9] Such models have been very useful in the description and design of protocols, including our own. They have not, however, led to much insight into the mechanisms involved, and *in vitro* studies of peritoneum and mesentery[10,11] have failed to account for more than a small fraction of the mass transfer resistance observed *in vivo*.

The concept of a distributed model is illustrated in Figure 1b. Drug absorption is considered here; however, reversing the direction is routine. We assume that drug diffuses from the peritoneal fluid through a capillary bed which, for simplicity, is regarded as being uniformly distributed in the tissue. The drug may bind to tissue constituents, or it may be metabolized in the tissue before it is absorbed by the flowing blood. If the drug is confined to the extracellular space or if it enters cells quite rapidly, the process may be described by the partial differential equation:

$$\frac{\delta C_T}{\delta t} = \frac{\delta}{\delta x} D \frac{\delta C}{\delta x} \quad -r_m \quad -r_a \quad (1)$$

| Rate of change of concentration in tissue | Spatial gradient of solute flux | Rate of metabolism | Rate of absorption |

From the Biomedical Engineering and Instrumentation Branch, Division Research Services, the Clinical Pharmacology Branch, National Cancer Institute, National Institutes of Health, Bethesda, Maryland and the Department of Chemical Engineering, University of Michigan, Ann Arbor, Michigan.

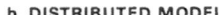

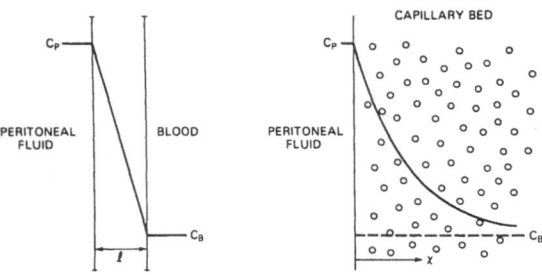

Fig. 1. Schematic diagrams showing the distinction between a membrane model of peritoneal transport and a model in which the blood capillaries are assumed to be distributed uniformly in the tissue.[3]

In equation (1) C is the diffusible concentration in the extracellular space, and D is the diffusivity in the tissue, which may be expressed

$$D = \frac{D_{void}\Psi}{\tau} \qquad (2)$$

where D_{void} is the diffusivity in the extracellular space, Ψ is the fraction extracellular space, and τ is known as the tortuosity. In the above we assume that transcellular pathways do not contribute to movement through tissue.

If we neglect metabolism in the tissue ($r_m = 0$) and assume that drug movement out of the tissue into the blood is limited by the capillary permeability, p, and capillary area per unit tissue volume, a, then

$$r_a = (pa)(C - C_B) \qquad (3)$$

where C_B is the concentration in the blood (or plasma). If c_p is the concentration in the peritoneal cavity, we can solve equation (1) at steady state with constant parameters to obtain

$$\frac{C - C_B}{C_p - C_B} = e^{\sqrt{\frac{pa}{D}}x} \qquad (4)$$

Equation (4) states that the concentration in the tissue approaches the concentration in the blood (or plasma) exponentially with distance away from the peritoneal surface and that the only parameter is the ratio of the pa-product to the intratissue diffusivity. The exponential decrease is shown by the curved line in Figure 1b.

If we compare the membrane model with the simple distributed model, we find that the mass transfer coefficient or permeability-area product (PA) for the peritoneal membrane is

$$PA = A\sqrt{D(pa)} \qquad (5)$$

so that the mass transfer coefficient can be calculated explicitly from the peritoneal surface area, the diffusivity in the tissue, and the pa-product for the capillaries.

Finally, if we examine peritoneal absorption of a solute that has transport limited by blood flow rather than by capillary permeability, than the "effective blood flow," Q, is

$$Q = A\sqrt{Dq} \qquad (6)$$

if the capillary blood flow per unit volume of tissue is q.

IMPLICATIONS

Nonreactive Solute

TISSUE CONCENTRATIONS

The plausibility of the distributed model requires that a declining concentration profile exists within the peritoneal tissue during absorption of a solute from the peritoneal cavity. In simple theory the concentration should decrease exponentially with distance from the peritoneal surface. Figure 2 shows a profile measured for polyethylene glycol-900 in the rat jejunum. The concentration profile is normalized by dividing the concentration in the extracellular space, C_{void}, by the concentration in the peritoneal cavity. We have not attempted detailed parameter estimation from this illustrative curve; however, there appears to be a least semiquantitative agreement with estimates made for a hexose based on equation (4) for parameter values[3]: D = 2.9 × 10^{-7} cm²/sec, p = 33 × 10^{-6} cm/sec, and a = 125 cm²/cm³.

Surprisingly, the shape and position of the steady-state concentration profiles are not expected to be strongly dependent on molecular weight. This may be concluded from Figure 3, which shows that the capillary permeability and diffusivity in water (and presumably in tissue)[12] decreases at about the same rate as molecular weight increases, so that their ratio, which determines the concentration profile, changes relatively little. The parameter (pa/D)$^{1/2}$ is expected to change only by a factor of 1.5 between urea and inulin despite almost a 100-fold increase in molecular weight. The time required to approach steady state (or pseudosteady state) would be expected to increase as molecular size increases.

DEPENDENCE OF PERITONEAL PERMEABILITY ON MOLECULAR WEIGHT

Examination of equation (5) in conjunction with Figure 3 for the PA product of the peritoneal membrane shows how PA would be expected to change with molecular weight. The capillary permeability varies as the -0.63 power of molecular weight, while the diffusivity in water varies as the -0.45 power of molecular weight. If we assume that the diffusivity in tissue is proportional to the diffusivity in water, then

$$PA \propto [(MW)^{-0.63} (MW)^{-0.45}]^{1/2}$$

$$PA \propto (MW)^{-0.54}$$

Thus, the PA product would be expected to be approximately inversely proportional to the square root of the molecular weight, in agreement with a variety of published studies.

INTERSPECIES SCALING

It is generally accepted that the peritoneal surface area is approximately the same as skin surface area.[13] The kinetic implications of this have been explored relatively little. Figure 4 shows the PA product (or clearance chosen under conditions to approximate the PA product) of urea and inulin in the rat, rabbit, dog, and human. Over this 350-fold range of body weight, the PA products for urea and inulin vary, respectively, as the 0.74 and 0.62 power of body weight. These values are in reasonable agreement with the value of 2/3 expected for surface area. This suggests that the intrinsic permeability of the peritoneum is similar among mammalian species.

The rate constant for the concentration change during absorption of solutes from the peritoneal cavity is PA/V_p, where V_p is the volume of fluid in the peritoneal cavity. Therefore, if the relative volume (ml/kg) is held the same between two species, the concentration would be expected to decrease more slowly in the larger species. The time scales can be made comparable by letting the volume vary as the 2/3 power of body weight. For example, the concentration in a peritoneal volume of 50 ml in a 250 g rat

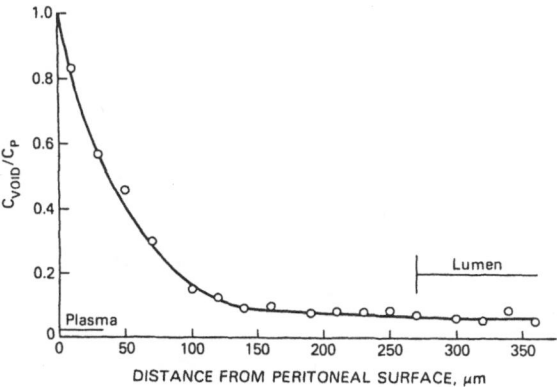

Fig. 2. Concentration profile of polyethylene glycol-900 in the jejunum of the rat.[3]

should follow approximately the same time course as the concentration in 2000 ml in a 60 kg human subject.

DISSOLVED GAS CLEARANCES

Figure 4 also shows dissolved gas clearance of hydrogen in the rat and rabbit and of carbon dioxide in the human. Dissolved gas clearances have been interpreted as measurements of effective blood flow to the peritoneum.[14] It is well recognized that these are considerably higher than clearances of hydrophilic solutes. The specific meaning of "effective blood flow" is indicated by equation (6), which

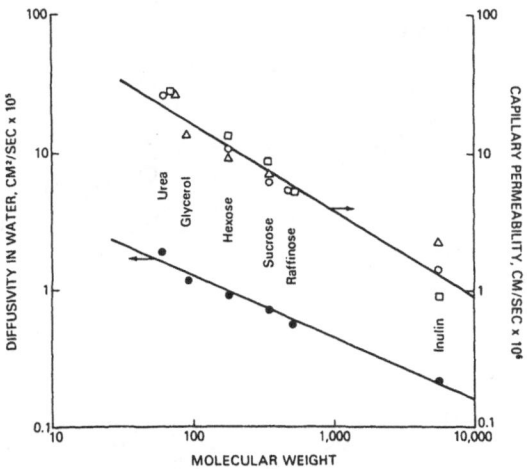

Fig. 3. Capillary permeability and aqueous diffusivity of a variety of solutes versus molecular weight.[3] ○ = cat legs; □ = human forearm; Δ = dog heart.

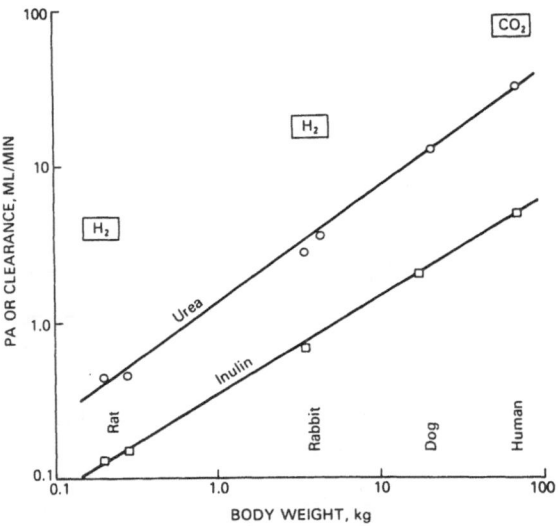

Fig. 4. Mass transfer coefficient or clearance for urea and inulin in the rat, rabbit, dog, and human. Clearance of dissolved hydrogen is also shown in the rat and rabbit, and carbon dioxide is also shown in the human.[3]

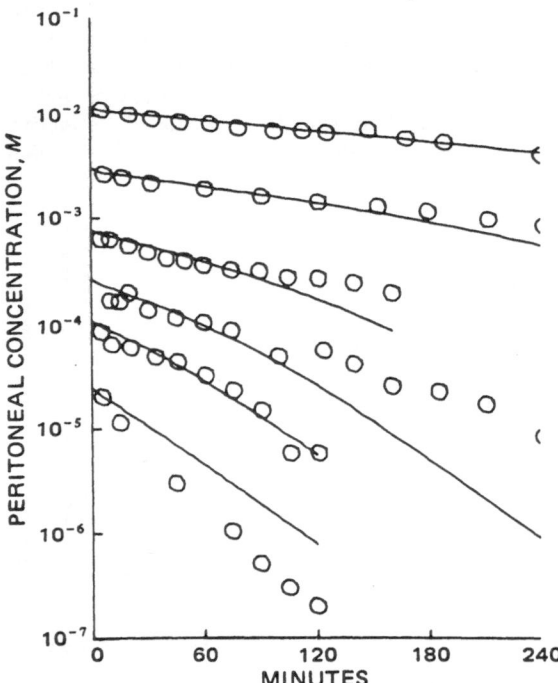

Fig. 5. Disappearance of 5-FU from the peritoneal cavity of the rat. The symbols represent experimental observations; the solid lines are model predictions.[2]

shows that the value is proportional both to the square root of the intratissue diffusivity, D, of the gas and the capillary blood flow per unit volume of tissue, q. Thus, the blood flow measured is "effective" in removing that gas, but would be expected to vary with the diffusivity of the gas, in agreement with the results of Collins.[15] Even if gas exchange is limited by blood flow at the tissue level, a gas with a higher diffusivity would be expected to show a larger effective blood flow than a gas with a lower diffusivity, because it can penetrate more deeply and, in effect, average over a larger tissue volume.

Reactive Solute

Most peritoneal transport studies with patients have been conducted with solutes that appear not to react chemically to any significant extent during their transport between the peritoneal cavity and the blood. One notable exception is the work of Maher et al.,[16] who reported that free fatty acid concentrations in peritoneal dialysate were greater than the concentrations in plasma water. They also noted a departure from the expected kinetics and inferred lipase-mediated release of fatty acids from tissue.

In the course of our preclinical studies of peritoneal absorption of 5-fluorouracil (5-FU) in the rat, we observed a striking concentration dependence of the rate of disappearance from the peritoneal cavity. The data are shown by the open circles in Figure 5. The relative rate of disappearance at low concentrations is 10-fold greater than the rate at high concentrations. This observation could be explained by chemical conversion of 5-FU in the tissues adjacent to the peritoneal cavity. Both anabolic and catabolic pathways are known to exist, and the enzymes that catalyze these are distributed widely in the body, including the abdominal organs.[2] We assumed that chemical conversion in the tissue represented a pathway for removal parallel to absorption by capillary blood. Nonlinearity of 5-FU metabolism has been documented in rat hepatocytes[17] with a Michaelis constant of 30 μM. This would be consistent with parallel mechanisms dominated by uptake into capillary blood at high tissue concentration, which saturate the effective enzyme capacity, and mechanisms dominated by metabolism at low tissue concentrations.

To check the plausibility of parallel pathways we included a saturable chemical reaction in equation (1) of the form

$$\tau_m = \frac{v_{max}C}{K_m + C} \qquad (7)$$

in which the parameters were chosen based on published *in vitro* studies with rat hepatocytes[17]: v_{max} = 71 nmol/min − cm³; K_m = 30 μM. Other parameters chosen were: A = 125 cm²; D = 1.2 × 10^{-6} cm²/sec; pa = 5 × 10^{-4} sec⁻¹. Further, we assumed that C_T = 0.6C.

The solid lines in Figure 5 represent the model simulations. Detailed refinement of parameter estimates was not attempted. In view of the very crude estimate of v_{max} and K_m and uncertainty in the other parameters, the model simulations have the correct qualitative and semiquantitative form. Considerably improved fits to the data can be obtained with suitable parameter adjustment.

INTERSPECIES SCALING

If the peritoneal PA product is calculated from the upper curve in Figure 5 for which 5-FU uptake by capillary blood dominates, a value of 0.25 ml/min is obtained. A value of 14 ml/min has been reported for cancer patients at high peritoneal fluid concentrations[18]—in the range expected for a 130 dalton solute.[1] If we compare the 230 g rats with 60 kg patients, the PA product is seen to vary as the 0.7 power of body weight, in agreement with the body-weight correlation discussed above for nonreactive solutes.

DISCUSSION

The simplified distributed model we have described has been shown to be consistent with a number of observations. These include the existence of a concentration gradient in rat jejunum, the variation of peritoneal permeability with the molecular weight of the diffusing species, and the variation of the PA product with body weight of the animal. The model also assists in the interpretation of dissolved gas clearances and predicts, perhaps counterintuitively, that the depth of penetration of small molecules at steady or pseudosteady state is not strongly influenced by molecular weight. Further, it provides a natural framework for the incorporation of chemical reactions that occur in the tissue.

The distributed model enables one to predict peritoneal transport characteristics from measurements of diffusivity in tissue, capillary permeability, and capillary surface area. It can also assist in the interpretation of data obtained in altered physiological states induced, e.g., by inflammation or pharmacologic manipulation. We expect that changes in capillary permeability and capillary surface area are

attenuated somewhat by the necessity for solute to diffuse through tissue. The square-root dependence of the peritoneal PA product on the capillary PA product suggests that doubling the latter would only be associated with a 41% increase in the former.

The effect of tissue edema associated with an increase in extracellular volume would be difficult to predict. The diffusivity in tissue would almost certainly increase because the extracellular space, ψ, would increase, and expansion of the extracellular matrix might increase D_{void}. On the other hand, the capillary spacing would increase, and this could lead to a decrease in the capillary surface area per unit tissue volume, which might not be offset by an increase in perfused capillary surface area or intrinsic capillary permeability.

Further speculation is not in order, but it is clear that hypertonic or hypotonic dialysate, peritonitis, hydrostatic pressure, and a variety of pharmacologic manipulations can influence peritoneal transport. The net change may be a result of more than one underlying mechanism. Consideration of the spatially distributed character of peritoneal transport can serve conceptually to integrate a variety of diverse mechanisms.

REFERENCES

1. Dedrick RL, Myers CE, Bungay PM, and DeVita VT: Pharmacokinetic rationale for peritoneal drug administration in the treatment of ovarian cancer. Cancer Treat Rep 62: 1, 1978
2. Collins JM, Dedrick RL, Flessner MF, and Guarino AM: Concentration-dependent disappearance of fluorouracil from peritoneal fluid in the rat: Experimental observations and distributed modeling. J Pharm Sci 71: 735, 1982
3. Dedrick RL, Flessner MF, Collins JM, and Schultz JS: Is the peritoneum a membrane? asaio J 5: 1, 1982
4. Flessner MF, Dedrick RL, and Schultz JS: A distributed model of peritoneal-plasma transport: Theoretical considerations. Am J Physiol 246: R597, 1984
5. Flessner MF, Dedrick RL, Fenstermacher JD, Blasberg RG, and Sieber SM: Peritoneal absorption of macromolecules. Chapter 7, this volume
6. Henderson LW, and Nolph KD: Altered permeability of the peritoneal membrane after using hypertonic peritoneal dialysis fluid. J Clin Invest 48: 992, 1969
7. Randerson DH, and Farrell PC: Mass transfer properties of the human peritoneum. asaio J 3: 140, 1980
8. Smeby LC, Wideroe T, and Jorstad S: Individual differences in water transport during continuous peritoneal dialysis. asaio J 4: 17, 1981
9. Garred LJ, Canaud B, and Farrell PC: A simple kinetic model for assessing peritoneal mass transfer in

chronic ambulatory peritoneal dialysis. asaio J 6: 131, 1983

10. Gosselin RE, and Berndt WO: Diffusional transport of solutes through mesentery and peritoneum. J Theoret Biol 3: 487, 1969

11. Nagel W, and Kuschinsky W: Study of the permeability of the isolated dog mesentery. Eur J Clin Invest 1: 149, 1970

12. Schultz JS, and Armstrong W: Permeability of interstitial space (rat diaphragm) to solutes of different molecular weights. J Pharm Sci 67: 696, 1978

13. Esperanca MJ, and Collins DL: Peritoneal dialysis efficiency in relation to body weight. J Ped Surg 1: 162, 1966

14. Aune S: Transperitoneal exchange II. Peritoneal blood flow estimated by hydrogen gas clearance. Scand J Gastroenterol 5: 99, 1970

15. Collins JM: Inert gas exchange of subcutaneous and intraperitoneal gas pockets in piglets. Respir Physiol 46: 391, 1981

16. Maher JF, Hirszel P, Hohnadel DC, Abraham J, and Lasrich M: Fatty acid removal during peritoneal dialysis: Mechanisms, rates and significance. asaio J 1: 8, 1978

17. Williams WM, and Kornhauser DM: Kinetics of 5-fluorouracil and uracil metabolism in rat liver. Fed Proc 38: 259, 1979

18. Speyer JL, Collins JM, Dedrick RL, Brennan MF, Buckpitt AR, Londer H, DeVita VT, and Myers CE: Phase I and pharmacological studies of 5-fluorouracil administered intraperitoneally. Cancer Res 40: 567, 1980

P. Hirszel, J.F. Maher, E. Chakrabarti, and R.R. Bennett

6

Maximal Peritoneal Pore Size Determined by Dextran Transport

SUMMARY

To assess peritoneal porosity, the clearance of neutral dextrans was measured in six rabbits using three dialysis solutions, zero, 1.5% and 4.25% dextrose. At all dextrose concentrations, clearances decreased as molecular mass increased up to about 50,000 daltons and then remained stable as molecular mass increased further. The low rate of transport of larger solutes is attributed to pinocytosis. When this is subtracted from the rate of transport by diffusion, the zero intercept for each dialysis solution was close to 50,000 daltons, suggesting that the maximal effective pore radius in 50 Å.

INTRODUCTION

Peritoneal permeability has traditionally been assessed by the clearance method, evaluating mass transport of solutes of differing sizes.[1] Mass transport results from a combination of diffusion and ultrafiltration. Mass transport by diffusion is retarded by resistances in the blood path, in the dialysate, and in the interstitium separating the membranocellular layers, as well as the intercellular channels. Accordingly, the relative clearance of solutes provides information about transport resistance through all

From the Nephrology Division, Department of Medicine, Uniformed Services University of the Health Sciences, Bethesda, Maryland, and the Nephrology Service, Department of Medicine, Walter Reed Army Medical Center, Washington, D.C.

layers and not the membranocellular pores alone. Two methods have been used to circumvent this problem. Firstly, isolated ultrafiltration has been achieved by instilling into dialysis fluid a solute concentration sufficient to eliminate the diffusion gradient. Curiously, these results show sieving of small solutes, attributed to ionic charge in some instances and unexplained in others.[2]

Alternatively, the transport of large solutes has been assessed. From these data the peritoneum appears to be highly porous. The test solutes vary in molecular geometry as well as molecular mass however, so the size-to-mass ratio is not predictable (Fig. 1). Moreover, the transport mechanism is assumed to be predominantly diffusion for all these substances, and many of these solutes are much smaller than the size of the pores of other capillary beds, such as the glomerulus.[3]

To circumvent the problems encountered in earlier studies, we evaluated peritoneal porosity by measuring the transport rates of dextrans. Polydispersed dextrans vary in molecular mass but not in configuration. They are large solutes of known dimensions, the range of which should encompass maximal pore size of the peritoneum. Transport was evaluated at different rates of ultrafiltration, attempting to assess the relative contributions of diffusion and of ultrafiltration and to estimate the sieving coefficient. Clearances were shown to decrease as solute size increased, and depended in part on the rate of ultrafiltration. When the dextran clearances were correlated with solute size, the maximal pore size of the peritoneum could be estimated.

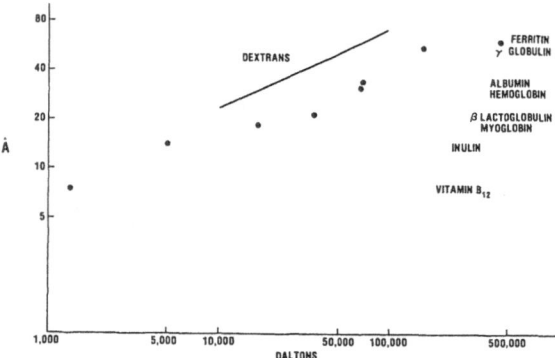

Fig. 1. The Stokes-Einstein radii of dextrans shown by the line correlate with molecular mass as Log n Å = 0.472 Log n daltons − 1.196. Other solutes do not show a predictable molecular radius as molecular mass varies.

MATERIALS AND METHODS

Studies were performed in six alert, lightly restrained female New Zealand white rabbits with slight modifications of a previously described technique.[4] Peritoneal dialysis was conducted by instilling through a percutaneously placed catheter 75 ml/Kg of dialysis solution. Based on prior study in these and other rabbits, the ultrafiltration rate had been calculated for dialysis solutions of known dextrose and osmolar composition. This ultrafiltration rate, added to the infused volume, gave an estimated dialysate volume at 60 minutes, at which time dialysate was drained as completely as possible for solute analysis. The drained volume was 61% of the calculated volume, with a variance of 17.4% of the mean at all osmolar concentrations.

In individual studies separated by several weeks, each animal was dialyzed with commercially prepared dialysis solutions containing 1.5% and 4.25% dextrose monohydrate and a dextrose-free solution consisting of sodium bicarbonate and sodium chloride with an osmolality equal to normal rabbit plasma. This salt solution does not change dialysate volume significantly,[5] whereas the 1.5% and 4.25% solutions induce ultrafiltration at rates of 0.17 and 0.54 ml/Kg/min, respectively.

Thirty minutes prior to dialysis 1.0 g/Kg of polydispersed neutral dextran 40 was injected intravenously. After 30 minutes, the dextran concentrations remained relatively stable, decreasing at a rate of <10%/h. Dextran 40 is a mixture the average molecular mass of which is 40,000 daltons, but the

range of which is 10,000–100,000 daltons. Plasma was sampled 30 minutes after dextran injection; dialysis was then commenced, and dialysate was drained as completely as possible after a 60-minute dwell in the peritoneum.

To verify the normal functioning of the peritoneum, clearances of urea and potassium were measured. To characterize permselectivity of the peritoneum, clearances of dextran fractions of known molecular dimensions were determined.

Before fractionation, dialysate samples were concentrated by filtration through an Amicon membrane with a 10,000 dalton porosity. No loss of dextran was detected by this filtration. The retentate and plasma samples were then processed by trichloroacetic acid precipitation and dialysis against a buffer of isotonic solution. Thereafter the samples were fractionated by filtration through a sephacryl 300 column. The collected fractions were then highly acidified and boiled. Anthrone was then added and the color reaction was quantified at 635 mμ in a Bausch and Lomb spectrophotometer. Because drainage was incomplete, the dialysate volumes calculated by isotope dilution were used for calculating clearances. Dialysate volume is a constant in the clearance equation, dialysate/plasma concentration ratio multiplied by volume per minute, (D/P) × (V/t). Thus, volume affects absolute clearances in a given experiment but not relative clearances of solutes of different size.

Sieving coefficients were calculated for each dextran fraction by determining the difference in dextran clearances at different rates of ultrafiltration $(C_1 - C_2)/(UF_1 - UF_2)$. Differences in clearances at the specific ultrafiltration rates were compared by Student's paired t test.

RESULTS

Clearances of urea and potassium were 520 and 812 μl/Kg/min, respectively, with 1.5% dextrose dialysis solution, each increasing by about 150 μl/Kg/min with hypertonic fluid, and decreasing comparably when dialysis fluid without glucose was used.

With 1.5% dextrose dialysis solution, mean clearances of dextrans (of all animals) ranged from 4.6 to 12.5 μl/Kg/min. As molecular mass increased from 17,000 to 50,000 daltons, clearances decreased linearly according to the regression, C = 13.2 μl/Kg/min − 0.00016 × daltons with a zero intercept at 83,000 daltons (Fig. 2). Above 50,000 daltons, dextran was cleared at a rather constant rate, 5.0 μl/Kg/

PERITONEAL CLEARANCE OF DEXTRANS CORRELATED WITH MOLECULAR MASS

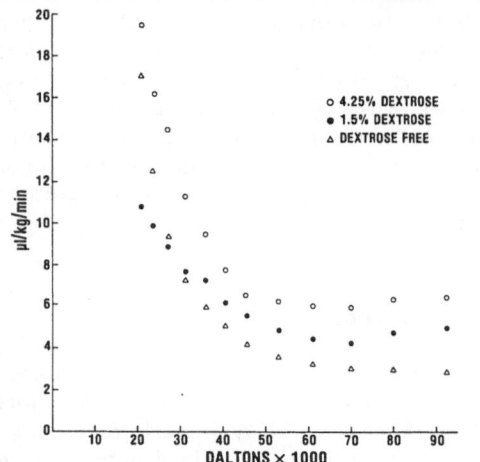

Fig. 2. Clearances of dextrans decrease as molecular mass increases up to about 50,000 daltons and thereafter are stable. The same correlation is observed at three rates of ultrafiltration, with 4.25%, 1.5% and zero dextrose dialysis.

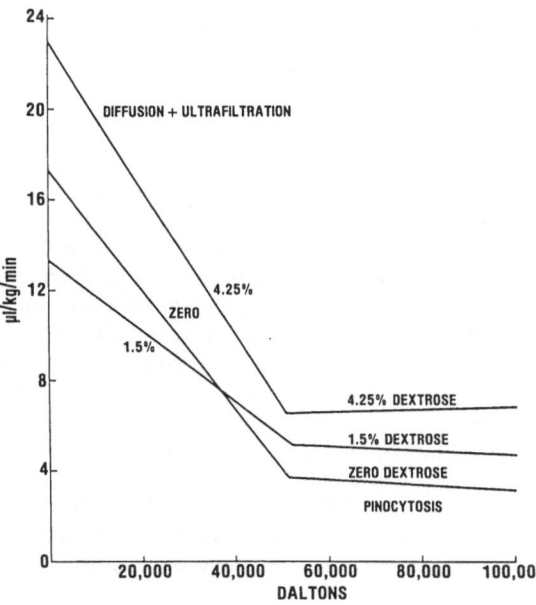

Fig. 3. Regression lines of dextran mass transport attributed to ultrafiltration and diffusion for three types of dialysis solutions each intercept the lines representing transport by pinocytosis at about 52,000 daltons or 50 Å.

min (C = 5.9 μl/Kg/min − 0.00001 × daltons). The zero clearance intercept exceeded 500,000 daltons. Below 53,000 daltons, the clearance of successive (alternate) fractions decreased significantly, but above this volume none of the values changed significantly.

With the glucose-free dialysis fluid, dextran clearances were 82% of the values with 1.5% dextrose dialysis fluid, but the relation of clearance to molecular mass was similar (Fig. 2). The lower clearance values were accounted for by a lower dialysate volume rather than a change in the dialysate/plasma concentration ratio. Above 50,000 daltons, the clearance was 3.6 μl/Kg/min, not significantly lower than with 1.5% dextrose dialysis fluid. Clearances of the larger dextrans were constant, C = 4.21 μl/Kg/min − 0.00001 × daltons, intercepting zero at 440,000 daltons. Below 50,000 daltons, however, clearances decreased more rapidly (C = 17.3 − 0.00026 × daltons), intercepting zero at 65,000 daltons.

When 4.25% dextrose dialysis fluid was used, clearances were 139% of the values with 1.5% dextrose dialysis solution (Fig. 2). Below 50,000 daltons, the clearances decreased according to the formula, C = 23.0 μl/Kg/min − 0.00032 × daltons, intercepting zero at 71,000 daltons. Above 50,000 daltons, dextran clearance averaged 6.4 μl/Kg/min

and were stable C = 6.2 μl/Kg/min + 0.000002 × daltons. Clearances of the larger dextrans were not significantly higher with 4.25% dextrose dialysis fluid than with either of the other dialysis solutions.

The declining slope of dextran clearance as molecular mass increased intercepted the rate of stable clearances of the larger dextrans (independent of molecular mass) at 53,000 daltons with 1.5% dextrose dialysis fluid and at 52,000 daltons with 1.5% dextrose dialysis fluid and at 52,000 daltons with each of the other two dialysis solutions (Fig. 3). When the molecular mass of the dextrans was converted to the Stokes-Einstein radius by the formula, Log n Å = 0.472 Log n daltons − 1.196, these intercepts were found to be close to 50 Å.

The modest differences in dextran clearances observed as the ultrafiltration rate was varied were used to calculate the sieving coefficient of each dextran fraction. The mean estimated sieving coefficient of the dextrans with this technique was 0.005. Because of the inaccuracy of this derived value at low rates of ultrafiltration, the sieving coefficient could not be correlated with molecular mass, however, because by linear regression the value changed by less than 0.004 over the range of dextran sizes studied.

DISCUSSION

By measuring the clearance of polydispersed dextrans, we have been able to assess peritoneal porosity. For large solutes such as the dextrans, the major impediment to mass transfer should be the intercellular gaps or pores, in contrast to small solutes that permeate these more readily but are relatively more restricted in traversing fluid films in the blood, dialysate, and peritoneal interstitium. Accordingly, a sharp decrement in mass transport would be anticipated as a uniform pore size was approached. These data did not demonstrate such a change, but rather indicated a steady decline in mass transport at all rates of ultrafiltration as dextran size increased, consistent with heteroporosity of the peritoneum.

A negative correlation of dextran clearance with molecular mass was evident at all rates of ultrafiltration. The declining slopes ended before reaching the zero intercepts, as a steady transport rate independent of size was observed at all rates of ultrafiltration. This slow rate of transport without size discrimination could represent diffusion through a few very large pores or more likely, pinocytosis, a biological process known to occur in transcapillary transport.

The rate of pinocytotic transport was not significantly different at the different rates of ultrafiltration. Nevertheless, the rate of pinocytotic transport appeared to depend in part on the ultrafiltration rate. This may be explained by the movement of dextrans to the cellular barrier by ultrafiltration and similar movement away from the cell after pinocytosis occurs. Indeed, convective transport across the peritoneal interstitium between two areas of pinocytotic transport would be in agreement with the data observed.

The intercept of the size-dependent transport with that attributed to pinocytosis occurred at nearly identical points on the abscissa, 52,000 daltons. This molecular mass is close to 50 Å, which is interpreted to be the maximal radius of the peritoneal pores.

The estimated peritoneal pore radius should be considered a functional dimension, not an anatomical measurement. Moreover, because only neutral dextrans were studied, no inference can be made about the effect of anionic charges of the membrane on transport of charged molecules. It is also anticipated but awaiting verification that peritoneal pore dimensions will increase when there is peritoneal inflammation.

ACKNOWLEDGMENT

This work was supported by the Uniformed Services University of the Health Sciences Protocol No. RO8318 and NKF/NCA Grant No. G18355. The opinions and assertions contained herein are the private ones of the authors and are not to be construed as official or reflecting the views of the Department of Defense or the Uniformed Services University of the Health Sciences. The experiments reported herein were conducted according to the principles set forth in the "Guide for the Care and Use of Laboratory Animals," Institute of Animal Resources, National Research Council, DHEW Pub. No. (NIH) 78–23.

REFERENCES

1. Maher JF: Characteristics of peritoneal transport: Physiological and clinical implications. Mineral Electrolyte Metab 5: 201, 1981
2. Nolph KD: Peritoneal anatomy and transport physiology. In Drukker W, Parsons FM, and Maher JF (Eds), Replacement of renal function by dialysis. The Hague: Martinus Nijhoff, 1983, p 440
3. Brenner BM, Bohrer MP, Bayliss C, and Deen WM: Determinants of glomerular permselectivity: Insights derived from observations in vivo. Kidney Int 12: 229, 1977
4. Maher JF, Hirszel P, and Lasrich M: An experimental model for study of pharmacologic and hormonal influences on peritoneal dialysis. Contrib Nephrol 17: 131, 1979
5. Maher JF, and Chakrabarti E: Ultrafiltration by hyperosmotic peritoneal dialysis fluid excludes intracellular solutes. Am J Nephrol 4: 169, 1984

M.F. Flessner, R.L. Dedrick, J.D. Fenstermacher,
R.G. Blasberg, and S.M. Sieber

7

Peritoneal Absorption of Macromolecules

SUMMARY

We have presented data quantifying both the absorption of fluid and solutes from the peritoneal cavity and the effective lymph flow rate of these substances to the blood. Peritoneal loss rate of macromolecules is dependent on IP pressure while the effective lymph flow rate has a much smaller value than the loss rate and is independent of IP pressure. Data has been presented showing the areas of local absorption and accumulation within peritoneal tissue. Macromolecular accumulation in specific peritoneal tissue depends on several factors, the most important of which is the presence or absence of lymphatics. We conclude from our studies that macromolecular agents injected IP will transport to the blood preferentially via the two major lymphatic systems draining the cavity (subdiaphragmatic and mesenteric). We further conclude that significant accumulation of such drugs will occur in the anterior abdominal wall and diaphragm, but that visceral tissues will have concentrations below one-tenth of the value at the peritoneum at positions beyond 1 mm from the peritoneum.

INTRODUCTION

Several promising Phase I trials have been completed in which antineoplastic agents have been

From the Biomedical Engineering and Instrumentation Branch, Division of Research Services, the Laboratory of Chemical Pharmacology, Division of Cancer Cause and Prevention, National Cancer Institute, National Institutes of Health, Bethesda, Maryland; and the Department of Neurological Surgery, SUNY, Stony Brook, New York.

dissolved in 2 L peritoneal dialysis solution and instilled into the cavity of patients with cancer restricted to the abdominal cavity.[1-4] This technique maintains a high concentration throughout the cavity, where most metastases from the primary tumor occur, and results in plasma concentrations from one to more than two orders of magnitude less than those in the peritoneal cavity. While most cancer drugs have molecular weights less than 500 daltons, there have been some clinical trials with cellular immunoadjuvants, and there are ongoing trials of the intraperitoneal administration of interferon.[5] Very little information is available concerning the transport of these substances into the tissue surrounding the cavity or from the tissue to the blood. It is therefore difficult to judge the efficacy or toxicity of macromolecular adjuvant therapy, based on fundamental pharmacokinetic principles.

Since the lymphatics form the primary route of macromolecular transport from the peritoneal cavity to the plasma,[6] the first topic addressed in this paper is the rate of lymphatic transport and its dependency on intraperitoneal pressure. The second topic is the local absorption of macromolecules into tissue surrounding the peritoneal cavity.

METHODS

Protocol A: Lymph Flow Rate Experiments

Twenty Sprague-Dawley female rats (210 ± 22 g) were anesthetized with an injection of sodium pentobarbital (60 mg/kg IM or IP). Each animal was placed in the supine position, and its temperature, monitored with a rectal probe, was maintained at 37

± 1°C with heat lamps. A multiholed catheter was inserted into the peritoneal cavity through the left abdominal wall at approximately right atrium level and secured with a purse stitch. This catheter was connected via a 3-way valve to a capillary manometer and to a reservoir whose height above the catheter determined the hydrostatic pressure in the peritoneal cavity. The right femoral vein and left femoral artery were each cannulated with PE-10 tubing. In some experiments the thoracic duct was cannulated proximal to the jugulosubclavian junction with PE-10 tubing. A portion of the prewarmed solution of 5% BSA in Krebs-Ringer (pH adjusted to 7.4) containing ^{125}I-fibrinogen or ^{51}Cr-red blood cells (RBCs was injected intraperitoneally (IP), with the remainder in the reservoir (volumes in the cavity varied from 30 to 60 ml). Arterial blood samples and peritoneal fluid samples were taken at 5, 15, 30, 60, 90, 120, 150, and 180 minutes after the IP injection. In thoracic duct-cannulated animals, lymph was collected for one hour prior to IP injection and every hour thereafter. Blood volume was monitored with ^{51}Cr-RBCs during the experiments in which ^{125}I-fibrinogen was used as the IP tracer or estimated from a measurement at the end of the experiment, when ^{51}Cr-RBCs were used. By carefully quantifying the amount of tracer transferred to the blood and collected from thoracic duct lymph, the effective rate of lymphatic transfer (L_{eff}) could be calculated. An observed fluid absorption (F_{obs}) was calculated by dividing the total amount of fluid absorbed from the peritoneal cavity by the duration of the experiment. Further details of the calculations and methods can be found in Flessner et al.[7]

Protocol B: Peritoneal Tissue Concentration by Quantitative Autoradiography

Female Sprague-Dawley rats (190–210 g) were anesthetized with sodium pentobarbital (60 mg/kg) via IM injection. Each animal was kept warm with heating lamps (37 ± 1.5°C). A multiholed peritoneal catheter was inserted through the lower lateral abdominal wall and secured with a purse stitch. It was later connected to a three-way valve and a capillary manometer (IP pressure monotor). Both femoral arteries were catheterized with PE-50 tubing: one for blood pressure monitoring and one for blood sampling. An experiment was begun with a 35 ml IP injection of a prewarmed (37°C) solution of Krebs-Ringer bicarbonate with 0.5% Evans Blue Dye and tracer amounts of ^{125}I-human serum albumin. The blue dye indicated the tissue areas of contact with

the dialysis fluid. Samples of peritoneal fluid and plasma were taken, and IP pressure readings were made at 5, 10, 15, 20, 30, 45, 60, 90, 120, 150, and 180 minutes after injection. Breathing rate, temperature, and blood pressure were monitored throughout the experiment. At the end of the experiment in rapid succession: the animal was decapitated; a laparotomy was performed and the fluid was drained; and the carcass was plunged into freon cooled to at least −70°C, and freon was poured directly into the peritoneal cavity. The animal was frozen within 40 to 60 seconds after decapitation and maintained in the frozen state until sections were collected. Fifty micron (50 μ)sections were obtained with an LKB-PMV 2250 cryomicrotome. Color photographs of the specimens were taken during sectioning for later comparison with the autoradiograms. The sections were either heat-dried or freeze-dried and were placed in a lead-lined cassette along with appropriate ^{125}I-tissue standards. A sheet of single-coated x-ray film was placed over them under darkroom conditions. After four weeks of exposure, the films were developed and analyzed with a computerized high-speed scanning microdensitometer. Tissue concentration gradients were determined from regional optical density measurements. Further details of the technique can be found in Flessner et al.[8]

RESULTS

Lymph Flow Rate

The animals in this study were divided into four groups. In the first group, the thoracic duct of each animal was cannulated and ^{125}I-fibrinogen was used as the tracer material. Figure 1 illustrates the typical peritoneal and plasma concentration profiles obtained in this group and is representative of all groups. The peritoneal concentration was always a relatively constant value, while the plasma concentration (corrected for loss from the plasma space) increased linearly with time. The total cumulative tracer CPM in thoracic duct lymph is also shown in the plot. In a subgroup of three rats, the IP pressure averaged 2.2–3.2 mm Hg and the observed fluid loss rate from the cavity (F_{obs} = tracer amount leaving the peritoneal cavity/time/average peritoneal concentration) was 20.3 ± 7.0 μ/min, while the effective rate of lymph flow (L_{eff} = tracer amount entering the blood/time/average peritoneal concentration) was 5.5 ± 2.1 μ/min. In another subgroup of four rats, the IP pressure was maintained at 4.3–4.4 mm Hg

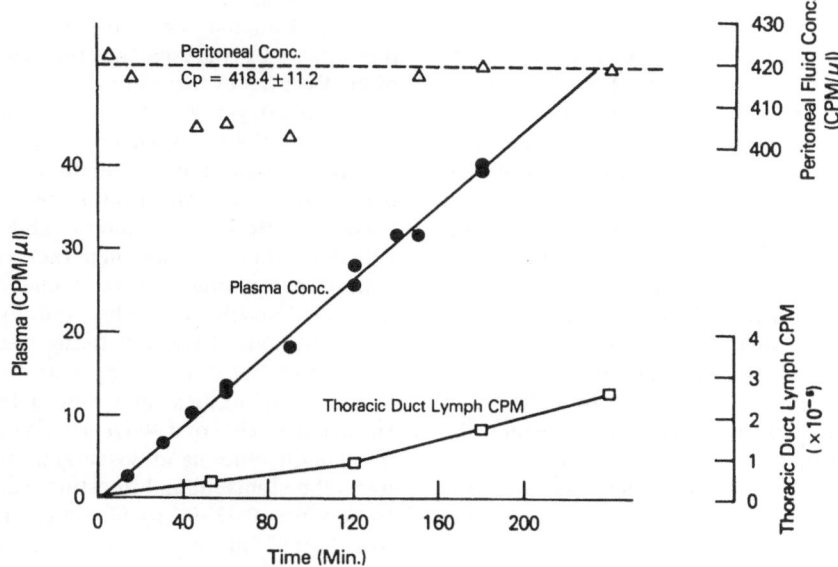

Fig. 1. Concentration of ^{125}I-fibrinogen in dialysis fluid and plasma and cumulative ^{125}I activity recovered in thoracic duct lymph during dialysis with a solution of ^{125}I-fibrinogen. Results are from a representative rat in which peritoneal pressure was maintained at 2.2 mm Hg.

and $F_{obs} = 86.9 \pm 17.2 \,\mu l/min$, while $L_{eff} = 5.8 \pm 1.5$ $\mu l/min$. The values of F_{obs} at the pressure ranges were significantly different ($p < 0.01$), while the values for L_{eff} did not differ. The average fraction of total peritoneal lymph flow transporting via the thoracic duct was 0.31 ± 0.20.

The second group of animals had intact thoracic ducts and were divided into a subgroup of four animals whose IP pressure averaged 2.2–2.9 mm Hg and a subgroup of three with IP pressure equal to 4.8–5.1 mm Hg. The IP tracer in this group was ^{125}I-fibrinogen. F_{obs} in the lower IP pressure subgroup was $34.9 \pm 5.9 \,\mu l/min$, which was significantly different from the average for the higher IP pressure of $58.7 \pm 7.3 \,\mu l/min$. Values of L_{eff} at the two pressure ranges were not significantly different: at the lower pressure, $L_{eff} = 3.1 \pm 1.6 \,\mu l/min$; at the higher pressure, $L_{eff} = 2.5 \pm 0.7 \,\mu l/min$.

In the third group, experiments were carried out with ^{51}Cr-RBCs in five animals with intact thoracic ducts. Intraperitoneal pressures averaged 1.8–3.2 mm Hg. The observed fluid loss rate from the cavity (F_{obs}) increased with increasing IP pressure and had an overall average of $21.9 \pm 5.6 \,\mu l/min$, while L_{eff} $= 2.6 \pm 1.2 \,\mu l/min$.

Because only 3–10% of the tracer lost from the peritoneal cavity was accounted for in the plasma and the thoracic duct lymph, two animals were used in a fourth group in order to assess this discrepancy in the tracer mass balance. After a three hour dialysis, all the tissues surrounding the peritoneal cavity were removed and analyzed separately for tracer content. In one animal in which the IP pressure was maintained at 2.9 mm Hg, the following amounts of tracer were obtained for each tissue (expressed as percent of the total amount of tracer absorbed from the peritoneal cavity): intestine, 9.9%; liver, 5.9%; stomach, 3.4%; retroperitoneal muscle, 4.3%; anterior abdominal wall, 27.4%; uterus, 3.8%; kidneys, 1.7%; spleen, 1.2%; diaphragm, 1.3%. The tracer concentrations were highest in the anterior abdominal wall and in the diaphragm, which were respectively, four and three times the concentration in the intestines. These very significant accumulations of tracer in peritoneal tissue prompted the further investigations of peritoneal tissue concentration gradients in order to define better the penetration of these substances into the tissue and to improve understanding of the underlying mechanisms of transport.

Peritoneal Tissue Concentrations

A total of six animals were used in the quantitative autoradiographic (QAR) studies. Two were dialyzed for two hours while the other four were dialyzed for three hours prior to sacrifice. The plasma and peritoneal fluid concentration profile of these experiments with ^{125}I-human serum albumin were similar to those of the fibrinogen study. Peritoneal concentration was a near-constant value for the three hours of dialysis, and plasma concentration (corrected for loss from plasma) increased linearly with time. Figure 2 displays concentrations in various peritoneal tissues versus the distance into the tissue from the peritoneum after three hours of dialysis. The zero on the abscissa represents the edge of the peritoneum. The tissue concentrations have been normalized by dividing each with the peritoneal fluid concentration at the beginning of the experiment (C_o). To the right of the tissue profiles are the average peritoneal fluid and plasma concentrations. Luminal concentrations within the intestines, as well as the concentration within the interior of the liver (all of these at three-hour dialysis time), are also displayed. Essentially the same results were obtained in the two-hour experiments.

In both the anterior abdominal wall and the diaphragm, the concentration profiles are nearly horizontal. Because the anterior abdominal wall has a thickness of 2–2.5 mm (diaphragmatic thickness = 1 mm), measurements were extended and the same horizontal profiles were observed. Fractional tissue concentrations (CPM/wet tissue weight/wet tissue weight/peritoneal fluid concentration) were very high in both tissues, and ranged from 0.7 at the surface to 0.9 beyond 400 μm from the peritoneum.

On the other hand, visceral tissues, such as the liver, the stomach, and intestine, varied in concentration from 0.22–0.33 μm at the peritoneal surface to 0.33–0.025 at 900 μm. The surface concentrations

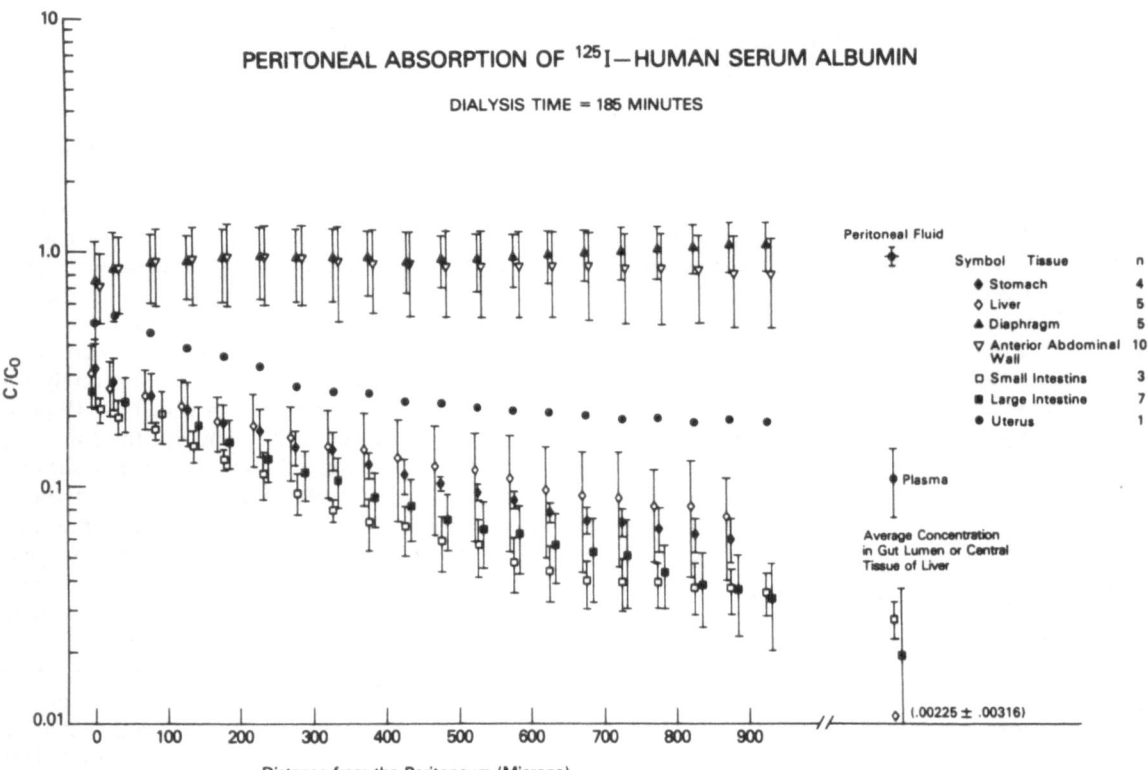

Fig. 2. Peritoneal tissue concentration profiles resulting from the absorption of ^{125}I-human serum albumin. Tissue concentration (based on wet tissue weight) divided by the initial peritoneal concentration versus distance in microns from the peritoneum. Tissue concentrations are expressed as the mean and standard deviation at each measurement interval.

in these organs corresponded to the estimated extracellular space in these tissues. Tissue gradients in uterine tissue were intermediate in concentration between the visceral and the parietal tissues.

DISCUSSION

The results demonstrate that the observed fluid loss rate (F_{obs}) from the peritoneal cavity is dependent on the intraperitoneal pressure. On the other hand, the effective lymph flow (L_{eff}), which transports protein from the tissues surrounding the cavity to the blood, is independent of the intraperitoneal hydrostatic pressure.

F_{obs} for the fibrinogen experiments in which thoracic duct lymph was collected was 34.8 ± 5.8 $\mu l/min$ at 2.2–2.9 mm Hg and 58.7 ± 7.3 $\mu l/min$ at 4.8–5.1 mm Hg. These results agree with Courtice and Steinbeck,[9] who found that after injecting 4 ml of plasma (IP pressure < 1 mm Hg) into the peritoneal cavity of a 200 g rat, the apparent loss rate was 38.0 $\mu l/min$ for the first hour and 20.4 $\mu l/min$ when averaged for three hours. Our results also correlate well with those of Zink and Greenway,[10] who experimented with cats. When their results are scaled to a 200 g rat by use of the factor (body wt)$^{0.7}$, an estimate of $F_{obs} = 26.6 \mu l/min$ for an IP pressure of 4.4 mm Hg is obtained. At 2.2 mm Hg, the scaled rate is 19.1 $\mu l/min$.

Henriksen et al.[11] have carried out a clinical study of protein absorption from ascitic fluid to the blood in eight cirrhotic patients. Their experimental design matched ours performed in rats. If the high and the low values are discarded, the effective lymph flow (based on the transport of labeled albumin or IgG) was 37.4 ml/h; this can be scaled by (body wt)$^{0.7}$ to be 0.6 ml/h in a 200 g rat. This value may be compared to the rate we found in the thoracic-duct intact rats—0.16 ml/h. Paralleling our results, they also observed that the peritoneal concentrations were relatively constant over time, and the corrected plasma concentration rose linearly with time.

To our knowledge, no one has previously examined macromolecular transfer into tissues surrounding the peritoneal cavity. Because of the ultimate application to cancer treatment, it was important to quantify concentrations of drug in the tissues, particularly in the gut, which has sensitive mucosal epithelial cells. From our results, it appears that the visceral tissues (except the layers close to the peritoneal surface) are not exposed to high concentrations during IP macromolecular drug delivery. On the

other hand, the abdominal wall and diaphragm tend to accumulate these substances. We conclude that convection dominates over diffusion in the transport of macromolecules into and through tissue, and that, once in the tissue, these substances will accumulate if not taken up by lymphatics.

Because the entire IP pressure is superimposed across its thickness, the abdominal wall is stretched and sustains an increase in its extracellular space.[13] The increase in extracellular space in turn increases the volume of distribution of the protein, which allows more protein to enter the tissue. The lymphatic system in skeletal muscle is known to be limited to fascial planes and there are few lymphatic capillaries in the muscle proper.[14] Therefore, the mechanism that removes protein from the interstitial space is diminished. All of these factors contribute to the accumulation of macromolecules in the anterior abdominal wall and are causes of the very high tissue concentrations displayed in Figure 2.

The diaphragm contains a specialized anatomical system that transports 60–80% of the peritoneal fluid taken up by lymphatics.[6] Casley-Smith[15] has demonstrated the mechanisism of uptake of particles and cells by stomata that communicate with lymphatic lacunae under the mesothelium. He demonstrated intracellular uptake by small (0.05 μm diameter) and large (0.1–1 μm diameter) vesicles, and further observed an increase in the size and density of the large vesicles with time. We conclude that the filling of lacunae and the accumulation of "storage-like" vesicles are the most likely causes of the high diaphragmatic concentration displayed in Figure 2.

The decreasing tissue concentration profiles in the liver, stomach, and intestines are due to well-developed lymphatic systems within these tissues. In the gut, there are plexi in each layer: mucosa, submucosa, and muscularis, and flow occurs from inner to outer plexi.[16] In the liver there are three systems of lymphatics: (1) capsular; (2) that associated with the hepatic vein; and (3) that associated with hepatic artery.[16] From our data we conclude that these systems have sufficient capacity to transfer fluid and solutes away from the tissue and to prevent significant accumulation.

REFERENCES

1. Jones RB, Collins JM, Myers CE, Brooks AE, Hubbard SM, Balow JE, Brennan MF, Dedrick RL, and DeVita VT: High-volume intraperitoneal chemotherapy with methotrexate in patients with cancer. Cancer Res 41: 55, 1981

2. Speyer JL, Collins JM, Dedrick RL, Brennan MF, Buckpitt AR, Londer H, DeVita VT, and Myers CE: Phase I and pharmacological studies of 5-fluorouracil administered intraperitoneally. Cancer Res 40: 567, 1980

3. Gianni L, Jenkins JF, Greene RF, Lichter AS, Myers CE, and Collins JM: Pharmacokinetics of the hypoxic radiosensitizers Misonidazole and Demethylmisonidazole after intraperitoneal administration in humans. Cancer Res 43: 913, 1983

4. Howell SB, Pfeifle CE, Wung WE, and Ohlsen RA: Intraperitoneal cis-diamminedichloroplatinum with systemic thiosulfate protection. Cancer Res 43: 1426, 1983

5. Knapp RC, St John E, and Bast RC: A review of intraperitoneal therapy of human ovarian carcinoma. Peritoneal Dial Bull 3: 59, 1983

6. Yoffey JM, and Courtice FC: Lymphatics, lymph, and the lymphomyeloid complex. London: Academic Press, 1970, p 206

7. Flessner MF, Parker RJ, and Sieber SM: Peritoneal lymphatic uptake of fibrinogen and erythrocytes in the rat. Am J Physiol 244: H89, 1983

8. Flessner MF, Fenstermacher JD, Blasberg RG, and Dedrick RL: Peritoneal absorption of macromolecules studied by quantitative autoradiography. Am J Physiol (in press)

9. Courtice FC, and Steinbeck AW: Absorption of protein from the peritoneal cavity. J Physiol (Lond) 114: 336, 1951

10. Zink J, and Greenway CV: Control of ascites absorption in anesthetized cats: Effects of intraperitoneal pressure, protein, and furosemide diuresis. Gastroenterology 73: 1119, 1977

11. Henriksen JH, Lassen NA, Parving H-H, and Winkler K: Filtration as the main transport mechanism of protein exchange between plasma and the peritoneal cavity in hepatic cirrhosis. Scand J Clin Lab Invest 40: 503, 1980

12. Schultz JS, and Armstrong W: Permeability of interstitial space of muscle (rat diaphragm) to solute of different molecular weights. J Pharm Sci 67: 696, 1978

13. Reed RK, and Wiig H: Compliance of the interstitial space in rats. I. Studies on hindlimb skeletal muscle. Acta Physiol Scand 113: 297, 1981

14. Pearson CM: Circulation in skeletal muscle. In Abramson DI (Ed), Blood vessels and lymphatics. New York: Academic Press, 1962, p 520

15. Casley-Smith JR: Endothelial permeability—the passage of particles into and out of diaphragmatic lymphatics. J Exp Physiol 49: 365,1964

16. Barrowman JA: Physiology of the gastrointestinal lymphatic system. Cambridge: Cambridge University Press, 1978, p 3

W.H. Boesken, H.C. Schuppe, A. Seidler, and P. Schollmeyer

8

Peritoneal Membrane Permeability for High and Low Molecular Weight Proteins (H/LMWP) in CAPD

SUMMARY

Peritoneal permeability was studied over the whole spectrum of serum proteins (10^4–10^6 daltons) to further evaluate membrane permeability and to compare it with the glomerular filtration barrier as well as with hemodialysis and hemofiltration membranes. Serum and PD-effluent concentrations of 11 different proteins as well as of creatinine, urea and potassium were determined in 13 patients with different glucose concentration and dwell times. During 20 episodes of peritonitis some of the proteins were determined daily for 2 to 3 wks, to study local immune responses. By SDS-PAGE analyses total peritoneal proteins were divided according to molecular size.

Total peritoneal protein losses averaged 9.6 ± 2.5 g/24 h, during peritonitis increasing to 19.2 (8–37) g/24 h. The ratio of LMWP to HMWP in the peritoneal effluent was higher when compared to serum. Effluent/serum (E/S) protein ratios decreased as a function of molecular weight, revealing a characteristic exponential profile. The peritoneum was different from most membranes mentioned above regarding higher HMWP- and lower LMPW-permeability. Individually different protein losses and peritonitis lead to parallel shifts of this profile. During and within 3 wks after peritonitis no local antibody production could be detected by daily measurement of IgG/transferrin response, or the IgM/d_2 macroglobulin ratio. Lysozyme, however, was produced locally during peritonitis. IgG dialysate/serum ratio under basal conditions but even more so during peritonitis was inversely proportional to peritonitis frequency. Individual IgG dialysate/serum values altered very little during CAPD up to 2 yrs. Two patients with terminal sclerosing peritonitis had the lowest peritoneal IgG-permeability.

Peritoneal protein excretion therefore is not only undesirable but LMWP may help in excretion of uremic toxins and sufficient HMWP response to produce IgG may protect or predict the individual susceptibility to peritonitis early in CAPD.

INTRODUCTION

Protein loss is one of the disadvantages of peritoneal dialysis.[1-3] Large quantities are lost with the dialysate. On the other hand, excretion of low molecular weight proteins (LMPW) and smaller peptides may indicate the removal of uremic toxins.[4] The presence of high molecular weight proteins (HMWP) may be required for humoral immune reactions. The present study was undertaken for several reasons: (1) Peritoneal permeability for HMW-serum proteins is well known.[5] Few data are available regarding LMW proteins (10,000–60,000 daltons). Completed protein permeability profiles may help us to understand the mechanisms of peritoneal dialysis. (2) Local antibody production, as known, i.e., for cerebrospinal fluids,[6] might be oper-

From the Department of Nephrology, Med. Univ. Klinik. Freiburg University Medical Hospital, Freiburg im Breisgau, Germany (FRG).

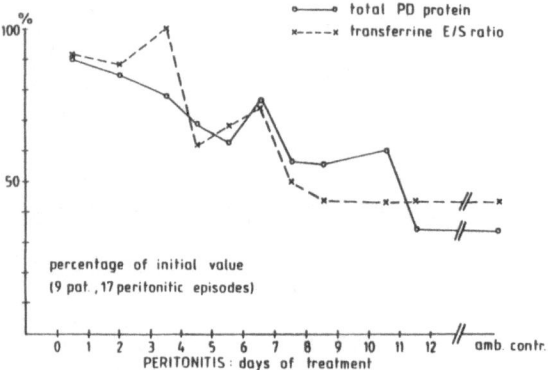

Fig. 1. Protein loss and membrane permeability during peritonitis. Total peritoneal protein (g/24 h) and transferrin permeability (E/S), expressed as percentage of maximal values on the first day of peritonitis. Mean values of 17 peritonitis episodes in nine patients.

ative also in the peritoneal cavity. To prove this hypothesis, clearances of cell derived lysozyme (Lys) and immunocompetent proteins (IgG, -M) were compared with inactive proteins of similar size—retinol binding protein (RBP), transferrin (Tf), and α_2 macroglobulin (α_2 M). (3) Peritoneal permeability was studied with regard to individual peritonitis incidence in order to find early parameters for exclusion of patients unsuitable for CAPD.

MATERIALS AND METHODS

Total protein was determined by standard TCA-biuret technique, as well as by tannin-ferric chloride technique according to Yatzidis.[7] The latter is more sensitive for detecting micromolecular proteins.[8] SDS-PAGE (sodium dodecylsulfate-polyacrylamide-gel-electrophoresis) was carried out as described before for urinary protein analysis.[9] Radial immuno-diffusion (RID) was used to quantify α_2 M, IgG, -M, Tf, alb, α_1 AT, α_1 GP, and RBP (LC-partigen, Behringwerke AG, Marburg, FRG). Lys was determined by a turbidimetric test (Lysomar, Behringwerke AG). Beta$_2$ microglobulin (β_2 M) was analyzed quantitatively by ELISA (Pharmacia AG, Frieburg). During stable CAPD the 24-h dialysate (3–5 bags) was studied in nine patients. One individual patient was analyzed during a four-day period with different glucose concentrations and different dwelling times. Additionally, 20 episodes of peritonitis were studied daily in nine patients up to 3 weeks. Total protein amounts per exchange (ex) and dialysate/serum ratios (E/S) (mean ± SD were calculated.

RESULTS

The peritoneal dialysate contained 9.6 ± 2.5 g protein/24 h, increasing to 19.2 (8–37) g/24 h during the early stages of peritonitis. Figure 1 documents the gradual decrease of protein losses, as well as of

Table 1. Proteins in Sera and Peritoneal Effluents.

Protein	Daltons	Dialysate (mg/ex)	Serum (mg/dl)	E/S
β_2 M (β_2-microglobulin)	12,000	15.0 ± 4.4	4.2 ± 0.4	0.189
Lys (lysozyme)	15,000	9.1 ± 2.7	3.7 ± 0.9	0.139
RBP (retinol-binding protein)	22,000	16.7 ± 4.0	19.4 ± 8.0	0.048
α_1 GP (acid glycoprotein)	40,000	84 ± 30	147 ± 21	0.027
α_1 AT (antitrypsin)	54,000	134 ± 44	277 ± 48	0.023
Alb (albumin)	67,000	1130 ± 395	2520 ± 765	0.023
Tf (transferrin)	79,000	54 ± 19	152 ± 72	0.020
IgG (immunoglobulin G)	156,000	306 ± 156	1310 ± 440	0.013
IgA (immunoglobulin A)	156,000	29.1 ± 12.3	201 ± 95	0.009
α_2 M (macroglobulin)	820,000	17.0 ± 13.8	273 ± 58	0.004
IgM (immunoglobulin M)	900,000	6.4 ± 4.7	149 ± 56	0.003
Total protein		1801.3 mg/ex		

Single protein analysis in peritoneal dialysate (mg/ex) and sera (mg/dl). Effluent/serum (E/S) ratios are a function of molecular weight. About 75% of total protein is detected by single protein analysis. ex = exchange.

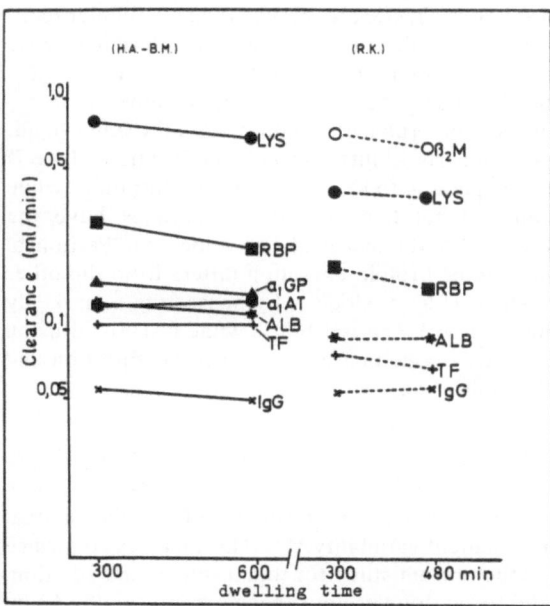

Fig. 2. Protein clearances (ml/min) as a function of dwell time. Left: Mean values of seven patients (H.A.-B.M.); right: Patient R.K. (mean of three peritoneal effluents).

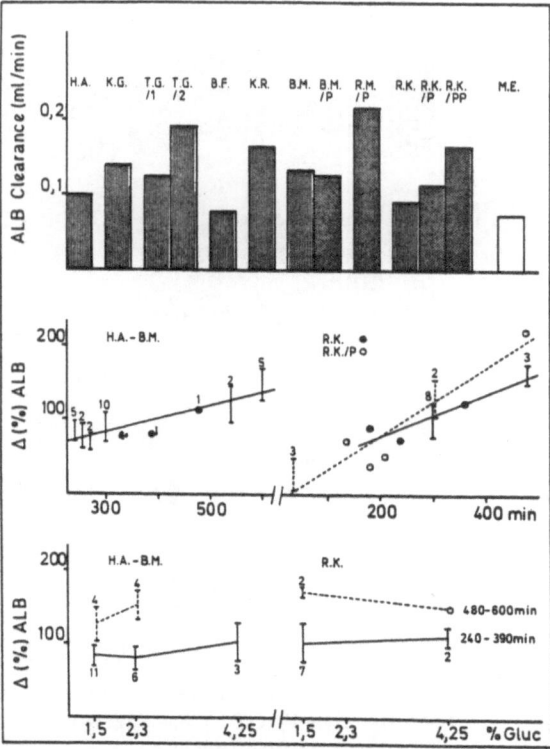

Fig. 3. Peritoneal albumin handling. Mean individual albumin clearance (ml/min) during CAPD (patients H.A., K.G., etc.) during CAPD-peritonitis (P) and during IPD (patient M.E.). Relative alteration of albumin excretion (Δ% Alb) is indicated in the case of increasing dwell time (min) respective glucose concentrations (% = g/dl), the latter subdivided for different dwell time (240–390 mm and 480–600 min). Mean values (± SD or range) and numbers of bags taken for calculation are indicated.

single protein permeability (Tf-E/S ratio) in relation to time of treatment.

By single-protein analysis about 75% of total protein could be identified. Table 1 lists the molecular size of the 11 protein molecules, the amount of protein per exchange, the respective serum level, as well as the E/S ratio of protein concentrations. E/S ratios decreased as an exponential function of molecular weight. Protein content per exchange depends on serum levels and molecular size. As shown before,[10] the amount of a single protein per exchange additionally is determined by dialysate dwell time. Small proteins reach their maximal dialysate concentration early; clearances decrease as a function of time (Fig. 2; i.e., RBP). Albumin, on the other hand, has the same clearance of about 0.1 ml/min after 300, 480, and 600 minutes, indicating that equilibrium has not been reached by this time. Glucose concentration had very little influence on peritoneal excretion of all proteins studied.

As shown in Figure 3, RBP excretion is not dependent on 1.5-2.3- or 4.25 g/dl dialysate dextrose concentrations, except for very long dwell times. The same figure, however, reveals peritoneal RBP loss increasing with time in a group of seven patients (H.A.-R.M.), as well in one patient on CAPD with-

out peritonitis (R.K.), but even more so with peritonitis complicating CAPD (R.K./P).

The distribution of protein species in CAPD effluent (Fig. 4, columns 2–4) differs from serum proteins (Fig. 4, column 1) by containing relatively higher quantities of the LMWP, but resembles urinary proteins in patients with glomerulopathies and renal insufficiency. Peritoneal lavage for pyogenic peritonitis due to intestinal perforation reveals a serum-like pattern (Fig. 4, columns 5 versus 1), probably due to serum leakage rather than to diffusion in to the peritoneum.

E/S ratios increase during peritonitis and lead to a parallel shift of the exponential permeability profile (Fig. 5), as shown before.[10] To study local

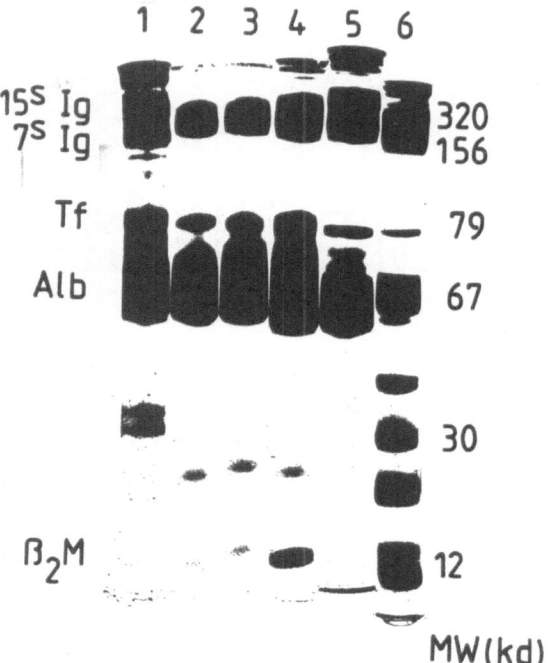

Fig. 4. Molecular weight analysis of peritoneal proteins (e-f) by SDS-PAGE. Characteristic contents (Ig, Tf, alb, β_2M) are indicated. 1 = serum proteins and 6 = glomerular and tubular proteinuria for comparison. 2–4 = CAPD effluents. 5 = peritoneal lavage for pyogenic peritonitis.

responses, i.e., antibody production, the permeability (E/S) of IgM as "early" antibody correlated with α_2M, a nonimmunocompetent protein of similar size (Fig. 6). No difference was seen during stable CAPD and peritonitis, disproving the hypothesis of local antibody secretion. The same has been shown for IgG in comparison to Tf,[10] while Lys is released locally,[10] probably from migrated cells.

E/S ratios of IgG were compared to the incidence of peritonitis episodes, revealing a significant reverse proportionality (Fig. 7). The IgG-E/S ratio turned out to be individually characteristic. Two patients with the highest peritonitis incidence (and eventually sclerosing peritonitis) had the lowest IgG-E/S values from the beginning of CAPD, remaining low during two years of treatment, despite frequent episodes of peritonitis.

Finally, peritoneal membrane permeability for proteins was compared with renal protein handling, as well as with artificial membranes (Fig. 5); Permeability for LMWP (30,000 daltons or less) (Fig. 5) is highest at the glomerular membrane, and lowest in

urine (Fig. 5), slope 4 versus 1), due to tubular reabsorption. Reduced E/S ratios in different disease states (3 = interstitial nephritis; 2 = transplant rejection) reflect tubular insufficiency rather than reduced glomerular permeability. On the other hand, protein permeability during hemofiltration (slope 7) is comparable to that of glomerular filtration, while conventional hemodialysis membranes have the lowest LMWP permeability (slope 6). Peritoneal membrane protein excretion differs from the other systems (Fig. 5, slope 5) by possessing a markedly higher HMWP permeability, while LMWP diffusion is restricted compared to glomerular filtration and hemofiltration.

DISCUSSION

Protein loss loss during CAPD exhibits a great interpatient variability.[13–15] This fact was confirmed by the present study for total protein, and additionally for various protein species, representing about 75% of total protein. Whereas dwell time and peritonitis augment the protein loss, dextrose concentration has little influence. Protein quantities measured by the Yatzidis technique[7] are about 30% higher when compared to standard biuret technique. This is due to LMWP present in the dialysate, which are underestimated by the biuret reaction.[8] E/S ratios for proteins of 10^4–10^6 daltons molecular weight were used to define peritoneal permeability. As far as possible, small proteins (10,000–60,000 daltons) were included in the study. With increasing molecular weight, permeability decreases markedly in the micromolecular range (10,000–30,000 daltons). The complete permeability profiles were exponential in character, even when plotted bi-logarithmically. Mean values for one patient and an additional group of seven patients under stable CAPD give identical profiles. However, marked parallel shift was noticed comparing long and short dwell times. The well known increase of protein loss during peritonitis shows a similar shift.[5, 14, 15] Profiles remain unchanged regarding immunoglobulins during acute peritonitis, as shown here for IgM in correlation with α_2M and in a previous study for IgG/Tf.[10] Lys obviously is locally released, as shown by Lys/RBP ratios.[10] The fact that the protein permeability (IgG-E/S ratio) decreases as a function of the peritonitis incidence, might be compared to a "protective ascites" containing high amounts of protein with local functions.[16]

Compared with other membranes and renal protein handling, peritoneal permeability profiles de-

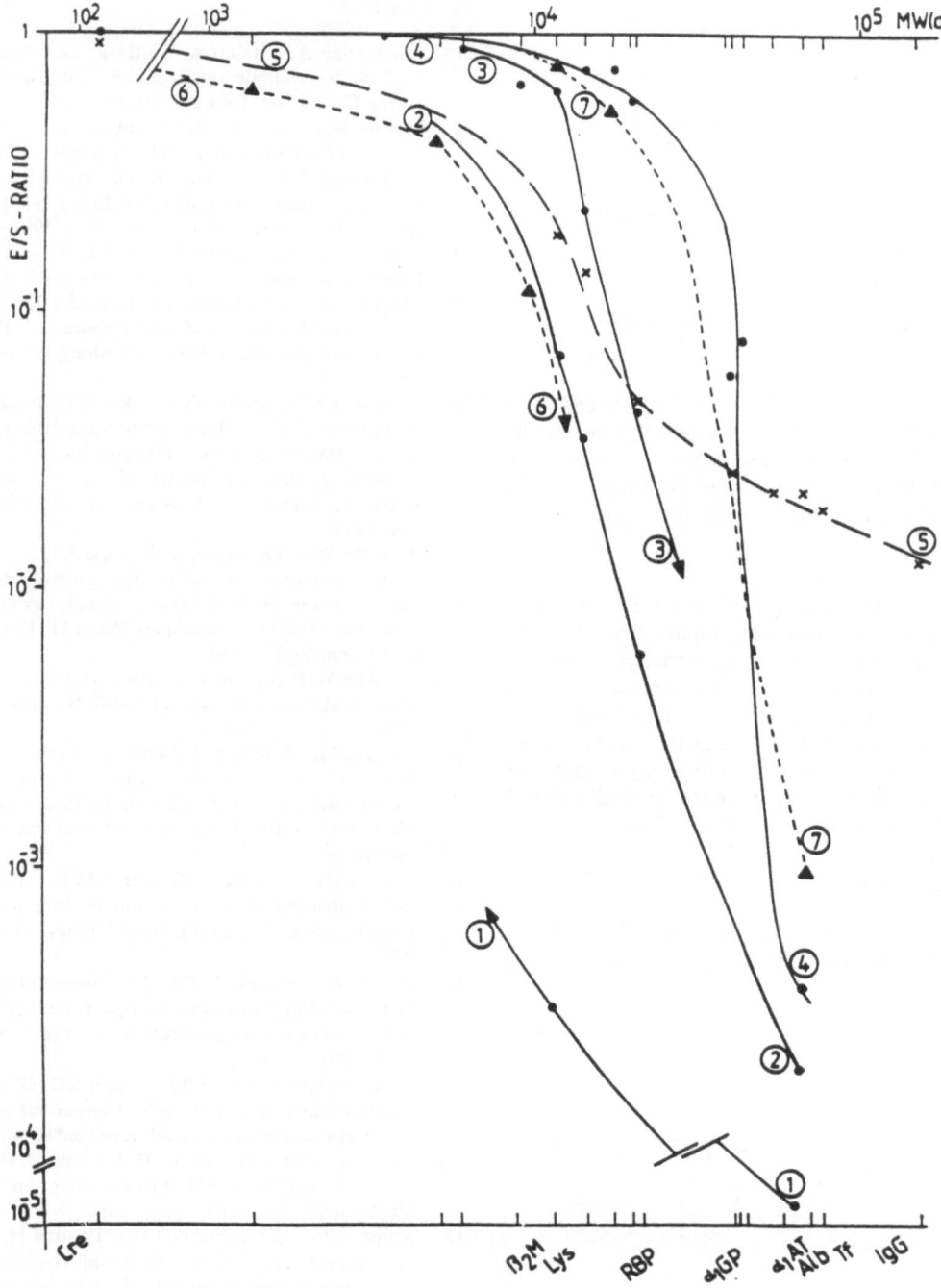

Fig. 5. Effluent/serum ratios (E/S) at the peritoneal membrane in comparison to renal protein handling and hemofiltration or hemodialysis membranes. 1 = normal kidney, final urine. 2 = mild transplant rejection. 3 = interstitial nephritis (E/S = fractional clearance, E/S-Cre = 1). 4 = glomerular membrane (E/S = sieving coefficient).[11,12] 5 = peritoneal membrane. 6 = hemodialysis (E/S = fractional clearance; manufacturers data). 7 = hemofiltration (E/S = sieving coefficient according to reference 17 and manufacturers data). For protein identification refer to Table 1.

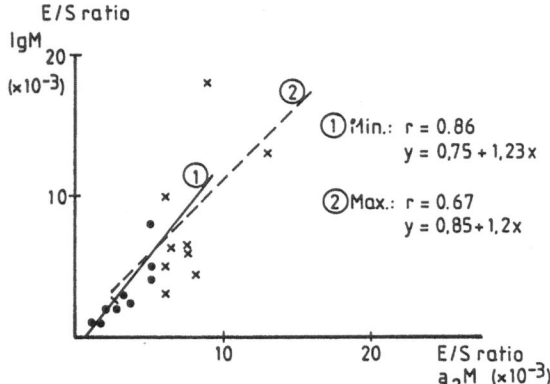

Fig. 6. Correlation of E/S ratios for IgM (900,000 daltons) and α_2M (820,000 daltons during stable CAPD (0 = Min.) and peritonitis (0 = Max.). Permeability of both proteins increased during peritonitis by the same proportion, disproving local IgM-secretion.

velop without a narrow "cut off" zone. Large-solute (>Alb) transfer is remarkably higher than the permeability of the glomerulus, hemodialysis and hemofiltration membranes. The transfer rate of small proteins (<Alb) appears slower than the glomerulus and hemofiltration, but surpasses the effectiveness of hemodialysis. The better removal of peptides and small proteins might contribute to the ability of the peritoneal membrane to control uremia.

ACKNOWLEDGMENT

Supported in part by grant Bo 378/12 from Deutsche Forschungsgemeinschaft, Bonn.

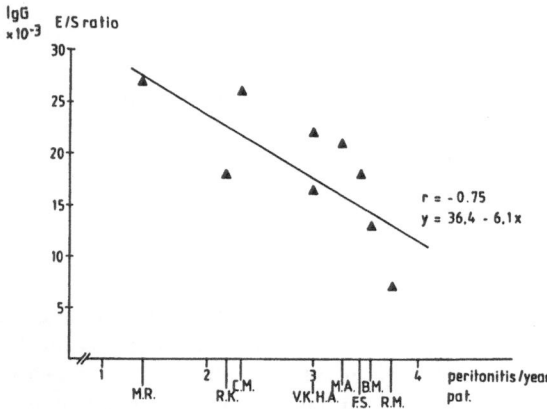

Fig. 7. IgG-E/S ratio is inversely correlated with individual peritonitis incidence.

REFERENCES

1. Giangrande A, Limido A, Cantu P, and Allaria P: SDS-Polyacrylamide electrophoresis of protein loss during CAPD. Ric Clin Lab 10: 117, 1980
2. Khanna R, Oreopoulos DG, Dombros N, Vas S, Williams P, Meema H, Husdan H, Ogilvie R, Zellerman G, Roncari DAK, Clayton S, and Itzatt S: CAPD after three years. Peritoneal Dial Bull 1: 24, 1980
3. Nolph KD: CAPD. Am J Nephrol 1: 1, 1981
4. Henderson LW, Cheung AK, and Chenoweth DE. Choosing a membrane. Am J Kidney Dis 3: 5, 1983
5. Blumenkrantz MJ, Gahl GM, Kopple JD, Kamdar AV, Jones MR, Kessel M, and Coburn JW: Protein loss during peritoneal dialysis. Kidney Int 19: 849, 1981
6. Felgenhauer K, Schliep G, and Rapid N: Evaluation of the blood-CSF barrier by protein gradients and the humoral immune response. J Neurol Sci 30: 113, 1976
7. Yatzidis H: New colorimetric method for quantitative determination of protein in urine. Clin Chem 23: 811, 1977
8. Boesken WH, Mamier A, and Ziupa J. Quantitative analysis of glomerular and tubular proteinuria: Critical evaluation of TCA-biuret, tannine-ferrichloride and Coomassie-blue techniques. Abstr 5th Eur Congr Clin Chem 1983, p 149
9. Boesken WH: Discelectrophoretic molecular weight analysis of urinary proteins. Contrib Nephrol 1: 143, 1975
10. Schuppe HC, Seidler A, Schollmeyer P, and Boesken WH: Peritoneal permeability for small proteins and immunoglobulins under CAPD. In Peters H (Ed), 32nd Coll Prot Biol Fluids. Oxford: Pergamon Press, 1984 (in press)
11. Galaske RG, Van Liew JB, and Feld LG: Filtration and reabsorption of endogenous low-molecular weight proteins in the rat kidney. Kidney Int 16: 394, 1979
12. Maack T, Johnson V, Kau ST, Figuereido J, and Sigulem P: Renal filtration, transport and metabolism of low-molecular weight proteins. A review. Kidney Int 16: 251, 1979
13. Popovich RP, Moncrief JW, Nolph KD, Ghods AJ, Twardowski Z, and Pyle WK: Continuous ambulatory peritoneal dialysis. Ann Intern Med 88: 449, 1978
14. Rubin J, Nolph KD, Arfania D, Prowant B, Fruto L, Brown P, and Moore H: Protein losses in CAPD. Nephron 28: 218, 1981
15. Katirtzoglou A, Oreopoulos DG, Husdan H, Leung M, Ogilvie R, and Dombros N: Reappraisal of protein losses in patients undergoing CAPD. Nephron 26: 230, 1980
16. Diskin CJ, and Ho G: The protective value of protein and complement in ascitic fluid. RI Med J 64: 521, 1981
17. Streicher E, and Schneider H: Stofftransport bei hämodiafiltration. Nieren- u Hochdruckkrankh 12: 339, 1983

R. Selgas, A.R-Carmona, M.E. Martinez, J. Conesa, M.P-Fontan, E. Huarte, O. Ortega, and L. S-Sicilia

9

Follow-up of Peritoneal Mass Transfer Properties in Long-term CAPD Patients

SUMMARY

To assess peritoneal diffusive transport, mass transfer coefficients were determined in 18 patients. After 3 to 4 yrs of CAPD there was a trend toward increased peritoneal permeability. Peritonitis changed peritoneal permeability in variable ways but usually only transiently. Direct correlations were identified between transport rates of varied solutes.

INTRODUCTION

The study of the physicochemical stability of the peritoneal membrane in patients on CAPD is one of the main concerns of all groups carrying out this type of dialysis, as evidenced by various papers published in recent years. These studies have commonly found short-term preservation of the permeability characteristics, or slight modifications.[1-6] The quantification of the peritoneal mass transfer coefficient (MTC) is currently regarded as the most accurate assessment of diffusive transport across this membrane.[1-6]

At the beginning of the sixth year of world-wide expansion of CAPD, we are able to assess mid-term evolution of this parameter. This paper reports serial MTC measurements in patients treated for up to four years with CAPD.

From C.S. La Paz, Madrid, Spain.

MATERIALS AND METHODS

Fifty-seven patients, 0.1–4 years on CAPD, were evaluated between one and eight times to determine peritoneal mass transfer coefficients for the following solutes: urea, creatinine, uric acid, inulin, glucose, and parathormone (PTH). The total number of studies performed was 176.

Assessment Procedure

The existence of peritonitis was ruled out by clinical, cytological, and bacteriological methods. No patient had a peritonitis episode for the four weeks preceeding the assessment. Antihypertensive drugs were withheld from the day preceding the procedure. Patients fasted during and prior to the test. The first exchange in the morning (as well as the immediately preceding one) was carried out with Dianeal 1.36% (anhydrous) dextrose. One hour before starting the exchange, the patients received 5 g inulin in 50 ml normal saline intravenously. Blood samples were collected upon commencing the dialysis fluid infusion and when dialysate was drained. Nine dialysate samples were taken, every 30 minutes, after four successive in-and-out pumpings of about 50 ml. The blood pressure and body weight were recorded both before and after the exchange. Urine and dialysate samples were collected over 24 hours for determination of residual renal function and solute generation rates.

Table 1. Mean (±SD) Baseline MTC
Values (ml/min).

	Value	Range	n
Urea	21.04 ± 4.8	(13.7 − 28)	n:18
Creatinine	9.74 ± 3.5	(4.6 − 17)	n:18
Uric Acid	10.02 ± 7.1	(1.8 − 25)	n:10
Parathyroid			
Hormone	1.16 ± 1	(0.5 − 4.2)	n:12
Inulin	2.1 ± 1.2	(0.5 − 4)	n:15

Analytical Procedures

Urea and creatinine were determined in an autoanalyzer. Uric acid was determined by the uricase method; glucose by glucose-oxidase method; inulin by the Walser method, corrected for glucose. For PTH quantification we used a commercial (IRE) kit with a specific antiserum for the 34–84 fragment of PTH.

Mathematical Model

For determination of MTC we used the model described by several authors, with two pools for

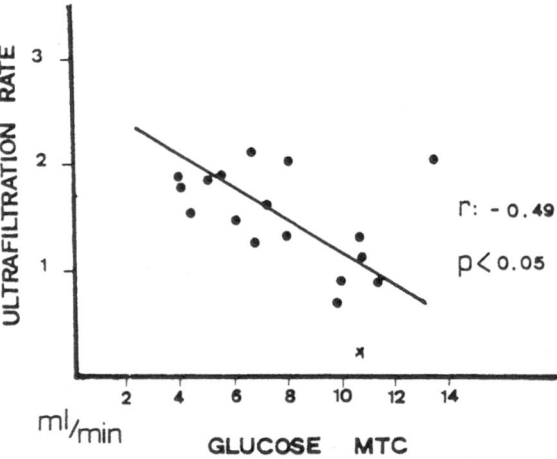

Fig. 2. Linear regression analysis for glucose MTC and 24 h ultrafiltration rate.

exchange: blood and dialysate. For sieving coefficient calculations we used 1 for the small molecules and 0.34 for the middle molecules. Integration of the differential equations and determination of MTC were carried out by the minimization of the 4th order quadratic error method of Runge-Kutta, with adaptation of the integration interval (subroutine DEF of the IBM PL-MATH library). The minimization was carried out as described by Powell (subroutine FMND of the same library). The integration interval was one minute, and the number of iterations to

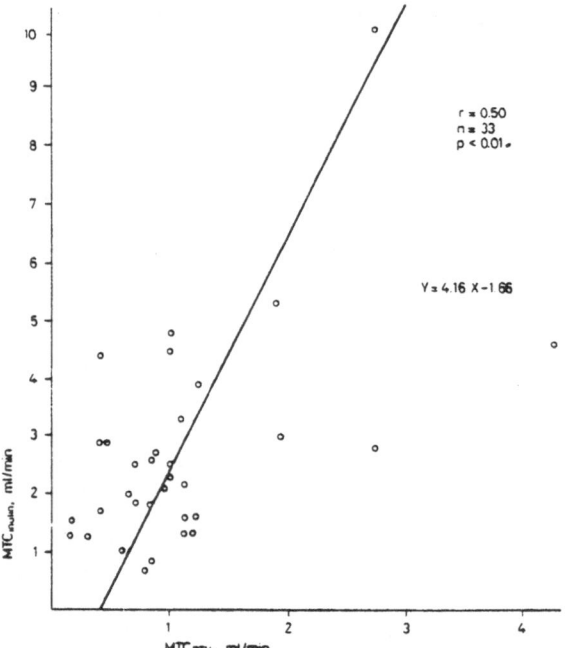

Fig. 1. Linear correlation between MTC_{inulin} and MTC_{PTH}.

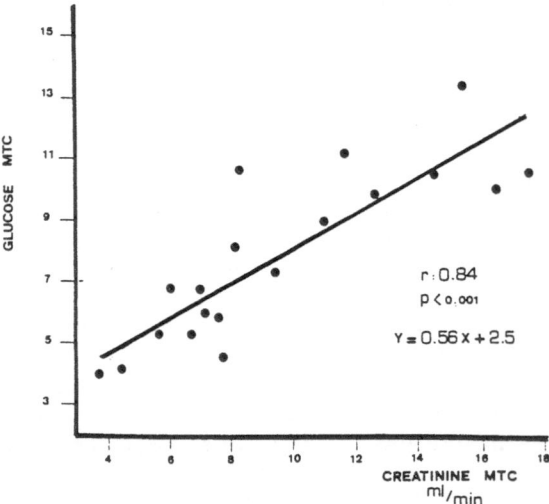

Fig. 3. Linear regression analysis for creatinine MTC and glucose MTC.

Table 2. MTC Changes after 3–4 years on CAPD.

	Urea	Creatinine	Uric Acid	Parathyroid Hormone	Inulin
Initial (ml/min)	18.5 ± 4.3	8.6 ± 3.6	7.8 ± 4	1.37 ± 1.5	2.08 ± 1.4
After 3–4 yrs (ml/min)	18.3 ± 4.7	9.8 ± 4.8	9.9 ± 6.3	1.78 ± 1.8	2.08 ± 1.4
	NS	$p < 0.01$	$p < 0.001$	$p < 0.05$	NS

achieve the minimum was four. Statistical analysis was performed with Student's t test for paired and nonpaired data.

RESULTS AND DISCUSSION

Table 1 shows the baseline mean values of MTCs in 18 patients studied during their first month in CAPD with no peritonitis episodes. These values showed no correlation with age, blood pressure, hematocrit, total protein, and albumin. Body surface and urea-MTC showed a linear direct relationship ($r = 0.47$; $p = 0.05$).

Figure 1 shows the relationship between inulin MTC and PTH MTC. Figures 2 and 3 show the linear regression analysis for creatinine MTC and glucose MTC and for 24 h ultrafiltration rate and glucose MTC. We also found a significant direct correlation between MTC values for urea and creatinine ($r = 0.62$), urea and uric acid ($r = 0.62$), uric acid and creatinine ($r = 0.85$), creatinine and PTH ($r = 0.63$), and uric acid and PTH ($r = 0.76$).

To examine the isolated effect of time on MTC values, we have studied the MTC evolution in 14 patients without peritonitis during 6–18 months. We found no change in seven patients (50%), corresponding to 56 patient-solutes (80%); increases in three patients (20%), nine patient-solutes (13%); and decreases in four patients (30%), corresponding to five patient-solutes (7%).

The effects of the first episode of peritonitis were followed in 13 patients studied after a 6-month maximal interval: MTC values of 27 patient-solutes (43%) showed no changes; 16 patient-solutes (29%) increased; and 16 patient-solutes decreased. The effects were quite variable, and three patients had permanent effects.

Multiple episodes of peritonitis caused the following effects in 12 patients: 83% showed changes—25 patient-solutes (50%) no changes, 14 patient-solutes (28%) increased, and 11 patient-solutes (22%) decreased. Three patients showed a permanent increase in some of their MTC values; two of these had a progressive loss of ultrafiltration capacity. One patient (who showed decreases) required an increase in the number of exchanges per day. Table 2 shows the MTC changes after 3–4 years of treatment (10 patients).

Evaluation of ultrafiltration capacity is possible by creatinine MTC. PTH and inulin have similar behavior across the peritoneum. Baseline peritoneal solute diffusivity is individual for each patient, as is the peritoneal response to injuries (time on CAPD, peritonitis). After four years on CAPD, there was a trend to increase peritoneal permeability. We believe it necessary to perform periodic evaluations of these parameters.

REFERENCES

1. Pyle W, Moncrief JW, and Popovich RP: Peritoneal transport evaluation in CAPD. In Moncrief JW, and Popovich RP (Eds), CAPD update. New York: Masson Publishing, 1981, p 32
2. Farrell PC, and Randerson DH: Membrane permeability changes in long-term CAPD. Trans Am Soc Artif Intern Organs 26: 197, 1980
3. Farrell PC: Peritoneal mass transfer. Peritoneal Dial Bull 2: 107, 1982
4. Nolph KD, Ghods AJ, and Brown PA: Effects of nitroprusside on peritoneal mass transfer coefficients and microvascular physiology. Trans Am Soc Artif Intern Organs 23: 210, 1977
5. Slingeneyer A, Canaud B, and Mion C: Permanent loss of ultrafiltration capacity of the peritoneum in long-term peritoneal dialysis: An epidemiological study. Nephron 33: 133, 1983
6. Rodriguez-Carmona A, Selgas R, and Martinez ME: Characteristics of the peritoneal mass transfer of parathormone in patients under continuous ambulatory peritoneal dialysis therapy. Nephron 37: 21, 1984

S.R. Ash, A.T.J. Bungu, and F.E. Regnier

10

Dependence of Middle Molecular Clearance on Protein Concentration of Peritoneal Fluid

SUMMARY

"Middle molecules" may be defined as substances which are dialyzable, but which dialyze very slowly. It is reasonable to assume that many of these are organic anions. Uremic serum has been studied by anion-exchange chromatography (DEAE-Sephadex, and HPLS) and shown to contain 12 to 15 separate peaks. *In vitro* dialysis of serum has shown that most of the anionic components of these peaks are highly protein bound, with molecular masses ranging from 180 to 300 daltons.

Outflow peritoneal fluid was collected from three patients on CAPD, after dwell times of 2 to 8 h. Anion exchange chromatograms indicated the presence of 12 to 15 peaks, with retention times similar to peaks of serum chromatograms. With the exception of one peak, all peaks were higher after 8 h than after shorter dwells (including vitamin B-12 and uric acid peaks). *In vitro* dialysis of peritoneal fluid samples demonstrated a high dialysance at one hour, but almost no dialysance at 2 to 4 h. It is concluded that the majority of anionic substances in peritoneal fluid are protein bound. This protein binding, rather than molecular weight, makes these substances fit the definition of "middle molecules." The exchange times of CAPD were appropriately chosen, to avoid limiting clearance of such substances. The protein which enters the peritoneal dialysate is important in maintaining clearance of these substances.

INTRODUCTION

The exchange times of CAPD (every 4–8 hours) were chosen originally to provide optimum removal of "middle molecules" with a minimum number of exchanges. It was postulated by Popovich et al.[1] that molecules of "middle molecular weight" (500–3000 daltons) would require at least 6–8 hours before reaching saturation levels in the peritoneum. Thus, the long dwell times of CAPD would not significantly interfere with clearance of such molecules, although they would, of course, diminish clearance for small solutes at the end of the dwell.

While the clinical effectiveness of CAPD can hardly be doubted, it has yet to be proven that the exchange time does in fact result in optimal middle molecular weight substance removal. The major difficulty in determining the clearance of the middle molecules is in consistency of the technique. The most widely utilized method of assay of uremic substances has been that of Bergström and Funck-Brentano and their coworkers.[2,3] This method involves filtration of uremic serum or peritoneal samples through an ultrafiltration membrane, chromatography on Sephadex (supposedly, for molecular

From Ash Medical Systems, Inc., West Lafayette, Indiana; World University School of Medicine, Santo Domingo, Dominican Republic; and School of Biochemistry, West Lafayette, Indiana.

weight discrimination), and a second chromatographic separation on DEAE-cellulose (an anionic exchange resin that separates peaks for different anions). This technique has demonstrated the presence of "middle molecule" peaks such as peak 7C in peritoneal dialysis fluid, but it has not allowed sufficient quantitation to demonstrate clearances of a rate of appearance of such peaks in peritoneal fluid. A difficulty with the Funck-Brentano method is that it yields information only on non protein-bound uremic substances. A large number of uremic substances such as hippurates and uric acid are partly protein bound,[4] thus their total concentration in fluid may exceed considerably the nonprotein portion.

Another difficulty with the method is the reliance on Sephadex columns for size exclusion and size discrimination. Solute-column interactions make interpretation of molecular weight of fractions difficult on Sephadex columns. In fact, many uremic substances in peaks thought to represent approximately 1000 daltons mw turned out, in fact, to include substances of approximately 200 daltons mw.[5] Filtration of biologic fluid through size-discriminating UF membranes also presents problems. The reflectance coefficient is dependent on ionic charge and other factors unrelated to molecular mass.

In 1983, we described a simpler method for the study of uremic substances than that of Bergstrom & Funck-Brentano.[7,8] This procedure allowed study of uremic substances in the presence of proteins. This method involved direct anion-exchange chromatography of the peritoneal fluid or uremic serum sample, without separation of the substances from proteins. From serum and peritoneal fluid samples, approximately 10 to 17 peaks were easily identified. Such peaks were clearly higher in uremic sera than normal sera, and the peaks in general decreased with dialysis. For size discrimination, we used a "double-diffusion" dialysis cell, in which 1 ml of serum or peritoneal fluid was sandwiched between two dialysis membranes (Fig. 1). Stationary distilled water was then placed opposite one membrane, and distilled water at 3 ml/min passed through the chamber opposite the other membrane. In these studies, the resultant mass transfer of peak substances across the two membranes indicated that most of the uremic and anion substances were in the range of 150–300 daltons. Furthermore, it was shown that the majority, if not all uremic anionic substances, were highly protein bound (70–90%). The rate of accumulation of such anionic substances in peritoneal fluid during CAPD exchanges, and the evidence for protein binding of these substances, is presented herein.

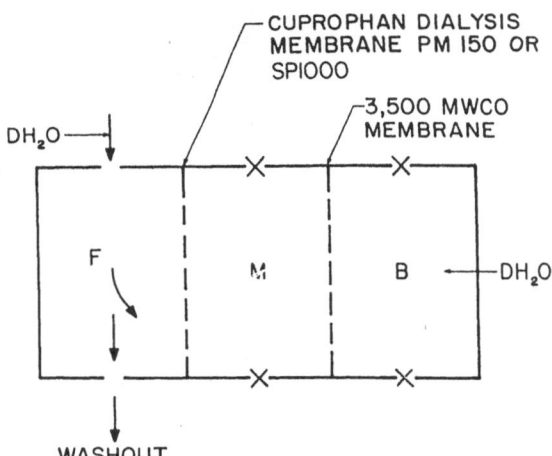

Fig. 1. Bidirectional diffusion cell-serum or peritoneal fluid placed in middle chamber. Distilled water in back chamber. Distilled water perfuses the front chamber at 3 ml/min. MWCO = molecular weight cut off (daltons).

METHODS

Samples and Sample Preparation for CAPD Fluid (Human)

Aliquots of peritoneal dialysate were obtained from two CAPD patients, each with residual renal creatinine clerance of 2–3 ml/min. Two liter volumes of 1.5% Dianal were used by these patients for four daily exchanges with dwell times of 2–8 hours. The Dianal bag was mixed thoroughly and 10 ml removed after completion of outflow. Samples were placed in capped vials, and refrigerated for less than one week (longer storage, or freezing, was shown to result in loss of certain peaks from the chromatographic analysis). The fluid was warmed to room temperature and placed directly in the chromatographic column, without filtration.

Chromatographic Conditions

Two liquid chromatographs were used: a Micrometrics Liquid Chromatograph, Model 7000 (Micrometrics Corporation, Norcross, VA) and a Varian Model 5000 Liquid Chromatograph (Varian Instrument Division, Palo Alto, CA). The mobile phase was a gradient of 0.01–1 M potassium phosphate buffer at pH 4.4 (KH_2PO_4 Monobasic: Matheson, Coleman and Bell, Norwood, OH). The anion

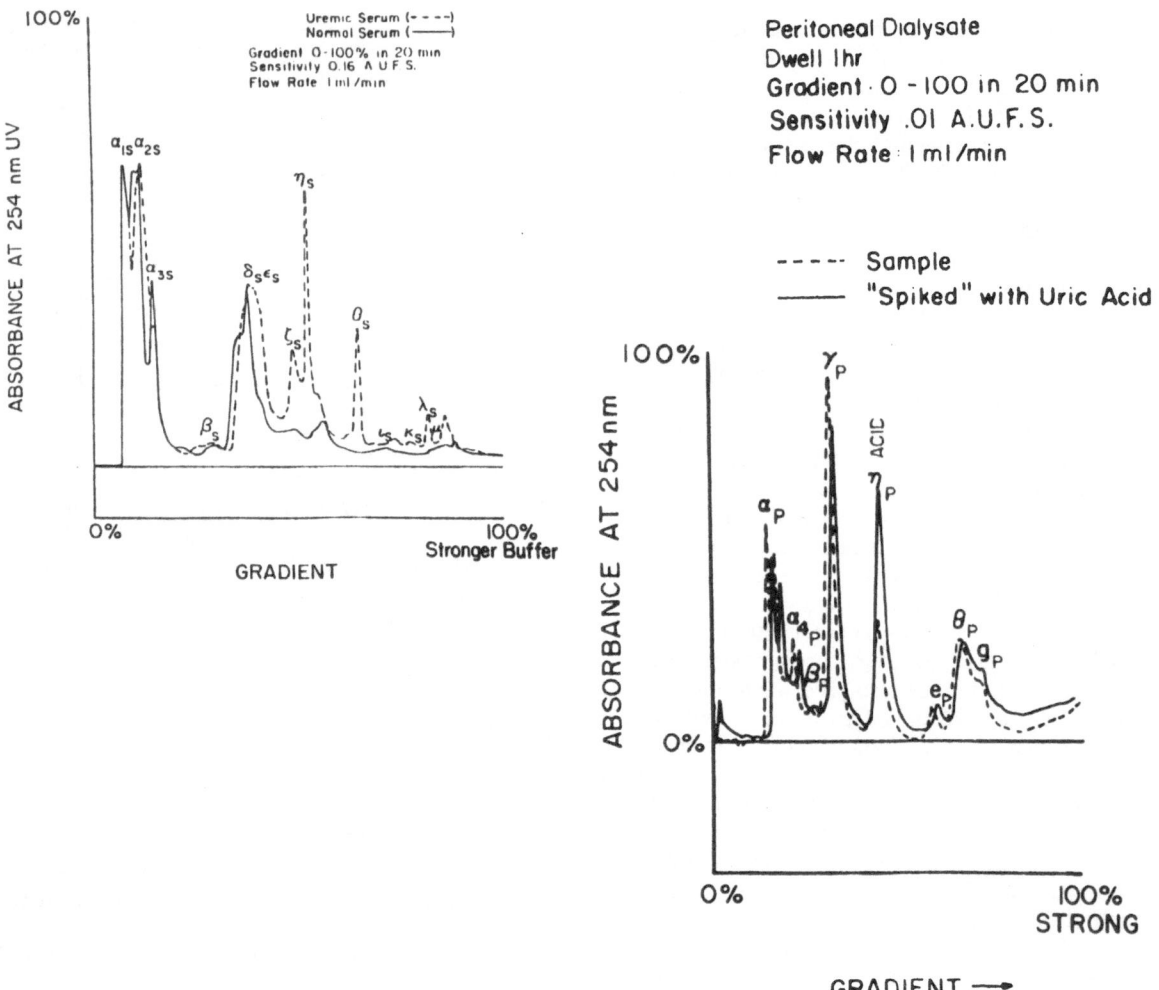

Fig. 2. (a) Predialysis chromatogram of serum. The separation pattern of uremic serum by direct anion-exchange chromatography. (b) Chromatogram of peritoneal dialysate. Separation pattern of peritoneal fluid (4 hour dwell), by anion exchange chromatography. Uric acid spike increases peak n.

exchange column used was a Synchropak AX 300 (Syn Chrom Inc., Linden, IN). The liquid chromatographic machines were equipped with Fischer Model 5000 recorders and UV detectors that measured absorbance at 254 nm. A linear mobile phase gradient ranging from 0–100% of the strong buffer was generated in 30 minutes with the Micrometric 7000, and 20 minutes with the Varian 5000. Flow rates were 1 ml/min in both cases.

Samples of either 10 or 100 μ L were introduced directly into anion exchange columns. Each sample was analyzed at least twice, according to the condi-

tions outlined above. Vitamin B_{12} and uric acid were chromatographed, both independently and in peak enrichment (spiking), to establish the general molecular weight of certain peaks.

Chamber Dialysance of Peritoneal Fluid

One ml samples of peritoneal fluid were placed in the middle chamber of four double diffusion cells (between the cellulosic membranes). One ml distilled water was placed in the back chamber. Distilled water was passed through from the chamber at

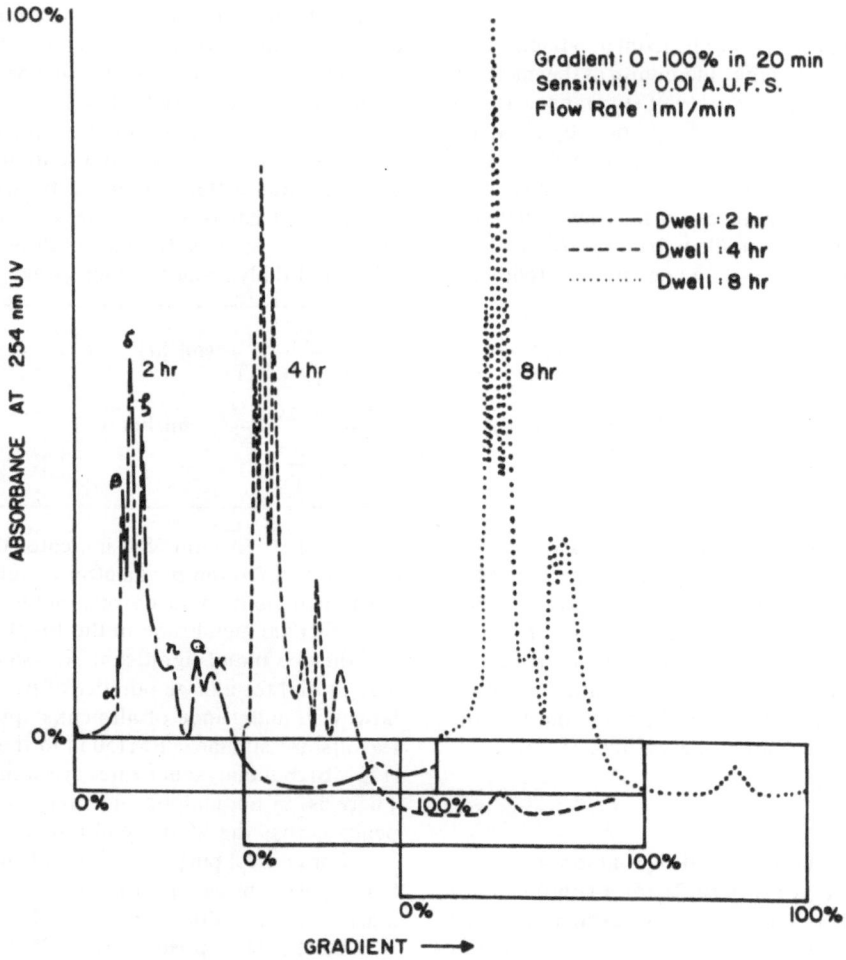

Fig. 3. Anion exchange chromatograms of 2 L of peritoneal fluid removed from one patient after dwells of 2, 6, and 8 hours.

3 ml/min, as shown in Figure 1. At 0, 1, 3, and 6 hours, dialysis was stopped, and the middle and back chamber sample removed from the cells. The samples were directly transferred to the anion exchange chromatographic columns. The area under curve (AUC) for peaks on the resulting chromatograms were measured by a mechanical integrator. This AUC was assumed to be proportional to the concentration of all substances in the peaks. Spectropor 3500 dalton cutoff membrane was always used for the membrane between the middle and back chambers (M-B membrane). Either SP1000 or Cuprophan PM 150 were used for the membrane between the middle and front membranes (M-F).

The purpose of the "double-diffusion" chamber was threefold.

1. To remove small molecules from the serum or peritoneal fluid, and from the back chamber fluid by dialysis of the samples against a large volume of distilled water. This was expected to lessen the interference of salt or small molecules with peaks of middle-size molecules.

2. To allow diffusion of "free" or unbound middle size molecules (less than 3500 daltons) from the middle to back chamber, demonstrating equilibrium concentration of "free" or unbound substances in the middle chamber.

3. To demonstrate the rate of transfer of substances across both the front and back membranes, thus allowing calculation of the maximal "dialysance" for a variety of substances across these membranes. This dialysance, by comparison to that of creatinine, should allow determination of effects molecular weight of transferable substances. Dialysance (ml/hr) was calculated for diffusion from middle to back (M-B) and middle to front (M-F) chambers by the following formulas:

$$\text{Dialysance } (M{\rightarrow}B)_t = \frac{\Delta C_B\, V_B}{(\overline{C}_M - \overline{C}_B) \times \Delta T} \quad (ml/hr) \tag{1}$$

$$\text{Dialysance } (M{\rightarrow}F)_t = \frac{\Delta C_m\, V_M + \Delta C_B\, V_B}{\dfrac{\overline{C}_M \times \Delta T}{2}} \quad (ml/hr) \tag{2}$$

Where D = dialysance; $\overline{C}$ = mean concentration (AUC) in chamber during time t; M = Middle chamber; B = Back chamber; V = volume of chamber; T = time interval (0–1 h, 1–3 h, 3–6 h). In this analysis, transfer of substances from middle to back chamber resulted in a positive dialysance. Transfer from middle to front resulted in a negative dialysance.

RESULTS

Figure 2a shows the direct anion exchange chromatograms obtained from uremic serum (predialysis). It is seen that anion exchange clearly defines a variety of peaks in uremic serum, and that most of the peaks are higher than those of normal serum. Chromatography of similar uremic serum samples on Sephadex G-10 or G-25 showed isolation of only 2 or 3 peaks. During a four hour hemodialysis of uremic patients, samples from the arterial line showed a decrease of the $\delta{-}\mu$ peaks to 50% of its original elevation. The α peaks decreased little during dialysis. This peak includes albumin and globulin.

Figure 2b shows anion exchange chromatographic peaks of peritoneal dialysate (obtained after a 4 hour dwell). A number of separate peaks are visible. Spiking the fluid with uric acid increased peak n. Spiking with creatinine increased peak α_4. Chromatography of peritoneal dialysate removed after 2, 4, and 8 hour dwells showed a continuing increase in all peak components with dwell time except peak n (Fig. 3). Similar results were found for repeat chromatograms of the two CAPD patients. The levels of most peaks were still increasing at 8

hours. Figure 4 indicates the anion exchange chromatograms obtained after chamber dialysis of peritoneal fluid, using SP1000 or PM150 membrane in the M-F position. In both uremic serum and peritoneal dialysate experiments, peaks rapidly rise in the back chamber and fall in the middle chamber in the first hour. After one hour, the size of all peaks changes extremely slowly. Separation of peaks by anion exchange is sufficient to allow calculation of AUC and dialysance for each peak.

Figures 5a and 5b indicate the calculated dialysance of anion peaks after chamber dialysis of peritoneal fluid (data corresponding to Figure 4). With SP1000 membrane in the M→F position (Fig. 5a), there is initial significant dialysance (of varying magnitude) for a large number of peaks. With time, however, dialysance of all peaks approaches zero. Results are similar if PM150 is in the M-F position (Fig. 5b), but dialysance rates are somewhat greater. There is an anomalous (+) dialysance for several peaks across the M-B membrane at 1–3 hours.

For control purposes, a double diffusion chamber experiment was performed using creatinine (20 mg/dl) in the middle chamber. SP 3500 membrane was in the M-B position and PM150 in the M-F position. Samples removed from the middle and back chambers at 0, 1, 3, and 6 hours were analyzed for creatinine. Dialysance across both membranes was found to be relatively constant, approximately 1.5 ml/hr.

During operation of the chamber dialysis cell, the fluids of the back chamber and middle chamber are effectively desalted. The initial concentration of sodium in the uremic serum sample in the middle chamber was 140 mEq, in one experiment. After 6 hours of dialysis, the final sodium concentration in the middle chamber was 33 mEq/L, and in the back chamber 26 mEq/L.

DISCUSSION AND CONCLUSIONS

To indicate the effective molecular size of uremic substances, we have used a membrane-diffusion test cell rather than size-exclusion chromatog-

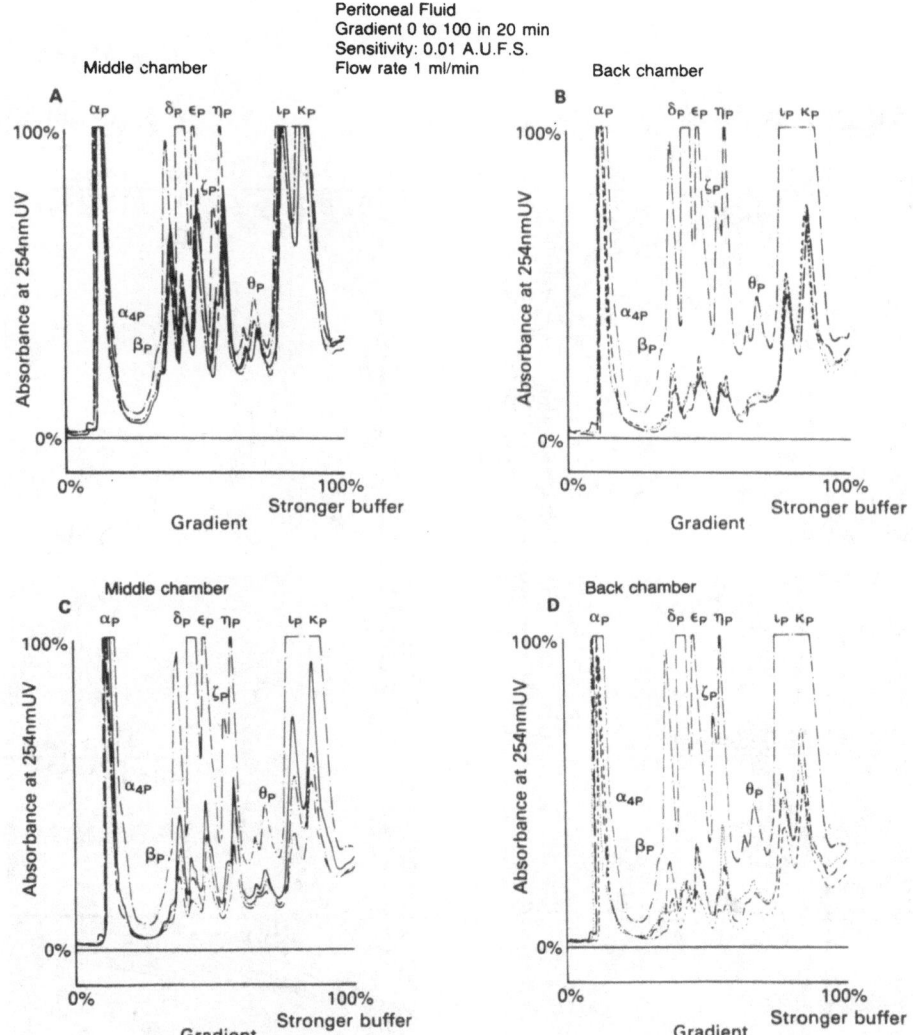

Fig. 4. (a) Separation pattern of peritoneal fluid, by anion-exchange chromatography of samples removed after 0, 1, 3 and 6 hours of dialysis in the middle chamber of the bidirectional diffusion cell (M-F membrane SP1000. M-B membrane SP3500). (b) Separation patterns of fluid from back chamber of bidirectional diffusion cell after 1, 3, and 6 hours of dialysis, same experiment as (a). (c,d) Same as (a) and (b), but with PM150 Cuprophan as M-F membrane.

raphy. Size exclusion chromatography may yield an inaccurate molecular weight. There are, of course, chemical interactions of anions with membranes (due to charge and solubility, for example), but these interactions would also be present during *in vivo* dialysis with cellulosic membranes. Therefore, the dialysance rates seen in the present study would be relevant to standard hemodialysis. Comparison of

the maximal (early) dialysance of individual peaks with that of creatinine, allows a calculation of effective molecular weight of peak components. Diffusion coefficient varies as $1/mw$,[2] up to 1000 daltons mw.[9] Up to the pore size of the membrane, dialysance is limited by the diffusion coefficient. The zero hour dialysance for uremic serum peaks α to μ were 0.3–1.75 ml/hr. (excepting anomalous dial-

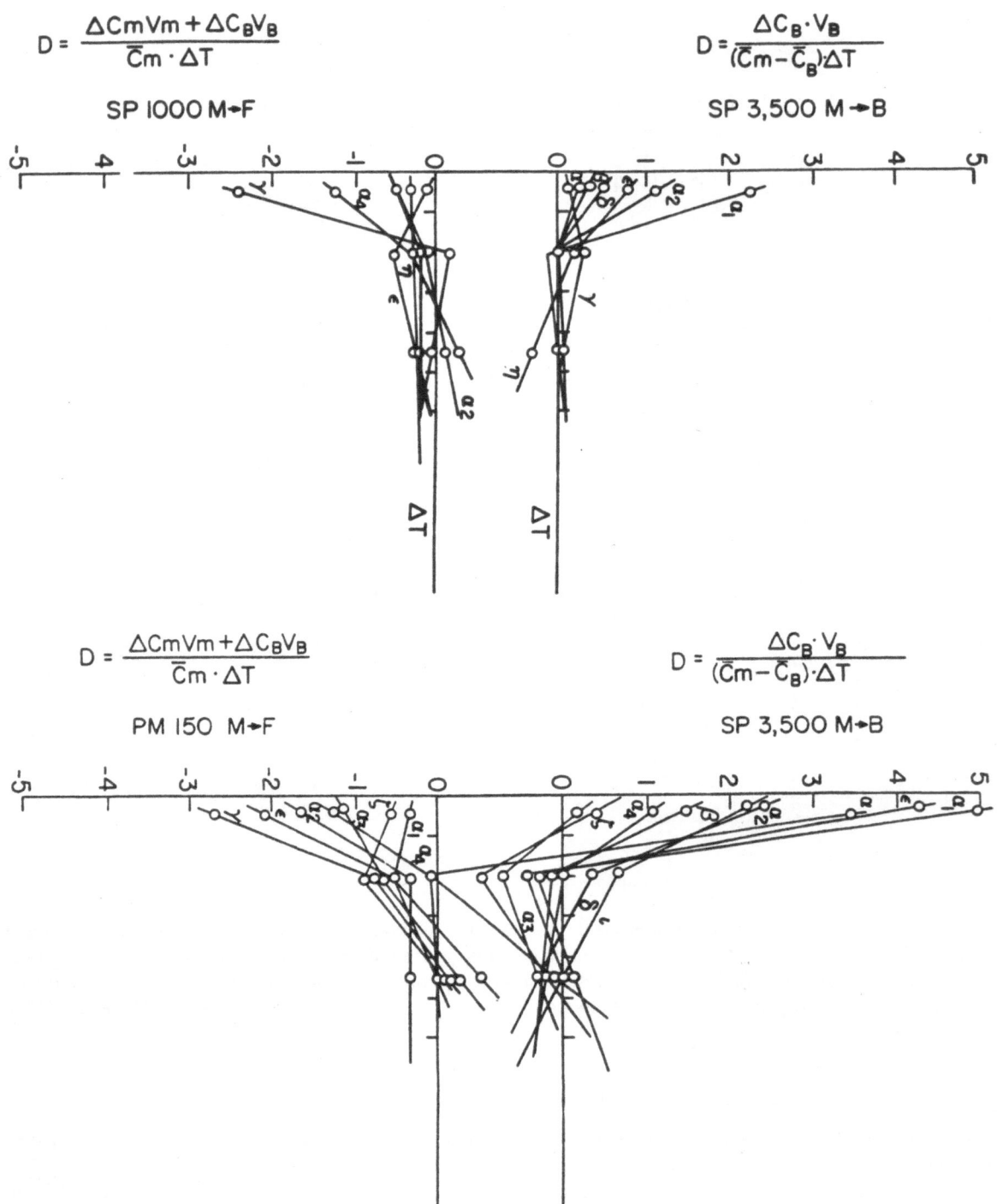

Fig. 5. (a) Dialysance of a variety of anion-exchange peaks of peritoneal fluid versus hours of residence in the bidirectional diffusion cell (from data on Figure 4a and b, M-F membrane SP1000). (b) Dialysance of a variety of anion-exchange peaks of peritoneal fluid versus hours of residence in the bidirectional cell (data of Figure 4, (c) and (d), M-F membrane PM150).

ysance behavior of 3 peaks on M-F membrane.) A calculated apparent molecular mass for the anionic substances in these peaks would be 186–218 daltons (from comparison to dialysance of creatinine). Dialysance of all peaks approached zero by six hours, indicating loss of gradient of freely diffusible substance and significant binding of peak substances to macromolecules (probably proteins).

In chamber dialysis of peritoneal fluid with PM150 in the M-F position, the zero hour dialysance of peaks ranged from 0.3–3.25 ml/hr. The apparently molecular weight of substances in these peaks would then be 97–218 daltons. Dialysance of all peaks approached zero late in dialysis, indicating significant protein binding of uremic substances onto macromolecules in peritoneal fluid, (as in uremic serum). The early, rapid dialysance of anionic substances from peritoneal fluid in the diffusion cell indicates a relatively small molecular weight of such substances. The deceleration of such dialysances represents evidence of protein binding.

In the present studies, it is apparent that most of the anionic peaks in peritoneal fluid are still rising at 8 hours of dwell (in two patients). The attainment of equilibrium concentration is considerably slower than that of urea and creatinine. For these small non-protein bound substances, 90% dialysate/plasma concentration ratios are obtained in about 1.5 and 3 hours, respectively. Thus, it appears that there are a variety of anionic organic compounds that transfer to peritoneal fluid at a rate slower than that of creatinine. Their kinetics would classify them as "middle molecules," or substances that dialyze slowly.[7] The exchange times of CAPD appear appropriate for allowing a continuous removal of these anionic, organic substances, since saturation is not attained at 8 hours. The molecular weights of such compounds, as determined by the double diffusion cell (above), appear to be in the 97–218 dalton range. Therefore, the transfer rates of these

substances would diminish by 3 hours dwell, as do the transfer rates of creatinine without protein binding. The protein binding of such substances probably regulates their clearance. With such protein binding, the free, dialyzable concentration of such substances is maintained at a low level in the dialysate, and the proteins operate as effective "sorbents." While protein loss of peritoneal dialysis is much maligned for its nutritional effects, it may have some beneficial chemical effects.

REFERENCES

1. Popovich P, Moncrief JW, Decherd JF, Bomar JB, and Pyle WK: The definition of a novel portable/wearable equilibrium peritoneal dialysis technique. Abstracts Am Soc Artif Intern Organs 5: 64, 1976
2. Bergström J, Fürst P: Uremic toxins. Kidney Int 13: (Suppl 8) S-9, 1978
3. Funck-Brentano JL, Man NK, Sausse A, Cueille C, Zinfraff J, Drueke T, Jungers P, and Billon JP: Neuropathy and middle molecule toxins. Kindey Int 7: S-352, 1975
4. Cohlmia JB, Whittier FC, and Grantham JJ: Similarity of the dialysance of endogenous aryl acids and o-iodohippurate (hippuran) in uremic man. Proc Clin Dial Transplant Forum 4: 224, 1974
5. Bergström J, Fürst P, and Zimmerman L: Separation and identification of uremic middle molecules. Introduction. Proc 8th Int Congr Nephrol 595, 8: 1981
6. Klein E, Holland F, and Ehrlich K: Membranes for isolating middle molecules in vitro and in vivo. Proc 8th Int Congr Nephrol 8: 618, 1981
7. Ash SR, Bungu ZTJ, and Regnier F: Anion exchange chromatography and double-diffusion cells for the study of middle molecules. Kidney Int 24: 250, 1983
8. Bungu ZTJ: Chromatographic techniques and bidirectional-diffusion cell in the separation and characterization of uremic middle molecules. Thesis, Purdue University, 1982
9. Einstein A: Elementare Theorie der Brownschen Schen Bewegunt. Electrochem 14: 235, 1908

K.D. Nolph

11

An International Survey of Ultrafiltration in CAPD

SUMMARY

Twenty-nine centers have participated in an international survey to document more clearly the incidence of impaired peritoneal ultrafiltration and factors associated with the problem. Ultrafiltration was significantly lower when certain brands of dialysis fluid were used. These dialysis solutions were also associated with higher rates of dextrose absorption.

INTRODUCTION

In March 1983, nephrologists from France, Canada, and U.S.A. met in Paris to review the problem of ultrafiltration (UF) loss in patients on continuous ambulatory peritoneal dialysis (CAPD) in France. The actuarial risk of losing some ultrafiltration in patients on CAPD in France has been reported to be 10% and 30% at 1 and 2 years respectively.[1] One series has documented ultimate transfer to hemodialysis from CAPD because of decreasing UF in 24% of patients.[1] Another study from France reported decreases in mean UF with hypertonic 2 L long dwell exchanges from 800–200 ml over 30 months CAPD.[2] There are other reports of losses of UF in French patients on CAPD.[3]

Loss of UF in patients on CAPD in North America has been reported infrequently.[4–7] In the U.S.A. CAPD Registry, less than 1.7% of 6,656 patients followed for 5,022 patient years have been transferred because of loss of UF.

Numerous centers are now participating in an international survey of UF to document more clearly areas where the loss of UF is more frequent.[8] The first results from this survey has been published, and the second report is in press.[8–9] This paper briefly summarizes the highlights of the second report.[9]

METHODS

Twenty-nine centers participated (France—20, U.S.A.—6, Canada—1, Greece—1, United Kingdom—1). A single exchange measurement was performed in each patient. On the morning of the clinic visit day the abdomen was drained as completely as possible and 2 L of a hypertonic exchange of the brand used by the patient instilled. The time from the end of instillation to the beginning of drainage was to be precisely 4 hours. Patients with a total cycle time exceeding 300 minutes were not included in the analyses.

The fresh bag and port clamp were weighed before instillation and the drain bag and port clamp weighed following drainage. The difference was reported as net UF. A sample of vigorously mixed dialysate was drawn for determination of glucose concentration within 2–4 hours of sampling. All studies were performed at least 10 days after the resolution of any peritonitis.

A form was completed by the participating center for each patient measurement. The timing of the cycle, the brand used, net UF, dialysis fluid, dex-

From the University of Missouri Health Sciences Center, H.S. Truman VA Hospital, and Dalton Research Center, Columbia, Missouri.

trose concentration, age, sex, date of initiation of CAPD, all brands of dialysis solution used for CAPD before the most recent one, the percent dextrose used, the buffer anion used in the dialysis solution, the number of episodes of peritonitis since starting CAPD, whether treatment of peritonitis included lavage with short cycles and/or acetate containing solutions, and the method for dialysate glucose concentration determination were all listed.

Data was processed by the University of Missouri computer network. Relationships were analyzed by correlations and linear regressions. Mean values were compared by the Student's t test and analysis of variance.

RESULTS

The characteristics of these 317 patients are summarized in Table 1. Table 2 summarizes the results in patients who had been exposed to only one brand of solution. Inflow dextrose concentrations are expressed as the actual concentration in solution. In North America it is customary to label the percent of hydrated dextrose. Concentrations are all expressed here according to the European custom (anhydrous). Drainage (outflow) dextrose concentrations and net UF values were lower (p < 0.001) in brands B and C as compared to brand A. Dextrose concentrations were also reduced in brand D (p < 0.03) as compared to brand A. The lower value of UF in brand D did not reach statistical significance with the small numbers represented.

Some patients were exposed to more than one brand of dialysis fluid. For example, in one center, 23 patients were maintained on an acetate solution until one month before the study, when they were switched to a lactate solution. The test was performed using the acetate solution. The acetate solu-

Table 1. Patient Characteristics (n = 317).

	Age (yrs)	Time on CAPD (mo)	Episodes of Peritonitis
Mean ± SD	56 ± 14	16 + 13	1.5 ± 2.1
Range	16–81	1–66	0–15

tion was brand B and the lactate solution was a modified brand B. Mean (±SEM) values for this group were 465 ± 67 ml of UF and 702 ± 35 mg/dl for dialysate dextrose concentration. Both means were lower (p < 0.001) than those in the patients using brand A only. Results with brand A were quite similar in Canada, the USA, England, and France.

Table 3 summarizes dextrose absorption rates for brand A in different countries, for brands B and D combined (the acetate solutions) in France, and for brand C (the European lactate) in France. Dextrose absorption was significantly higher in the latter two groups compared to those using brand A.

A number of methods were used to determine glucose concentrations in the different centers. No correlation with choice of method was seen. Significant correlations (p < 0.001) are summarized in Table 4. UF correlated positively with dialysate dextrose but inversely with dextrose absorption, choice of buffer (assigning arbitrarily 1 for lactate, 2 for acetate, and 3 for a combination of acetate and lactate), and with time on CAPD. The inverse correlation with time on CAPD was primarily related to a progressive decrease in UF in patients using non-brand A solutions. There was a positive correlation of the number of peritonitis episodes with time on CAPD. There were no significant correlations of UF or dialysate dextrose concentration with patient age or peritonitis rates. Mean ages, peritonitis rates, and

Table 2. Results According to Brand.

Brand	Producer	Buffer	N	Inflow Dextrose (mg/dl)	Outflow Dextrose (mg/dl)	Net UF
A	Travenol	lactate	220	3860	1073	728
B	Aguettant	acetate	53	4000	667*	532*
C	Fresenius	lactate	19	4250	701*	503*
D	Assistance Publique	acetate	5	4500	807†	548

* p < 0.001 from Brand A.
† p < 0.03 from Brand A.
N = Number of Patients.

Table 3. Dextrose Absorption.

	Mean g/Exchange (±SEM)	N
Brand A, Canada	46 ± 1	31
Brand A, USA	46 ± 1	61
Brand A, England	46 ± 2	19
Brand A, France	49 ± 1	118
Brands B and D, France	64 ± 2*	42
Brand C, France	68 ± 1*	19

* p < 0.001 from Brand A Groups.

times on therapy were similar for groups using different brands.

DISCUSSION

This report summarizes highlights of the second detailed report of the international survey. The first report noted reduced dialysate dextrose concentration and UF in patients using acetate buffered solutions.[8] The second report now extends the association between low dextrose and low UF to lactate solutions other than brand A. A wide degree of scatter was anticipated in such a mass survey. It was hoped that trends would emerge to stimulate further research. Several impressions have already surfaced.

Mean values for UF are significantly lower in some patients in France. Lower UF values are associated with lower concentrations of dialysate dextrose and greater dextrose absorption during exchanges. Most interestingly, lower values are associated with the use of solutions other than brand A. In fact one of the French centers originally reporting progressive loss of UF with time on CAPD has reanalyzed the data to find that the association was in patients using a brand other than brand A.[10]

Centers using a North American brand other than brand A are now participating in the survey.

Table 4. Significant Correlations
(p < 0.001).

Variables	r Value
UF vs dialysate dextrose	0.24
UF vs dextrose absorption	−0.57
UF vs buffer	−0.26
UF vs time on CAPD	−0.20
peritonitis vs time on CAPD	0.55

The lactate solution produced in Europe (brand C) is represented only in small numbers. Centers in Germany are now participating in this survey to expand these numbers. Preliminary results in 22 patients yield results very similar to brand A. Low values with brand C in France may involve center factors.

Original suspicions that the problem might relate to acetate exposure are complicated by the observations with brand C. Perhaps multiple factors are involved. Impurities in salts, different water preparation procedures, and differences in containers and in tubing must all be evaluated. It is not known whether this rapid dextrose absorption represents a subtle membrane injury. Rapid dextrose absorption and loss of UF are characteristic of acute peritonitis.[11–12]

It is not known whether there is any link to early loss of UF and rapid dextrose absorption with eventual sclerosing peritonitis. Most cases of sclerosing peritonitis reported have been exposed to intermittent peritoneal dialysis with acetate solution and/or CAPD with brands, B, C, or D.[13–18]

The observations in this survey are meant to suggest areas for future definitive investigations. If it is true that losses of UF and sclerosing peritonitis are not seen with the same frequency in different regions and with the same frequency in groups of patients using different solutions, then ideally the positive factors should be identifiable and the problems preventable.

INTERNATIONAL SURVEY TEAM

Coordinating Centers

K. Nolph, L. Ryan, H. Moore: *University of Missouri Health Sciences Center, H.S. Truman VA Hospital, and Dalton Research Center, Columbia, MO.* **M. Legrain, J. Rottembourg, B. Issad, M. Montassine:** *Groupe Hospitalier, Pitie-Salpetriere, Paris, France.* **Mion, A. Slingeneyer, J. Bouzigue:** *Hopital Saint Charles, Montpellier, France.* **D. Oreopoulos, R. Khanna, S. Clayton:** *Toronto Western Hospital, Toronto, Canada.*

Other Centers

P. Dandoz, J. Walls: *Leicester General Hospital, Leicester, England.* **D. Dubois, B. Temperville, E. Lehoussel:** *Hopital Ecole de la Croix-Rouge Francaise, Bois-Guillamme, France.* **C. Wone, S. Savariaud:** *Hopital Saint-Andre, Bordeaux, France.* **J. de Fremont, A. Fournier, M. Fourre:** *Centre Hos-*

pitalier Universitaire, Amiens, France. **J. Chanliau,
M. Kessler, D. Hamsau:** *Unite d'Entrainement a'la
Dialyse a' Domicile, Centre Hospitalier Regional,
Nancy, France.* **P. Lebon, E. Kernaonet, D. Hamsau:** *Centre Hospitalier Le Mans, France.* **J.
Bouchet, J. Montoriol, J. Derck:** *Hopital Pellegrin,
Bordeaux, France.* **B. Faller, J. Marichal, S. Lallemand:** *Centre Hospitalier General L. Pasteur,
Colmar, France.* **J. Sabatier, F. Berthoux:** *Centre
Hospitalier Universitaire de St. Etienne, Hopital
Nord, Saint Pries en Jarey, France.* **R. Guibersteau,
A. Talin D'Eyza, N. Millet:** *Centre Hospitalier General, Bourges, France.* **J. Ryckelynck, P. Mignot, M.
Roland:** *Centre Hospitalier Universitaire Clemenceau, Caen, France.* **P. Collin, J. Denis, A. Gabard:**
Centre Hospitalier Cholet, France. **B. Monnier, H.
Duplay, M. Novembri:** *Hopital Pasteur, Nice,
France.* **G. Janin, E. Beverey, M. Braillon:** *Hospital
des chanaux, Macon, France.* **C. Verger, J.
Vantelon, N. Bataille:** *Centre Hospitalier de
Pontoise, Pontoise, France.* **C. Michel, F. Mignon,
J. Denis:** *Centre E.P.C.A., Hopital Tenon, Paris,
France.* **P. Schohn, H. Jahn, D. Gautheron:** *Hospices Civils de Strasbourg, Strasbourg, France.* **Y.
Berland, M. Olmer, M. Genier:** *Hopital de la Conception, Marseille, France.* **P. Rilbe, G. Balit, C.L.
Boissard:** *Centre Hospitalier Regional, Angers,
France.* **A. Katirtzoglou, G. Digenis:** *Hippocratean
Hospital, 2nd Department of Medicine, University
of Athens, Athens, Greece.* **C. Feldman, C. Elwood:**
Satellite Dialysis, Palo Alto, CA. **J. Raimondo, H.
Ziemek:** *Lankenau Hospital, Philadelphia, PA.* **K.
Lempert, F. Whittier, M. Fragale:** *West Virginia
University Medical Center, Morgantown, WV.* **C.
Charytan:** *Booth Memorial Satellite Dialysis Facility, Flushing, NY.* **N. Shusterman, G. Morrison,
C. Moffitt:** *Hospital of the University of Pennsylvania, Philadelphia, PA.*

REFERENCES

1. Slingeneyer A, Canaud B, and Mion C: Permanent loss of ultrafiltration capacity of the peritoneum in long term-term peritoneal dialysis: An epidemiological study. Nephron 33: 133, 1983
2. Faller B, and Marichal JF: Loss of ultrafiltration in CAPD: Clinical data. In Gahl GM, Kessell M, and Nolph KD (Eds), Advances in peritoneal dialyis: Proceedings of the 2nd international symposium on peritoneal dialysis. Amsterdam: Excerpta Medica, 1981, p 227
3. Verger C, Brunschvicg O, LeCharpentier Y, Lavergne A, and Vantelon J: Structural and ultrastructural peritoneal membrane changes and permeability alterations during CAPD. Proc Eur Dial Transplant Assoc 18: 199, 1981
4. Oreopoulos DG, and Khanna R: Complications of peritoneal dialysis other than peritonitis. In Nolph KD (Ed), Peritoneal dialysis. The Hague: Martinus Nijhoff, 1981, p 309
5. Nolph KD, and Pyle WK: NIH CAPD Patient Registry Report: Population demographics and outcomes for the period 1/1/82–12/31/82. Published 4/15/83
6. Rubin J, Nolph K, Arfania D, Brown P, and Prowant B: Follow-up of peritoneal clearances in patients undergoing continuous ambulatory peritoneal dialysis. Kidney Int 16: 619, 1979
7. Rubin J, Nolph KD, Popovich RP, Moncrief JW, and Prowant B: Drainage volumes during continuous ambulatory peritoneal dialysis. asaio J 2: 54, 1979
8. An International Cooperative Study: Factors affecting ultrafiltration in continuous ambulatory peritoneal dialysis. First Report. Peritoneal Dial Bull 4: 14, 1984
9. A Survey of Ultrafiltration in Continuous Ambulatory Peritoneal Dialysis. Second Report. Peritoneal Dial Bull (in press)
10. Faller B, and Marichal JF: Loss of ultrafiltration in CAPD: A role for acetate. Peritoneal Dial Bull 4: 10, 1984
11. Rubin J, Ray R, Barnes T, and Bower J: Peritoneal abnormalities during infectious episodes of continuous ambulatory peritoneal dialysis. Nephron 29: 124, 1981
12. Verger C, Luger A, Moore H, and Nolph KD: Acute changes in peritoneal morphology and transport properties with infectious peritonitis and mechanical injury. Kidney Int 23: 823, 1983
13. Ghandi VC, Hymayun HM, Ing TS, Daugirdas JT, Jabolow VR, Iwatsoki S, Gers P, and Hano JE: Sclerotic thickening of the peritoneal membrane in maintenance peritoneal dialysis patients. Arch Intern Med 140: 1201, 1980
14. Rottembourg J, Gahl G, Poignet JL, Mertani E, Strippoli P, Langlois P, Tranbaloc P, and Legrain M: Severe abdominal complications in patients undergoing continuous ambulatory peritoneal dialysis. Proc Eur Dial Transplant Assoc 20: 236, 1983
15. Schmidt RW, and Blumenkrantz MJ: Peritoneal sclerosis: A "sword of Damocles" for peritoneal dialysis. Arch Intern Med 141: 1265, 1981
16. Slingeneyer A, Mion C, Mourad G, Canaud B, Faller B, and Béraud JJ: Progressive sclerosing peritonitis: A late and severe complication of maintenance peritoneal dialysis. Trans Am Soc Artif Intern Organs 29: 633, 1983
17. Bradley JA, McWhinnie DL, Hamilton DNH, Starnes F, MacPherson SG, Seywright M, Briggs JD, and Junor BJR: Obstructive peritonitis after CAPD. Lancet 2: 113, 1983
18. Bradley JA, Hamilton DNH, McWhinnie DL, Briggs JD, and Junor BJR: Sclerosing peritonitis after CAPD. Lancet 2: 572, 1983

L.C. Smeby, T.-E. Widerøe, S. Mjaaland, and K. Dahl

12

Changes in Ultrafiltration and Solute Transport During CAPD

SUMMARY

Measurements of solute equilibration and mass-transfer-area coefficients for urea and creatinine during normal CAPD routines are less sensitive than ultrafiltration volumes (long dwell exchanges) in revealing peritoneal membrane' changes. These clinical results are supported by calculations based on the use of pore theory in kinetic modeling of peritoneal dialysis. Calculations also indicate that the resistance of unstirred fluid layers may be an important factor in maintaining the ultrafiltration characteristics during CAPD. Long term reductions in the ultrafiltration volume for patients with a relatively 'tight membrane' (low permeability) in the early stages of CAPD, can usually also be detected by increased solute equilibration, at least for those above 200 to 300 daltons. Changes in the peritoneum of patients with early development or an initially high permeability 'membrane,' can only be detected through routine volume measurements or special experiments using large (>1000 daltons) tracer molecules. Our experience shows that the latter group of patients also are more likely to develop serious problems with water removal during long term CAPD treatment.

From the Institute of Biophysics and Department of Nephrology, University of Trondheim, Trondheim, Norway.

INTRODUCTION

Long term effects of continuous ambulatory peritoneal dialysis (CAPD) on the morphology and mass transfer properties of the peritoneum remain unresolved. Several groups have studied changes in solute transport during CAPD, but the results are conflicting.[1-4] Measurements of ultrafiltration capacity appear to reveal membrane changes in some patients during long-term CAPD,[4-7] and preliminary ultrastructural studies of the peritoneum appear to confirm that the morphology of the human peritoneal membrane is altered in patients treated with CAPD.[8,9] However, to our knowledge, there are no unified studies linking structural membrane changes to mass transfer assessment in these patients. Such studies would be of great value in the prediction and possible prevention of 'the detrimental pathology that may develop during CAPD. A better understanding of the morphological alterations leading to mass transfer changes could also give clues to pharmacological manipulations of the transport properties of the peritoneum.

The aim of this study was to measure any changes in solute and water transport during CAPD, and to compare these results with an analysis based on a mathematical model linked to structural alterations in the peritoneal membrane,[4,10] taking into account changes in "equivalent pore radius," effective membrane area/diffusive length, and the transport resistance of "unstirred fluid layers" on the dialysate side of peritoneal membranes.

MATERIALS AND METHODS

Patient Selection and Clinical Measurements

Seven patients with a mean age of 44 ± 13 years were selected for this investigation. All patients used instillations of 2 L dialysis fluid (Dianeal, Travenol Laboratories, Halden, Norway) and noted ultrafiltration volume (UF), dwell-time (T), and the initial dextrose concentration in dialysate (Gi) for each exchange from the start of CAPD. After the initial training period, the patients came into the hospital for routine monthly measurements of general biochemistries (only urea, creatinine, uric acid, and glucose measurements are included here). For comparative purposes, data from each patient were grouped into two periods separated by at least six months of CAPD treatment. Each period comprised three consecutive months, giving mean solute values based on three measurements in blood and 4–5 hours dwell times. Average UFs for both periods were computed from the patients' records of long dwell exchanges (8–10 hours). The individual need for dextrose in the dialysis solution varied, but only measurements with equal Gi were used in the comparison of results from one period to the other. These selection criteria resulted in 20–60 volume measurements as the basis for individual mean ultrafiltration values in each period. Data recorded during the last week before peritonitis and for the next month thereafter were not included in this study. Statistical evaluation of differences between means were based on unpaired t-distribution tests.

Model Calculations

The basic compartmental model used in this, study has been described elsewhere.[4, 10] It is sufficient to note that solute (Js) and water (Jv) transport were based on Equations (1) and (2):

$$Js = MP (Cp - Cd) + Jv (1 - \sigma) Cm \qquad (1)$$
$$Jv = Lp (\Delta P - \Sigma (\sigma \cdot \Delta \pi)) \qquad (2)$$

where

MP = total diffusive transport coefficient
Cp = plasma concentration
Cd = instillate concentration
Cm = (Cp + Cd)/2
Lp = hydraulic permeability
σ = reflection coefficient
ΔP = hydraulic pressure gradient
$\Delta \pi$ = osmotic concentration gradient

Estimates of the total diffusive transport coefficient, the reflection coefficient and the hydraulic permeability can be obtained employing instillate (Cd) and plasma (Cp) concentrations together with measured drainage volumes (Vd) in various experimental or curve fitting procedures,[4, 10–12] but such methods do not relate mass transfer properties to structural features of the peritoneal barrier. The so-called "pore theory" was developed in an attempt to relate solute and volume flow across biological membranes to the mean pore radius (Rp) and the relative pore area (Ap/A) of such membranes.[13] Further refinement of this method can be employed to show that

$$Lp = (Ap/\Delta X) \cdot (Rp^2/8 \, \mu) \qquad (3)$$
$$Pm = (Ap/\Delta X) \cdot D/K_1 \cdot Sd \qquad (4)$$
$$\sigma = 1 - K_2/K_1 \cdot Sf - RTVs \cdot (Pm/Lp) \qquad (5)$$

where

Pm = "membrane" diffusivity
Rp = equivalent pore radius
Ap = effective pore area = $Nx \cdot \pi \cdot Rp^2$; Nx = number of pores
ΔX = effective diffusional length
μ = fluid viscosity
D = "free" diffusion coefficient
$Sd = (1 - q)^2$; $Sf = (2 - Sd) \cdot Sd$; $q = Rs/Rp$
Rs = effective solute radius
Vs = solute molar volume; RT = gas constant $\cdot$ temperature
K_1, K_2 = constants related to q[14]

Similar theories[15] can also be employed to establish equivalent pore radii and the relative transport contribution of "small and large pores" in membranes with more than one pore population. Assuming that overall diffusive transport through blood capillaries, basement membranes, interstitium, and mesothelium (see Fig. 1) can be simulated by a composite membrane with a given "equivalent pore radius," the total diffusive mass transfer resistance (Rt) can be written as

$$Rt = Rf + 1/Pm \qquad (6)$$

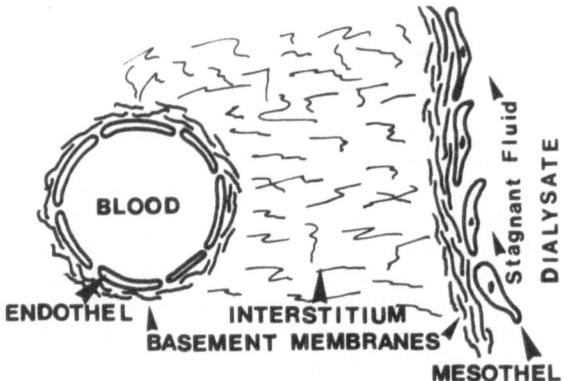

Fig. 1. Schematic representation of the peritoneal "membrane."

where Rt = 1/Mp and Rf represent the transport resistance of "unstirred fluid layers" on the dialysate side of the mesothelium (Fig. 1). This fluid layer will not have a significant effect on hydraulic permeability or the reflection coefficient, but will lead to a concentration gradient within the dialysate compartment and hence reduce diffusive transport for "small" molecules such as urea, creatinine, and glucose.

To obtain an initial estimate of the equivalent mean pore radius of the peritoneal barrier, it was assumed that Rf was negligible for solutes >10,000 daltons, and that the mass transfer contribution of the "large pore population" (Rp = 180–300 Å)[15] was small for solutes <20,000 daltons. Using previously obtained values for the reflection coefficient for a solute with molecular weight of 15,000 daltons,[4, 10] together with the above outlined theories, gave an equivalent pore radius of 47–55 Å, which corresponds well to measured values of the small pore population of capillaries in the stomach region.[15] Such calculations also gave the effective number of pores/diffusional length (Ap/ΔX = Nx · π · Rp²/ΔX), which was used with Rp to calculate Pm for a range of solutes. The difference between calculated Pm and estimates of Mp[4, 10] was then employed in calculations (equation 6) of the resistance of "unstirred fluid layers" (Rf). Keeping Rf constant, while changing Rp or Nx/ΔX, then gave a series of values for Mp, Lp, and σ, which were used in the compartmental model to study changes in solute and water transport due to variations in the equivalent pore radius and the pore area/diffusional length of the peritoneum during CAPD.

Measurements of the commonly used mass-transfer-area-coefficient (MTC) were based on a simplified kinetic model[16] giving Equation 7:

$$\ln[\{Vd(Cp - Cd) \mid t = T\}/\{Vd(Cp - Cd) \mid t = 0\}] =$$

$$-\int_0^T MTC/Vd \cdot dt \qquad (7)$$

Using MTC/Vd = constant, yields a simple expression that can be employed with measured Cp, Cd, and Vd to find MTCs for various solutes.

RESULTS

Table 1 shows the mean (±SD) equilibration of solutes between instillate and blood for 4–5 hour dwell times, and the mean (±SD) ultrafiltration volume (ml) for long dwell exchanges (T = 8–10 hours) in all seven patients. Urea (%), creatinine (%), and uric acid (%) during the first (I) and second (II) period of measurements were calculated as Cd (4–5 hours)/Cp · 100%, while the glucose rest (%) was estimated from Cd (4–5 hours)/Cd (T = 0) · 100%. The differences between mean values in period I and II is given by Δ: Only Δ with · (p < 0.05) or · · (p < 0.01) indicate significant differences between the two periods.

The mass-transfer-area coefficients (MTC, equation 7) for creatinine and uric acid, based on measurements in plasma and 4–5 hour instillates, are given in Table 2. Mean (±SD) values for each patient in period I and II were calculated using concentrations and the corresponding 4–5 hour dialysate volumes. Δ refer to differences between means as in Table 1. MTC-values for urea are not included in this table due to the fact that instillate/plasma equilibrations for T = 4–5 hours were close to 100%, which makes estimates of MTC unreliable or impossible (see equation 7). It should be noted that only MTC for uric acid in one patient (L.G.) was significantly different (p < 0.05) from one period to the other, while four of the seven patients showed significant differences in solute equilibration for uric acid (Table 1). The basic mass transfer parameters used in model simulations are given in Figure 2. Mp (L/hour) and σ (Fig. 2a) for solutes with different molecular weights (mol wt) were taken from previous investigations,[4, 10] while Pm (L/hour) were calculated as described above. Rf% (Fig. 2b) shows the relative diffusive mass transport contribution of "unstirred fluid layers" expressed as a percentage of the total diffusive resistance Rt (hour/L). These calculations gave a mean effective pore radius of

48.3 Å. The difference between full and broken lines for Rt (mol wt >10,000) shows the effect of the large pore system, which contributes about 10% of the total pore area.[15]

The effects of changes in mean pore radius and the number of pores/diffusional length (Nx, Ap = Nx · π · Rp²) on net ultrafiltration volumes for different dwell times are shown in Figure 3. Curve O refers to the basic transport parameters for the peritoneum as given in Figure 2, while ±R corresponds to a ±50% change in Rp for a given number of pores (Nx). ±Nx are the results of ±50% changes in Nx/ΔX when Rp is 48.3 Å (reference value). All curves were calculated with instillations of 2 L dialysis solution containing dextrose 22.5 g/L. Figure 4 shows calculated correlations between changes in the ultrafiltration volume (ΔUF, ml) for long dwell exchanges (T = 9 hours) and the solute equilibration (ΔSE%) for T = 4 hours. Changes in mean pore radius with a given number of pores/ΔX results in curves indicated by the broken lines, while variations in Nx/ΔX are given by the full lines. C and B refer to changes in percentage equilibration for creatinine and a solute of 1355 daltons, while G is the result for percentage glucose rest as defined above (Table 1).

DISCUSSION

Routine assessments of peritoneal mass transfer have frequently been used in studies related to the long term viability of the peritoneum during CAPD.[3,4,6,16] Clinical results (Table 1)[4,7] show that long dwell ultrafiltration volumes are more sensitive to changes in peritoneal "membranes" than estimates of mass-transfer-area coefficients or measured equilibration between blood and instillates for solutes <500 daltons. Accurate measurements of solute permeability must either be based on experiments with short dwell times or the use of large (>1000 daltons) tracer molecules. Protein concentrations in drained dialysate are usually so low that routine analysis has a ±50% variability for the same fluid sample, and any lymphatic drainage, even less than 0.5 ml/min, will have a significant effect on mass transfer evaluation based on protein measurements. These factors together with our experience that water removal frequently becomes a clinical problem while solute transport is adequate,[7] supports the use of long dwell ultrafiltration volumes as the best parameter for routine assessment of possible changes in peritoneal membranes during CAPD.

Table 1. Mean (±SD) equilibration (Cd[T = 4–5 hours]/Cp · 100%) for urea, creatinine and uric acid, the glucose rest percent (Cd[T = 4–5 hours]/Cd[T = 0] · 100%) in drained fluid and the mean (±SD) ultrafiltration volume (T = 8–10 hours) during two periods (I and II) of 3 months. The difference between the means of the two periods, separated by at least 6 months of CAPD treatment, is given by Δ.

Patient	Urea (%)			Creatinine (%)			Uric Acid (%)			Glucose Rest (%)			Ultrafiltration (ML)		
	I	II	Δ	I	II	Δ	I	II	Δ	I	II	Δ	I	II	Δ
I.Aa.	99 ± 4	101 ± 1	+2	79 ± 10	81 ± 5	+2	66 ± 8	75 ± 4	+9	26 ± 7	32 ± 3	+6	335 ± 31	330 ± 34	+5
B.B.	99 ± 5	98 ± 3	-1	86 ± 6	81 ± 6	-5	75 ± 3	68 ± 2	-7*	23 ± 2	28 ± 4	+5	330 ± 38	451 ± 32	+121**
I.T.	101 ± 9	103 ± 4	+2	77 ± 11	80 ± 10	+3	63 ± 4	76 ± 5	+13**	27 ± 7	19 ± 7	-8	484 ± 39	394 ± 33	-90**
L.G.	98 ± 1	100 ± 4	+2	88 ± 2	93 ± 9	+5	80 ± 2	90 ± 3	+10**	18 ± 1	12 ± 7	-6	195 ± 41	52 ± 45	-143**
A.F.	97 ± 5	90 ± 1	-7*	78 ± 9	69 ± 1	-9	72 ± 9	60 ± 3	-12*	25 ± 4	33 ± 3	+8	69 ± 36	158 ± 49	+89**
P.S.	103 ± 3	104 ± 2	+1	97 ± 3	98 ± 5	+1	94 ± 6	94 ± 8	0	6 ± 5	7 ± 4	+1	10 ± 47	-175 ± 61	-185*
AM.S.	98 ± 5	102 ± 4	+4	85 ± 4	87 ± 3	+2	86 ± 6	83 ± 5	-3	16 ± 4	16 ± 2	0	643 ± 51	552 ± 38	-91*

* p < 0.05.
** p < 0.01.

Table 2. Mean (±SD) mass-transfer-area coefficients (MTC ml/min) for creatinine and uric acid based on measured concentrations and volumes for T = 4–5 hours during two periods (I and II) separated by at least 6 months of CAPD. Individual differences in mean values between the two periods are given by Δ.

Patient	Creatinine (ml/min)			Uric Acid (ml/min)		
	I	II	Δ	I	II	Δ
I.Aa.	12.2 ± 3.9	14.7 ± 2.0	+2.5	8.9 ± 2.5	11.9 ± 1.3	+3.0
B.B.	14.0 ± 3.4	11.2 ± 2.0	−3.8	9.6 ± 1.1	7.6 ± 0.5	−2.0
I.T.	14.1 ± 6.1	15.3 ± 5.6	+1.2	9.4 ± 4.2	12.5 ± 1.9	+3.1
L.G.	18.7 ± 1.8	23.7 ± 5.0	+5.0	14.3 ± 0.6	24.9 ± 4.1	+10.6*
A.F.	13.6 ± 3.1	9.8 ± 0.3	−3.8	9.8 ± 2.3	7.6 ± 0.6	−2.2
P.S.	36.1 ± 17.7	38.7 ± 18.6	+1.6	27.1 ± 5.6	31.3 ± 8.8	+4.2
AM.S.	16.0 ± 2.4	17.1 ± 2.0	+1.1	15.5 ± 3.1	14.9 ± 3.0	−0.6

* $p < 0.05$.

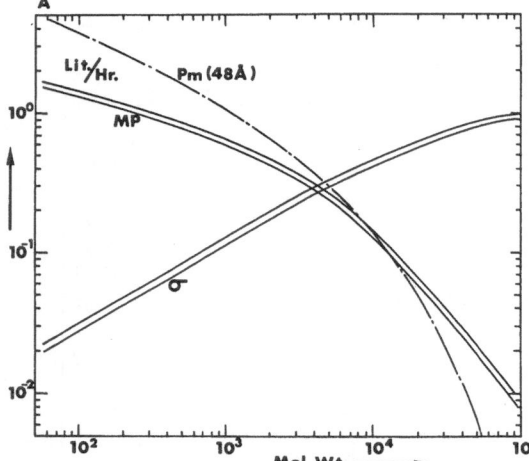

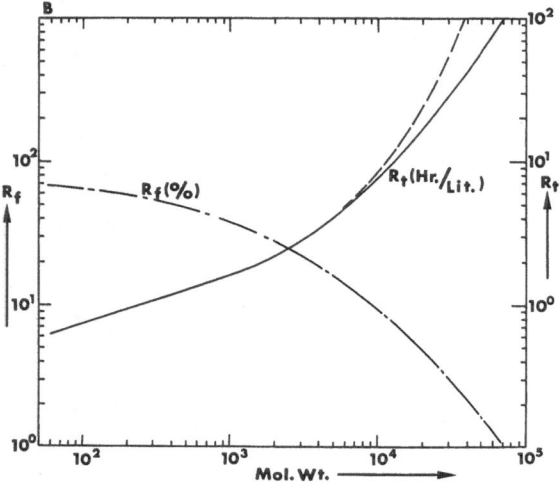

Fig. 2. (A) shows the "observed" diffusional transport parameter MP (L/hour), the calculated "membrane" diffusivity Pm (L/hour) (see text), and reflection coefficient (σ) based on an effective mean pore radius of 48.3 Å for substances with different molecular weights (mol wt). (B) gives "observed" (full lines) and calculated (broken lines) diffusional mass transfer resistance Rt (hour/L) and the relative contribution of stagnant fluid layers (Rf %) for substances with different mol wt.

As suggested by Figure 1, the peritoneal barrier is a complex "membrane" consisting of the capillary wall, basement membranes, the interstitium, mesothelium, and an unstirred fluid layer adjacent to the mesothelial cells. The pore theory has been widely used to correlate structural features to transcapillary water and solute transport. Estimates of small and large pore populations in different capillaries fall in the range of 45–80 Å and 180–300 Å respectively, with an increasing proportion of large pores toward the venous end.[15] Studies on normally hydrated dense tissues suggest an effective mean pore radius of about 250 Å for the interstitium, which should not restrict movement of water and solutes (<35 Å) significantly. However, changes in the hydration of the interstitium will have an effect on the diffusive length and hence vary the term Ap/ΔX in the expressions for water and solute transport (Equations 1–5). The contribution of the mesothelium to overall transport resistance of the peritoneal barrier is uncertain. An intact cellular layer will re-

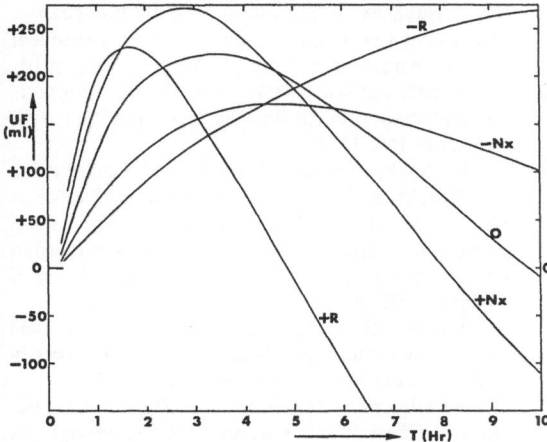

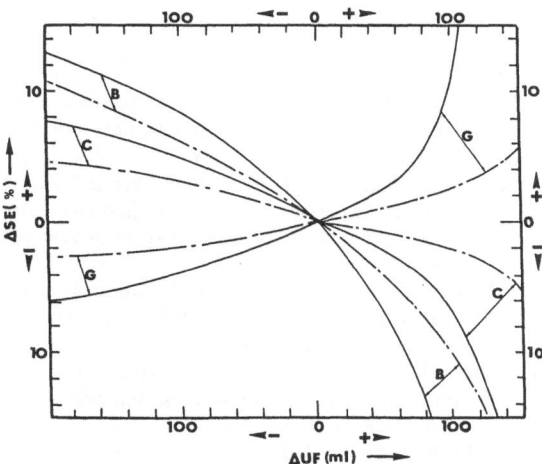

Fig. 3. Net ultrafiltration volume UF (ml) as a function of dwell time T (hours) for peritoneal "membranes" with different mean pore radii or different number of pores/diffusional length. All calculations were based on instillations of 2 L dialysis fluid with a dextrose concentration of 22.5 g/L. 0 refer to the basic membrane properties given in Figure 2, while ±R corresponds to ±50% variations in pore radius, and ±Nx refer to similar changes in the number of pores/diffusional length.

Fig. 4. Calculated correlation between changes in long dwell (T = 9 hours) ultrafiltration volume Δ UF (ml) and the corresponding change in solute equilibration Δ SE (%) for T = 4 hours. O-values refer to calculations using the basic transport parameters in Figure 2. C and B are solute equilibrations for creatinine and vitamin B_{12}, while G refers to the glucose rest (%) (calculated as given in text of Table 1). Broken lines correspond to results obtained by varying the pore radius, keeping the number of pores/diffusional length constant, while the full lines refer to variations in number of effective pores/ diffusional length (Rp constant).

duce the effective pore area, and mesothelial cells appear to resist solute and water flux during peritoneal dialysis.[17] Cellular degeneration or loss of mesothelial cells has been observed in CAPD patients,[8,9] and the mesothelium is therefore probably an important factor in long term changes leading to reduced ultrafiltration capacity for some CAPD patients.

The resistance of unstirred fluid layers will be dependent on anatomical features of the peritoneal cavity as well as the clinical routines during CAPD. Rapid fluid cycling can influence Rf (Equation 6), and hence measurements of MTCs based on short exchanges can give values that are higher than those encountered during normal CAPD routines. Our results (Fig. 2) indicate that Rf contributes more than 50% of the total mass transfer resistance for solutes of <300 daltons, and this could in fact be a positive factor. A reduction in Rf would lead to a more rapid absorption of glucose and hence more problems with ultrafiltration during long dwell exchanges. It could be that the rapid loss of the osmotic gradient and the "poor" ultrafiltration characteristics observed in children on CAPD[18] are partly due to a low Rf

caused by a smoother surface in the peritoneal cavity of these patients.

The calculations in Figures 3 and 4 show that a given change in mean pore radius or the effective number of pores/diffusional length have a much more pronounced effect on ultrafiltration volumes than on solute transfer. Differences in Ap/ΔX lead to greater changes in ΔSE for given values of ΔUF than the corresponding changes due to variations in Rp. However, a given difference in pore radius (i.e., ±50%, Figure 3) leads to greater variations in ultrafiltration than similar variations in pore area/ diffusional length. It should be noted that loss of area or reduction of pore radius (leading to increased UF for T = 8–10 hours) has a more pronounced effect on solute transfer (ΔSE) than increases in Rp or Ap/ ΔX. This is illustrated by the increasing gradient of the curves for ΔSE versus ΔUF (Fig. 4) when the ultrafiltration volume for long dwell exchanges increases.

REFERENCES

1. Finkelstein FO, Kliger AS, Bastl C, and Yap P: Sequential clearance and dialysance measurements of chronic peritoneal dialysis patients. Nephron 18: 342, 1977
2. Rubin J, Nolph KD, Arfania D, Brown P, and Prowant B: Follow up of peritoneal clearances in patients undergoing continuous ambulatory peritoneal dialysis. Kidney Int 16: 619, 1979
3. Farrell PC, and Randerson DH: Membrane permeability changes in long term CAPD. Trans Am Soc Artif Intern Organs 26: 197, 1980
4. Smeby LC, Widerøe TE, and Jorstad S: Individual differences in water transport during continuous peritoneal dialysis. asaio J 4: 49, 1981
5. Faller B, and Marichal JF: Loss of ultrafiltration in continuous ambulatory peritoneal dialysis. In Gahl GM, Kessel M, and Nolph KD (Eds), Advances in peritoneal dialysis: Proceedings of the 2nd international symposium on peritoneal dialysis. Amsterdam: Excerpta Medica, p 227
6. Slingeneyer A, Canaud B, and Mion C: Permanent loss of ultrafiltration capacity of the peritoneum on long term peritoneal dialysis. Nephron 33: 133, 1983
7. Widerøe TE, Smeby LC, Mjaaland S, Dahl K, Berg KJ, and Wessel-Aas T: Long term changes in transperitoneal water transport during continuous ambulatory peritoneal dialysis. Nephron (in press)
8. Dobbie JW, Zaki M, and Wilson M: Ultrastructural studies on the peritoneum with special reference to chronic ambulatory peritoneal dialysis. Scott Med J 26: 213, 1981
9. Verger C, Brunschvigg O, LeCarpentier Y, Lavergne A, and Vantelon J: Peritoneal structural alterations on CAPD. In Gahl GM, Kessel M, and Nolph KD (Eds), Advances in peritoneal dialysis: Proceedings of the 2nd international symposium on peritoneal dialysis. Amsterdam: Excerpta Medica, 1981, p 10
10. Smeby LC, and Wideroe TE: Kinetics of continuous ambulatory peritoneal dialysis. Proc Eur Soc Artif Organs 6: 156, 1979
11. Popovich RP, Pyle WK, Moncrief JW, Decherd JF, and Brooks S: Preliminary verification of the low dialysis clearance hypothesis via a novel equilibrium peritoneal dialysis technique: Second Australasian conference on heat and mass transfer. University of Sydney, 1977, p 217
12. Randerson DH: Continuous ambulatory peritoneal dialysis—a critical appraisal, PhD thesis. University of New South Wales, Sydney, 1980
13. Pappenheimer JR, Renkin EM, and Borrero LM: Filtration, diffusion and molecular sieving through peripheral capillary membranes. Am J Physiol 167: 13, 1951
14. Verniory A, DuBois R, Decoodt P, Gassee JP, and Lambert PP: Measurements of the permeability of biological membranes. J Gen Physiol 62: 489, 1973
15. Granger DN, and Perry MA: Permeability characteristics of the microcirculation. In Mortillaro NA (Ed), The physiology and pharmacology of the microcirculation. New York: Academic Press, 1983, p 143
16. Garred LJ, Canaud B, and Farrell PC: A simple kinetic model for assessing peritoneal mass transfer in CAPD patients. asaio J 1983, 6: 131
17. Maher JF, and Chakrabarti E: Ultrafiltration by hyperosmotic peritoneal dialysis fluid excludes intracellular solutes. Am J Nephrol 4: 169, 1984
18. Popovich RP, Alexander SR, Pyle KW, Balfe JW, Posenthal DA, and Moncrief JW: Kinetics of peritoneal dialysis in children, In Moncrief JW, and Popovich RP (Eds), CAPD update. New York: Masson Publishing, 1981, p 227

T.E. Widerøe, L.C. Smeby, S. Mjåland, and K. Dahl

13

Prediction of Changes in Transperitoneal Water Transport During CAPD—A Prospective Study

SUMMARY

Nine patients were observed prospectively during 14 to 40 mo of CAPD seeking to detect subclinical changes in ultrafiltration volume and to correlate these with changes in the peritoneal membrane or biochemical or clinical parameters. Highly significant changes in ultrafiltration volume occurred that were not detected by routine clinical assessment. Five patients had a reduction in ultrafiltration associated with a higher rate of dextrose absorption than occurred in four patients with an increase in the ultrafiltration rate.

INTRODUCTION

Loss of ultrafiltration capacity during treatment with CAPD can occasionally be a clinical problem,[1-3] although not observed by all.[4,5] Several factors such as varying plasma osmolality, fluid intake, dialysate composition and drainage routines, the incidence of peritonitis, and the types of diseases treated, could account for reported changes in transperitoneal water transport. Accurate dialysis protocol and changes based on differences between weekly or monthly averages are necessary to investigate this problem.

Loss of daily ultrafiltration volume during peritonitis in patients on CAPD has been reported.[6-9]

We previously described changes in peritoneal membrane permeability during peritonitis; these changes only partially returned to "normal" values after recovery.[6,7] However, others have not found a correlation between incidence of peritonitis and loss of ultrafiltration volume during long-term CAPD treatment.[3] Measurements of solute transport have not revealed any deterioration of the peritoneal membrane during CAPD,[11,12] but this observation is not necessarily synonymous with an invariable peritoneum.[6,13]

The aim of the present study was to detect subclinical changes in ultrafiltration in patients during long-term CAPD treatment, and to evaluate if any changes in ultrafiltration volume were caused by changes in the "peritoneal membrane" or could be correlated to biochemical and clinical parameters.

METHODS

Patients

Nine patients from 19–56-years-old (mean 41 years) were selected for this investigation and observed prospectively during CAPD treatment for 14–40 months (mean 23 months) (Table 1). None had previously been through any intraperitoneal surgery. One patient (patient 1) was anephric, the others were anuric or oliguric. A modified Tenckhoff catheter with one Dacron cuff was introduced to the peritoneal cavity through a minor laparatomy. The daily cycling procedure for dialysate was four to six

From the Department of Nephrology and Institute of Biophysics, University of Trondheim, Trondheim, Norway.

exchanges of 2 L (Table 1). Plastic bags with lactate buffered dialysis fluid were used (Dianeal®, Travenol Industries, Halden, Norway). In the diabetic patients, all insulin was administered into the dialysis solution.

Procedure of Investigation

Initial glucose concentration in dialysate, drained volume, and dwell-time for each exchange, together with daily measurements of fluid intake, body weight and blood pressure, were recorded for each patient on a special form. These data were fed into an Apple II computer with 48k RAM and double disc system (Apple Computer Inc., Cupertino, CA, USA) for data reduction and storage. A specially designed BASIC program was used for statistical evaluation and printing of selected data.

At the start of CAPD, the drained ultrafiltration volume (ΔV) and initial glucose concentration in the dialysis solution (G_D) was variable due to differences in hydration and also in the time needed to adapt each patient to the CAPD routines. Changes in ΔV in this unstable period were not studied, and the first month with stabilized G_D was used as a time reference. The reference month (see Fig. 1) had to be chosen individually, dependent on the different time before reaching a stable period. Mean values for one month were compared in each patient. The reference month and two other months were compared in each patient. These two months were also depicted individually and correlated to the different time-dependent changes in ΔV. The mean values for daily

fluid intake were also recorded for the same months (Figs. 1A & 1B).

During each episode of peritonitis, the daily changes in ΔV were calculated (% of mean values) for exchanges during one month using the same G_D and the same dwell times as during the peritonitis period (Table 2). Ultrafiltration values during one week before and after peritonitis were excluded from the data used to compute long-term changes. Statistical evaluation of differences between means was based on an unpaired t-distribution test.

RESULTS

Four patients were hospitalized for a total of six episodes of culture positive peritonitis (Table 1). They were all treated with antibiotics parenterally or orally the first day and into the peritoneal cavity for 10–14 days. Cephalothin was most widely used initially, and the antibiotic was adjusted according to the antibiogram and treatment response. The following bacterial growths were found: *Staphylococcus epidermidis*, *Staphylococcus aureus*, *Streptococcus viridans*, and *Klebsiella*. No symptoms or signs or culture-negative peritonitis occurred. Eight re-implantations of new catheters were needed; three because of peritonitis and five because of catheter dislocations.

Figure 1A shows changes in ΔV by stable G_D for short and long dwell times together with the changes in daily fluid intake in the five patients where the UF capacity was reduced during CAPD treatment. The

Table 1. Clinical Details of 9 Patients in the Study.

# Patient	Diagnosis	Episodes of Peritonitis (number)	Long-term Changes in Daily UF (↑ increase, ↓ decrease)	# Daily Exchanges	Observation Time (months)
1	Oxalosis		↓	6	14
2	Diabetic nephropathy	2	↓	5	14
3	Diabetic nephropathy		↓	5	27
4	LCAT* deficiency	1	↓	4	23
5	Nephrosclerosis		↓	5–6	26
6	Juvenile nephronophthisis		↑	4	14
7	Juvenile nephronophthisis		↑	4	23
8	Polycystic renal disease	1	↑	4	26
9	Glomerulonephritis	2	↑	4	40

* LCAT = Lecithin-cholesterol acyltransferase.

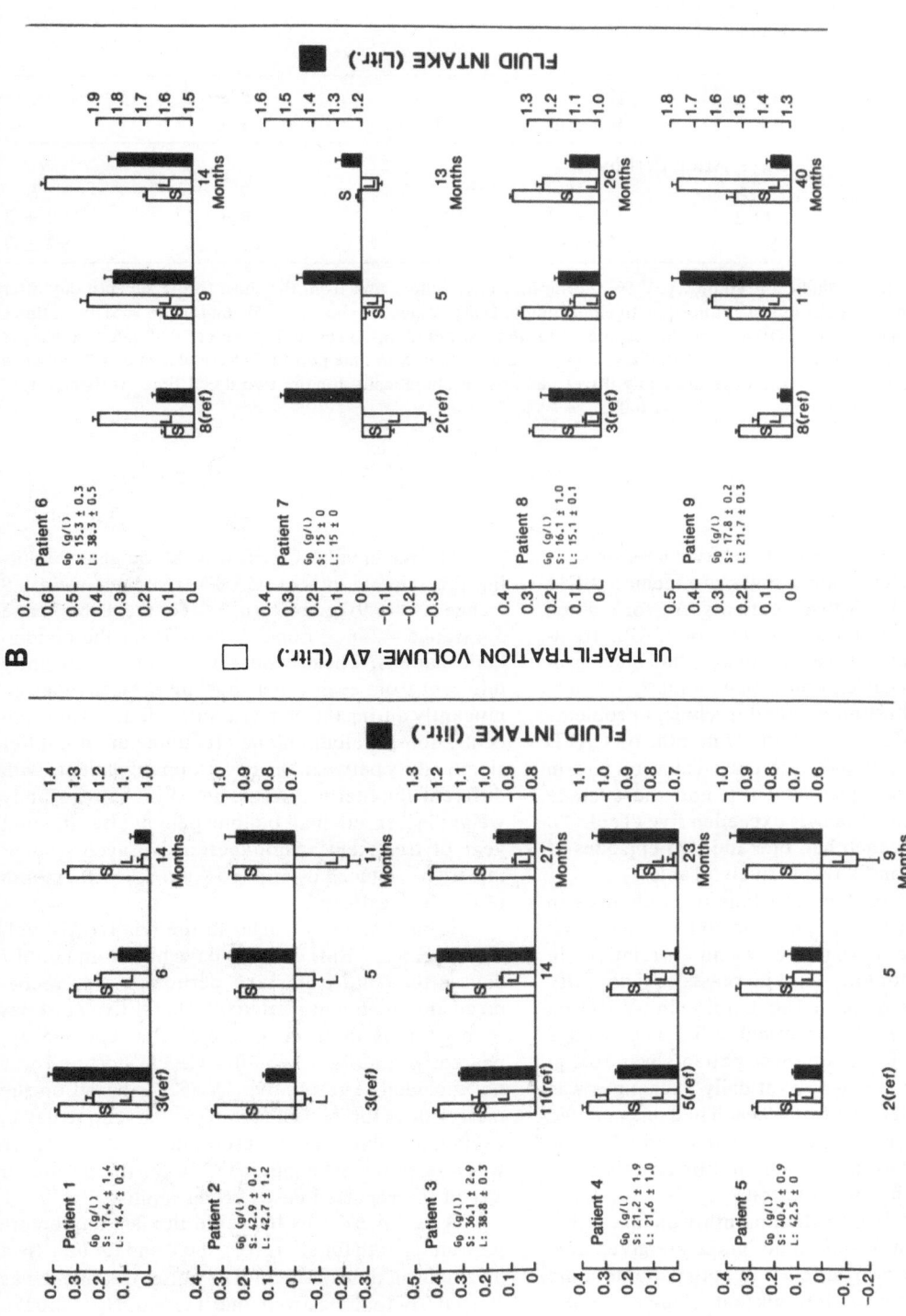

Fig. 1 (A) Time correlated changes in ultrafiltration volume (ΔV) for long (8–10 hours) and short (4–5 hours) dwell times and for daily fluid intake in five patients with decreasing UF capacity during 14–27 months of CAPD treatment (monthly mean ± SEM). The reference month (ref) is compared with two later months in each patient. Initial dextrose concentration in dialysis fluid (G_D) is given for short and long dwell times. The number of months on the abscissa represents time after start of CAPD treatment. (B) The same time correlated changes, as shown in (A), in four patients with increasing ultrafiltration capacity during 14–40 months of CAPD treatment. (L = long dwell time. S = short dwell time.)

Table 2. Relative Daily Ultrafiltration Volume (%).

| Dwell Time (hours) | Days Before Peritonitis | | | |
	−4	−3	−2	−1
4– 5	101 ± 3	101 ± 3	100 ± 2	96 ± 2*
8–10	100 ± 2	100 ± 9	97 ± 3	83 ± 1**
	Days After Peritonitis				
	3	4	5	6	7
4– 5	99 ± 1	102 ± 2	102 ± 2	100 ± 1	100 ± 3
8–10	97 ± 3	99 ± 3	110 ± 4***	101 ± 10	99 ± 2

Relative (mean ± SEM) daily UF volume (ΔV %) during four days before and from the third to the seventh day after diagnosis (day 0) of five episodes of culture-positive peritonitis. Daily values for short (n = 5) and long (n = 5) dwell times are given. Individual baselines (100%) are the mean Δ-V for the last month up to seven days before day 0, for exchanges with the same initial glucose concentration in dialysate G_D as during the given time period. Differences in Δ-V% between the days before and between the days after day 0 were compared statistically for the two dwell times respectively.
* p < 0.05   ** p < 0.025   *** p < 0.005.

reference month is compared with two later periods in each patient. The values given are mean ± SEM for one month. In all these patients, ΔV for a given G_D decreased within the first year on CAPD treatment. All changes were significant, but most pronounced for long dwell times. In patients 2, 3, and 5, reduced ultrafiltration resulted in clinical problems with water overload during 14–27 months on CAPD treatment. The average reference value for G_D in these five patients was 33.2 g/L and the average number of daily exchanges exceeded five (Table 1). Patients 2 and 4 each had one and two episodes of diagnosed peritonitis respectively (Table 1).

No correlation between long-term changes in ΔV and in fluid intake could be found. Figure 1B shows the same measurements and correlations in four patients with long-term increased UF capacity during CAPD treatment. The increase in ΔV started within one year on CAPD by stable G_D. The average reference value for G_D in these patients was 16.3 g/L, and the average number of daily exchanges was four (Table 1). Patients 8 and 9 each had one and two episodes of diagnosed peritonitis respectively. The long-term changes in ΔV could not be correlated to fluid intake in this patient group.

In Figure 2, intermittent monthly changes (p < 0.025–0.995— in ΔV and fluid intake are given during one period in two patients. In both patients some correlations between intermittent changes in ΔV and fluid intake could be observed. These variations in UF capacity and fluid intake were not seen clinically.

The mean values for fasting blood glucose during the third month on CAPD treatment were 8.9 (range 4.2–16.9) mmol/L (n = 6) for the diabetic and 5.4 (range 4.2–6.5) mmol/L (n = 7) for the nondiabetic patiens. These values were not significantly different from each other, nor did they change significantly during the observation period. Serum concentrations of albumin and creatinine did not differ significantly between the two groups of patients with different long-term changes in ΔV. The lean body weight increased in all but one patient after the first year of treatment. Antihypertensive agents could mostly be reduced or omitted within the first month of CAPD treatment.

Table 2 shows changes in the relative UF volume (mean ± SEM) during 4 days before and until 7 days after culture positive peritonitis was recognized and treatment started (day 0) for five episodes of peritonitis in three patients. One episode appeared within one week after CAPD start and was not included. The relative ΔV (%) is based on the mean values for the last month (=100%) up to day 0, excluding values for the preceeding 7 days. There was no significant change in G_D during this period for any of the reported cases of peritonitis.

A fall in ΔV was found on the last day before peritonitis both for short (p < 0.05) and for long (p < 0.025) dwell times. The fifth day after treatment was started, ΔV for long dwell time increased (p < 0.005). The dwell time was reduced the first 3 days during peritonitis, and hence ΔV from this period could not be compared.

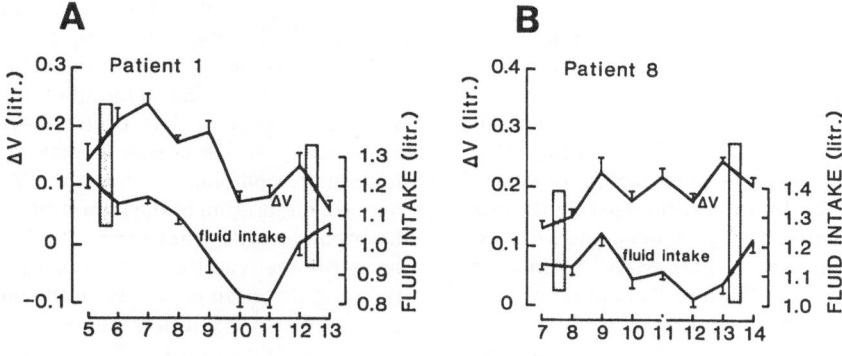

Fig. 2. Intermittent changes in daily ultrafiltration volume (ΔV) and fluid intake during one period in patient 1 (A) and in patient 8 (B). Between the hatched areas, correlations between changes in ΔV and fluid intake can be seen. The values are the mean ± SEM of daily measurements during one month.

Although most changes were intermittent, lasting only a few months, the patients developed progressive increases or decreases in ΔV that could not be directly attributed to changes in osmotic and hydraulic forces. These changes in volume were most distinct for long dwell times. For patients with continued decrease in ΔV, the main fall in ultrafiltration for short dwell times occurred early and then more or less stabilized at a low level, while ΔV for long dwell times continued to fall, often over periods lasting more than a year.

DISCUSSION

We have demonstrated highly significant changes in water transport for all patients evaluated. In our daily routine, we were aware of such changes only in three patients who had clinical UF problems. The early start of these continuous changes in ΔV, and the intermittent changes between monthly averages, were only revealed when the data were analyzed statistically. Due to daily variations, a realistic assessment of UF capacity must be based on a large number of exchanges, and we therefore compared monthly averages for each patient.

Individual differences in average G_D are relatively large, even at the early stages of CAPD treatment (Fig. 1). This can be explained by differences in permeability of the peritoneal "membrane" when entering the dialysis treatment,[6] which could be im-

portant for prediction of long-term changes in UF behavior during CAPD treatment.

In this study, monthly changes in ΔV showed some correlation with changes in fluid intake (Fig. 2). However, it was not possible to decide whether change in ΔV or in fluid intake was the effector. There was no general correlation between fluid intake and long-term changes in ΔV. All but one patient gained body weight progressively during this study, but no correlation with fluid balance or plasma albumin concentrations could be found. Blood pressure remained stable and the use of antihypertensives was unchanged in all patients during the observation period.

Figure 1 shows that UF volumes are smaller for long than for short dwell times, indicating reabsorption of water from the peritoneal cavity during longer dwell times. Most of the dextrose is absorbed within 5 hours.[6] It could therefore be suggested that the increased water reabsorption during 5–10 hours after dialysis fluid instillation is mainly due to increased hydraulic permeability, while the diffusional effects on water transport (i.e., dextrose concentration) should be most important for short exchanges. The smaller variations in UF volume for 4–5 hours dwell time could therefore be a combined result of changing rate of dextrose absorption (diffusion) and modified hydraulic permeability.

It is suggested that long-term changes in ΔV as observed in this study, relate to changes in the peritoneal barrier, and that loss of UF capacity during

CAPD ordinarily results from an increasingly permeable peritoneal barrier. We have previously described individual variations in water kinetics and changes during peritonitis in patients on CAPD,[6,7,13] and this study supported earlier suggestions that problems with fluid balance for CAPD patients mainly are due to increased permeability of the peritoneal barrier. The long-term increased ultrafiltration that was found in four patients could be caused by changes leading to a less permeable "membrane" or to a reduction in effective "membrane" area. This could give slower absorption of dextrose, at least for short exchanges, as well as decreased water flux and an intraperitoneal volume peak operative during longer dwell times.[6,7,13] Reduced permeability could be related to fibrosis or sclerosis of the endothelial basal membrane and of the interstitium, or to a state of vasoconstriction with increased transport resistance across the "membrane."[16,17]

The long-term changes in monthly averages for ΔV were mostly independent of periods with clinical peritonitis. However, changes in daily ΔV appeared the day before peritonitis was diagnosed (Table 2). This was most significant for long dwell times and could be used as an early sign of peritonitis. During peritonitis, the peritoneal barrier becomes more "open," the intraperitoneal volume peak appears earlier, and water reabsorption is more rapid. All decreases in UF volume found in this study appeared to be most significant for long dwell times, compatible with the above discussion of a peritoneum changing to a more "open" membrane with an early intraperitoneal volume peak and small drainage volumes for long dwell times. Changes in the vasculature, in the interstitium and in the mesothelial cell layer can be important factors related to changes in water transport across the peritoneal membrane.

Short-term changes in the permeability of the peritoneum can be caused by vasoconstriction or vasodilatation,[16,17] but this is not a plausible explanation for the ongoing changes in ultrafiltration as seen in this study. The mesothelial cell layer has been suggested to be an important barrier both for water transport and solute diffusion,[18] and in patients losing daily ultrafiltration during time on CAPD and during episodes of peritonitis, patchy or total destruction of the mesothelium has been found.[2]

Rapid water movement across the interstitial space caused by high initial dextrose content in the dialysis solution can also in the long term have an effect on the transport properties of the interstitial matrix. It is generally acknowledged that changes in the interstitial content of complex polysacharides lead to great changes in diffusive and hydraulic permeability.[19,20] The hydraulic conductivity of subcutaneous tissue has been shown to increase dramatically during edema formation,[21] and a high fluid intake combined with a low ΔV could lead to increased hydration of the interstititum, aggravating the problem with water removal. Vasodilatation of the peritoneal capillaries caused by high osmolality,[22] and its possible effects on the mesothelial cell layer may also result in increased permeability and loss of daily ultrafiltration (Table 1). Patients with an initial "open" membrane who need a high glucose solution and more frequent exchanges could therefore develop more serious problems with ultrafiltration after some time on CAPD.

Whether different diseases act differently on the membrane permeability cannot be concluded from this study, but it should be noted that patients suffering from metabolic diseases such as diabetics (two), primary oxalosis (one), lecithin-cholesterol-acyltransferase (LCAT) deficiency (one), and heavy atheromatosis (one), all lost ultrafiltration during CAPD treatment. The practical implication of these observations may contribute to reduce problems with loss of UF capacity during CAPD treatment or to allow calculation of the daily UF volume needed when the drained exchange volume decreases. It seems reasonable to use as low a dextrose concentration in dialysis fluid as possible from the start of CAPD treatment. To maintain needed UF volume in patients with decreasing drainage volume, the long dwell exchange during the night should be omitted. If necessary, a short exchange (<4 hours) can be included during the day, and was successfully done in three of the patients in this study.

In conclusion, this study shows that highly significant changes in monthly average UF volumes occur more frequently and much earlier than clinically observed in these nine patients. Individual differences in peritoneal permeability when the patients enter the CAPD program and factors such as dialysis fluid composition, rate of exchange during each day, peritonitis, and perhaps different diseases can be important factors when evaluating prospectively the long-term maintenance of daily ultrafiltration in CAPD patients.

ACKNOWLEDGMENT

This work was supported by a grant from Travenol Laboratories A/S, Norway.

REFERENCES

1. Faller B, Marichal JF: Loss of ultrafiltration in continuous ambulatory peritoneal dialysis: Clinical data. In Gahl GM, Kessel M, and Nolph KD (Eds), Advances in peritoneal dialysis: Proceedings of the 2nd international symposium on peritoneal dialysis. Amsterdam: Excerpta Medica, 1981, p 227

2. Verger C, Brunschvicg O, Le Charpentier Y, Lavergne A, and Vantelon J: Peritoneal structure alterations on CAPD. In Gahl GM, Kessel M, and Nolph KD (Eds), Advances in peritoneal dialysis: Proceedings of the 2nd international symposium on peritoneal dialysis. Amsterdam: Excerpta Medica, 1981, p 10

3. Slingeneyer A, Canaud B, and Mion C: Permanent loss of ultrafiltration capacity of the peritoneum in long-term peritoneal dialysis: an epidemiological study. Nephron 33: 133, 1983

4. Nolph KD, Sorkin M, Rubin J, Arfania D, Prowant B, Fruto L, and Kennedy D: Continuous ambulatory peritoneal dialysis: Three-year experience at one center. Ann Intern Med 92: 609, 1980

5. Khanna R, Oreopoulos DG, Dombros N, Vas S, Williams R, Meema HE, Husdan H, Ogilvie R, Zellerman G, Roncari DAK, Clayton S, and Izatt S: Continuous ambulatory peritoneal dialysis after three years: Still a promising treatment. Peritoneal Dial Bull 4: 24, 1981

6. Smeby LC, Widerøe T-E, and Jörstad S: Differences in volume transport during continuous peritoneal dialysis. asaio J 4: 17, 1981

7. Smeby LC, Widerøe T-E, Svartås TM, and Jörstad S: Changes in water removal due to peritonitis during continuous peritoneal dialysis. In Gahl GM, Kessel M, and Nolph KD (Eds), Advances in peritoneal dialysis: Proceedings of the 2nd international symposium on peritoneal dialysis. Amsterdam: Excerpta Medica, 1981, p 287

8. Raja RM, Kramer MS, Rosenbaum JL, Bolisay C, and Krug M: Contrasting changes in solute transport and ultrafiltration with peritonitis in CAPD patients. Trans Am Soc Artif Intern Organs 27: 68, 1981

9. Rubin J, Ray R, Barnes T, and Bower J: Peritoneal abnormalities during infectious episodes of continuous ambulatory peritoneal dialysis. Nephron 29: 124, 1981

10. Katirtzoglou A, Oreopoulos DG, Husdan H, Leung M, Ogilvie R, and Dombros N: Reappraisal of protein losses in patients undergoing continuous ambulatory peritoneal dialysis. Nephron 26: 230, 1980

11. Rubin J, Nolph K, Arfania D, Brown P, and Prowant B: Follow-up of peritoneal clearances in patients undergoing continuous ambulatory peritoneal dialysis. Kidney Int 16: 619, 1979

12. Farrell PC, and Randerson DH: Membrane permeability changes in long term CAPD. Trans Am Soc Artif Organs 26: 197, 1980

13. Smeby LC, and Wideröe T-E: Kinetics of continuous ambulatory peritoneal dialysis. Proc Eur Soc Artif Organs 6: 156, 1979

14. Daugirdas JT, Ing TS, Gandhi VC, Hano JE, Chen W-T, and Yuan L: Kinetics of peritoneal fluid absorption in patients with chronic renal failure. J Lab Clin Med 95: 351, 1980

15. Wayland H: Transmural and interstitial molecular transport. In Legrain M (Ed), Continuous ambulatory peritoneal dialysis. Amsterdam: Excerpta Medica, 1980, p 18

16. Maher JF: Characteristics of peritoneal transport: Physiological and clinical implications. Mineral Electrolyte Metab 5: 201, 1981

17. Nolph KD, Miller FN, Pyle WK, Popovich RP, and Sorkin MI: An hypothesis to explain the ultrafiltration characteristics of peritoneal dialysis. Kidney Int 20: 543, 1981

18. Gosselin RE, and Berndt WO: Diffusional transport of solutes through mesentery and peritoneum. J Theoret Biol 3: 487, 1962

19. Fox JR, and Wayland H: Interstitial diffusion of macromolecules in the rat mesentery. Microvasc Res 18: 255, 1979

20. Aukland K, and Nicolaysen G: Interstitial fluid volume: Local regulatory mechanisms. Physiol Rev 61: 556, 1981

21. Guyton AC, Scheel K, and Murphree D: Interstitial fluid pressure III. Its effect on resistance to tissue fluid mobility. Circ Res 19: 412, 1966

22. Miller FN, Nolph KD, Joshua IG, Wiegman DL, Harris PD, and Andersen DB: Hyperosmolality, acetate, and lactate: Dilatory factors during peritoneal dialysis. Kidney Int 20: 397, 1981

C. Ronco, D. Borin, A. Brendolan, L. Bragantini,
S. Chiaramonte, M. Feriani, A. Fabris, and G. La Greca

14

Influence of Blood Flow and Plasma Proteins on UF Rate in Peritoneal Dialysis

SUMMARY

Factors that limit the rate of peritoneal ultrafiltration were evaluated *in vivo* and by *in vitro* studies with a hollow fiber dialyzer. With continued ultrafiltration plasma protein concentrations increased, offsetting the osmotic gradient, thereby decreasing the rate of fluid flux. Because the filtration fraction was high, the concentration of protein in the venous end of the capillary reached a point where filtration ceases. The low peritoneal blood flow appeared to limit the ultrafiltration rate.

INTRODUCTION

The rate of ultrafiltration in peritoneal dialysis depends highly on the dextrose concentration in the dialysis solution. Other forces contribute to the generation of the global transmembrane pressure in the peritoneum. However, the osmotic gradient, which generates a pressure of several hundred mm Hg (1 mOsm = 15 mm Hg), is certainly the most important factor.[1] Even in the presence of such a tremendous pressure gradient (the TMP generated by a 2.5% dextrose solution averages 1000 mm Hg), the ultrafiltration coefficient K (Qf/TMP) of the peritoneal membrane appears to be very small in comparison with other dialysis membranes, producing a low amount of ultrafiltrate per minute. The aim of this study was to evaluate the possible factors limiting the ultrafiltration rate (Qf) and particularly: demonstration of the influence of the plasma protein concentration on Qf; demonstration that filtration pressure equilibrium occurs in the peritoneal capillary; calculation of the protein concentration leaving the capillary; calculation of the real UF rate for a certain applied TMP and the relative filtration fraction; calculation of the effective peritoneal capillary blood flow and demonstration that the low UF rate in peritoneal dialysis depends primarily on the limited blood flow passing through the peritoneal capillary network.

We assume that the systemic protein concentration and the inlet capillary protein concentrations are identical; however, we must consider a physiological dilution of the blood in the microvasculature. A high inlet protein concentration near the arterial side of the capillary might induce filtration pressure equilibrium and further reduce ultrafiltration. For these purposes we studied the kinetics of ultrafiltration during rapid 2L exchanges of a 30 L IPD session to examine the instantaneous movement of water through the peritoneal membrane. The peritoneal surface area and the peritoneal membrane permeability should not be limiting factors; the surface area is calculated to be in the range of 1–2 m² and the suspected limited number of pores is enough to permit an adequate clearance of small and middle molecules (the sieving coefficient for these solutes is similar to that of other membranes.[2–5] In our opinion the factor primarily affecting the peritoneal UF rate is the low blood flow in the capillary network, and

---

From the Department of Nephrology, St. Bortolo Hospital, Vicenza, Italy.

we will try to demonstrate this concept. Comparison with a hollow fiber hemofilter at a low blood flow (for example CAVH treatment) and various TMP allows us to hypothesize that filtration pressure equilibrium at high filtration fractions may occur in the peritoneal capillary, influenced by plasma protein concentrations in the system.[6]

METHODS

The approach to the problem consists in both *in vivo* and *in vitro* studies.

In Vivo Studies

Hourly measurement of ultrafiltration in three patients during successive IPD sessions carried out with rapid 2 L exchanges, zero dwell time and dextrose 2.5% were studied for control with a 1.5% dextrose solution. The IPD sessions were carried out in basal conditions, after acute dehydration by extracorporeal ultrafiltration (-2.5 Kg) and after restoration of normal body hydration by IV saline infusion. Peritoneal ultrafiltration rate was measured according to the formula

$$Qf = \frac{(Vd_o - Vd_i) + (RV_2 - RV_1)}{\text{Time of one exchange}} \quad (1)$$

where Vd_o and Vd_i are the outlet and inlet volumes of fluid and RV_1 and RV_2 are the residual intraperitoneal volumes of fluid before and after the exchange,

measured by the dilution of a nondiffusible radioisotope (^{131}I RISA). Venous blood samples were taken at the beginning and the end of each session for measurement of glucose, electrolytes, total plasma proteins, and hematocrit. Systemic blood values were considered identical to the capillary inlet concentration.

In Vitro Studies

Measurements of ultrafiltration, filtration fraction, and protein concentration in the arterial and venous blood lines of a circuit with a hollow fiber hemofilter (Amicon 20) were performed utilizing different blood flows and transmembrane pressures. This was done to obtain a protein concentration able to generate an oncotic force which equalizes a certain hydrostatic pressure, and to show that filtration pressure equilibrium is achieved inside the fibers.

FIRST EXPERIMENT

The blood was pumped through the circuit in single pass from the arterial to the venous line. The ultrafiltrate was collected and measured over a fixed period of time. Different blood flows were planned: 50, 100, 150, and 200 ml/min. Several TMP were applied: from 20–1200 mm Hg. An arterial blood sample was taken before each experiment. A venous sample for each period of time in which a stable pressure was applied (10 minutes), was drawn. Hematocrit and total plasma proteins were measured in each sample. Figure 1 depicts the circuit.

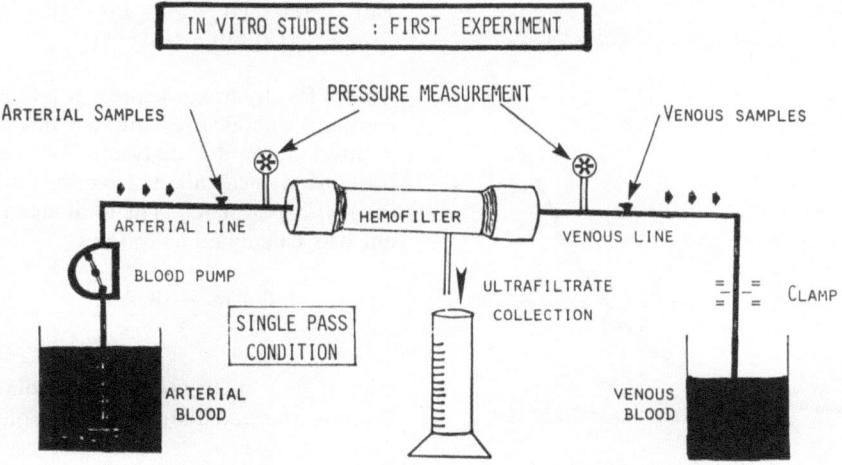

Fig. 1. Ultrafiltration circuit.

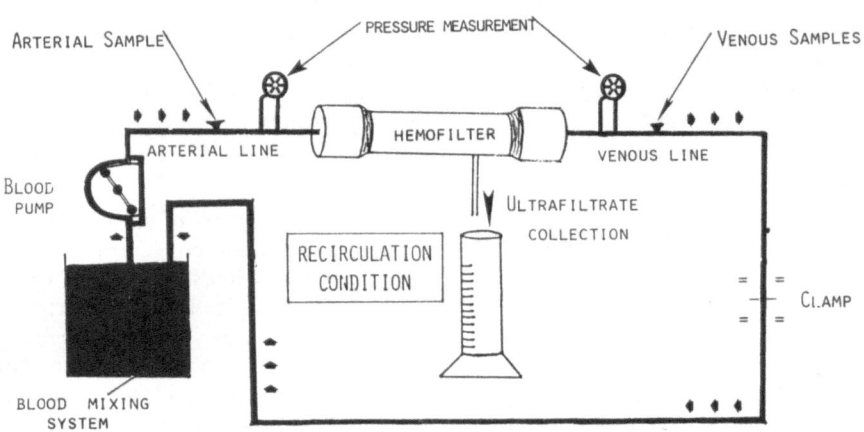

Fig. 2.   Circuit for blood recirculation and ultrafiltration.

SECOND EXPERIMENT

The blood was pumped and recirculated in the same circuit (Fig. 2); a stirrer allowed for continuous mixing of the arterial and venous blood in the container. The same blood flows and TMP described above were used. For each blood flow and TMP, the blood was recirculated to the point when no more ultrafiltrate was produced; at that point, arterial and venous samples were drawn for plasma protein concentration and hematocrit measurement. Each group of experiments was performed three times. The protein concentration at the same blood flow and TMP were compared between first and second experiment. When the two protein concentrations were identical, the condition of filtration pressure equilibrium was considered achieved in the single pass condition.

CALCULATIONS

The peritoneal TMP was calculated according to the formula:

$$TMP = (Pb - Pi) - (\pi b - \pi i) + (Oi - Op) + (Pi - Pd) - (\pi i - \pi d) + (Od - Oi) \qquad (2)$$

where: P = hydrostatic pressure; O = osmotic pressure; π = oncotic pressure; b = blood; p = plasma; i = interstitium; d = dialysate. The capillary oncotic pressure was calculated from the curve obtained by *in vitro* experiments. The total mean osmotic gradient was calculated as follows:

$$\frac{dOsm_I + dOsm_O}{2} - pOsm \qquad (3)$$

where: d = dialysate and p = plasma. Filtration fraction was calculated with the following formula

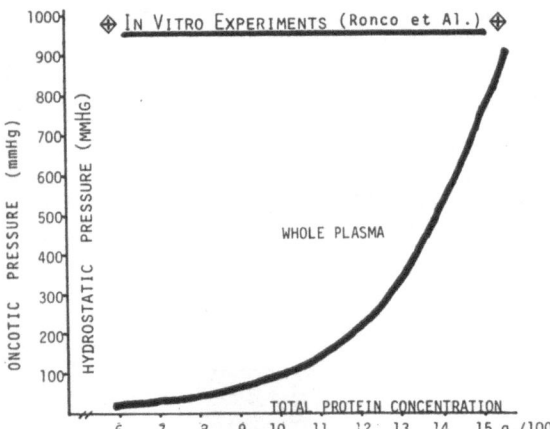

Fig. 3.   Correlation of plasma protein equilibrium and pressure.

$$FF = 1 - \frac{\text{protein inlet concentration}}{\text{protein outlet concentration}} = Qf/Qp \qquad (4)$$

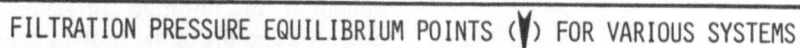

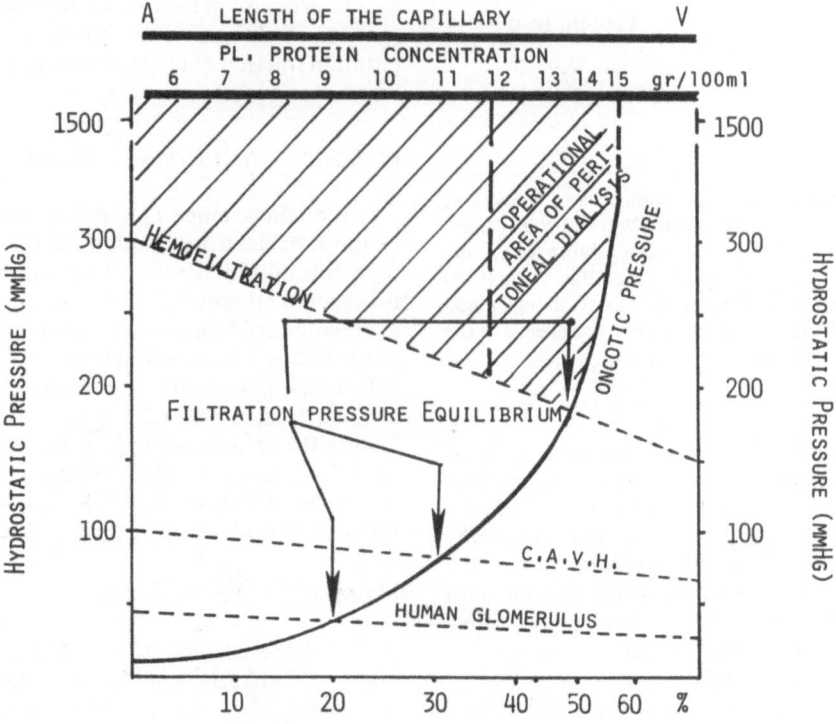

Fig. 4. Filtration pressure equilibrium points.

where: protein inlet concentration is the systemic protein concentration, while the protein outlet concentration is calculated from the curve obtained from *in vitro* experiments (Fig. 3), in the assumption that filtration pressure equilibrium occurs in the capillary (Fig. 4). Peritoneal plasma flow (Qp) was measured as Qf/FF and the effective peritoneal capillary blood flow (Qb) was calculated as

$$Qp \times \frac{1}{1 - Ht} \qquad (5)$$

RESULTS

The peritoneal UF rate showed a significant decrease (from 10.5 to 7.1 ml/min) during a 6 hour session. A parallel increase in plasma protein concentration (from 6.5 to 7.8 g/dl) was noted. After acute dehydration (−2.5 Kg), achieved by a 4 hour session of continuous A-V hemofiltration, Qf showed

stable low values during a 6 hour peritoneal dialysis (4.5 ± 1.2 ml/min). The starting plasma protein concentration was 7.9 g/dl (due to ultrafiltration) and remained 8.0 g/dl at the end of the dialysis. After fluid reinfusion, the protein concentration decreased to 6.6 g/dl, and the UF rate was restored to 9.9 ml/min. It must be noted that other parameters changed during the experiment, such as hematocrit, blood viscosity, plasma osmolality and mean arterial pressure; however, the most important changes concerned the plasma protein concentration. Tables 1 and 2 show the values for venous protein concentration obtained in the first *in vitro* experiment and in the second one. Since there is no difference between the total protein concentrations measured in the venous blood both in single pass and recirculation conditions at the same TMP, the hypothesis that filtration pressure equilibrium is achieved inside the fibers during a single passage of the blood was proved. These two experiments led us to draw the

Table 1. *In Vitro* Results: First Experiment.

TMP (mm Hg)	Venous Plasma Protein (g/dl)
25	7.0
50	7.5
75	8.0
100	9.4

Blood flow (single pass) was 50 ml/min. The same values were obtained for blood flows of 100–150 and 200 ml/min. Utilizing another artificial membrane (Cuprophan), the same values were obtained only for blood flows below 100 ml/min showing an increase less important with high blood flows. The total protein concentration in the plasma at the beginning of the experiment was 6 g/dl.

nomogram depicted in Figure 3, which can be used *in vivo* for the calculation of the outlet plasma protein concentration. In fact there is high evidence for a similar behavior of the peritoneal capillary and the polysulphone hollow fiber: the permeability coefficient for several solutes in the small and medium molecular weight range was not significantly different between the two membranes; the velocity of the blood stream inside the capillary was calculated to be very low and comparable to the lowest blood flow used *in vitro*; the TMP applied to the peritoneal capillary membrane is very high and acting along the complete length of the capillary.

On the basis of these considerations we may strongly suppose that, in the peritoneal capillary, the

Table 2. *In Vitro* Results: Second Experiment.

TMP (until QF = 0)	Protein (g/dl)*
50	7.5
100	9.5
200	10.4
400	12.6
600	13.5
800	14.2
1000	14.7
1200	14.9

* Arterial and venous protein concentration when UF ceased. There is no difference between the total protein concentrations measured in the venous blood in condition of single pass and recirculation at the same TMP.

condition of filtration pressure equilibrium is achieved and the outlet protein concentration must be proportional to the oncotic pressure able to equalize the pressure generated by the dialysis solution. In these conditions we may calculate the peritoneal filtration fraction obtained with a certain transmembrane pressure.

FILTRATION FRACTION CALCULATION

With the average TMP of 760 mm Hg generated by the 2.5% dextrose solution and the average measured ultrafiltration rate of 8.1 ml/min, being the average inlet protein concentration 6.8 g/dl, the average outlet protein concentration resulted (13.9 g/dl) with a filtration fraction of 52%. The same calculation gave a filtration fraction of 43% in the subjects treated with 1.5% dextrose solution. In our studies the peritoneal filtration fraction ranged from 38–54%. This can be considered quite a stable range of values, which is very high in comparison with other treatments.

BLOOD FLOW CALCULATION

With the calculated filtration fractions, we were able to calculate the average blood flow in the peritoneal capillary system, available for fluid and solute exchange with the dialysis solution. The average plasma flow calculated in our patients was 16 ml/min. This value, corrected for an average hematocrit of 31%, showed an average blood flow, effective for the peritoneal dialysis exchange, of 22.4 ml/min. In all calculations, the blood flow ranged from 12.5–32 ml/min.

DISCUSSION

From our results there is good evidence that a poor blood flow is the factor primarily limiting the UF rate in peritoneal dialysis. Our calculations are necessarily made with some approximations, but there is good evidence that the peritoneal capillary systems may be compared roughly with a hollow fiber hemofilter used at very low blood flow and very high TMP. All the calculations were sustained by the assumption that filtration pressure equilibrium was achieved in the peritoneal capillary, as in the polysulphone hollow fiber. The influence of plasma protein concentration may be explained by approaching the filtration pressure equilibrium point due to higher inlet protein concentrations.

The high values obtained for the filtration fraction suggest that the peritoneal membrane has a high efficiency in removing water from the blood, and the small amounts of ultrafiltrate achievable, even in the presence of a tremendous TMP, is due to the poor blood flow available for peritoneal dialysis.

REFERENCES

1. La Greca G, Biasioli S, and Ronco C: Peritoneal dialysis. Milano: Wichtig Editore, 1982, p 85

2. Pappenheimer JR: Passage of molecules through capillary walls. Physiol Rev 33: 378, 1953

3. Nolph KD: The peritoneal dialysis system. Nephrol 17: 44, 1978

4. Karnovsky MJ: The ultrastructural basis of capillary permeability studies with peroxides as a tracer. J Cell Biol 35: 213, 1967

5. Maher JF: Acceleration of peritoneal mass transport by drugs and hormones. Artif Organs 3: 224, 1979

6. Lauer A, Saccaggi A, Ronco C, Belledonne M, Glabman S, and Bosch JP: Continuous arteriovenous hemofiltration in the critically ill patient. Ann Intern Med 99: 455, 1983

C. Verger, L. Larpent, and M. Dumontet

15

Prognostic Value of Peritoneal Equilibration Curves in CAPD Patients

SUMMARY

In some still unprecise circumstances CAPD results in alterations of peritoneal permeability. Using equilibration curves for glucose it is possible to predict the type of peritoneal damage associated with these alterations and therefore to propose an appropriate therapy.

When a decreased volume drainage is observed on CAPD: If it is associated with hyperpermeability it is probable that reversible lesions are present and temporary interruption of CAPD may help recovery towards a normal peritoneum. If peritoneal ultrafiltration is decreased and if associated with hyperpermeability to glucose it may be the result of a reduced exchange surface due to either multiple adhesions or encapsulating peritonitis (even if asymptomatic). Thus CAPD must definitely be stopped and systematic laparotomy must be considered.

INTRODUCTION

Patients on CAPD may separate into different groups; most do well after several years on CAPD; a smaller group may lose UF capacity without clinical evidence of severe visceral pathology; while a third group has been described that may develop sclerosing encapsulating peritonitis. As this last complication is the most severe, we felt it important to investigate a simple method for its early detection. We present here a graphic means by which early detection of peritoneal membrane damage in CAPD patients may be achieved.

METHODS

Equilibration curves (EC) were determined with 1.5% and 4.25% dextrose (hydrated) dialysis solutions, buffered with lactate during a 6 hour dwell time (from beginning of inflow to beginning of drainage). Sodium, urea, and glucose were measured every 30 minutes in the dialysate, as well as in plasma at the beginning and end of the dwell time. Plasma urea was estimated as the mean of its concentration at the beginning and end of the dwell time. Curves were best fitted for dialysate to plasma urea ratio versus time to define the urea equilibration curve. Similarly, the ratio of dialysate glucose concentration to the initial dialysis fluid glucose concentration versus dwell time were made to define the glucose equilibration curve. Net UF after drainage was calculated from the difference between the drainage and initial bag weights.

Glucose was determined by the glucose dehydrogenase method on a GEMSAEC analyzer. Sodium determination was made on a IL 243 flame emission photometer. Urea and plasma proteins were measured with a SMA II apparatus (diacetyl monoxime for urea and biuret reaction for protein):

From the Service de Medecine Interne et Nephrologie, et Laboratoire de Biochimie. Centre Hospitalier Rene Dubos, 95301 Pontoise, France.

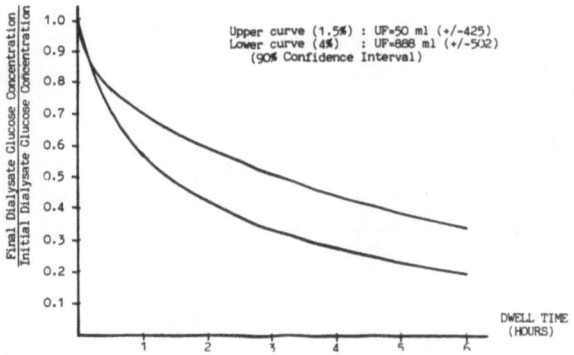

Fig. 1. Normal glucose ECs with 1.5% and 4% dextrose dialysis solutions (mean of 30 different CAPD patients).

Fig. 2. Normal urea ECs with 1.5% and 4% dextrose dialysis solutions (mean of 30 different CAPD patients).

in the dialysate samples, protein was determined by a turbidimetric method using trichloracetic acid.

One hundred and twenty ECs were determined in 42 CAPD patients: 30 of them had 40 laparotomies during catheter placement and/or its removal: 30 peritoneal biopsies, taken from the mesentery, were examined under light and electron microscopy.

Sixty EC (30 with 1.36% and 30 with 3.86% (anhydrous) dextrose dialysis solution) were determined in 30 patients during the first 6 months of CAPD treatment: these first measurements were considered baseline: at each time (every 30 minutes) mean values were calculated and the 90% confidence intervals determined using student tables.

In the remaining 60 measurements, EC values at comparable times were graphically compared to baseline values. When possible, changes in EC were correlated with the data obtained at laparotomy, and this group comprises the study group.

RESULTS

Control Group (I)

Baseline values were obtained from 30 patients. Large interpatient variations were observed. With 1.5% dextrose dialysis solution baseline UF was 50 ml (±426 ml). With 4.25% dextrose dialysis fluid, mean UF was 888 ml (±502 ml). The same large variations were observed for glucose and urea ECs. However, for normals, we were able to define a normal EC area with 90% confidence intervals from 30 minute samples: this normal area is shaded in all

figures and has been called the standard equilibration curve area (SECA). Glucose tended to decrease more rapidly with 4.25% dextrose dialysis fluid than with 1.5% dextrose (Fig. 1); a similar difference was observed for urea equilibration (Fig. 2), which was faster with 4.25% dextrose dialysis fluid. Therefore when comparing EC, identical dextrose concentrations must be used.

Study Group (II) (12 patients)

In group IIa, seven patients had UF and ECs in the normal range. Laparotomy and peritoneal biopsy were identical to those observed in control subjects. However, some patients had increased

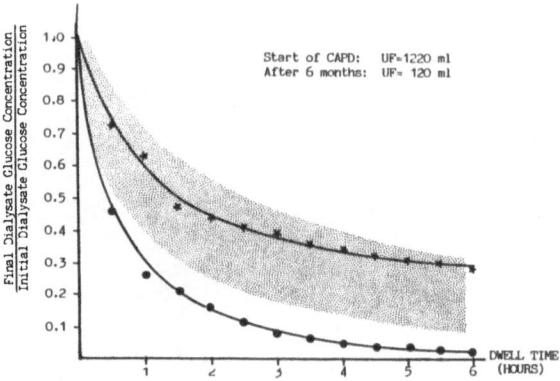

Fig. 3. Decreased UF due to hyperpermeable peritoneum. Glucose EC (with 4% dextrose dialysis solution).

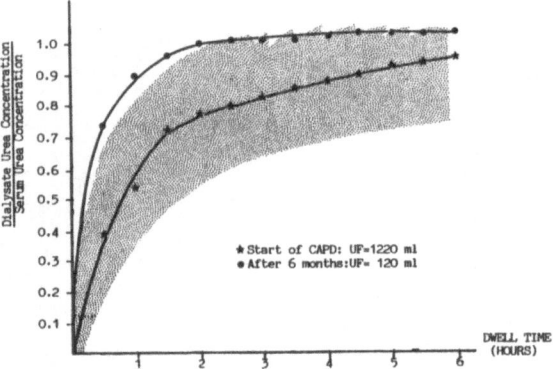

Fig. 4. Decreased UF due to hyperpermeable peritoneum. Urea EC (with 4% dextrose dialysis solution).

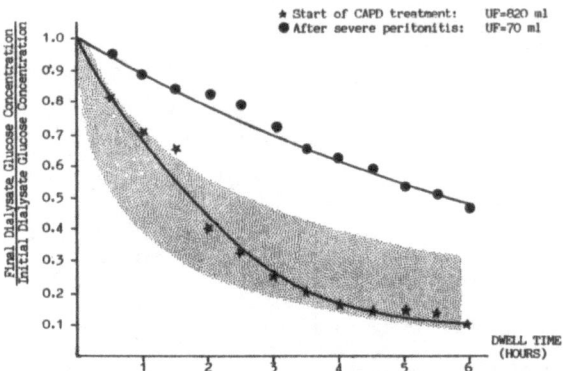

Fig. 6. Decreased UF due to reduced peritoneal area following multiple adhesions after peritonitis. Glucose EC (with 4% dextrose dialysis solution).

submesothelial fibrosis, which is common in uremic patients as well as in CAPD patients.

In group IIb, five patients had UF below the normal range. In two cases this occurred spontaneously with no history of peritonitis; in the first case, one week after initiation of CAPD in a patient using Travenol Dianeal® solution; and in the other case, after 6 months of treatment in a patient using Fresenius solutions (Figs. 3 & 4). In the other three cases the loss of UF appeared 1–3 years after the beginning of treatment. In these patients all the ECs were similar to those in Figures 3 and 4, showing a more rapid decrease in glucose concentration and faster equilibration of dialysate urea over the six hour exchange. No abnormalities were observed in this

group during laparotomy, but on light and electron microscopy, severe abnormalities of the mesothelial cells were present and large gaps were observed between junctions; in the other there was complete mesothelial desquamation frequently associated with moderate hypervascularization.

Only one patient could be studied after interruption of CAPD. In this patient the peritoneal catheter was left in place while she was on hemodialysis, thus allowing ultrafiltration and equilibration curves to be regularly followed. The results show a continuous improvement in UF that correlated with a lower glucose absorption over a six month period (Fig. 5). At the end of this period, the catheter was removed and laparotomy was performed; the peritoneal cavity was absolutely normal without any adhesions. On light microscopy, the peritoneal membrane was normal with a continuous layer of mesothelial cells.

In group IIc, two patients presented with UF below the normal range associated with EC showing a high dialysate glucose concentration for the whole six hour exchange. At the same time, urea EC showed a slower equilibration than normal.

Case 1 was a 40-year-old female on CAPD for three months. At the time of initiation of treatment her UF was normal and glucose EC was in the SECA (Fig. 6). She developed peritonitis, but did not call the medical staff and came to the outpatient clinic three weeks later, with three weeks of continuous peritonitis! She was rapidly treated by local antibiotics with the maintenance of four exchanges per day, but she did not recover normal UF, which remained below 100 ml after a 6-hour dwell with 4.25% dextrose dialysis solution. Her EC for glucose moved

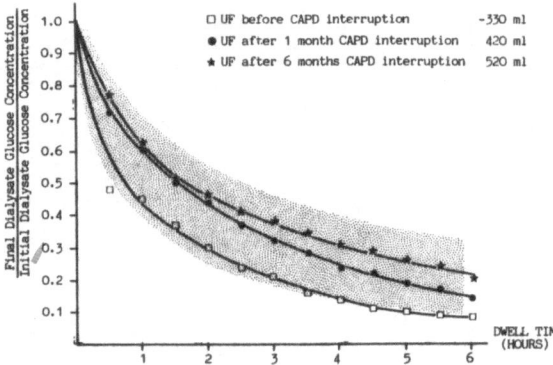

Fig. 5. Recovery of normal peritoneal UF after temporary hemodialysis. Glucose EC (with 4% dextrose dialysis solution).

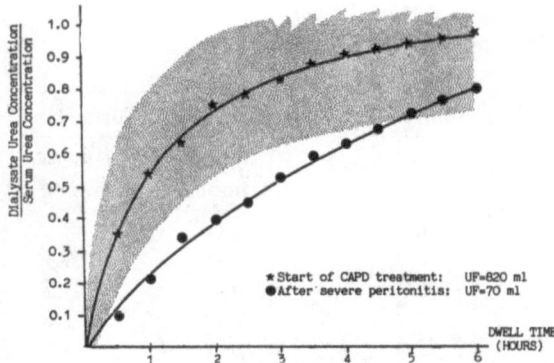

Fig. 7. Decreased UF due to reduced peritoneal area following multiple adhesions after peritonitis. Urea EC (with 4% dextrose dialysis solution).

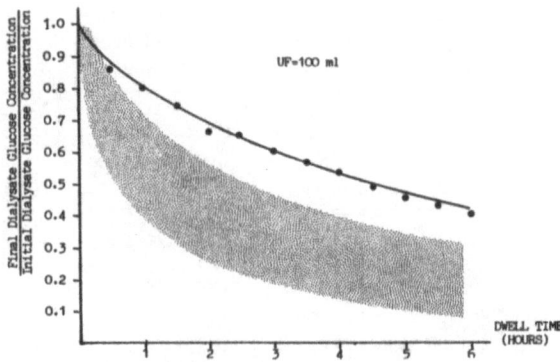

Fig. 8. Decreased UF due to reduced peritoneal area following encapsulating peritonitis. Glucose EC (with 4% dextrose dialysis solution).

above the SECA (Fig. 6), whereas it moved under it for urea (Fig. 7). Both results were obviously in favor of a hypopermeable peritoneum. Although she did not suffer abdominal pain, and because we suspected severe peritoneal disease, we decided to perform a systematic laparotomy when removing the catheter; laparotomy showed multiple adhesions with all intestinal loops being stuck together, and it was not possible to separate them from each other. No peritoneal biopsy was possible.

Case 2 was a 45-year-old male who had been treated with Travenol Dianeal solutions for four years; he had eight short duration episodes of peritonitis during the first three years (Figs. 8 & 9). Only the first two episodes of peritonitis were treated with 48 hours of continous lavage with dialysate containing acetate as buffer. The other episodes were treated with four exchanges per day with Travenol Dianeal solutions. During the last year, UF decreased and blood urea levels increased dramatically. The EC suggested fibrosis or loss of surface area as in case 1, and a systematic laparotomy was performed. It showed a typical encapsulating peritonitis. The capsule was opened, and inside this fibrotic bag the intestinal loops were relatively free, but numerous adhesions were also present. Biopsy of the fibrotic encapsulating tissue showed that it was composed of collagen fibrils containing a few fibroblasts, with the outer part showing signs of fibrinoid degeneration. A peritoneal biopsy was also performed on the mesentery, which looked macroscopically normal. On light microscopy, however, no mesothelium was present on the surface, which appeared to be made up of 40 μ thick fibrotic tissue.

This was confirmed by scanning electron microscopy, which showed a completely denuded peritoneum.

DISCUSSION

The main structures involved in transperitoneal solute exchange have been clearly described in the last few years.[1] Peritoneal permeability depends upon the mass transfer area coefficient (MTAC), which depends on solute molecular size, anatomical resistances to transport, and the peritoneal area available for exchange.[2] A delicate equilibrium must be present to obtain both good clearances and nor-

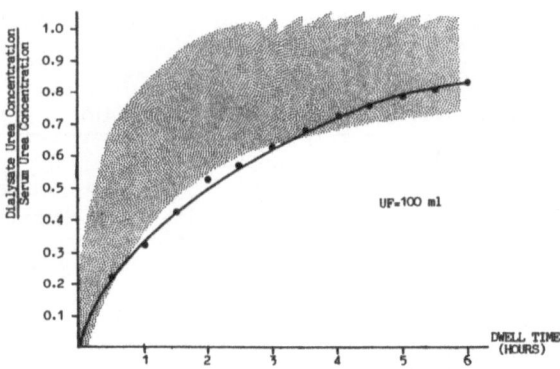

Fig. 9. Decreased UF due to reduced peritoneal area following encapsulating peritonitis. Urea EC (with 4% dextrose dialysis solution).

Table 1. Dialysate Glucose and Sodium Concentrations during a 6 Hour Dwell Time in Three CAPD Patients with Different Types of Peritoneal Permeability. (3.86% Dianeal Solution—2 L Exchange).

Time (min)	Normal		Hyperpermeability		Loss of Surface	
	Sodium (mmol/l)	Glucose (mmol/l)	Sodium (mmol/l)	Glucose (mmol/l)	Sodium (mmol/l)	Glucose (mmol/l)
0	134	201	133	196.1	133	203
30	125	153	131	94.7	133	175.5
60	120	134	132	90.2	132	163.2
90	118	116.7	132	73.7	132	151.6
120	117	102.1	133	59.0	132	135.6
150	116	90.9	134	48.5	132	133.0
180	117	84.8	135	41.0	132	122.9
210	117	78.12	135	32.8	132	115.6
240	118	73.26	136	27.8	132	108.1
270	118	69.48	136	22.8	133	100.1
300	119	65.52	136	21.0	133	83.0
330	120	62.16	136	18.2	133	88.2
360	121	58.8	137	16.1	133	81.8
Vol drained:	3000 ml		1900 ml		2030 ml	

mal UF. Hence, the peritoneal membrane must be sufficiently permeable to allow easy passage of uremic toxins from the blood through the different structures toward the peritoneal cavity; but it must also be resistant enough to prevent rapid absorption of glucose so that its high concentration in the peritoneal cavity develops the necessary osmotic pressure to obtain a normal UF. Ergo, any change in "pore" diameter or total peritoneal surface area should induce variations in the kinetics of urea, glucose, and water.

Loss of UF has been investigated these last years by French authors,[3–6] and more recently by a multicenter study conducted by Nolph and co-workers.[7] The exact cause of observed decreased UF is still under investigation, but it has been shown to be associated with hyperpermeability to glucose. We first suggested that mesothelial alterations could be the responsible physiological mechanism,[3] and this was later confirmed by an animal study.[8] Our present data agree with the hypothesis that loss of UF, associated with a hyperpermeable peritoneum, is mainly due to mesothelial alterations, and may be reversible.

On the other hand, the more severe complication—sclerosing encapsulating peritonitis—has

Table 2. Peritoneal Permeability Alterations.

Type	Dialysate Dextrose Decrease	Dialysate Urea Equilibration	Volume Drained	Dialysate Sodium Decrease	Peritoneal Status
I	Normal	Normal	Normal	Yes	Normal
II	Normal	Normal	Low	Yes	Leakage
III	Normal	Normal	Low	No	Early adhesions or
IV	Rapid	Rapid	Low	No	Reversible mesothelial alterations and/or hypervascularization
V	Slow	Normal or Slow	Low	No	Numerous adhesions or sclerosing peritonitis

been observed during CAPD.[9, 10] In these cases there is an important reduction in the available surface for peritoneal solute exchange; the same conditions are realized when multiple adhesions are present. It is not surprising that a loss of UF is present in these cases even with a high dextrose concentration in the peritoneal cavity; nothing can go through the structures separating blood vessels from dialysate, neither solutes of any size nor water.

Decreased UF with poor glucose absorption was reported by Wu et al. in 1984.[11] They suggested it should be associated with reduced dialysing surface, but they did not state whether laparotomy had been performed. In the same period, Slingeneyer[12] in France also observed a decreased UF in patients with encapsulating peritonitis, and suggested it should be associated with high dialysate glucose concentration. The present work confirms these authors' hypotheses, demonstrating an obvious correlation between ECs and the type of membrane alterations.

When using hypertonic solutions, dialysate sodium concentrations tend to decrease during the dwell time in normally filtrating subjects (Table 1); this is due to the passage of hypotonic water from blood vessels toward the peritoneal cavity. Therefore, dialysate sodium decreases reflect efficient UF. Hence, if there is a true loss of filtration, dialysate sodium does not decrease. In the case of dialysate leakage, either in the abdominal wall or outside, the low drainage volume is associated with a normal sodium decrease.

Therefore, by comparing graphically urea and glucose EC to our SECA, and using dialysate sodium concentratons as an index of water removal, it is possible to define five types of peritoneal permeability. These are summarized in Table 2, along with their corresponding anatomical lesion.

It is worth pointing out that our patient with sclerosing encapsulating peritonitis had no mesothelium on the mesenteric peritoneum. This suggests that the first step for peritoneal sclerosis would be desquamation of mesothelial cells with hyperpermeability, and that the unprotected tissues would adhere to each other as is a natural tendency in these circumstances.[13] At this step a decrease in UF is still present, not related to absorption of glucose and low peritoneal osmotic pressure but due to a decrease in exchange surface. The ultimate step would be the appearance of the encapsulating process. If this is true, it is of particular importance to stop CAPD at the stage of hyperpermeability, as these abnormalities seem to be reversible.

REFERENCES

1. Miller FN: The peritoneal microcirculation. In Nolph KD (Ed), Peritoneal dialysis. Martinus Nijhoff, 1981, p 42
2. Henderson LW: The problem of peritoneal membrane area and permeability. Kidney Int 3: 409, 1973
3. Verger C, Brünschvicg O, Le Charpentier Y, Lavergne A, and Vantelon J: Structural and ultrastructural peritoneal membrane changes and permeability alterations during continuous ambulatory peritoneal dialysis. Proc Eur Dial Transplant Assoc 18: 199, 1981
4. Faller B, and Marichal JF: Loss of ultrafiltration in continuous ambulatory peritoneal dialysis. Clinical data. In Gahl GM, Kessel M, and Nolph KD (Eds), Advances in peritoneal dialysis: Proceedings of the 2nd international symposium on peritoneal dialysis. Amsterdam: Excerpta Medica, 1981, p 227
5. Slingeneyer A, Canaud B, and Mion C: Permanent loss of ultrafiltration capacity of the peritoneum in long-term peritoneal dialysis: An epidemiological study. Nephron 33: 133, 1983
6. Faller B, and Marichal JF: Loss of ultrafiltration in continuous ambulatory peritoneal dialysis: A role of acetate. Peritoneal Dial Bull 4: 10, 1984
7. Nolph KD, Ryan L, Moore H, Legrain M, Mion C, and Oreopoulos DG: Factors affecting ultrafiltration in continuous ambulatory peritoneal dialysis. First report of an international cooperative study. Peritoneal Dial Bull 4: 14, 1984
8. Verger C, Luger A, Moore HL, and Nolph KD: Acute changes in peritoneal morphology and transport properties with infectious peritonitis and mechanical injury. Kidney Int 23: 823, 1983
9. Slingeneyer A, Mion C, Mourad J, Conaud B, Faller B, and Beraud GG: Progressive sclerosing peritonitis: A late and severe complication of maintenance peritoneal dialysis. Trans Am Soc Artif Intern Organs 29: 633, 1983
10. Rottembourg J, Gahl GM, Poignet JL, Mertani E, Strippoli P, Langlois P, Carmbaloc P, and Legrain M: Severe abdominal complication in patients undergoing continuous ambulatory peritoneal dialysis. Proc Eur Dial Transplant Assoc 20: 236, 1983
11. Wu G, Khanna R, Oreopoulos DG, and Vas SI: Incidence and pathogenesis of ultrafiltration failure among CAPD patients. Kidney Int 25: 262, 1984
12. Slingeneyer A: Une complication grave de la dialyse peritoneale: la peritonite progressive encapsulante. A propos de six case. Memoire CES de Nephrologie. Faculte de Medecine de Montpellier (FRANCE), 1983
13. Ryan GB, Grobety J, and Majno G: Postoperative peritoneal adhesions. A study of the mechanisms. Am J Pathol 65: 117, 1971

U. Coli, G. Bazzato, S. Landini, A. Fracasso,
F. Righetto, F. Scanferla, and P. Morachiello

16

Role of Peritoneal Membrane Hydration in UF Capacity of Patients on CAPD

SUMMARY

Of 72 uremic patients who entered our CAPD program, 11 showed a reduction or loss of ultrafiltration capacity (UF) of the peritoneal membrane (PM). Treatment with a high oral dose of furosemide (F) was used to stimulate residual urine output. Seven responded to drug administration with a significant increase in urine volume (UV), Na excretion and, within a week attained their dry body weight (BW).

In the remaining four patients F given either orally or intraperitoneally (IP) was ineffective, and fluid removal was obtained only by hemofiltration (HF).

In both groups an increase in the UF capacity of PM was noted when the patient reached the dry BW, either by pharmacological or technical methods.

These results support the assumption that overhydration of the PM plays a major role in maintaining the UF process.

INTRODUCTION

Increasing clinical experience has shown that CAPD is an effective modality of treatment for uremic patients in the short and intermediate term. Nevertheless, long-term CAPD patients, even with normal peritoneal clearances, are often not able to maintain satisfactory water and electrolyte balance.

This condition may be seen also in patients in whom daily bag exchanges are performed mostly with hypertonic solutions. Furthermore, reduction or complete loss of UF capacity of the peritoneal membrane is one of the most frequent causes for drop-out from CAPD.

The aim of this study was to evaluate the effectiveness of diuretic therapy with high dose furosemide (F) to control water and electrolyte balance, either by activating the residual urine output, or by direct effect of this agent on the peritoneal membrane (PM) through its administration into the abdominal cavity. In addition, CAPD patients who appeared refractory to F, were evaluated after occasional hemofiltration (HF), which was also used to reach the patient's dry body weight (BW). Intraperitoneally, F, acetate, and lactate as buffers were subsequently tested in these subjects to compare the PM behavior with the use of these different substances. This composite protocol allowed us to assess the systemic and local action of F per se on the PM and the role of overhydration on UF capacity.

PATIENTS AND METHODS

Of 72 CAPD patients, 11 (15%) had reduction or loss of the UF capacity of the PM. They had been on CAPD from 16–54 months (average 27.2) and had progressive water and salt retention with a mean BW increase of 7.3 ± 0.6 Kg.

The clinical picture included ankle edema, inability to control blood pressure, and intercurrent

From the Nephrology and Dialysis Departments, Umberto I Hospital, Venice-Mestre, Italy.

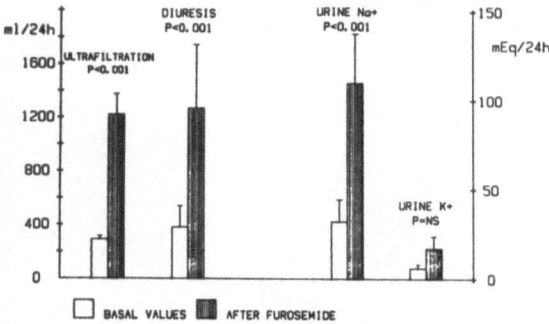

Fig. 1. Peritoneal UF, diuresis, and natriuresis before and after high-dose diuretics in seven patients (mean ± SD).

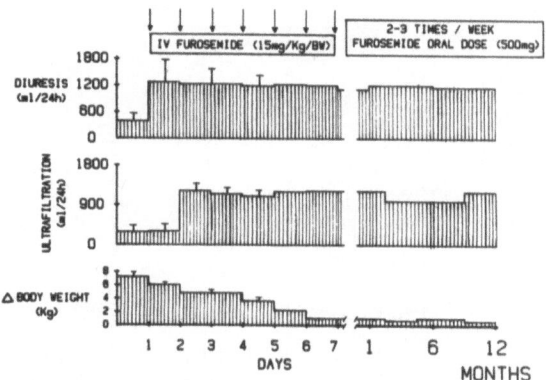

Fig. 2. Effect of high-dose diuretics on seven CAPD patients with reduction of peritoneal UF (mean ± SD).

dyspnea. The schedule of bag exchange was modified with 4–5 daily hypertonic solutions (2 L 4 g/dl dextrose, four times a day and 1 L during the night). The usual composition of dialysate was: Na^+ 135–137, K^+ 0–1, Ca^{++} 4, Mg^{++} 0.5–1, Cl^- 103.5, acetate 38.5 mEq/L using our double bag system described elsewhere.[1]

Acetate was temporarily substituted at the same concentration as lactate to assess its effect on UF capacity in "nonresponders." The incidence of peritoneal infection was not different from the overall average (one episode/18.2 pt/month) of our CAPD population. The residual renal creatinine clearance ranged between 0.7–7 ml/min, with an average 3.5 ml/min.

The investigation was carried out during hospitalization, by administering a high dose of F (15 mg/Kg/day) IV and measuring daily urine volume (UV), UF, Na, urea, creatinine, phosphorus, uric acid removal with dialysate, and protein losses. Routine lab data were performed under basal conditions and every 2–3 days during the observation period. In order for nonresponders to reach their dry BW, HF treatment was performed, and the same lab tests as above were carried out. These subjects were also studied after IP administration of F (40 mg/L) with different osmolality and buffers solutions, when volume overloaded and after dehydration.

RESULTS

Among our 11 patients, seven responded to F therapy as shown by a significant increase in urine volume (UV) from 380 ± 154 to 1270 ± 475 ml/24 h

($p < 0.001$) and in Na excretion, from 32 ± 10 to 110 ± 28 mEq/24 h ($p < 0.001$) (Fig. 1). A BW decrease mean of 1.2 ± 0.3 Kg/day was observed in these patients.

After reaching dry BW, we observed a progressive increase in the UF capacity of the PM: significant fluid removal was already seen in the third day of diuretic therapy (from 288 ± 123 to 1220 ± 154 ml/24 h) ($p < 0.001$) (Fig. 2), leading to ideal BW within a week, and subsequent return to a dialysis schedule of one or two hypertonic bags/day.

Subsequently, the patients were discharged, and at home they have been taking an oral dose of F (500 mg) two or three times a week. No side effects were observed, while satisfactory water and electrolyte balance was maintained. The four nonresponders, in whom residual UV and UF remained unchanged either by oral or IP administration of F,

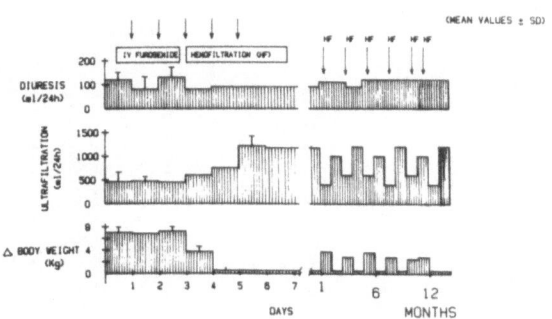

Fig. 3. Effect of high-dose diuretics and hemofiltration on four CAPD patients with reduction of peritoneal UF.

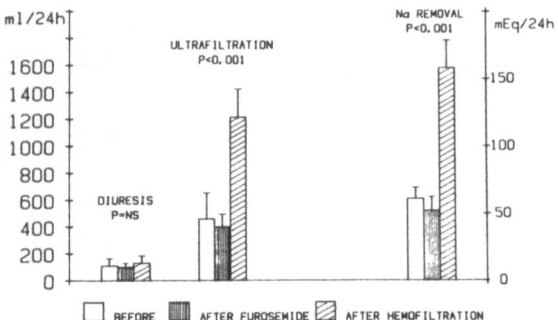

Fig. 4. Diuresis, peritoneal UF, and Na removal with dialysate before, during high-dose diuretics, and after hemofiltration in four CAPD patients (mean ± SD).

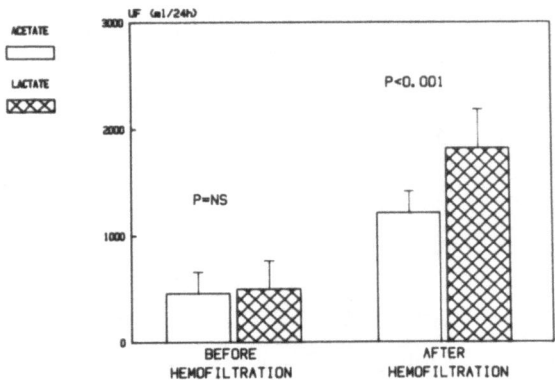

Fig. 6. Effect of different "buffers" on peritoneal UF in four nonresponders to oral/IV diuretic administration.

were treated by HF therapy (Amicon 20), using a subclavian catheter (Uldall type) inserted after drug therapy failure (Figs. 3–5). The mean BW decrease/ HF session was 3.5 Kg, which permitted the four patients to reach their dry BW. Thereafter we observed a significant progressive increase in the UF capacity of the PM from 460 ± 192 to 1215 ± 202 ml/ 24 h ($p < 0.001$), associated with an increase in Na removal from 61 ± 8 to 158 ± 20 mEq/24 h ($p < 0.001$) (Fig. 4). A further increase of UF (1820 ± 350 ml/24 h) ($p < 0.001$) was seen by adding 40 mg/L of F to dialysate (Fig. 5). After dehydration, the change to lactate dialysis solutions promoted a marked increase in UF compared to acetate (1610 ± 242 ml/24 h) ($p < 0.001$) (Fig. 6). Water and electrolyte balance

was stable during the period of 12 months observation in all 11 patients allotted to our protocol.

Only two subjects needed a HF session every 40 days to maintain their dry BW, which after every treatment resulted in an increase of peritoneal UF (Fig. 3). Indeed, either before or after F therapy and/ or HF, we did not observe any significant changes in urea, creatinine, phosphorus, uric acid removal with dialysate, nor in protein loss (Table 1).

It is important to outline that blood lab data and solute removal in all our patients remained essentially stable during the whole period of investigation (Tables 1 & 2), indicating an unchanged effectiveness in the peritoneal diffusive capacity, despite the alteration in UF.

DISCUSSION

The reduction or loss of the UF of the PM is a frequent complication in long-term CAPD patients. It has been reported that there is a direct relationship between the reduction of UF capacity and the duration of CAPD treatment.[2,3] Certainly the longer the period the patients have been treated, the greater the number of hypertonic bags necessary to maintain water and electrolyte balance. This condition has been claimed to be responsible for PM alteration as well as for metabolic disorders, consequent on the large amount of dextrose absorption.

Several investigators have suggested, however, that the loss or reduction of the UF capacity of the PM may be related to the high incidence of peritonitis, while others relate this to the duration of CAPD

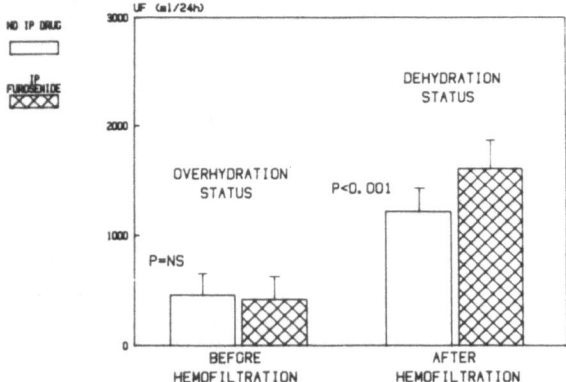

Fig. 5. Effect of intraperitoneal furosemide (40 mg/L) on peritoneal UF in four nonresponders to oral/IV diuretic administration.

Table 1. Solute Removal (g/week) with Dialysate in 11 CAPD Patients with Impaired PM UF (Mean ± SD).

| | Basal Values (11 pts) | After Diuretic Administration | | After Hemofiltration Session (In 4 'Not Responders' pts to Diuretic) |
		Responders (7 pts)	Not Responders (4 pts)	
BUN	57 ± 19	58 ± 16	56 ± 15	59 ± 12
Creatinine	8.9 ± 2	8.6 ± 3	8.8 ± 2.5	8.9 ± 2.2
Uric Acid	3.8 ± 1	4.1 ± 1.2	3.7 ± 1.0	3.8 ± 0.8
P	3.4 ± 1	3.3 ± 0.9	3.8 ± 0.8	3.7 ± 1.0
Protein (g/day)	9.8 ± 4	10.3 ± 3.5	9.7 ± 2.4	8.9 ± 3.0
P	NS	NS		NS

treatment. The long-term irrigation of the peritoneum with hyperosmolar solutions may injure the peritoneum. It has also been reported that the use of acetate instead of lactate as buffer, or other still unknown factors, may be implicated in this alteration even though clear evidence has not yet been presented.[2-6]

Of our 11 patients, seven demonstrated a significant increase in diuresis and natriuresis after high oral/IV dose of F, which allowed them to regain dry BW.

On the other hand, restoration of UF capacity of the PM, which occurs later than the diuretic phase, suggests that this is not a local direct effect of F if given by IV or oral routes. However, a direct action of F has been observed on the mesothelium when intraperitoneally administered.[7] In fact, it is well established that F does not affect, by vascular means, peritoneal UF and Na removal, since its peritoneal clearance is negligible.[8,9] The recovery of UF capacity may be due to dehydration of the interstitial space of the PM, promoting better physical hydraulic forces involved in the UF process. In fact, this condition is clearly observed when the PM structures gain their normal status of hydration.[10] Also, it is well known that during episodes of peritonitis, and in patients with loss of UF capacity, the PM is more permeable to dextrose, with a consequent rapid dissipation of the osmotic gradient necessary to maintain an adequate peritoneal UF.[11]

Moreover, in patients with reduction or loss of the UF capacity, peritoneal biopsies show a disappearance of mesothelium, associated with a reduction in the thickness of the submesothelial tissue.[12] Poor response to F of residual renal function did not allow the four nonresponders to increase their diuresis with F by IV/oral or IP routes.

In the days following treatment with HF, when dry BW was attained, we noted an increase in the UF capacity of the PM. Similarly, when they were

Table 2. Lab Data before and after Diuretics and HF in 11 CAPD Patients with Reduced Peritoneal UF (Mean ± SD).

		Before	After Diuretics	After Hemofiltration
Creatinine	mg/dl	9.5 ± 1.5	9.3 ± 1.2	9.4 ± 0.9
Uric Acid	"	6.2 ± 1.3	6.1 ± 1.5	6.4 ± 0.9
Urea	"	115 ± 29	120 ± 25	118 ± 30
PO_4^{--}	"	4.4 ± 1.2	4.2 ± 1.4	4.3 ± 1.5
Ca^{++}	"	9.6 ± 0.7	9.7 ± 1.2	9.1 ± 1.1
Na^+	mEq/l	139 ± 3.2	141 ± 3.9	139 ± 2.6
K^+	"	4.6 ± 0.8	4.7 ± 0.8	4.7 ± 0.7
P			NS	NS

given IP F or treated with lactate solutions, better UF was achieved, supporting other reports.[3,7,13] These results also support our assumption that improvement of the physical–chemical status of PM is achieved with normalization of its hydration either obtained by F or by HF.

The interstitium of the PM, which includes a network of watery channels among collagen fibers and mucopolysaccharides, had its physical–chemical structure modified by both therapies for fluid removal. This condition allowed recovery of the UF capacity of the PM, apparently by reducing dextrose transfer from the peritoneal cavity into the bloodstream.

It must also be stressed that during the period of observation after achieving the dry BW, the patients' dialysis schedules were reduced to only one to two hypertonic exchanges, with satisfactory water balance. Only two of the four nonresponders needed further HF sessions to maintain their dry BW, which resulted in regular UF capacity. Lactate fluids seem preferable in these patients for its greater removal of fluid, compared to acetate solutions of the same osmolality.

F administration and HF treatment achieved the same result, which was to keep dry BW stable in our CAPD patients, who have continued peritoneal therapy. This suggests that the reduction of UF was functional and thus reversible, rather than a permanent structural alteration.

CONCLUSIONS

Our data suggest how important it is to evaluate the PM physical–chemical status in patients with reduction or loss of UF capacity. The therapeutic approaches proposed for CAPD patients with reduced UF may lead to these preliminary conclusions: (1) F therapy (IV/oral) allows responders satisfactory BW control with simultaneous recovery of peritoneal UF; (2) occasional HF sessions leading to dry BW induce the nonresponders to restore UF capacity of the PM; (3) the response of PM to IP F after dehydration is of great speculative relevance and suggests an active mechanism for this diuretic agent, outlining a local functional alteration of the PM when UF is impaired; (4) lactate seems to promote better UF at dry BW, compared to acetate, in long-term CAPD patients, probably by virtue of its lesser vasodilatory action. We think that both these therapeutic modalities, normalizing PM hydration and water and electrolyte balance, play an important

role in UF in CAPD patients. In fact, the PM, if altered by overhydration, may be normalized either by forced diuresis or by conventional HF, leading to a complete recovery of its UF capacity.

REFERENCES

1. Bazzato G, Landini S, Coli U, Lucatello S, Fracasso A, and Moracchiello M: A new technique of continuous ambulatory peritoneal dialysis (CAPD): Double-bag system for freedom to the patient and significant reduction of peritonitis. Clin Nephrol 6: 251, 1980
2. Faller B, and Marichal JF: Loss of ultrafiltration in continuous ambulatory peritoneal dialysis: Clinical data. In Gahl GM, Kessel M, and Nolph KD (Eds), Advances in peritoneal dialysis: Proceedings of the 2nd international symposium on peritoneal dialysis. Amsterdam: Excerpta Medica, 1981, p 227
3. Faller B, and Marichal JF: Loss of ultrafiltration in continuous ambulatory peritoneal dialysis: A role for acetate. Peritoneal Dial Bull 1: 10, 1984
4. Farrell PC, and Randerson DH: Membrane permeability changes in long-term CAPD. Trans Am Soc Artif Intern Organs 26: 197, 1980
5. Slingeneyer A, Canaud B, and Mion C: Permanent loss of ultrafiltration capacity of the peritoneum in long-term peritoneal dialysis: An epidemiological study. Nephron 33: 133, 1983
6. Arifie MM: Failure of ultrafiltration in patients on CAPD. Peritoneal Dial Bull (Suppl) 3: 38, 1983
7. Grzegorzewska A, and Baczyk K: Influence of furosemide added to peritoneal dialysate on the volume of residual diuresis and urinary excretion of uric acid. 4° Donau symposium fur nephrologie, varna 5–7 Oktober 1979. Verlag Carl Bindernagel, Friedberg Hesen 92, 1980
8. Boutron HF, Brocard JF, Singlas E, Charpentier B, and Fries D: Pharmacokinetic of furosemide in CAPD. In Gahl GM, Kessel M, and Nolph KD (Eds), Advances in peritoneal dialysis: Proceedings of the 2nd international symposium on peritoneal dialysis. Amsterdam: Excerpta Medica, 1981, p 90
9. Scarpioni L, Ballocchi S, Bergonzi G, Fontana F, Poisetti P, and Zanazzi MA: High dose diuretics in continuous ambulatory peritoneal dialysis. Peritoneal Dial Bull 4: 177, 1982
10. Wayland H: Transmural and interstitial molecular transport. In Legrain M (Ed), Continuous ambulatory peritoneal dialysis. Amsterdam: Excerpta Medica, 1979, p 18
11. Raja RM, Kramer MS, Rosenbaum JL, Bolisay C, and Krug M: Contrasting changes in solute transport and ultrafiltration with peritonitis in CAPD patients. Trans Am Soc Artif Intern Organs 27: 68, 1981
12. Verger C, Brunschvicg O, LeCharpentier Y, Lavergne A, and Vantelon J: Structural and ultra-

structural peritoneal membrane changes and permeability alterations during continuous ambulatory peritoneal dialysis. Proc Eur Dial Transplant Assoc 18: 199, 1981

13. Maher JF, Shea C, DiSanzo F, and Cassetta M: Effect of intraperitoneal diuretics on solute transport during hypertonic dialysis. Clin Nephrol 7: 96, 1977

14. Feriani M, Biasioli S, Chiaramonte S, Fabris A, Pisani E, Ronco C, and LaGreca G: Anatomical bases of peritoneal permeability: A reappraisal. Anatomy of peritoneum. Int J Artif Organs 5: 345, 1982

C. Ronco, D. Borin, A. Brendolan, L. Bragantini,
S. Chiaramonte, M. Feriani, A. Fabris, and G. LaGreca

17

Studies on Peritoneal UF Loss: The UF Coefficient (K) as an Index of the PM Filtration Efficiency

SUMMARY

The ultrafiltration rate progressively decreased during an IPD session of 40 L carried out with rapid exchanges of 2.5% dextrose solution. Several factors vary during the session causing a decrease in the global transmembrane pressure and consequently in ultrafiltration rate. In these conditions while K calculated as Qf/ΔOsm seems to vary, the coefficient K, calculated as Qf/"real" TMP appears to be constant. The blood pressure plasma protein concentration, hematocrit and blood viscosity may influence ultrafiltration rate in peritoneal dialysis.

INTRODUCTION

Loss of ultrafiltration (UF) capacity is one of the major complications of peritoneal dialysis treatment.[1] Several factors have been hypothesized to explain this phenomenon.[2] An increased amount of protein loss with rapid absorption of dextrose from the solution (suggesting an increased permeability to the osmotic agent) and a rapid dissipation of the osmotic gradient may be the most common cause.[3] If glucose absorption is not enhanced and clearances of several solutes are reduced, loculation of fluid, loss of surface area, or sclerosing peritonitis may be supposed.[4]

In our opinion, several problems in this field need to be clarified. First of all the method of meas-

uring UF and the IP residual volume. It is impossible to measure UF without taking into account the highly variable residual volume in the peritoneum. Furthermore, in the absence of peritoneal biopsy or serial clearance studies, we need a reliable coefficient of UF that is easy to calculate and able to furnish standardized information concerning the PM filtration efficiency. Up to now the UF coefficient (K) has been considered fallacious and less useful than in hemodialysis.[5] We would like to emphasize that K is calculated as the ratio between UF rate (Qf, ml/min) and the osmotic gradient generated by the dialysis solution (ΔOsm). The assumption is that the osmotic excess of the dialysis solution should be the major component for the transperitoneal pressure gradient, other forces operating in the system being negligible. This coefficient appears unstable and rapidly variable even in the same subject measured within a few hours. Since this is not likely to occur, we tried to calculate a new coefficient of UF, stable and dependent only on the actual characteristics of the peritoneum.

The aim of this study was to evaluate the influence of several factors on the generation of the "real" peritoneal transmembrane pressure (TMP) and UF rate, in order to make precise the calculation of K. Factors such as plasma protein concentration (TP), mean arterial pressure (MAP), hematocrit (Ht), blood viscosity (m) and plasma osmolality (POsm) might greatly influence the peritoneal TMP, and render the osmotic gradient only one of the pressures acting on the peritoneal membrane. This hypothesis suggests that the calculation of K as Q_f/

From the Department of Nephrology, St. Bortolo Hospital, Vicenza, Italy.

Δ Osm may not be correct and proposes the calculation of K as Q_f/TMP.

The demonstration of a stable value for K, even in the presence of different UF rates, would allow us to define a constant relationship between the UF rate and the "real" TMP. This would also allow us to define the PM UF at a certain pressure, avoiding fallacious evaluation of a temporary reduction in UF (due to modifications of various pressure components and not to membrane failure).

The observation of a reduction in Q_f with constant K means a parallel reduction in the forces applied to the membrane. A reduction of Q_f with reduction of K may suggest some alterations in the membrane or loss of surface area. Under these conditions, K becomes an index of the PM filtration capacity and an interesting parameter to follow in the same patient as time on CAPD goes by.

METHODS

Ten patients were studied during successive IPD 40 L sessions with 2 L exchanges ($Qd = 5$ L/h), dwell time of zero, and a solution with 2.5% dextrose. The UF rate was calculated as follows:

$$Qf = \frac{(Vd_o - Vd_i) + (Rv_2 - Rv_1)}{\text{exchange time}} \qquad (1)$$

where Vd_o and Vd_i were the outlet and inlet fluid volumes, and Rv_1 and Rv_2 were the residual IP volumes before and after the exchange, measured by the dilution of a nondiffusible radioisotope ([131]RISA). Venous blood samples for measurement of hematocrit (Ht), total proteins (TP), albumin, plasma osmolality (POsm), glucose, electrolytes, and whole blood viscosity were drawn from a peripheral vein at the beginning and at the end of each treatment session. Samples were taken from inflow and outflow dialysis solutions for measurement of glucose, sodium, osmolality, and protein.

The capillary hydrostatic pressure was calculated on the basis of MAP according to the Starling principle and the Hagen-Poiseuille law. The capillary oncotic pressure was measured by the Pappenheimer nomogram.[6] The peritoneal TMP was calculated according to the following formula:

$$TMP = (Pb - Pi) - (\pi b - \pi i) + (Oi - Op) + $$
$$(Pi - Pd) - (\pi i - \pi d) + (Od - Oi) \qquad (2)$$

where: P = hydrostatic pressure; O = osmotic pressure; π = oncotic pressure; b = blood; p = plasma; i = interstitium; d = dialysate.[7]

The UF coefficient K was calculated as Qf/TMP. The following were carried out in succession: (1) measurement of Qf during a 40 L PD session with evaluation of K and TMP (all the factors contribut-

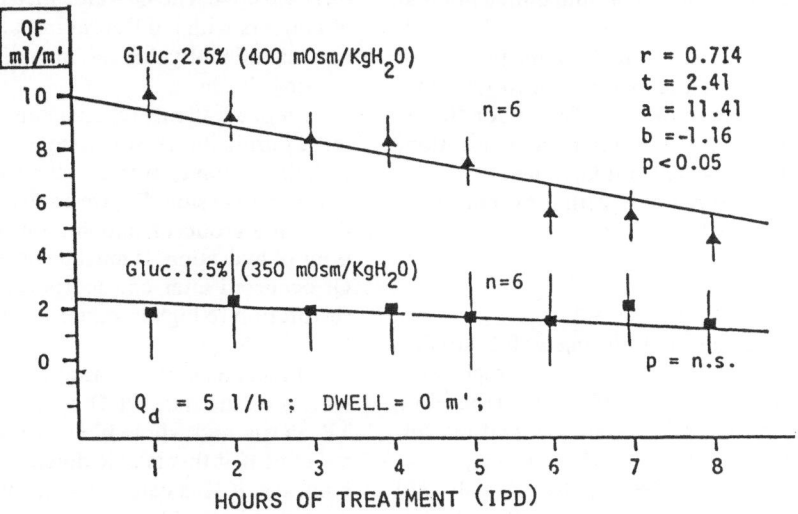

Fig. 1. Progressive loss of UF rate with time.

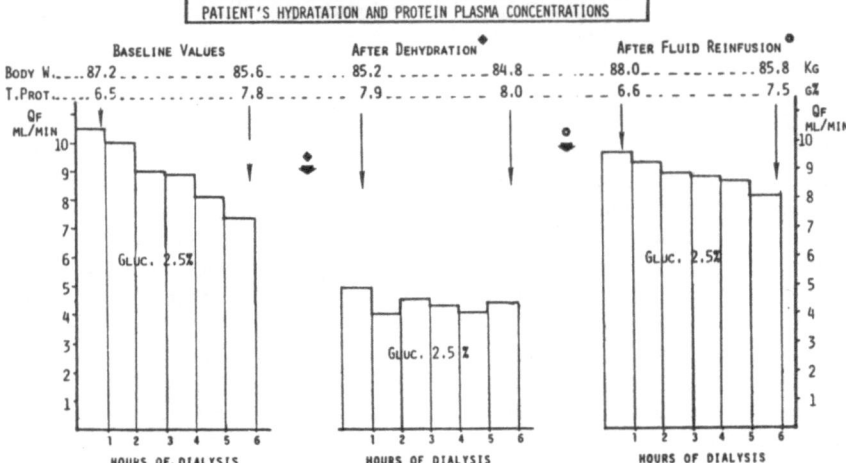

Fig. 2. Effect of dehydration on UF rate with a constant osmotic stimulus.

ing to TMP) at the beginning and at the end of the session, with Qf measured as the average hourly value; (2) hourly measurement of Qf during different PD sessions in the same patients under (a) steady state, (b) drug-induced hypotension (nonvasodilator drugs—in each patient significant MAP reduction was induced [−30 mm Hg]), (c) increased systemic protein concentration (IV infusion of 50g of albumin), (d) increased systemic hematocrit (IV infusion of 500 ml of packed red blood cells), (e) after dehydration (a four-hour session of extracorporeal UF), and (f) after a reinfusion of fluid until a point at which the original body weight was reached—all these studies were carried out in the same patients in order to determine whether variations in Qf could occur in the same patient under different conditions of arterial blood pressure, protein concentration, hematocrit, and viscosity; (3) hourly measurement of Qf in two groups of patients with different initial plasma osmolality.

RESULTS

The hourly measured Qf during a 40 L session showed a significant decrease from an average value of 10.1 to 6.2 (p < 0.05). During this session (baseline condition), the studied parameters showed the following variations: MAP = 120→95 mm Hg; TP = 6→7,2 g/dl; Ht = 23.8→25.9%; pOsm = 300→320 mOsm/Kg; whole blood viscosity = 4.6→5.5 cps. According to these variations, the calculated TMP

changed from 990 to 675 mm Hg, and since a parallel decrease in Qf was registered, the UF coefficient (K) remained stable during the session (0.01→0.0097) (Fig. 1).

Qf behaved differently in the same patient, with MAP constantly higher than 120 mm Hg (9.9→6.5) or with MAP lowered by drugs constantly less than 85 mm Hg (7.1→5.3). After 500 ml of packed red blood cells, Qf decreased in the same patients (7.6→5.5 ml/min) from the baseline values (9.7→7.1 ml/min). A parallel increase in viscosity was noted (3.7–4.6 cps). The Qf value measured in two groups of patients with a different initial plasma osmolality was significantly higher in patients with a lower starting POsm.

In one patient, replacement fluid was administered during the session to maintain POsm and body weight constant; in this patient Qf remained stable during the session. Figure 2 shows the Qf behavior in the same group of patients during different conditions of hydration. It must be noted that reduction of Qf occurred after extracorporeal dehydration, and restoration to higher values of Qf occurred after IV fluid reinfusion.

Figure 3 shows the range of influence of several factors on the ratio Qf/Osm. It is evident that MAP, TP, POsm and whole blood viscosity may alter the value of K if this is calculated as Qf/ΔOsm. On the contrary, if K is calculated as Qf/"real TMP" (Fig. 4), it remains stable. Figure 5 shows the values of UF coefficients for different membranes. It should be

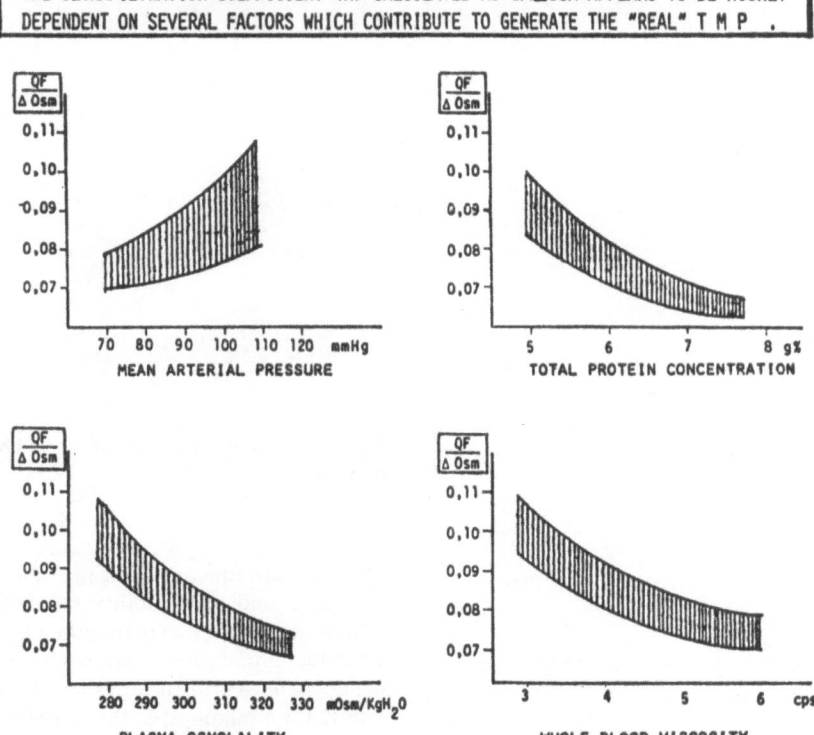

Fig. 3. Effect of arterial blood concentration, plasma protein concentration, plasma osmolality, and blood viscosity on the relationship Qf/ΔOsm.

noted that there is a very low value for the PM UF coefficient.

DISCUSSION

Calculation of the peritoneal UF coefficient, reliable and stable in the same subject over a prolonged period of time, offers an index of PM status and filtration capacity. Up to now, K has been calculated as Qf/ΔOsm, emphasizing the maximal role of the osmotic force of dialysis solutions, while considering the other forces negligible. Since TP, MAP, Ht, blood viscosity, and POsm have been demonstrated to influence the ratio Qf/ΔOsm, the UF coefficient should be recalculated as Qf/TMP (where TMP includes all the forces operating in the system). This offers a more reliable index of PM filtration capacity, and K becomes more stable and more useful to follow in the same patient over time. This

coefficient should be corrected for body surface area to be comparable among different subjects.

The studied factors here have a relatively small influence on the UF rate in comparison to the osmotic pressure. A possible explanation for this phenomenon may be that there are two steps for the transport of water through the peritoneal membrane: (1) water movement across the capillary wall to and from the interstitium; (2) water movement across the peritoneal mesothelium to the peritoneal cavity from the interstitium. In summary, these forces may act in concert to change the hydration of the interstitial tissue. The high osmotic force of the dialysis solution can finally act on the water trapped in the interstitium. Factors contributing to an increase in the interstitial water content could increase Qf, while factors reducing the hydration of the interstitium could decrease Qf (Fig. 6).

The UF coefficient (K) for the peritoneal membrane appears to be very small in comparison with

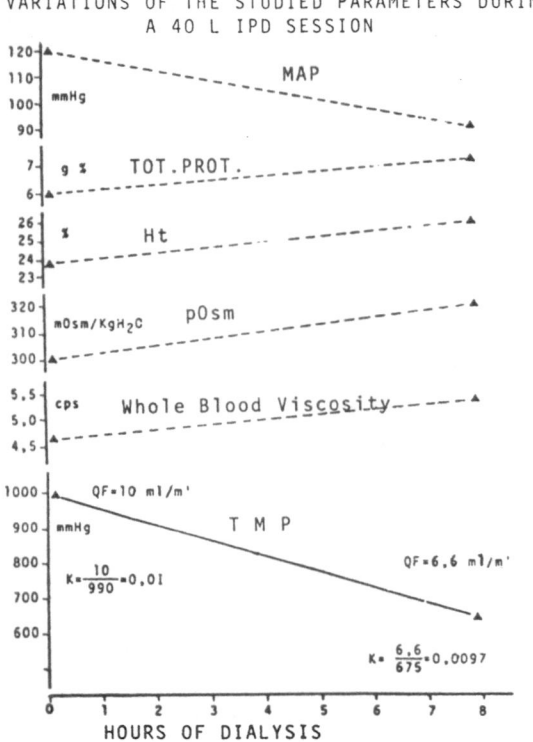

VARIATIONS OF THE STUDIED PARAMETERS DURING A 40 L IPD SESSION

Fig. 4. Effect of UF dialysis on parameters that affect TMP and Qf.

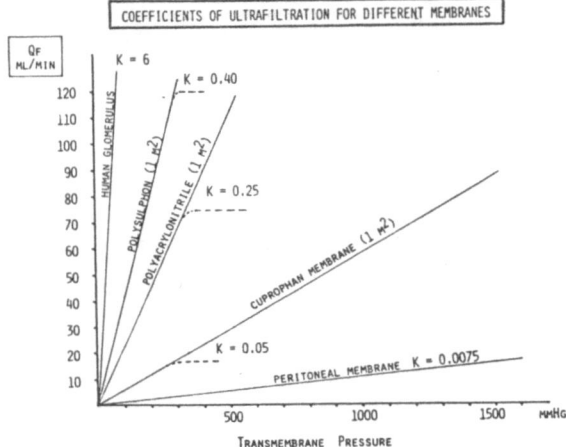

COEFFICIENTS OF ULTRAFILTRATION FOR DIFFERENT MEMBRANES

Fig. 5. Correlation of Qf and TMP for various membranes.

other membranes, even at the same estimated surface area and permeability characteristics. In our opinion, a possible explanation may be the very low effective blood flow that perfuses the peritoneal capillary network. In other words, when we calculate K for a membrane, the function $K_{(TMP)}$ is stable and linear only under condition of unlimited blood flow and membrane surface area. K for the perito-

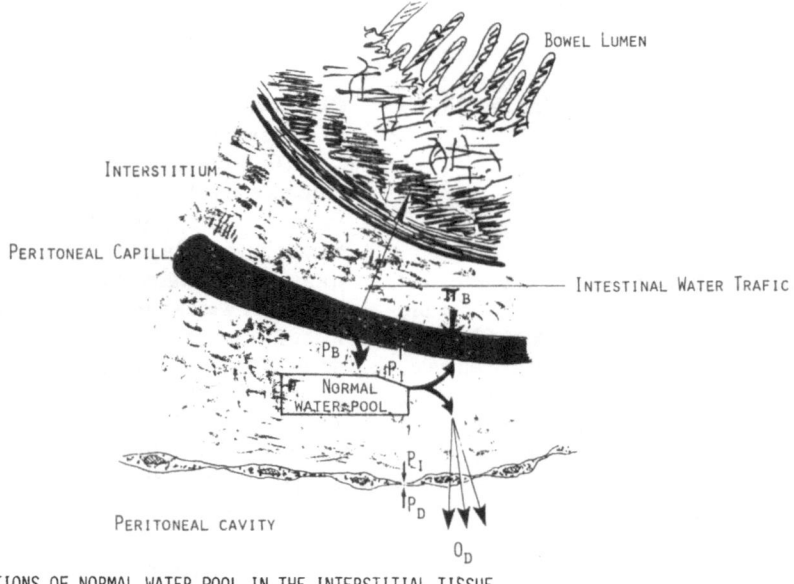

CONDITIONS OF NORMAL WATER POOL IN THE INTERSTITIAL TISSUE

Fig. 6. The relationship of the peritoneal capillary to surrounding tissues and spaces.

neal membrane is always calculated under conditions of a limited range of blood flows. Therefore, only K as calculated on TMP determinants should be useful as a parameter of filtration capacity in the same patient over a period of time.

REFERENCES

1. Slingeneyer A, Canaud B, Mion C: Permanent loss of ultrafiltration capacity of the peritoneum in long-term peritoneal dialysis: An epidemiological study. Nephron 33: 133, 1983

2. Faller B, and Marichal JF: Loss of ultrafiltration in CAPD: Clinical data. In Gahl GM, Kessel M, and Nolph KD (Eds), Advances in peritoneal dialysis: Proceedings of the 2nd international symposium on peritoneal dialysis. Amsterdam: Excerpta Medica, 1981, p 227

3. Nolph KD, Ryan L, Moore H, Legrain M, Mion C, and Oreopoulos DG: Factors affecting ultrafiltration in continuous ambulatory peritoneal dialysis. Peritoneal Dial Bull 1: 14, 1984

4. Slingeneyer A, Mion C, Mourad G, Canaud B, Faller B, and Béraud JJ: Progressive sclerosing peritonitis: A late and severe complication of maintenance peritoneal dialysis. Trans Am Soc Artif Intern Organs 29: 633, 1983

5. LaGreca G, Biasioli S, and Ronco C: Peritoneal Dialysis. Milano: Wichtig, 1982, p 85

6. Pappenheimer JR: Passage of molecules through capillary walls. Physiol Rev 33: 387, 1953

7. Nolph KD: The peritoneal dialysis system. Contrib Nephrol 17: 44, 1978

J.F. Maher, P. Hirszel, E. Chakrabarti, and R.R. Bennett

18

Increased Peritoneal Ultrafiltration Due to Amphotericin B Augmented Sodium Transport

SUMMARY

In rabbits, intraperitoneal instillation of amphotericin B significantly increased the peritoneal ultrafiltration rate in response to 1.5% dextrose dialysis fluid from 0.18 ml/Kg/min, without changing the osmotic gradient or the solute permeability of the peritoneum. Unlike other causes of increased ultrafiltration, amphotericin B increased mass transport of sodium (from 13 to 36 μEq/min) and ultrafiltrate sodium concentration. The raised sodium concentration may prevent back diffusion of water. Alternatively, amphotericin B may open new channels in the peritoneal membrane allowing the ultrafiltration of an isotonic sodium solution.

INTRODUCTION

Loss of ultrafiltration capacity is being recognized with increasing frequency as a complication of peritoneal dialysis of considerable importance.[1] The mechanism of this abnormality is only partially understood. In some instances it has been associated with increased solute permeability and rapid dissipation of the osmotic gradient that is required to

---

From the Nephrology Division, Department of Medicine, Uniformed Services University of the Health Sciences, Bethesda, Maryland, and the Nephrology Service, Department of Medicine, Walter Reed Army Medical Center, Washington, D.C.

promote ultrafiltration (UF). In others, UF is retarded despite maintenance of the gradient.

Previous studies of the effect of drugs on peritoneal transport have focused on agents that affect solute transport, predominantly vasodilators.[2] Indeed, minimal changes in the UF rate per milliosmole of osmotic gradient are offset by more rapid loss of the gradient when vasodilators are added locally or act preferentially on the mesenteric vasculature. Hence, net UF does not change.[3,4] Exceptions are dopamine, which is believed to raise capillary hydrostatic pressure, and secretin, which increases the capillary UF coefficient.[4,5]

To explore further the effect of drugs on the peritoneum, we have evaluated the effect of surface active agents, including amphotericin B. The polypeptide fungicide, amphotericin B, was found to increase fluid movement significantly (from 0.18 to 0.31 ml/Kg/min) across the peritoneum while influencing solute transport only minimally.[6] Because dextrose transport did not change, the UF rate per milliosmole of gradient increased. When given intravenously, amphotericin B was ineffective despite a comparable concentration, suggesting that this slowly diffusible agent acts on the mesothelial side of the filtration barrier.[7]

In the absence of a diffusion gradient, sodium only partially accompanies water during peritoneal UF, a phenomenon that may relate to restriction of cationic charges, but is not fully explained.[8] The hyponatric ultrafiltrate would thereby represent a sodium gradient retarding UF or promoting back filtration. Accordingly, the effect of amphotericin B on mass transport of sodium during peritoneal dialysis with 1.5% dextrose dialysis fluid was examined. Amphotericin B significantly increased mass transport of sodium, suggesting that this mechanism contributes to the augmentation of UF induced by the drug.

MATERIALS AND METHODS

Studies were performed in 13 alert, lightly restrained female New Zealand white rabbits by a previously described technique.[9] In brief, 75 ml/Kg of 1.5% dextrose dialysis fluid was instilled intraperitoneally into supine animals over the course of 4 minutes. A tracer amount of [203]Hg-labeled autologous protein was added to the dialysis solution before instillation to allow determination of dialysate volume and UF rate by indicator dilution. Dialysate was sampled at the completion of instillation and at 12-minute intervals after the midpoint of the infusion for an hour thereafter for measurement of solute concentrations. Plasma was sampled immediately preceding dialysis.

Mass transport of sodium was calculated as dialysate sodium concentration multiplied by dialysate volume, minus instilled sodium (dialysis solution concentration multiplied by volume). Ultrafiltrate sodium concentration was calculated as mass transport of sodium divided by UF rate.

Each animal underwent control dialyses before and after experimental dialyses in which amphotericin B was added to the dialysis fluid before instillation, in a dose of 0.5–25 mg/Kg. Values from experimental dialyses were compared to controls by Student's t test.

The changes in sodium transport indices were compared to those that resulted when the UF rate was varied by changing dextrose concentration and adding dimethyl sulfoxide (DMSO) in 10 rabbits[10] and by using hypertonic dextrose dialysis fluid in 6 rabbits.

RESULTS

During control dialyses with 1.5% dextrose dialysis fluid, the dialysate sodium concentration decreased from 97.5% of plasma sodium concentration to 92.5% after 60 minutes IP dwell. With IP amphotericin B the decline in dialysate/plasma sodium concentration was less (Fig. 1). This was not

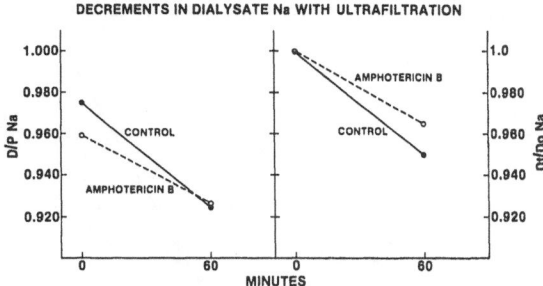

Fig. 1. The decrease in dialysate/plasma sodium concentration ratio (D/P Na) that occurs with a 60-minute dwell of 1.5% dextrose dialysis solution is not as pronounced when amphotericin B is added intraperitoneally (left half). The 60-minute dialysate/initial dialysis fluid sodium concentration ratio therefore decreases less with the addition of amphotericin B.

accounted for by the sodium content of the amphotericin solution. After 60 minutes IP dwell, the dialysate sodium concentration decreased to 95% of the initial dialysis fluid concentration with 1.5% dextrose solution, but decreased less (to 96.5%) when amphotericin B was added.

Although these differences in sodium concentration were only modest, amphotericin B increased

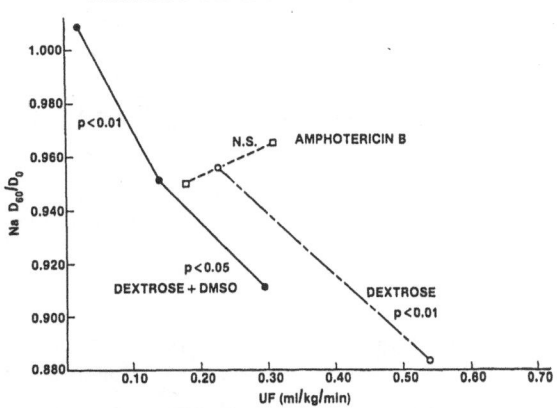

Fig. 2. The 60-minute dialysate/initial dialysis solution sodium concentration ratio is plotted as a function of UF rate. When the UF rate increases with added dextrose and DMSO or with hypertonic dextrose, the dialysate sodium decreases significantly. Amphotericin B raises the UF rate without decreasing dialysate sodium.

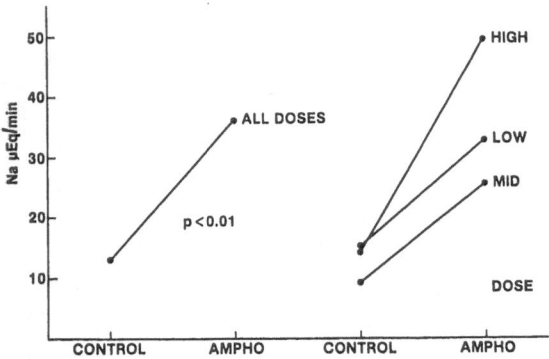

EFFECT OF AMPHOTERICIN B ON PERITONEAL MASS TRANSPORT OF Na

Fig. 3. Mass transport of sodium is increased significantly when amphotericin B is added to peritoneal dialysis fluid. In paired studies this effect was detected at all dose ranges employed, i.e., low (below 1 mg/Kg), mid (5.5 to 8.0 mg/Kg), and high (above 10 mg/Kg).

the UF rate. When the UF rate is increased by raising the osmotic gradient with DMSO or hypertonic dextrose, the dialysate sodium decreases further. This contrasts with the increment in sodium concentration observed when amphotericin B raises the UF rate (Fig. 2).

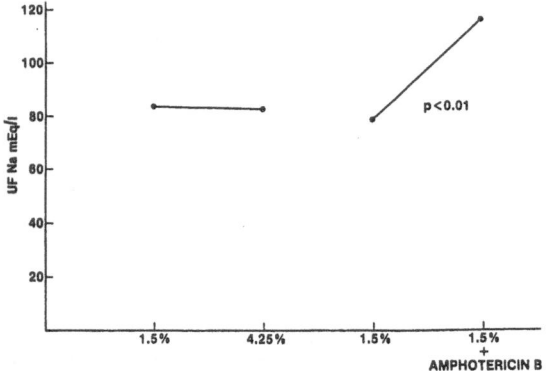

EFFECT OF AMPHOTERICIN B ON PERITONEAL ULTRAFILTRATE Na CONCENTRATION

Fig. 4. The concentration of sodium in peritoneal ultrafiltrate (mass transport of sodium by convection divided by UF rate) is slightly more than half that of plasma water sodium concentration and is unchanged by increasing the UF rate by hypertonic dextrose dialysis fluid. The addition of amphotericin B to peritoneal dialysis fluid promotes ultrafiltration of a fluid with a higher sodium concentration.

Despite the absence of an appreciable sodium gradient, sodium mass transport occurs during UF. When amphotericin B is added intraperitoneally, mass transport of sodium increases significantly, from 13–36 μ Eq/Kg/min, a change detected at all doses employed (Fig. 3).

The calculated sodium concentration in peritoneal ultrafiltrate is approximately 80 mEq/l, a value that does not change as the UF rate increases with hypertonic dextrose. When the UF rate is increased by adding amphotericin B, however, the sodium concentration in the ultrafiltrate increases significantly, approaching plasma concentration (Fig. 4).

DISCUSSION

The appreciable increase in the rate of osmotically induced UF associated with intraperitoneal amphotericin B is associated with an increase in mass transport of sodium. This is not due to an overall increase in permeability or peritoneal surface area, nor to nonspecific irritation and inflammation, because these changes would increase clearance of all solutes, which does not occur with amphotericin B.[6] Moreover, amphotericin B does not affect the osmotic gradient.[7] Hence, the UF coefficient increases.

The solubilizing agent and buffer used to prepare amphotericin B solutions (sodium desoxycholate and sodium phosphate) did not account for the change in sodium transport, since the quantity of sodium added was always less than 0.1 mEq/Kg and the concentration in the solution was much less than that of the dialysis fluid to which it was added.

Most drugs that affect peritoneal transport rates influence both the rate of solute movement by diffusion and the rate of water movement by ultrafiltration.[2] Because of more rapid dissipation of the osmotic gradient owing to augmented dextrose transport, the increased UF is recognized only as an increase in the UF coefficient, i.e., fluid movement per osmotic gradient.

It is unusual, therefore, for a drug to affect UF but not clearances, as amphotericin B does.[6] Nolph et al.[11] have postulated that UF and diffusion occur through different loci in the capillary wall. The pharmacological separation of effects on these two processes adds credence to the concept that the resistances to each mechanism of transport differ. Because amphotericin B, a slowly diffusible peptide, is ineffective from the vascular side,[7] it suggests that a barrier on the mesothelial surface is affected by the drug.

Amphotericin B creates channels in membranes that allow permeation by electrolytes, uncharged solutes, and water.[12] Such channels do not affect diffusive transport since clearances do not increase. This suggests that the pore area for diffusion is not appreciably increased by amphotericin B, and that the major determinant of diffusion, the concentration gradient, is unaffected.

On the other hand, this study confirms earlier observations that sodium transport is retarded during UF and demonstrates that, with amphotericin B, sodium accompanies ultrafiltrate water more readily.[8, 13] This is in accord with the creation by amphotericin of new channels through the membranes to allow isotonic ultrafiltrate.

Alternatively, amphotericin B could modify existing channels for UF to allow sodium to accompany water. When sodium transport is retarded during UF, the hyponatric ultrafiltrate creates a concentration gradient for sodium to follow by diffusion. Until this concentration disequilibrium is corrected, however, the osmolality of dialysate adjacent to the UF barrier is diluted, retarding the rate of fluid movement. Amphotericin B would therefore increase the rate of UF by augmenting sodium transport.

For selected patients that have diminished UF capacity, amphotericin B could be a useful additive to dialysis fluid because it selectively augments the rate of peritoneal UF. Since the effect was seen at the lowest dose studied, 6.7 μg/ml of dialysis solution (0.5 mg/Kg), amphotericin B might be used for short intervals without major toxicity. The duration of this effect remains to be established. Certainly, it should represent the prototype of other safer drugs that should be explored experimentally and clinically for this indication.

ACKNOWLEDGMENT

This work was supported by the Uniformed Services University of the Health Sciences Protocol No. RO8318. The opinions and assertions contained herein are the private ones of the authors and are not to be construed as official or reflecting the views of the Department of Defense or the Uniformed Services University of the Health Sciences. The experiments reported herein were conducted according to the principles set forth in the "Guide for the Care and Use of Laboratory Animals," Institute of Animal Resources, National Research Council, DHEW Pub. No. (NIH) 78-23.

REFERENCES

1. Oreopoulos DG, and Khanna R: Complications of peritoneal dialysis other than peritonitis. In Nolph KD (Ed), Developments in nephrology 2. Peritoneal dialysis. The Hague: Martinus Nijhoff, 1981, p 309
2. Maher JF: Characteristics of peritoneal transport: Physiological and clinical implications. Mineral Electrolyte Metab 5: 201, 1981
3. Maher JF, and Hirszel P: Augmentation of peritoneal clearances by drugs. In Legrain M (Ed), Continuous ambulatory peritoneal dialysis. Amsterdam: Excerpta Medica, 1980, p 42
4. Hirszel P, Lasrich M, and Maher JF: Augmentation of peritoneal mass transport by dopamine. Comparison with norepinephrine and evaluation of pharmacologic mechanisms. J Lab Clin Med 94: 747, 1979
5. Maher JF, Hirszel P, and Lasrich M: Effects of gastrointestinal hormones on transport by peritoneal dialysis. Kidney Int 16:130, 1979
6. Maher JF, Hirszel P, Bennett RR, and Chakrabarti E: Amphotericin selectively increases peritoneal ultrafiltration. Am J Kidney Dis 4: 285, 1984
7. Maher JF, Hirszel P, Bennett RR, and Chakrabarti E: Augmentation of peritoneal hydraulic permeability by amphotericin B: Locus of action. Peritoneal Dial Bull 4: 229, 1984
8. Ahearn DJ, and Nolph KD: Controlled sodium removal with peritoneal dialysis. Trans Am Soc Artif Intern Organs 28: 423, 1972
9. Maher JF, Hirszel P, and Lasrich M: An experimental model for study of pharmacologic and hormonal influences on peritoneal dialysis. Contrib Nephrol 17: 131, 1979
10. Maher JF, and Chakrabarti E: Ultrafiltration by hyperosmotic peritoneal dialysis fluid excludes intracellular solutes. Am J Nephrol 4: 169, 1984
11. Nolph KD, Miller FN, Pyle K, Popovich RP, and Sorkin MI: An hypothesis to explain the ultrafiltration characteristics of peritoneal dialysis. Kidney Int 20: 543, 1981
12. Andreoli TE, Dennis VW, and Weigl AM: The effect of amphotericin B on the water and nonelectrolyte permeability of thin lipid membranes. J Gen Physiol 53: 133, 1969
13. Maher JF, Hohnadel DC, Shea C, DiSanzo F, and Cassetta M: Effect of intraperitoneal diuretics on solute transport during hypertonic dialysis. Clin Nephrol 7: 96, 1977

J. Rottembourg, J.L. Gallego, M.C. Jaudon, and J.P. Clavel

19

Serum Concentration and Peritoneal Transfer of Aluminum during Treatment by CAPD

SUMMARY

The evolution of aluminum (Al) serum levels was studied in 43 patients treated by CAPD during a 2 yr follow-up, with varying aluminum exposure. Serum levels and peritoneal transfer of Al were studied in 22 patients. Al concentration in the dialysis fluid was very low (range = $0.25 - 0.30 \, \mu$mol/L). Patients were divided into three groups. Transfer of Al from the patient to the dialysate was observed in all patients. In group 1, patients exclusively treated by CAPD and who have never received aluminum-containing phosphate binders (ACPB), the mean serum Al concentration was stable in a safe normal range ($0.60 \pm 0.28 \, \mu$mol/L) with a very low peritoneal transfer. In group 2, the oral administration of ACPB in patients exclusively treated by CAPD induced a slow and progressive increase of serum Al concentration despite an increase in Al excretion through the peritoneal route. In group 3, patients previously treated by hemodialysis and receiving ACPB, the high serum Al levels before CAPD treatment were rapidly reduced on CAPD, with a higher removal of Al through the peritoneal membrane.

INTRODUCTION

Positive aluminum (Al) balance is considered a causative agent and/or a contributing factor of some complications in patients with end stage renal dis-

ease (ESRD) such as dialysis dementia,[1,2] renal osteodystrophy,[3,4] and anemia.[5] Al intoxication among nondialyzed patients with ESRD has been reported after long-term consumption of aluminum containing phosphate binders (ACPB).[6-8] In dialyzed patients, mainly hemodialyzed patients, sources of Al are a high Al dialysis fluid concentration and/or chronic consumption of ACPB.[8,10] Evolution of serum Al levels in patients undergoing CAPD remains controversial.[11-15] A multicenter report of acute and severe Al intoxication in relation to contaminated dialysis fluid has recently appeared.[16] Our present study was conducted to investigate the peritoneal transfer of Al in patients treated by CAPD under varying exposure to Al.

MATERIAL AND METHODS

Fifty normal healthy subjects of both sexes not taking ACPB served as controls for Al serum determination. Forty-three patients treated for at least two years by CAPD were divided into three groups from which 22 participated in the investigation. These 22 patients (13 males, 9 females) gave informed consent for the study. Their mean age at the beginning of CAPD was 56.04 ± 13.44 years (range 32–81 years). Primary renal diseases were chronic glomerulonephritis in eight, diabetic nephropathy in seven, chronic interstitial nephropathy in five, and nephropathy of unknown origin in two patients.

The patients were divided into three groups (Table 1). Group I included nine patients who had been treated before the study by CAPD exclusively dur-

From the Department of Nephrology and Laboratory of Biochemistry, Groupe Hospitalier Pitie-Salpetriere, Paris, France.

Table 1. Patient Characteristics.

Group	Patients M = Male F = Female	Mean ± SD Age (range) Yrs	Primary Renal Disease*	Mean ± SD Duration of CAPD before the Study (mo)	Mean ± SD Duration of Previous Treatment on Hemodialysis (mo)	Al (mg/day) Intake during CAPD
I	9 (6M, 3F)	53.3 ± 12.1 (32–75)	ND 4 NIC 2 GNC 1 UN 2	13.3 ± 7.4 (3–27)	—	—
II	7 (3M, 4F)	59.7 ± 15.2 (32–81)	ND 2 NIC 3 GNC 2	10 ± 5.6 (1–19)	—	863 ± 428
III	6 (4M, 2F)	55.8 ± 12 (37–74)	GNC 5 ND 1	3 ± 4.1 (1–12)	75.8 ± 38.9 (27–144)	791 ± 750

* GNC = glomerulonephritis; ND = diabetic nephropathy; NIC = chronic interstitial nephritis; UN = nephropathy of unknown origin.

ing a mean period of 13.3 ± 7.4 months and had never received ACPB. Group II included seven patients also treated exclusively by CAPD during a mean period of 10 ± 5.6 months but who received ACPB to control serum phosphate. Group III included six patients previously treated by hemodialysis (HD) for a mean period of 75.8 ± 38.9 months (two on home dialysis treatment) and who had received ACPB during HD and CAPD. These patients had been transferred from HD therapy to CAPD because of cardiovascular instability in three, vascular access problems in one, and personal choice in two patients. The Al compound used to control serum phosphate during CAPD treatment was exclusively Al hydroxide in capsules (1 g $Al(OH)_3$ = 346 mg or 12.7 mmol of Al).

Aluminum Investigation

METHODS OF MEASUREMENT OF ALUMINUM

Measurements of Al in serum, urine, dialysis fluid, and peritoneal dialysate were performed by electrothermal atomic absorption spectrometry using an atomic absorption spectrometer (Model 370, Perkin Elmer) equipped with a graphite furnace (HGA 74).[18] Details of the technique are given elsewhere.[19]

SERUM ALUMINUM MEASUREMENTS

The 43 patients, divided in three groups (in which 22 participated in the investigation), from the beginning of CAPD treatment had serial serum Al determinations at least every six months. Food intake or fecal Al were never measured.

PERITONEAL MASS TRANSFER PROTOCOL

Studies were performed during a 24-hour period three times at three-month intervals. During the six-month period required for the study, the patients were on a four-bag exchange schedule, which consisted of three bags with 1.5% dextrose concentrations and one bag with a concentration between 3.8–4.5%. Aluminum peritoneal transfer equals the daily inflow volume (L) multiplied by dialysis fluid Al concentration minus the daily outflow volume multiplied by dialysate Al concentration. The mass transfer is positive when a gain is observed, and is negative when there is removal. The residual renal clearance corrected for body surface area and the peritoneal clearance of creatinine were calculated as previously described using a multiparameter SMAC Technicon analyzer.[20] Plasma proteins were measured using the biuret method. Urine and dialysate proteins were determined using the sulphosalicylic acid method.

Table 2. Biological Parameters, Peritoneal and Residual Renal Creatinine Clearances.

	Group I	Group II	Group III
Number of Patients	9	7	6
Number of Determinations	27	20	17
Serum creatinine (μmol/L)	890 ± 200	1013 ± 360	1130 ± 120
Serum protein (g/L)	58.0 ± 5.0	66.0 ± 6.5	64.0 ± 4.5
Serum albumin (g/L)	30 ± 6	34 ± 4	32 ± 3
Hemoglobin (g/dl)	10.8 ± 1.8	9.5 ± 1.2	9.6 ± 1.5
Serum calcium (mmol/L)	2.48 ± 0.16	2.40 ± 0.12	2.46 ± 0.07
Serum phosphorus (mmol/L)	1.65 ± 0.30	1.85 ± 0.30	1.86 ± 0.26
Alc phosphatase (UI/L)	102 ± 60	130 ± 80	110 ± 60
Protein losses (g/day), in dialysate	8.4 ± 3.5	5.7 ± 2.1	4.8 ± 1.6
Peritoneal creatinine clearance (ml/min)	4.7 ± 1.0	4.6 ± 0.6	4.2 ± 1.0
Residual renal creatinine clearance (ml/min)	3.0 ± 2.1	1.6 ± 2.2	0.16 ± 0.30

RESULTS

Biological Parameters

The results are summarized in Table 2. Some differences occur between the groups, but no variation was observed in each group during the study period. Total serum protein and serum albumin were lower in group I than in group II and III, while protein losses through the dialysate were higher in group I compared to the other groups. There was no difference between the groups in peritoneal creatinine clearances. Residual renal function was stable around 3 ml/min in group I, lower in group II, and negligible in group III.

Evolution of Al Serum Levels

The mean serum Al level in the normal control group was 0.34 ± 0.08 μmol/L (range 0.18 ± 0.48 μmol/L). The evolution of the serum Al in 43 patients treated at least two years by CAPD is shown in Figure 1. In group I (17 patients exclusively treated by CAPD, never exposed to ACPB), there was a slow but regular increase in serum levels slightly over the concentration in the control groups: 0.38 ± 0.12 μmol/L at start, 0.51 ± 0.16 μmol/L at one year, 0.59 ± 0.18 μmol/L at two years. In group II (19 patients exclusively treated by CAPD, regularly exposed to Al through ACPB), serum Al level was 0.66 ± 0.29 μmol/L at the start and increased to the value of 1.51 ± 0.46 μmol/L after one year of treatment, and 1.71 ± 0.52 μmol/L after two years on CAPD. On the other hand, in group III (seven patients previously treated by HD during a mean period of 60 months and transferred to CAPD and exposed during HD and CAPD periods to ACPB), the mean serum Al value at the time of transfer was 3.84 ± 0.76 μmol/L, which decreased to 2.12 ± 0.80 μmol/L after one year of CAPD and to 1.75 ± 0.76 μmol/L after two years of treatment.

Peritoneal Mass Transfer

AL CONTENT IN THE DIALYSIS FLUID

The Al content of the dialysis fluid of the three brands routinely used were similar (Table 3). The mean Al content of the 1.5% dextrose concentration was 0.27 ± 0.07 μmol/L. The mean Al content of the high dextrose concentration was 0.29 ± 0.09 μmol/L.

SERUM AL CONCENTRATION

During study of peritoneal mass transfer, the serum Al concentration in the three groups remained stable. Mean serum Al level in group I was 0.60 ± 0.28 μmol/L, in group II 2.08 ± 0.80 μmol/L, and 2.40 ± 0.70 μmol/L. Mean values are statistically different ($p < 0.01$) between group I and the two other groups, but not between group II and III.

THE AL CONTENT OF THE DIALYSATE

Al content of dialysate for each group was statistically different. The concentrations remained stable during the study period in group I and II, and increased in group III, reaching 1.03 ± 0.25 μmol/L at the end of the study (Table 4).

The aluminum concentration of the dialysate outflow was always higher than that in the fresh dialysis fluid (Table 4) indicating a transfer of Al from the body fluids into the dialysate. There was a statistically significant correlation between the serum Al concentration and the Al dialysate concentration (r = 0.518, p < 0.01).

AL REMOVAL

The daily Al removal through the peritoneum was very low in group I, but much higher in the two other groups (Table 4). The values in group III were higher than in group II, although the differences between serum Al concentration of group II and III were not statistically different (Table 4).

RENAL AL EXCRETION

Renal excretion was low in group I and II and almost negligible in group III (Table 4). Urinary Al concentration was stable but there was a significant correlation with the residual renal function expressed by the creatinine clearance (r = 0.438, p < 0.004).

DISCUSSION

As for dialysis membranes, transfer of Al across the peritoneum is mainly determined by the concentration gradient between the free (diffusible) Al in serum and the dialysate.[21,22] Accordingly, the amount of Al removed by peritoneal dialysis will depend mainly on the plasma Al concentration. Negative Al transfer requires dialysis fluid Al concentration below the free (diffusible) plasma Al concentration, which is estimated to be around 20–40% of total plasma Al.[12,22,23] The possibility of a reverse situation with positive Al transfer is well illustrated by the recently reported severe acute Al intoxication occurring in patients treated by CAPD using dialysis fluid with a very high Al concentration.[16]

Serum Al concentration depends on different factors, such as Al exposure before and during the dialysis, including Al concentration in dialysis fluid, the consumption of ACPB, the endogenous loss of aluminum through the gastrointestinal tract, and the residual renal function. The multiple factors involved in Al loading and Al removal through various routes can easily explain the large variations observed in serum Al levels of patients treated by CAPD.[11-13,15]

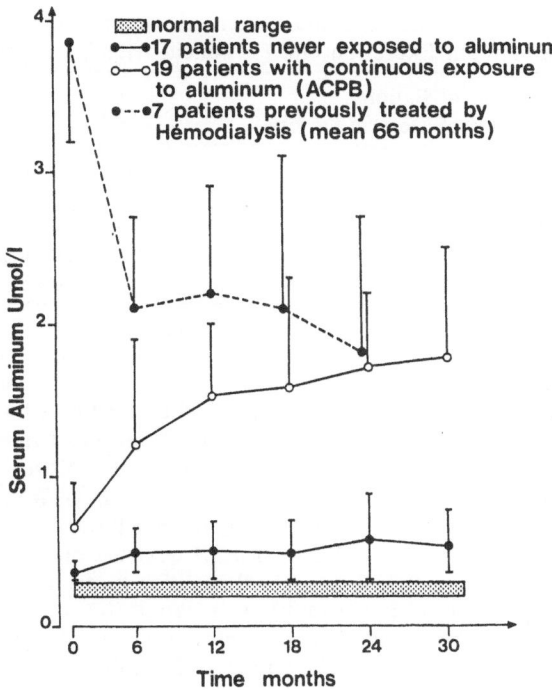

Fig. 1. Evolution of serum Al levels (μ mol/L) during the first two years of treatment by CAPD. Group I (●————●): patients exclusively treated by CAPD and who never received ACPB. Group II (○————○): patients exclusively treated by CAPB and receiving ACPB. Group III (●– – – –●): patients previously treated by hemodialysis and receiving ACPB. The shaded area represents the normal range.

Table 3. Aluminum Concentration of the Dialysis Solutions.

Origin	Number of Bags Tested	Value (m + 1 SD) μ mol/L
Aguettant		
1.5% dextrose	12	0.25 ± 0.04
4.0% dextrose	2	0.28 ± 0.07
Assistance Publique**		
1.5% dextrose	26	0.26 ± 0.07
4.5% dextrose	2	0.28 ± 0.09
Travenol Dianeal***		
1.5% dextrose	18	0.29 ± 0.09
3.86% dextrose	2	0.31 ± 0.09

* Lyon, France.
** Paris, France.
*** Deerfield, IL.

Table 4. Dialysate and Serum Aluminum Concentrations and Urinary Aluminum Excretion and Peritoneal Aluminum Transfer (Mean ± SD).

Number of Patients	9	7	6
Number of Determinations	27	20	17
Serum (μmol/L)	0.60 ± 0.28	2.08 ± 0.80	2.40 ± 0.78
Dialysate (μmol/L)	0.33 ± 0.06	0.47 ± 0.10	0.89 ± 0.19
Urine (μmol/day)	0.38 ± 0.47	0.37 ± 0.54	0.10 ± 0.27
Dialysate (μmol/day)	0.50 ± 0.50	2.00 ± 1.16	5.46 ± 2.49
Total daily removal (μmol/day)	0.88 ± 0.66	2.37 ± 1.24	5.56 ± 2.15

In patients exclusively treated by CAPD, who have never received ACPB (group I), serum Al values remain very low (0.60 ± 0.28 μmol/L). Nevertheless, the mean Al concentration in the dialysate in the three studies was slightly higher than the average Al concentration of the fresh 1.5% dextrose dialysis fluid, suggesting a very small negative transfer. Al concentration in the outflow is about 50% of the serum Al concentration (Table 4), a value which is higher than the usually estimated 20–40% free diffusible fraction. Different factors can explain such surprising results. The low serum protein levels around 58 g/L observed in this group (Table 2) can contribute to increase the free diffusible fraction of serum Al. The high peritoneal protein losses observed in this group allow Al removal bound to protein through the drainage fluid. Finally, as for other molecules, diffusion should not be considered the only mechanism involved in peritoneal transfer. A sieving effect in relation to transperitoneal UF can also apply to aluminum and explain a higher Al concentration in the outflow than that expected from diffusion alone.[24]

In group I (never exposed to extra sources of aluminum), the mean daily aluminum removal, including by the urine and the peritoneal routes, reached 0.88 ± 0.66 μmol/day, a value slightly above the daily urine excretion, 0.6 ± 0.3 μmol/day, found by Kaehny et al. in normal subjects.[25] Such Al removal contributes to the stabilization of Al serum concentration around values considered to be safe,[8,13] although higher than in the controls. In this group, renal Al excretion almost equals Al removal through the dialysate, illustrating the beneficial effect of persisting residual renal function during the first year of treatment by CAPD.[18]

The oral administration of ACPB to patients treated by CAPD increases serum Al concentrations despite a large increase in Al excretion through the peritoneum (and likely also by the intestinal route).

It is unknown if an equilibrium between the Al intake from various sources including ACPB and the peritoneal aluminum removal will be obtained and if serum Al concentration will stabilize for a very long period.

In patients of group III (previously treated by hemodialysis and receiving ACPB), the evolution of the Al serum level is the opposite of that observed in group III. The high serum Al concentrations decreased rapidly during the first months of treatment by CAPD and more slowly later. The Al concentration in peritoneal dialysate and the Al removal through the peritoneal route were much higher in group III than in group II (Table 4). A higher Al tissue content in group II in relation to long-standing Al exposure is likely. The exact reason for such a situation remains unclear. It can be expected that tissue Al content in group III was higher than in group II, because of a longer Al exposure. For this reason, more rapid transfer from the body cells into the plasma and from the plasma into the peritoneum without significant change in serum Al levels can be observed during the dialysis procedure. Accurate kinetic studies with serial serum Al determinations during and after stopping dialysis might clarify this situation. Our results agree with the recent report by Gokal et al.,[13] who also observed a decrease in serum Al levels in a few patients treated by CAPD when serum values were high at the start of treatment, and a moderate increase in patients not receiving ACPB and with normal serum levels at the onset of CAPD.

Much attention should be paid to the dialysis fluid Al concentration used for intermittent or continuous peritoneal dialysis to avoid positive peritoneal transfer and chronic aluminum loading, especially in patients starting with low serum Al values. Our data suggest that an Al content of the dialysis fluid below 0.30 μmol/L can be considered safe. Such Al concentrations are lower than those of the dialysis fluid used by Sorkin et al.[17] and Gokal et al.[13] to treat patients by CAPD. The Al levels in the dialysis fluid and in the serum are not the only factors which can influence Al transfer across the peritoneal membrane. Gacek et al.[26] demonstrated that slight fluctuation in dialysis fluid pH can cause dramatic changes in aluminum dialyzability through artificial membranes. This could also be, as suggested by Gilli et al.,[27] an important factor in Al transfer through the peritoneum. The usual pH (5.5–6) of commercial dialysis solutions can favor a positive Al transfer across the peritoneum.

In conclusion, in patients on CAPD, positive or negative transfer of Al through the peritoneum was observed in relation to Al concentration in dialysis fluid and in serum, and perhaps with tissue Al concentration. Despite very low dialysis fluid Al concentration, patients are at risk of increasing serum Al concentration as soon as they take ACPB. Control of serum Al levels in such patients is justified even if serum Al does not reflect aluminum stores in uremic patients.[28, 29] In patients with high serum levels, large amounts of Al can be removed through the peritoneal route.

ACKNOWLEDGMENTS

This study was supported by a grant from the Association pour l'Utilisation du Rein Artificiel. More complete results were published by the same authors in Kidney International 25: 919–924, 1984. We thank Mr. C. Debrun for secretarial assistance and all the nurses and staff of Pavillon de la Grille for technical assistance.

REFERENCES

1. Alfrey AC, Legendre GR, and Kaehny WD: The dialysis encephalopathy syndrome. Possible aluminum intoxication. N Engl J Med 294: 184, 1976
2. Balvarte HJ, Gruskin AB, Hinder LB, Foley CM, and Grover WD: Encephalopathy in children with chronic renal failure. Proc Clin Dial Transplant Forum 7: 95, 1977
3. Berlyne GM, Ben-Ari J, Pest D, Weinberger J, Stern N, Gilmore GR, and Levine R: Hyperaluminaemia from aluminium resins in renal failure. Lancet 2: 494, 1970
4. Drueke T: Dialysis osteomalacia and aluminum intoxication. Nephron 26: 207, 1980
5. O'Hare JA, and Murnaghan DJ: Reversal of aluminum-induced hemodialysis anemia by a low-aluminum dialysate. N Engl J Med 306: 654, 1982
6. Boukari M, Rottembourg J, Jaudon MC, Galli A, Clavel JP, and Legrain M: Influence de la prise prolongée de gels d'alumine sur les taux sériques d'aluminum chez les patients atteints d'insuffisance rénale chronique. Nouv Presse Med 5: 85, 1978
7. Eliott HL, MacDougall AI, Fell GS, Gardiner PHE, and Willams ED: Dialysis encephalopathy: Evidence implicating aluminum. Dial Transplant 9: 1027, 1980
8. Fleming LW, Stewart WK, Fell GL, Halls DJ: The effect of oral aluminum therapy on plasma aluminum levels in patients with chronic renal failure in an area with low water aluminum. Clin Nephrol 17: 222, 1982
9. Pierides AM: Dialysis dementia, osteomalacia, fractures and myopathy: A syndrome due to chronic aluminum intoxication. Int J Artif Organs 5: 206, 1978
10. Sideman S, and Manor D: The dialysis dementia syndrome and aluminum intoxication. Nephron 31: 1, 1982
11. Calderaro V, Oreopoulos DG, Mesma HE, Ogilvie R, Husdan H, Khanna R, Quinton C, Murray T, and Carmichael D: The evolution of renal osteodystrophy in patients undergoing CAPD. Proc Eur Dial Transplant Assoc 17: 533, 1980
12. Gilli P, Farinelli A, Fagioli F, De Bastiani P, Buoncristiani U: Serum aluminum levels in patients on peritoneal dialysis. Lancet 2: 742, 1980
13. Gokal R, Ramos JM, Ellis HA, Parkinson I, Sweetman V, Dewar J, Ward MK, and Kerr DNS: Histological renal osteodystrophy and 25 hydroxycholecalciferol and aluminum levels in patients on continuous ambulatory peritoneal dialysis. Kidney Int 23: 15, 1983
14. Smith DB, Lewis JA, Burk JS, and Alfrey AC: Dialysis encephalopathy in peritoneal dialysis. JAMA 244: 365, 1980
15. Wolf A, Graf H, Pinggera WF, Stumvoll HK, and Meisinger W: Serum aluminum and continuous ambulatory peritoneal dialysis. Ann Intern Med 92: 130, 1981
16. Cumming AD, Simpson G, Bell D, Cowie J, and Winney R: Acute aluminium intoxication in patients on CAPD. Lancet 1: 103, 1982
17. Sorkin MI, Nolph KD, Anderson HD, Morris JS, Kennedy J, Prowant B, and Moore H: Aluminum mass transfer during continuous ambulatory peritoneal dialysis. Peritoneal Dial Bull 1: 91, 1981
18. Rottembourg J, Issad B, Gallego JL, Degoulet P, Aime F, Gueffaf B, Legrain M: Evolution of residual renal function in patients undergoing maintenance haemodialysis or continuous ambulatory peritoneal dialysis. Proc Eur Dial Transplant Assoc 19: 397, 1982
19. Clavel JP, Jaudon MC, and Galli A: Dosage de l'aluminium dans les liquides biologiques par spectrométrie d'absorption atomique en four graphite. Ann Biol Clin 36: 33, 1978
20. Clavel JP, Jaudon MC, and Galli A: Dosage de l'aluminium sérique: Nouvelle estimation des valeurs usuelles. Ann Biol Clin 40: 51, 1982

21. Graf H, Stummvoll HK, and Meisinger W: Dialysate aluminium concentration and aluminum transfer during haemodialysis. Lancet 1: 46, 1982

22. Graf H, Stummvoll HK, Meisinger W, Kouarik J, Wolf A, and Pinggera WF: Aluminum removal by hemodialysis. Kidney Int 19: 587, 1981

23. Berlyne GM: Plasmapheresis, aluminium and dialysis dementia. Lancet 2: 1155, 1978

24. Nolph K, Miller FN, Pule WK, Popovich R, and Sorkin M: An hypothesis to explain the ultrafiltration characteristics of peritoneal dialysis. Kidney Int 29: 543, 1981

25. Kaehny WD, Hegg AP, and Alfrey AC: Gastrointestinal absorption of aluminum from aluminum containing antacids. N Engl J Med 296: 1389, 1977

26. Gacek EM, Babb AL, Uvelli DA, Fry DL, and Scribner BH: Dialysis dementia: The role of dialysate pH in altering the dialyzability of aluminum. Trans Am Soc Artif Intern Organs 25: 409, 1979

27. Gilli P, Debastiani P, Fagioli F, Buoncristiani U, Carobi C, Stabellini N, Squerzanti R, Rosati G, and Farinelli A: Positive aluminium balance in patients on regular peritoneal treatment: An effect of low dialysate pH? Proc Eur Dial Transplant Assoc 17: 219, 1980

28. Cundy T, and Kanis JA: Serum aluminium measurements in renal bone disease. Lancet 2: 1168, 1983

29. Verbeelen D, Smeyers-Verbeke J, Sennesael J, and Massart DL: Serum aluminium measurements in renal bone disease. Lancet 2: 1169, 1983

G. Panarello, D. Schinella, P. Quaia, and F. Tesio

20

Calcium Peritoneal Mass Transfer in CAPD

SUMMARY

We studied the influence of two different dialysis fluids, calcium concentrations (7 mg/dl in period A, and 8 mg/dl in period B) on calcium peritoneal mass transfer (CaPMT) in 6 CAPD patients. CaPMT was calculated over 24 h and during single exchange periods. Higher CaPMT occurred in period B for both 24 h and single exchange studies. An inverse correlation between CaPMT and ultrafiltrate volume (UFV) was found. Collected data suggest that ultrafiltration strongly opposes positive CaPMT in CAPD. Net removal from the body can be avoided by providing CAPD dialysates containing 8 mg/dl, at least for 2.5% and 4.25% dextrose solutions.

INTRODUCTION

CAPD is accepted worldwide for treatment of end-stage renal failure. So-called renal osteodystrophy is present in the majority of patients with chronic renal failure. Recent reports provide increasing evidence that the course of renal osteodystrophy is not reversed by CAPD.[1,2] Mechanisms claimed to affect bone lesion evolution in CAPD patients are peritoneal loss of calcium,[3] of vitamin D and D-binding protein,[4] inadequate removal of phosphorus,[3] and effects of magnesium,[5] and aluminum absorption.[6] Other factors (parathyroid hormone[7] and calcitonin peritoneal losses[8]) have uncertain pathophysiological significance.

From the Division of Nephrology, Stabilimento Ospedaliero USL n11, Pordenone, Italy.

Reduced intestinal calcium absorption occurs in patients with renal failure,[9] and increased calcium intake and added vitamin D metabolites are required to maintain metabolic balance. With hemodialysis treatment, net calcium gain occurs at every dialysis session when dialysate calcium levels exceed the diffusible concentration in plasma by 1.5–2 mg/dl.[10] In CAPD patients, constant calcium loss,[3] substantial equilibrium,[11] and net calcium gain[12] have been reported. The purpose of this study was to evaluate calcium peritoneal mass transfer (CaPMT) in continuous peritoneal dialysis patients. We also compared the peritoneal calcium gain induced by two different levels of calcium in dialysis fluid. The role of other factors affecting CaPMT in CAPD is discussed.

METHODS

Six patients (3 males, 3 females, mean age of 57 years) maintained on CAPD for a mean time of 13 months were studied. All patients were anuric. Three patients were taking the same amount of aluminum hydroxide for all the study period in order to maintain the serum phosphorus level lower than 5 mg/dl. No oral calcium salts or vitamin D metabolites were taken throughout the study and for three months before. CAPD was performed as described by Oreopoulos et al.[3] Informed consent was given by all patients.

The study involves two six-month periods; all patients performed CAPD with dialysate containing 7 mg/dl Ca (Dianeal®, Travenol, Italy) in period A and 8 mg/dl Ca (Bieffe, Italy) in period B. Peritoneal

Table 1. 24-Hour Study.

Indices	Period A	P	Period B
CaPMT (mg/24 h)	37.4 ± 7.9	0.004	109 ± 12.3
Serum Ca (mg/dl)	9.64 ± .51	ns	10.17 ± .41
Serum albumin (g/dl)	3.44 ± .2	ns	3.53 ± .14
UFV (ml/24 h)	1271 ± 171	ns	1116 ± 194

PMT = Peritoneal mass transfer; UFV = ultrafiltrate volume.

clearances evaluated bimonthly in every patient were unchanged throughout the study period. CaPMT was calculated both in 24-hour periods (n = 40) and in single exchanges with 1.5% (n = 77), 2.5% (n = 61), and 4.25% (n = 30) dextrose dialysis solutions. Serum and dialysate calcium concentrations and albumin levels were determined by routine laboratory methods adapted for the Technicon AutoAnalyzer (Technicon Instruments Corporation, Tarrytown, NY). The mass transfer of calcium was calculated by the net amount removed per exchange from the amount instilled:

Mass transfer (PMT) =
Dialysate concentration instilled ×
Dialysate volume instilled −
Dialysate concentration drained ×
Dialysate volume drained.

Ultrafiltration volume (UFV) =
Dialysate volume drained −
Dialysate volume instilled.

A positive net transfer therefore represents the amount gained from the patient and a negative net transfer the amount removed. Data are shown as mean ± SEM using the mean value for all determinations of each patient to exclude possible bias due to biological variance. Statistical analysis was performed with the Student's t test, regression analysis, and one-way analysis of variance.

RESULTS

Mean values of CaPMT, Ca, albumin and UFV for 24-hour studies in both A and B periods are showed in Table 1. CaPMT values were lower in period A (p = 0.004). Differences were not found for Ca, albumin and UFV values between A and B periods. No differences were found for albumin and Ca values for single-exchange studies throughout the same period or between A and B period. As shown in Table 2, CaPMT significantly increased in period B for 1.5% (p = 0.04) and 2.5% (p = 0.02) dextrose dialysate concentrations, but not with 4.25% dextrose bags (p = 0.1). UFV was not different in either period A or B for the same dextrose dialysis fluid concentration. UFV increased (A: F < 0.001; B: F < 0.001) and CaPMT decreased as dextrose concentration increased in both A and B periods (A: F = 0.001; B: F = 0.01).

Table 2. CaPMT and UFV in Single-Exchange Study.

Indexes	Bag Dextrose (g/dl)	Period A	P	Period B
CaPMT (mg)	1.5	19.8 ± 4.9	0.04	46.1 ± 8.7
	2.5	5.4 ± 3.3	0.02	22.6 ± 3.5
	4.25	−1.8 ± 8.1	ns	11.9 ± 11.1
		F = 0.001		F = 0.01
UFV (ml)	1.5	100 ± 77	ns	−108 ± 130.5
	2.5	483 ± 63	ns	309 ± 154
	4.25	705 ± 202	ns	762 ± 209
		F < 0.001		F < 0.001

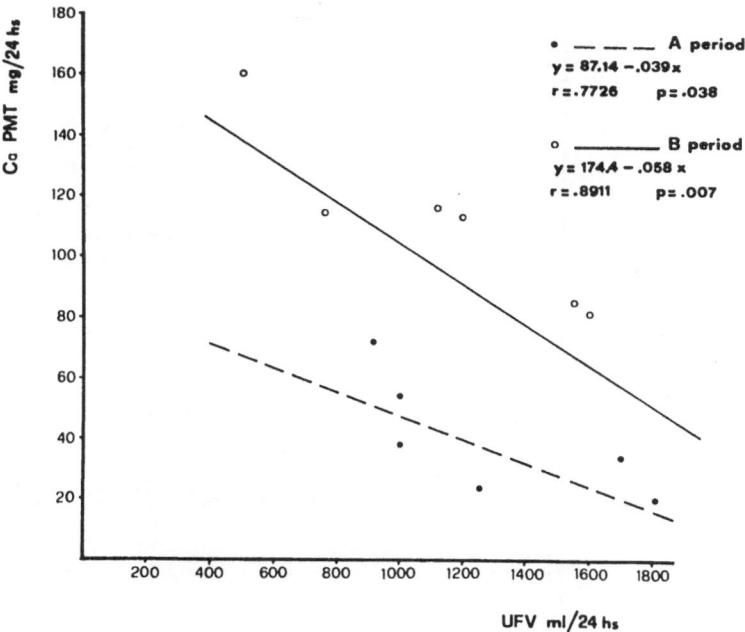

Fig. 1. CaPMT/UFV in 24-hour study.

UFV at different dextrose dialysate concentrations are shown in Table 2. An inverse correlation between CaPMT and UFV was found in both periods for both 24-hour and single-exchange studies (Figs. 1 and 2).

DISCUSSION

Negative mass transfer detected by Oreopoulos et al.[3] was due to low calcium concentration in dialysate (6 mg/dl). Different data reported by Parker and Nolph[11] and Delmez et al.,[5] both using 7 mg/dl calcium dialysis solution concentration, may be due to different UFV values. Parker and Nolph[11] also reported a negative correlation between serum calcium and peritoneal mass transfer. We also correlated these parameters in a previous study in CAPD patients using a 6 mg/dl calcium dialysate, but that correlation disappeared when calcium concentration in dialysate was increased to 7 mg/dl.[12] In this study in period A, we found CaPMT lower than in period B using a dialysate different only for Ca concentration. Therefore, we believe dialysate Ca concentration is the main factor affecting CaPMT.

Since we found that 8 mg/dl Ca dialysis solution almost constantly provided positive peritoneal calcium balance, we think it mandatory to raise calcium concentration in dialysate to 8 mg/dl at least in 2.5% and 4.25% dextrose dialysis fluids. In our study, serum calcium and albumin levels did not affect CaPMT. Mechanisms claimed to affect evolution of bone lesions in CAPD patients (e.g., peritoneal losses of vitamin D and D binding protein,[4] PTH[7] and calcitonin,[8] inadequate removal of magnesium,[5] or aluminum absorption,[6] do not actually contribute importantly or have a limited role in worsening of renal osteodystrophy.[4-8]

The role of CaPMT in uremic bone lesion evolution has been confirmed by several clinical reports.[1,2,13,14] CAPD patients with constantly negative peritoneal Ca balance show progressive renal osteodystrophy,[1,13] while in patients with 7 mg/dl calcium dialysis fluid concentration, no significant deterioration[2] or improvement[14] in bone lesions is reported, in spite of long-term vitamin D and/or calcium salt therapy.[1,2,13,14]

Recently Oren et al.[15] reported that 1,25 (OH) vitamin D_3 treatment plays an important role in the pathogenesis of kidney stones in CAPD patients

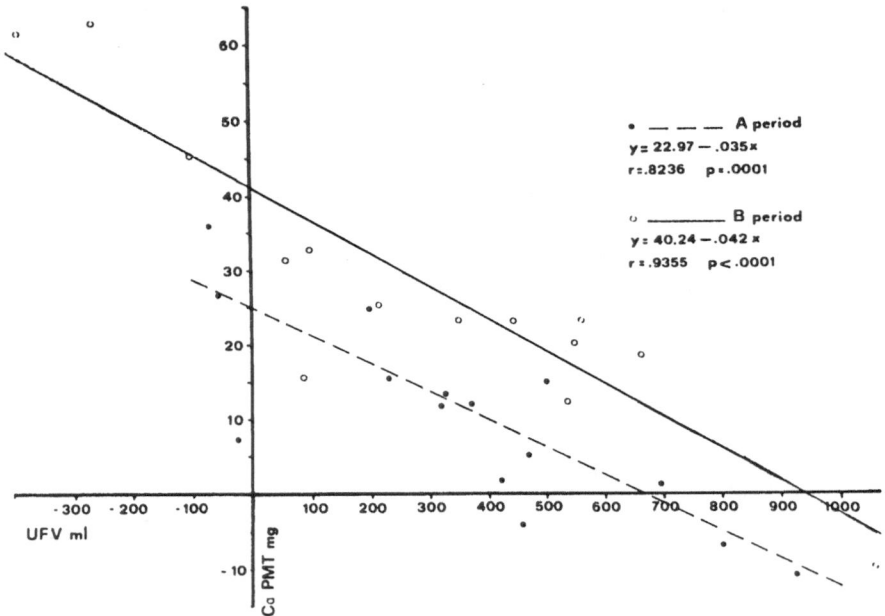

Fig. 2. CaPMT/UFV in single-exchange study.

with maintained diuresis. Long-term calcium salt therapy is expensive and not well accepted by many patients because of its side effects on the alimentary tract. The peritoneal route for positive calcium balance in CAPD patients appears to be safe (hypercalcemia in period B was never detected), and may reduce vitamin D metabolite requirements. Last but not least, patient acceptance and good dialysis treatment expenditure might be decreased, since oral Ca salts may not be required.

REFERENCES

1. Digenis G, Khanna R, Pierratos A, Meema HE, Rabinovic S, Pettit J, and Oreopoulos DG: Renal osteodystrophy in patients maintained on CAPD for more than three years. Peritoneal Dial Bull 3: 81, 1983
2. Zucchelli P, Fusaroli M, Casanova S, Fabbri L, and Catizone L: Renal osteodystrophy in CAPD patients. In La Greca G, Biasioli S, and Ronco C (Eds), Peritoneal dialysis. Milano: Witchig Editore, 1982, p 406
3. Oreopoulos DG, Robson M, Faller B, Ogilvie R, Rapoport A, and de Veber GA: Continuous ambulatory peritoneal dialysis: A new era in the treatment of chronic renal failure. Clin Nephrol 11: 125, 1979
4. Aloni Y, Shani S, and Chaimovitz C: Losses of 25 hydroxyvitamin D in peritoneal fluid: Possible mechanism for bone disease in uremic patients treated with chronic ambulatory peritoneal dialysis. Mineral Electrolyte Metab 8: 82, 1983
5. Delmez JA, Slatopolsky E, Martin KJ, Gearing BN, and Harter HR: Minerals, vitamin D, and parathyroid hormone in continuous ambulatory peritoneal dialysis. Kidney Int 21: 862, 1982
6. Cannata JB, Junior BJR, Briggs JD, Fell GS, and Beastall G: Effect of acute aluminium overload on calcium and parathyroid hormone metabolism. Lancet 1: 501, 1983
7. Schinella D, Panarello G, and Quaia P: Una valutazione della dialysance peritoneale del PTH in CAPD. Giorn Piemont Nefrol S1: 235, 1982
8. Martinez ME, Miguel JL, Gomez P, Selgas R, Salinas M, Gentil M, Mateos F, Montero JL, and Sanchez Sicilia L: Plasma calcitonine concentration in patients treated with chronic dialysis: Difference between hemodialysis and CAPD. Clin Nephrol 19: 250, 1983
9. Coburn JW, Hartenbower DL, Brickman AS, Massry SG, and Kopple JD: Intestinal absorption of calcium, magnesium and phosphorus in chronic renal insufficiency. In David DS (Ed), Calcium metabolism in renal failure and nephrolithiasis. New York: John Wiley, 1977, p 77
10. Mirahmady KS, Duffy BS, Shinaberger JH, Jowsey J, Massry SG, and Coburn JW: A controlled evalua-

tion of clinical and metabolic effects of dialysate calcium levels during regular hemodialysis. Trans Am Soc Artif Intern Organs 17: 118, 1971

11. Parker A, and Nolph KD: Magnesium and calcium mass transfer during continuous ambulatory peritoneal dialysis. Trans Am Soc Artif Intern Organs 26: 194, 1980

12. Panarello G, Schinella D, Quaia P, Camurri C, and Tesio F: Bilancio peritoneale di calcio in CAPD. Giorn Piemont Nefrol S1: 221, 1981

13. Calderaro V, Oreopoulos DG, Meema HE, Ogilvie R, Husdan H, Khanna R, Quinton C, Murray T, and Carmichael D: The evolution of renal osteodystrophy

in patients undergoing continuous ambulatory peritoneal dialysis (CAPD). Proc Eur Dial Transplant Assoc 17: 533, 1980

14. Gokal R, Ramos JM, Ellis HA, Parkinson I, Sweetman V, Dewar J, Ward MK, and Kerr DNS: Histological renal osteodystrophy, and 25 hydroxycholecalciferol and aluminum levels in patients on continuous ambulatory peritoneal dialysis. Kidney Int 23: 15, 1983

15. Oren A, Husdan H, Cheng PT, Khanna R, Pierratos A, Digenis G, and Oreopoulos DG: Calcium oxalate kidney stones in patients on continuous ambulatory peritoneal dialysis. Kidney Int 25: 534, 1984

A. Abramov, A. Khavilov, and V. Favorov

21

Changes in Plasma Protein Spectra after IP Injection of Hypertonic and Isotonic Solutions*

SUMMARY

Peritoneal dialysis was carried out in Wistar rats using Tyrode solution or processed sea water of 1200 mmol/L hypertonicity and the changes in concentration of the components of the plasma protein spectrum were evaluated. After a 6 h dwell, Tyrode solution was associated with a 5.9% decrease in the albumin zone while sea water induced a 4.1% increase. These changes were more marked after a second exchange and were associated with reciprocal changes in other protein components, most notably the ceruloplasmin and transferrin zones. It is concluded that hypertonic solutions including sea water can be used for dialysis and cause only minimal plasma protein imbalance.

INTRODUCTION

Protein losses remain a fundamental problem in clinical peritoneal dialysis. They vary from 0.5–4.5 g/L, and the total loss reaches 20–200 g during a 24–48 hour cycle. Protein loss can increase tremendously during peritonitis.[1] Modern technology makes it possible to decrease significantly this unfavorable phenomenon.[2] Protein losses increase as the volume and tonicity of the dialysing solution are raised. The velocity of protein transport into dialy- sate correlates with the concentration of proteins, as shown by determinations of immunoglobulin M and G concentrations in both dialysate and blood plasma.[2] The rates of resorption and transudation of proteins in the peritoneal cavity relate inversely to the molecular weights of the proteins. The transport rate was higher for low-molecular-weight proteins such as albumin and transferrin and lower for high-molecular-weight immunoglobulins.[3] Based on these observations, we may suppose that the tonicity of solution will affect not only the amount of total protein loss, but also the protein composition of dialysate and plasma. We investigated the changes in protein spectra in plasma of rats after IP injections of isotonic and hypertonic solutions.

METHODS

Seventy Wistar line rats were used in the study, 10 animals in each series. Isotonic Tyrode solution of 300 mOsm/L and hypertonic sea-water solution of 1200 mOsm/L were injected intraperitoneally (IP) in a dose of 50 ml/100 g body weight, using sterile technique. Three injections were made at six-hour intervals. Blood was sampled from the neck vein of ether-anesthetized rats at six hours postinjection.

Tris was purchased from "Sigma" (U.S.A.), acrylamide,methylene-bis-acrylamide, Coomassi R-250, and TEMED from "Reanal" (Hungary), and other reagents of the chemical purity grade were obtained from v/o "Sojuzglavreactive."

Acrylamide was recrystallized from ethylacetate and bis from acetone before using. Analytical

From the Department of Physiology and Pharmacology, Institute of Marine Biology, Far East Science Center, USSR Academy of Science, Vladivostok, USSR.
* Not presented at Symposium.

disc-electrophoresis was performed according to the usual procedure in Tris-chloride-buffer system.[4] Densitometry of washed gels was made on a "Joice Loeble" scanner, and band intensities were determined by an integrator.

The entire protein spectrum was separated into 13 zones to quantify changes in protein proportions. R_T values[5] of different proteins[6] are given in parentheses: albumin zone (1.63–1.89, albumin); the I postalbumin zone (1.50–1.63, α_1-globulins); the II postalbumin zone (1.34–1.50, α_2-globulins); the III postalbumin zone (1.18–1.34, ceruloplasmin); the IV postalbumin zone (1.05–1.18, β-globulins); transferrin zone (1.0, β-globulins and transferrin); the I posttransferrin zone (0.86–0.92, complement proteins); the II posttransferrin zone (0.75–0.86, β-fraction IgA, haptoglobins); the III posttransferrin zone (0.63–0.75, immunoglobulins, haptoglobins); the IV posttransferrin zone (0.55–0.63, IgA, IgG, IgM); fast immunoglobulins zone (0.10–0.55, α_2- and β-globulins; the II start zone (0.03–0.10, α_2-macroglobulins, IgM); the I start zone (0.00–0.03, IgG, α-lipoproteins). Electrophoresis was carried out in triplicate, and statistical significance of results was determined by Student's t-test.

Sea water was sterilized by UF through 0.2 μm pore nitrate cellulose filter "Synpor" (CSSR) and subsequent UV-filtration in a flow-through system. Sea water was standardized by sodium content determined by flame photometry.

RESULTS

The main variations in plasma protein concentrations occurred in the albumin and haptoglobin fractions. Accordingly, the entire spectrum was divided into 13 zones, and the intensity of each zone, but not that of a discrete protein band, was determined to quantify the protein changes. The results are listed in Table 1. Six hours after injection of the solutions, sea water increased the albumin zone by 4.1%, but Tyrode solution decreased this portion by 5.9% while it increased immunoglobulin by 29.3%. The most obvious alterations in the protein spectrum were obtained six hours after the second injection. Sea-water injection caused an increase in the albumin zone by 22.4% compared to the control, but markedly diminished portions of the third and the fourth postalbumin zones, of transferrin, and of the second, third, and fourth posttransferrin zones. On the contrary, the Tyrode solution injections decreased the albumin zone by 19.4% but increased the ceruloplasmin and transferrin zones by 48.4 and

Table 1. The Changes in Plasma Protein Spectra of Rats after Multiple Injections of Isotonic Tyrode Solution (300 mOsm/L) and Hypertonic Sea Water Solution (1200 mOsm/L) in Relative Percent (Mean ± SEM).

Protein Zone	First Injection		Second Injection		Third Injection		Control
	Sea Water	Tyrode	Sea Water	Tyrode	Sea Water	Tyrode	
1	25.04 ± 0.69	22.63 ± 0.81	29.45 ± 0.33	19.39 ± 0.56	29.36 ± 1.15	29.50 ± 0.32	24.06 ± 0.08
2	4.90 ± 0.08	4.50 ± 0.11	5.67 ± 0.33	7.41 ± 0.15	3.32 ± 0.17	3.44 ± 0.16	5.56 ± 0.01
3	4.13 ± 0.12	4.04 ± 0.36	5.49 ± 0.11	6.51 ± 0.19	2.56 ± 0.20	5.62 ± 0.17	5.30 ± 0.01
4	1.60 ± 0.11	2.26 ± 0.16	2.07 ± 0.10	2.85 ± 0.07	1.47 ± 0.13	1.45 ± 0.15	3.43 ± 0.02
5	3.68 ± 0.04	3.84 ± 0.10	1.87 ± 0.10	3.77 ± 0.12	1.15 ± 0.09	0.99 ± 0.12	2.54 ± 0.03
6	6.72 ± 0.20	7.29 ± 0.22	6.17 ± 0.11	8.94 ± 0.19	6.17 ± 0.19	6.35 ± 0.57	6.70 ± 0.02
7	5.70 ± 0.07	5.48 ± 0.07	5.60 ± 0.18	6.08 ± 0.17	7.69 ± 0.17	6.63 ± 0.13	4.41 ± 0.01
8	6.51 ± 0.08	6.46 ± 0.13	6.85 ± 0.06	6.39 ± 0.11	7.55 ± 0.11	8.01 ± 0.29	7.37 ± 0.01
9	5.18 ± 0.08	5.21 ± 0.15	6.14 ± 0.12	3.87 ± 0.15	7.70 ± 0.25	6.26 ± 0.13	6.56 ± 0.01
10	5.09 ± 0.09	5.28 ± 0.15	4.98 ± 0.11	5.80 ± 0.07	5.69 ± 0.47	5.05 ± 0.08	5.90 ± 0.01
11	23.01 ± 0.34	25.13 ± 0.26	19.51 ± 0.59	21.48 ± 0.37	18.97 ± 0.41	20.43 ± 0.32	20.99 ± 0.09
12	4.62 ± 0.14	4.13 ± 0.07	3.06 ± 0.13	4.60 ± 0.04	4.78 ± 0.12	3.75 ± 0.12	2.35 ± 0.02
13	3.82 ± 0.18	3.57 ± 0.07	3.08 ± 0.34	2.92 ± 0.25	4.19 ± 0.22	2.91 ± 0.14	4.84 ± 0.02

33.4%, respectively. After the third injection, the changes in protein spectrum were less pronounced.

DISCUSSION

To enhance the possible effect of changes in the plasma protein spectrum, the isotonic Tyrode and hypertonic sea water solutions were injected IP three times. Sea water is a naturally equilibrated hypertonic solution wherein the proportion of the main cations is approximately the same as in blood plasma.[7] Intravenous sea water injection has not produced overt pathological effects on organisms studied.[8] An additional reason to use sea water is that the salt composition of Tyrode solution makes it impossible to prepare a hypertonic solution of 1200 mOsm/L tonicity.

Thus, isotonic Tyrode solution and hypertonic sea water solution injected IP caused different changes in blood plasma proteins. The hypertonic solution increased and isotonic solution diminished the portion of protein-containing albumin which provides most of the oncotic pressure of plasma.[9] It is pertinent that injections of hypertonic solution induced quantitatively smaller deviations in protein proportions than did isotonic solution. Accordingly, it may be assumed that hypertonic solutions, includ-

ing sea water, can be used for dialysis in treating peritonitis and exogenous poisoning and should induce minimal plasma protein imbalance.

REFERENCES

1. Berlyne GM, Jones H, Hewitt V, and Nibwarangkur S: Protein loss in peritoneal dialysis. Lancet 1: 738, 1964
2. Blumenkrantz MJ, Gahl G, Kopple J, Kamdar A, Jones M, Kessel M, and Coburn J: Protein losses during peritoneal dialysis. Kidney Int 19: 593, 1981
3. Szabo G, and Magyar Z: Absorption and transport of protein from the peritoneal cavity. Acta Med Acad Sci Hung 30: 303, 1973
4. Davis BI: Disc electrophoresis. II. Method and application to human serum proteins. Ann NY Acad Sci 121: 404, 1964
5. Evans IH, and Quick DT. Polyacrilamide gel electrophoresis of spinal-fluid proteins. Clin Chem 12: 28, 1966
6. Putman FW: The plasma proteins, VI. New York: Academic Press, 1975, p 27
7. Dietrick G: General oceanography. New York: Interscience, 1963, p 6
8. Shakhnazarova AB, and Lukash NV: Sea water and its application in medicine. Moscow: Medicina, 1969, p 7
9. Squire RG, Moser P, O'Konski CT: The hydrodynamic properties of bovine serum albumin monomer and dimer. Biochemistry 7: 4261, 1958

K.L. Heim, C.E. Halstenson, C.M. Comty, and G.R. Matzke

22

Pharmacokinetics of Cefotaxime during CAPD

SUMMARY

Pharmacokinetics of cefotaxime have been studied in five patients undergoing CAPD. Given IV the t 1/2 was 2.12 h and Cl_p was 91 ml/min, C_{CAPD} contributing only 1.7 ml/min. The distribution space was 0.19 l/Kg. With IP administration the values differed somewhat, possibly because of the effect of residual dialysate. The metabolite, desacetyl cefotaxime, had a t 1/2 of about 24 h. Dialysate concentrations of the drug and its metabolite were detectable for at least 18 h.

INTRODUCTION

CAPD has become an increasingly important alternative for the treatment of patients with ESRD. Peritonitis is often a serious adverse complication of CAPD. Although the organisms isolated from CAPD patients with peritonitis include multiple gram-positive and gram-negative bacteria, the most frequent isolates are *Staphylococcus epidermidis*, *Staphylococcus aureus*, and *Enterobacteriaceae*.[1] Cefotaxime, a new third generation cephalosporin, has a broad spectrum of activity, including both gram-positive and gram-negative organisms.[2,3] In addition, its primary metabolite, desacetyl cefotaxime, has been shown to be approximately 1/4–1/8 as active as cefotaxime and more active than cefazolin,

cefamandole, or cefoxitin.[4,5] Furthermore, synergy has been noted for up to 76% of organisms evaluated with the combination of cefotaxime and desacetyl cefotaxime.[3–5] Thus, cefotaxime may be of potential use in CAPD patients who develop peritonitis.

The pharmacokinetics of cefotaxime in patients undergoing CAPD have not been rigorously assessed. The purpose of this study was to quantitate cefotaxime and desacetyl cefotaxime in plasma, peritoneal dialysate fluid, and urine after administration of single IV and IP doses of cefotaxime. The following pharmacokinetic parameters of cefotaxime were determined: elimination rate, elimination half-life, volume of distribution, total body clearance, peritoneal clearance, and the bioavailability of IP administered cefotaxime.

METHODS

Five patients with no known hypersensitivity to cephalosporins participated in the study after written informed consent was granted. All subjects had been on CAPD for at least three months and none had peritonitis in the three months prior to the study. Each patient had a physical examination and laboratory screening profile before and after the study. Patients were excluded if they had unstable renal function, or if they had participated in an investigational drug trial or received any antimicrobial agent during the four weeks preceding the study. Demographic information is listed in Table 1.

All patients had an indwelling Tenckhoff catheter. The CAPD exchange schedule for each patient was 2 L of 2.5% dextrose peritoneal dialysis solution

From the Drug Evaluation Unit, Regional Kidney Disease Program, Department of Medicine, Hennepin County Medical Center, and the College of Pharmacy and School of Medicine, University of Minnesota, Minneapolis, MN.

Table 1. Patient Demographic Characteristics.

Patient	Age (Years)	Weight (kg)	Height (Inches)	Sex	Diagnosis
1	63	67.7	67	F	Polycystic kidney disease
2	70	74.1	70	M	Unknown etiology
3	59	72.7	67	M	Diabetic nephropathy
4	67	56.4	64	F	Unknown etiology
5	54	82.7	68	F	Hypertensive nephrosclerosis
Mean ± SD	62.6 ± 6.3	70.7 ± 9.7	67.2 ± 2.2		

(Dianeal®, Travenol Laboratories, Deerfield, IL) every 6 hours. A single 2 g dose of cefotaxime was infused intravenously over a five-minute period. In addition, each patient received a 2 g dose of cefotaxime instilled intraperitoneally as the first exchange of the day. The two doses were separated by at least 72 hours. Blood samples were collected just prior to 0.08, 0.16, 0.25, 0.5, 1, 1.5, 2, 2.5, 3, 4, 6, 8, 12, 15, 18, 24, 36, 48, 60, and 72 hours after the start of the intravenous infusion from a heparin lock placed in a forearm vein in the contralateral arm. Blood samples were drawn from a heparin lock just prior to instillation of the intraperitoneal dose 0.25, 0.5, 1, 2, 4, 6, 8, 10, 12, 15, 18, 24, 30, 36, 48, 60, and 72 hours after instillation. Total dialysate outflow was collected and measured with each exchange during both of the 72-hour study periods. Total urinary output was also collected and measured during both of the 72-hour study periods. Plasma, dialysate, and urine samples were stored at −70°C until analysis.

The concentrations of cefotaxime and desacetyl cefotaxime in plasma, dialysate, and urine were determined by a modification of the HPLC technique of Chamberlain et al.[6] The between-day coefficients of variation in plasma and dialysate for cefotaxime were 11.8 and 15.9%, and for desacetyl cefotaxime were 9.1 and 10.2%, respectively.

Data Analysis

The decline in cefotaxime plasma concentrations after IV administration in each patient was biexponential. Therefore, the plasma concentration time profile was analyzed in terms of the following equation:

$$C_t = Ae^{-\alpha t} + Be^{-\beta t} \qquad (1)$$

where C_t is the concentration in serum at time t, A, and B are the intercepts, and α and β are the disposi-

tion rates obtained from the first and second phases respectively of the plot of log cefotaxime concentration in plasma versus time.

Standard curve stripping procedures were used to obtain initial estimates of the parameters. Final estimates were obtained by nonlinear regression analysis with the program KINA on a Control Data Digital Computer (University Computing Center, University of Minnesota, Minneapolis, MN). All plasma cefotaxime concentrations were weighted according to their reciprocal squared concentrations during the computer fitting procedure. The appropriate equations for the biphasic decay of log plasma concentration versus time after the termination of the five-minute intravenous infusion were used in analyzing the results of the computer analyses.[7] The steady state volume of distribution (V_{ss}), the half-life of the alpha and beta phase ($t\frac{1}{2}\alpha$ and $t\frac{1}{2}\beta$, respectively), and the total body clearance (Clp) were calculated by standard techniques.

The elimination rate (k) of cefotaxime after IP administration and desacetyl cefotaxime, after IV and IP administration, were determined by nonlinear regression analysis of the post absorption/distribution plasma concentration time data. The half-life of the elimination phase was calculated as:

$$t\frac{1}{2} = 0.693/k \qquad (2)$$

The area under the cefotaxime and desacetyl cefotaxime plasma concentration time curve ($AUC|_0^x$) was calculated using the linear trapezoidal method with extension utilizing the elimination rate constant. The area under the moment curve ($AUMC|_0^x$) for each compound was calculated as described by Gibaldi and Perrier.[8]

The bioavailability of cefotaxime (F) was calculated as:

$$F = \frac{AUC_{IP}^{0 \rightarrow \infty}}{AUC_{IV}^{0 \rightarrow \infty}} \cdot \frac{Dose_{IV}}{Dose_{IP}} \qquad (3)$$

where $Dose_{IP}$ is the amount administered in the first dialysis bag minus the amount recovered in the first dialysate effluent. The steady state volume of distribution (V_{ss}) of cefotaxime following IP administration was calculated using the noncompartmental method described by Perrier and Mayersohn.[9]

Total body clearance (TBC) of cefotaxime was calculated as:

$$TBC = F\,Dose/AUC\big|_o^\infty \qquad (4)$$

The CAPD clearance of cefotaxime and desacetyl cefotaxime following IV and IP administration was calculated as:

$$C_{CAPD} = Ad^{t_1 \to t_2}/AUC^{t_1 \to t_2} \qquad (5)$$

where Ad = the amount of drug recovered in the dialysate and $AUC^{t_1 \to t_2}$ equals the area under the plasma concentration/time curve during the same time interval.

The pharmacokinetic parameters of cefotaxime and desacetyl cefotaxime following IV and IP dosing of cefotaxime were analyzed by paired Student's t test. Statistical significance for all tests were assessed at the p = 0.05 level.

RESULTS

The cefotaxime and desacetyl cefotaxime plasma concentration time profiles following IV and IP administration are depicted in Figures 1 and 2. The plasma concentrations of cefotaxime and desacetyl cefotaxime following IP administration of cefotaxime are lower than those observed after IV administration. However, the time above the MIC_{90} for most susceptible organisms is approximately the same when cefotaxime is given IV or IP (Fig. 3).

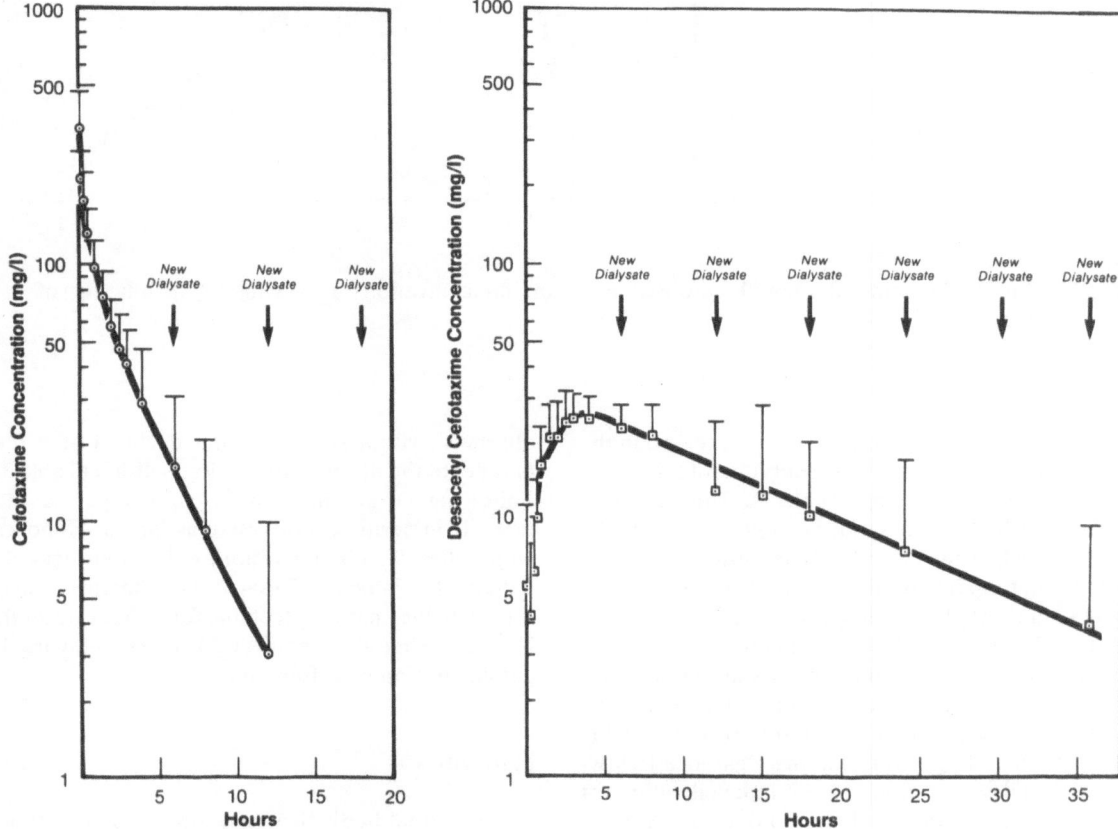

Fig. 1. Cefotaxime and desacetyl cefotaxime serum concentrations following IV administration of 2 g cefotaxime.

128

Heim, et al.

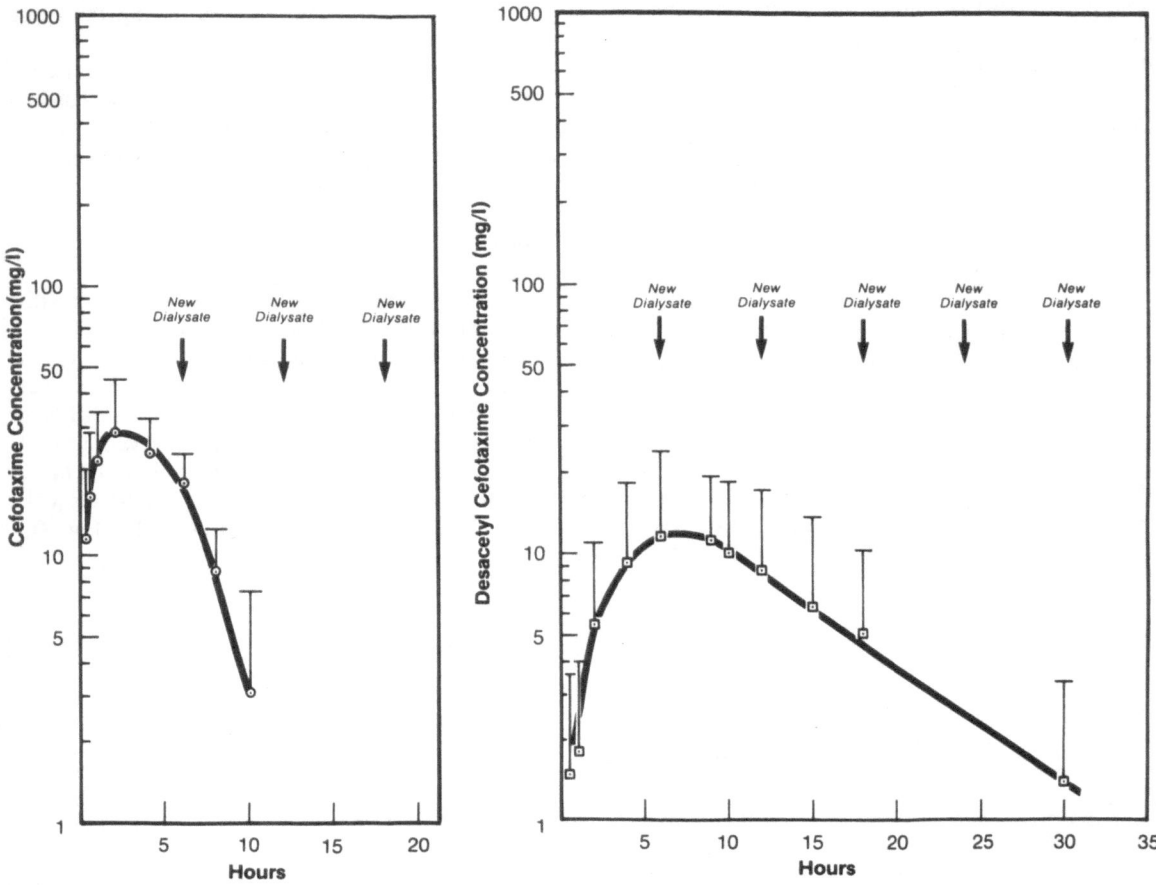

Fig. 2. Cefotaxime and desacetyl cefotaxime serum concentrations following IP instillation of 2 g cefotaxime.

No significant differences were observed in the half-life of cefotaxime or desacetyl cefotaxime following IV and IP dosing (Table 2). The desacetyl cefotaxime half-life was significantly longer than the cefotaxime half-life. No significant differences were noted in cefotaxime total body clearance and steady state volume of distribution after IV and IP administration. The CAPD clearance of cefotaxime following both routes of administration was significantly less than the total body clearance. However, the CAPD clearance of cefotaxime following IP dosing was significantly greater than the clearance following IV administration. The bioavailability of cefotaxime following IP administration was 78.0% ± 25.7 (mean ± SD).

The maximum peritoneal dialysate concentrations of cefotaxime and desacetyl cefotaxime were observed within six hours and declined at a rate parallel to the plasma elimination half-life (Table 3). Following IV administration, cefotaxime was detectable in peritoneal dialysate as long as 18 hours, while after IP administration, cefotaxime was detectable for 24 hours. Desacetyl cefotaxime in peritoneal dialysate was detectable for 48 hours after the IV cefotaxime dose and for 24 hours following IP administration of cefotaxime.

DISCUSSION

The total body clearance, steady state volume of distribution, and terminal half-life of cefotaxime were 91.0 ml/min, 0.19 L/kg, and 2.1 hours following IV administration of cefotaxime. Similar results for these pharmacokinetic parameters were observed following IP administration. These pharmacokinetic values of cefotaxime are comparable to previous reports by our group and others in patients with ESRD not yet on dialysis.[10, 11] It has been demonstrated that as creatinine clearance decreases, cefotaxime renal and plasma clearance decrease and cefotaxime half-life increases.[10] The cefotaxime total body clearance in these patients also agrees well with the only previous assessment in CAPD patients.[12]

The CAPD clearance of cefotaxime following IP administration was significantly greater than that calculated following IV administration. The clearance data following both routes are similar to previous reports.[12, 13] The greater CAPD clearance following IP cefotaxime instillation may however be artifactual, due to incomplete drainage of dialysate from the peritoneal cavity with the first exchange. Despite these differences, the CAPD clearance of cefotaxime after IV and IP administration was minimal in comparison with total body clearance (1.9% and 16.2%, respectively). The CAPD clearance of desacetyl cefotaxime following IV and IP administration of cefotaxime was 2.9 and 3.0 ml/min, respectively. Plasma clearance could not be calculated since desacetyl cefotaxime was not administered.

After IV and IP administration, cefotaxime and desacetyl cefotaxime are detectable in dialysate fluid for at least 18 hours. Synergy between cefotaxime and its primary metabolite,[3-5] coupled with the persistence of detectable concentrations, makes cefotaxime a potentially useful antibiotic for the treatment of peritonitis in CAPD patients. The plasma concentration time profiles of cefotaxime and desacetyl cefotaxime after IV administration of cefotaxime to CAPD patients are similar to those observed in nondialysis patients with ESRD. The plasma concentrations of cefotaxime and desacetyl

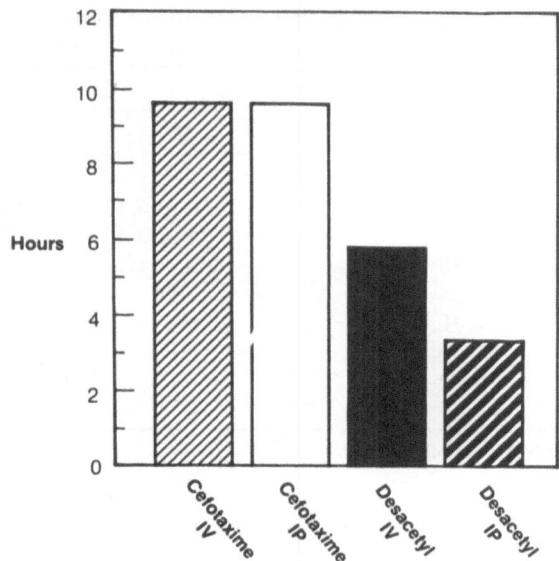

Fig. 3. Duration of time that serum concentrations were equal to or exceeded the MIC_{90} for susceptible organisms. These data assume no synergy.

cefotaxime following IP administration of cefotaxime are lower than those after IV administration. However, the time above the cefotaxime MIC_{90} for most susceptible organisms is approximately the same whether cefotaxime is given IV or IP.

Cefotaxime may be utilized for the treatment of systemic infections in CAPD patients at the dosages recommended for nondialyzed ESRD patients, since the pharmacokinetic parameters in these groups are similar. The use of the IP route for cefotaxime may require increased dosage due to decreased bioavailability of this route relative to IV administration.

Table 2. Pharmacokinetic Parameters (Mean ± SD).

	Cefotaxime		Desacetyl Cefotaxime	
	IV	IP	IV	IP
$t\frac{1}{2}$ (h)	2.12 ± 1.24	4.43 ± 4.03	23.78 ± 27.17	33.39 ± 41.92
Cl_p (ml/min)	91.0 ± 34.6	79.9 ± 35.4	—	—
C_{CAPD} (ml/min)	1.7 ± 0.5	12.6 ± 8.4*	2.9 ± 0.8	3.0 ± 1.2
V_{ss} (L/kg)	0.19 ± 0.04	0.30 ± 0.14	—	—
F (%)	—	78.02 ± 25.66	—	—

* $p < 0.05$.

Table 3. Peritoneal Dialysate Effluent Concentrations (mg/L, Mean ± SD in Dialysate Outflow from the Indicated Dwell Period).

Exchange Time	Cefotaxime		Desacetyl Cefotaxime	
	IV	IP	IV	IP
0–6	16.8 ± 6.1	252.7 ± 161.0	10.4 ± 5.3	22.7 ± 6.7
6–12	2.1 ± 3.4	14.0 ± 7.1	8.1 ± 2.9	7.5 ± 3.4
12–18	0.5 ± 1.1	1.3 ± 2.3	5.6 ± 3.6	2.5 ± 1.7
18–24	ND*	2.2 ± 4.8	3.6 ± 4.6	1.9 ± 1.5
24–30	ND	ND	2.0 ± 3.6	ND
30–36	ND	ND	1.7 ± 3.9	ND
36–42	ND	ND	1.3 ± 2.9	ND
42–48	ND	ND	1.2 ± 2.6	ND

* ND = nondetectable.

ACKNOWLEDGMENT

This paper was supported in part by a grant from Hoechst-Roussel Pharmaceuticals, Inc.

REFERENCES

1. Peterson PK, and Keane WF: Infections in chronic peritoneal dialysis patients. In Remington JS, and Swartz MN (Eds), Current clinical topics in infectious disease (in press)
2. Jones RN, and Thornsberry C: Cefotaxime: A review of in vitro antimicrobial properties and spectrum of activity. Rev Infect Dis 4(suppl): S300, 1982
3. Limbert M, Seibert G, and Schrinner E: The cooperation of cefotaxime and desacetyl-cefotaxime with respect to antibacterial activity and β-lactamase stability. Infection 10: 97, 1982
4. Neu HC: Antibacterial activity of desacetyl alone and in combination with cefotaxime. Rev Infect Dis 4(suppl): S374, 1982
5. Jones RN, Barry AL, and Thornsberry C: Antimicrobial activity of desacetylcefotaxime alone and in combination with cefotaxime: Evidence of synergy. Rev Infect Dis 4(suppl): S336, 1982
6. Chamberlain J, Coombes JD, Dell D, Fromson JM, Ings RL, MacDonald CM, and McEwen J: Metabolism of cefotaxime in animals and man. J Antimicrob Chemother 6(suppl A): 69, 1980
7. Wagner JG: Linear pharmacokinetic equations allowing direct calculation of many needed pharmacokinetic parameters from the coefficients and exponents of polyexponential equations which have been fitted to the data. J Pharmacokin Biopharm 4: 443, 1976
8. Gibaldi M, and Perrier D: Pharmacokinetics. New York: Marcel Dekker, 1982
9. Perrier D, and Mayersohn M: Noncompartmental determination of the steady-state volume of distribution for any mode of administration. J Pharm Sci 71: 372, 1982
10. Matzke GR, Abraham PA, Halstenson CE, O'Connell MB, Miller KW, Puri S, and Keane WR: Pharmacokinetics of cefotaxime in patients with various degrees of renal function. Drug Intell Clin Pharm 18: 507, 1984
11. Ings RMJ, Fillastre JP, Godin M, Leroy A, and Humbert G: The pharmacokinetics of cefotaxime and its metabolites in subjects with normal and impaired renal function. Rev Infect Dis 4(suppl): S379, 1982
12. Matousovic K, Moravek J, Vitko S, Prat V, Horcickova M, Novak Z, Kuklik R, Krebs V, Janken J, and Hatala M: Pharmacokinetics of intravenous and intraperitoneal cefotaxime in patients undergoing CAPD. 13th International Conference on Chemotherapy (unpublished)
13. Schurig R, Kampf D, Spieber W, Weihermuller K, and Becker H: Cefotaxime pharmacokinetics in peritoneal dialysis: Abstracts 2nd international symposium on peritoneal dialysis. Berlin, 1981, p 59

M.C. Rogge, P.G. Welling, C.A. Johnson, and S.W. Zimmerman

23

Multiple Dose IP Vancomycin Kinetics during CAPD

SUMMARY

Kinetics of vancomycin were studied in five noninfected CAPD patients given repeated IP doses. More than 60% of the first dose was absorbed and absorption from later exchanges was slightly lower. The volume of distribution increased for 18 h but plasma concentrations were maintained by repeated dosing.

INTRODUCTION

Because peritonitis associated with CAPD is generally caused by gram-positive organisms,[1] vancomycin is recommended as a suitable antibiotic for the treatment of this disease.[2] Despite widespread use, relatively little is known about vancomycin pharmacokinetics during CAPD. As a result, dosing of this drug has been based largely upon clinical experience and observation. For the treatment of CAPD-associated peritonitis, vancomycin has been administered both intravenously and intraperitoneally. Nielsen et al.[3] examined the peritoneal transfer of vancomycin in 11 noninfected patients treated with intermittent peritoneal dialysis (IPD). Following a 1 g intravenous (IV) dose at the beginning of dialysis, a peak plasma concentration of 29 μg/ml was obtained. During dialysis, the peritoneal clearance of vancomycin was 6.1 ml/min with a plasma half-life of 18 hours. During intraperitoneal (IP) dosing with 25 and 50 μg/ml of vancomycin, peak plasma levels ranged from nondetectable to 8.5

μg/ml, and 5.1–21.5 μg/ml, respectively. Since the clearance characteristics of the peritoneal membrane change during peritonitis,[4] the application of these data to infected patients is unknown.

Ayus et al.[5] and Magera et al.[6] have reported on the peritoneal pharmacokinetics of IV vancomycin in six patients with peritonitis being treated with IPD. The plasma half-lives observed were 9.2 days[5] and 8.6 days.[6] IP vancomycin concentrations following the IV dose were variable, but generally exceeded for several days the minimum inhibitory concentrations for most gram-positive pathogens that cause CAPD peritonitis.

The peritoneal transport of IP vancomycin during CAPD was first reported by Pancorbo and Comty.[7] Four noninfected patients were given a 1 g IP dose at the beginning of a six hour dialysis exchange. At the end of the exchange, the mean plasma level was 23.7 μg/ml. During the six-hour dwell period, 53.6% of the dose was absorbed. The mean volume of distribution (V_D) of vancomycin was 0.43 1/kg. During subsequent exchanges containing no vancomycin, the observed plasma half-life was 66.9 hours, with a peritoneal clearance of 2.4 ± 0.8 ml/min. More recently, Bunke et al.[8] reported on the kinetics of IP vancomycin following a single 10 mg/kg dose to six noninfected CAPD patients. At the end of a four-hour dwell, the mean plasma vancomycin concentration was 6.3 μg/ml. During the four hours, 65% of the dose was absorbed. Computer modeling of the plasma data led to predicted sustained steady-state plasma concentrations of between 11 and 14.8 μg/ml from an IP loading dose of 30 mg/kg and a daily IP maintenance dose of 7 mg/kg. However, multiple dose experiments were

From the Schools of Pharmacy and Medicine, University of Wisconsin, Madison, Wisconsin.

not performed to test these predicted values. The study reported here was conducted to determine the pharmacokinetics of vancomycin following an IP loading dose and three subsequent maintenance doses.

METHODS

Patient Selection

Five noninfected patients on CAPD therapy were selected for the study. All patients were males, 32 to 63 years old (mean 50 years), weighing 64–119 kg (mean 87.8 kg). They were receiving no other antibiotics at the time of the study. Informed consent was obtained from all patients.

Drug Administration

During the study all patients received dialysate containing 1.5% dextrose. Each exchange was 2 L, and dwell times were six hours. For the first exchange, 1000 mg of vancomycin (Eli Lilly & Co.) was added to the dialysis solution. The dialysis solution was infused over 10 minutes. Simultaneous blood and dialysate samples were obtained at 0, 0.25, 0.5, 0.75, 1, 2, 3, 4, 5, and 6 hours. Blood was obtained through an indwelling forearm catheter; dialysate was removed through a three-way stopcock attached to the peritoneal catheter. Prior to sample withdrawal, the dialysate in the peritoneal cavity was mixed by means of a 50 ml syringe (Fig. 1). At six hours, the dialysate was drained and replaced with 2 L of fresh dialysis fluid containing 50 mg of vancomycin. The third and fourth exchanges

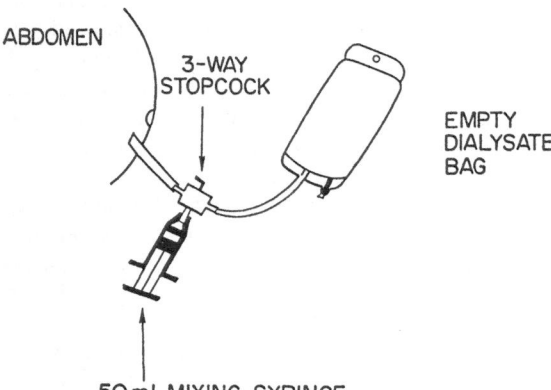

Fig. 1. Apparatus for mixing and withdrawing dialysate samples.

were performed in a similar manner. Additional blood and dialysate samples were obtained at 6.5, 7, 8, 10, 12, 13, 14, 15, 18, 19, 20, 21, and 24 hours. An aliquot of drained dialysate was obtained after each exchange. Plasma was separated from blood by centrifugation. All plasma and dialysate was stored at −20°C until assayed. All assays were performed within two weeks of the clinical study.

VANCOMYCIN ASSAY

Plasma and dialysate vancomycin concentrations were determined by a microbiological assay. The test organism was *Bacillus subtilis* ATCC 6633. Plasma standards were prepared from pooled human plasma. Dialysate standards were prepared from antibiotic-free drained dialysate obtained prior to the study. A linear standard curve was generated over a vancomycin concentration range of 0.5–100 μg/ml ($r^2 = 0.998$). Samples from the first dialysate exchange were diluted 20 times in sterile water. The assay was unaffected by pH over the range of 5.0–7.5.

PHARMACOKINETIC CALCULATIONS

Drug absorption from the peritoneal cavity was determined by subtracting the amount of vancomycin recovered in the dialysate from the amount initially instilled. The body volume of distribution for vancomycin (V_D) was approximated from equation 1:

$$V_D = \frac{A}{C_{peak}} \qquad (1)$$

where A = amount absorbed (mg), and C_{peak} = the peak plasma concentration obtained during the dwell. The data presented in this paper are expressed as mean ± SD.

RESULTS

No adverse effects from vancomycin administration were observed during the study. Mean plasma vancomycin concentrations during the four dialysis exchanges are shown in Figure 2. A peak concentration of 9.1 μg/ml was achieved following the loading dose. Declining vancomycin concentrations in dialysate during the first six hours are shown in Figure 3. Mean absorption of the loading dose was 63.7 ± 7.3%. At the end of six hours, the dialysate vancomycin concentration was approximately 17-fold higher than the plasma concentration, indicat-

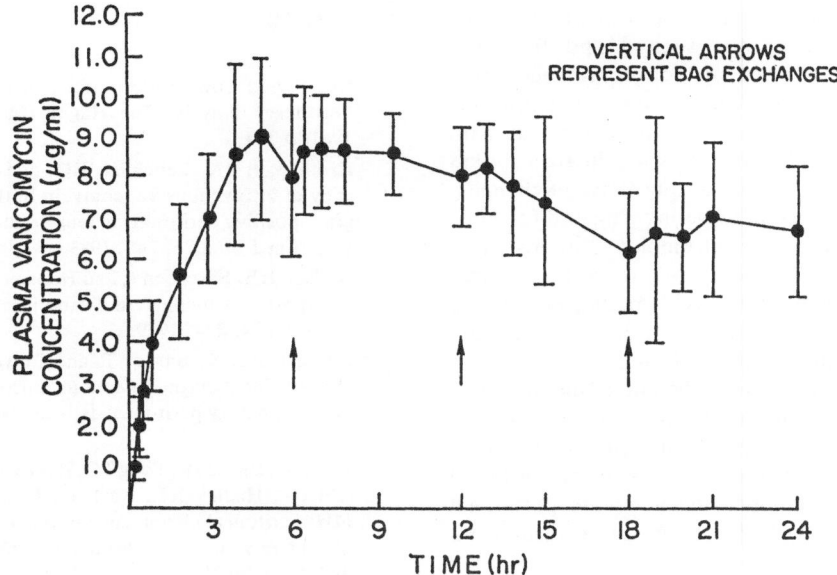

Fig. 2. Plasma vancomycin concentrations (mean ± SD).

ing that plasma-dialysate equilibrium had not been achieved.

While there was some fluctuation, the plasma concentrations during exchanges 2, 3, and 4 remained relatively constant. Mean absorption of the maintenance doses was 57%.

The V_D for vancomycin was determined during each dwell period. The values for exchanges 1–4 were 83.3 ± 26.1, 94.5 ± 15.1, 134.0 ± 55.4, and 128.0 ± 40.0 L respectively.

DISCUSSION

Staphylococcus aureus and *S. epidermidis* continue to be responsible for the majority of cases of CAPD-associated peritonitis. As a result, vancomycin is used widely in the treatment of this disease. This study has demonstrated that vancomycin can be administered safely and effectively via the intraperitoneal route. An IP dose of 1000 mg produced plasma concentrations within six hours that are therapeutic for most strains of susceptible organisms.[9] For resistant strains, especially methicillin-resistant *S. aureus*, larger doses should be employed.

The peak plasma vancomycin concentration of 9.1 μg/ml and the 64% absorption of the loading dose obtained in this study are in agreement with the data of Bunke et al.[8] Pancorbo and Comty,[7] however, reported a peak plasma concentration of 23.7

μg/ml and 54% absorption following a 1000 mg dose. The reason for this inconsistency is unclear; however, there were marked differences in observed distribution volumes. In addition, Pancorbo and Comty[7] employed a radioimmunoassay, while Bunke et al.[8] and the present study determined vancomycin concentrations by microbiological methods. In all three studies, relatively small patient populations were used.

As has been reported previously,[10] wide variations in distribution volumes were noted in this

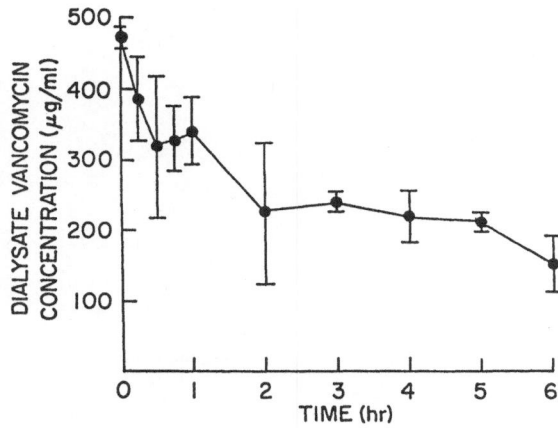

Fig. 3. Dialysate vancomycin concentrations during first exchange (mean ± SD).

study. Of interest was the apparent increase in V_D that occurred during the second and third exchanges. While drug absorption continued during these exchanges, observed plasma concentrations did not increase. These data are consistent with continued penetration of vancomycin from blood into extravascular tissues during these exchanges. This observation needs to be investigated further.

The maintenance doses employed in this study provided dialysate vancomycin concentrations that were therapeutic for most CAPD-pathogens. Bunke et al.[8] demonstrated a rapid decline in dialysate vancomycin concentrations during the exchanges following the loading dose, when no IP maintenance dose was used. Addition of a maintenance dose to the dialysate, in a concentration equal or similar to the plasma concentration obtained from the initial loading dose, should provide adequate peritoneal fluid concentrations and prevent loss of drug from the plasma into dialysate.

In conclusion, therapeutic systemic concentrations of vancomycin can be achieved by IP administration to CAPD patients. The plasma concentration can be controlled by the concentration of drug in dialysate and the length of the dwell. IP drug administration can be done quickly and, in most cases, by the patient at home. Such an approach may reduce hospitalization for the purpose of IV vancomycin administration. Since these data were obtained from noninfected patients, the effects of peritonitis on vancomycin pharmacokinetics need to be examined.

ACKNOWLEDGMENTS

Supported by a grant from Eli Lilly and Co., Indianapolis, IN.

REFERENCES

1. Vas S, and Low D: Peritonitis. In Nolph KD (Ed), Peritoneal dialysis. The Hague: Martinus Nijhoff, 1981, p 344

2. Krothapalli RK, Senekjian HO, and Ayus JC: Efficacy of intravenous vancomycin in the treatment of gram-positive peritonitis in long-term peritoneal dialysis. Am J Med 75: 345, 1983

3. Nielsen HE, Sorensen I, and Hansen HE: Peritoneal transport of vancomycin during peritoneal dialysis. Nephron 24: 274, 1979

4. Rubin J, Ray R, Barnes T, and Bower J: Peritoneal abnormalities during infectious episodes of continuous ambulatory peritoneal dialysis. Nephron 29: 124, 1981

5. Ayus JC, Eneas JF, Tong TG, Benowitz NL, Schoenfeld PY, Hadley KL, Becker CE, and Humphreys MH: Peritoneal clearance and total body elimination of vancomycin during chronic intermittent peritoneal dialysis. Clin Nephrol 11: 129, 1979

6. Magera BE, Arroyo JC, Rosansky SJ, and Postic B: Vancomycin pharmacokinetics in patients with peritonitis on peritoneal dialysis. Antimicrob Agents Chemother 23: 710, 1983

7. Pancorbo S, and Comty C. Peritoneal transport of vancomycin in 4 patients undergoing continuous ambulatory peritoneal dialysis. Nephron 31: 37, 1982

8. Bunke CM, Aronoff GR, Brier ME, Sloan RS, and Luft FC. Vancomycin kinetics during continuous ambulatory peritoneal dialysis. Clin Pharmacol Ther 34: 631, 1983

9. Cunha BA, and Ristuccia AM: Clinical usefulness of vancomycin. Clin Pharm 2: 417, 1983

10. Matzke GR, McGory RW, Halstenson CE, and Keane WF: Pharmacokinetics of vancomycin in patients with various degrees of renal function. Antimicrob Agents Chemother 25: 433, 1984

G.D. Morse, D.M. Janicke, R.F. Cafarell, M.A. Apicella,
W.J. Jusko, R.C. Venuto, and J.J. Walshe

24

IP Administration of Moxalactam during CAPD

SUMMARY

The pharmacokinetics of moxalactam were studied in eight patients on continuous ambulatory peritoneal dialysis. Patients received moxalactam intravenously (IV) and intraperitoneally (IP) in 1.0 g or 2.0 g dosages. Serum, dialysate and urine samples were obtained for 72 hours. Moxalactam absorption from the peritoneal cavity was 88 ± 2.1% of that administered. Mean peak serum concentration after the 2.0 g IP dose was 98.4 ± 25.6 μg/ml and remained >29 μg/ml after 24 hours. The 1.0 g IP dose gave a peak level of 20.9 ± 8.9 μg/ml and remained >7 μg/ml at 24 hours. Diarrhea developed in all patients receiving the 2.0 g dose. No side effects were noted after 1.0 g. Based on these results 1.0 g of moxalactam given IP every 24 hours should be adequate to treat susceptible organisms causing local or systemic infections in CAPD patients.

INTRODUCTION

Bacterial peritonitis in patients on CAPD is primarily caused by Staphylococci and aerobic gram-negative bacilli.[1] Initial antibiotic therapy is frequently empiric. Moxalactam is an extended-spectrum cephalosporin with increased activity against Staphylococci; it is a potentially useful alternative antibiotic for CAPD peritonitis.[2]

From the Departments of Pharmacy and Medicine, State University of New York at Buffalo, Buffalo, New York.

Administration of antibiotics for CAPD peritonitis evolved from initial reports, which favored parenteral therapy, to more recent experiences, which stressed the role of IP administration.[3,4] Rational use of IP administration requires knowledge of the pharmacokinetic characteristics of individual antibiotics following IP instillation. The purpose of this study was to investigate the clinical pharmacokinetics of moxalactam in noninfected CAPD patients and describe preliminary dosing guidelines.

MATERIALS AND METHODS

Subjects

Eight adult ESRD patients participating in the CAPD program at the Erie County Medical Center were enrolled in this study. Patients were excluded from the study on the following basis: a history of recent infection, having received antibiotic therapy within two weeks prior to the study period, a history of penicillin or cephalosporin allergy, abnormal coagulation parameters, or a hematocrit <20%. All patients were functionally anephric (Cl_{cr} < 3 ml/min). Informed consent was obtained from all patients prior to initiating the study. Demographic data are presented in Table 1.

Study Design

A randomized, crossover study design was utilized whereby each subject was to receive both an

Table 1. Patient Characteristics.

Patient Number	Sex	Age (yrs)	Weight (Kg)	Diagnosis	CAPD Duration (months)
1	M	47	87.3	Hypertensive nephrosclerosis	11
2	M	70	64.1	Chronic glomerulonephritis	11
3	M	71	57.3	Obstructive uropathy	16
4	M	61	65.9	Unknown etiology	13
5	M	59	77.3	Amyloidosis	16
6	F	35	59.1	Sclerosing glomerulonephritis	5
7	M	71	57.3	Obstructive uropathy	19
8	M	73	63.6	Unknown etiology	3

Demographic data describing CAPD patients who received moxalactam.

IV and IP dose of moxalactam with a 1–2 week washout period between doses. Patients were studied in the CAPD unit for the first 12–24 hours and then on an ambulatory basis for the remaining sample collection period. Prior to moxalactam administration, a complete blood count, serum electrolyte, creatinine, glucose, and blood urea nitrogen concentrations and prothrombin time were determined. Throughout the study period, all urine excreted was measured and aliquots stored at −70°C.

Intravenous Administration

Following a 10-minute gravity-fed infusion of 2 L dialysis fluid (Dianeal® 137 with 1.5% dextrose) into the peritoneum, a single 1.0 g or 2.0 g dose of moxalactam (Eli Lilly Co., Lot No. 6CM31A) was administered over 2–4 minutes through an indwelling venous catheter. During the initial 24-hour period, dialysis fluid exchanges were made approximately every six hours. Blood samples (5 ml) were collected in nonheparinized Vacutainers® from an indwelling venous catheter in the arm contralateral to the infusion site at 0, 0.08, 0.25, 0.5, 0.75, 1, 2, 4, 6 (end of first dialysis cycle), 7, 9, 12 (end of second dialysis cycle), 24, 48, and 72 hours after drug administration. Peritoneal dialysate (5 ml) was collected after discarding the first 7 ml (peritoneal catheter volume) at 0, 0.25, 0.5, 0.75, 1, 2, 4, 6, 7, 9, and 12 hours after drug administration. Dialysis fluid exchanges continued on a six-hour basis, with the volume of each exchange recorded and an aliquot taken.

IP Administration

A single 1.0 g or 2.0 g dose of moxalactam (Eli Lilly Co., Lot No. 6CM31A) was admixed with the first 2 L dialysis fluid. The dialysis fluid was then introduced into the peritoneal cavity by gravity infusion over 10 minutes. Blood and dialysis fluid samples were collected as described.

Drug Analysis

Blood was allowed to clot at room temperature and serum was obtained by centrifugation. Serum and dialysate samples were placed in dry ice within one hour of collection and then stored at −70°C until assayed. However, dialysate samples that were collected on an ambulatory basis were stored at room temperature for up to 12 hours prior to freezing.

The concentration of moxalactam in serum and dialysate was determined by high pressure liquid chromatography analysis. The mobile phase consisted of 9% methanol/91% 0.1 M phosphate buffer at pH 7.0. Separation was obtained on a Whatman RAC ODS column at a flow rate of 3.0 ml/min, and was detected at a wavelength of 280 nm by a Waters 441 Detector.

A 50:50 epimer mixture of moxalactam (Lilly Research Laboratories) was used as the analytical standard. Serum standards were prepared in blank pooled plasma, and the dialysate standards were prepared in 0.1 M phosphate buffer at pH 7.0. Standards (1.56–100 μg/ml) were run in duplicate and peak areas determined by integration. If necessary, samples were diluted to be within the range of the standard curve.

Moxalactam was extracted from serum and dialysate by a modification of the method of Ziemniak et al.[5] Initially, 500 μl of 0.07 M KCl-HCl buffer at pH 1.0 was added to 500 μl of sample. Protein precipitation was then carried out by the addition of 200 μl of concentrated HCl. Ethyl acetate (3.0 ml) was added and then the drug was back extracted into 0.1 M phosphate buffer, pH 8.0, following shaking (5 min) and centrifugation (1000 × g; 5 min). Prior to injection of the sample onto the column, the phosphate buffer fraction was partially evaporated under nitrogen (28°C; 20 min) to remove residual ethyl acetate, which was found to interfere with the chromatography. Cephacetrile (Ciba-Geigy), used as the internal standard, was added with the ethyl acetate and subsequently eluted after moxalactam.

The intraday relative standard deviation of the 50 μg/ml moxalactam plasma standard was 2.6 ± 0.05% (n = 4). The corresponding intraday values for the 6.25 μg/ml concentration was 6.4 ± 0.02% (n = 5). The interday relative standard deviation of moxalactam plasma standards was 5.1 ± 2.49% (n = 6) at 50 μg/ml and 6.4 ± 0.41% (n = 6) at 6.25 μg/ml. Measured recovery of moxalactam from plasma was 59.8 ± 1.97% for the 50 μg/ml (n = 4) plasma standard and 59.1 ± 5.41% for the 6.25 μg/ml (n = 4) plasma standards.

Pharmacokinetic Analysis

Noncompartmental analysis was used to calculate the time-average pharmacokinetic parameters describing the disposition of moxalactam.[6] Lagrange polynomial interpolation of the serum moxalactam concentrations versus time, and subsequent integration of the fitted polynomial over each experimental time interval, was used to calculate the area under the serum concentration-time curve (AUC).[7] Residual AUC was determined from the quotient of the final concentration-time point (Cp) and terminal slope (k_e).

The apparent serum clearance (CL) and the peritoneal dialysis clearance (CLPD) for moxalactam were determined by the equations 1 and 2:

$$CL = F \: Dose/AUC \qquad (1)$$

$$CLPD = XPD|_6^{24}/AUC|_6^{24} \qquad (2)$$

where, $XPD|_6^{24}$ equals the amount of drug recovered in the dialysis fluid from 6–24 hours, dose equals the administered dose, and F equals the fraction of moxalactam systemically absorbed (see below). The volume of distribution (V_d) was calculated as the product of CL and k_e.

The fraction of moxalactam systemically absorbed (F) following IP administration was calculated as the ratio of the AUC following IP and IV dosing, with the assumption that clearance remained constant during each part of the study:

$$F = AUC \: IP/AUC \: IV \qquad (3)$$

The F was also calculated based on the amount of drug recovered in the dialysate following IP administration:

$$F = Dose \: IP - XPD \: at \: 6.0 \: h/Dose \: IP \qquad (4)$$

where, XPD at 6 hours is the drug recovered in the dialysate following a six-hour dialysis cycle. Half-life (t½) was determined from the terminal slope, which was calculated by least-squares regression analysis.

RESULTS

Subjects

Physical and biochemical evaluation of all subjects at the time of entry into each study period did not reveal clinical or microbiologic evidence of bacterial peritonitis. All laboratory examinations were within expected limits for patients with chronic renal failure. Three patients who received a 2.0 g dose of moxalactam (IV and IP) developed diarrhea approximately 24 hours following administration. The diarrhea was not associated with abdominal discomfort and lasted less than 24 hours. Patient No. 3 withdrew when diarrhea developed after the IV dose. Patients No. 4 and 5 received 1.0 g IV and IP and successfully completed both phases of the study. Patients No. 6, 7, and 8 received 1.0 g IP only without adverse effects.

Pharmacokinetics

Representative serum and dialysate concentration-time profiles of moxalactam following a 2.0 g and 1.0 g IP dose are shown in Figures 1 and 2. Mean moxalactam serum concentrations following a 2.0 g IP dose were 98.4 ± 36 μg/ml at 6 hours (peak values) after administration and 35.4 ± 7.8 μg/ml at 24 hours. A 1.0 g dose yielded mean moxalactam serum concentrations of 44.7 ± 3.9 μg/ml at six hours, and 20.9 ± 8.9 μg/ml at 24 hours.

Mean moxalactam dialysate concentrations at 0.5 hours were 466 ± 23 μg/ml and 310 ± 90 μg/ml for the 2.0 g and 1.0 g doses, respectively. Mean moxalactam dialysate concentrations at 24 hours were 11.4 ± 7.9 μg/ml (2.0 g) and 7.88 ± 3.2 μg/ml (1.0 g). Individual patient serum and dialysate data are summarized in Table 2.

Moxalactam absorption was evaluated in four patients with mean bioavailability (F) values of 80 ± 22%. Application of equation 4 to the seven patients

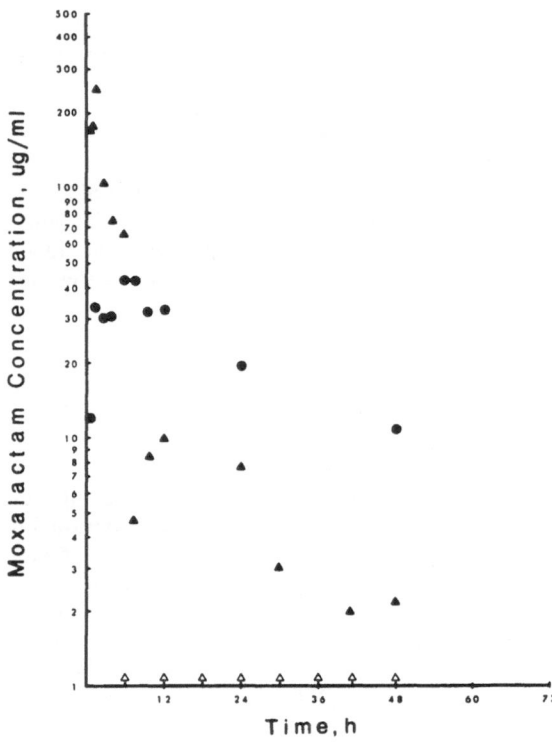

Fig. 1. Serum and dialysate concentration-time profile of moxalactam for Patient No. 1 after a 1.0 g IP dose of moxalactam (serum = ●, dialysate = ▲).

Fig. 2. Serum and dialysate concentration-time profile of moxalactam for Patient No. 1 after a 2.0 g IP dose of moxalactam (serum = ●, dialysate = ▲).

Table 2. Moxalactam Concentration Following IP Administration.

Dose	Patient Number	Serum (μg/ml) Peak	Serum (μg/ml) 24 h	Dialysis Fluid (μg/ml) 0.5 h	Dialysis Fluid (μg/ml) 24 h
2.0 g					
	1	72.7	29.8	483	5.82
	2	124.0	40.9	450	17.00
	3	*	*	*	*
	X̄	98.4	35.4	466	11.40
1.0 g					
	4	46.1	11.6	437	3.61
	5	48.3	33.0	349	9.10
	6	39.8	19.0	202	11.30
	7	41.3	QNS	313	9.77
	8	48.2	19.9	252	5.61
	X̄	44.7	20.9	310	7.88
	± S.D.	3.9	8.9	90	3.20

* Patient No. 3 withdrew following IV dose. QNS—insufficient quantity for analysis. Moxalactam, serum, and dialysate concentrations following a 2.0 g or 1.0 g IP dose.

who received an IP dose yielded F values of 85.6 ± 9.3%. Serum clearance of moxalactam was 12.7 ± 31 ml/min and peritoneal dialysis clearance (1.87 ± 0.9 ml/min) contributed only 15%. The mean V_d of moxalactam was 0.29 ± 0.1 L/Kg, and serum half-life was 17.7 ± 2.7 hours. Individual patient pharmacokinetic parameters are presented in Table 3.

DISCUSSION

Intraperitoneal antibiotic administration is used increasingly as the preferred treatment of bacterial peritonitis in CAPD patients.[3,4] It has been assumed that providing high antibiotic concentrations within the peritoneal cavity is beneficial when treating a "localized" infection of the peritoneum. In fact, the significance of peritoneal fluid antibiotic concentrations and their role in treating this infection has yet to be determined. However, this is the rationale behind maintaining elevated dialysate antibiotic concentrations throughout therapy via the addition of antibiotics to every dialysis exchange.

In the present study IP moxalactam was well absorbed and attained serum and dialysate concentrations exceeding the minimum inhibitory concentrations for susceptible organisms. For example, the MIC-90 levels for *S. marcescens* and *E. coli* are usually less than 1 μg/ml while that of *S. aureus* is 6 μg/ml or less. In our patients the 24-hour serum and dialysate levels after 1 gm of moxalactam IP were 20 μg/ml and 8 μg/ml, respectively. The extensive absorption of IP moxalactam is consistent with other studies that examined IP antibiotic administration.[1,8-11] Previous reports described antibiotic movement across the peritoneal membrane as "unidirectional." Those authors noted good absorption following IP administration but minimal drug removal by peritoneal dialysis. Closer consideration of pharmacokinetic principles may explain this phenomenon.

The IP administration presents a high concentration of unbound drug to the peritoneal surface. This unbound (free) drug is available for diffusion across the mesothelial and endothelial barriers into the systemic circulation. Upon entry into the vascular space, antibiotics bind to plasma proteins to varying degrees based on individual physicochemical properties unique to each drug.[12] The plasma concentration of unbound antibiotic becomes the driving force for drug distribution into peripheral body compartments (Fig. 3). The volume of drug distribution in the body is a function of individual drug characteristics, and along with extraperitoneal

Table 3. Pharmacokinetic Parameters of Moxalactam.

Patient Number	Cl (ml/min)	Cl_{pd} (ml/min)	V_d (l/Kg)	t (1/2) (h)
1	10.0	1.16	0.14	14.5
2	9.1	1.23	0.23	18.4
3	12.6	1.20	0.25	13.3
4	15.9	2.98	0.37	17.6
5	15.7	2.78	0.31	18.2
6	15.2	3.18	0.42	20.9
7	10.0	1.45	0.26	17.6
8	11.0	1.12	0.32	20.8
$\overline{X}$	12.7	1.87	0.29	17.7
± S.D.	3.1	0.90	0.10	2.7

Pharmacokinetic parameters obtained following IP administration.

clearance mechanisms, determines the plasma concentrations achieved following a given dose of IP antibiotic. The combined effects of antibiotic distribution and plasma protein binding tend to lessen the concentration of unbound drug, which ultimately creates the diffusion gradient for drug transfer back into the peritoneal cavity. The net result is unimpeded drug absorption followed by minimal removal from the circulation.

These observations bring forth questions with regard to current treatment regimens for CAPD peritonitis that include the addition of antibiotics to dialysis fluid throughout the entire period of therapy. The data presented in this paper with regard to

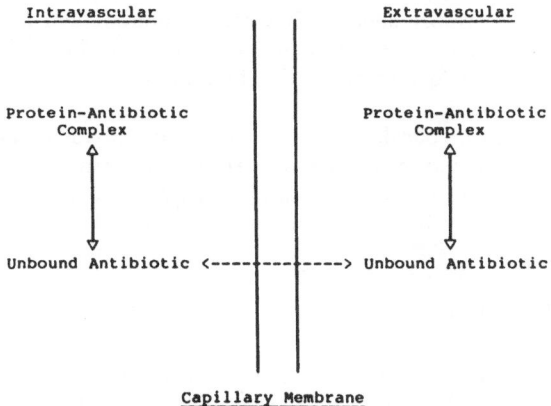

Fig. 3. The unbound (free) antibiotic concentration in serum provides the driving force for extravascular drug distribution.

moxalactam are similar to those for other beta-lactam antibiotics and suggest that less frequent dosing may be advisable.[10, 11, 13] Despite the low peritoneal clearance, dialysate antibiotic concentrations exceed the MIC for susceptible pathogens. Administration of antibiotics on a once-daily basis would avoid continuous exposure to potentially toxic antibiotics, require less frequent injections into dialysis fluid, avoiding potential contamination, and reduce drug expense incurred during treatment.

The advantages of this alternative method may be outweighed by possible dose-related side effects. Although most single-dose antibiotic studies in noninfected CAPD patients report minimal drug-related toxicity, this study describes a dose-related gastrointestinal side effect secondary to moxalactam. All patients who received a single 2.0 g dose either IV or IP developed diarrhea on the second study day. This problem was avoided when the dose was decreased to 1.0 g. Other studies in dialysis patients used a 1.0 g dose of moxalactam without related side effects.[14, 15] Biliary excretion of elevated moxalactam concentrations or the combined effect of elevated serum and dialysate moxalactam concentrations permeating the bowel may explain the dose-related diarrhea. The diarrhea subsided on the third study day in all three patients without further gastrointestinal problems, suggesting a dose-response relationship.

Numerous antibiotic studies in noninfected CAPD patients have extrapolated their results to make recommendations for treatment of peritonitis. The possible compounding variables during bacterial peritonitis—such as changes in membrane permeability, increased protein concentration in dialysate, etc.—may alter the pharmacokinetic behavior that is observed in the noninfected patient. We therefore suggest that data in noninfected patients be used as a guideline to establish dosing regimens for further evaluation in patients with CAPD peritonitis.

From our data it appears that 1.0 g moxalactam IP administered once daily results in serum and dialysate concentrations that appear adequate to treat local as well as systemic infection for 24 hours.

REFERENCES

1. Bunke CM, Aronoff G, Breier ME, Sloan RS, and Luft FC: Vancomycin kinetics during continuous ambulatory peritoneal dialysis. Clin Pharmacol Ther 34: 631, 1983

2. Fitzpatrick BJ, and Stardiford HC: A comparative evaluation of moxalactam: antimicrobial activity, pharmacokinetics, adverse reactions and clinical efficacy. Pharmacotherapy 2: 197, 1982

3. Rubin J, Rogers WA, Taylor HM, Everett ED, Prowant BF, Fruto LV, and Nolph KD: Peritonitis during continuous ambulatory peritoneal dialysis. Ann Intern Med 92: 7, 1980

4. Gokal R: Peritonitis in continuous ambulatory peritoneal dialysis. J Antimicrob Chemother 9: 417, 1982

5. Ziemniak JA, Chiarmonte DA. Miner DJ, and Schentag JJ: HPLC determination of D and L moxalactam in human serum and urine. J Pharm Sci 71: 399, 1982

6. Jusko WJ: Guidelines for collection and pharmacokinetic analysis of drug disposition data. In Evans WE, Schentag JJ, and Jusko WJ (Eds), Applied pharmacokinetics. San Francisco: Applied Therapeutics, Inc, 1980, p 639

7. Yeh KC, and Kwan KC: A comparison of numerical integrating algorithms by trapezoidal, Lagrange, and Spline approximation. J Pharmacokinetics Biopharmaceutics 6: 79, 1978

8. Somani P, Shapiro RS, Stockard H, and Higgins TT: Unidirectional absorption of gentamicin from the peritoneum during continuous ambulatory peritoneal dialysis. Clin Pharmacol Ther 32: 113, 1982

9. Pancorbo S, and Comty C: Pharmacokinetics of gentamicin in patients undergoing continuous ambulatory peritoneal dialysis. Antimicrob Agent Chemother 19: 605, 1981

10. Bunke CM, Aronoff G, Breier ME, Sloan RS, and Luft FC: Cefazolin and cephalexin kinetics in continuous ambulatory peritoneal dialysis. Clin Pharmacol Ther 33: 66, 1983

11. Jansen A, Pelz K, Keller E, Schollmeyer P, and Hoppe-Seyler G: Plasma levels of cefoperazone after intraperitoneal application. Clin Pharmacol Ther (Abstract) 33: 235, 1983

12. Gwilt PR, and Perrier D: Plasma protein binding and distribution characteristics of drugs as indices of their hemodialyzability. Clin Pharmacol Ther 24: 154, 1978

13. Singlas E, Boutron HF, Merdjan H, Brocard JF, Pocheville M, and Fries D: Moxalactam kinetics during chronic ambulatory peritoneal dialysis. Clin Pharmacol Ther 34: 403, 1983

14. Aronoff G, Sloan R, Mong S, Luft FC, and Kleit SA: Moxalactam pharmacokinetics during hemodialysis. Antimicrob Agent Chemother 19: 575, 1981

15. Srinivasan S, and Neu HC. Pharmacokinetics of moxalactam in patients with renal failure and during hemodialysis. Antimicrob Agent Chemother 20: 398, 1981

SECTION II

Technology Access, Solutions

H.A. Frank

25

Experimental and Clinical Origins of Peritoneal Dialysis for Renal Failure

SUMMARY

The experimental and clinical origins of peritoneal dialysis have been reviewed. Shortly after
World War II understanding of acute renal failure, of
fluid and electrolyte balance and dialysis reached a
level that encouraged clinical application of peritoneal dialysis. This achieved the first survival attributed to control by peritoneal dialysis of the effects of
acute renal failure. Subsequent developments in the
dialysis procedure have been reviewed.

INTRODUCTION

I am not undertaking an official history, but will
describe briefly our experiences with peritoneal
dialysis in the setting of the 1940s. Unfortunately,
my colleagues, Drs. Arnold Seligman and Jacob
Fine are no longer alive. We three worked together
during World War II, studying shock and war injuries under the auspices of the U.S. Office of Scientific
Research and Development. Reports from the field
during the Italian campaign described the occurrence of anuria and uremia in soldiers who had
seemed to have recovered from shock and the other
initial effects of injury. An incorrect physiological
notion persisting from World War I, that shock was a

From the Department of Surgery and the Charles A.
Dana Research Institute, Beth Israel Hospital and Harvard
Medical School, Boston, Massachusetts.

deficit specifically in plasma volume due to a generalized increase in capillary permeability (a notion,
incidentally that we in our laboratory were disproving by means of new radioisotopic methods), led to
an underutilization of whole blood and also to an
inadequate preparation for transfusion therapy in
the American armed forces of this theater.[1] Therefore, transfusion mismatch reaction must be added
to shock as a cause of renal shutdown in these
soldiers, and there were other causes, such as the
crush injuries studied so well by Bywaters[2] among
civilians during the bombings of London, and the
widespread use of sulfonamides among civilians
and soldiers. Physiological studies in the field
and postmortem observations in military and civil-
ian hospitals established two key points: that the
mortality rate in post-traumatic anuria was greater
than 90%, but that the renal lesions seemed potentially reversible, if survival time could be extended
sufficiently.[3-7]

Our group undertook to extend survival by
extrarenal dialysis. The two classic papers by Putnam[8] and by Abel, Rowntree, and Turner[9] in the
early 1900s were primarily pharmacological studies,
but they indicated the possibility of substitution for
renal glomerular function by extracorporeal hemodialysis, or *in vivo* dialysis via the peritoneal membrane. We were only vaguely aware of Dr. Kolff's
work at the time,[10] and it does not really bear on our
present story, but I must acknowledge my admira-
tion for his effective clinical research during the
hostile occupation of his country.

Table 1. Chemical Composition
(g/L) of Peritoneal Dialysis Fluid.

NaCl	7.25
KCl	0.2
CaCl$_2$ (anhyd.)	0.1
MgCl$_2$ · 6H$_2$O	0.2
NaH$_2$PO4	0
NaHCO$_3$	1.5
Dextrose	10.0
Gelatin	10.0
Final pH	7.4

We chose to apply dialysis via the peritoneal membrane. In designing our dialysis fluid we turned to James Gamble's[11] studies of the composition of the extracellular fluid, for we shared his view that restoration of the electrolyte composition of the extracellular fluid is more essential to the immediate survival of an anuric animal or patient than is the correction of azotemia. An example of fluid composition is shown in Table 1. Because nearly all of our patients were severely overhydrated, we made the dialysis fluid hypertonic, using 1% colloid as well as 1% dextrose in order to avoid the irritant effect of a more concentrated dextrose solution. We prepared and sterilized these solutions in large carboys by hand, with care to separate the bicarbonate from the remaining constitutents during the heating process. Since it was evident that failure to retrieve the infused peritoneal fluid would vitiate the dialysis, we gave attention at the outset to the method of peritoneal drainage, and chose the sump drain principle, with which we were familiar in surgery.

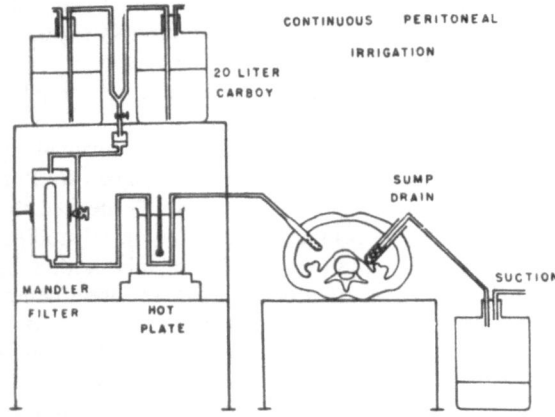

Fig. 1. Diagram of our initial system for peritoneal dialysis by continuous flow.

Our experimental work was done in dogs.[12] After bilateral nephrectomy and placement of peritoneal irrigation tubes under general anesthesia, the animals were allowed to awaken and to become severely uremic; by 72 hours, untreated dogs began to die. We determined optimal peritoneal irrigation flow rate for maximum urea clearance (25–50 ml/min) and achieved an urea clearance averaging 24 ml/m^2/min, which is 41–48% of average renal urea clearance in the dog. Intermittent irrigation corrected azotemia and acidosis and maintained survival for periods many days longer than had been achieved previously. The animals were released to run about and eat normally during intervals between irrigation periods. No dog died of uremia. Clearance by means of irrigation of segments of intestine was also tested and found to be too low to be useful.

As we entered upon our experimental work we found references in the European literature of two decades earlier, to both experimental and clinical attempts to correct uremia by peritoneal dialysis. Several of these authors are noted here together with later American reports.[13–17] Inadequacies in fluid composition or of peritoneal flow volumes limited the effectiveness of these efforts. Jonathan Rhoads, a leading academic surgeon, was fully cognizant of the fluid and electrolyte considerations, but applied the method in only a small number of patients, all irreversibly uremic.[15] The Wear group reported inability to correct acidosis by the solutions they used[16]; one of their patients recovered following the spontaneous release of a transient bladder obstruction and was the only survivor among the 13 patients treated by all of the investigators listed here.

Nevertheless, our successful experience in the laboratory encouraged clinical application. We constructed Gamble columns and set up our irrigation system (Fig. 1).[18] The whole system was homemade (Fig. 2). The first patient was a woman with bilateral ureteric obstruction due to ovarian carcinoma. Urea clearances of 13–16 ml/min were achieved, with chemical and clinical improvement. Because the neoplastic process produced intestinal as well as ureteral obstruction, we had the opportunity to test gastrointestinal suction drainage and irrigation of an isolated ileal segment. These were ineffective for solute clearance mechanisms. We calculated that over 10 feet of small bowel as an isolated segment would have been required to supply 10% of normal renal urea clearance. The patient whose course is shown in Figure 3 was the first recorded recovery from acute renal failure that can be attributed to peritoneal dialysis.[20] He was admitted to our hospital intensely uremic, acidotic, and edematous, after

10 days of anuria due to sulfathiazole intoxication. His favorable response to peritoneal dialysis is charted here, as well as the onset of renal recovery. As we see, for 3–4 days after urine output returned, he remained dependent on peritoneal dialysis for nitrogenous excretion. He went on to full recovery.

By 1948, the Mayo Clinic was able to collect 101 cases of renal insufficiency in whom peritoneal lavage was undertaken.[20] In only 63 of these patients was the renal lesion considered reversible, and 32 (51%) of these recovered. Our own final clinical report was given in September, 1948.[21] It emphasized the importance of integration of systemic management with dialysis. We modified the original sump drain catheters to provide a flexible shaft that could be led into the pelvis and used both for inflow and outflow (Fig. 4). By this time we had become convinced that uremia could be consistently controlled and that the dominant residual problem was that of bacterial invasion of the peritoneal cavity. We achieved systems that entirely excluded skin, air, or other extrinsic contamination, but could not prevent the entry of enteric organisms, and returned to dog experiments in which we demonstrated the transmural migration of radioactively tagged *E. coli* through the intact intestinal wall under circumstances of peritoneal irritation.[22] Although the solution used for peritoneal dialysis did not provoke bacterial entry in normal dogs during irrigation periods of two weeks and longer, bacterial entry did occur after four days of peritoneal irrigation in uremic dogs,[23] but could be prevented by the oral administration of nonabsorbable antibiotics active against coliform organisms.

Our own work in this field ended in this period of "handcraft." Our experience and that of others including Kop[24] in Holland, Grollman et al.[25] in Texas, Doolan et al.[26] in U.S. Naval Hospitals had clearly established the appropriate compositions of dialysis fluids, the continuing efficacy of properly conducted peritoneal dialysis—the clinical outcome which was of course dependent upon the underlying disease or injury, and the requirements for concurrent systemic management of fluids, electrolytes, and nutrition. In fact, the improved systemic management of acute renal failure that emerged from this experience often eliminated the need for the dialysis procedure.[27]

For later years I will venture to mention names only with the diffidence of a distant onlooker. According to Mr. Patrick T. McBride,[28] historian of our Bulletin, the next step, here dated 1959, is primarily due to M.H. Maxwell.[29] The rubber-glass-steel era was replaced by bio-acceptable plastics, and off-the-

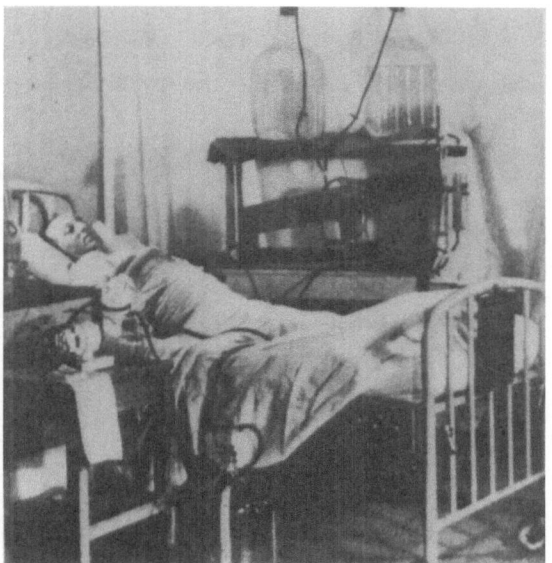

Fig. 2. Photograph of peritoneal irrigation system in operation for patient in Figure 3.

shelf equipment and solutions were developed that made peritoneal dialysis convenient, widely available, and relatively routine. At the same time, the dominant clinical need shifted from the acute problems of the wartime setting to those of chronic and end-stage renal disease. In the hands of Boen,[30]

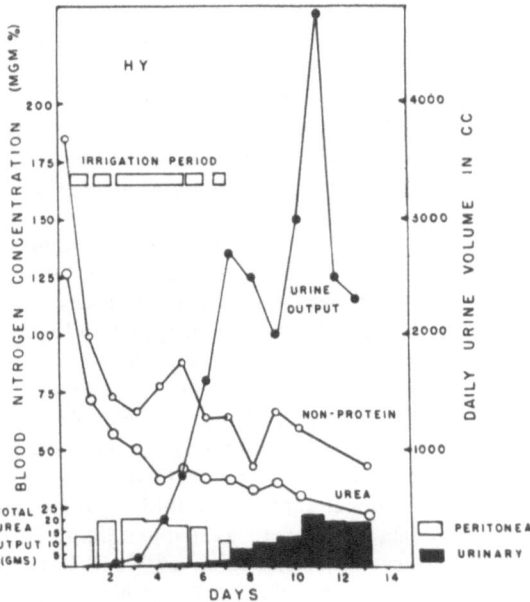

Fig. 3. Correction of azotemia and recovery of urine output in the first case of acute renal failure successfully treated by peritoneal dialysis.

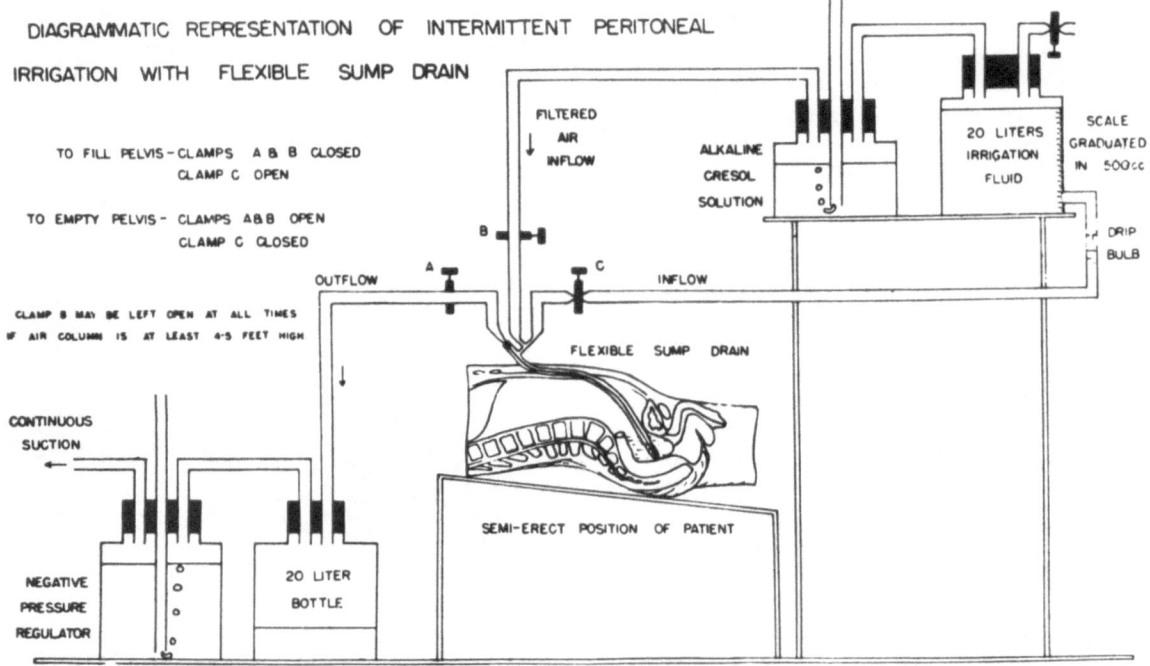

DIAGRAMMATIC REPRESENTATION OF INTERMITTENT PERITONEAL
IRRIGATION WITH FLEXIBLE SUMP DRAIN

Fig. 4. Modified system for peritoneal dialysis by alternating inflow and outflow.

Mion et al.,[31] Burns et al.,[32] and their many colleagues, methods for long-term intermittent peritoneal dialysis were developed and applied.

The date 1968 is noted for the introduction by Tenckhoff and Schechter[33] of a well-tolerated chronically implanted peritoneal catheter, which with modifications by them and others facilitated intermittent dialysis in hospital or at home. Subsequently we saw the more continuous ambulatory exchange proposed and conducted successfully by Popovich, Moncrief, Oreopoulos, and others.[34, 35] The time intervals in these steps are rather typical of bio-mechanical innovation, which is characterized by the interdependence of conceptual and methodological factors, and often awaits the development of new materials. We may note, for example, that John Gibbon had worked out the physiological requirements for cardiopulmonary bypass surgery in animal experiments by 1937, but did not achieve successful clinical application until 1953, when appropriate materials were available. Similarly, Dr. Kolff observed arterialization of blood during its passage through the tubing of his artificial kidney in 1944, but a satisfactory membrane oxygenator was not developed experimentally until 1956 or applied clinically until 1958.

I look forward to learning whether peritoneal infection remains a problem. In our shorter treatment periods under hospital supervision, skin and other external sources of bacterial invasion could be eliminated, but the problems for chronic dialysis are obviously more difficult. In closing, from the perspective of 40 years, it is pleasing to observe that peritoneal dialysis is now a standard treatment for chronic renal insufficiency, and has matured to the stage of being evaluated not only in physiological and mechanical terms but by the quality of life it provides.[36]

REFERENCES

1. Beecher HK, and Altschule MD: Medicine at Harvard. The First Three Hundred Years. New Hampshire: University Press of New England, 1977, p 506
2. Bywaters EGL: Ischemic muscle necrosis. Crushing injury, traumatic anuria, compression syndrome: a type of injury seen in air raid casualties following burial beneath debris. JAMA 124: 1103, 1944
3. Burnett CH, Shapiro SL, Simeone FA, Beecher HK, Mallory TB, and Sullivan ER: Renal function studies in the wounded. Surgery 22: 856, 1947
4. Lucké B: Lower nephron nephrosis: renal lesion of crush syndrome of burns, transfusions, and other

conditions affecting lower segments of nephrons. Mil Surgeon 99: 371, 1946

5. Lauson HD, Bradley SE, and Cournand A: The renal circulation in shock. J Clin Invest 23: 381, 1944

6. Oliver J, MacDowell M, and Tracy A: The pathogenesis of acute renal failure associated with traumatic and toxic injury. Renal ischemia, nephrotoxic damage and ischemuric episode. J Clin Invest 30: 1305, 1951

7. Trueta J, Barclay AE, Daniel PM, Franklin KJ, and Prichard ML: Studies of the renal circulation. Springfield, IL: CC Thomas, 1947

8. Putnam TJ: The living peritoneum as a dialyzing membrane. Am J Physiol 3: 548, 1923

9. Abel JJ, Rowntree LG, and Turner BB: On removal of diffusible substances from circulating blood of living animals by dialysis. J Pharmacol Exp Ther 5: 275, 1914

10. Kolff WJ, and Van Noordwijk J: The artificial kidney. Kampen, Holland: JH Kok NV, 1946

11. Gamble JL: Chemical anatomy, physiology, and pathology of extracellular fluid. Lecture Syllabus, Harvard Medical School, 1942

12. Seligman AM, Frank HA, and Fine J: Treatment of experimental uremia by means of peritoneal irrigation. J Clin Invest 25: 211, 1946

13. Ganter G: Über die Bieseitigung giftiger Stoffe aus dem Blut durch Dialyse. Munch Med Wochschr 70: 1478, 1923

14. Heusser H, and Werder H: Untersuchungen über peritonealdialyse. Beitr Klin Chir 14: 38, 1927

15. Rhoads JE: Peritoneal lavage in the treatment of renal insufficiency. Am J Med Sci 196: 642, 1938

16. Wear JB, Sisk IR, and Trinkle AJ: Peritoneal lavage in the treatment of uremia. J Urol 39: 53, 1938

17. Rosenak SS, and Oppenheimer GD: An improved drain for peritoneal lavage. Surgery 23: 832, 1948

18. Fine J, Frank HA, and Seligman AM: The treatment of acute renal failure by peritoneal irrigation. Ann Surg 124: 857, 1946

19. Frank HA, Seligman AM, and Fine J: Treatment of uremia after acute renal failure by peritoneal irrigation. JAMA 130: 703, 1946

20. Odel HM, Ferris DO, and Power MH: Peritoneal lavage as an effective means of extrarenal excretion. Am J Med 215: 63, 1950

21. Frank HA, Seligman AM, and Fine J: Further experiences with peritoneal irrigation for acute renal failure. Ann Surg 128: 561, 1948

22. Schweinburg FB, Seligman AM, and Fine J: Transumural migration of intestinal bacteria. A study based on the use of radioactive Escherichia coli. N Engl J Med 242: 747, 1950

23. Schweinburg FB, Frank HA, Heimberg F, and Fine J: Transmural migration of intestinal bacteria during peritoneal irrigation in uremic dogs. Proc Soc Exp Biol Med 71: 150, 1949

24. Kop PSM: Peritoneale dialyse. Kampen Holland: Drukkerij JH Kok NV, 1948

25. Grollman A, Turner LB, and McLean JA: Intermittent peritoneal lavage in nephrectomized dogs and its application to the human being. Arch Intern Med 87: 379, 1951

26. Doolan PD, Murphy WP Jr, Wiggins RA, Carter NW, Cooper WC, Watten RA, and Alpen EL: An evaluation of intermittent peritoneal lavage. Am J Med 26: 831, 1959

27. Strauss MB: Acute renal insufficiency due to lower nephron nephrosis. N Engl J Med 239: 695, 1948

28. McBride PT: Pioneers in peritoneal dialysis—Morton Maxwell. Peritoneal Dial Bull 4: 58, 1984

29. Maxwell MH, Rockney RE, Kleeman CR, Twiss MR: Peritoneal dialysis. JAMA 170: 917, 1959

30. Boen ST: Kinetics of peritoneal dialysis: comparison with artificial kidney. Medicine 40: 243, 1961

31. Boen ST, Mion CM, Curtis FK, and Shilepetar G: Periodic peritoneal dialysis using the repeated puncture technique and an automatic cycling machine. Trans Am Soc Artif Intern Organs 10: 409, 1964

32. Burns RO, Henderson LW, Hager EB, and Merrill JP: Peritoneal dialysis. Clinical experience. N Engl J Med 267: 1060, 1962

33. Tenckhoff H, and Schechter H: A bacteriologically safe peritoneal access device. Trans Am Soc Artif Int Organs 14: 181, 1968

34. Popovich RP, Moncrief JW, Nolph KD, Ghods AJ, Twardowski AJ, and Pyle WK: Continuous ambulatory peritoneal dialysis. Ann Intern Med 88: 449, 1978

35. Atkins RC, Thomson NM, and Farrell PC (Eds): Peritoneal Dialysis. Melbourne: Churchill Livingstone, 1981, p 313

36. Churchill DN, Morgan J, and Torrance GW: Quality of life in end-stage renal disease. Peritoneal Dial Bull 4: 20, 1984

S.R. Ash, D.J. Carr, D.E. Blake, and J.A. Thornhill

26

The Sorbent Suspension Reciprocating Dialyzer for Use in Peritoneal Dialysis

SUMMARY

The greatest cost of peritoneal dialysis is in the preparation, packaging, and shipping of sterile dialysis fluid. CAPD and CCPD represent attempts to support patients on the minimal volumes of such dialysis fluid. Sorbent chemicals which regenerate dialysate could decrease the shipping weight of disposables, while allowing much higher dialysate flows.

A plate dialyzer with screen supports has been designed which can operate with a thick sorbent suspension on the screen side (SSRD). The sorbent suspension contains charcoal, covalently-bound urease, calcium-loaded zeolites, and hydrogen-loaded cation exchangers. Alteration in pressure of the sorbent suspension propels 200 ml of peritoneal dialysate into and out of the dialyzer (through a single central port), where it lies directly across the membrane from the sorbent suspension. In tests of the SSRD on dogs with BUN 50–60 mg/dl and plasma creatinine 6 mg/dl, the clearances, of urea and creatinine were 80–100 ml/min, phosphorus was 50, and K was 20 ml/min for 4 hours. These clearances are high enough to maintain low concentrations of urea, creatinine, phosphorus and K in the peritoneal dialysate. Protein is not removed, and calcium and bicarbonate are returned to the animal. Ultrafiltration ranged from 0.2–0.8 L/h. Protein re-moval is entirely avoided. The sorbent suspension need not be sterile. If sorbent components can be made at moderate cost, the SSRD may be a simple, cost effective method of intermittent peritoneal dialysis.

INTRODUCTION

The sorbent suspension reciprocating dialyzer (SSRD) is a parallel plate dialyzer with a suspension of sorbents surrounding the membrane packages. A central port allows both inlet and exit of biologic fluid in response to pressure changes within the sorbent suspension. The membrane packages of the SSRD thus act as a pump, allowing removal and return of small volumes (100–300 ml) of fluid through a single access without need for valves or a blood pump.[1] The sorbent suspension contains approximately 7% charcoal, 20% calcium-sodium loaded zeolite, 15I U/ml urease, and 0.5% methyl cellulose (1500 cps) by weight. This suspension is kept in a fluid state by bidirectional motion of the suspension between the membrane packages. The sorbent suspension functions to keep the concentration of uremic substances low at the membrane surface, and allows urea and creatinine efficiency of approximately 50% during 3–4 hour dialysis with the SSRD.[2] A theoretical analysis of stagnant diffusion within reciprocating dialyzer membrane packages has indicated that this efficiency is within 10–20% of the maximum possible. This analysis also indicated that the highest efficiency is obtained by "square wave" filling, in which the dialyzer is filled and emptied in the minimum amount of time.[3]

From Ash Medical Systems, Inc., and the Small Animal Clinic, School of Veterinary Medicine, Purdue University, West Lafayette, Indiana.

During hemodialysis with the SSRD, the calcium-sodium loaded zeolite results in an ion balance which is appropriate for the conditions of renal failure.[4] Bicarbonate and calcium are returned to the blood, with inflow-outflow concentration changes of 5–10 mEq/L and 1–2 mEq/L, respectively. Sodium and potassium removal are modest, with concentration changes of approximately 5 mEq/L and 2 mEq/L, respectively. These ion balances would be appropriate for many patients on hemodialysis and also many patients on peritoneal dialysis. The sorbent suspension of the SSRD attains this ion balance without the need for reinfusion of buffered cations, as in the Redy[R] system,[5] and without the need for multiple sorbent columns as described by Klein et al.[6] or Kablitz et al.[7]

The SSRD was initially envisioned as a hemodialyzer, with single-needle access, complete self-containment, and ease of operation. A 1.4 m[2] surface area SSRD would allow 80–100 ml/min urea and creatinine clearances, at a blood flow rate of 200 ml/min.[2] This clearance is slightly less than generally obtained with hollow fiber hemodialysis and thus, an increased time of dialysis would be necessary. In return for slightly longer time on dialysis, however, the patient would be offered mobility and self-operation of the single-needle dialyzer.

Since peritoneal dialysis is a longer procedure than hemodialysis, the need for portability and patient mobility during the procedure is even greater. If the SSRD were utilized as an intermittent peritoneal dialyzer, the 10–12 hour duration of this dialysis period would be more tolerable, In addition, if a machine were developed with appropriate monitoring, the night-time hours might be utilized for dialysis, as proposed in the past for automatic cycling machines.[8,9]

In use of the SSRD as a peritoneal dialyzer, the abdomen need not be completely emptied during each cycle. Several investigators have tested continuous flow peritoneal dialysis or rapid cycling machines. In one design, a continuous flow of peritoneal dialysate is passed through a sorbent column, at a slow rate.[9] In another sorbent system, approximately 200 ml of peritoneal fluid is removed from the peritoneal cavity, passed through a dialyzer, and returned to the peritoneum. Utilizing this system (with a tank for urea and phosphate removal, and a charcoal column for creatinine removal), urea clearances may be obtained which are as high or higher than standard peritoneal dialysis schedules.[7] With a cycle volume of 200–300 ml, and a 60-second cycle, the SSRD would exchange 12–18 L/h into and out of the abdomen. This paper describes the application of the SSRD to peritoneal dialysis in the dog. It appears that this utilization of the SSRD is feasible and practicable.

METHODS

Dialyzer Construction

The SSRD is a single access, parallel plate dialyzer specifically designed for sorbent suspension in the dialysate. The construction has been thoroughly described in two previous publications.[1,2] The model with the highest mass transfer coefficient obtained so far has been the "modified pyramidal support" dialyzer, which includes molded, polyethylene pyramid-shaped supports in the dialysate space. These pyramids allow sorbent suspension to flow between them, and also limit membrane expansion to produce a thin, flat blood column at the full expansion. One central port allows blood inflow and outflow. Peripheral slots allow sorbent suspension inflow and egress. An expanded view of the modified pyramidal support SSRD is given in Figure 1a. For use in peritoneal dialysis, a 30 membrane package SSRD was constructed. The surface area was 0.7 m[2], and the fill volume was 100 ml. After air testing and compliance testing, as previously described, the dialyzer was ready for animal tests.

An alternative dialyzer design was the "Z-fold" dialyzer (Fig. 1b). In this dialyzer, the cellulose membrane is folded between screen supports. A single blood port and sorbent suspension port are opposite each other on the package. The surface area of this dialyzer was 1.1 m[2].

Animal Model of Uremia

A healthy mongrel female dog was anesthetized and a 3/4 nephrectomy performed as previously described.[10] Three weeks later, under general anesthesia, a peritoneal catheter was implanted, just left of midline and half way between the umbilicus and symphysis pubis. The catheter used was the "column disc catheter," developed at Purdue University.[9] This catheter was chosen over the Tenckhoff catheter, because of its higher outflow rate and more reproducible drainage characteristics. A 1 m "transfer set" was attached to the catheter.

After placement of the peritoneal catheter, 2 L of peritoneal dialysis fluid was placed in the abdomen (1.5% Dianeal including 1000 units of heparin). This solution was exchanged twice daily by draining the abdomen, attaching a 2 L bag of Dianeal to the

PYRAMIDAL
SUPPORT
SSRD

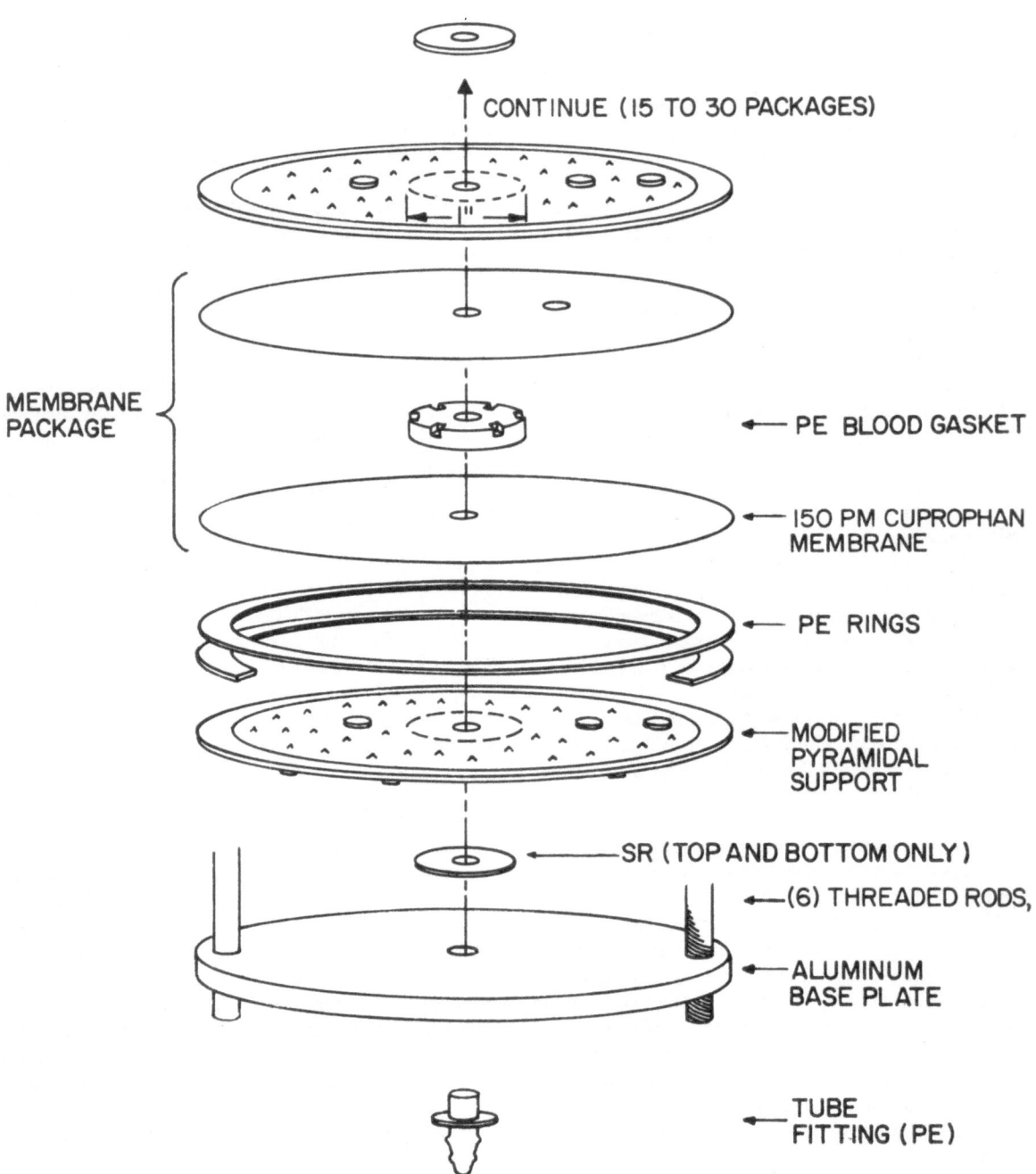

CONTINUE (15 TO 30 PACKAGES)

MEMBRANE
PACKAGE

PE BLOOD GASKET

150 PM CUPROPHAN
MEMBRANE

PE RINGS

MODIFIED
PYRAMIDAL
SUPPORT

SR (TOP AND BOTTOM ONLY)

(6) THREADED RODS,

ALUMINUM
BASE PLATE

TUBE
FITTING (PE)

A

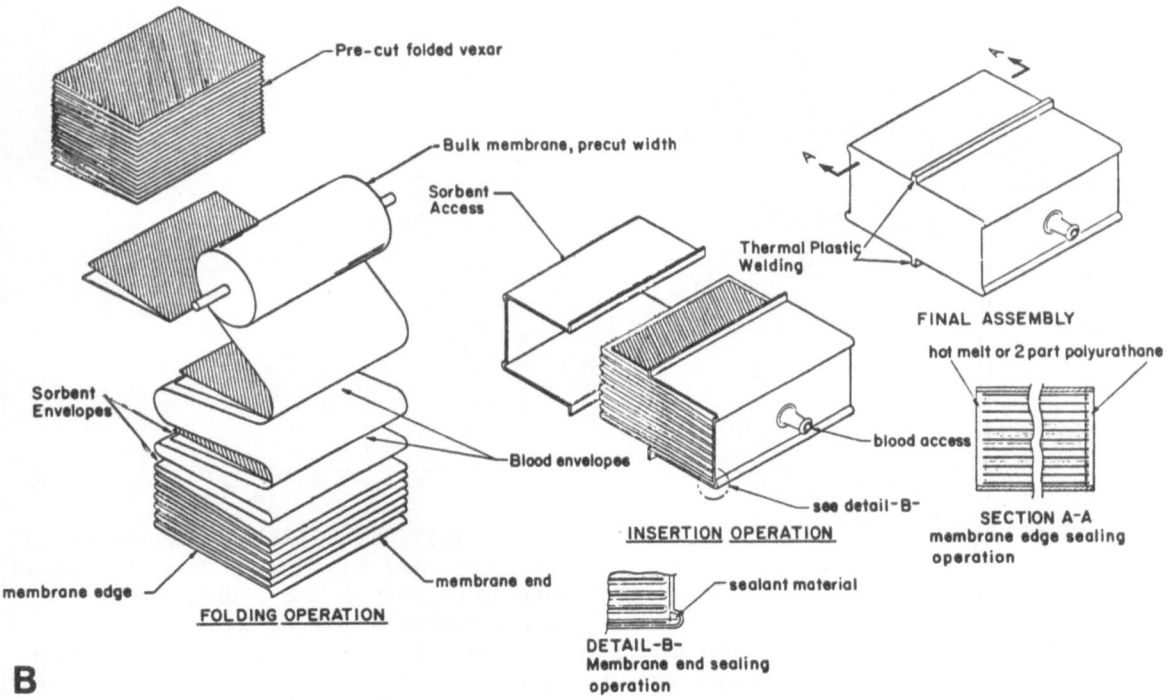

B

Fig. 1. (*a*) Expanded view of construction of the modified pyramidal support SSRD. Polyethylene supports with pyramidal projections separate each membrane package. After assembly, the entire membrane package is pressure-sealed between the base plate and the top plate, and placed in a rigid case. (*b*) The "Z-fold" SSRD design with screen supports.

"transfer set," and infusing under gravity. After infusion, the bag was rolled up and placed under the elastic bandages around the abdomen. On drainage, approximately 1400–1500 ml was obtained. The method of exchange was similar to that of CAPD. For initiation of dialysis with the SSRD, residual 1.5% Dianeal (placed in the abdomen the night before) was used as the primary fluid.

Just before dialysis, a stomach tube was advanced through the oropharnyx of the animal; 20 g of urea and 10 g of creatinine were introduced (in 500 ml water). This allowed a further increase in serum creatinine and BUN concentrations.

Sorbent Suspension

The sorbent suspension was essentially similar to that tested in hemodialysis experiments.[4] Suspended in 2 L of water were: 450 g of F-82 zeolite (loaded with 60% calcium, 40% sodium); 30,000 I.U. urease (covalently bound to silica); 30 g H-loaded IRP (for pH adjustment); 140 g powdered charcoal

(Mallinckrodt, USP), and 10 g Methocel (1500 cps, for suspending properties). The final volume of the suspension was 2.4 L. The ammonium absorbing capacity of zeolite in the suspension is equivalent to 15 g urea nitrogen, when the perfusate concentration is 3000 μM/L.

Dialysis Procedures

Before use, the SSRD was air pressure tested and the dialysate space was filled with saline. A compliance test was then performed using sterile saline. Volume and pressure were recorded, up to 200 mm Hg. The dialyzer was then sterilized using Betadine® (PVP-iodine). Betadine (60 ml) was placed in the membrane package, and then washed from the inside of the membrane package using syringes of sterile saline. When a faint yellow color remained, the absorbent suspension was placed in the dialysate case. Several cycles of sterile saline into and out of the membrane package resulted in a clear effluent. The sorbent suspension was not ster-

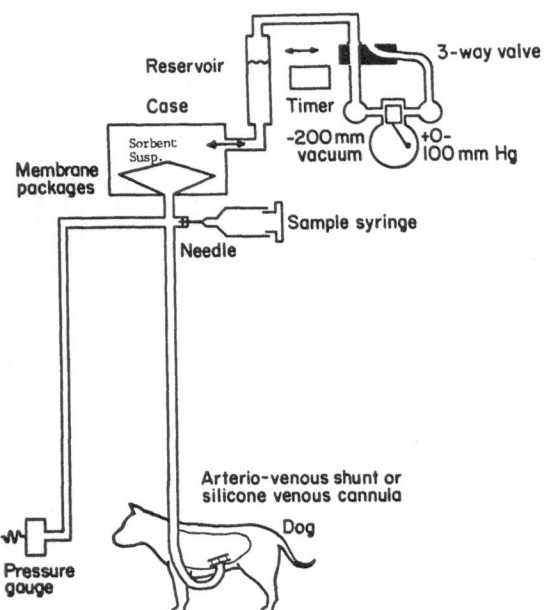

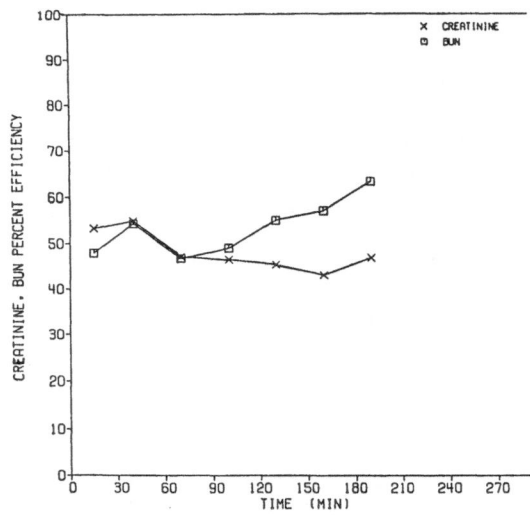

A

Fig. 2. Animal test set up for peritoneal dialysis. Pressure in reservoir is cycled between +200 and −100 mm Hg.

Fig. 3. (*a*) Efficiency of removal of creatinine and urea, comparing inflow and outflow of peritoneal fluid of the SSRD. Time of dialysis is shown on horizontal axis. (*b*) Blood and dialysate (inflow and outflow) urea nitrogen concentrations during peritoneal dialysis with SSRD. (*c*) Blood and peritoneal (inflow and outflow) creatinine concentrations during peritoneal dialysis with SSRD.

ilized, and contained 0–5 bacteria/ml. The dialyzer was attached to the column disc catheter by means of a 1/8" ID silicone tube (steam sterilized). A graduated cylinder was then attached to the dialysate case and the cylinder was one-half filled with sorbent suspension, as demonstrated in Figure 2. The top of the graduated cylinder was closed, and a 1/2" ID tube connected to a threeway electric valve. A pressure vacuum pump generated +100 mm Hg and −200 mm Hg alternately at the three-way valve. The cycle time of the valve was controlled by an electronic timer. Inflow time (negative pressure) was set to 48 seconds, outflow to 12 seconds.

A four-way connector within the silicone tubing was utilized for collection of inflow and outflow samples, and for measurement of pressure transients. Inflow samples were obtained by means of a syringe and needle through a rubber stopper on the four-way connector at the end of inflow. For outflow samples, the entire effluent of the dialyzer was collected in a sterile vinyl bag. This was performed by clamping the silicone tube between the four-way connector and the animal, and opening the four-way connector into the vinyl bag. After mixing the con-

tents of the bag, a sample was drawn utilizing a small syringe and needle through the rubber stopper of the bag. The dialyzer was then placed on negative pressure and the remaining fluid in the bag drawn into the dialyzer. Subsequently this fluid was returned to the dog. Pressure transients recorded at the four-way connector monitored the adequacy of flow, and also indicated the cessation of flow as the membrane package reached compliance limits during the cycle.

Inflow and outflow samples were analyzed for urea, creatinine, potassium, sodium, bicarbonate (base excess), and calcium. Inflow and outflow samples were obtained approximately every 30 minutes during the dialysis.

RESULTS

During peritoneal dialysis with the pyramidal support dialyzer, the average fill volume was 100 ml, and the cycle time 1 minute. Figure 3a illustrates the efficiency of removal of urea and creatinine from the peritoneal fluid. The initial inflow concentration of urea nitrogen was 48 mg/dl, and of creatinine was 4.5

Dialysate Inflow to SSRD
Dialysate Outflow from SSRD
Patient (blood)
Pre and Post Slurry
BUN (mg%)
Time (min)
100
90
80
70
60
50
40
30
20
10
0
0
30
60
90
120
150
180
210

3B

Dialysate Inflow to SSRD
Dialysate Outflow from SSRD
Patient (blood)
Pre and Post Slurry
Creatinine (mg%)
Time (min)
14
13
12
11
10
9
8
7
6
5
4
3
2
1
0
0
30
60
90
120
150
180
210

3C

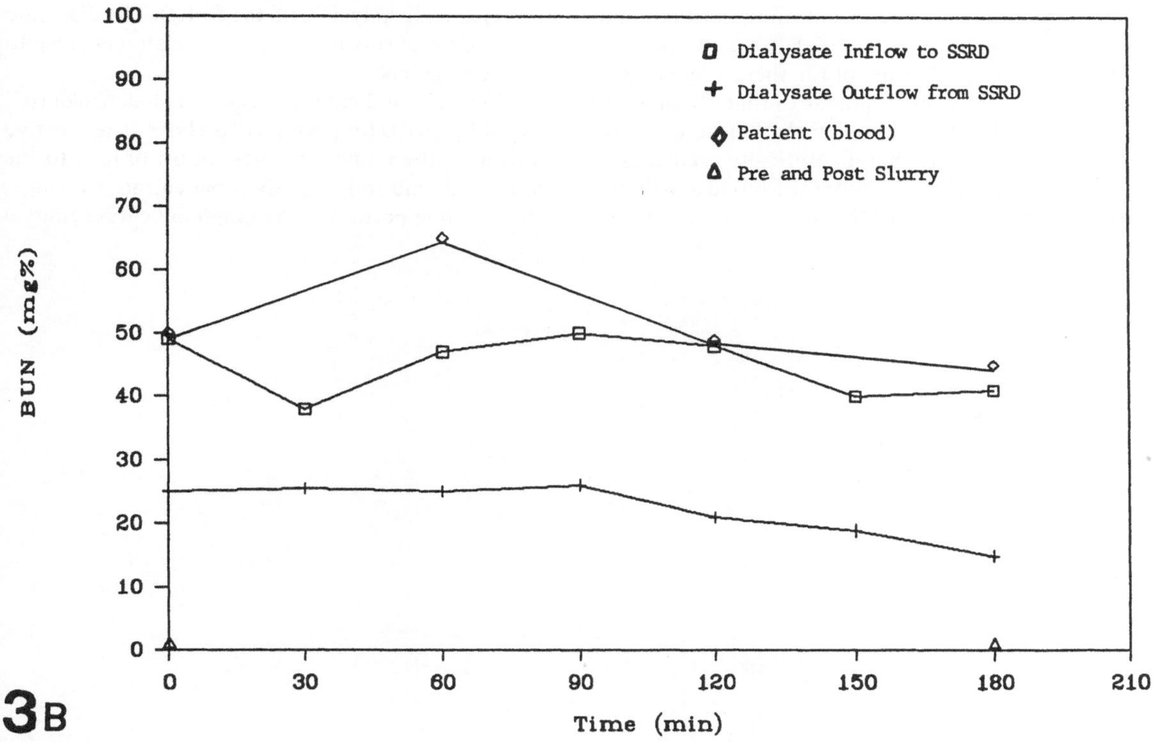

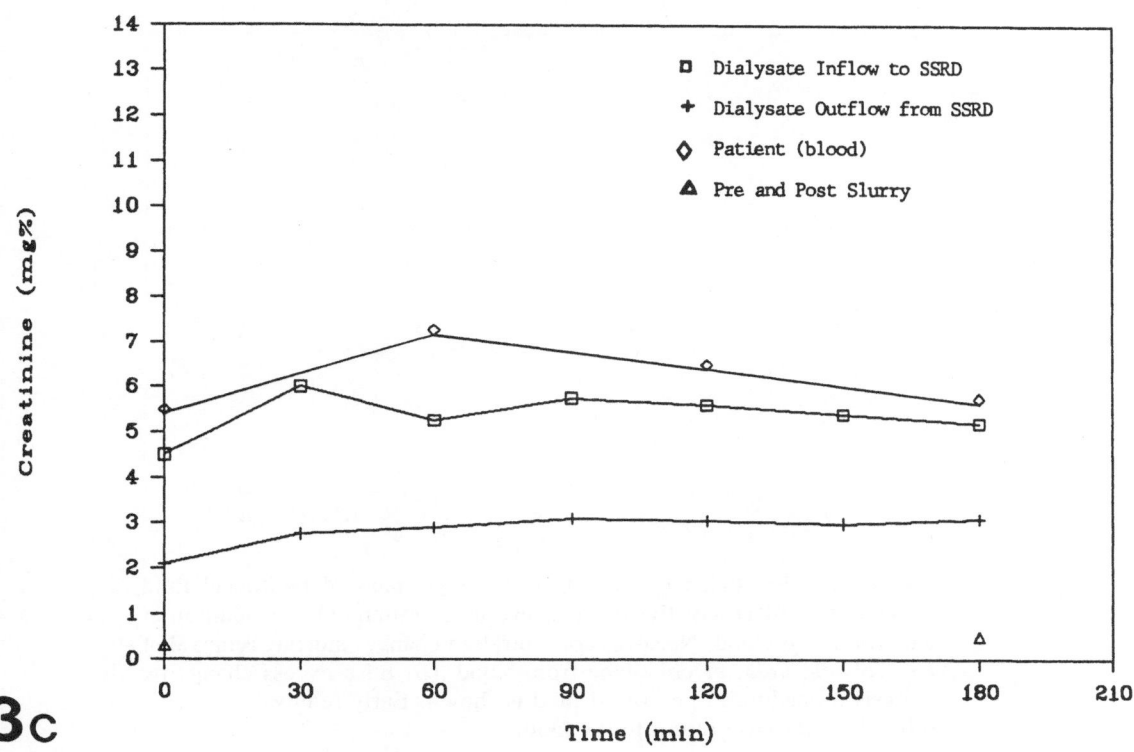

mg/dl. The final inflow concentrations of urea and creatinine were 41 mg/dl and 5.0 mg/dl, respectively. Efficiency of removal for these compounds was approximately 50%, similar to that obtained in use of the SSRD for hemodialysis. These efficiencies are also similar to that theoretically predicted.[3]

Figure 3 (b and c) illustrates the blood and dialysate concentrations of BUN and creatinine during

the peritoneal dialysis with the SSRD. The dialysate levels of these substances stayed relatively close to the blood levels.

Figure 4a indicates the chemical balance during use of the SSRD for peritoneal dialysis. The positive portion of the graph indicates return of ions to the peritoneal fluid and a positive concentration change. The negative portion of the graph indicates removal

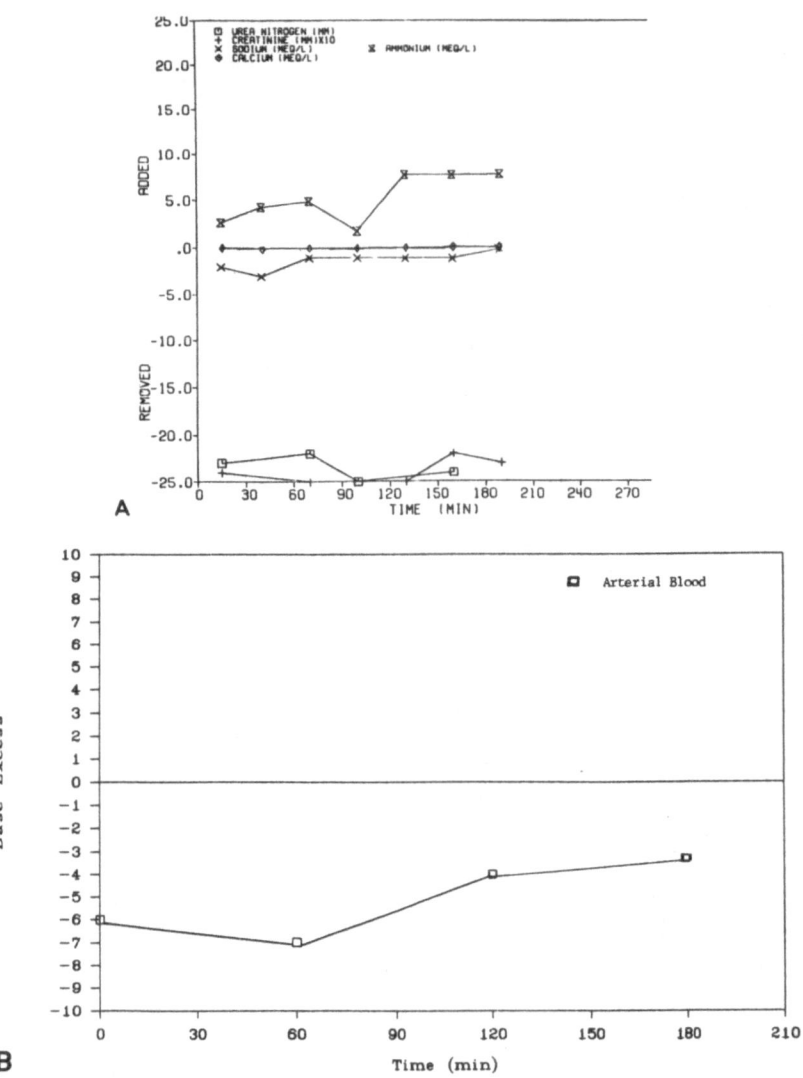

Fig. 4. (*a*) Ion balance resulting from single pass of peritoneal fluid through the SSRD. Positive changes in concentration indicate addition of electrolytes to blood. Negative concentration changes indicate removal of electrolytes, urea, or creatinine from blood. (*b*) Base excess change by dialysis procedure in peritoneal fluid is shown. Early removal of base is offset by later base return to the fluid.

of ions from the peritoneal fluid and a negative concentration change. There is a marked change in urea nitrogen during treatment of the fluid by the SSRD. Figure 4b indicates a large return of bicarbonate (normal base excess change of 25 mEq/L) by the SSRD. In addition, there is a modest removal of calcium, sodium, and potassium. These results are similar to those that occur with treatment of blood by the SSRD,[4] with the exception of the late increase in bicarbonate return and removal, rather than return of calcium. The inflowing peritoneal dialysate was somewhat lower than blood in bicarbonate and higher in acetate. This acetate functioned to keep the pH less than that of blood, even when large amounts of bicarbonate were returned up to the third hour. Efficiency of phosphate removal was approximately 40% throughout dialysis.

During treatment with the SSRD, the outflow pH of the dialyzer rose to 8.26 after 180 minutes. This coincided with the large recorded change in bicarbonate return. At no time did the animal show any evidence of discomfort, even during the highest pH change. Following and during the peritoneal dialysis procedure, there was no evidence of peritonitis nor of cloudy peritoneal fluid. The animal remained alert and appeared normal during treatment.

Three more peritoneal dialysis experiments were performed with two-fold dialyzers. The overall ion balances were similar to those of the modified pyramidal support dialyzer above. The fill volume was 200 ml, and cycle time 1 minute. The clearances were increased, of course, in proportion to the flow rate and membrane surface area. Urea and creatinine clearance averaged 80–100 ml/min, phosphate clearance averaged 50 ml/min, and K clearance averaged 70 ml/min (a lower K zeolite was utilized). As a result of these higher clearances, the dialysate concentrations diminished.

DISCUSSION AND CONCLUSIONS

The requirements for a peritoneal dialysate regenerating system are remarkably similar to those of a hemodialysis system. The biologic fluid must be perfectly sterile, and a high flow of peritoneal fluid must enter and exit from the dialyzer each minute to maintain a high clearance rate. All of the peritoneal fluid need not be drained during each cycle.

Small volume, rapid cycle peritoneal dialysis offers excellent clearance for small molecules due to surprisingly good mixing within the peritoneum. The SSRD functions as a peritoneal dialyzer with a clearance of approximately 1/2 of its perfusion rate. An SSRD treating 200 ml/min (with approximately 1.4 m² surface area) clears approximately 100 ml/min of urea or creatinine. With this clearance, the concentration of uremic substances in the dialysate is kept low, and peritoneal clearance approximates that obtained with nonregenerative dialysis systems at high dialysate flow rates.

In spite of the use of nonsterile sorbent suspension, there appears to be no toxicity or irritation associated with the use of the SSRD. The membranes of the SSRD apparently function to prevent bacterial contamination of peritoneal fluid, as do the membranes on the standard hemodialyzer. A membrane package sterilized by ethylene oxide would be more convenient than one sterilized by Betadine. The ion balance of the SSRD appears to be appropriate for patients in renal failure. A mild calcium return is possible with higher calcium loading of the zeolite. Bicarbonate and calcium return should result in mild hypercalcemia and correction of acidosis of patients in renal failure.

From the present study, it appears that the SSRD would be useful as an intermittent peritoneal dialyzer (possibly a night-time dialyzer) for those patients for whom peritoneal dialysis is indicated. The SSRD would offer some mobility, especially with a portable system for control of the pressure-vacuum system. Besides the apparently high small molecule clearances, there are other potential advantages of regenerating dialysate peritoneal systems. Protein removal should be essentially zero. The clearance of larger molecules of slower clearance (such as phosphate) should be greater than with CAPD or CCPD. A variety of larger osmotic agents could be used efficiently, since their removal across the cellophane membrane might be minimal. The bulk of dialysate sorbents and water might be provided in nonsterile form. In addition, shipping weight of sorbents would be less than for presterilized dialysis fluid. Disadvantages include the cost of supplying a dialyzer and sorbents, and the need to provide osmotic agent for each dialysis treatment. The device should be relatively easy to set up, and its disposable dialysate and sorbent components would obviate the need for resterilization procedures, as presently used with intermittent peritoneal dialysis machines.

REFERENCES

1. Barile RG, Wang NL, Blake DE, Belcastro PF, Gupta S, Regnier FE, Thornhill JA, Kessler DP, and

Ash SR: A reciprocating, single-needle hemodialyzer with bidirectional flow of sorbent suspension. Artif Organs 6: 267, 1982

2. Ash SR, Barile RG, Wilcox PG, Wright DL, Thornhill JA, Dhein CR, Kessler DP, and Wang NL: The sorbent suspension reciprocating dialyzer: A device with minimal sorbent saturation. asaio J 4: 28, 1981

3. Wang NHL, Kessler DP, and Ash SR: Mass transfer characteristics of a sorbent-based reciprocating dialyzer. Chem Eng Com 5: 347, 1980

4. Ash SR, Barile RG, Thornhill JA, Sherman JD, and Wang NHL: In vivo evaluation of calcium-loaded zeolites and urease for urea removal in hemodialysis. Trans Am Soc Artif Intern Organs 26: 111, 1980

5. Gordon A, Better OS, Greenbaum MA, Marantz LB, Gral T, and Maxwell MH: Clinical maintenance hemodialysis with a sorbent-based low-volume dialysate regeneration system. Trans Am Soc Artif Intern Organs 17: 253, 1971

6. Klein E, Holland FF, Eberle K, Morton SC, and Cabasso I: Sorbent-filled hollow fiber for hemopurification. Trans Am Soc Artif Intern Organs 24: 127, 1978

7. Kablitz C, Stephen RL, Duffy DP, Jacobsen SC, Zelman A, and Kolff WJ: Technological augmentation of peritoneal urea clearance: Past, present and future. Dial Trans 9: 741, 1980

8. Banks G: Maintenance peritoneal dialysis as an alternative for the patient with end-stage renal failure. Clin Digest 6: 1, 1978

9. Maxwell MH, Gordon A, and Lewin AJ: Sorbent-based regenerative peritoneal dialysis system. Proc 11th Annu Contractors' Conf Artificial Kidney Program, NIAMDD, DHEW Publ No (NIH) 79-1442, 1978, p 54

10. Ash SR, and Thornhill JA: Animal models of renal failure. CRC Press, 1984

11. Ash SR, Johnson H, Hartman J, Granger J, Koszuta JJ, Sell S, Dhein CR, Blevins W, and Thornhill JA: The column disc peritoneal catheter: A peritoneal access device with improved drainage. asaio J 3: 109, 1980

S.Z. Trooskin, R.A. Harvey, A.P. Donetz, and R.S. Greco

27

Application of Antibiotic Bonding to CAPD Catheters

SUMMARY

The techniques of non-covalently bonding anionic antibiotics using cationic surfactants were applied to the problem of CAPD catheter infection. Pretreatment of silicone elastomer catheter segments with 5% tridodecylmethylammonium chloride (TDMAC) increased the bonding of ^{14}C-penicillin from 0.09 μg/cm to 181 μg/cm. Elution rates of bound ligands in dialysis solution were studied. after 1 week, 50% of the TDMAC remained bound. Of the bound penicillin, 85% was lost in the first few hours, but 6 μg/cm remained bound after 4 days in dialysis solution.

Rats underwent insertion of CAPD catheters. Exit sites were innoculated with 1×10^8 Staphylococcus aureus. At sacrifice, 3 days post-insertion, 58.8% of rats receiving sterile control catheters had positive intraperitoneal catheter tip cultures, while 12.5% of those receiving TDMAC-penicillin bonded catheters had positive catheter tip cultures ($p < 0.006$).

Anionic antibiotics may be bonded to CAPD catheters using a cationic anchor. Antibiotic bonding decreased catheter infection in an animal model.

From the Department of Surgery, University of Medicine and Dentistry, Rutgers Medical School, New Brunswick, New Jersey.

INTRODUCTION

CAPD is now a standard method of treating end-stage renal failure. Nearly every patient who undergoes CAPD experiences peritonitis during the course of treatment. In spite of recent improvements in delivery systems and careful attention to sterile technique, the incidence of peritonitis remains one episode every 6–12 treatment months.[1-3] Peritonitis is the most common cause of CAPD failure and morbidity. Although uncomplicated peritonitis necessitates an average annual hospital stay of only four days per patient per year,[1] 2.3% of episodes of peritonitis result in death.[4] Transcatheter and pericatheter migration of bacteria account for over two-thirds (66%) of episodes of peritonitis.[5,6] It is, therefore, not surprising that the most common microorganisms responsible for peritonitis are skin flora.

We have described the noncovalent bonding of anionic antibiotics using cationic surfactants to prevent infection in implantable devices. These techniques were originally applied to infection prevention in Dacron and polytetrafluoroethylene prosthetic vascular graft materials.[7,8] More recently, we have described the application of antibiotic bonding to the problem of hyperalimentation catheter-related infections.[9] Hyperalimentation catheters are constructed of polyethylene or silicone elastomer. CAPD catheters are constructed of silicone elastomer and have either a Dacron or polytetrafluoro-ethylene cuff for suturing to the peritoneum. The application of antibiotic bonding to CAPD catheter-related infections, therefore, represents a logical application of this technology.

MATERIALS AND METHODS

[14]C-TDMAC and ^{14}C-benzylpenicillin were obtained from Amersham Corporation. Peritoneal dialysis catheters were obtained from the Quinton Corporation. Silicone elastomer tubing was purchased from Dow Corning Corporation. Tridodecylmethylammonium chloride was obtained from Polysciences, Inc., and benzylpenicillin from Sigma Chemical Company. Dialysis solution was obtained from Travenol Laboratories, Inc.

Radiochemical Assays

BONDING OF ^{14}C-PENICILLIN

Standard CAPD catheters made of silicone elastomer were cut into 0.5 cm segments and were submerged in a solution of 5% tridodecylmethylammonium chloride (TDMAC) and 95% ethanol. Following incubation for 30 minutes, the catheter segments were drained, air dried for a minimum of one hour at room temperature, and washed in five changes of distilled water using a Vortex mixer. After air drying, catheter segments were incubated for one hour at room temperature with benzylpenicillin 10 mg/ml containing 0.25 μCi ^{14}C-penicillin. Catheter segments were air dried and washed in five changes of distilled water and subjected to liquid scintillation counting to determine the quantity of bound antibiotic.

ELUTION OF BOUND LIGANDS IN THE PRESENCE OF DIALYSIS SOLUTION

Catheter segments of silicone elastomer that had been previously radiolabeled with either ^{14}C-TDMAC or TDMAC-bonded ^{14}C-penicillin were incubated at room temperature in 5 ml glass screw-cap bottles containing 4 ml 2.5% Dianeal solution. The dialysis solution was kept in motion by inverting the bottles five times per minute using a rotary mixer. At various time intervals, the catheter segments were removed and drained. Catheter segments were then processed for liquid scintillation counting to deter-

mine the amount of bound TDMAC or radiolabeled penicillin remaining on the segment.

In Vivo Studies

Male Sprague-Dawley rats (Charles River) weighing 250–400 g were utilized in this study. They were housed in individual cages and maintained on a standard rodent chow and water diet. At operation, 33 rats underwent a 1.5 cm incision in the left lower quadrant. The peritoneum was entered and 4 cm of silicone elastomer tubing (o.d. = 0.37 in) was inserted in the peritoneal cavity. The abdominal incision was closed in layers with 4-0 silk sutures. The catheter was secured to the external oblique fascia and tunneled posteriorly to exit the skin in the midline between the forelimb girdles. All catheters were connected to a small animal swivel mechanism (Instech Laboratory) that allowed free movement. Prior to closure of the posterior midline, the exit site was inoculated with 1.0 ml phosphate-buffered saline containing 1×10^8 Staphylococcus aureus. Animals in Group I underwent insertion of untreated sterile control catheters. Animals in Group II received TDMAC-penicillin bonded catheters. TDMAC pretreatment was carried out prior to sterilizing the catheters. TDMAC pretreated and control untreated catheters were individually packaged and subjected to steam sterilization at 15 lb (1.02 atm (ca. 101.3 kPa)) and 120°C for 15 minutes. Group II TDMAC pretreated catheters were incubated in 10 mg/ml/cm of penicillin solution prior to catheter insertion. Catheters were connected to a continuous infusion of sterile Ringer's lactate solution at a rate of 1.5 ml/h for three days. On the third postinsertion day, the animals were sacrificed with a lethal dose of intraperitoneal nembutal and the intraperitoneal catheter tip was removed via sterile right upper quadrant laparotomy incision. The catheter tips were cultured using semiquantitative techniques on mannitol salt agar plates. More than ten colonies per plate were considered a positive catheter tip culture result.

RESULTS

Radiochemical Assays

BONDING OF ^{14}C-PENICILLIN

TDMAC increased the bonding of ^{14}C-penicillin to silicone elastomer catheter segments from 0.09 μg/cm in untreated catheters to 181 μg/cm in bonded catheters.

ELUTION OF BOUND TDMAC
AND PENICILLIN IN THE PRESENCE
OF DIALYSIS SOLUTION

The stability of bound ^{14}C-TDMAC and ^{14}C-penicillin to silicone elastomer segments was evaluated *in vitro* by prolonged incubation in dialysis solution. Incubation was interrupted at various times and the amount of radiolabeled surfactant was determined. Figure 1 shows a semilogarithmic plot of the ^{14}C-TDMAC remaining on the silicone elastomer catheter segments as a function of time. Although there is an initial rapid loss of TDMAC from the CAPD catheter over the one-week period of study, the bonding of the TDMAC to the catheter was relatively stable. Approximately 50% of the surfactant remained bound to the catheter after the one-week incubation period. Figure 1 also shows the semilogarithmic plot of the ^{14}C-penicillin remaining on the silicone elastomer as a function of time. The data can be fit by two straight lines, suggesting that the dissociation of the radiolabeled penicillin occurs by two concurrent first order processes with different rate constants. The initial elution is rapid, with nearly 85% of the total ^{14}C-penicillin dissociated during the first few hours. By 24–28 hours, more than 95% of the radiolabeled penicillin had left the catheter. A significant amount of radiolabeled penicillin (6 μg/cm) remained bound after four days in dialysis solution.

In Vivo Study

In Group I (untreated control catheters), 8 of 17 animals had positive intraperitoneal catheter tip cultures (58.8%). In Group II (TDMAC-penicillin bonded), 3 of 16 had positive catheter tips (12.5%). The difference between the number of colonized catheter tips in Groups I and II was highly significant ($p < 0.006$).

DISCUSSION

Our laboratory has shown that a number of anionic antibiotics, including the cephalosporins and the penicillins, can be noncovalently bound to the surfaces of Dacron, polytetrafluoroethylene, polyethylene and silicone elastomer using a variety of cationic surfactants.[7–10] Although most of the previous work with this technique has been applied to infection in vascular grafts, the present work demonstrates that it may also be applied to infectious problems related to peritoneal dialysis catheters. It

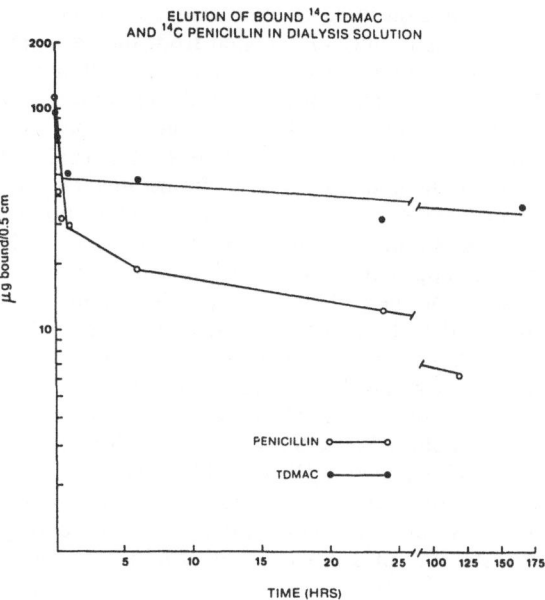

Fig. 1. Elution of bound ligands is biphasic with an initial rapid elution phase and a second slower elution rate. The bound TDMAC is more stable in dialysis solution than the bound penicillin.

has been shown that the surfactant TDMAC when applied with ethanol as a solvent bonds firmly to both the silicone elastomer (catheter surfaces) and to Dacron and polytetrafluoroethylene (cuff materials). It has been previously shown that increasing the concentration of the surfactant in the solvent increased the amount of TDMAC bonded to the silicone elastomer catheters.[10] This, in turn, allows bonding of greater quantities of antibiotic. The bonding and elution characteristics of both the surfactant and the penicillin to silicone elastomer tubing are qualitatively similar to those described for polytetrafluoroethylene and Dacron vascular grafts.[7,8] The only differences in bonding are quantitative. Dacron and polytetrafluoroethylene bond approximately ten times more antibiotic than silicone elastomer. This difference is most likely related to the greater porosity of Dacron and polytetrafluoroethylene vascular grafts. The more surface area is available for contact with the bonding surfactant, the more surfactant will be bound to the Dacron and polytetrafluoroethylene and, therefore, the more antibiotic that will also be bound. Since the silicone elastomer is nonporous, lesser amounts of the surfactant and antibiotic may be bound.

The elution studies demonstrated that the bound antibiotic is rapidly dissociated from the catheter. The amount of antibiotic remaining after 48 hours, although only a small fraction of the total originally bound, is above the minimum inhibitory concentration (0.1 μg/ml) for these bacteria.[11] Although the antibiotic rapidly dissociates, the surfactant TDMAC is relatively stable when incubated in dialysis solution. At the end of the one-week study period, approximately 50% of the surfactant remained on the catheter. Our previous studies examining the elution rate of TDMAC incubated in plasma have revealed that more than 60% of the TDMAC remained bound to silicone elastomer catheters after two weeks of incubation.[10] This desirable characteristic of long-term TDMAC adherence to silicone elastomer may be useful in treating catheter colonization occurring with episodes of peritonitis. Current studies in progress are examining the long-term stability of TDMAC applied to silicone elastomer in dialysis solution, as well as after intraperitoneal implantation in experimental animals. It may be possible to "recharge" TDMAC-treated dialysis catheters with antibiotic by direct catheter perfusion with the appropriate anionic antibiotics, such as other penicillins or cephalosporins. This could be easily carried out by simply adding the antibiotic to the dialysis solution. Recent studies completed by our laboratory offered support for the concept of catheter "recharging." TDMAC-pretreated polytetrafluoroethylene and Dacron segments, when implanted into a rat muscle pouch, will bond appreciable amounts of both locally instilled and intravenously administered antibiotics.[11,12]

Antibiotic bonding offered added protection against catheter tip colonization in animals with catheter exit site bacterial innoculation. This treatment resulted in a decrease in the number of intraperitoneal catheter infections from 58.8% to 12.5% in the face of bacterial exit site challenge. It is hoped that antibiotic bonding will prove useful in both preventing early acquired dialysis catheter tract infections, as well as inhibiting catheter colonization during bouts of peritonitis. The use of chronic ambulatory peritoneal dialysis is increasing. The problem of peritonitis in terms of morbidity, mortality, and dialysis failure may be well addressed by the use of a peritoneal dialysis catheter that is more resistant to infection. The ultimate role of antibiotic bonding in achieving this goal must be determined by clinical trials.

ACKNOWLEDGMENT

Supported in part by National Heart, Lung and Blood Institute Grant No. ROI HL 24252.

REFERENCES

1. Kurtz SB, Wong VH, Anderson CF, Vogel P, McCarthy JT, Mitchell JC III, Kumar R, and Johnson WJ: Continuous ambulatory peritoneal dialysis: Three years' experience at the Mayo Clinic. Mayo Clinic Proc 58: 633, 1983
2. Oreopoulos DG, Khanna R, and Vas SI: Peritonitis in patients on CAPD. In Gahl GM, Kessel M, and Nolph KD (Eds), Advances in peritoneal dialysis: Proceedings of the 2nd international symposium on peritoneal dialysis. Amsterdam: Excerpta Medica, 1981, p 261
3. Williams C: University of Toronto collaborative dialysis group: CAPD in Toronto—An overview. Peritoneal Dial Bull 3(Suppl): S6, 1983
4. Fenton SSA: The problem of peritonitis—Peritonitis-related deaths among CAPD patients. Peritoneal Dial Bull 3(Suppl): S9, 1983
5. Oreopoulos D, Vas S, and Khanna R: Prevention of peritonitis during continuous ambulatory peritoneal dialysis. Peritoneal Dial Bull 3(Suppl): S18, 1983
6. Wu G: University of Toronto collaborative dialysis group: A review of peritonitis episodes that caused interruption of CAPD. Peritoneal Dial Bull 3(Suppl): S11, 1983
7. Greco RS, and Harvey RA: The role of antibiotic bonding in the prevention of vascular prosthetic infections. Ann Surg 195: 168, 1982
8. Greco RS, Harvey RA, Smilow PC, and Tesoriero JV: Prevention of vascular prosthetic infection by a benzalkonium-oxacillin bonded polytetrafluoroethylene graft. Surg Gynecol Obstet 155: 28, 1982
9. Trooskin SZ, Harvey RA, and Greco RS: Prevention of catheter sepsis by antibiotic bonding. Surg Forum 34: 132, 1983
10. Trooskin SZ, Donetz AP, Harvey RA, and Greco RS: Prevention of catheter sepsis by antibiotic bonding (unpublished)
11. Harvey RA, Tesoriero JV, and Greco RS: Noncovalent bonding of penicillin and cefazolin to dacron. Am J Surg 147: 205, 1984
12. Harvey RA, Alcid CV, and Greco RS. Antibiotic bonding to polytetrafluoroethylene with tridodecylmethylammonium chloride. Surgery 92: 504, 1982

K. Ota

28

Clinical Experience in CAPD Using Flame-Lock Connecting Device: A Group Study

SUMMARY

The Flame-Lock CAPD system was used in 60 end-stage renal failure patients. Incidence of peritonitis was 1 per 16.7 patient-months overall. However, excluding those caused by tunnel infection, the incidence decreased to 1 per 22.4 patient-months. Device failure occurred once per 747 exchanges, and the majority of them were related to the overheating of the joint. Only five episodes were considered to be responsible for the development of peritonitis. From these results it is concluded that the Flame-Lock CAPD (Terumo Corp., Tokyo, Japan) system is useful in treating ESRD patients. The advantages of the system are: 1. Perfect sterilization, 2. Rapid and fail-safe connection, 3. No complicated apparatus. The disadvantages are: 1. Instability of heating condition, 2. Damage to plastic by overheating, 3. Carmelization of glucose.

INTRODUCTION

To eliminate peritonitis is the most important prerequisite for wide spread application of CAPD. A completely new fail-safe connecting device named Flame-Lock (Terumo Corp, Tokyo, Japan) has been

---

From the Flame-Lock Study Group, Kidney Center, Tokyo Women's Medical College. 10 Kawada-cho, Shinjuku-ku, Tokyo 162, Japan.

developed and examined clinically. This report presents the results of a group study conducted from September, 1981, to May, 1984, using this system.

MATERIALS AND METHODS

Structure of Flame-Lock CAPD System

The Flame-Lock CAPD system consists of a soft plastic bag containing dialysate, transfer tube, and peritoneal catheter. There are two joints in the dialysate line, namely a titanium joint and a bag-ceramic joint. The former connects catheter to transfer tube and the latter connects transfer tube to the dialysate line extending from the bag (Fig. 1). The structure of the former is similar to other connectors used for the same purpose; however, the latter, known as the Flame-Lock connecting device, has special construction and characteristics.

The details of the device are reported elsewhere,[1] but an outline of the structure and function is summarized here. The bag-ceramic joint consists of a ceramic male part and nickel-plated brass as female part. The former is attached to the transfer tube and the latter is attached to the tube on the bag side. Inside both of the joints, silicone 0 rings are equipped to assure water-tight connection. Furthermore, on the ceramic side of the joint, a sleeve screw nut is furnished to reinforce the connection. The bag, including the bag joint, is disposable.

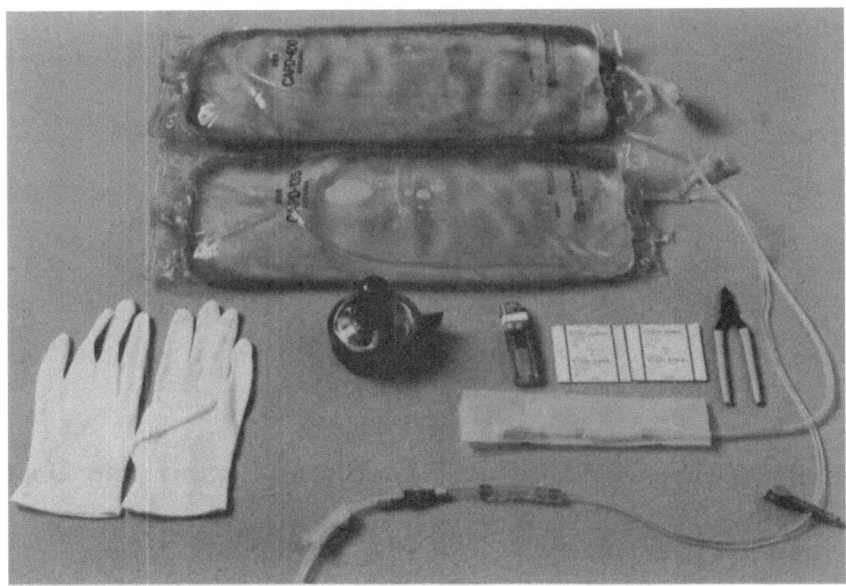

Fig. 1. Flame-Lock CAPD system.

Procedure of Connection and Disconnection of Flame-Lock Device

At the time of connection, both parts of the joint are heated over an alcohol lamp for approximately 20 seconds. The difference in heat expansion between ceramics and brass makes it possible to insert the ceramic part into the brass part and at the same time they are sterilized. After 1–2 minutes of cooling by dialysate passing inside the joint, the brass shrinks and holds the ceramic part of the joint firmly. Then the sleeve screw nut is advanced to cover the junction. At the time of disconnection, the sleeve screw nut is retracted and the exposed joint is heated again to detach the connection (Figs. 2 & 3).

PATIENTS

Sixty end-stage renal failure patients (42 males and 18 females), age range 21–74 years, with an average age of 45.1 ± 13.1 yrs, took part in the study. The duration on CAPD treatment ranged from 1–26 months, with a mean of 10.8 ± 5.9 months, providing a total experience of 651 patient-months. More than half of their initial renal diseases were chronic glomerulonephritis (37 cases: 61%), followed by diabetic nephropathy (8 cases: 13%), nephrosclerosis (3 cases: 5%), and polycystic kidney (2 cases: 3%)

(Table 1). The treatments of the patients before entering the study were hemodialysis (31 cases: 53%), conservative therapy (15 cases: 25%), intermittent peritoneal dialysis (12 cases: 20%), and CAPD using another system (2 cases: 3%).

RESULTS

Patient and Technical Survival

Among 60 patients entered in the study, 51 were still on the CAPD treatment. Eight patients discontinued the treatment and switched to hemodialysis due to repeated peritonitis. The causative organisms were *Staphylococcus aureus* in three cases, and others were one each of *Pseudomonas cepacia*, *Enterobacter aglomerous*, *Candida*, and unknown cause. The route of introduction of organisms into the peritoneal cavity was ascribed to tunnel infection in two cases of peritonitis caused by *Staphylococcus aureus*. One patient died of brain hemorrhage 212 days after the start of CAPD.

Incidence of Peritonitis

Peritonitis developed 39 times in 26 cases. Among them, ten episodes were from tunnel infection and five were directly related to device failure.

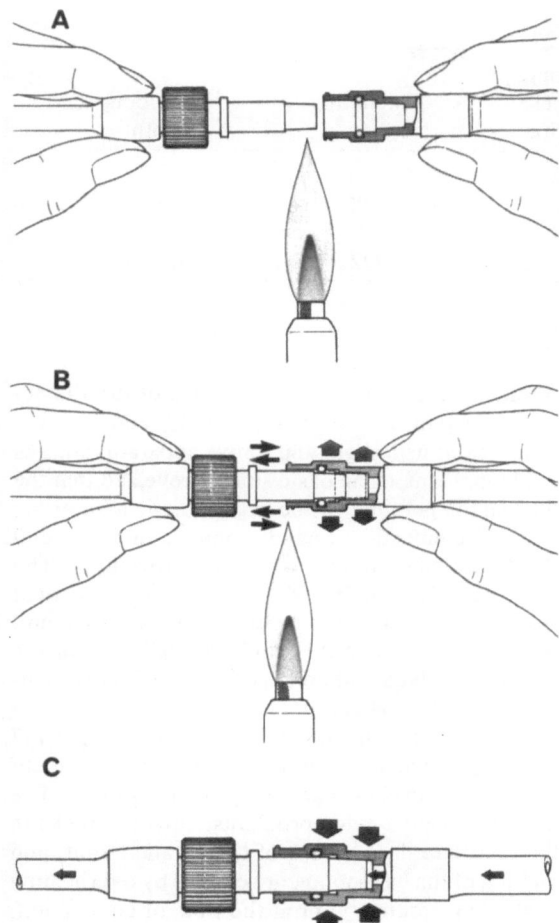

Fig. 2. Procedure of connection and disconnection. (*a*) heating and sterilization, (*b*) connection and disconnection, (*c*) cooling and shrinkage.

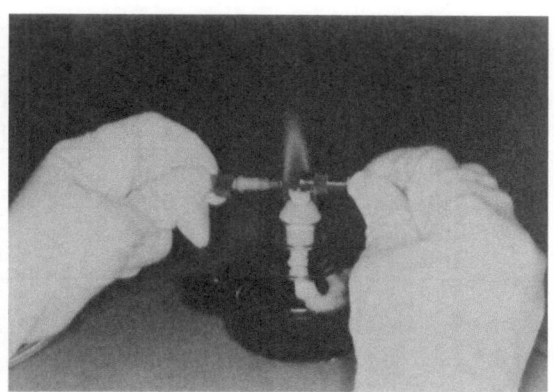

Fig. 3. Connecting bag-ceramic joint.

Four patients had three episodes, while five cases had two. The remaining 17 had only one episode of peritonitis. The incidence of peritonitis was 1 per 16.7 patient months for all cases; however, it decreased to 1 per 22.4 patient months if the peritonitis directly related to tunnel infection was excluded (Table 2).

Organisms found in the dialysate are listed in Table 3. As for side effects and complications, hypopotassemia was observed in eight, and catheter trouble in five. Four patients complained of constipation and abdominal distension, respectively. Forty-five complications were noted among 60 patients (Table 4).

Troubles in the Connecting Device

Troubles originated from the connecting device among 79,200 exchanges (Table 5). As is obvious

Table 1. Primary Renal Diseases.

	Total	Male	Female	%
Chronic glomerulonephritis	37	28	9	61
Diabetic nephropathy	8	6	2	13
Nephrosclerosis	3	2	1	5
Toxemia in pregnancy	2		2	3
Polycystic kidney	2		2	3
Malignant hypertension	1	1		2
Acute glomerulonephritis	1	1		2
Nephrotic syndrome	1	1		2
Autoimmune nephritis	1	1		2
Chronic pyelonephritis	1	1		2
Unknown	3	2	1	5
Total	60	43	17	100

Table 2. Number of Episodes and Incidence of Peritonitis.

	Total	Excluding Tunnel Infection	Excluding Drop-outs	Excluding Both
Patients	60	60	52	52
Patient-mo	651	651	596	596
Episodes	39	29	26	18
Incidence/pt-mo	1/16.7	1/22.4	1/22.9	1/33.1

from this table, the most frequently encountered trouble was obstruction of the bag-ceramic joint caused by caramelized glucose residue (35 times: 33.0%), followed by a break of the ceramic joint (20 times: 18.9), and a crack in the dialysate line (16 times: 15.1%). The total rate of connecting device troubles were 106 times among 79,200 exchanges. The incidence was once per 747 exchanges.

DISCUSSION

The most frequent cause of drop-out from CAPD programs is peritonitis. The incidence reported by Oreopoulos et al.[2] was 1 per 7.3 patient months, and in the European Dialysis and Transplant Registry, more than 60% of the patients on CAPD experienced peritonitis within a year.[3]

There are several reports[4-6] on devices or techniques contrived to reduce the incidence of peritonitis in CAPD treatment. Many of them, however, are troublesome or require special apparatus of consid-

erable weight. The main advantages of the Flame-Lock system is to provide rapid and reliable connections using light and simple apparatus such as an alcohol lamp. The basic studies revealed that the surface temperature of the bag–ceramic joint at the time of connection and disconnection is around 200°C, which is enough to assure sterilization.[1] The incidence of peritonitis of 1 episode per 16.7 patient months is considered to be low, taking into account the situation that in this study group many of the doctors involved had no experience in CAPD treatment prior to this study.

On the other hand, device troubles of 1 per 747 exchanges, which means once in 187 days for patient repeating four exchanges daily, is not so low. The majority of the device problems, such as cracks in the dialysate line, breaks of the ceramic joint, and melting of the bag tubing, are caused by overheating of the bag-ceramic joint at the time of connection.

Table 3. Organisms Found in Dialysate.

S. aureus	7
S. epidermidis	5
S. species	3
Enterobactes agglomerous	2
Pseudomonas	2
E. coli	1
Candida	1
Micrococcus	1
Klebsiella oxytoca	1
Bacillus	1
Streptococcus species	1
Culture negative	14
Total	39

Table 4. Complications.

	No. of Cases
Hypertriglyceridemia	16
Tunnel infection	10
Hypercholesterolemia	6
Hypo HDL cholesterolemia	3
Lumbago	2
Hypotension	1
Hydrocele	1
Obesity	1
Inguinal hernia	1
Subcutaneous edema	1
Ileus	1
Intraperitoneal hemorrhage	1
Exit erosion	1
Total	45

Table 5. Connecting Device Problems.

Obstruction of joint	35
Break of ceramic joint	20
Crack in dialysate line	16
Transfer tube	(9)
Bag tube	(7)
Loose connection	16
Bag-ceramic joint	(8)
Titanium joint	(8)
Overheating of bag tubing	14
Difficult to detach (Bag-ceramic joint)	3
Leakage from joint	2
Total	**106**

(Total exchanges = 79,200; incidence of trouble = 1/747.)

However, there are only five instances of peritonitis caused by device troubles. Organisms found in the dialysate at the time of peritonitis are not different from those found in patients using other connecting devices. Other side effects and complications are similar to those observed in patients treated with CAPD using other systems.

CONCLUSION

The Flame-Lock CAPD system proved its clinical utility in 60 end-stage renal failure patients. The incidence of peritonitis was low, and the majority of device failures could be eliminated by education.

REFERENCES

1. Ota K, Suzuki T, Sudo N, and Takemoto M: A simple and foolproof connecting device for CAPD. Artif Organs (in press)
2. Oreopoulos DG, Robson M, Faller B, Ogilvie R, Rapoport A, and deVeber GA: Continuous ambulatory peritoneal dialysis: A new era in the treatment of chronic renal failure. Clin Nephrol 11: 125, 1979
3. Jacobs C, Broyer M, Brunner FP, Brynger H, Donckerwolcke RA, Kramer P, Selwood NH, Wing AF, and Blake PH: Combined report on regular dialysis and transplantation in Europe, XI, 1980. Proc Eur Dial Transplant Assoc 18: 4, 1981
4. Maiorca R, Cantaluppi A, Cancarini GC, Scalamogna A, Broccoli R, Graziani G, Brasa S, and Ponticelli C: Prospective controlled trial of a Y-connector and disinfectant to prevent peritonitis in continuous ambulatory peritoneal dialysis. Lancet 2: 642, 1983
5. Ash SR, Horswell R Jr, Heeter EM, and Bloch R: Effect of the Peridex® filter on peritonitis rates in a CAPD population. Peritoneal Dial Bull 3: 89, 1983
6. Hamilton R, Adams P, Burkart J, Disher B, Dillingham G, and Crater C: Feasibility of a sterile splice for connection in continuous ambulatory peritoneal dialysis. Trans Am Soc Artif Intern Organs 29: 623, 1983

R.J. Bielawa, K.L. Carr, and G.G. Bousquet

29

Intraluminal Thermosterilization Using a Microwave Autoclave

SUMMARY

This paper discusses the application of microwave heating to achieve a sterile CAPD connection and thereby minimize the incidence of peritonitis.

In essence a small amount of dialysate is trapped within the mated connector which, in turn, is held within a microwave coupler, creating in effect, a microwave autoclave which produces intraluminal thermosterilization for surface organisms, such as *S. aureus, S. epidermidis, E. coli* and *Candida albicans,* including spore-forming bacilli and viruses.

The prototype microwave system has proven to be very effective as a sterilizing device, achieving dialysate temperatures in excess of 138°C.

INTRODUCTION

The reported instances of peritonitis varies between 1 in 6 and 1 in 14 patient months and is generally a function of the age of the program, patient compliance, and patient selection. The generally accepted infection sites and the percentage of cases of peritonitis attributed to each site are shown in Table 1. Of these, the connector is responsible for 50–90% of peritonitis, and the tunnel or exit site for 5–20%. The bowel is also an important source, but bloodborne infection and ascending infection from the

From M/A-Com, Inc., Burlington, Massachusetts, and St. Joseph's Hospital, Lowell, Massachusetts.

vagina to Fallopian tubes are probably responsible for less than 1% of peritonitis.

Table 2 lists the organisms generally responsible for peritonitis and the frequency of occurrence, which is highly variable from center to center. Because the greatest percentage of peritonitis incidents is associated with the connector, the ideal situation would be to eliminate the connection altogether, for as the number of connections increases so does the incidence of peritonitis.

METHODS

Efforts to reduce or eliminate peritonitis associated with the connector fall into three major types. These are listed in Table 3. The first of these is asepsis. To this end, various connectors have been designed. Various chemicals, iodine in nature, have been added as a prophylaxis or an attempt toward sterilization. Bacterial filters have been introduced into the system, which has reduced the incidence of peritonitis; however, the filters are bulky, costly, and rarely last longer than three weeks. If one considers the incidence of postoperative infections under ideal conditions in the best of centers (which is approximately 1%), one can see that asepsis is not the total answer.

The second type is mechanical exchanges, whereby human hands are removed from the system. Examples of this type of device are the DuPont Splicing Device and the Trav-X-Change. Again, this

Table 1. Infection Sites.

1. Connector and bag
2. Tunnel and exit site
3. Bowel
4. Blood borne
5. Ascending from vagina to Fallopian tubes

Table 3. Methods of Prevention.

1. Asepsis
   Variable connectors
   Chemical—iodine
   Bacterial filter
2. Mechanical exchange—no human hands
3. Intraluminal thermal sterilization using microwave energy

is not a sterilization procedure but more an aseptic procedure.

The third type is the one we are concerned with here. The device was developed by M/A-COM, Inc. of Burlington, Massachusetts, and uses microwave technology to sterilize the connector. In essence, it is a microwave autoclave that produces intraluminal thermosterilization against organisms, such as *S. aureus*, *S. epidermidis*, *E. coli*, and *Candida albicans*, including spore-forming bacilli and viruses.

RESULTS

The prototype system shown in Figure 1 also provides for the mechanical mating of the connec-

Table 2. Peritonitis Causing Organisms and Frequency of Occurrence.

Staphylococcus Epidermidis *Staphylococcus Aureus* *Streptococcus Species*	65–75%

Enterobacteriaceae
  Proteus Species
  E. Coli
  Klebsiella Species
  Enterobacter Cloacae
Acinetobacter Species
Pseudomonas Species
	25–30%

Serratia Species *Bordetella Bronchiseptica* *Pasteurella* *Corynebacterium (Diphtheroids)* *Candida Albicans* *Nocardia Asteroides* *Aspergillus Species* *Fusarium Species* *Actinomyces Species* *Pitrosporum Ovale* *Rhodotorula Species* *Mycobacterium Fortuitum*	<5%

tor. The male and female ends of the connector are placed in "nests" (Fig. 2). The tubing is clamped near the connector; the male connector or "spike," is automatically aligned and moved forward, trapping a small amount of liquid within the mated connector. A microwave antenna surrounds the mated connector, and the sterilization process begins. After the sterilization is completed, the clamps are released in such a fashion as to discharge any pressure into the dialysate solution rather than into the patient.

The connector material used is transparent to microwave energy, while the dialysate, on the other hand, absorbs the microwave energy. Because the clamping arrangement holds the liquid at a constant volume, the pressure inside the connector increases, allowing the liquid temperature to rise well above the normal boiling temperature of 100°C. Initial tests on the prototype device indicated that the solution temperature exceeded 138°C. Figure 3 is a graph of the boiling temperature of water as a function of pressure. Figure 4 is a plot of time required

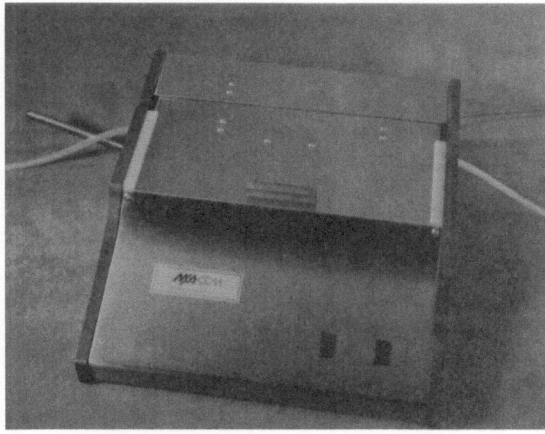

Fig. 1. The prototype system for the mechanical mating of the connector.

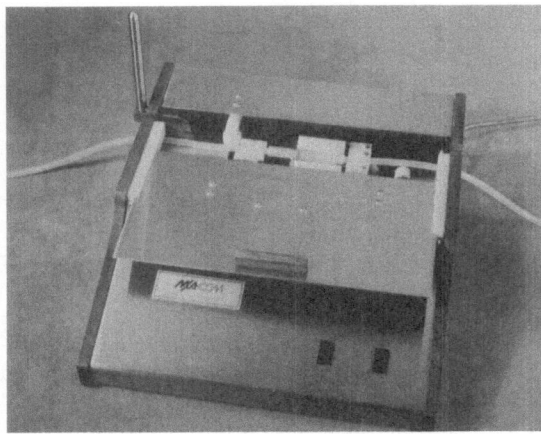

Fig. 2. The male and female ends of the connector are placed in "nests."

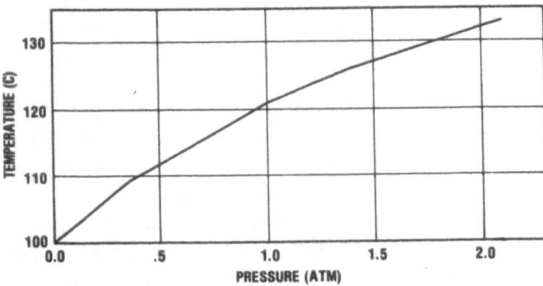

Fig. 3. Pressure differential versus boiling temperature.

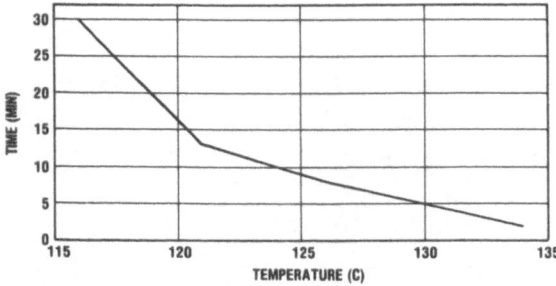

Fig. 4. Clinical sterilization time versus temperature.

Table 4. Benefits.

1. Intralumenal sterilization
2. Reduction of exhange time to less than 4 minutes
3. Lower cost—no need for disposables, including filtration
4. If peritonitis occurs, look at other sites—tunnel, etc.

to achieve clinical sterilization as a function of temperature.

Cultures were prepared (i.e., bacteria, including spore form) in a supporting media conducive to their growth. These samples were placed in the Microwave Sterilizer for 4.5 minutes at an average power of 15 W. During this time, the temperature of the solution (as determined through the use of heat-sensitive indicators) exceeded 138°C. The various solutions were examined at the end of seven days, and it was determined that the solutions were sterile—that is, all forms of bacteria, including spores, were destroyed.

DISCUSSION

The present prototype unit (Fig. 4) could be significantly reduced in size and weight. It is our intention, for example, to modularize the construction, separating the power supply from the basic unit. In addition to weight and size reduction, this will allow the unit to operate from a 12 V source, such as the cigarette lighter in an ordinary automobile. Also, elimination of the automatic mating feature for those patients not in need of this feature would result in a very compact portable model that could be easily carried in a briefcase. The major benefits of this system are enumerated in Table 4. They include intraluminal sterilization, reduction of exchange time, and lower costs. There is no need for disposables, including filter. With this technique the origin of peritonitis should be more easily located. Moreover, it can be used by blind patients.

R.P. Popovich, J.W. Moncrief, "P" A.J. Sorrels-Akar,
C. Mullins-Blackson, and K. Pyle

30

The Ultraviolet Germicidal System: The Elimination of Distal Contamination in CAPD

SUMMARY

The UV germicidal system will eliminate peritonitis associated with bag exchanges in CAPD. Catheter infections represent a significant problem which must be solved if the overall peritonitis rate is to be drastically reduced. UV radiation at a dosage of 45,000 μW sec/cm² disinfects bio-burdens of organisms in excess of those resulting from touch contamination.

INTRODUCTION

Peritonitis is the most significant medical complication associated with peritoneal dialysis.[1] Figure 1 outlines the sources of potential contamination. These are (1) the primary connection site, which is interrupted approximately 120 times per month during dialysis solution exchange; (2) injection of medications; (3) the transfer set/catheter connection, which is interrupted approximately once a month; (4) catheter exit site and tunnel; (5) endogenous sources such as diverticulitis.

The organisms associated with peritonitis and the relative frequency of occurrence are illustrated in Figure 2. Approximately two-thirds of the organisms are gram positive, and the microbial origins of all organisms are listed in Table 1.[3] Skin represents the most likely primary source of contamination. However, airborne contamination is a secondary source for the most common organisms associated with peritonitis, namely *Staphylococcus epidermidis (S. epidermidis)* and *Staphylococcus aureus (S. aureus)*. This mechanism could thwart even the most rigorous aseptic technique designed to eliminate touch contamination. These data, along with the fact that the primary connection site is interrupted so frequently by manual manipulation, led to the development of a connection system that would reduce microbial bio-burden at the primary connection site.

CONCEPT AND METHOD DEVELOPMENT

The fundamental concept in the development of the primary connection system is illustrated in Figure 3. It must be assumed, under a worst case basis, that both the spike and bag port can become contaminated by touch and/or airborne sources during a typical bag exchange. This is illustrated by Step 1 in Figure 3. The basic concept is to isolate the contaminated regions (Step 2), resterilize the isolated zone (Step 3), and finally, complete the connection and proceed with the exchange (Step 4).

From the University of Texas at Austin, and the Acorn Research Laboratory, Austin, Texas.

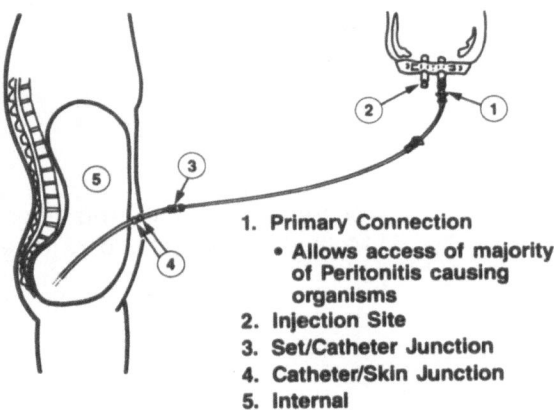

1. **Primary Connection**
   • **Allows access of majority of Peritonitis causing organisms**
2. **Injection Site**
3. **Set/Catheter Junction**
4. **Catheter/Skin Junction**
5. **Internal**

Fig. 1.   Potential sources of peritonitis.

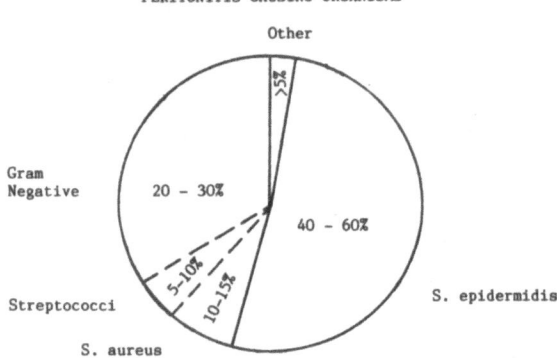

PERITONITIS CAUSING ORGANISMS

Fig. 2.   Incidence distribution of organisms causing peritonitis.

There are numerous methodologies to resterilize or inactivate the microorganisms in Step 3. These include heat, radiation, and toxic chemicals. Each has its respective advantages. A list of criteria was prepared that must be fulfilled by the method selected (Table 2). Ultraviolet (UV) radiation was the method that best fit the criteria and was selected as the antimicrobial agent.

Ultraviolet radiation is invisible to the eye and lies just above the visible range in the energy spectrum. It is an important component of nature. Ultraviolet radiation can be generated by passing an electric current between two electrodes in a mercury vapor. The electron flow ionizes the mercury atoms, which emit photons in the ultraviolet range with a maximum at 2537 Å. This radiation causes significant alterations in the DNA molecule, as outlined in Figure 4. The alterations interfere with normal metabolic and reproductive functions.

Microbial inactivation by ultraviolet radiation is a statistical phenomenon. The probability that a microbe will be inactivated depends upon the energy absorbed and the relative sensitivity of the organism to UV radiation. Once these factors are established, one can utilize probability theory to predict the outcome.

CONNECTION SYSTEM AND HARDWARE

The connection system consists of a molded bag port with a membrane and a "transfer set" spike, which transmits UV radiation. Both the spike and the bag port fit into opposite ends of a closed chamber (Fig. 5A). The chamber is surrounded by a convoluted bulb that emits UV radiation. The chamber serves two purposes: (1) it prevents further touch

Table 1.   Microbial Origins of Gram-Positive Cocci.

Type	Primary Origin	Secondary Origin
S. Epidermidis	Skin, nose	Airborne Mouth/pharynx Large intestine Vagina
S. Aureus	Skin, nose	Same as above
Streptococci Group A	Skin	Mouth/pharynx Nose
Group D *Viridans*	Large & small intestine Mouth/pharynx	Skin

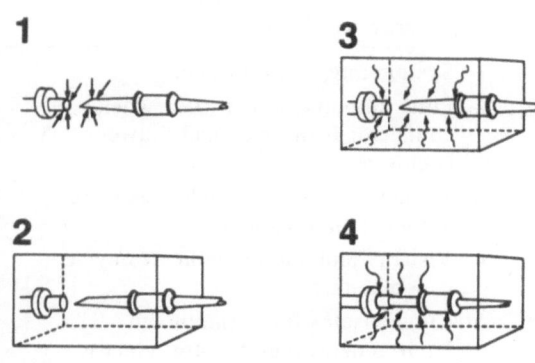

Fig. 3. Conceptual steps in connector sterilization.

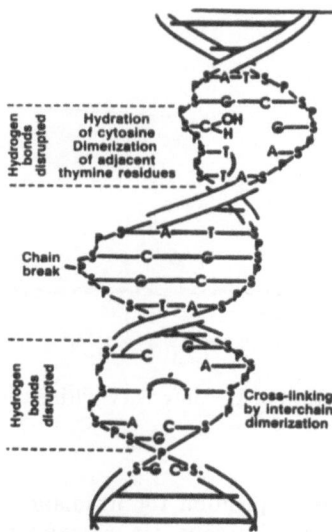

(Courtesy of R.A. Deering and Scientific American.)

Fig. 4. Effect of UV radiation on DNA molecule.

contamination of the spike and bag port, and (2) it irradiates the contaminated portions with UV light. Following microbial inactivation, the bag is spiked *inside* the closed chamber, thus preventing further contamination (Fig. 5B). The connection is then removed from the chamber and covered with a sliding shield cover that is part of the "transfer set" (Fig. 5C). Materials were chosen that had both the proper mechanical properties and acceptable transmission of UV radiation at 254 nm over the intended product life. The solution container is a one-usage component. The "transfer set" was designed to function for approximately six months.

The device was designed to deliver a consistent dosage of UV energy adequate to inactivate any conceivable bio-burden associated with bag exchanges. This was accomplished by a dosimeter within the device that read the UV intensity within the closed chamber and integrated the intensity over time until the predetermined dosage was reached according to the relationship in Equation (1):

$$\text{Dosage} = \int \text{Intensity dt} \qquad (1)$$

Table 2. Criteria for Antimicrobial Method.

1. Consistent, reproducible microbial inactivation
2. Portable
3. Minimize patient involvement
4. No toxic residual
5. Reasonably rapid
6. Fail-safe in the event of patient error

The system is thus capable of accommodating variations in both environment and power required to run the unit. A typical intensity versus time profile for a one-minute exposure is illustrated in Figure 6. The device is activated by placing the connection system in a drawer and closing the drawer. The cycle is automatically started and completed when integrated dosage of $600,000 \, \mu$ Watt-sec/cm^2 is reached. The device is portable, with power being supplied by either a wall adaptor or a battery pack. Battery life is approximately 20 exchanges between recharges.

The device includes a set of "nests" that will receive analogous flanges on the bag port and "transfer set" spike. These nests align the compo-

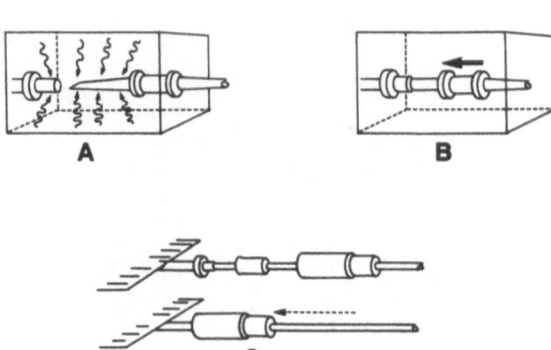

Fig. 5. The UV connection system.

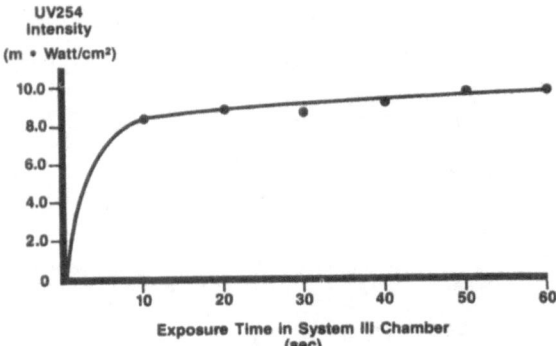

Fig. 6. Correlation of UV intensity with exposure time.

Table 3. Hardware Features.

1. System integrates dosage.
2. Fully automatic—activates when connector is inserted and drawer is closed.
3. Visually and audibly indicates error if cycle is interrupted.
4. Visually and audibly indicates cycle is complete.
5. Compensates for variations in environment, temperature, electric power.
6. Can be run on rechargeable battery pack.

nents in the proper position for irradiations and puncturing via a set of springs. Upon completion of the UV cycle, the "nest" can be advanced by moving a lever outside the chamber, thus puncturing the bag port in a closed environment (Fig. 7). The lever provides a mechanical advantage that assists in opening and closing the bag port–spike connection. Hardware features are summarized in Table 3. A photograph of the complete apparatus is presented in Figure 8.

RESULTS

When a population of microorganisms is subjected to a dosage of UV radiation they are not all inactivated at once, but rather a fraction are inactivated in each increment of time. The fraction that survive after a given time increment is a function of exposure time, intensity of the radiation, and the sensitivity of the organism, as expressed by Equation (2)[4]:

$$\frac{N}{N_0} = e^{-KIt} \qquad (2)$$

**IRRADIATION WITH
SPIKE ADVANCEMENT**

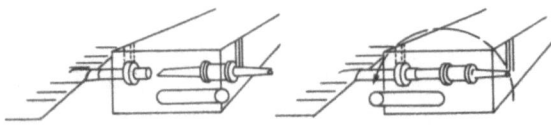

Fig. 7. Operation of the UV sterilization chamber.

where

N_0 = microbial population initially present

N = microbial population present after exposure time t

K = constant related to organism

I = intensity of radiation

The form of Equation (2) suggests that a straight line will be achieved if the logarithm of surviving organisms is plotted as a function of exposure time. The dosage is a measure of incident UV energy per unit area of exposed surface (the intensity multiplied by exposure time) and is usually expressed in units of microwatt seconds per square centimeter (μW sec/cm^2).

Many hundreds of *in vitro* tests were performed using prototype UV germicidal systems. Figure 9 illustrates the relative sensitivity of three organisms using the suggested plot of logarithm population versus time. Three nearly straight lines result. The radiation intensity was constant at 500 μW/cm^2. Note that the organism most commonly associated with peritonitis in CAPD (*S. epidermidis*) is higly UV-sensitive. A population of approximately 10,000 organisms was totally inactivated after an exposure time of less than 10 seconds. *Candida albicans (C. albicans)*, on the other hand, is a highly UV-resistant organism and represents an extreme challenge.

Table 4 gives the effect of UV intensity on microbial kill. For a given organism, the same overall dose was applied in each test. The intensity and times of exposure were varied accordingly. The results indicated that dosage, regardless of how applied, had the same effect on reducing bio-burden. These results conform to the Bunsen-Rescol reciprocity law, which states that dosage is a function of

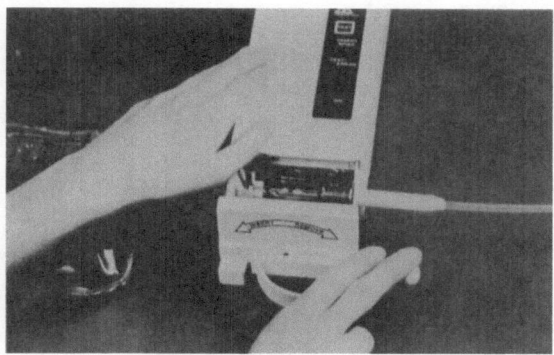

Fig. 8. The UV system.

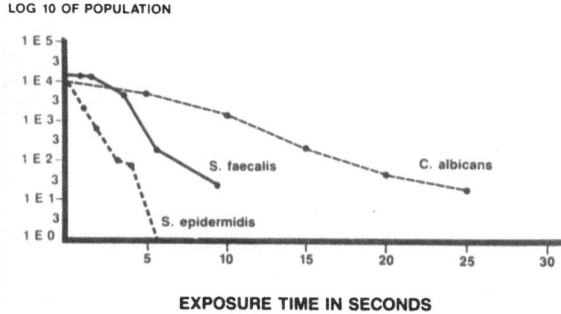

Fig. 9. Relative sensitivity of test organisms versus exposure time.

total energy and does not depend on the absolute values of either the intensity or time.[5] Note also the higher dose required (45,000 μW sec/cm²) to achieve approximately 99.9% kill with *C. albicans* relative to *S. epidermidis* (6,000 μW sec/cm²).

Table 5 gives the percent kill and shows that this was not effected by temperature within the range of 5–35°C. Results from these and other initial tests and IU transmission of connectors were used to establish the dosage of 600,000 μW sec/cm² supplied by the germicidal chamber.

Final *in vitro* testing of the actual components was performed by the following method. A suspension of *C. albicans* in spent Dianeal® (Travenol Laboratories Deerfield, IL) was placed into the lumen of spikes and irradiated in the UV chamber. Under these conditions, *C. albicans* was consistently disinfected at a rate of $10^{5.5}$ (316,228) organisms/spike during each full UV cycle. This value was calculated using the most probable numbers method.

A literature review was completed on the relative germicidal effectiveness of UV radiation on other microorganisms more commonly associated with peritonitis, such as *S. epidermidis*, *S. aureus*, and *S. faecalis*. These values are shown in Figure 10 as a relative comparison to the kill rate for *C. albicans*.

Additional *in vitro* testing was performed by "touch contaminating" the spike with the hand. Twenty-seven subjects each touch-contaminated a spike by rolling the spike between the thumb and index finger. Each subject also performed a negative control (no touch) and a positive control (no irradiation). Each subject also touch-contaminated a spike that was used to determine the bio-burden of the subject's fingers. Bio-burden ranged from 0 to 3080 organisms, with an average of 170.9 organisms/unit. All test units and negative controls were subjected to a complete UV cycle. Spikes were subsequently advanced into media-filled containers and incubated.

The results of the "touch contamination" tests are illustrated in Table 6. None of the test units (subjected to UV radiation) exhibited growth of or-

Table 4. Effect of UV Radiation Intensity on Microbial Kill.

Intensity μW/cm²	*S. epidermidis* 6000 μW sec/cm²		*S. faecalis* 8000 μW sec/cm²		*C. albicans* 45000 μW sec/cm²	
	N	% kill	N	% kill	N	% kill
0	8.8E4	0	1.7E4	0	8.1E4	0
200	2.9E1	99.7	3.0E1	99.8	9.6E0	99.9
375	2.9E0	99.9	9.2E0	99.9	1.2E1	99.9
750	6.7E0	99.9	1.3E1	99.9	2.1E0	99.9
1500	8.0E1	99.1	1.2E1	99.9	5.8E1	99.9
6000	<1.0E0	99.9	1.3E2	99.3	6.3E0	99.9

Table 5. Microbial Kill by UV Radiation with Changing Temperature.

Temp °C	UV Dose μW sec/cm²	Starting Population	Surviving Population	% Kill
S. Epidermidis				
5	3,000	4.4E3	8.6E0	99.8
15	3,000	4.2E4	1.0E0	99.9
22	3,000	1.2E5	4.8E0	99.9
35	3,000	8.6E4	7.7E1	99.9
S. Faecalis				
5	3,900	1.9E3	9.1E1	95.2
15	3,900	8.9E3	8.6E0	99.9
22	3,900	1.9E4	1.4E1	99.9
35	3,900	3.0E3	1.9E0	99.9
C. Albicans				
5	22,500	7.7E4	1.2E1	99.9
15	22,500	4.8E4	3.1E1	99.9
22	22,500	7.1E4	1.0E0	99.9
35	22,500	2.1E5	3.3E0	99.9

ganisms, indicating complete disinfection. Twenty-two of the positive controls (no UV irradiation) showed growth. It is interesting to note that the subjects with no positive control growth showed lower than average bio-burden levels (less than 10 organisms). None of the negative controls (no touch) exhibited growth.

DISCUSSION

The UV Germicidal System is capable of disinfecting bio-burdens in excess of 100,000 highly UV-resistant organisms during its one-and-one-half minute cycle. Since "touch contamination" represents a bio-burden significantly less than 10,000 organisms, the system will eliminate peritonitis associated with routine bag exchanges if the proper technique is followed. This will result in a lowered incidence of peritonitis in CAPD, which will, in turn lower the cost, decrease hospitalization days, ease the burden on the nursing staff, increase the potential patient pool, reduce the drop-out rate, ease patient fear, and assist diagnosis of auxiliary problems.

Preliminary results of a trial of the germicidal system in Austin showed a 25% decrease in the peritonitis rate for a 12-month period with and without the use of the UV System. The peritonitis rate of the test group (1.59 episodes/yr) was 32% less than

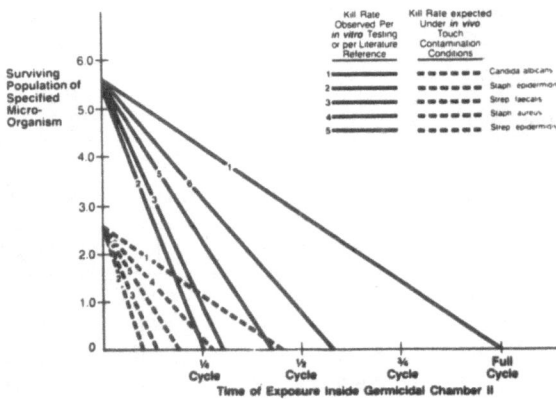

Fig. 10. Survival curves of microorganisms undergoing UV irradiation.

Table 6. Touch Contamination Test.

Study	# Studies	# Positive Growth
Test Units (touch & irradiation)	27	0
Positive Controls (no irradiation)	27	22
Negative Controls (no touch)	27	0

all other patients not on UV (2.34 episodes/yr). However, the results are not statistically significantly different with the small number of patients (10) in the test study. Nevertheless, the patients all expressed a marked decrease in their fears and anxieties associated with peritonitis, which greatly enhanced their quality of life on CAPD.

Finally, we were able to pinpoint catheter exit site and tunnel infections as the causative agent in several patients on the UV system who continued with high peritonitis rates. In two cases catheters were replaced without evidence of exit site or tunnel infections because of repeated peritonitis episodes (we knew the problem could not be related to bag exchange procedures). Both catheters were culture-positive following removal, and the peritonitis episodes ceased with implantation of new catheters. These preliminary results strongly suggest that catheters are the source of a significant percentage of the episodes of peritonitis in CAPD.

REFERENCES

1. Nolph KD (Ed): Peritoneal dialysis. The Hague: Martinus Nijhoff, 1981

2. Isenberg HD, and Painter BG: Indigenous and pathogenic microorganisms in humans. In Manual of clinical microbiology, 3rd Ed. Washington, D.C.: American Society of Microbiology, 1980, p 25

3. Jawatz E, Melnick JL, and Adelberg EA: Normal microbial flora of the human body. In Review of medical microbiology, 13th Ed. Lange Medical Publications, 1978, p 260

4. Abbot WE, and Shea P: Treatment of temporary renal insufficiency (uremia) by peritoneal lavage. Am J Med Sci 211: 312, 1946

5. Doolan PD, Murphy WP, Wiggins RA, Carter NW, Cooper WD, Watten RH, and Alpen EI: An evaluation of intermittent peritoneal lavage. Am J Med 26: 831, 1959

W.P. Reed, P.D. Light, and K.A. Newman

31

Biofilm on Tenckhoff Catheters: A Possible Source for Peritonitis

SUMMARY

The inner portion of peritoneal catheters that had been removed from seven CAPD patients for a variety of reasons were examined. Biofilm was identified on all catheters. In patients that were clinically free of infection, catheters also showed coccoid forms and the majority grew *Staphylococcus epidermidis* from at least one segment. The colonization of indwelling Tenckhoff catheters may serve as a potential source for peritonitis.

INTRODUCTION

Peritonitis is one of the main problems complicating the use of implantable peritoneal catheters for CAPD. Breaks in techniques allowing transluminal entry of microorganisms are most frequently suggested as the mechanism of contamination.[1] While these infections will clear with appropriate antibiotics in some patients, rapid recurrence after the cessation of therapy has also been observed.

A parallel experience has occurred with long-term central venous (Hickman) catheters in our cancer patients requiring chemotherapy.[2] Initially we assumed that bacteremia was the result of careless technique allowing introduction of microorganisms into the catheter lumen as an isolated event. Eventually it became apparent that some patients behaved as if the catheter were a bacterial reservoir, since repeated episodes of infection occurred with the same organism. Usually the bacteremia developed only at times when chemotherapy or disease activity rendered patients profoundly granulocytopenic. During periods when white cell counts were normal, patients remained afebrile.

Recently we have begun to examine all Hickman catheters with electron microscopy at the time of explantation undertaken either for infection or at the completion of therapy. We have been able to demonstrate a biofilm layer, often containing coccoid forms, as a possible source of repeated bacteremia, along the luminal surface of all catheters examined.[3] The current investigation was undertaken to determine whether similar biofilm deposits could be detected on the luminal surface of explanted Tenckhoff catheters.

MATERIALS AND METHODS

All catheters were inserted and removed under local anesthesia in the outpatient operating room. The linea alba was identified through a transverse incision just inferior to the umbilicus and opened longitudinally to expose the peritoneum. The catheter was directed into the pelvis through an incision in the peritoneum just large enough to accommodate the diameter of the tubing. The peritoneum was tightened about the catheter with a 2-0 polyglactin purse-string suture, following which a water-tight

From the University of Maryland School of Medicine, Baltimore, Maryland.

Table 1. Survey of Catheters Removed from 7 Patients.

Patient	Culture Results	EM Results	Reason Removed	Clinical Status
1	*S. epidermidis*	Biofilm + cocci	Preferred hemodialysis	Well
2	No growth	Biofilm + cocci	Mechanical failure	Well
3	*S. epidermidis*	Biofilm	Repeated infections	Well on antibiotics
4	No growth	Biofilm	Preferred hemodialysis	Well
5	*S. epidermidis* (1/8 sections)	Biofilm	Preferred hemodialysis	Well on antibiotics
6	*E. coli*	Biofilm—no cocci	Infection	Septic
7	*Enterobacter cloacae*	Biofilm + WBC	Repeated infections	Recovering on antibiotics

closure of the linea alba to outer aspect of the deep cuff was formed using interrupted circumferentially placed 2-0 polyglactin sutures. The outer end of the catheter was drawn through a subcutaneous tunnel to a separate exit site, positioning the superficial cuff at least 4 cm inside this opening.

Catheters were removed for fungal peritonitis, repeated episodes of peritonitis, cloudy drainage not clearing with appropriate antibiotic therapy, mechanical catheter failure, renal transplantation, or patient dissatisfaction with CAPD as a dialysis mode. Removal was accomplished by exposing and dividing the catheter between the two cuffs, taking care to exclude the potentially colonized exit site and external catheter from the operative field. Once the catheter was divided, it was relatively easy to follow the tubing down to the deep cuff and detach this cuff from the abdominal fascia by sharp dissection. The inner cuff and catheter could then be withdrawn in a sterile manner for culture. After the fascia was closed with 2-0 polyglactin, and the skin and subcutaneous tissues with 4.0 polyglactin, the exit site could be enlarged to expose and detach the external cuff, completing the removal procedure.

The isolated inner portion of the catheter was divided under sterile conditions into six segments. Half of these segments were vortexed to dislodge bacteria and cultured by standard microbiological techniques. Half were fixed in pH 7.2 cacodylate buffer and stored at 4°C until scanning electron microscopy could be accomplished.

RESULTS

Since April 1979, 67 patients have participated in the program of CAPD at the University of Maryland Hospital. In addition, 15 patients have been maintained by weekly peritoneal dialysis through Tenckhoff catheters for variable periods of time when vascular access problems or hemorrhagic complications dictated interruption of hemodialysis. Currently, there are 38 patients still on CAPD. The remaining patients discontinued this form of dialysis because of multiple infections (8), bowel perforation (3), cardiac-related death (3), hydrothorax (3), mechanical failure (1), transplantation (4), or patient preference for hemodialysis (7). Catheters removed

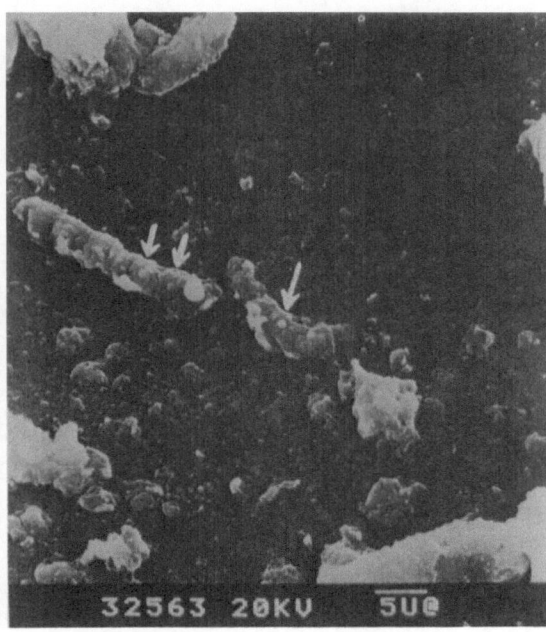

Fig. 1. Coccoid profiles (arrows) on biofilm deposits (Patient #1).

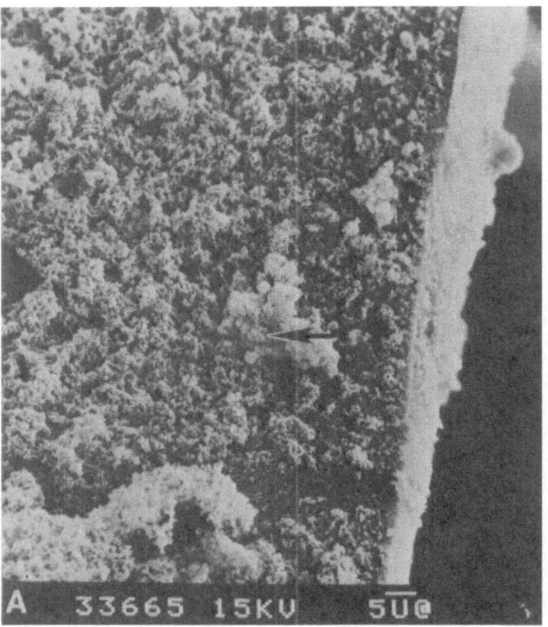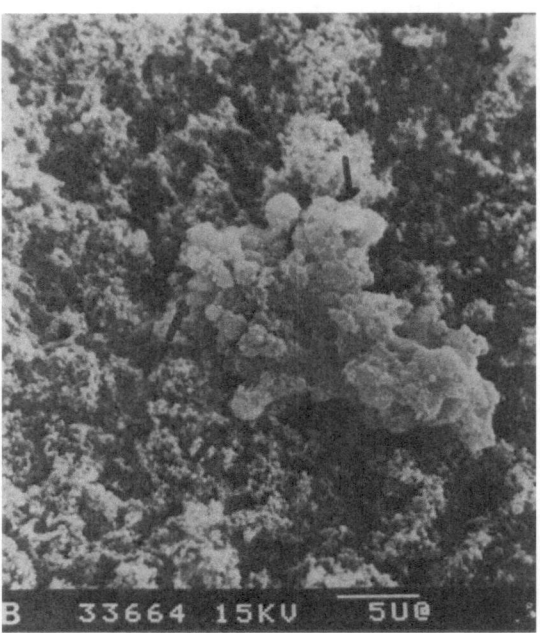

Fig. 2. (*a*) Coccoid forms (arrow) on typical fluffy biofilm (Patient #2). (*b*) Closer view of coccoid forms.

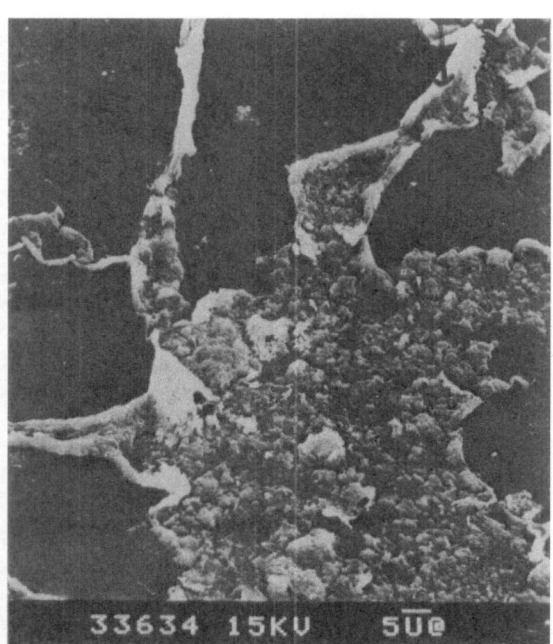

Fig. 3. Well developed biofilm without bacterial profiles (Patient #6).

from seven patients have been studied. Three of these were removed because of patient preference for hemodialysis, one for mechanical failure, and three because of repeated infections, one of which was probably due to biliary tract disease (Patient #6).

All catheters examined demonstrated biofilm, whether there was active infection or not (Table 1). In patients who were clinically well, catheters also showed coccoid forms, and 2/3 of them grew *Staphylococcus epidermis* from at least one segment of the catheter. The two patients with gram-negative organisms on culture also demonstrated biofilm, but neither showed any definite forms suggestive of microorganisms.

Figures 1 and 2 demonstrate the typical biofilm containing coccoid forms that were seen in clinically well patients whose catheters were removed for mechanical reasons or because the patient expressed a preference for hemodialysis. Figures 3 and 4 are from patients with clinical infection. Both catheters again demonstrate biofilm, but bacterial forms could not be identified in either. White cells, which are clearly different from the coccoid forms, are abundant in one of these catheters.

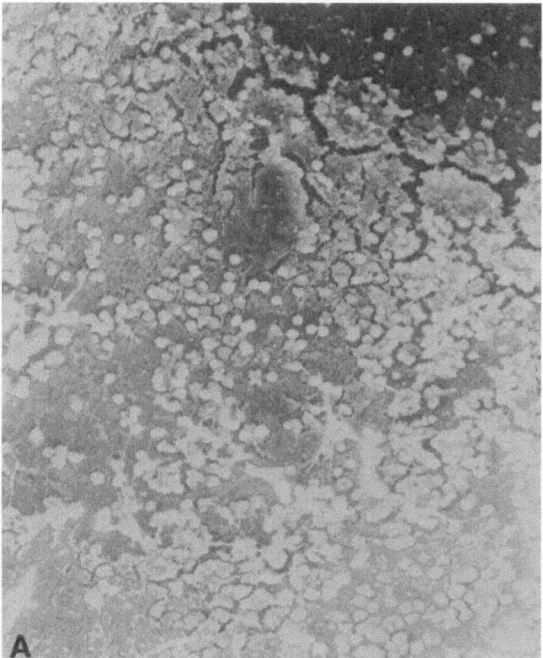 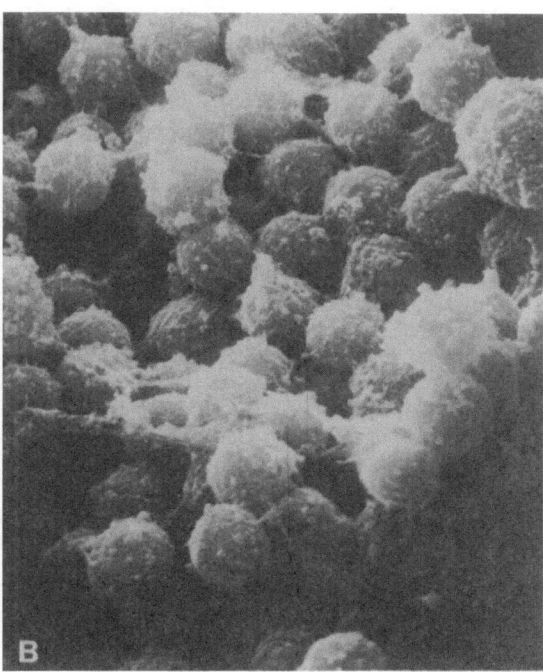

Fig. 4. (*a*) White cells on biofilm in patient with peritonitis (Patient #7). (*b*) Closer view of white cells.

DISCUSSION

Prolonged transcutaneous access to a body space is always associated with the potential risk of infection. Since the tubing used for access interrupts the integrity of the protective epidermis, microorganisms will have a route of entry, either transluminally or around the catheter, as long as it remains in place. In addition, a foreign substance may act as a refuge from host defenses for bacteria that have gained entry through sites quite independent of the material itself. It is not surprising, therefore, that peritonitis should be one of the commonest complications of prolonged peritoneal access for dialysis.[1]

The Dacron cuff surrounding long-term implantable catheters of the Hickman-Tenckhoff type effectively seals the outer surface against bacterial invasion, but protection of the lumen against contamination continues to depend upon technical precision in the preparation of solutions and in tubing changes. This lumen seems particularly susceptible to colonization with coagulase negative staphylococci, as evidenced by the increased prevalence of Staphylococcus epidermidis as a causative agent of bacteremia in granulocytopenic patients with indwelling catheters.[4-6]

One characteristic of coagulase negative Staphylococci that appears to aid in the attachment of these organisms to catheters is their production of an extracellular film or slime[7,8] The appearance of such a film on all catheters examined suggests colonization by coagulase negative Staphylococci, although this does not establish such an event by any means.

Of interest is the fact that coccoid forms or positive cultures for *Staphylococcus epidermidis* were only obtained in patients who were clinically well. This finding implies that catheter colonization by these organisms seldom produces clinical infections and may even have a protective role in limiting the establishment of more pathogenic species. This is consistent with our findings in previous studies[3] on Hickman central venous catheters, where colonization by *Staphylococcus epidermidis* did not appear to produce clinical symptoms unless host resistance had been lowered by chemotherapy or disease.

We conclude that there is evidence for colonization of the luminal surface of long-term indwelling

Tenckhoff peritoneal catheters. This colonization may serve as a potential source for peritonitis but may also be present in clinically healthy patients. The role that biofilm plays in the development of or resistance to peritonitis remains to be elucidated.

REFERENCES

1. Gloor HJ, Nichols WK, Sorkin MI, Prowant BF, Kennedy JM, Baker B, and Nolph KD: Peritoneal access and related complications in continuous ambulatory peritoneal dialysis. Am J Med 74: 593, 1983
2. Reed WP, Newman KA, DeJongh C, Wade JC, Schimpff SC, Wiernik PH, and McLaughlin JS: Prolonged venous access for chemotherapy by means of the Hickman catheter. Cancer 52: 185, 1983
3. Tenney JH, Reed WP, Newman KA, Costerton JW, Moody MR, Wade JC, and Schimpff SC: Clinical significance of sessile microorganisms on silicone intravenous catheters removed from cancer patients (unpublished)
4. Wade JC, Schimpff SC, Newman KA, and Wiernik PH: Staphylococcus epidermidis: An increasing cause of infection in patients with granulocytopenia. Ann Intern Med 97: 503, 1982
5. Begala JE, Maher K, and Cherry JD: Risk of infection associated with the use of Broviac and Hickman catheters. Am J Infect Control 10: 17, 1982
6. Lowder JN, Lazarus HM, and Herzig RH: Bacteremias and fungemias in oncologic patients with central venous catheters. Changing spectrum of infection. Arch Intern Med 142: 1456, 1982
7. Peters G, Locci R, and Pulverer G: Adherence and growth of coagulase-negative staphylococci on surfaces of intravenous catheters. J Infect Dis 146: 479, 1982
8. Christensen GD, Simpson WA, Bisno AL, and Beachy EH: Notes: Experimental foreign body infections in mice challenged with slime producing staphylococcus epidermidis. Infect Immunol 40: 407, 1983

C. Smith

32

CAPD: One Cuff vs Two Cuff Catheters in Reference to Incidence of Infection

SUMMARY

The incidence rates of peritonitis, exit site infection and catheter tunnel infection in two regions of California were compared in relation to the number of peritoneal dialysis catheter cuffs. Tunnel infections were considerably less frequent with double cuff catheters than with single cuff catheters. Peritonitis and exit site infections were not appreciably different with either catheter.

INTRODUCTION

BMA Oakland (BMAO) is a free-standing CAPD unit that began in June 1980. In over 600 months of experience, 33 patients have been trained successfully. Our peritonitis rate has improved through the years and now stands at one episode every 36 patient months. Exit site and tunnel infection rates continue to be the same as or below the national average. BMAO uses only single cuff catheters that are surgically inserted using a midline incision, with the single cuff sutured into the fascia at the midline.

There has been a longstanding controversy in the peritoneal dialysis field over which CAPD catheter is superior. This study is based not on the type of catheter used, but solely on how many cuffs on the catheter, and compares the infection rates with each.

METHODS

Fifteen Northern California and ten Southern California units were polled by questionnaire to determine which catheter was used, how many cuffs were on the catheter, how was the catheter inserted, the percentage of erosions through the skin of the second cuff, current peritonitis data, current exit site infection data, and current tunnel infection data.

RESULTS

The average experience in each unit was 296 patient months. The average number of patients per unit was 15.8. Patients were treated with either continuous ambulatory peritoneal dialysis (CAPD), intermittent peritoneal dialysis (IPD), or continuous cycling peritoneal dialysis (CCPD). The types of catheters included the Tenckhoff single cuff, Tenckhoff double cuff, Toronto Western single cuff, Toronto Western double cuff, and the Life-cath double cuff catheters. Only one unit polled had switched from single cuff to double cuff catheters, due to a new nephrologist's preference, and not because of statistical data or infection problems.

In Northern California, 73% of the catheters were inserted surgically, the other 27% using a trocar and catheter insertion by the nephrologist. In Southern California, 100% of the catheters were in-

From the BMA Dialysis Unit of Oakland, Oakland, California.

182   Smith

Table 1. Rates of Infection (per Patient Month) in Southern and Northern California.

	Peritonitis	Exit Site Infection	Tunnel Infection
Southern California	9.4	20.9	61.6
Northern California	9.9	22.0	59.3
Average	9.65	21.45	60.45

serted surgically. No unit in Northern California kept any records of erosions of the second cuff, infections due to erosions, erosions due to infection, nor loss of catheter due to erosions. In Southern California, 24% of the second cuffs eroded, but no infection-related data were kept. One unit had recently switched from double cuff to single cuff catheters due to 100% erosions associated with 100% exit site infections.

There were insufficient data collected to compare trocar insertion to surgical insertion for infection rates. Of the 25 units, two kept no peritonitis data, six kept no exit site infection data, and seven kept no tunnel infection data. Definitions of infection agreed upon by all 25 units were as follows:

Peritonitis

1. Cloudy effluent, dialysate WBC greater than 50/mm³
2. Abdominal cramping or pain
3. May or may not have
   A. Positive culture
   B. Fever
   C. Nausea and/or vomiting
   D. Diarrhea
4. Exit site and tunnel clear, clean and dry

Exit Site Infection

1. Redness around exit and/or
2. Tenderness around exit and/or
3. Hardened cellulitis knot around exit and/or
4. Usually accompanied with purulent drainage
5. May or may not have a positive culture
6. Tunnel easily palpable
7. Dialysate clear

Table 2. Rates of Infection (per Patient Month) Using Single or Double Cuff Catheters.

	Peritonitis	Exit Site Infection	Tunnel Infection
Single Cuff	12.1	18.7	24.2
Double Cuff	9.65	21.45	60.45

Tunnel Infection

1. Redness along entire tract and/or
2. Hardness along entire tract and/or
3. Bogginess along entire tract and/or
4. Pain along tract
5. Purulent drainage easily expressed from entire tract
6. Dialysate clear

Northern California infection data were tallied first. With regard to peritonitis, one unit kept no data, two units (still very young) had no cases to report, and 12 units offered current data (three units using single cuff catheters and nine units using double cuff catheters). Units using single cuff catheters had one case every 12.1 patient months, and those using double cuff catheters had one case every 9.9 patient months. Regarding exit site infection, five units kept no data, two units had no cases to report, and eight units offered current data (three units using single cuff catheters and five units using double cuff catheters). With single cuff catheters there was one case every 18.7 patient months, and with double cuff catheters there was one case every 22.0 patient months. As far as tunnel infection was concerned, six units kept no data, three units had no cases to report, and six units offered current data (three units using single cuff catheters and three units using double cuff catheters). For single cuff catheters the incidence was one case every 24.2 patient months, and for double cuff catheters it was one case every 59.3 patient months.

All ten of the Southern California units in this study use double cuff catheters. Therefore double cuff infection data were tallied to find an average. Infection rates were found as shown in Table 1. Then collective double cuff data were compared to single cuff infection data (Table 2). Then collective double cuff infection data were compared to single cuff infection data. Results are shown in Table 2.

CONCLUSION

These data show marginal differences between the two catheters when comparing them for peritonitis rates, less than 2.5 months difference, and exit site infection rates, less than 3 months difference. The most significant data appears when comparing the two catheters for rates of tunnel infection, with over 36 patient months difference in favor of double cuff catheters. Tunnel infections, which at BMAO leads to immediate catheter removal and termination of CAPD for a minimum of four weeks, are decreased greatly when using double cuff catheters of any kind.

F.M. Parsons, A.M. Brownjohn, J.H. Turney, G.A. Young, J. Young, I.H. Ahmed-Jushuf, J. Gibson, and S. Coltman

33

Profound Reduction in Peritonitis in CAPD Using Travenol System IIR Connectors and Betadine®

SUMMARY

In continuous ambulatory peritoneal dialysis a method of sterilizing the connector between the 2 L bag and transfer set with povidone-iodine has been developed along with double clamping of the transfer set. There was a profound reduction in the incidence of peritonitis which fell from 1 attack per 19 patient weeks to 1 attack per 376 patient weeks.

INTRODUCTION

In the mid-1960s we used once weekly peritoneal dialysis with a trocath inserted for each session of 40 hourly exchanges with minimal peritonitis.[1] On instituting twice weekly peritoneal dialysis in 1978, using a Tenckhoff catheter, each session consisting of 24 hourly exchanges, a high incidence of peritonitis occurred. This was traced to bacterial contamination at the end of the Tenckhoff catheter. Infection from this entry site was eradicated by thorough soaking of the end of the catheter and its connector with 10% povidone-iodine (Betadine®) before and after each session. As in the earlier series, the inci-

From the Renal Research Unit, The General Infirmary, Leeds, United Kingdom.

dence of peritonitis in this intermittent technique then became low, in keeping with that found by others. Following the introduction of CAPD in 1980 a high incidence of peritonitis recurred. Furthermore, we gained the impression that the incidence increased (but it was not statistically significant) when the connector to the 2 L bag was changed from a Travenol spike system to the Travenol IIR system, which is a luer connector with a two-start screw lock device. We investigated the possibility of applying to the Travenol IIR connector the povidone-iodine technique, which had proved so successful in eradicating infection at the end of the Tenckhoff catheter.

METHODS

Radiographic examination of the Travenol IIR connector revealed large air spaces within the screw part of the connector (Fig. 1), the full extent being displayed using radio opaque contrast medium (Fig. 2). Radiological examination also demonstrated one of the major disadvantages of a rigid male/female connector, for the female part fills with potentially infected air on disconnection (Fig. 3). In the Travenol IIR connector the female part is attached to the transfer set, which is probably a greater bacterial hazard than in the spike system, where the female part is the port of the dialysis bag, which is discarded at each exchange. On reconnecting the Travenol IIR

183

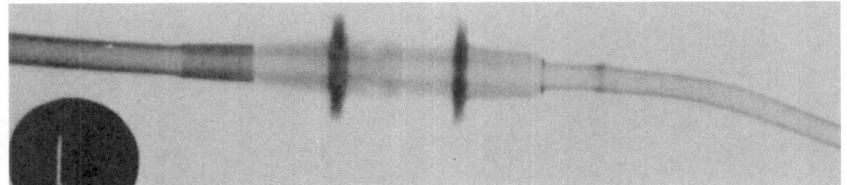

Fig. 1. Radiograph of Travenol IIR connector. (In this and subsequent radiographic figures 2 L bag to left and peritoneal cavity to right. All X-rays are reversal films).

system this pocket of air is "trapped" in the lumen of the connector (Fig. 4) and enters the abdominal cavity on inflow of fresh dialysis fluid.

First we tried immersing the opened connector in 10% povidone-iodine, but after reconnection and storing at 37° C for several hours the connector could not be unscrewed by hand. This did not occur after spraying the connector with 5% povidone-iodine using nitrogen as the propellant (marketed as "Betadine® Aerosol Spray"). In practice we train our patients to spray the connector attached to the 2 L fresh bag of dialysis fluid because it is a fixed point (Fig. 5). Assembling the connector disperses the povidone-iodine over both male and female surfaces of the Travenol IIR screw, where it is trapped by the locking device (Fig. 6) for the total exchange time. On disconnection a very small quantity of the povidone-iodine is sucked into the female luer connector, which will enter the abdominal cavity at the next exchange (Fig. 7).

In cooperative patients this spray technique is used on alternate exchanges, but the poorly compliant patient is instructed to use the spray at each exchange. Patient acceptance of the spray procedure is probably close to 100%, for it is simple, not time-consuming, and requires no alteration to existing apparatus. The Travenol IIR system uses a clamshell that clips onto the connector after assembly, the inbuilt sponge being saturated with povidone-iodine. It is doubtful whether this clamshell has any major antimicrobial activity in CAPD so we only change it daily, respraying the sponge with 5% povidone-iodine at each exchange. This saves about $920/year, less about $60 for the total cost of the povidone-iodine.

Whilst undertaking the above radiographic studies it was noted that the on/off roller clamp applied to the transfer set was sometimes difficult to operate and occasionally did not completely occlude the PVC tube. Observation of the patients revealed the same problem, and when the roller clamp was not fully occluded air was sucked into the transfer tube during normal respiration. As this air will enter the peritoneal cavity, it could be a potential source of infection; this hazard must be prevented. We now insist that all our patients use two port clamps during each exchange; one is applied to the port of the 2 L bag and the other is applied to transfer set. Patients are trained to vary the site of application of the clamp on the transfer set to prevent damage. The major advantage of the port clamp is that it only has two positions—fully on or fully off. Full compliance on the part of the patients in using two port clamps and the roller clamp is easy to achieve. We cannot overemphasize the importance of the double clamping technique of the transfer set in order to prevent potentially contaminated air entering the peritoneal cavity.

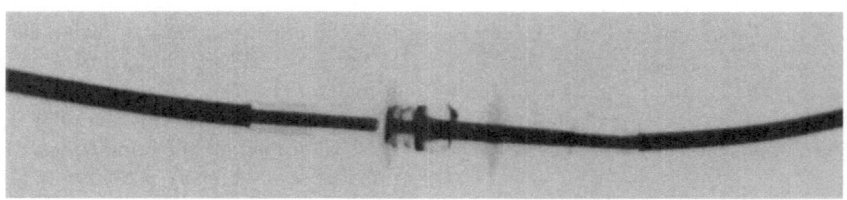

Fig. 2. Lumen of tubing, connector, and screw union filled with radio opaque contrast liquid.

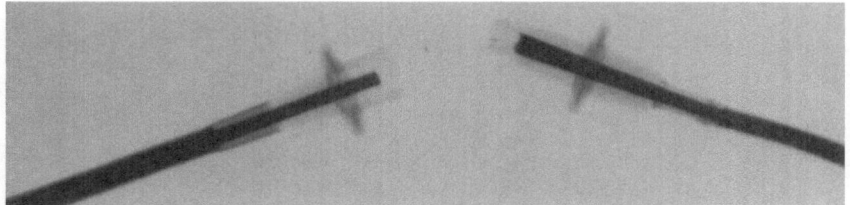

Fig. 3. Female luer (on right) fills with air on disconnection.

RESULTS

On introducing the povidone-iodine spray and extra clamping procedure we only had 12 patients on treatment, an inadequate number for a controlled trial, so all patients were trained in the new techniques during November and December, 1982. Table 1 gives the results of the peritonitis incidence thought to arise from contamination of the connector and patient errors in the home before and after the new procedures were introduced. The peritonitis incidence before the spray and extra clamping procedures were introduced (June to November, 1982, Table 1) was high at 1 per 19 patient weeks. After the new procedures were instituted there were two episodes of peritonitis in the first six-month period (November 1982 to April 1983) and one episode in each of the two following six-month periods, to give an average incidence of peritonitis of only 1 per 376 patient weeks (7.2 patient years). Two of these incidents (one in the second and one in the third six-month period) were almost certainly caused by patient error. One patient used a bag that he knew was leaking, whilst the second accidently disconnected at the transfer set/Tenckhoff catheter union. Both patients failed to report these errors to the unit until peritonitis developed within two days of the episode. However, neither of these attacks of peritonitis resulted from a breakdown in the povidone-iodine sterilizing and extra clamping procedures. Ignoring these two errors, which allows a more comprehensive assessment of the new techniques, the peritonitis rate fell to 1 per 1129 patient weeks (21.7 patient years). As the peritonitis rate fell so dramatically, it was deemed unethical to embark on a controlled trial when more patients entered the program. All our patients on CAPD (age range 23–74 years) used the new techniques so there was no patient selection and they came from most social classes present in the UK.

During the period under review (June 1982 to April 1984), peritonitis arose from other causes, but these were not under the control of the patient. Two "exit site" infections led to peritonitis. Three patients developed peritonitis from readily identifiable surgical causes: two had a strangulated hernia, whilst the third had an accidental perforation of bowel at the time of renal transplantation. In an earlier assessment,[3] our highest incidence of peritonitis followed insertion of the Tenckhoff catheter, 26% being followed by peritonitis. A radical review of the surgical procedures used at that time was undertaken and, as a result of the action taken, the incidence of peritonitis from this cause has now fallen to insignificant levels.

DISCUSSION

We have modified the Montpellier classification of the etiology of peritonitis in CAPD[4] into three main groups:

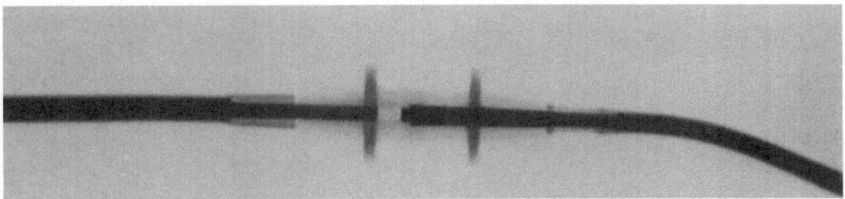

Fig. 4. On reconnection of Figure 3 air trapped in connector.

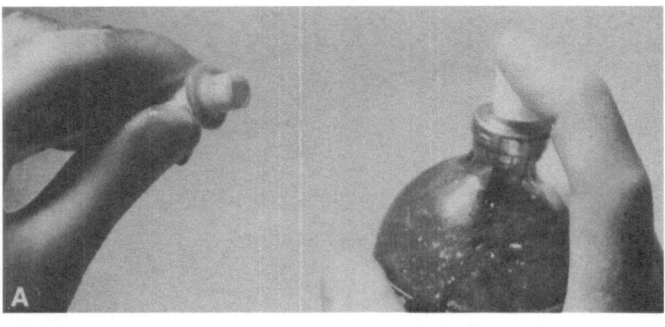
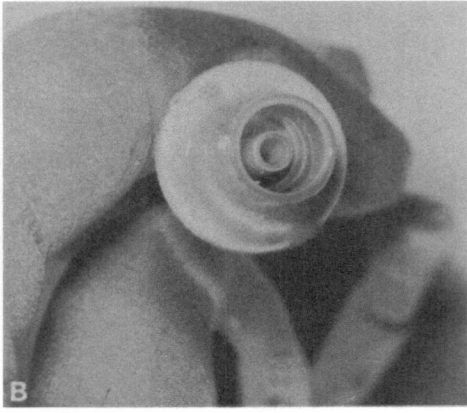

Fig. 5. Povidone-iodine spray. Note pool of povidone-iodine in female screw of Figure 5(*b*).

1. *Patient responsibility.* This includes the care of the connector attached to the 2 L bag, inspection of the bag for manufacturing faults, and care of the exit site and the integrity of the screw connector between transfer set and catheter. One manufacturer (Travenol, UK, personal communication) has estimated that one faulty bag per 10,000 is dispatched from their factory. A patient using four exchanges per day is, therefore, likely to encounter one faulty bag per 6.8 years, which is significant if the aim is to reduce the incidence of peritonitis to one attack per 6–10 years. If, inadvertently, a patient uses a faulty bag, this must be reported to the center, where a decision on the need for a prophylactic course of antibiotics is made. Exit site problems should always be referred to the center for further advice. A disconnection at the transfer set and catheter union is, in our experience, very likely to cause peritonitis, and a prophylactic course of antibiotics is given.

2. *Center responsibility.* This includes peritonitis arising from bacterial contamination at the time of catheter insertion and during the changing of the transfer set, which in our unit is performed in the hospital by trained CAPD nurses. The latter is done with full aseptic precautions using a 10% povidone-iodine soak of the titanium connector and the end of the catheter. Since the introduction of this technique, we are confident that no case of peritonitis has arisen on changing the transfer set.

3. *Intraabdominal complications.* Only those septic conditions directly resulting from peritoneal dialysis are included under this heading. Such conditions would include a strangulated incisional hernia arising from inserting the catheter or adhesions causing obstruction. Other surgical conditions should be listed, but few arise as a result of dialysis.

   It is accepted that in many cases of CAPD peritonitis the exact entry site of bacteria cannot be

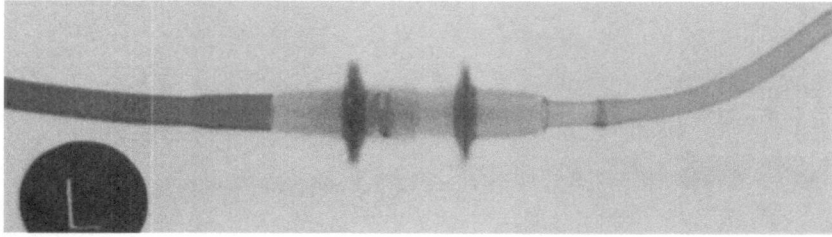

Fig. 6. Connector assembled after spraying with povidone-iodine (to which radio opaque contrast medium had been added).

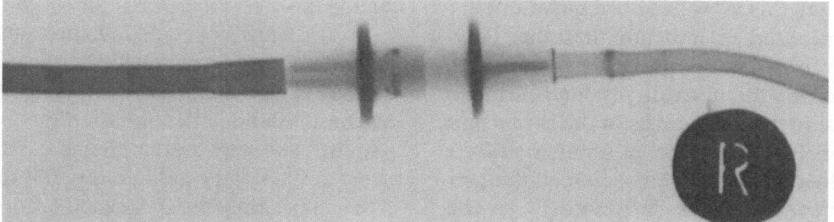

Fig. 7. As for Figure 6, after disconnection and reconnection. Note contrast medium in lumen of right hand connector.

proven, but it can usually be deduced from the history given by the patient. Ideally, CAPD should be undertaken as a "closed" procedure in order to prevent bacterial contamination. It is normal pharmaceutical practice when adding drugs to sterile intravenous fluids to use laminar sterile airflow cabinets in a specially designed room containing only one operator who wears sterile clothing and gloves.[5] This is necessary to prevent ingress of air contaminated with bacteria. Atmospheric "dust" in a domestic environment is composed mainly of desquamated skin scales.[6,7] Some 237 to 17,000 skin scales are liberated into the atmosphere by the human body every minute,[8] and many of these contain viable bacteria.[9] Skin scales are electrostatically attracted to the plastic connectors as used in CAPD.[10] It is, therefore, not surprising that peritonitis frequently complicates CAPD, as it is impossible to use laminar sterile airflow cabinets in the home with the patient wearing sterile clothing and gloves.

The problem is compounded by the frequency of exchanges. A patient undertaking four exchanges per day breaks into the otherwise "closed" CAPD system 1460 times a year. Thus, in addition to the possibility of contamination from skin scales, one error per year made by the patient (which is only 0.07% of the total exchanges) may also lead to peritonitis. As few patients, if any, can maintain this level of proficiency, it must be assumed that the chances of peritonitis are great. The high incidence of skin organisms (*Staphylococcus epidermidis* and *Staphylococcus aureus*) causing peritonitis[11] indirectly confirms the importance of air-borne contamination by skin scales.

The initial aim of these investigations was to demonstrate that adequate sterilization of the connector attached to the 2 L bag would reduce the incidence of peritonitis. Povidone-iodine was chosen as it kills most bacteria and fungi within 60 seconds[12] and bacterial resistance does not de-

Table 1. Incidence of Peritonitis before and after Introducing Povidone-Iodine Spray and Extra Clamping Procedure.

Povidone-Iodine Spray and Extra Clamping Procedure	Before	After		
	6/82–11/82	11/82–4/83	5/83–10/83	11/83–4/84
Episodes of Peritonitis	15	2	1	1
Number of Patients (Range)	10–16	9–18	13–21	21–23
Treatment (Patient Weeks)	285	274	413	579
Peritonitis Incidence/ Patient Weeks	1/19	1/137	1/413	1/579
Average Peritonitis Incidence/Patient Weeks	1/19	1/376		

velop,[13,14] although this view has been questioned.[15] Our radiographic studies indicate that the Travenol IIR screw connector is particularly suited to povidone-iodine, for the agent is retained throughout the exchange in the air pockets in the screw part of the connector. It is, however, possible that if the two halves of the connector were reversed the procedure would be even more satisfactory, as the female luer, which sucks in povidone-iodine on disconnection, would then be discarded with the bag. We have not observed any deleterious reaction from the small amount of povidone-iodine that enters the peritoneal cavity as a result of the female luer being attached to the transfer set. With the high dextrose content of dialysis fluid, the iodine will be of minimal consequence except in situations where there is a "lavish use of povidone-iodine,"[16] resulting in high levels of plasma iodine, for this may cause hypothyroidism. A small fraction of the polyvinylpyrrolidone molecule will be dialyzed into the patient and will remain. After spraying, the connector remains brown-stained for several exchanges, suggesting that the plastic absorbs povidone-iodine that could be still active against bacteria. If this is so, then less frequent spraying may be possible, thereby reducing the intraperitoneal dose.

Other methods of sterilizing the connector attached to the 2 L bag have been described. The "Hong Kong" connector[17] uses chlorhexidine and an ingenious "closed-bag" technique. This reduced the incidence of peritonitis attributable to a connection failure to zero in 11.5 patient years. Even more remarkable was that these excellent results were obtained in very inferior home environments. The modified Perugia system, using a Y-connector filled with sodium hypochlorite as the sterilizing agent, reduced the incidence of peritonitis in a controlled trial from 1 per 11.3 patient months to 1 per 33 patient months.[18] In a controlled trial, the Travenol UV spike sterilizer also significantly reduced the incidence of peritonitis (Travenol Laboratories, Deerfield, IL personal communication). Povidone-iodine has also been advocated in spike contamination with a reduction in peritonitis rate.[19]

The lower incidence of peritonitis in intermittent peritoneal dialysis than in CAPD could be due to the more frequent and continuous dilution of opsonins in CAPD.[20] This makes it imperative to prevent bacteria entering the CAPD system during an exchange.

These findings, along with those recorded here, when the peritonitis rate was reduced from 1 per 19 patient weeks to 1 per 376 patient weeks after intro-ducing the povidone-iodine spray and double clamping of the transfer set, all indicate quite conclusively that some method of sterilizing the connector to the 2 L bag is now mandatory in CAPD. Unfortunately, all these methods depend on the compliance of the patient, who may be tempted occasionally to take a short cut and very deliberately fail to use the advocated sterilizing procedure or ignore all previous training. It would seem the right time for manufacturers of CAPD equipment to design a tamper-proof connector that can only be manipulated by a simple manually operated machine that can undertake 100% perfect exchanges with an automatic built-in sterilizing system. The on/off clamp on the transfer set must be redesigned to be always 100% occlusive when in the off position. These modifications should remove the possibility of patient error to give 100% reliability with a further reduction in peritonitis.

REFERENCES

1. Moriarty MV, and Parsons FM: Intermittent peritoneal dialysis. Br J Urol 38: 623, 1966
2. Mion CM: Practical use of peritoneal dialysis. In Drukker W, Parsons FM, and Maher JF (Eds), Replacement of renal function by dialysis, 2nd Ed. The Hague: Martinus Nijhoff, 1983, p 457
3. Parsons FM, Ahmed-Jushuf IH, Brownjohn AM, Coltman SJ, Gibson J, Young GA, and Young JB: Preventing peritonitis. Lancet 2: 907, 1983
4. Slingeneyer A, Mion C, Beraud JJ, Oules R, Branger B, and Balmes M: Peritonitis, a frequently lethal complication of intermittent and continuous ambulatory peritoneal dialysis. Proc Eur Dial Transplant Assoc 18: 212, 1981
5. Report of Working Party on the addition of drugs to intravenous fluids. Health Services Division, DHSS, London, 1976
6. Davies RR, and Noble WC: Dispersal of bacteria on desquamated skin. Lancet 2: 1295, 1962
7. Clark RP: Skin scales among airborne particles. J Hyg (Camb) 72: 47, 1974
8. May KR, and Pomeroy NP: Bacterial dispersion from the body surface. In Hers JFP, and Winkler KC (Eds), Airborne transmission and airborne infection. Utrech: Oosthoek Publishing, 1973, p 426
9. Noble WC, and Davies RR: Studies on the dispersal of Staphylococci. J Clin Pathol 18: 16, 1965
10. Holmes CJ, and Allwood MC: The potential for contamination of intravenous infusions by airborne skin scales. J Hyg (Camb) 79: 417, 1977
11. Gokal R, Ramos JM, Francis DMA, Ferner DE, Goodship TH, Proud G, Bint AJ, Ward MK, and Kerr DNS: Peritonitis in continuous ambulatory peritoneal dialysis. Lancet 2: 1388, 1982

12. Saggers BA, and Stewart GI: Polyvinyl-pyrrolidone-iodine: an assessment of antibacterial activity. J Hyg (Camb) 62: 61, 1964

13. Houang ET, Gilmore OJA, Reid C, and Shaw EJ: Absence of bacterial resistance to povidone iodine. J Clin Pathol 29: 752, 1976

14. Prince HN, Nonemaker WS, Norgard RC, and Prince DL: Drug resistance studies with topical antiseptics. J Pharm Sci 67: 1629, 1978

15. Parrott PL, Terry PM, Whitworth EN, Frawley LW, Coble RS, Wachsmuth IK, and McGowan JE Jr: *Pseudomonas aeruginosa* peritonitis associated with contaminated poloxamer-iodine solution. Lancet 2: 683, 1982

16. Gavin LA, Eitan NF, Cavalieri RR, and Schmidt WR: Hypothyroidism induced by continuous ambulatory peritoneal dialysis. West J Med 138: 562, 1983

17. Clark RD: Peritonitis prevented in continuous ambulatory peritoneal dialysis by using the Hong Kong connection. Br Med J 288: 353, 1984

18. Maiorca R, Cantaluppi A, Cancarini GC, Scalamogna A, Broccoli R, Graziani G, Brasa S, and Ponticelli C: Prospective controlled trial of a Y-connector and disinfectant to prevent peritonitis in continuous ambulatory peritoneal dialysis. Lancet 2: 642, 1983

19. West L: Does a five-minute Betadine soak of a contaminated spike provide effective decontamination? Peritoneal Dial Bull 3: 102, 1982

20. Keane WF, Comty CM, Verbrugh MD, and Peterson PK: Opsonic deficiency of peritoneal dialysis effluent: a risk factor for peritonitis in continuous ambulatory peritoneal dialysis. Kidney Int 25: 539, 1984

M. Dratwa, F. Collart, and L. Smet

34

CAPD Peritonitis and Different Connecting Devices: A Statistical Comparison

SUMMARY

The incidence of peritonitis in 33 CAPD patients using the Reverse, i.e., Travenol Luer-Lock, connecting devise was compared to that in 20 patients using the Spike system. By life table analysis the probability of acquiring peritonitis was not different with the two techniques.

INTRODUCTION

Peritonitis remains the major complication of CAPD, and new preventive technology, such as connectors, bacteriostatic filters, or sterilizing devices, are continuously put on the market. To evaluate these modifications of technique and to assess their efficacy, a statistically valid method for comparing infection rates is necessary. Such a method, based on life-table analysis, was proposed by Randerson and Farrell[1] and Pierratos et al.[2] We used the latter to evaluate the effect on peritonitis risk of a new connecting device (Travenol Luer-Lock or Reverse system) proposed in 1981 as an easier and safer alternative to the original Spike system used in Belgium since 1978. It must be stressed that, although no proof of its greater safety has been offered, the Reverse system is presently used by one-third of Belgian CAPD patients.

From the Department of Nephrology, Brugmann University Hospital, Brussels, Belgium.

PATIENTS AND METHODS

The data for analysis was obtained from a single CAPD unit (B.U.H.) involving 33 patients treated between January 1979 and December 1983, with a cumulative patient experience of 40.5 years. The titanium adapter was adopted for all patients in the end of 1979. Peritonitis was defined as rebound tenderness and cloudy dialysate characterized by leucocyte counts in excess of $100/mm^3$. Twenty patients (mean age 61.7 ± 2.0 years) used the Spike system (Fig. 1A) beginning in July 1981. Thirteen out of 15 new patients (aged 57.9 ± 4.1) began CAPD with the Reverse system (Fig. 1B).

The Reverse system has two major features: (1) the set-to container attachment, a simple twist luer-lock connector, employs the same double-barrier of protection as the titanium catheter adapter, and (2) the solution bag outlet port contains a detachable seal freed by flexing the port several times. This eliminates the need to spike the solution container, thus reducing the chance of touch contamination. The peritonitis rate was calculated by means of life-table analysis using the first episode of peritonitis as described by Pierratos et al.[2] In this analysis, the probability of developing peritonitis is calculated by first determining a crude incidence:

$$\lambda = \frac{\text{number of peritonitis episodes}}{\text{number of patient-months at risk, in time interval } \tau}$$

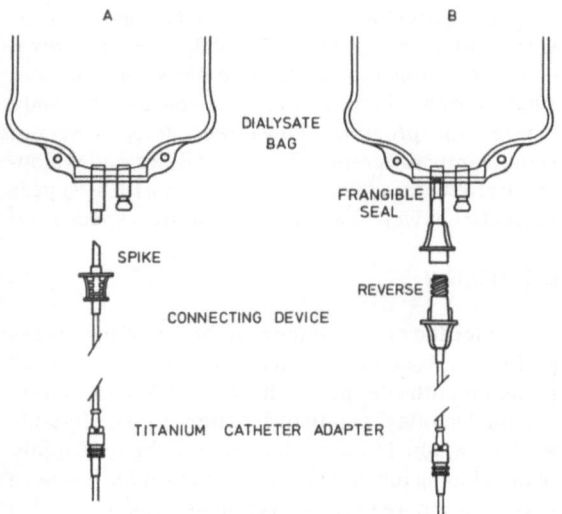

Fig. 1. CAPD systems evaluated in the study. (*A*) Spike and (*B*) Reverse, which is characterized by a frangible seal at the bag outlet and a Luer-lock connection.

The cumulative probability of peritonitis is determined by $P = 1 - e^{-\Sigma\lambda\tau}$ over the time of study. One month intervals were used for analysis of data and daily peritonitis rate for life table estimates.[3] The cumulative probability of contracting peritonitis resulted in a curve exponentially approaching one for each group of patients. This curve was then fitted by least squares linear analysis, using the formula $P = 1 - e^{-\bar{\lambda}\tau}$, where $\bar{\lambda}$ is the average monthly incidence of peritonitis for the group.

Comparison of the peritonitis probability of patients using the Reverse system to that of patients using the Spike was achieved by comparing the two peritonitis probability curves or life-tables with log-rank test,[3] and $\bar{\lambda}$ of the two groups were also compared by Mann-Witney nonparametric U test. In addition, to detect the possibility that a change in the

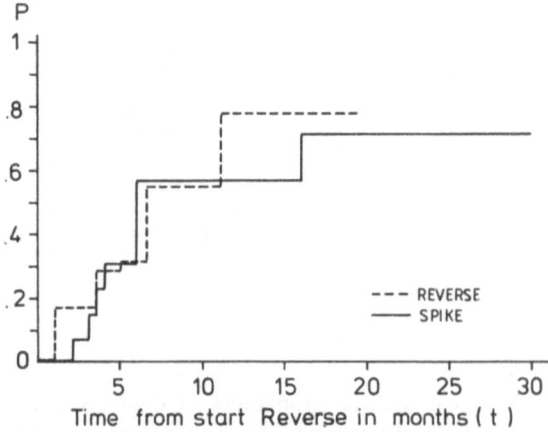

Fig. 2. Life table for time to first infection since the introduction of Reverse (7/5/82). P = probability of developing peritonitis.

performance of our CAPD unit with time might have overshadowed a change induced by the new connecting device, we also compared the peritonitis probability curves for each calendar year included in the period of study.

RESULTS

Table 1 presents the bacteriologic findings obtained by culturing the peritoneal effluents in the 14 first peritonitis episodes developed by 20 patients using the Spike and in the five first episodes contracted by patients using the Reverse system. Three episodes were culture-negative. These results are similar to those reported by most centers and do not seem to be influenced by the type of connecting device.

Figure 2 shows the life-table analysis for time to first infection from July 5, 1981, when the first patient began CAPD using the Reverse connecting device. By 20 months, the probability of developing

Table 1. Bacteriologic Findings in First Episodes of Peritonitis Expressed as Percent of Positive Cultures (N = 19).

		Spike (n = 14)	Reverse (n = 5)
Gram +	*Staphylococcus epidermidis*	29	60
	Staphylococcus aureus	7	0
	Streptococcus sp.	21	0
Gram −	*Pseudomonas sp.*	14	20
	Corynebacterium sp.	14	0
	Escherichia coli	14	0
	Enterobacter sp.	0	20

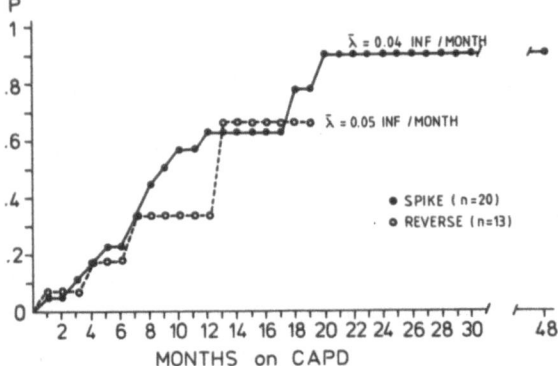

Fig. 3. Cumulative probability of developing the first episode of peritonitis for patients using either connecting device from the start of CAPD in B.U.H. (calculated by linear least squares analysis). P = probability of developing peritonitis.

peritonitis was 0.72 for the Spike group and 0.78 for the Reverse group, a difference not statistically significant when the two curves were compared using the log-rank test.

Figure 3 shows the peritonitis probability curves in patients using the Spike and in those using the Reverse system since their first day on CAPD. The two curves and the overall incidence rates ($\bar{\lambda}$) of the two groups were not significantly different (0.04 infections/month for the Spike versus 0.05 for the Reverse).

The peritonitis probability curves for the first episode for the three groups of patients large enough

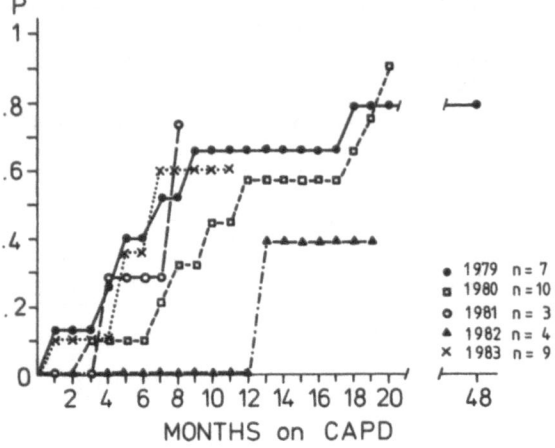

Fig. 4. Cumulative probability of developing the first episode of peritonitis according to calendar year of starting CAPD (linear least squares analysis). P = probability of developing peritonitis.

to be compared according to their calendar year of entry into the program (1979, 1980, 1983) are shown in Figure 4 together with the curves for 1981 and 1982, during which a total of seven patients only entered the program. The three curves were not significantly different. The probabilities of developing the first episode of peritonitis within the first year of treatment were 0.66, 0.57, and 0.61, respectively.

DISCUSSION

Since the most common method used to express peritonitis risk (calculation of the elapsed number of patient months per peritonitis episode) is inaccurate and inadequate for statistical comparisons, life-table analysis applied to the calculation of the probability of developing the first episode of peritonitis has been used to compare two connecting devices. Using this method, we found no significant difference in our unit between the peritonitis risk curves for the Spike or the Reverse system. This lack of improvement that could have derived from the use of the Reverse type of connection was confirmed by the absence of difference in peritonitis probability curves for calendar years before and after the introduction of the Reverse system. In addition, this shows that the performance of our staff and patients has not changed since the start of our CAPD program and remains satisfactory.

Although it should be stressed that this is not a randomized nor controlled study, and only included a small group of patients, we can reasonably conclude that the Reverse system does not reduce the risk of peritonitis and that its higher price (N.B. the price of the Spike system has just been increased to reach that of the Reverse) might not be justified for this purpose. Nevertheless, it may be useful for patients afflicted with tremor or hand weakness, for whom the Spike connection seems more difficult.

REFERENCES

1. Randerson DH, and Farrell PC: Analysis of peritonitis in CAPD. In Gahl GM, Kessel M, and Nolph KD (Eds), Advances in peritoneal dialysis: Proceedings of the 2nd international symposium on peritoneal dialysis. Amsterdam: Excerpta Medica, 1981, p 265
2. Pierratos A, Amair P, Corey P, Vas S, Khanna R, and Oreopoulos DG: Statistical analysis of the incidence of peritonitis on continuous ambulatory peritoneal dialysis. Peritoneal Dial Bull 2: 32, 1982
3. Peto R, Pike MC, Armitage P, Breslow NE, Cox DR, Howard SV, Mantel N, McPherson K, Peto J, and Smith PG: Design and analysis of randomized clinical trials requiring prolonged observations of each patient II. Analysis and examples. Br J Cancer 35: 1, 1977

U. Buoncristiani, C. Carobi, M. Cozzari, and N. DiPaolo

35

Clinical Application of a Miniaturized Variant of the Perugia CAPD Connection System

SUMMARY

The Perugia "Y" shaped connection system for CAPD has been modified by decreasing the tubing length and repositioning the clamp from the tubing to the catheter, itself. Clinical evaluation of this miniaturized system shows excellent patient acceptance and a low rate of peritonitis, i.e., one per 42.2 patient-months.

INTRODUCTION

The development of the "Y" autosterilizing CAPD connection with disinfectant[1] and its subsequent clinical application have greatly improved the clinical results of this dialysis technique, due to dramatic reduction in the peritonitis rate.[2-4] In addition, the esthetic acceptance has been significantly improved with respect to the original CAPD system; the new variant avoids the need of permanently wearing the rolled bag by adopting a small prosthesis filled with disinfectant. In order to further improve the esthetic acceptance while maintaining and possibly improving the high level of safety achieved, we have designed and experimented with a miniaturized version of the "Y" shaped prosthesis.

From the Dialysis Units, Perugia and Siena, Italy.

MATERIAL AND METHODS

The Prosthesis

The new prosthesis consists of a miniaturized "Y" shaped plastic tube, the main characteristics of which (Fig. 1) are: the reduced size total length (8 cm); that both branches are short, as the extension for the outflow is stored apart under disinfectant between the exchanges and connected to the outflow branch only during the exchanges; and that the clamp that closes the access to the peritoneal cavity has been moved from the prosthesis directly to the catheter.

Operational Guidelines

These are essentially the same as for the original Perugia system[1,2] except that the extension for the outflow must be connected and disconnected to and from the outflow branch of the prosthesis, respectively, at the beginning and end of each exchange.

Clinical Experience

Nineteen patients, (6 males, 13 females) aged from 18 to 74 years (mean 52.3 years) were treated with CAPD, using the miniaturized prosthesis for a

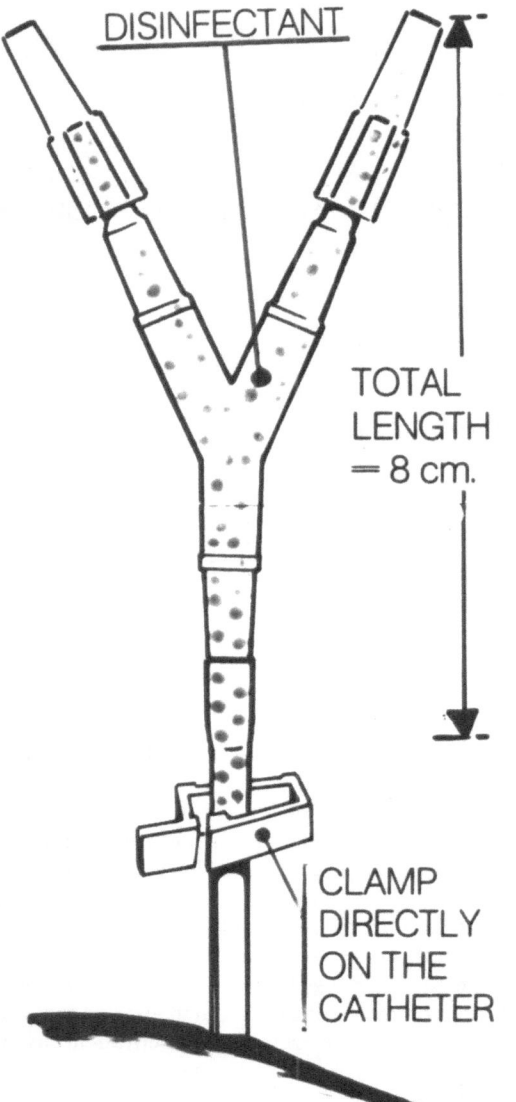

Fig. 1. The miniaturized prosthesis (total length 8 cm), with the clamp directly on the catheter; both branches of the "Y" are short, with the outflow-extension stored apart in disinfectant between exchanges.

total of 717 months (7 to 54, average 37.7 months). Patient selection was based solely on spontaneous choice, mostly conditioned by esthetic reasons.

The probability of remaining free of peritonitis up to any point in time and that of developing peritonitis were calculated according to the method of Pierratos et al.[5]

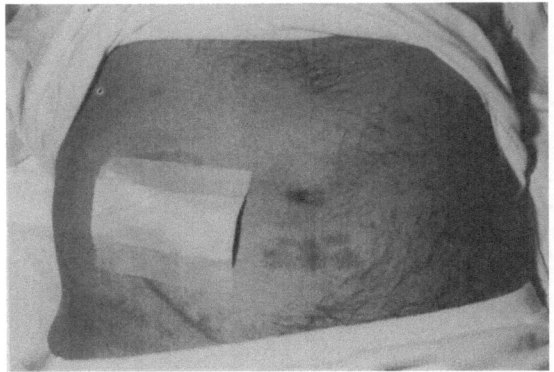

Fig. 2. Concealing the miniaturized prosthesis under a small dressing.

RESULTS

Acceptance

In spite of the small, added task of connecting and disconnecting the outflow extension to the miniaturized prosthesis at each exchange, this modification was universally welcomed with enthusiasm, due to the reduced size of the prosthesis. This enabled its concealment under a small bandage (Fig. 2), thus eliminating every inferiority complex during the diverse situations of social or private life (i.e., the possibility of wearing close-fitting clothes or bathing costumes or of enjoying sexual intercourse) (Figs. 3 and 4). Moreover, the marked smallness enabled the prosthesis to be easily placed in a colostomy bag in order to avoid any risk when bathing or swimming (Fig. 5).

Peritonitis

The total number of peritonitis episodes registered during the entire study period of 717 patient-months was 17, three of which could be considered almost certainly aseptic using the criteria based on our original diagnostic protocol described elsewhere.[2] The total incidence of bacterial peritonitis is equal to one case every 51.2 patient-months, a rate of one every 42.2 months when aseptic peritonitis is included. More than half of the patients remained free from peritonitis. Only four patients were affected more than once, three of whom were affected twice and two three times (Table 1). No statistically significant differences were evident between the two groups with respect to treatment duration or to mean age.

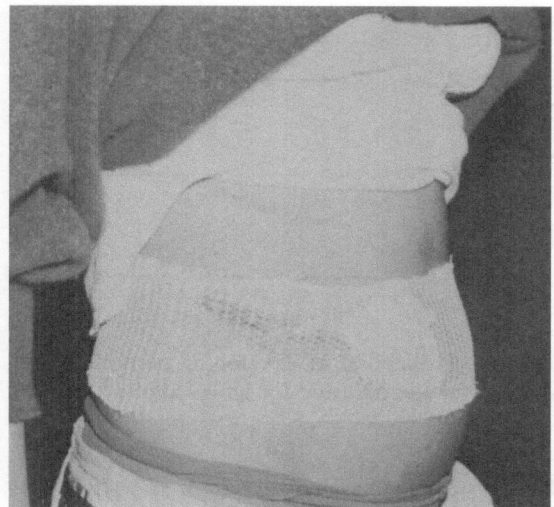

Fig. 3. Due to its reduced size the prosthesis is easily concealed under close-fitting clothes.

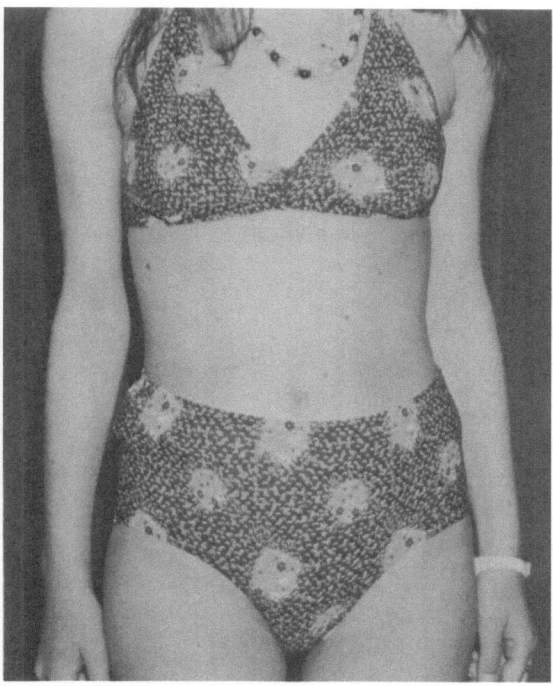

Fig. 4. The smallness of the prosthesis enables the patients to freely wear bathing costumes (even a bikini).

The probability of being infection-free is reported in Figure 6. The median time to the first infection is approximately 3.5 months for both curves. The data for both the first and subsequent episodes are almost identical. The probability of experiencing the first episode at each time over the 36 months of the study is shown by the curve reported in Figure 7: it is equal to 0.19, 0.38, and 0.54, respectively, in the first, second, and third years. The probability of developing peritonitis is not significantly different when calculated for all episodes.

With regard to the outcome, 16 patients are still on CAPD, two have changed to hemodialysis (one because of persistent tunnel infection and one because of loss of ultrafiltration unrelated to peritonitis), and one died due to cerebrovascular accident.

DISCUSSION

Our original Perugia CAPD connection system has already been successful[2-4] in its efficacy in overcoming the two main limitations of the standard CAPD system, i.e., the low rate of acceptance due to esthetic problems, and the permanently high peritonitis rate. This twin goal was achieved by adoption of the "Y" shaped prosthesis, which eliminated the need of wearing the bag and enabled use of a disinfectant (Amuchina, hypochlorite produced by partial electrolysis; Amuchina S.p.A., Genoa, Italy) for sterilization of the connection site.

Soon after the beginning of our experience we were able to offer our patients a miniaturized version of the prosthesis in order to improve further the acceptance of the technique from an esthetic point of view. In fact, the difference between the cumbersome and humiliating need to wear a bag with the standard system suggests that our miniaturized prosthesis improves our previous experience. There is now the possibility of concealing the system under

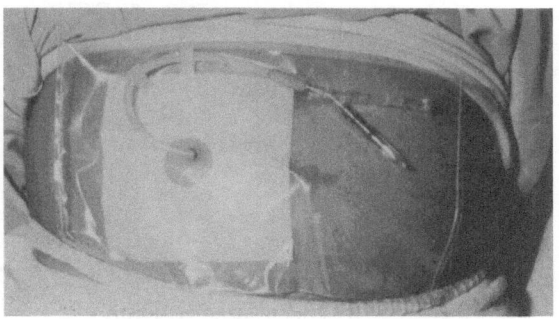

Fig. 5. Easy location of the small prosthesis into a colostomy bag for bathing or swimming.

Table 1. Peritonitis Rate and Characteristics.

Etiology	
Staph. aureus	8
Strept. viridans	1
Enterococcus	2
E. coli	1
Pseudomonas aeruginosa	1
Enterobacteriaceae	1
Patients unaffected	10
Patients affected	9
One time	5
Two times	3
Three times	1
Treatment duration (months)	
Unaffected	36.4*
Affected	39.2*
Age (years)	
Unaffected	47.4*
Affected	51.7*

* Difference not statistically significant

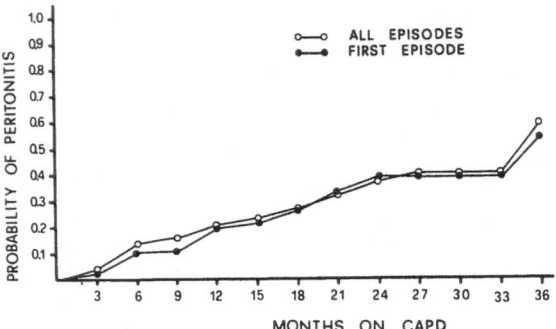

Fig. 7. Probability of developing peritonitis, calculated for the first and for all episodes.

a small dressing or colostomy bag and this eliminates almost every psychological problem, restoring the pleasure of again wearing close-fitting clothes or bathing costumes, and also the pleasure of enjoying an almost completely normal life-style with regard to every kind of activity: work, sports, social and sexual relations.

Moreover, the adoption of the mini ''Y'' has not reduced safety. On the contrary, the peritonitis incidence in this group of patients, no matter how expressed (i.e., as number of episodes per patient-month, or as probability of remaining peritonitis-free or of developing peritonitis), is significantly lower than that still currently reported by the most experienced centers,[5-7] and is also lower than in our cumulative experience.[2] It must be underlined that in four instances it was possible to establish a clear relationship with definite causal factors (tunnel infection or breaks in technique, such as cutting of the catheter). These very good results were obtained despite introducing an additional step in the procedure—the connection-disconnection of the outflow extension to and from the outflow branch of the prosthesis. The success must be essentially attributed to a further improvement in the safety of the system, which consists of the displacement of the clamp that controls access to the peritoneal cavity from the prosthesis directly to the catheter. In this way the catheter remains closed even if there is disconnection of the prosthesis, so that the abdominal cavity is safely excluded from potential external contamination. In fact, evidence is lacking for a substantial role of other possible factors. One can only speculate about the contributory, marginal influence of better compliance due to the motivation by spontaneous choice of the patient for this particular type of prosthesis. Perhaps the age difference between the present group and our cumulative group of the previous report: 49.4 years versus 57.4 years contributes, since the two subgroups do not differ significantly in age. The treatment duration was significantly longer in the present study, 37.7 months versus 12.3 months in the previous study, but the affected and unaffected subgroups did not differ in duration.

The present experience thus not only conclusively confirms the previously reported[2-4] advantages of the Perugia system in terms of esthetic acceptance and safety, but also shows that these

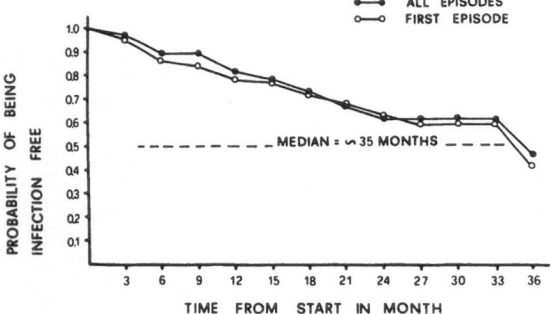

Fig. 6. Probability of being infection free, calculated both for the first and for all episodes.

advantages can even be further improved, thus establishing the basis for wider application of CAPD.

REFERENCES

1. Buoncristiani U, Bianchi P, Cozzari M, Carobi C, Quintaliani G, and Barbarossa D: A new safe simple connection system for CAPD. Int J Nephrol Urol Androl 1: 50, 1980
2. Buoncristiani U, Cozzari M, Quintaliani G, and Carobi C: Abatement of exogenous peritonitis risk using the Perugia CAPD system. Dial Transplant 12: 14, 1983
3. Maiorca R, Cantaluppi A, Cancarini GC, Scalamogna A, Broccoli R, Graziani G, Brasa S, and Ponticelli C: Prospective controlled trial of a Y-connector and disinfectant to prevent peritonitis in continuous ambulatory peritoneal dialysis. Lancet 2: 642, 1983
4. Mileto G, Pellegrino E, and Consolo F: CAPD in Sicily: Decrease in peritonitis rate with the use of the Perugia system. Peritoneal Dial Bull 3: 161, 1983
5. Pierratos A, Amair P, Corey P, Vas SI, Khanna R, and Oreopoulos DG: Statistical analysis of the incidence of peritonitis on continuous ambulatory peritoneal dialysis. Peritoneal Dial Bull 2: 32, 1982
6. Williams CC: CAPD in Toronto: An overview. Peritoneal Dial Bull 3: S6, 1983
7. Prowant B, Ryan L, and Nolph KD: Six years of experience with peritonitis in a CAPD program. Peritoneal Dial Bull 3: 199, 1983

A. Cantaluppi, A. Scalamogna, L. Guerra,
C. Castelnovo, G. Graziani, and C. Ponticelli

36

Peritonitis Prevention in CAPD: Efficacy of a Y-Connector and Disinfectant

SUMMARY

An open trial of the Y connector system for peritoneal dialysis has been carried out in 62 patients and the results compared to those in 18 patients using the standard spike connector for dialysis fluid exchanges. The incidence of peritonitis was lower (14.5%) with the Y connector, and the interval until peritonitis occurred was longer. Diabetic patients had a higher frequency of infection. When this group was excluded the peritonitis rate was one episode every 110.2 patient-months in the Y connector group. Technical accidents with the system were infrequent and inconsequential except for transient pain. CAPD treatment was continued by 80% of these patients after 10.1 months.

INTRODUCTION

Continuous ambulatory peritoneal dialysis (CAPD) is now considered an effective way to treat patients with end-stage renal disease,[1,2] and its use is increasing throughout the world.[3] However, despite continuous progress, peritonitis remains the major serious complication, and many patients have to drop out of CAPD programs because of repeated episodes of peritonitis.[3]

From the Divisione di Nefrologia, Ospedale Maggiore Policlinico, Milano, Italy.

The technique most commonly used for prevention of peritonitis is that of Oreopoulos et al.[1] To reduce further the risk of dialysis fluid contamination, some modifications of the original system have been suggested.[4-6] Buoncristiani et al. used a Y-shaped set filled with the disinfectant sodium hypochlorite solution during the dwell time,[7,8] and a sizeable reduction in peritonitis incidence occurred. Since June 1981 to December 1982 we have used a modified Y-connector. We could confirm, in a randomized controlled study in two centers, the superiority of the Y-system when compared to the standard Oreopoulos technique.[9]

During the controlled trial we have gained a lot of experience in the use of the Y-connector and in the past 17 months we have continued the use of this connector in an open study.

PATIENTS AND METHODS

From January 1, 1983 to May 31, 1984, all new patients referred to our hospital for CAPD were trained to use the Y-connector, while patients already on treatment continued with the standard or the Y-system. Moreover, if patients who were using the standard bag-exchange method had one or two episodes of peritonitis, they were shifted to the Y-set treatment. This occurred in eight cases. We decided to make this change because the superiority of the Y-set over the standard connector had become evident from a previous controlled study.[9] Therefore, our cumulative experience refers to two groups of patients.

Group A. Eighteen patients (8 female, 10 male; mean age 54.7 ± 11.4 years, range 37 to 75 years) used the Travenol spike connector with the standard bag-exchange method.[1] The total experience was 222 patient-months (mean ± SD, 11.9 ± 4.9 months, range 3 to 17 months). No patient in this group had diabetes mellitus.

Group B. Sixty-two patients (22 female, 40 male; mean age 53.1 ± 16.8 years, range 13 to 78 years) seven of whom were insulin-dependent diabetics and used the experimental Y-Solution Transfer Set (Travenol, Lessines). The total experience was 617 patient-months (mean ± SD, 10.1 ± 5.4 months, range 1 to 17 months).

The experimental device has been already described.[9] It consists of three tubes linked by a Y-connection (Fig. 1). The shortline (B) is connected to the titanium adaptor of the peritoneal catheter by means of a 'Luer-lock' (A) and is provided with a roller clamp (G). At the end of the inlet tube (C) there is a spike protected by a cap (D). A screw plug (F) closes the outlet tube (E). Between exchanges the connector is filled with sodium hypochlorite solution between roller clamp G and caps D and F. For the exchange procedure, after removal of cap D, which is placed in a tank containing hypochlorite solution, the spike of the inlet tube C is connected to the outlet port of a new plastic bag containing dialysis fluid. Screw plug F is removed from outlet tube E and placed in the disinfectant tank; the outlet tube is secured to the edge of a graduated cylinder. The disinfectant agent and the killed bacteria are then washed out of the Y-set through outlet tube E with 100 ml of fresh dialysis solution. Inlet tube C is then clamped and roller clamp G is opened, allowing discharge through outlet tube E of the used solution from the abdomen. This maneuver provides an additional washing of the Y-set before inflow of fresh dialysis fluid, completely removing the disinfectant. When the abdomen is empty, the outlet is clamped and the inlet tubing opened, allowing the fresh dialysis fluid to flow into the peritoneal cavity. After the inflow phase, roller clamp G is closed, the empty bag is disconnected, and the disinfectant solution is poured into the transfer set, using tube C as a siphon. Finally, spike cap D and screw plug F are retrieved from the disinfectant tank and put back on the inlet and outlet tubes.

The disinfectant solution used (Amuchina, Amuchina SpA, Genova) is hypochlorite produced by partial electrolysis of a concentrated sodium chloride solution. It is used in a dilution containing 6

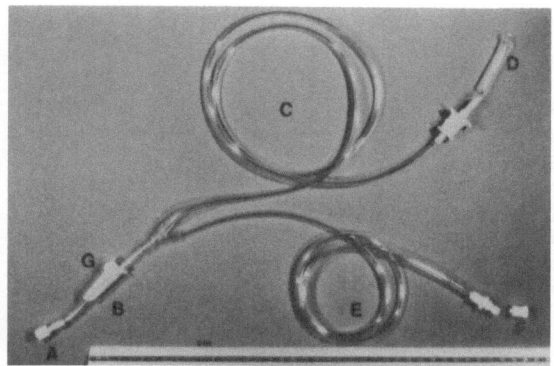

Fig. 1. Y-solution transfer set.

× 10³ ppm of available free chlorine. The sterilizing effectiveness of this solution has been demonstrated by Buoncristiani et al.[10]

The peritoneal access consisted of a double-cuff Tenckhoff catheter with a titanium connector (Baxter Travenol, Deerfield, IL). The same kind of bag was used for both groups (Viaflex, Travenol). In group A, 13 patients were treated with 4 exchanges/day, and five patients with 3 exchanges/day; in group B, 48 patients were treated with 4 exchanges/day, and 14 with 3 exchanges/day. The dialysis set was changed every 8 weeks by a skilled nurse.

The diagnosis of peritonitis was based on the presence of two of the following three findings: abdominal pain, dialysate white-cell counts over $100/mm^3$, and positive dialysate cultures.

For the two groups, which are comparable in age, dialysis duration, and number of exchanges per day, the number and frequency of peritonitis episodes, and the percentage of affected patients were evaluated by Yates' corrected chi-square test. Life-table analysis, according to the Kaplan-Meier method, was used to calculate the probability that peritonitis would develop in a patient within a given time. We took into account all the episodes of peritonitis and used the log-rank test to compare the probability curves of the two groups.[11]

RESULTS

Peritonitis

In group A, over 222 patient months, (peritonitis developed in 13 (72%) of the 18 patients, and in group B, over 617 patient-months, only 9 of 62 patients had episodes of peritonitis (14.5%) ($\chi_c^2 = 20.5$; $p < 0.0001$). There were 19 episodes of peritonitis in

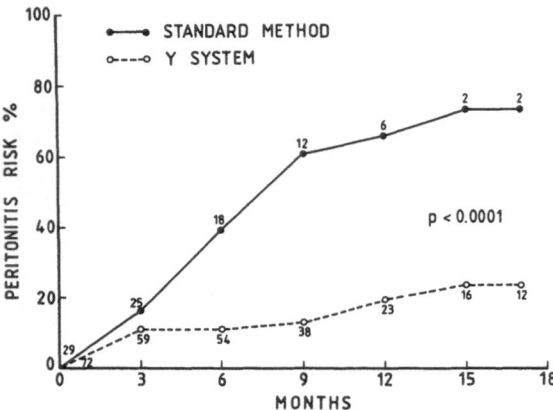

Fig. 2. Peritonitis probability curves for group A (solid line) and group B (broken line). Numbers indicate patients at risk at each time point.

group A and 11 in group B. The incidence of peritonitis during the period of the study was one episode every 11.7 patient-months in group A and one episode every 56.1 patient-months in group B. The peritonitis probability curves differed significantly between the groups (Fig. 2: $\chi^2 = 19.7$; $p < 0.0001$). When we exclude from group B the seven diabetic patients adding insulin to the bags, the incidence of peritonitis in this group was one episode every 110.2 patient-months (i.e., about every 10 patient-years). Indeed, in diabetic patients, over 66 patient-months, peritonitis developed in four (57%) of the seven patients. There were six episodes of peritonitis and the incidence of peritonitis was one episode every 11 patient-months. In the eight patients initially treated with the standard technique and then shifted to Y-set treatment after 1 to 2 episodes of peritonitis, the peritonitis rate fell from one episode every 4.5 patient-months to one episode during 51 patient-months.

Table 1. Organisms Causing Peritonitis.

	Group A	Group B
Staphylococcus epidermidis	13	4
Staphylococcus aureus	1	3
Streptococci	1	1
Enterobacter cloacae	—	2
Pseudomonas aeruginosa	1	1
Acinetobacter	1	—
Serratia marcescens	1	—
No growth	1	—

Dialysate cultures were carried out for all the peritonitis cases. No bacteria could be grown for one patient in group A; 79% of group A and 73% of group B had gram-positive infections, and 16% and 27%, respectively, gram-negative infections (Table 1).

In group A, one episode of *Pseudomonas* peritonitis was due to skin-exit-site infection and two episodes of *Staph. epidermidis* peritonitis were due to leaks, from administration set and Tenckhoff catheter, respectively. In group B, two episodes of *Staph. aureus* peritonitis were due to skin-exit-site infection.

Technical Accidents with the Y-Connector

The B line disconnected from the Y-connection eight times because of defective sticking in one batch of devices. No peritonitis developed in these patients. There was accidental introduction of the disinfectant solution into the abdomen in nine patients. The patients experienced sudden abdominal pain that disappeared after two or three rapid bag-exchanges. There were no changes in the biochemical findings nor loss of ultrafiltration capacity in these patients.

Outcome of Patients

Group A. Three patients died during the follow-up (two myocardial infarction and one rupture of thoracic aorta aneurysm), and eight patients were shifted to Y-set treatment because of frequent peritonitis episodes; seven patients continue CAPD treatment.

Group B. Six patients died during the follow-up (two pneumonia, two myocardial infarction, one miliary tuberculosis, and one cardiac failure), five patients received a renal transplant, and two patients were transferred to hemodialysis (one patient left CAPD at his own request, and the other one had to be removed because of skin-exit-site infection due to *Staph. aureus* with secondary peritonitis); 49 patients continue CAPD treatment.

DISCUSSION

Peritonitis is the major disadvantage of CAPD. It is generally considered the most frequent complication and cause of drop-out, can cause disability, protein loss, increased time in the hospital, and in the most severe cases may threaten life. Thus intensive effort should be made to reduce the frequency of this complication.

Since the introduction of the technique of Oreopoulos et al.,[1] an encouraging fall in the frequency of peritonitis has been reported,[12,13] but peritoneal infection rates of one episode every 10 to 14.1 patient-months are still being reported.[14,15] Modifications of the original technique, such as double-bag technique,[4] in-line bacteriologic filters,[5] and OZ-connector,[6] have been suggested to reduce the frequency of peritonitis. With these modifications, the incidence of peritonitis ranges between one episode every 17–18 patient-months. The possibility of further reducing the incidence of peritonitis by using a Y-set filled with a disinfectant agent was shown by Buoncristiani et al. in an open study.[8]

The principle of Buoncristiani et al.[8] system is the sterilization of the connection site between the administration set and the bag with a disinfectant agent that, after the connection has been made, can be completely discharged to the outside through an outflow branch. In addition to the disinfectant effect, the flushing of the Y-connector reduces the risk of contamination.[7] Additional advantages of the Y-set are that it frees the patient from the bag during the dwell time and that the volume of dialysis solution can be adapted to the anatomical and clinical condition of the patient (e.g., reduced volume requirement in children). Finally the fact that sterile gauzes and connector shields are not needed, makes the Y-system cheaper than the standard Oreopoulos technique.

In a prospective controlled trial performed in two centers we have shown that the peritonitis rate in patients treated with the Y-system was much lower than that in patients using the standard method, and life table analysis showed a significantly reduced incidence of peritonitis in the group treated with the Y-connector system.[9] During the past 17 months we have continued the use of the Y-connector in an open study and, possibly due to the experience gained during the controlled study, we have obtained even better results (one episode every 33 patient-months in the controlled study).

In contrast with previous papers reporting a peritonitis incidence in diabetic patients similar to that of nondiabetic subjects,[16–18] in our experience the results in diabetic patients (one episode of peritonitis every 11 patient-months) were much worse than those in nondiabetic patients (one episode of peritonitis every 110.2 patient-months). One possible explanation for this discrepancy is the small number of diabetic patients in our CAPD population, but more probably the much higher incidence of peritonitis is due to the maneuver of adding insulin to the bags. Indeed, the consequences of this potentially contaminating act cannot be prevented by the sterilization and flushing of the connection site obtained with the Y-connector.

In our study none of the 62 patients in the Y-system group had to be dropped from the CAPD program because of peritonitis. Moreover, eight patients using the standard bag-exchange method with a high rate of peritonitis were able to continue CAPD after transfer to the Y-system with the peritonitis incidence dropping from one episode every 4.5 patient-months to one episode every 51 patient-months.

One possible complication of the Y-system is accidental introduction of the disinfectant agent into the peritoneum. In our patients this complication occurred nine times in more than 70,000 exchanges. It was immediately followed by severe abdominal pain, but after two or three rapid bag-exchanges the pain was eliminated without any other consequence, not surprisingly since the disinfectant agent, Amuchina, was found to be innocuous in experimental animals.[10]

In conclusion, these results confirm that the Y-connector with disinfectant is a simple, safe, and economical system that is extremely effective in reducing the rate of peritonitis in patients on CAPD.

REFERENCES

1. Oreopoulos DG, Khanna R, Williams P, and Vas SI: Continuous ambulatory peritoneal dialysis-1981. Nephron 30: 293, 1982
2. Levey AS, Harrington JT: Continuous peritoneal dialysis for chronic renal failure. Medicine 61: 330, 1982
3. Wing AJ, Broyer M, Brunner FP, Brynger H, Challah S, Donckerwolcke RA, Gretz N, Jacobs C, Kramer P, and Selwood NH: Combined report on regular dialysis and transplantation in Europe, XIII, 1982. Proc Eur Dial Transplant Assoc 20: 5, 1983
4. Bazzato G, Coli U, Landini S, Fraeasso A, Moracchiello P, Righetto F, and Scanferla F: Continuous ambulatory peritoneal dialysis with double bag system: 40 months experience of better patient rehabilitation. In 54th Hahnemann Symposium (Venice, 1982)
5. Slingeneyer A, and Mion C: Peritonitis prevention in continuous ambulatory peritoneal dialysis: Long term efficacy of a bacteriological filter. Proc Eur Dial Transplant Assoc 19: 388, 1982
6. Oreopoulos DG, Vas SI, and Khanna R: Prevention of peritonitis during continuous ambulatory peritoneal dialysis. Peritoneal Dial Bull 3: S18, 1983
7. Buoncristiani U, Bianchi P, Cozzari M, Carobi C, Quintaliani G, and Barbarossa D: A new safe simple

connection system for CAPD. Int J Nephrol Urol Androl 1: 50, 1980

8. Buoncristiani U, Cozzari M, Quintaliani G, and Carobi C: Abatement of exogenous peritonitis risk using the Perugia CAPD system. Dial Transplant 12: 14, 1983

9. Maiorca R, Cantaluppi A, Cancarini GC, Scalamogna A, Broccoli R, Grazianig, Brasa S, and Ponticelli C: Prospective controlled trial of a Y-connector and disinfectant to prevent peritonitis in continuous ambulatory peritoneal dialysis. Lancet 2: 642, 1983

10. Buoncristiani U, Bianchi P, Barzi AM, Quintialiani G, Cozzari M, and Carobi C: An ideal disinfectant for peritoneal dialysis (high efficient, easy to handle and innocuous). Int J Nephrol Urol Androl 1: 45, 1980

11. Peto R, Pike MC, Armitage P, Breslow NE, Cox DR, Howard SV, Mantel N, McPherson K, Peto J, and Smith PG: Design and analysis of randomized clinical trials requiring prolonged observation of each patient. II. Analysis and examples. Br J Cancer 35: 1, 1977

12. Nolph KD, Prowant B, Sorkin MI, and Gloor H: The incidence and characteristics of peritonitis in the fourth year of a continuous ambulatory peritoneal dialysis program. Peritoneal Dial Bull 1: 50, 1981

13. Khanna R, Oreopoulos DG, Dombros N, Vas S, Williams P, Meema HE, Hudson H, Ogilvie R, Zellerman G, Roncari DAK, Clayton S, and Izatt S: Continuous ambulatory peritoneal dialysis (CAPD) after three years: Still a promising treatment. Peritoneal Dial Bull 1: 24, 1981

14. Prowant B, Ryan L, and Nolph KD: Six years of experience with peritonitis in a CAPD program. Peritoneal Dial Bull 3: 199, 1983

15. Williams CC, and the University of Toronto Collaborative Dialysis Group: CAPD in Toronto—An overview. Peritoneal Dial Bull 3: S6, 1983

16. Amair P, Khanna R, Leibel B, Pierratos A, Vas A, Meema E, Blair G, Chisolm L, Vas M, Zingg W, Digenis G, and Oreopoulos D: Continuous ambulatory peritoneal dialysis in diabetics with end-stage renal disease. N Engl J Med 306: 625, 1982

17. Flynn CT: Long-term continuous ambulatory peritoneal dialysis. Proc Eur Dial Transplant Assoc 20: 700, 1983

18. Rottembourg J, El Shahat Y, Agrafiotis A, Thuillier Y, de Groc F, Jacobs C, and Legrain M: Continuous ambulatory peritoneal dialysis in insulin-dependent diabetic patients: A 40-month experience. Kidney Int 23: 40, 1983

C. Rotellar, J.F. Winchester, S.R. Ash, T.A. Rakowski,
W.F. Barnard, and E. Heeter

37

Long-Term Use of Unidirectional Bacteriologic Filters to Reduce Peritonitis Frequency in CAPD

SUMMARY

We report the long term (up to 24 months) use of
a 0.22 μ, 270 cm^2 membrane bacteriologic filter on
the frequency of peritonitis in 33 patients considered
to be at high risk for developing peritonitis. The
frequency of peritonitis in 20 patients (in 325 patient-
months) before the filter was placed was one in 3.38
months, and this was reduced (over 250 patient-
months) to one in 5.95 months, a decrease of 49.9%
($p < 0.001$). In all 33 patients the cumulative probability of peritonitis was significantly reduced and
the mean crude incidence ($\overline{\lambda}$) of peritonitis was reduced from 0.265 to 0.134 ($p < 0.01$). This confirmed
that the filter reduced the incidence of peritonitis
and that the use of the filter maintained the reduction
of peritonitis up to 24 months. Bacteria and spores
introduced into dialysis fluid by touch contamination are trapped on the inflow surfaces of the filter,
which reduced the probability of peritonitis and
drop-outs from CAPD.

INTRODUCTION

Bacterial peritonitis remains the most important complication of continuous ambulatory peritoneal dialysis (CAPD).[1,2] Mion et al.[3] introduced a

From Georgetown University, Washington, D.C. and
Purdue University, Lafayette, Indiana.

bacterial rejecting filter into a large unselected population of patients undergoing intermittent peritoneal
dialysis and demonstrated a reduction in the incidence of peritonitis. Additionally, Slingeneyer and
Mion[4] have demonstrated that the bacterial rejecting
filter could also substantially reduce the incidence of
peritonitis in CAPD patients in a largely unselected
population of patients. We have previously shown
that in a high risk group of patients on CAPD that the
short-term use of a bacterial filter substantially reduced the incidence and cumulative probability of
peritonitis.[5] The present study extends the experience of long-term use of the bacterial filter between
the dialysis bag and delivery line in high risk patients
followed for up to 2 years.

PATIENTS AND METHODS

Thirty-three patients (mean age 49.7 $\pm$ 14.9
years) considered to be at high risk for developing
peritonitis entered the study. Patients were considered to be at high risk of developing peritonitis when
they had a frequent history of peritonitis (equal to
one episode of peritonitis every 3 months), were
visually impaired, or had poor manual dexterity and
technique, and the elderly. Twenty patients had a
history of frequent peritonitis before the introduction of the bacterial filter and the other 13 patients
had entered the study at the same time as they began
CAPD. Throughout the study the use of betadine

spike barriers (wraps) was discontinued in those patients who had used them previous to the study. The bacterial filter was changed every 14 days by nursing personnel using an aseptic technique. The bacterial rejecting filter (Peridex CAPD filter, Millipore Corp., Bedford, MA) is a membrane filter comprising three stacks of double membrane filtering units with support structure.[5] The surface area of the filter is 270 cm², the filter has an external diameter of 9.3 cm and width of 1.9 cm. By use of one-way check valves the filter is designed to filter inflow fluid and bypass outflow fluid.

An episode of peritonitis was defined as cloudy fluid, greater than 100 WBC/ml of peritoneal dialysate, and/or systemic and abdominal symptoms. Each episode of peritonitis was recorded as were the organisms involved. Peritonitis was treated in a standard manner with oral cephalosporin and intramuscular and intraperitoneal aminoglycoside, increasing the frequency of exchanges to 6/day and changing antibiotics depending on the sensitivity of the microbial species.

The data were analyzed by a modification of the method of Peirratos et al.[6], $p = 1 - e^{-\lambda t}$, where $\lambda =$ the crude incidence of peritonitis per month and t = months at risk. The cumulative probability of infection per month was derived from the expression probability (p), $p = 1 - e^{-\Sigma \lambda t}$; the mean λ $(\overline{\lambda})$ was derived after linearization of the probability curves using least squares linear regression analysis derived from the following expression: $\mathrm{Ln}\,(1 - p) = \overline{\lambda}$. Probability curves were also constructed for visual comparison of patient groups. Statistical comparison of the raw data was made by Mann Whitney "U" test for nonparametric statistics. The probability curves were subjected to linear regression analysis and compared by Fisher F test.

RESULTS

The results in terms of peritonitis frequency are shown in Figure 1. In the 20 patients with a previous history of frequent peritonitis (Group I) there were a total of 96 episodes of peritonitis prior to introduction of filter over a cumulative total of 320 patient-months (one episode of peritonitis every 3.38 patient-months). After introduction of the filter, the

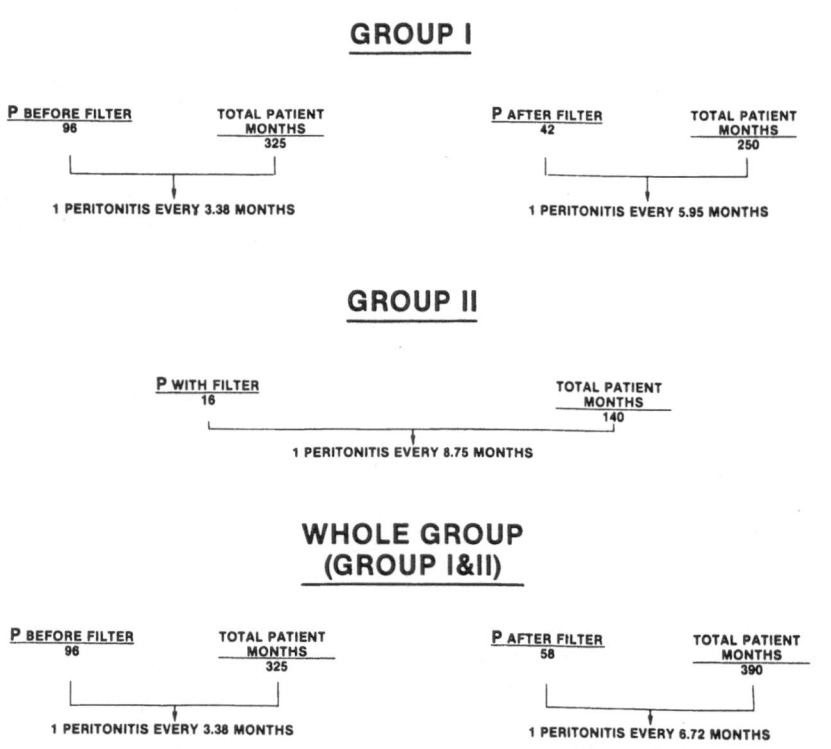

Fig. 1. Frequency of peritonitis before and after use of the bacteriologic filter.

crude incidence of peritonitis was reduced to one episode every 5.95 patient-months (42 episodes in a cumulative total of 250 patient-months). This is equivalent to a reduction of peritonitis incidence of approximately 49.9%. In 13 patients considered at high risk (Group II) of developing peritonitis, started simultaneously on CAPD and the filter, there was a recorded incidence of peritonitis of one episode every 7.5 months (16 episodes of peritonitis in 140 cumulative patient-months). Combining groups I and II (33 patients) the incidence of peritonitis was reduced from one episode every 3.38 months to one episode every 6.72 months.

Figure 2 shows the cumulative probability curves for the development of peritonitis, and linearization of the probability curves for derivation of $\bar{\lambda}$. There was a decrease of $\bar{\lambda}$ from 0.265 to 0.134, giving a reduction in the incidence of peritonitis of 49.9% ($p < 0.001$).

DISCUSSION

Continuous ambulatory peritoneal dialysis is now an established treatment for end-stage renal disease since its introduction by Popovich and col-

leagues.[1] However, peritonitis remains the single most important complication of CAPD and is responsible for considerable morbidity in the CAPD patient and accounts for approximately one fifth of the drop-outs from CAPD both in the United States and Europe.[7,8] We and others have previously shown that bacterial filters remove bacterial touch contaminants introduced during the exchange procedure and that filters have a positive culture rate of between 20 and 25%.[4,5] We and others have shown that the bacterial filters do reduce the peritonitis rate,[4,5] and in the present study, in a population defined as high risk patients, the long-term use of unidirectional filter decreased the mean incidence of peritonitis approximately by 49% ($p < 0.001$). In addition, the drop-out rate from our CAPD program due to development of bacterial peritonitis in the filter users has been 12%. This is less than the national average.[7]

The major criticism of the use of bacterial filters has been raised by Shaldon et al.,[9] who have suggested that long-term use of bacterial filters allow passage of bacterial pyrogens or other products to cross the filter membrane from the contaminated side and generate interleukin-1 production in the

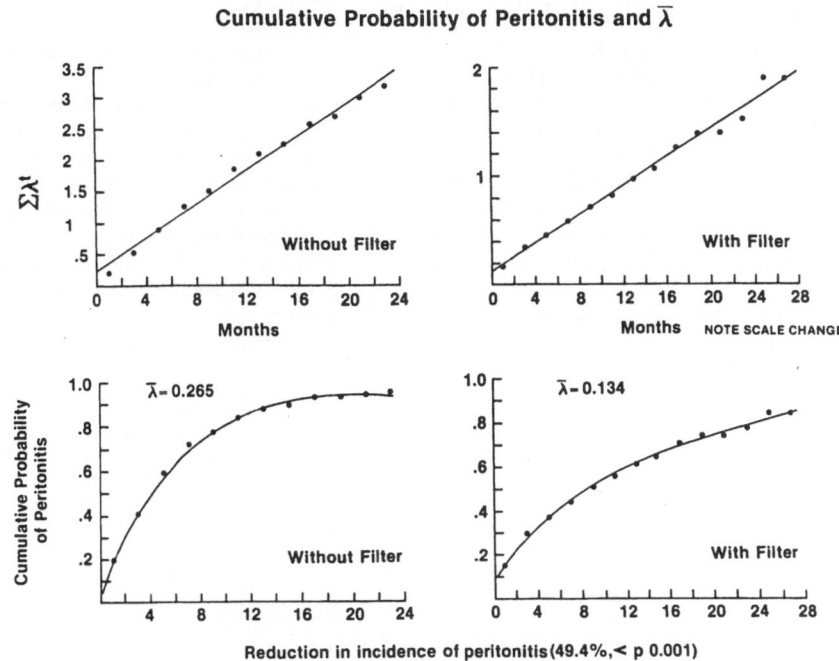

Cumulative Probability of Peritonitis and $\bar{\lambda}$

Reduction in incidence of peritonitis (49.4%, < p 0.001)

Fig. 2. Cumulative probability of peritonitis with and without bacteriologic filter.

peritoneum. This in turn may be associated with the development of sclerosing peritonitis. Sclerosing encapsulating peritonitis is a well-described phenomenon seen particularly in Europe.[10-12] Several other etiologies for sclerosing encapsulating peritonitis have also been put forth.[12, 13]

In our view there is little evidence to support the hypothesis of Shaldon et al. in patients using bacterial filters since not every patient using bacterial filters has developed sclerosing peritonitis, the patients involved have been situated predominantly in Europe, and patients who have never used bacterial filters have developed sclerosing peritonitis. In our own group of patients none have symptoms or signs of sclerosing encapsulating peritonitis, nor have they developed symptoms associated with pyrogen production into the peritoneum.

We feel that the bacterial rejecting filter has several advantages for CAPD patients, particularly those at high risk for developing peritonitis, and since the incidence of peritonitis can be reduced, the drop-out rate from peritonitis is reduced. Potentially, the cost of peritonitis and hospitalization may also be lowered.

REFERENCES

1. Popovich RP, Moncrief JW, Nolph KD, Ghods AJ, Twardowski JJ, and Pyle WK: Continuous ambulatory peritoneal dialysis. Ann Intern Med 88: 449, 1978
2. Oreopoulos DG, Robson M, Izatt S, Clayton S, and deVeber G: A simple and safe technique for continuous ambulatory peritoneal dialysis (CAPD). Trans Am Soc Artif Intern Organs 24: 484, 1978
3. Mion C, Slingeneyer A, Liendo-Liendo C, Perez C, and Despaux E: Reduction in incidence of peritonitis (P) associated with continuous ambulatory peritoneal dialysis (CAPD). Proc Dial Transplant Forum 9: 9, 1979
4. Slingeneyer A, and Mion C: Peritonitis prevention in continuous ambulatory peritoneal dialysis: Long term efficacy of a bacteriological filter. Proc Eur Dial Transplant Assoc 19: 388, 1983
5. Winchester JF, Ash SR, Bousquet G, Rakowski TA, Barnard WF, Heeter E, and Haley S: Successful peritonitis reduction with a unidirectional bacteriologic CAPD filter. Trans Am Soc Artif Intern Organs 29: 611, 1983
6. Pierratos A, Amair P, Corey P, Vas SI, Khanna R, and Oreopoulos DG: Statistical analysis of the incidence of peritonitis in continuous ambulatory peritoneal dialysis. Peritoneal Dial Bull 2: 32, 1982
7. The National Institutes of Health, CAPD patient Registry: Patient population demographic and selected outcome measure for the period January 1, 1981 through December 31, 1982. Report Number 83: 1, 1983
8. Broyer M, Brunner FP, Brynger H, Donckerwolcke RA, Jacobs C, Kramer P, Selwood NH, and Wing AJ: Combined report on regular dialysis and transportation in Europe XII, 1981. Proc Eur Dial Transplant Assoc 19: 2, 1983
9. Shaldon S, Koch KM, Dinarello CA, and Quellhorst E: Pathogenesis of sclerosing peritonitis in CAPD. Abstracts Am Soc Artif Intern Organs 13: 55, 1984
10. Slingeneyer A, Mion C, Mourad G, Canaud B, Faller B, and Beraud JJ: Progressive sclerosing peritonitis: A late and severe complication of maintenance peritoneal dialysis. Trans Am Soc Artif Intern Organs 29: 633, 1983
11. Bradley JA, McWhinnie DL, Hamilton DNH, Starnes F, MacPherson SG, Seywright P, Briggs JD, and Junor BJR: Sclerosing obstructive peritonitis after continuous ambulatory peritoneal dialysis. Lancet 2: 113, 1983
12. Rottembourg J, Gahl GM, Poigalt JL, Bertani E, Strippoli P, Langlois P, Tranbaloc P, and Legrain M. Severe abdominal complications in patients undergoing continuous ambulatory peritoneal dialysis. Proc Eur Dial Transplant Assoc 20: 236, 1983
13. McWhinnie DL, Bradley JA, Hamilton DNH, MacPherson SG, Smith WGJ, Briggs JD, and Junor BJR. Sclerosing peritonitis—a further complication of continuous ambulatory peritoneal dialysis. Peritoneal Dial Bull 4: S41, 1984

P. Amair, O. deCamejo, O. Domínguez, and M. Boissiere

38

Skin Reaction Against the Catheter: An Explanation for Exit Site Infection in CAPD

SUMMARY

To define the possible mechanisms involved in the production of skin exit site infection in patients on CAPD, a histological evaluation of the skin around the catheter exit site was performed in nine patients.

In all but one patient foreign body granulomata were found, and in six an inert refringent material was circled by the granulomata. This inert material is similar to the catheter material. This suggests that skin reacts against the catheter to produce foreign body granulomata that may be the cause of the exit site infection.

INTRODUCTION

Exit site infection frequently complicates continuous ambulatory peritoneal dialysis (CAPD) and may cause peritonitis or catheter loss.[1,2] The etiology of this infection remains controversial. To define further the possible mechanisms involved in the development of exit site infection, we conducted a histologic evaluation of the skin around the catheter at the exit site, in patients on CAPD.

_____

From the Servicio de Nefrología y Trasplante Renal y Servicio de Dermatología y Hospital Universitario de Caracas, Caracas, Venezuela.

METHODS

Nine patients (aged 18–62 years) were maintained on CAPD during a period ranging from 5 to 24 months. All were using a one-cuff catheter or a two-cuff catheter with the external cuff shaved and the catheter laterally placed. The mean catheter life was 13 ± 6 months. Two types of material were sent for histologic evaluation. One was a block containing the catheter and the surrounding skin at the exit site obtained during catheter replacement in three patients with fungal peritonitis. The other was a block containing only the skin and the subcutaneous tissue adjacent to the catheter exit site obtained in six patients during resection of granulomatous lesions with chronic discharge at the catheter exit site. The catheter was left in place.

All tissue blocks were fixed in formalin and processed in an autotechnicon. Thereafter, they were embedded in paraffin and cut on a rotary microtome. All sections were stained with hematoxylin-eosin, PAS (fungi), Fite-Faraco (acid fast bacilli), or Giemsa and Gram (parasites and bacteriae) stains.

RESULTS

The clinical findings are shown in Table 1. All six patients with chronic skin reaction had positive cultures for Staphylococcus epidermidis. Foreign

Table 1. Clinical Findings.

| Patient | Duration of Catheter Implantation (Months) | Material Removed | | Removal Reason |
		Skin Exit Site	Skin Exit Site Plus Catheter	
1	12	—	Yes	Peritonitis
2	14	—	Yes	Peritonitis
3	14	—	Yes	Peritonitis
4	20	Yes	Yes	Exit site*
5	6	Yes	—	Exit site*
6	24	Yes	—	Exit site*
7	20	Yes	—	Exit site*
8	5	Yes	—	Exit site*
9	7	Yes	—	Exit site*

* Chronic skin reaction and exit site discharge.

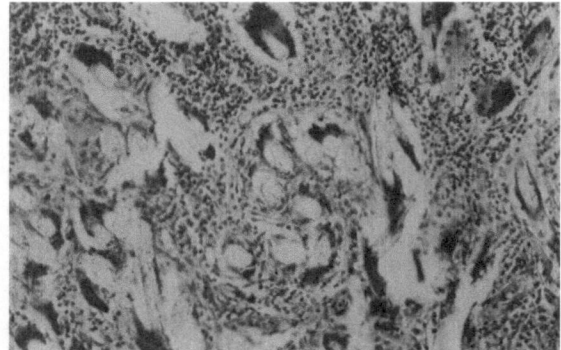

Fig. 1. Inert refringent material encircled by foreign body granulomata.

body granulomata were found in eight patients, and in six of them inert refringent material was circled by the granulomata (Fig. 1). This material is similar to the microscope appearance of the catheter and different from the cuff microscopic appearance (Fig. 2). In two cases, the catheter was clearly invaded by the skin. Other microscopic findings included: hemorrhage, fibrosis, and polyphormonuclear leucocyte infiltration in all patients; an eosinophilic reaction was found in five (Tables 2 & 3).

DISCUSSION

Exit site infection is a troublesome complication and may be life-threatening if it causes peritoni-

Table 2. Histologic Findings.

| Patient | Foreign Body Granulomata | Inert Material | Hemorrhage | Infiltration | | |
				Neutrophil	Mononuclear	Eosinophil
1	+ + + +	+ + + +	+ + +	+	+ + + +	+ +
2	+	No	+ + + +	+ + + +	+ + + +	No
3	+ + + +	+ + +	+ + + +	+	+ + + +	+ + +
4	No	No	+ + +	+ + +	+ + + +	No
5	+	+	+ + + +	+ + + +	+ + + +	No
6	+ + + +	+ + + +	+ + +	No	+ + + +	No
7	+ + +	No	+ + +	+	+ + + +	+ +
8	+ +	+ +	+ + +	+	+ + + +	+ +
9	+	+	+ + +	+	+ + + +	+ +

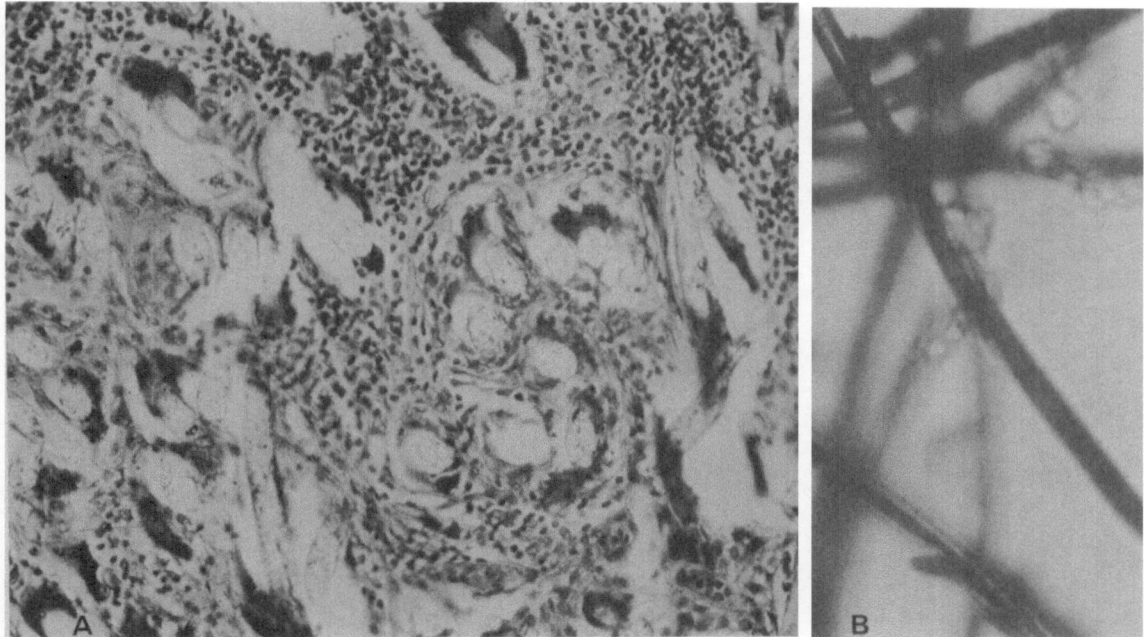

Fig. 2. (*a*) inert refringent material and (*b*) catheter cuff material.

Table 3. Summary of Histologic Findings.

	Number	%
Foreign body granulomata	8	88
Inert material	6	66
Hemorrhage	9	100
Fibrosis	9	100
Mononuclear infiltration	9	100
Polymorphonuclear infiltration	6	66
Eosinophilic infiltration	5	55
Mucoid degeneration	1	11

tis or catheter loss.[2] The cause of the exit site infection still remains unknown[1] and efforts to prevent it have been discouraging.[3] Our results show that the catheter promotes a skin reaction that may be due directly to the catheter or to changes in its biocompatibility derived from continuous exposure to antiseptic solutions. This reaction is manifested by foreign body granulomata, mononuclear infiltrate, hemorrhage and fibrosis, and subsequently secondary infection that affects the catheter exit site. A more careful study should be conducted to determine the origin of such a reaction and thus avoid these complications.

REFERENCES

1. Gloor HJ, Nichols WK, Sorkin MI, Prowant BF, Kennedy JM, Baker B, and Nolph KD: Peritoneal access and related complications in continuous ambulatory peritoneal dialysis. Am J Med 74: 593, 1983
2. Vas SI: Indications for catheter removal of the permanent peritoneal catheter. Peritoneal Dial Bull 1: 145, 1981
3. Nichols WK, and Nolph KD: A technique for managing exit site and cuff infection in Tenckhoff catheters. Peritoneal Dial Bull 3: 54, 1983

V.L. Poirier, B.D.T. Daly, K.A. Dasse,
C.C. Haudenschild, and R.E. Fine

39

Elimination of Tunnel Infection

SUMMARY

Because tunnel infection often underlies peritonitis and also contributes directly to morbidity of
CAPD patients, a systematic study of percutaneous
access materials has been undertaken. Porous biomaterials became infiltrated with serum and later
with round cells and fibroblasts. Percutaneous
porous polytetrafluoroethylene implants then developed a collagen seal that inhibited downward epidermal migration. The tight seal is a barrier to
infection and the implants performed adequately for
more than a year recommending their long-term performance in dialysis patients.

INTRODUCTION

Extraluminal bacterial invasion of the peritoneum (tunnel infection) has been recognized as a
contributor to the development of peritonitis during
continuous ambulatory peritoneal dialysis (CAPD).
It has been estimated that tunnel infection has been
the primary cause of 10 to 15 percent of these documented incidents. Our laboratories have been studying the response of the living system in contact with

From the Department of Cardiothoracic Surgery,
St. Elizabeth's Hospital and Tufts University School of
Medicine, the Departments of Physiology and Pathology,
Boston University School of Medicine, Boston, and Ther-
medics Inc., Woburn, Massachusetts.

a foreign object that penetrates the integument. The
primary failure modes of these devices can be cate-
gorized into three general areas: extrusion due to
marsupialization, extrusion due to infection and abscess formation, and extrusion due to avulsion.

Historically, conduits of percutaneous devices
have been smooth or rough textured surfaces and
their survival in animals has been measured in
months.[1-4] Smooth-surfaced conduits invariably
developed wet sinuses by the process of marsupialization. Sinus tract formation also occurred with
rough-textured devices. In these systems, initial epidermal bonding to the textured material occurred,
but cell maturation and surface migration were
thought to lead to repeated disruption of the seal.
Both types of conduits ultimately failed due to infection. Improved device survival was achieved when
various methods of strain relief were applied to reduce forces at the skin surface. However, consistent
long-term survival through this historic development phase did not occur.

Six years ago we began the systematic development of a percutaneous access device based on the
hypothesis that a mature collagen-biomaterial seal
would inhibit epidermal downgrowth and eliminate
sinus tract formation.[4-6] This hypothesis was supported by the observation that percutaneous porous
polytetrafluoroethylene (PTFE) implants developed
a collagen seal extending into the pores that inhibited downward epidermal migration.[2]

Eighteen basic biomaterials were screened *in
vitro* to evaluate their potential utilization at the

dermal-prosthetic interface. Human skin fibroblast growth, morphology, and biocompatibility in response to each material were evaluated. Of these, 14 porous material types/configurations were further evaluated *in vivo* to determine tissue ingrowth, bond strength, collagenase and nonspecific protease activity, the effects of coating materials with fibronectin, and the effects of prewetting porous materials prior to implant. Eighty-six skin-penetrating prostheses were then implanted in pigs. Ten configurations were evaluated with five types of materials. Six prostheses were explanted after 351 ± 33 days and demonstrated a stable sinus formation. Mature collagen was present at the biomaterial/dermis sinus termination point, providing support to our hypothesis that collagen will inhibit epidermal downgrowth. Twenty-one devices are currently being tested (for periods between 245 days and 721 days).

MATERIALS AND METHODS

The level I *in vitro* analysis of 18 coded biomaterials consisted of evaluating 180 samples (ten per group) in 0.5 ml of growth medium containing approximately 20,000 human skin fibroblasts. These cells (CCL76) were obtained from the American Type Culture Collection and had reached the 22nd passage when the experiment was initiated. The test chambers were placed in an incubator at 37° C and gassed with 5 percent CO_2, 95 percent air. Cells were examined on a daily basis and fed on days 4 and 8. The focus of attention was on examination to determine the extent to which the cells polarized and underwent spreading. The test was continued for 11 days to allow the cells to reach confluency.

The level II evaluation consisted of implanting 14 porous material types/configurations to determine tissue ingrowth. Biomaterial samples were placed in reaction cast sheets of polyurethane elastomers, 1.5 cm × 6.0 cm × 1.5 mm thick. A cavity, 1.0 cm × 5.0 cm × 1.0 mm deep was molded in the center of the specimen carrier. Test samples of the porous biomaterials were bonded into the cavity with pressure-sensitive adhesives with the porous side of the samples facing outwardly. Samples were ethylene oxide sterilized and implanted in miniature pigs and rabbits, in either a subdermal or intermuscular position, for time periods from 14 to 365 days.

Porous biomaterials were prewetted prior to implant by placing samples in a vacuum container. Once the strips were inserted, the container was closed and evacuated for approximately 5 minutes.

The container was then backfilled with saline and the samples removed. PTFE and carbon impregnated PTFE were evaluated with four different surface treatments: control (untreated strips), strips wetted with saline under vacuum, strips wetted with ethanol and rinsed in saline under vacuum, and saline-ethanol-benzylkonium-chloride air-dried overnight and rinsed with sterile saline under vacuum. All strips had the same porosity (11:1 expansion ratio).

Excised samples of biomaterial/tissue were placed in lactated Ringer's solution and tested within 2 hours. Tissue adherence was determined by using a Model 1130 Instron Tester, equipped with a 0 to 500 g load cell. Approximately 1 cm of tissue was separated from the smooth polyurethane backing to enable clamping into the upper Instron jaw. Crosshead speed was maintained at a constant 5 cm/minute separation rate. Each adhesion test was measured on a chart recorder and conducted until complete separation of the biologic lining from the 5 cm strip of material occurred. Quantitative values were calculated by dividing the average force (in grams) of separation by the specimen width (in centimeters).

Methods of enzyme assays for collagenase and nonspecific proteases (collagen degrading activity) and surface treatment of porous biomaterials with pure lyophilized fibronectin have been previously described.[7]

Histologic examinations of tissue samples to determine tissue ingrowth were carried out by excising test specimens en bloc. Sections from several areas of the specimens were stained by hematoxylin and eosin for evaluation on the general architecture and inflammation. A reticulum stain was utilized to evaluate early connective tissue fibers, the Masson-Trichrome stain was used to evaluate collagen; and the Verhoff von Geison stain was used for elastin.

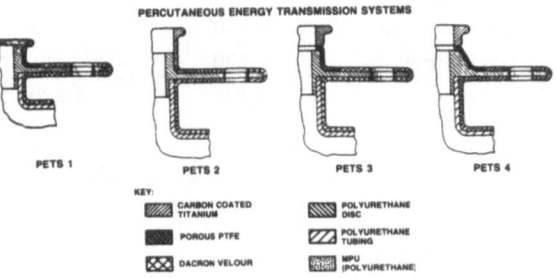

Fig. 1. PETS iterations designed for flange located in deep subcutaneous tissue.

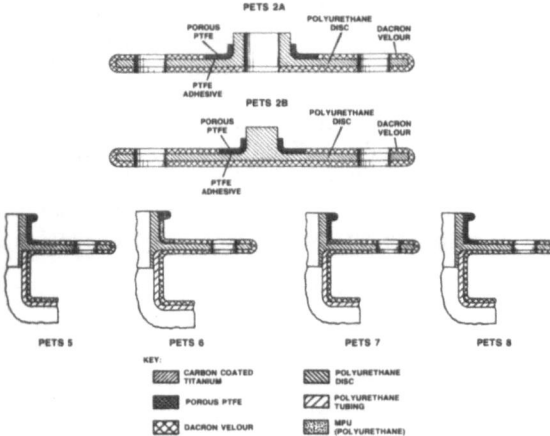

Fig. 2. PETS iterations designed for flange located in a superficial subcutaneous plane.

Table 1. Level I Evaluation.

Material	Mean Number of Cells/cm²	± Standard Deviation
EG-60D-PE	21,960	5,780
EG-70D-PE	19,240	4,800
EG-60D-C-PE	18,560	3,260
DF-80A	16,340	3,560
DF-80A-C	14,000	6,080
EG-60D	11,640	2,760
DF-80A-PE	10,840	3,840
EG-60D-C	10,160	2,680
EG-80A-C-PE	9,440	4,100
DF-80A-C-PE	9,320	2,520
EG-80A-C	7,220	2,120
EG-80A-PE	7,160	3,120
EG-80A	5,060	2,260
Teflon	4,600	3,200
EG-70D	3,280	1,040
PVC-Dibutyl Tin Dilaurate	2,740	3,540
Butyl Rubber	1,620	
Polystyrene	1,540	1,880
Control	27,520	4,020

EG—Extrudable Grade Polyurethane—Thermedics Inc.
DF—Lacquer Polyurethane—Thermedics Inc.
PE—Plasma Etched Surface.
C—Carbon Filled.
PVC—Poly Vinyl Chloride.
Control—Petri Dish.
80A, 60D, 70D,—Shore Hardness.

Ground substance was evaluated with periodic acid Schiff. Where appropriate, transmission electron microscopy was used.

The level III evaluation consisted of implanting 86 prostheses that penetrate the integument. Ten configurations have been evaluated as shown in Figures 1 & 2. These have been previously described in detail.[8,9] The initial design consisted of five components. The basic structural component was a semirigid polyurethane skirt, positioned at the subdermal level, with an integral neck 10 mm in diameter extending perpendicularly to the skirt. External to the neck was a flanged, carbon-coated titanium insert at the epidermal level. Porous biomaterials were positioned along the neck and 6 mm onto the skirt to interface at the dermal and subdermal levels. A flexible polyurethane conduit was attached beneath the skirt and extended through deeper tissues. The remainder of the skirt and conduit was covered with Dacron velour. The carbon-coated insert was intended to minimize reaction at the epidermal level, the porous biomaterial to encourage a collagen collar to form and inhibit epidermal downgrowth, and the Dacron velour to promote rapid, tenacious bonding in deeper tissues. Strain relief was imparted at three levels by the skin flange, subcutaneous skirt, and tunneling in the deeper tissues.

RESULTS

Results of the level I evaluation are shown in Table 1. The most critical component of the prosthesis is the interface material that crosses the integument. Several factors are important in choosing this material. The material must be biocompatible and nontoxic; it must maintain cell viability; and it must be structured with the correct pore size and pore geometry. Our level I evaluation was designed to determine cell viability and compatibility with the biomaterial. Our results clearly demonstrate that there are several materials that can be used for this critical component. Cell counts in excess of 10,000 cells/cm² are considered acceptable. It is also interesting to note that, in this test, plasma etched surfaces maintained better cell viability than nonplasma etched surfaces. Carbon filled material was of secondary importance.

In the level II evaluation, 14 porous material types/configurations were evaluated *in vivo* to determine: tissue ingrowth; bond strength; collagenase and nonspecific protease activity; and the effects of prewetting porous materials prior to implant. Test strips were implanted for a period of 3 months in the flank of the miniature pig in a subdermal location. The test strips were excised *en bloc* and evaluated for enzymatic activity. Table 2 shows the results of the assays for collagenase and nonspecific protease conducted on the tissue immediately adjacent to the biomaterial surface. The only significant differences observed in these analyses were for the collagenase. The nonspecific proteases were all within a few units of the control. There was wide variance in the results. However, there appeared to be some correlation between these results and the degree of cellularity observed histologically at the tissue-biomaterial interface. Of interest, the stripped Dacron velour was superior to the standard Dacron velour; i.e., less enzymatic activity was present. In terms of the histologic results, Dacron velour was compared to the same material that had the finish stripped off and to the same material that had the fibers overcoated with Biomer polyurethane. Proplast was also evaluated as a potential material for use on the skirt. The tissue reaction to each of these materials was similar, qualitatively, but significantly different, quantitatively. All of the materials produced a fi-

brocellular reaction, but of varying degrees and thicknesses. The cellular component consisted of fibroblasts, focal round cell infiltration, and a giant cell reaction about the fibrils. The degree of vascularity varied. Stripped Dacron velour had a mild round cell and giant cell infiltration, with thinner capsulation, and the collagen fibers could be seen to wrap around the fibrils in several sections.

In terms of the histologic results between Gore-Tex (W.L. Gore, Elkton, MD (5:1) and Impra (Tempe, AZ) (11:1), there appeared to be very little difference. The tissue encapsulating each material was between 1.5 and 3 mm in thickness and was quite cellular with moderate vascularity and scattered round cell infiltration. The cellularity was increased near the surface of the material with scattered areas of moderate inflammation. In general, the capsule surrounding the Impra was thinner, contained more collagen, and was less cellular with less vascularity when compared to GoreTex. The pores of the Impra had far more cellular infiltration than the GoreTex. The cells penetrated two thirds of the material and the superficial cells were actively producing collagen; capillary ingrowth was also

Table 2. Level of Collagenase Activity Level of Nonspecific Proteases Activity (3 Months).

Material	Collagenase (units)	Nonspecific Protease (units)
Gortex (5:1)	354	114
Gortex-F (5:1)	96	71
Impra (11:1)	280	84
Impra-F (11:1)	600	89
Proplast	145	72
PMS 40–100	100	82
PMS EG-60D-F	125	70
PMS EG-60D	131	79
Dacron Velour-Stripped	100	86
Dacron Velour-Biomer	168	68
Dacron Velour-Tecoflex	173	89
Dacron Velour-Standard	121	83
Tecoflex Felt	316	75
Tecoflex Felt-F	150	65
Control Epidermis	74	74

F—Fibronectin.
(5:1) and (11:1)—Expansion ratio.
PMS—Sintered titanium sphere; 40 to 100 micron pore size.
PMS EG-60D—Bonded titanium spheres with urethane.
Stripped—Finish removed.
Dacron Velour-Biomer, overcoated with urethane.

214   Poirier, et al.

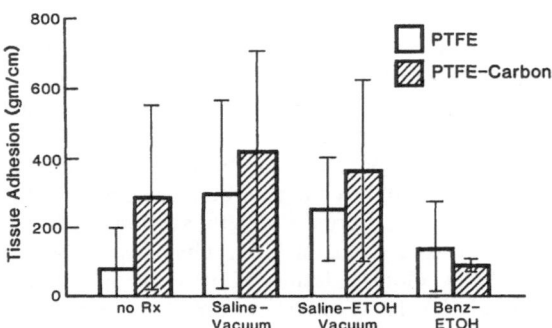

Fig. 3. Tissue adhesion.

carbonized PTFE since this material is hydropho-
bic. Each of the strips indicated in Figure 3 were
evaluated following 6 weeks of implantation in a
subdermal position in the rabbit for the purpose of
tissue bonding and for histologic appearance. Although the results were variable, partially due to the
small sample size, tissue adhesion to the wetted
PTFE and PTFE-carbon appeared to exceed that
observed to the control (untreated) strips. In fact,
the saline wetted samples had a mean tissue adhesion approximately three times greater than the
standard, unwetted controls. Pre-wetting porous
materials enhances the cell infiltration and bond
strength.

Bond strength testing of tissue to biomaterial
was carried out on 17 materials. Results are shown in
Table 3. Although the data obtained varied considerably, we are still able to make general statements.
Impra (11:1) is superior to GoreTex (5:1); fibro-
nectin-coated surfaces do not improve bond strength;
velour that has its finish stripped is superior to the
as-received Dacron velour; and the highest bond

present in these. Fibronectin did not improve the
histologic appearance of these implanted materials.
What did occur, however, was a very intense superficial angiogenic stimulus. A large number of capillaries formed near the biomaterial surfaces and
appeared to be oriented toward the pores.

Studies were carried out to evaluate various
methods of wetting the surface of the PTFE and the

Table 3. Bond Strength (g/cm).

Material	Implant Duration (Days)				
	14	28	42	60	90
Gortex (5:1)	100	27	7	33	1.0
Gortex-F (5:1)	20	54	91		3.0
Impra (11:1)		66			85
Impra-F (11:1)					40
Dacron Velour		207	224	270	585
Dacron Velour-Stripped					614
Dacron Velour-Biomer					120
Proplast					149
PMS (35–95)	210	221	180		230
PMS (17–34)	250	86	78		
Dacron-Tecoflex					69
PMS-60D (40–100)					7
PMS-60D-F (40–100)					19
Polyethylene		46			
Impra (19:1)		34			
Impra (38:1)		58			
PMS (100–200)		46			

(5:1)—Expansion Ratio.
F—Fibronectin.
Stripped—Finish Removed.
PMS (35–95)—Sintered Titanium Spheres with a Pore Size of 35–95 microns.
Dacron—Tecoflex—Dacron Velour Overcoated with Tecoflex Polyurethane.
PMS-60D (40–100)—Titanium Spheres Bonded with Polyurethane.

strength and most consistent results were obtained from the Dacron velour samples.

The level III study consisted of implanting 86 skin-penetrating prostheses in miniature pigs. Ten configurations were evaluated with five types of materials. This study has been previously described in detail.[7–13]

Clinically, a superficial sinus developed around every system. The sinus first appeared as a narrow space between the epidermis and urethane conduit which gradually widened superficially as the epidermal edge turned inward. By 2 months the sinus usually widened to between 0.5–1.0 mm and was filled with dark compact keratin and debris. The skin edge tightly approximated this keratinous ring. The origin of the sinus, however, gradually widened until 3 to 4 months postimplantation, with little change after that time. In those systems surviving 1 year, this sinus reached approximately 2–4 mm in width. Nevertheless, the depth of the sinus was limited, permitting system survival.

In those systems explanted at one to 2 months, the extent of coverage with squamous epithelium (epidermalization) along the PTFE and Dacron velour was variable with regard to the duration of implantation. The sinus stopped at points varying between the angled or radial portion of the PTFE to near the termination of the PTFE at the PTFE-Dacron velour junction with one exception—where the sinus terminated on the vertical portion of the PTFE. In contrast, in the system removed at 6 months and in all of the 1 year systems, sinus termination was at the PTFE-Dacron velour junction.

Results from the electively removed systems have been previously described; however, a brief review will be presented for completeness.[14] Histologic examination of the systems electively removed at 1 and 2 months demonstrated a well-defined sinus termination point on the PTFE. Here, the epidermal cells lining the sinus ended abruptly at a point where granulation tissue had extended into the PTFE pores. This new connective tissue was cellular with large numbers of round cells and fibroblasts near the PTFE surface, sometimes penetrating the pores. However, only the first three to five cells below the PTFE surface appeared viable. The number of cells deep within the pores were few, and these cells were pyknotic. Only an occasional polymorphonuclear leukocyte was present. The sinus was filled with ground substance and necrotic cells. The collagen abutting the PTFE near the sinus termination point occasionally appeared oriented towards the opening of the PTFE pores. A collagen stain has demonstrated the presence of some loose collagen

within these pores as early as 1 month postimplant, and electron microscopy has confirmed this. The Dacron velour demonstrated the typical foreign body giant cell and fibroblastic reaction around its fibers. Within the granulation tissue surrounding the prosthesis there were multiple accumulations of inflammatory round cells, and the collagen that was present was more delicate than the relatively coarse bundles of collagen in the dermis.

The histologic picture observed in the one system electively removed at 6 months was significantly different from those removed at the 1 to 2 month period and all the 1 year systems appeared similar to the 6 month system. In these systems, the sinus terminated at or just beyond the PTFE-Dacron velour junction and was lined by a thin layer of epidermal cells. Occasionally, areas of mature granulation tissue could be seen where epidermal atrophy may have occurred due to pressure from the keratin in the sinus or where epidermal migration was never completed. In addition, small areas of acanthotic epidermis were sometimes seen, especially at the superficial portion of the sinus. The tissue abutting the epidermal lining consisted of mature connective tissue with essentially no inflammation, and the collagen, except for a small rim of thin delicate fibers along the lining, appeared architecturally similar to that seen in the dermis. This appearance continued to the PTFE-Dacron velour junction. There, the sinus terminated abruptly. Examination of multiple sections of the PTFE-Dacron velour junction from these long-term systems demonstrated occasional small areas of acute and chronic inflamation with necrosis. However, the absence of the pronounced foreign-body giant-cell reaction about the Dacron velour and at the junction was remarkable and distinguished these systems from those removed earlier.

Table 4 lists a summary of the results obtained thus far as a function of development time and initi-

Table 4. 1978–1984.

| Group | Implant Survival (Days) | |
	Mean	Range
I	28	27–56
II-A	66	26–99
II-B	70	33–238
II-C	278	84–371
II-D	355	322–377

21 currently on test (from 245–721 days).

ation of system improvements in terms of materials and geometric configuration. As shown, system longevity is increasing with improved materials, implant techniques, and animal care.

DISCUSSION

It is clear from our results that all the porous materials are subsequently infiltrated with round cells and fibroblasts. Even in our earliest specimens, where the sinus tract terminated on the vertical or radial portions of the system, the pores exposed to the sinus were filled with serum and necrotic cells. As soon as a system is implanted, epidermal cells begin to migrate, each seeking to surround itself completely with other epidermal cells. The granulation tissue, which forms near the surface, provides an ideal bed over which these cells can migrate. Their initial contact with the porous material must occur within the first week or two after implantation, and the serum, fibrin, and cells within the pores form an ineffectual barrier to epidermal migration. By 4 weeks, however, some loose collagen is present within the material sinuses further down. This is a consistent finding. By 2 months the collagen in the granulation tissue surrounding the prosthesis increases and appears relatively mature but is still loose. The sinus reaches a variable position on the horizontal portion of the porous material but measures only 0.5–1 mm in width at its superficial origin. However, in reality, the sinus has only progressed a few millimeters in 2 months time. We believe some inhibition of sinus development must have occurred. The best explanation for our observations is that the collagen at and within the pores inhibits or delays sinus progression, but does not stop it completely. Over time, the relatively weak tissue material bond is broken down by one or more factors which likely include epidermal cell and bacterial collagenases, nonspecific proteases, and/or shear from the mismatch between the viscoelastic properties of the prosthesis/tissue. The alignment of the collagen formed near the sinus termination point probably reflects these mechanical stresses.

Between 2 months and 6 months, there were no explanted PETS systems available for histologic analysis. However, the sinus at the skin surface widened progressively so that by 3 to 4 months, it ranged between 1 and 4 mm in transverse diameter. At the same time, we know that in most systems, the sinus had already extended to a position on the horizontal portion of the prosthesis. It seems reasonable to conclude that the sinus progression was even

slower during this period, although in the one system electively explanted at 6 months, the sinus had reached the PTFE-Dacron velour junction without evidence of infection or inflammation. It is likely, therefore, that although the sinus reaches this junction in a majority of systems by 2 to 6 months, its progress is slowed sufficiently to allow the connective tissue around the Dacron velour to mature. The key to the success of the current system, therefore, has been that it has retarded epidermal migration long enough to permit the tissue–velour interaction to mature.

By 6 months, the connective tissue abutting the epidermis lining the sinus is similar to dermis. The connective tissue at the PTFE-Dacron velour interface has a similar appearance. The typical chronic foreign body type of inflammation seen about the Dacron velour earlier has virtually disappeared, and mature collagen bundles appear to completely envelop the Dacron fibrils. This interface appears to be more or less stable for periods of 1 year or longer. Although the reasons for this are unclear, it is possible that the wicking potential of the Dacron velour fibril is retarded by the tight envelopment of mature collagen and the ability of this collagen to "turn off" epidermal migration and enzymatic degradation.

CONCLUSIONS

A retrospective analysis of all electively removed systems has supported the "collagen inhibition to epidermal downgrowth" hypothesis. Based on our results, we believe that adequate performance in animals for durations in excess of 1 year is sufficient to demonstrate the potential for long-term performance in humans.

ACKNOWLEDGMENTS

Supported by contract No. 1-HV-8-2919 from the Devices and Technology Branch, DHVD-NHLBI-NIH, Bethesda, Maryland.

REFERENCES

1. Von Recum AF: Applications and failure modes of percutaneous devices: A review. J Biomed Mater Res 18: 323, 1984
2. Winter GD: Transcutaneous implants, reactions of the skin-implant interface. J Biomed Mater Res 5: 96, 1974

3. Robinson WH, and Daly BDT: Percutaneous leads for artificial hearts and other prosthetic devices. In Szycher M, and Robinson W (Eds), Synthetic biomedical polymers: Concepts and practices. Westport: Technomic, 1980, p 211

4. Daly BDT, Szycher M, Poirier VL, Robinson WJ, Haudenschild CC, and Cleveland RF: A method of establishing permanent percutaneous energy transmission. Surgery 88: 148, 1980

5. Hasting WL, Aaron GL, Denicris G, Wessler PR, Pons AB, Rayzeca D, Olsen DB, and Kolff WK: A retrospective study of 8 calves surviving 5 months in pneumatic total artificial heart. Trans Am Soc Artif Intern Organs 27: 71, 1981

6. Von Recum AF, and Park JB: Permanent percutaneous devices. Bioeng 5: 37, 1981

7. Daly BDT, Szyeher M, Worthington M, Quimby FW, Warren RG, Robinson WJ, Haudenschild CC, Lewis MB, and Scheller CE: Development of percutaneous energy transmission systems. Annual Report No. NHLBI-NO1-HV-8-2919-5, 1983. Available from National Technical Information Service, Springfield, VA.

8. Daly BDT, Worthington M, Scheller CE, Szycher M, Haudenschild CC, Poirier VL, and Cleveland RJ: Percutaneous energy transmission systems. Trans Am Soc Artif Intern Organs 26: 244, 1980

9. Daly BDT, and Dasse KA: Development and in vivo testing of a chronic percutaneous prosthesis. Artif Organs 7: 454, 1983

10. Daly BDT, Szychr M, Worthington M, Robinson WJ, Quimby FW, Warren RG, Robinson WJ, Haudens-

child CC, Lewis MB, and Scheller CE: Development of a percutaneous energy transmission system. Annual Report No. NHLBI-NO1-HV-8-2929-1, 1979. Available from National Technical Information Service, Springfield VA.

11. Daly DBT, Dasse K, Haudenschild CC, Lesis MB, Poirier VL, Scheller C, Szycher M, Warren R, and Worthington M: Development of a percutaneous energy transmission system. Annual Report No. NHLBI-NO1-HV-8-2919-2, 1980. Available from National Technical Information Service, Springfield VA.

12. Daly BDT, Blitz Al, Clay W, Dasse KA, Dempsey DJ, Dewire P, Huadenschild CC, Hopkins RE, Kayne HL, Lewis MB, Poirier VL, Robinson WJ, Szycher M, and Worthington M: Development of a percutaneous energy transmission system. Annual Report No. NHLBI-NO1-HV-8-2929-3, 1981. Available from National Technical Information Service, Springfield, VA.

13. Daly BDT, Szycher M, Worthington M, Quimby FW, Warren RG, Robinson WJ, Haudenschild CC, Lewis MB, and Scheller CE: Development of a percutaneous energy transmission system. Annual Report No. NHLBI-NO1-HV-8-2919-4, 1982. Available from National Technical Information Service, Springfield. VA.

14. Daly BDT, Dasse KA, Haudenschild CC, Clay W, Szycher M, Ober NS, and Cleveland RJ: Percutaneous energy transmission systems: Long-term survival. Trans Am Soc Artif Intern Organs 29: 526, 1983

A.S. Levey, G.M. Simon, J. McCauley, T.J. Smith,
S.I. Cho and J.T. Harrington

40

Successful Peritoneal Catheter Placement after Major Abdominal Surgery or Peritonitis

SUMMARY

Experience with peritoneal catheters in 13 patients with prior abdominal surgery or peritonitis, a high risk group, was compared to 20 patients without prior complications. Intraperitoneal hemorrhage and drainage failure were more frequent in the high risk group. Catheter failure was least likely with curled Tenckhoff catheters. Nevertheless, with present techniques, more than 90% of high risk patients can anticipate successful catheter placement.

INTRODUCTION

Previous major abdominal surgery or peritonitis usually are considered to be relative contraindications for permanent peritoneal catheter placement. Despite this widespread impression, there are few quantitative estimates of the incidence of complications and likelihood of success after catheter insertion in patients with such a history. In our total experience, 13 of 33 patients (40%) treated with continuous ambulatory peritoneal dialysis (CAPD) had a past history of either major abdominal surgery or peritonitis unrelated to prior peritoneal dialysis.

These patients were highly motivated, however, to initiate CAPD because of their medical conditions or personal preferences for the lifestyle provided by this form of therapy. In view of the limited information on the risk of catheter insertion and our patients' strong motivations, we recommended CAPD. In order to provide quantitative data on the risk of serious early complications, we review our experience with permanent peritoneal catheter insertion for CAPD. In an earlier report, we compared the outcomes of catheter insertion in patients with and without a history of major abdominal surgery and peritonitis.[1] In this study, we report our experience with a larger number of patients with a longer duration of follow-up. We conclude that prior abdominal surgery and peritonitis do not prohibit successful catheter placement and are not absolute contraindications to peritoneal dialysis.

METHODS

CAPD was introduced at New England Medical Center in 1980. Since then, 33 patients have undergone 45 attempts at permanent peritoneal catheter placement (18 men, 15 women, ages 20 to 72 years). Twenty-three patients transferred to CAPD from hemodialysis; in 10 patients, CAPD was the initial form of dialysis. Selection of patients was based solely on their desires and our assessment of their overall suitability for home dialysis. No patients

From the Nephrology Division, Department of Medicine, and the Departments of Nursing and Surgery, Tufts University School of Medicine and New England Medical Center, Boston, Massachusetts.

were denied CAPD because of prior abdominal surgery or peritonitis.

Patients were hospitalized one day prior to catheter implantation. None had evidence of a clinically significant defect of coagulation or platelet aggregation. Platelet counts, prothrombin times and partial thromboplastin times were normal in all patients. Bleeding times, when measured, also were normal. In patients receiving hemodialysis, the last heparin dose was administered more than 12 hours prior to surgery. No patients were receiving anticoagulant drugs or inhibitors of platelet aggregation.

The peritoneal catheter was inserted in the midline position as described by Tenckhoff.[2] Surgery was performed in the operating room using local anesthesia. In some patients with multiple previous operations, lysis of extensive intraperitoneal adhesions or lateral catheter placement sometimes was required. Hernias were repaired prior to or at the time of catheter insertion. We used 22 straight and 18 curled Tenckhoff catheters, four column-disc catheters, and one Toronto-Western Hospital catheter. Dialysate was infused into the peritoneal cavity and drainage was tested and found to be adequate in all patients prior to completion of surgery. Afterwards, the peritoneal cavity was irrigated three times daily with 500 ml Dianeal® containing 1500 units heparin. Dialysate was blood tinged after surgery and usually cleared within 3 days. If the effluent contained gross blood or fibrin clots, the heparin dose was increased. Unless complications arose, patients were discharged on the third hospital day and training for CAPD began 3 days later. In statistical analysis, significance was tested by chi-square analysis; a p value of <0.05 was considered significant.

RESULTS

Major Surgery or Peritonitis Not Associated with CAPD

For this study, patients with previous major abdominal surgery or peritonitis not associated peritoneal dialysis were considered at high-risk for complications of catheter placement. There were 13 patients so defined in our "high-risk" group. The remaining 20 patients comprised our "low-risk" group. We compared the outcomes of catheter placement in patients in the high-risk and low-risk groups.

Among the 13 high-risk patients, 11 had a past history of major abdominal surgery, including bi-

lateral nephrectomy in three, cholecystectomy in three, hysterectomy in two, cesarean delivery in two, ureteral reimplantation in two, and ileal loop urinary diversion, suprapubic prostatectomy, aorto-iliac bypass, and appendectomy with open drainage in one patient each. The patients had undergone from one to six operations each (26 operations total). Two patients had prior episodes of peritonitis unrelated to peritoneal dialysis. One patient had a ruptured pancreatic pseudocyst with diffuse chemical peritonitis and shock. Another patient with systemic lupus erythematosus previously had suffered a prior episode of fever, abdominal pain, and diarrhea thought to be due to peritonitis. Neither patient had undergone surgery or peritoneal lavage for treatment of peritonitis. The reasons for selecting CAPD in the high-risk group included vascular access failure in five patients, ischemic heart disease in two, and personal lifestyle preferences in six.

Transplantation, Minor Surgery, or Peritonitis Associated with CAPD

A total of 21 patients (from both the high-risk and low-risk groups) had undergone transplantation, minor abdominal surgery (herniorraphy, uncomplicated appendectomy, unilateral nephrectomy), or had an episode of peritonitis while on CAPD prior to another catheter insertion. Nine of 13 patients in the high-risk group, compared to 12 of 20 patients in the low-risk group, had a history of one or more of these events (p = NS). We also analyzed the effect of these events on outcomes of subsequent catheter placement.

Serious Early Complications

Within the first week after surgery, there were 13 serious complications of catheter placement in eight patients. Complications included five episodes of intraperitoneal hemorrhage in four patients and six instances of drainage failure in six patients. (Some patients had more than one complication.)

Intraperitoneal hemorrhage was defined as the presence of gross blood in the dialysate. In patients with hemorrhage, packed cell volume in dialysate effluent ranged from 3 to 22%. The onset of hemorrhage was within one day in four instances and after 6 days in one case. Treatment included blood transfusions (3–8 U/patient), peritoneal lavage with dialysate containing heparin (3,000–10,000 U/L) to prevent blood clotting within the catheter and catheter thrombectomy if necessary. With these measures, all clotted catheters were reopened. Two catheters were removed because of persistent bleeding after two and seven days; bleeding was due to lysed peritoneal adhesions and subsided thereafter. In one instance, bleeding stopped spontaneously after four days, but subsequently the catheter failed to drain and was removed. In the remaining two cases, bleeding subsided after 3 and 6 days; subsequently the catheters remained functional. Thus, intraperitoneal hemorrhage led to catheter removal in three of five instances. There were no other serious complications of intraperitoneal hemorrhage.

Drainage failure was defined as incomplete drainage of dialysate requiring catheter replacement or abandonment of CAPD. Three instances of drainage failure occurred within one day due to malposition of one curled and two straight Tenckhoff catheters. The remaining three instances of drainage failure occurred within one week and appeared to be due to migration of three straight Tenckhoff catheters. Five of the six catheters were removed. The remaining patient refused catheter removal and transferred to intermittent peritoneal dialysis, but continued to experience incomplete dialysate drainage.

Three other catheters were removed within the first month after implantation. In two instances, patients were unable to cope with the home dialysis regimen and did not complete their training. One patient developed a recurrence of Pseudomonas peritonitis which had preceded catheter insertion. These events were *not* considered to be complications of catheter insertion *per se*.

Overall, intraperitoneal hemorrhage and dialysate drainage failure occurred in 11 of 45 catheter insertions (24%), in 8 of 33 patients (24%), and collectively were the cause of 9 of the 12 instances of early catheter removal. In subsequent analyses, we examine the incidence of complications in patients with and without a history of prior abdominal surgery or peritonitis. Because some patients underwent repeated attempts at catheter insertion, we also compare the likelihood of successful catheter placement in both groups. For this analysis, we defined successful catheter insertion as normal catheter function two weeks after surgery.

Outcomes of Catheter Placement

First, we compared the outcomes of catheter placement in the high-risk and low-risk patients. Table 1 demonstrates the probabilities of drainage failure or hemorrhage and of successful catheter placement in both groups. There were no differences in the incidence of peritonitis, exit site or tunnel infections, dialysate leaks or hernia after catheter placement.

LOW-RISK GROUP

Twenty low-risk patients underwent 24 catheter placements (Table 1). Three patients (15%) had three instances (13%) of drainage failure due to catheter malposition in one patient and presumed migration in two. Each patient refused subsequent attempts at catheter insertion. The probability of success in the low-risk group, therefore, was 21 of 24 catheters (87%) in 17 of 20 patients (85%).

HIGH-RISK GROUP

Thirteen high-risk patients underwent 21 attempts at catheter insertion. There was a higher risk of complications of catheter placement in this group (Table 1). There were three instances of drainage failure in three patients resulting from catheter migration in one patient and malposition due to adhesions in two patients. The five instances of intraperitoneal hemorrhage occurred in four patients in the high-risk group. Overall there were eight serious complications (38%) in five high-risk patients (38%).

Table 1. Outcomes of Catheter Placement.

	n	Drainage Failure or Hemorrhage n (%)	Success n (%)
Patients	33		
Low risk	20	3 (15%)	17 (85%)
High risk	13	5 (38%)	12 (92%)
Catheter Placements	45		
Low risk	24	3 (13%)	21 (87%)
High risk	21	8 (38%)*	15 (71%)

* $p < 0.05$.

Four of the five high-risk patients with serious complications eventually achieved successful catheter function. In two patients with intraperitoneal hemorrhage, catheters were functional for 27 and 32 months. In one patient with drainage failure due to migration of a straight Tenckhoff catheter, a curled Tenckhoff catheter was inserted and has remained functional for 24 months. In another patient who suffered from two instances of hemorrhage and one episode of drainage failure due to malposition of a straight Tenckhoff catheter, insertions of a Toronto-Western Hospital and a column-disc catheter were not followed by serious complications and led to successful function for 13 and 3 months respectively. In the remaining patient, two attempts at catheter placement were complicated by drainage failure and hemorrhage. She refused a third attempt.

Overall, 15 of 21 catheter insertions (71%) were successful in high-risk patients. In these 15 instances, catheter function and peritoneal solute and water transport were adequate for CAPD, except in one patient with previous Candida peritonitis in whom ultrafiltration was impaired. At present, 10 of the 15 catheters continue to function normally after an average of 18 months. The duration of function prior to removal of the remaining five catheters was 10 months. Although the risk of serious early complications was increased with previous major abdominal surgery or hemorrhage, successful catheter placement was eventually achieved in 12 of 13 patients (92%).

IMPACT OF TRANSPLANTATION, MINOR SURGERY, AND PERITONITIS ASSOCIATED WITH CAPD

We also analyzed the effect of a prior history of transplantation, minor surgery, and peritonitis associated with CAPD on the outcome of subsequent catheter insertion. These events were examined separately because we considered the risk of extensive intraperitoneal adhesions after these procedures to be less than after the major surgical procedures in the high-risk group. The incidence of intraperitoneal hemorrhage or drainage failure did not differ between patients with and without a history of one or more of these events (Table 2).

DISCUSSION

Intraperitoneal hemorrhage and drainage failure were the most important serious complications of peritoneal catheter insertion in our patients and were the most common causes of removal of the

catheter soon after its implantation. In our experience, the risk of these complications is 38% in patients with previous major abdominal surgery or peritonitis unrelated to peritoneal dialysis, compared to only 13% in patients without a history of these events ($p < 0.05$). By contrast, a past history of transplantation, minor surgery, or peritonitis related to peritoneal dialysis was not associated with a higher risk of complications. Our findings not only confirm the conventional teaching that major abdominal surgery and peritonitis lead to a higher risk of early serious complications, but also provide a quantitative estimate of the degree of risk.

Despite the fact that the risk for complications is higher, all but one of the high-risk patients, subsequently underwent successful catheter placement. Thus more than 90% of high-risk patients eventually were able to perform CAPD. We conclude therefore that these risk factors are not absolute contraindications to successful peritoneal dialysis. For patients with previous major surgery or peritonitis, the decision to attempt catheter insertion requires assessment of the patients' motivations for choosing peritoneal dialysis as well as discussion of the additional risk of catheter placement. For patients highly motivated to perform CAPD, we continue to recommend attempts at catheter implantation.

Our experience also illustrates potential advantages of different peritoneal catheters. In our

Table 2. Transplantation, Minor Surgery, or Peritonitis with CAPD.

Number with Potential Risk Factor*		Number with Drainage Failure or Hemorrhage†	p‡
Transplantation	18	5	NS
Minor surgery	15	2	NS
CAPD Peritonitis	6	1	NS
Any of the above	30	6	NS

* Forty-five catheters were inserted. For example, in 18 cases, transplantation preceded catheter insertion; in 27 cases, it did not.

† There were 11 instances of drainage failure and hemorrhage. For example, there were five complications in the 18 cases with prior transplantation; there were six complications in the 27 cases without transplantation.

‡ Value for χ^2 was calculated for each 2×2 contingency table. For example,

	Complication	No Complication
Transplantation	5	13
No Transplantation	6	21

patients drainage failure due to catheter migration and malposition occurred after insertion of 5 of 22 straight Tenckhoff catheters (23%), compared with only one of 18 curled Tenckhoff catheters (6%) ($p < 0.05$). Moreover, Rottembourg and Oreopoulos and their colleagues also reported a lower incidence of drainage failure from catheter migration with curled Tenckhoff or Toronto Western Hospital catheters.[3,4] As a result of these findings, we now routinely use the curled Tenckhoff catheter for CAPD.

In our patients massive intraperitoneal hemorrhage after catheter insertion occurred only in patients with previous major abdominal surgery or peritonitis. We hypothesize that hemorrhage was due to deliberate or inadvertent lysis of adhesions during catheter placement. We found that subsequent placement of column-disc catheters, which do not require creation of an intraperitoneal pathway,[5] did not lead to bleeding in two patients who previously had suffered intraperitoneal hemorrhage. We now use the column-disc catheter in high-risk patients if adhesions prevent easy placement of a curled Tenckhoff catheter. Ash and colleagues also have described successful placement of the Tenckhoff catheter in patients with adhesions by using a peritoneoscope to guide catheter insertion.[6]

Using presently available techniques, more than 90% of high-risk patients selecting CAPD can anticipate successful catheter placement. Further studies must determine the relative advantages of the wide variety of catheters now available for peritoneal dialysis.

REFERENCES

1. Levey AS, Simon GM, McCauley J, Smith TJ, Cho SI, and Harrington JT: Outcome of peritoneal catheter placement in the high-risk patient. Peritoneal Dial Bull 3(Suppl 4): 112, 1984

2. Tenckhoff H: Chronic peritoneal dialysis manual, Chapt 8. Seattle, University of Washington School of Medicine, 1974, p 23

3. Rottembourg J, Jacq D, Vonlanthen M, Issad B, and El Shahant Y: Straight or curled Tenckhoff peritoneal catheter for CAPD. Peritoneal Dial Bull 1: 123, 1981

4. Ponce SP, Pierratos A, Izatt S, Mathews R, Khanna R, Zellerman G, and Oreopoulos DG: Comparison of the survival and complications of three permanent peritoneal dialysis catheters. Peritoneal Dial Bull 2: 82, 1982

5. Ash SR, Slingeneyer A, and Schardin KE: Peritoneal access using the column-disc catheter. Perspectives Peritoneal Dial 1: 9, 1983

6. Ash SR, Handt AE, and Bloch R: Peritoneoscopic placement of the Tenckhoff catheter: Further clinical experience. Peritoneal Dial Bull 3: 8, 1983

O. Domínguez, P. Amair, R. Fernández, and M. Boissiere

41

Reduction of Complications with Bedside Lateral Placement of Catheter for CAPD

SUMMARY

A bedside technique for lateral placement of CAPD catheters is described. Catheters with a single internal cuff are used, fixing it to the posterior rectus aponeurosis and opening the peritoneum with a small incision.. The internal cuff is covered with the anterior rectus muscle and the anterior aponeurosis. The skin exit site is made in a straight line with the peritoneal entry site.

Using this technique, 40 catheters have been implanted, without incisional hernia, and only two early leakages occurred that closed spontaneously after 10 days on IPD. There have been no catheter related deaths.

The technique described here, is an easy and safe procedure which reduces catheter complications.

INTRODUCTION

Catheter complications are frequent causes of patient dissatisfaction and discontinuation of peritoneal dialysis. The particular complications are early dialysate leakage, incisional herniae, and external cuff extrusion.[1] In an attempt to decrease the incidence of these complications, we have designed a bedside technique for lateral placement of chronic peritoneal catheters for CAPD.

From the Servicio de Nefrología y Trasplante Renal Hospital Universitario de Caracas, Caracas, Venezuela.

TECHNIQUE

Oral intake is not permitted for 2 hours before the operation. Systemic antibiotics cephalosporin 1 g and tobramycin 75 mg are administered intravenously 60 minutes before surgery. The premedication consists of meperidine hydrochloride and diazepam given intramuscularly. Only one-cuff catheters or two-cuff catheters with the external cuff shaved are used.

At bedside, under aseptic conditions and local anesthesia with 2% lidocaine, a 5 cm incision, lateral to the umbilicus, is performed. The anterior rectus aponeurosis and the anterior rectus muscle are opened longitudinally. Two reference sutures (black silk 00), are placed on the posterior rectus aponeurosis, separated by the catheter's diameter; using scissors, a small incision is made between the reference sutures and the peritoneum is opened. The catheter is introduced using a rigid guide into the culdesac. The peritoneum is closed if necessary, and the internal cuff is fixed to the posterior rectus aponeurosis with the reference sutures. Two liters of dialysate are infused to test leakage and catheter patency. The dialysate is drained, then the anterior rectus muscle and the anterior rectus aponeurosis are closed separately, with resorbable material, in an ascending fashion, over the internal cuff. The patency of the catheter is checked again with the rigid guide. The skin exit site is approached by a subcutaneous tunnel of 3 cm, in straight line to the peritoneal entry site, and parallel to the abdominal mid-line, thus avoiding angulation of the catheter

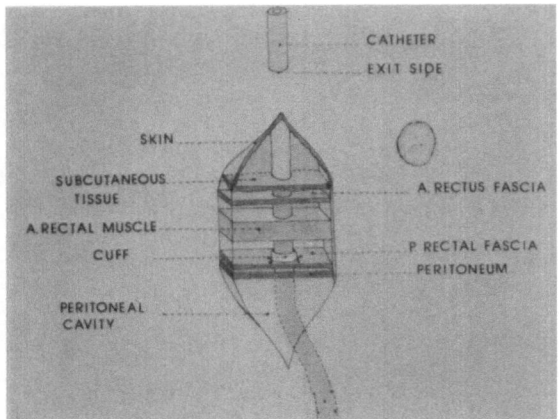

Fig. 1. Diagram representing catheter pathway.

(Fig. 1). The patency and location of the catheter are checked again with the rigid guide; subcutaneous tissue and skin are closed. A titanium adapter is attached immediately and CAPD started. Figure 2 illustrates the final aspect of the procedure.

RESULTS

Forty catheters have been implanted using this technique. The mean catheter life is 15 ± 6 months, ranging from 3–28 months. No incisional herniae have occurred and early leakage was observed only in two cases, both receiving steroids. In both patients the leakage closed spontaneously after 10 days on intermittent peritoneal dialysis. Exit site infection occurred in six cases. A total of five catheters were removed: four because of peritonitis and one for exit site infection. In another five patients, the catheters were removed after renal transplantation.

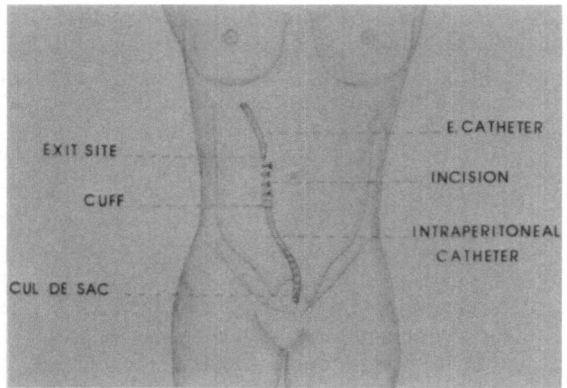

Fig. 2. Representation of completed catheter insertion.

There have been no catheter related deaths or catheter extrusions.

DISCUSSION

The lateral placement of chronic peritoneal catheters has been adopted as the preferable technique in patients on CAPD.[2] The technique described in this report for lateral placement of peritoneal catheters differs from others previously published[3,4] in that only catheters with one internal cuff are used, avoiding outer cuff extrusion or infection. The fixation of the cuff on the posterior rectus aponeurosis, and its coverage with the anterior rectus muscle and the anterior rectus aponeurosis offer more layers to prevent leakage or incisional herniae. Furthermore, the avoidance of a large peritoneal incision markedly reduces the probabilities of leakage.

Finally, the skin exit site is straight in line with the peritoneal entry site, and allows the use of external procedures to correct catheter migration at the bedside.[5] The frequency of exit site infection in our patients was only 15%, no different from other previous reports in which two-cuff catheters were used.[1,3] All but one of these patients responded to local treatment or resection of the affected skin without catheter replacement as proposed by Nichols and Nolph.[6] In conclusion, the present technique for lateral placement of chronic peritoneal catheters is a safe and easy procedure that can contribute to CAPD success because of reduction of early and late complications.

REFERENCES

1. Gloor HJ, Nichols WK, Sorkin MI, Prowant BF, Kennedy JM, Baker B, and Nolph KD: Peritoneal access and related complications in continuous ambulatory peritoneal dialysis. Am J Med 74: 593, 1983
2. Helfrich GB, and Winchester JF: What is the preferable technique for peritoneal catheter implantation? Peritoneal Dial Bull 2: 132, 1982
3. Helfrich GB, Pechan BW, Alijani MR, Barnard WF, Rakowski TA, and Winchester JF: Reduction of catheter complications with lateral placement. Peritoneal Dial Bull 3: S2, 1983
4. Nghiem DD: A technique of catheter insertion for uncomplicated peritoneal dialysis. Surg Gynecol Obstet 157: 574, 1983
5. Dans R, Young J, Diamond D, and Bourke E: Management of chronic peritoneal catheter malfunction. Am J Nephrol 2: 85, 1982
6. Nichols WK, and Nolph KD: A technique for managing exit site and cuff infection in Tenckhoff catheters. Peritoneal Dial Bull 3: 54, 1983

G. Shilipetar and M. Riggins

42

Microcomputer Peritoneal Programmer in Service of Acute Peritoneal Dialysis

SUMMARY

A microcomputer peritoneal programmer is described. It allows control of peritoneal fluid instillation volume and rate, includes an alarm system, provides data printouts and facilitates patient care. It is especially recommended for control of fluid balance in patients undergoing peritoneal dialysis for acute renal failure.

INTRODUCTION

Microcomputers can be useful in hospital settings because they provide rapid, accurate computational capabilities at an affordable price.[1] One example of this integration of technology and medicine is the microcomputer peritoneal programmer (MCPP) recently developed at the University of Washington Hospital in Seattle.

The programmer replaces an automatic cycling machine that was part of the hospital's "closed" peritoneal dialysis system. This "closed system" was pioneered two decades ago by a team of hospital researchers who were concerned about the incidence of infection resulting from the open system.[2,3] They substituted 40 L glass bottles of irrigation fluid for the smaller containers used in the "open system." Since 1963, over 10,800 acute peritoneal dialysis procedures have been performed using that closed that closed system at the University of Washington Hospital; not one case of infection has been reported.

Now, with the development of the programmer, the authors have further refined the unique and effective closed system. Their programmer controls and monitors the dialysis cycles, collects more accurate patient data, displays these data on its front panel and features an extensive alarm system.

MATERIALS AND METHODS

General Description

MCPP is a microprocessor based system. The microprocessor, by means of metering pumps, valves, liquid sensors, and other integral parts of this system monitors and controls the functions of above devices. This microprocessor and its support circuitry make up a set of six circuit boards (Fig. 1).

The computer or CPU board (central processing unit) is the central element of the system. On this board the microcomputer chip Z-80 (Zilog) resides along with its associated memory. The memory element consists or 4096 bytes of ROM (read only memory), which contains the control program itself, and 256 bytes of RAM (random access memory), which

From the University of Washington Hospital, Seattle, Washington.

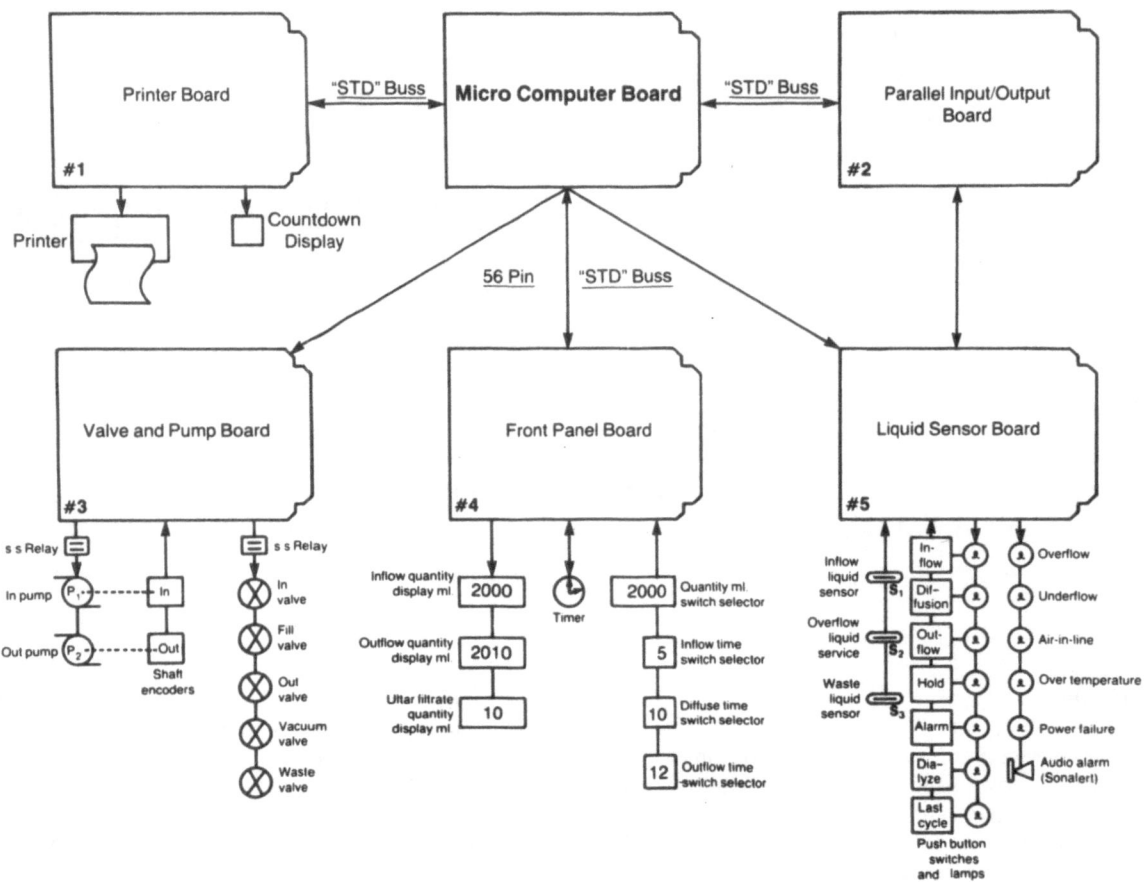

Fig. 1. Micro-computer boards

is used as a scratch pad for storing fluid totals, timing information, etc. The remaining five circuit boards are directly controlled by the computer's main board which provides the necessary interfacing for monitoring and controlling the entire dialysis procedure.

MCPP Monitors and Controls
Dialysis Cycles

A specially designed PVC administration set (Dravon Medical Inc., Clackamas, OR) is used in the procedure with the programmer. The set includes a 2.5 L overhead plastic bag and two identical pump headers used for assembly of metering pumps (Cole-Palmer, Chicago, IL) P_1 and P_2 (Fig. 2). Each pump header is made of Silastic and is 15 cm long, 6.35 mm OD and 3.18 mm ID. These dimensions and fluid temperature (36.5–37.5°C) are crucial to the accuracy of fluid to be transferred since each full revolu-

tion of either pump, with such pump header, will carry a quantity of exactly 0.833 ml.

Liquid sensors S_1, S_2, and S_3 are attached to the administration set. These sensors detect either air or fluid in the tubing. After the sterile dialysis fluid, which rests on the heater in a 40 L glass bottle B_1, reaches body temperature and the sterile disposable administration set has been attached to the programmer's integral parts, the system is ready to be primed.

One hundred milliliters of dialysis fluid is used to purge the air from the administration set followed by attachment of the patient to the set.

The programmer accurately measures the fluid's transfer as follows. As the fluid is pumped from the 40 L glass bottle B_1 into the administration set's overhead 2.5 L plastic bag, it passes through open mode of pinch valve V_1 and metering pump P_1. Both metering pumps P_1 and P_2 have shaft encoders

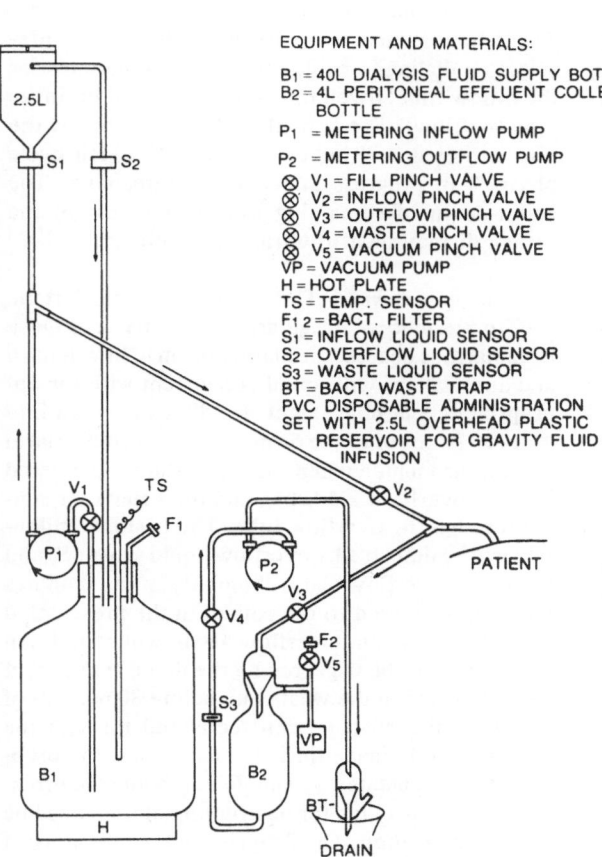

EQUIPMENT AND MATERIALS:

B₁ = 40L DIALYSIS FLUID SUPPLY BOTTLE
B₂ = 4L PERITONEAL EFFLUENT COLLECTION
     BOTTLE
P₁ = METERING INFLOW PUMP
P₂ = METERING OUTFLOW PUMP
⊗ V₁ = FILL PINCH VALVE
⊗ V₂ = INFLOW PINCH VALVE
⊗ V₃ = OUTFLOW PINCH VALVE
⊗ V₄ = WASTE PINCH VALVE
⊗ V₅ = VACUUM PINCH VALVE
VP = VACUUM PUMP
H = HOT PLATE
TS = TEMP. SENSOR
F₁₂ = BACT. FILTER
S₁ = INFLOW LIQUID SENSOR
S₂ = OVERFLOW LIQUID SENSOR
S₃ = WASTE LIQUID SENSOR
BT = BACT. WASTE TRAP
PVC DISPOSABLE ADMINISTRATION
SET WITH 2.5L OVERHEAD PLASTIC
     RESERVOIR FOR GRAVITY FLUID
     INFUSION

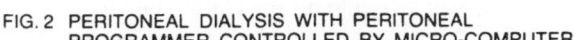

FIG. 2 PERITONEAL DIALYSIS WITH PERITONEAL
PROGRAMMER CONTROLLED BY MICRO-COMPUTER

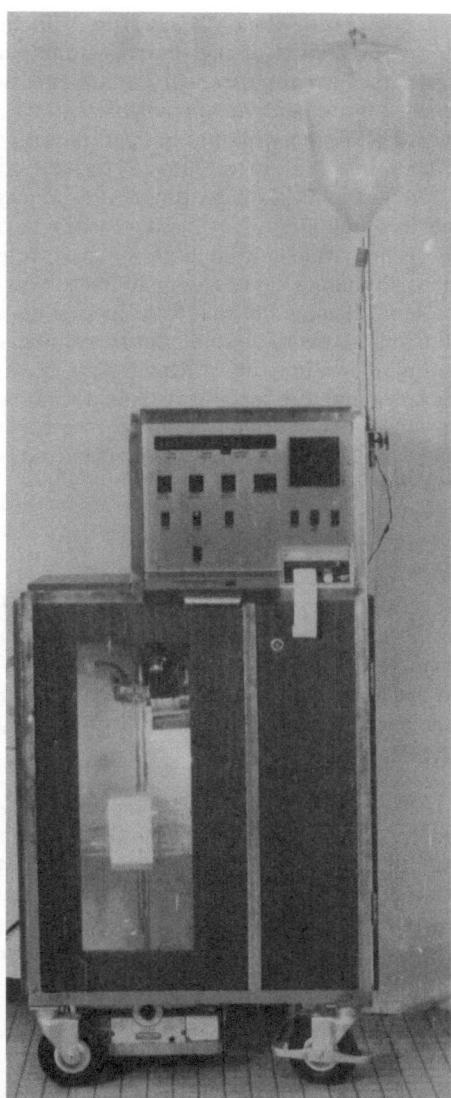

Fig. 2. Peritoneal dialysis with peritoneal programmer controlled by micro-computer

that transfer the number of full pump revolutions to the computer board. This information is then stored in memory.

After the overhead 2.5 L bag is filled with the preselected volume of fluid to be used per cycle and the "dialyze" button at the front of the programmer is pressed, the monitoring will automatically start by microcomputer.

This means the pinch valve V_2 will open, allowing the fluid to flow by gravity to the patient for a preset infusion time (inflow). If the infusion time selected is too generous, as soon as the last milliliter from the bag crosses the liquid sensor S_1, it will trigger the pinch valve V_2 to close and the time left for infusion will be erased. The dwell cycle time will start. After expiration of dwell-time (diffusion), the programmer will switch to the drainage time (outflow) by triggering the pinch valve V_3 to open, which will allow the peritoneal effluent to drain by gravity into the specially designed 4 L peritoneal effluent collection bottle B_2 (Lab Glass Inc., Vineland, NJ). Upon completion of the drainage time cycle (outflow), the programmer will initiate the closure of pinch valve V_3 and the opening of valves V_4 and V_5, allowing the metering pump P_2 to pump peritoneal effluent into the waste. Pump P_2 has the same characteristics as P_1 as far as function is concerned. As the last milliliter of effluent crosses through the waste line attached liquid sensor S_3, the programmer will initiate simultaneously the following information; display on the front panel of screen a cumulative record of fluid infused, effluent removed and plus-or-minus ultrafiltrate; print on tape information about this specific cycle and cumulative data as well; and switch to the next cycle. This will continue until the "last cycle" control button is pressed and that cycle is completed.

FRONT PANEL CONTROL BUTTONS AND DISPLAYS

The front panel (Fig. 3) allows the medical staff to set cycle controls and to scan data quickly. It features quantity, time buttons and screen display; an alarm system, a fluid temperature control and a small printer. A brief description of the controls and displays follows.

Quantity selector and screen display. Quantity selecting switch (quantity cycle, ml) allows staff to dial-in any desirable amount of dialysis fluid from 50 to 2500 ml to be used for the patient per cycle. The screen displays show continuous cumulative record of fluid infused (inflow, total, ml), efflu-

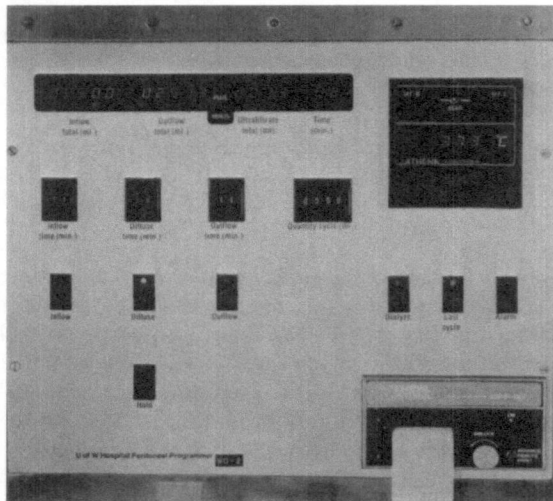

Fig. 3. Front panel

ent collected (outflow, total, ml) and the ± difference (± ultrafiltrate total, ml).

Cycle time switch selectors and display. These time switch selectors allow the staff to preselect by dialing-in cycle time values in minutes for the inflow time, dwell time (diffusion) and drainage time (outflow). The lighted push buttons below the time switches will indicate, when lit, which cycle phase is in progress and minutes remaining. The count-down of remaining time is located on the screen display next to ultrafiltrate volume.

Alarm systems. The programmer can alert the staff to a number of irregularities. When one of these irregularities occurs, the alarm button light will flash and audio alarm will sound concurrent with the appropriate cycle phase light. It will also switch into "Hold" status until the problem is corrected. Alarm conditions include when too much fluid is delivered into the overhead 2.5 L bag and fluid starts streaming through the overflow tube. The first few milliliters will be detected by overflow liquid sensor S_2 and initiate an overflow alarm. Similarly, if the fluid has not been delivered to the patient in the preselected amount of time an underflow alarm will sound. An alarm will also be triggered by the liquid sensor S_3 if air is detected in the waste line before 80 percent of the fluid infused has been recovered through the preselected drainage time. In such cases, the problem can be remedied by simply extending the drainage time or checking for obstruction of drainage line or patient position. The dialysis fluid temperature of 38.5° C will also initiate the alarm condition.

Temperature controller. This unit turns the heater on and off to maintain the dialysis fluid at body temperature (36.5–37.5° C).

Printer. This unit provides a tape print-out throughout the dialysis procedure. It prints cycle number, cycle volumes in milliliters infused, recovered and the plus-or-minus difference. It also prints cumulative volumes infused, recovered and the plus-or-minus difference (ultrafiltrate) (Fig. 4). If any alarm occurs during the procedure, it will also indicate on the tape through a coding system (A-1, A-2, A-3).

RESULTS AND DISCUSSION

The MCPP functions more effectively than the automatic cycling machine in several ways. First, it ensures a more accurate dialysis fluid measurement and a permanent record of data. When the cycling machine was used, one measurement check was the falling level of liquid in the 40 L glass bottles. Although the bottles were well marked, off-side visual checks were likely to contain a certain percentage of inaccuracy.

The computational ability of the programmer combined with the precise design of the tubing set eliminates this guesswork. It also eliminates the need for expensive bed scales. Lab testing of the programmer's measuring process has shown the error range to be within 1 percent. Second, the programmer's alarm system constantly checks for machine errors or problems. It never suffers from fatigue or attention lapses. It can react instantly in an emergency, putting the machine on "hold" until staff correct the problem. Also, it provides a permanent alarm record on the print-out tape.

Third, the front panel provides continuous, easy-to-read data about the dialysis cycle. With one glance at the displays, we know what cycle the machine is in, how much fluid is inflowing or outflowing, and how much time is left in a particular cycle. Also, the printout tape provides a permanent data record. This may be critical after a power loss, which will erase the cumulative amounts on the panel displays.

Fourth, the programmer makes patient care easier for staff. They can leave the patient's room knowing that the programmer is monitoring the dialysis and that the alarm system will alert them to any problem. Because some felt initial "computer anxiety," the hospital offered several hours of training in the use of the programmer. Now staff report that they greatly prefer the programmer to the old cycling machine.

Finally, the programmer is as cost effective as the cycling machine although it functions more effectively. And as staff time decreases, cost effectiveness may increase.

CONCLUSION

MCPP has been in service for the past 15 months, and has been used in over 500 acute peritoneal dialyses; it has demonstrated technologically superior performance over the previous device. We can now direct more accurate amounts of fluid to a diverse patient population and maintain better records. Medical staff time involvement has decreased, and with the need for a bed scale now obsolete, the cost effectiveness has increased. The alarm systems

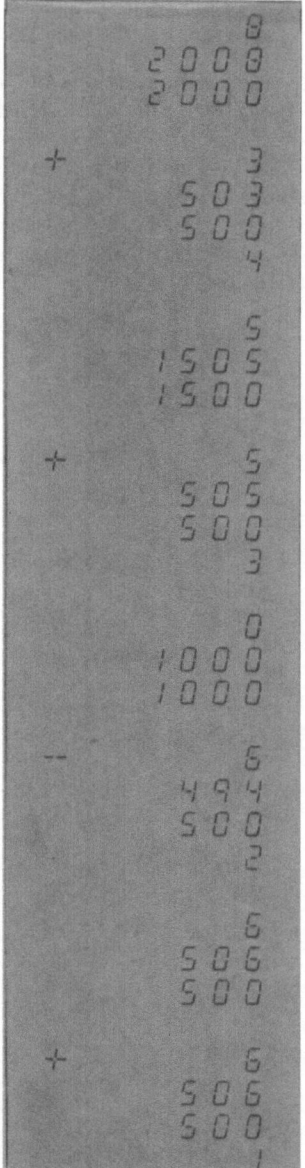

Fig. 4. Print-out tape

of the programmer have contributed to patient safe treatment by alerting staff to any discrepancies. We would strongly recommend for the patient with acute renal failure where peritoneal dialysis is recommended, the use of such a "closed-system" with the dialysis fluid stored in large containers over the use of the "open system" with small containers. Patient safety and avoidance of peritonitis should never be compromised for the staff's convenience.

ACKNOWLEDGMENTS

The authors would like to thank University of Washington Hospital's Administration for approving this development, specifically Jack Murray for his support. Thanks are also due to Louise Rasmussen for assistance in typing the manuscript and to dialysis technicians Rene Colobong, Steve Bentz, and Herman Washington for their assistance during the time of testing.

REFERENCES

1. Microcomputers in clinical applications. In Issues in health care technology, Vol 1. ECRI, Plymouth Meeting, PA, July 1983, Chapt 4.9
2. Boen ST, Mion CM, Curtis FK, and Shilipetar G: Periodic peritoneal dialysis using the repeated puncture technique and an automatic cycling machine. Trans Am Soc Artif Intern Organs 10: 409, 1964
3. Tenckhoff H, Boen ST, and Shilipetar G: Preparation of peritoneal dialysis fluid. Hosp Pharm 2: 7, 1967

J.F. Winchester, L.D. Stegink, S. Ahmad, M. Gross,
M. Hammeke, A.M. Horowitz, J.F. Maher, V. Pollak, T. Rakowski,
M. Schreiber, S. Singh, P. Somani, and D. Vidt

43

A Comparison of Glucose Polymer and Dextrose as Osmotic Agents in CAPD

SUMMARY

Dialysis solutions containing a mixture of glucose oligosaccharides (average molecular mass 710 daltons) derived from starch, were compared with 1.5% or 4.25% dextrose-containing dialysis fluids in single exchanges in 88 patients on continuous ambulatory peritoneal dialysis (CAPD). Dialysis fluid osmolality, net ultrafiltration and dialysate-to-plasma solute ratios for urea and creatinine were determined during a single 2 L exchange over 1 to 10 hours dwell time. In addition, absorption of the dextrose and oligosaccharides was investigated. Net ultrafiltration (mean ± SEM) was comparable for an 8 hour dwell time (1086 ± 169 ml for 4.25% dextrose solution and 1081 ± 100 ml for 8% polymer solution). In addition, clearances of urea and creatinine were nearly identical for the 4.25% dextrose and 8% glucose polymer solutions, as were the dialysate-to-plasma concentration ratios for urea and creatinine. Both dextrose and glucose oligosaccharides were absorbed within 2 hours of starting dialysis. Although few adverse effects were observed during glucose polymer single exchanges, absorbed oligo-

From Georgetown University, Washington, D.C.; University of Iowa, Iowa City, Iowa; University of Washington, Seattle, Washington; Medical College of Ohio, Toledo, Ohio; St. Joseph's Hospital, Omaha, Nebraska; Abbott Laboratories, North Chicago, Illinois; Uniformed Services University of the Health Sciences, Bethesda, Maryland; Veterans Administration Hospital, Cincinnati, Ohio; and Cleveland Clinic, Cleveland, Ohio.

saccharides were eliminated slowly from the blood (half-life of 20 hours) suggesting a limited use for this particular preparation of glucose oligosaccharides for CAPD.

INTRODUCTION

Patients with renal insufficiency have several metabolic derangements, the more important of which involve glucose[1,2] and lipid metabolism.[3] While dialysis may modify these abnormalities, abnormal values often do not return to normal. For example, lipid abnormalities do not improve with intermittent hemodialysis[4] or intermittent peritoneal dialysis (IPD).[5] Dextrose-based dialysis solutions are cheap, safe and effective. Further, the rapid absorption of dextrose provides a source of energy in malnourished patients. However, the use of dextrose-based dialysis solutions may further complicate the abnormalities present in patients with renal insufficiency. For example, hyperglycemia and hyperosmolality may complicate IPD,[6] while obesity and hyperlipidemia may result from the use of dextrose-containing dialysis fluids for the maintenance of continuous ambulatory peritoneal dialysis (CAPD) patients.[7] The use of dextrose solutions may also be associated with an ultrafiltration of limited duration because of the rapid absorption of dextrose.[7,8] More recently, a dextrose-derived compound (5-hydroxymethylfurfural) has been implicated in the reduction of peritoneal ultrafiltration.[9] Thus, the disadvantages of dextrose-based solutions have resulted in a search for alternative

Table 1. Oligosaccharide Distribution in Dialysis Solution.

Number of Dextrose Residues	%
G1*	ND†
G2	0.65
G3	27.5
G4	14.9
G5	35.3
G6	13.3
G7	ND
G8–G12	5.0
>G12	3.4

* The values refer to the number of glucose residues per oligosaccharide: G1 = glucose, G2 = maltose, etc.
†ND = Not detected.

osmotic agents for dialysis solutions. Alternative agents investigated include amino acids,[10] glycerol,[11] polyanions,[12] gelatin,[13] and xylitol.[14] Each of these products has a theoretical advantage over dextrose, but none has yet proved useful for long term maintenance CAPD.

Solutions of glucose oligosaccharides, derived from the acid hydrolysis of corn starch, are widely used in Europe and the United States as oral nutritional supplements.[15] A solution of fractionated glucose oligosaccharides suitable for use in peritoneal dialysis has recently been prepared (Abbott Laboratories, North Chicago, IL). This preparation contains oligosaccharides with chain lengths ranging

Table 2. Patient Characteristics.

	No.	%
Sex		
Male	65	74
Female	23	26
Age 46.3 years		
range 20–79 years		
Primary Diagnosis		
Chronic glomerulonephritis	23	26
Diabetic nephropathy	21	24
Interstitial nephritis	12	14
Nephrosclerosis	11	12
Polycystic renal disease	9	10
Hypertensive renal disease	5	6
Miscellaneous	7	8

from 2 to 15 glucose units, with an average molecular mass of 710 daltons (G4) (Table 1). Seventy-eight percent of the oligosaccharides in this preparation range in size from 2 to 7 glucose units, 5% are from 8 to 12 glucose units in size and 3.4% of the oligosaccharides are of 13 glucose units or larger in size. The preparation also contains trace quantities of organic salts and solvents. Most of the glucose units are linked by alpha-1,4-glucosidic bonds, but some alpha-1,6 linkages are present. Theoretically the larger size of the oligosaccharides relative to glucose should limit their rate of absorption from the peritoneal cavity and provide more sustained ultrafiltration. To test this hypothesis, we studied the effect of peritoneal dialysis solutions containing different concentrations of this oligosaccharide preparation in a series of single CAPD exchanges in comparison with dialysis solutions containing 4.25 percent dextrose.

MATERIAL AND METHODS

Eighty-eight patients undergoing intermittent peritoneal dialysis or CAPD participated in this multi-center study after giving full, written, and informed consent. The study was approved by the appropriate Institutional Review Boards at all institutions from which patients participated. The patient characteristics are shown in Table 2. All patients were treated as outpatients and no restrictions were made as to diet, fluid intake, or medications.

Study Technique

All patients had a Tenckhoff catheter in place and had been stabilized on peritoneal dialysis. The study consisted of two treatment periods separated by 24 hours. During the control period a single exchange of 4.25% dextrose dialysis solution was instilled into the peritoneal cavity. The test period consisted of a similar single exchange using one of the oligosaccharide preparations. Thirty patients received the oligosaccharide solution first, followed by the control dextrose solution (Dianeal®, Travenol Laboratories, Deerfield, IL or Inpersol®, Abbott Laboratories, North Chicago, IL). The remainder of the patients were studied in reverse order.

The test dialysis solution containing oligosaccharides was prepared from Inpersol® dialysis solution not containing dextrose, to which the oligosaccharide preparation was added to make a final solution providing 2 to 8% oligosaccharides (58 patients). Alternatively the patients received a premixed solution of Inpersol® dialysis solution containing 8% oligosaccharides (30 patients). Dwell times varied from 1 to 10 hours. After each study period, continuous dialysis with standard Inpersol® or Dianeal® dialysis solutions was carried out until the next study period. For the exchange immediately preceding the initiation of the control and test periods, all patients were requested to use 1.5% dextrose solutions.

Selection of the oligosaccharide concentration and dwell period were made from a centralized treatment schedule. The assigned dwell time for control and test periods was identical for each patient. Blood and dialysate samples for determination of endogenous solutes, free glucose, and oligosaccharide-bound glucose were obtained from each patient: immediately before each exchange, every 2 hours thereafter for the duration of the dwell period, and at 24 hours after the exchange. In two patients, serum samples were obtained for a 80 hour period after a single exchange using the 8% oligosaccharide solution.

Blood samples were drawn through an indwelling needle placed in an antecubital vein and serum was separated by centrifugation. Dialysate samples were obtained by draining 200 ml dialysate into the empty bag attached to the patient and aspirating 15 ml dialysate for analysis. The remaining dialysate was instilled back into the peritoneal cavity. All samples were stored at −20°C until analyzed.

At the conclusion of each control and test exchange, dialysate was collected and the volume carefully measured. The volume of dialysate samples drawn for analytical purposes was added to the volume drained from the peritoneal cavity at the end of the dwell to obtain the total volume recovered. The volume of the instilled fluid (weight of bag full minus weight of bag empty) was subtracted from the final volume to obtain net ultrafiltration volume.

Patients were monitored for changes in vital signs (temperature, blood pressure, pulse rate, and respiration rate) as well as symptoms and untoward effects.

Peritoneal Dialysis Solution

The peritoneal dialysis solutions tested contained a mixture of glucose oligosaccharides with a mean chain length of four glucose units (Table 1). A 5% solution of the oligosaccharide preparation was approximately isotonic with human blood, whereas the osmolality of an 8% solution was calculated to be 357 mOsm/kg. The calculated osmolar concentra-

Table 3. Chemical Composition of Glucose Polymer Dialysis Solution.

	Premix	Admix	
Glucose Polymer (%)	8%	8%	5%
pH	5.2	5.2	
Na (mEq/L)	132.0	117.5	123.0
Cl (mEq/L)	102.0	90.0	95.0
Ca (mEq/L)	3.5	3.1	3.5
Mg (mEq/L)	1.5	1.3	1.5
Lactate (mEq/L)	35	31	34
Dextrose (mg/dl)	0	0	0

tions for the control dextrose solutions were as follows: Inpersol® or Dianeal® with 1.5% dextrose, 346 mOsm/kg; Inpersol® or Dianeal® with 4.25% dextrose, 485 mOsm/kg. The electrolyte composition and pH of the premixed solution of glucose oligosaccharides were identical to that of Inpersol® with dextrose (Table 3).

Analytic Methods

Dialysate to plasma (D/P) concentration ratios for urea nitrogen and creatinine were calculated without correction for ultrafiltration. Endogenous solutes were determined from samples obtained at the end of the exchange rather than midpoints since it was assumed that this represented the maximal total solute concentration.

Serum and dialysate were analyzed for concentrations of BUN, creatinine, sodium, chloride, potassium, phosphorus, and glucose as well as osmolality by routine laboratory methods. Determinations of free and total (after acid hydrolysis) glucose were carried out as described by Andersen et al.[16] The difference between the total and free glucose values represented the amount of oligosaccharides present in the sample.

Peritoneal clearances for the control dextrose and the test oligosaccharide exchanges were calculated and compared. Clearance per exchange (ml/min) was calculated as dialysate/plasma concentration times drainage volume/total exchange time.

Statistics

Unpaired or paired t-tests and Pearson correlation coefficients were applied to test the null hypothesis, where appropriate. Due to the small number of patients treated with any one concentration of glucose polymer at a given dwell time, any statements

MEAN NET ULTRAFILTRATION VOLUMES AT DIFFERENT DWELL TIMES USING GLUCOSE POLYMER (G.P.) AND DEXTROSE SOLUTIONS

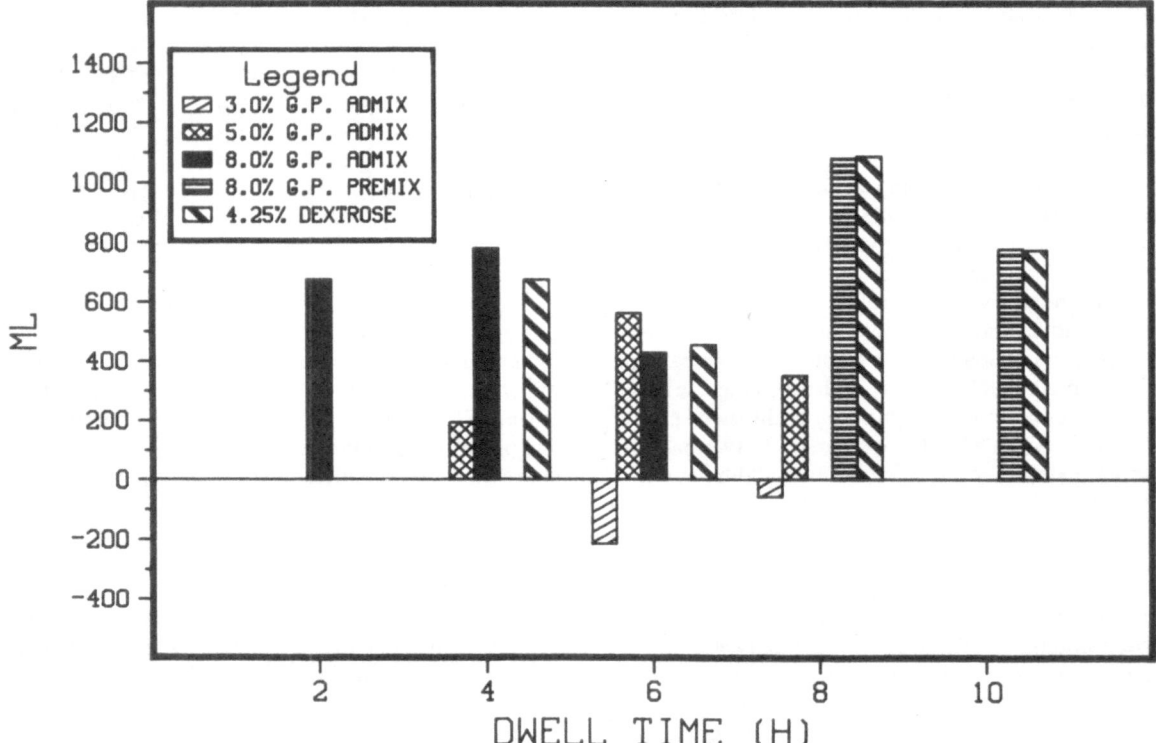

Fig. 1. Mean net ultrafiltration volumes achieved with glucose polymer solutions of different concentrations and with 4.25% dextrose solution in relation to duration of intraperitoneal dwell are shown.

regarding comparisons were based on individual trends.

RESULTS

Ultrafiltration

The net ultrafiltration volume was measured in all patients and comparisons were made between oligosaccharide and dextrose exchanges in the same patient. There was great variation in results from individual patients, particularly with longer dwell times. Figure 1 gives the net ultrafiltration volumes for 4.25% dextrose solution as well as for 3, 5, and 8% solutions of glucose oligosaccharides in relation to total dwell time. Comparable ultrafiltration volumes were achieved with peritoneal dwell times of 8 to 10 hours with 4.25% dextrose and 8% oligosac-

charide solutions. The mean ($\pm$ SEM) net drainage volumes for 4.25% dextrose at 8 hours and 10 hours were 1086 ± 169 ml and 773 ± 119 ml, respectively. For the 8% solution of oligosaccharides, the 8 hours and 10 hours net ultrafiltration volumes were 1081 ± 100 ml and 777 ± 84 ml, respectively. The mean net drainage volumes for 3 and 5% solutions of oligosaccharides were substantially lower over an 8 hour dwell time. Negative net ultrafiltration (minus 56 ml) was only seen with the 3% solution of oligosaccharide; when the 5% solution of glucose oligosaccharides was used a net ultrafiltration volume of 350 ± 96 ml was observed over an 8 hour period.

Figures 2 and 3 show the dialysate to plasma concentration ratios for urea and creatinine respectively, for 4.25% dextrose exchanges in comparison to exchanges using 3, 5, and 8% solutions of oligosaccharides. Urea nitrogen and creatinine equilib-

MEAN UREA NITROGEN DIALYSATE/PLASMA (D/P) RATIO
FOR GLUCOSE POLYMER (G.P.) AND DEXTROSE EXCHANGES

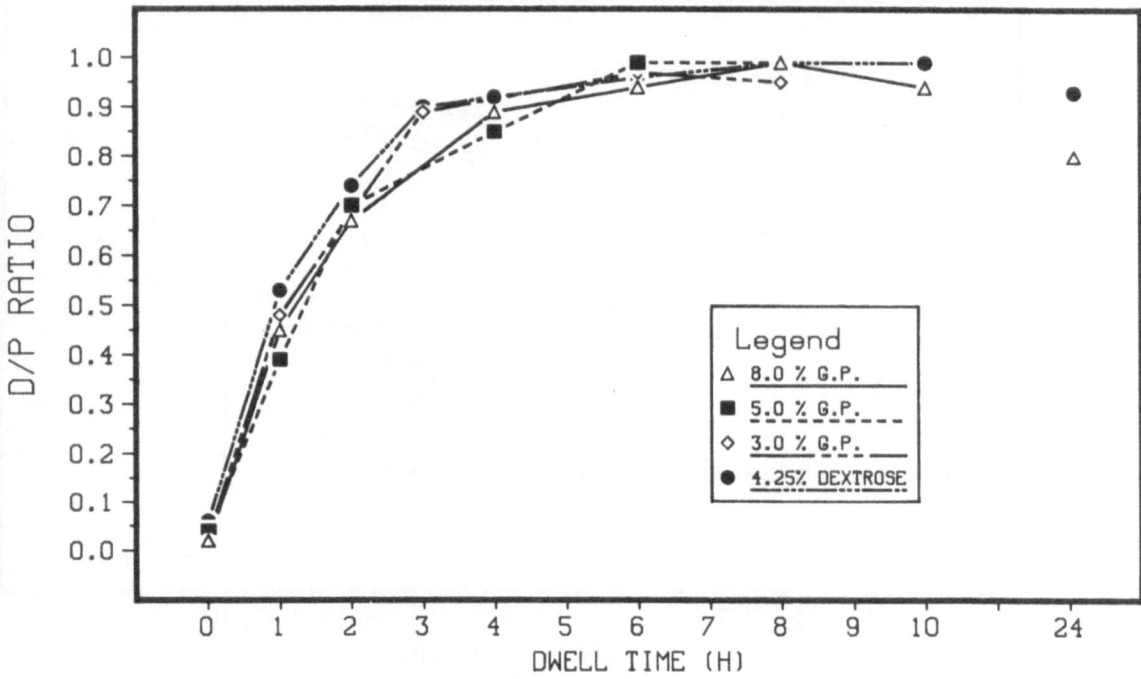

Fig. 2. The dialysate/plasma concentration ratio of urea is shown in relation to intraperitoneal dwell duration for 4.25% dextrose and for glucose polymer solutions.

rium were reached between 6 and 8 hours dwell time for both types of solution. The mean serum urea nitrogen concentration for the 4.25% dextrose exchange was 59.9 ± 7.4 mg/dl and for exchanges using 5 and 8% solutions of premixed oligosaccharide solution were 68 ± 9.3 and 60.2 ± 8.9 mg/dl, in comparison to 5 and 8% glucose oligosaccharide premix exchanges of 12.4 ± 1.5 and 9.8 ± 1.5 mg/dl, respectively, for an 8 hour dwell.

Table 4 shows the mean clearances of urea nitrogen and creatinine at 6 and 8 hour dwell times for 4.25% dextrose and glucose oligosaccharide solutions. Except for the 3% oligosaccharide solution, which was associated with decreased urea and creatinine clearances, there were no significant differences between 4.25% dextrose and the 5 and 8% oligosaccharide dialysis solutions.

Figure 4 shows mean dialysate osmolality values for oligosaccharide and dextrose exchanges. Osmolality fell more rapidly with the dextrose solutions than with the oligosaccharide solutions. At the

end of 8 hours however, almost identical osmolality values were seen for 4.25% dextrose, 5% oligosaccharide and 8% oligosaccharide solutions.

Figure 5 shows the mean dialysate concentrations of free and oligosaccharide-bound glucose in patients treated with either 8% oligosaccharide solution (top panel) or 4.25% dextrose solution (bottom panel). In each case, data were also obtained after a subsequent exchange with 4.25% dextrose starting 24 hours after the original test exchange. When 4.25% dextrose was used as the test solution (bottom panel), dialysate concentrations of free glucose fell from a mean initial value of 4040 mg/dl to 1254 mg/dl at 4 hours and 449 mg/dl at 10 hours. No oligosaccharide-bound glucose was detected at any time. Similar results were obtained during a subsequent exchange (at 24 hours) using the 4.25% dextrose solution. When the 8% oligosaccharide solution was used as the test solution (top panel), the initial dialysate concentration of free glucose was 4 mg/dl and the oligosaccharide-bound glucose concentration

MEAN CREATININE DIALYSATE/PLASMA (D/P) RATIO
FOR GLUCOSE POLYMER (G.P.) AND DEXTROSE EXCHANGES

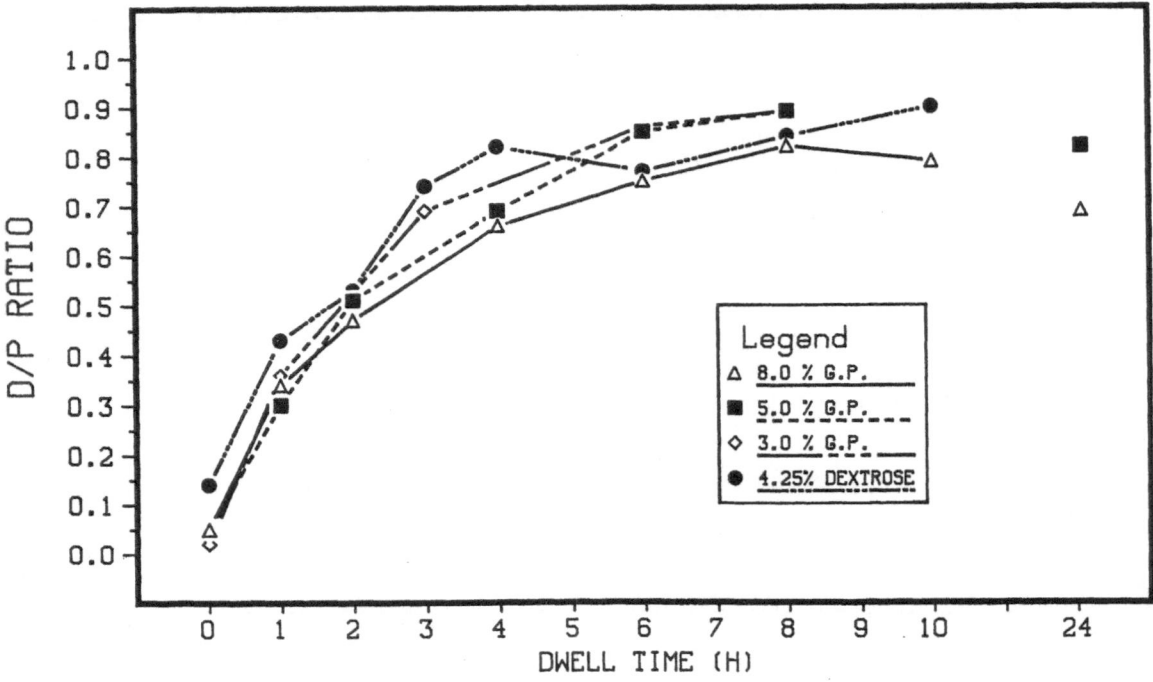

Fig. 3. The dialysate/plasma concentration ratio of creatinine is shown in relation to the duration of intraperitoneal dwell for 4.25% dextrose and for glucose polymer solutions.

Table 4. Comparison of Peritoneal Solute Clearance for Glucose Polymer and Dextrose Exchanges.

	Dwell time (hours)	CCr (ml/min)	Curea (ml/min)
4.25% D	6	6.41 ± 0.42	6.90 ± 0.23
	8	5.08 ± 0.19	5.72 ± 0.31
3% P	6	4.45 ± 0.35*	5.00 ± 0.60*
	8	3.60 ± 0.20*	3.90 ± 0.20*
5% P	6	5.60 ± 0.49	6.57 ± 0.67
	8	4.73 ± 0.18	4.60 ± 0.26
8% P	6	6.33 ± 0.58	7.03 ± 0.61
	8	5.47 ± 0.26	6.52 ± 0.25

Results are expressed as mean ± SEM.
* $p < 0.05$ compared to dextrose at same dwell time.
D = dextrose, P = glucose polymer.
CCr = Creatinine clearance, Curea = Urea clearance.

was 7693 mg/dl. Concentrations of oligosaccharide-bound glucose decreased with increasing dwell time, falling to a mean value of 3418 mg/dl at 4 hours and 1761 mg/dl at 10 hours. In contrast, free glucose concentrations in the dialysate increased slowly and then leveled off reaching a value of 118 mg/dl at 4 hours and 108 mg/dl at 10 hours when the 8% oligosaccharide solution was used. Dialysate samples examined during the subsequent exchange (at 24 hours) with 4.25% dextrose solution did not contain detectable quantities of oligosaccharide-bound glucose, although oligosaccharides were still present in plasma (see Fig. 6).

Figure 6 shows plasma free and oligosaccharide-bound glucose concentrations in patients treated with either 8% oligosaccharide (top panel) or 4.25% dextrose solutions (bottom panel). In each case, plasma analyses were also carried out during a subsequent exchange (at 24 to 34 hours) with the 4.25% dextrose solution. In patients treated with the 4.25% dextrose solution (bottom panel), mean

MEAN DIALYSATE OSMOLALITY VALUES
FOR GLUCOSE POLYMER (G.P.) AND DEXTROSE EXCHANGES

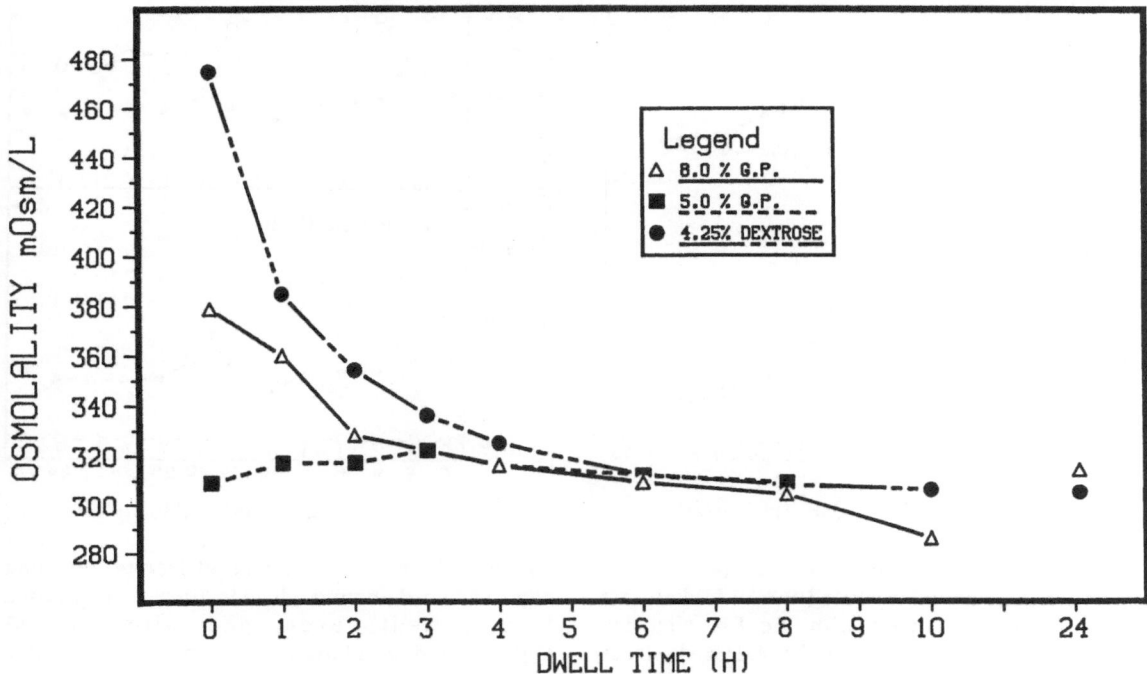

Fig. 4. Mean dialysate osmolality decreased more rapidly when 4.25% dextrose dialysis solution was used than when glucose polymer was employed as the osmotic agent.

plasma glucose values increased slightly over baseline values after 1 to 3 hours dwell time and then returned to baseline values. No oligosaccharide-bound glucose was detected. When patients were treated with the 8% oligosaccharide solution (top panel), plasma glucose concentrations also increased slightly at 1 hour and then returned to baseline. However, plasma levels of oligosaccharide-bound glucose increased rapidly with increasing dwell times, reaching a mean value of 552 mg/dl at 10 hours during treatment with the oligosaccharide solution. The oligosaccharide-bound glucose was cleared slowly from the plasma despite subsequent exchanges using the 4.25% dextrose solution. Plasma oligosaccharide-bound glucose concentration was 365 mg/dl at 24 hours and 254 mg/dl at 48 hours after a single exchange with the 8% oligosaccharide solution. Thus, oligosaccharides were not efficiently cleared from plasma by subsequent exchanges with 4.25% dextrose solutions.

Table 5 shows plasma and dialysate free and oligosaccharide-bound glucose values in a single patient who was given a second exchange using the 8% oligosaccharide solution 24 hours after a first exchange with the oligosaccharide-based solution. Oligosaccharides accumulating in the plasma after the first exchange were not completely cleared after 24 hours, the time at which the second exchange was initiated. As a result, plasma oligosaccharide concentrations increased to even higher values during the second exchange with the 8% solution of oligosaccharides. These data indicate a very slow metabolism and clearance of absorbed oligosaccharides in patients with renal insufficiency.

The slow clearance of oligosaccharides from the plasma of patients treated with the 8% oligosaccharide solution led us to measure plasma oligosaccharide concentrations in two additional patients for up to 80 hours following a single exchange with the 8% oligosaccharide solution. These data (Table 6)

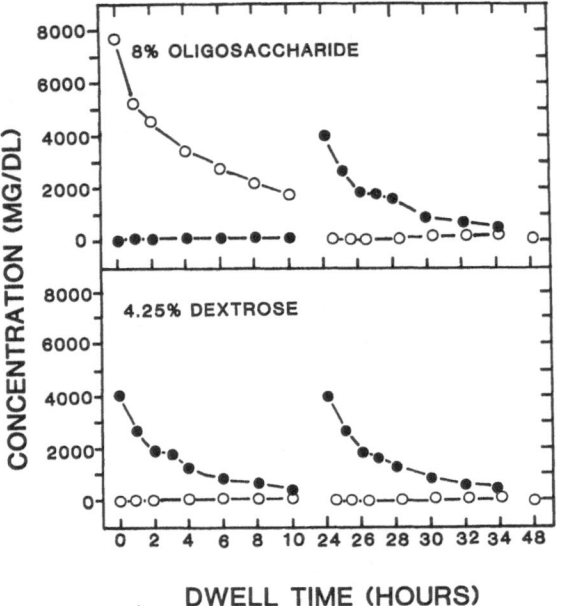

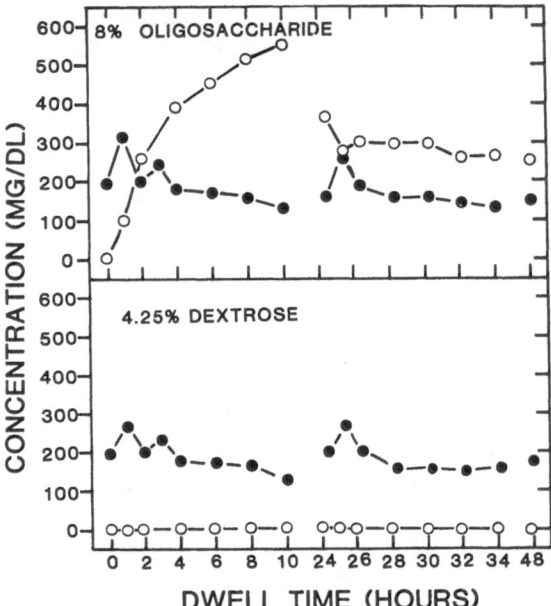

Fig. 5. Mean concentrations of free (●——●) and oligosaccharide-bound glucose (○——○) in dialysate from patients exchanged with the 8% oligosaccharide solution (top panel) and a 4.25% dextrose solution (bottom panel). In each case, dialysate analyses were also carried out during a subsequent exchange with 4.25% dextrose starting 24 hours after the initial test exchange.

Fig. 6. Mean concentrations of free (●——●) and oligosaccharide-bound glucose (○——○) in plasma from patients exchanged with the 8% oligosaccharide solution (top panel) and a 4.25% dextrose solution (bottom panel). In each case, plasma analyses were also carried out during a subsequent exchange with 4.25% dextrose starting 24 hours after the initial test exchange.

indicate that at least 80 hours are required to clear oligosaccharide-bound glucose from the blood (calculated half-life was 20 hours) after a single exchange with an 8% oligosaccharide solution, despite dialysis treatment with dextrose-based solutions during the interval.

A fall in serum sodium from 136 mEq/L to 128 mEq/L was observed after 10 hour dwell when using the admixed oligosaccharide solution (starting sodium concentration 128 mEq/L). Serum osmolality, however, did not change (310 mOsm/L at the start and 302 mOsm/L after 10 hour dwell). The oligosaccharides present in serum between 10 hours and 48 hours (n = 2) were principally maltose, maltotriose, maltotetraose, and maltopentaose (G2 to G5 in size). No oligosaccharides greater then 5 glucose units in size (G5) were detectable in serum. A similar distribution of oligosaccharides was observed in the dialysate after an 8 to 10 hour dwell, indicating that most

oligosaccharides greater than G6 units had been split into smaller units. Side effects were minimal (Table 7).

DISCUSSION

We have demonstrated that comparable ultrafiltration volumes are achieved with 4.25% dextrose and 8% glucose oligosaccharide solutions over a dwell time of 8 to 10 hours, with a lower ultrafiltration volume being achieved with 3 and 5% oligosaccharide solutions over the same dwell time. Similarly clearance values for uremic compounds were nearly identical for both 4.25% dextrose and 8% oligosaccharide solutions, as were the dialysate-to-plasma concentration ratios for urea and creatinine. When the 3% oligosaccharide solution was used, however, a decrease in urea nitrogen and creatinine

Table 5. Plasma and Dialysate Free and Oligosaccharide-Bound Glucose Concentrations in a Single Subject Given Two Exchanges with the 8% Oligosaccharide Preparation at 24 Hour Intervals.

Time (hours)	Plasma (mg/dl)		Dialysate (g/L)	
	Free	Bound	Free	Bound
0	96	0	0.005	7.89
2	119	252	0.04	4.81
4	100	309	0.06	3.89
6	140	416	0.08	3.05
8	128	436	0.10	2.42
10	100	446	0.10	1.83
24	135	421	0.005	8.12
26	169	497	0.06	5.17
28	137	703	0.08	4.07
30	175	600	0.09	3.30
32	131	693	0.11	2.91
34	115	801	0.11	2.51

Table 6. Mean Free and Oligosaccharide-Bound Glucose in Plasma of Two Subjects after a Single Exchange with the 8% Oligosaccharide Solution.

Time (hours)	Free Glucose (mg/dl)	Oligosaccharide-Bound Glucose* (mg/dl)
0	105	0
5	127	334
10	126	357
24	153	260
32	166	232
48	136	170
56	154	101
72	109	48
80	107	0

* Oligosaccharide-bound glucose is the total glucose value obtained after acid hydrolysis minus the free glucose.

clearances were observed. The results with the 3% oligosaccharide solution were not surprising. Solutions with a lower concentration of dextrose give lower clearance values than values obtained with a 4.25% dextrose dialysis solution as well.[17] As expected, a rapid fall in dialysate osmolality was observed for the 4.25% dextrose solution, and maintenance of osmolality was more prolonged with the oligosaccharide solution. However, at the end of an 8 hour dwell time almost identical osmolality values were seen for the 4.25% dextrose and 5% glucose oligosaccharide solutions. The loss of osmolalilty from the glucose polymer solutions reflected the hydrolysis of larger oligosaccharides

within the peritoneal cavity to small oligosaccharides and the transfer of oligosaccharides of G2 to G5 size from the peritoneal cavity. This is supported by the finding that the major oligosaccharides present in plasma are of G2 to G5 size.

The persistence of glucose oligosaccharide concentrations in the plasma up to 72 hours after a single exchange with the oligosaccharide-based solution probably reflects the slow breakdown of maltose (G2) and maltotriose (G3). Maltose and maltotriose are end products of the metabolism of the larger oligosaccharides by serum and tissue enzymes. Maltase activity is high in renal tissue,[18] but is absent in human plasma.[19,20] Thus, these compounds would be metabolized less well in the absence of functioning kidneys. For example, infused maltose is cleared slowly from rabbit plasma after nephrectomy[21] indi-

Table 7. Reported Untoward Effects.

Symptom	Onset	Duration	Dialysis Solution	Dwell Time
Dry mouth	30 min	2.5 h	4% Polymer	4 h
"Funny taste"	4 h	?	5% Polymer	8 h
Weakness	2 h	30 min	8% Polymer	3 h
Feeling full	4 h	10 min	8% Polymer	8 h
Abdominal discomfort	4 h	?	8% Polymer	8 h
Mild thirst	6 h	?	8% Polymer	10 h
Abdominal distention	6 h	?	8% Polymer	10 h
Abdominal cramps	Start	15 min	4.25% dextrose	8 h
Vomiting, belching	?	?	4.25% dextrose	10 h

cating a major role of the kidney in maltose metabolism. Although the long term effects of maltose and maltotriose persistence in plasma are unknown, we did observe a slight fall in serum sodium (although this is likely to be due to the relatively lower starting dialysis fluid sodium concentration used in the admixed solutions (128 mEq/L).

Interestingly, serum free glucose concentrations changed little after exchanges using the oligosaccharide solutions. This contrasts with a rise in blood glucose observed when dextrose-based solutions were used. We are unable to comment on possible long term effects of oligosaccharide preparations on lipid metabolism since our studies were brief. However, the potential energy load from a single exchange of an 8% solution of oligosaccharides is approximately twice that of 4.25% dextrose solution (assuming complete metabolism of the oligosaccharides). Thus, synthesis of lipid might be increased due to the increased energy intake.

The oligosaccharide solutions used for single exchanges in peritoneal dialysis patients were well tolerated, but the particular formulation chosen for study may not be useful in the long term in view of the persistence of oligosaccharides in plasma up to 72 hours after a single exchange. It is possible that a preparation combining glucose oligosaccharides of higher molecular weights along with other osmotic agents, for example amino acids, may be useful as an alternative to standard dextrose solutions.

REFERENCES

1. Horton ES, Johnson C, and Lebovitz HE: Carbohydrate metabolism in uremia. Ann Intern Med 68: 83, 1968
2. Spitz IM, Rubenstein AH, Bersohn I, Abrahams C, and Lowry C: Carbohydrate metabolism in renal disease. Q J Med 39: 201, 1970
3. Bagdade JD, Porte D Jr, and Bierman EL: Hypertriglyceridemia, a metabolic consequence of chronic renal failure. N Engl J Med 279: 181, 1968
4. Lindner AL, Charra B, Sherrard DJ, and Scribner BH: Accelerated atherosclerosis in prolonged maintenance hemodialysis. N Engl J Med 290: 697, 1974
5. Chan MK, Varghese Z, Persaud JW, Baillod RA, and Moorhead JF: Hyperlipidaemia in patients on maintenance haemodialysis and peritoneal dialysis: The relative pathogenetic roles of triglyceride production and triglyceride removal. Clin Nephrol 17: 183, 1982
6. Boyer J, Gill N, and Epstein FH: Hyperglycemia and hyperosmolality complicating peritoneal dialysis. Ann Intern Med 67: 568, 1967
7. Oreopoulos DG, Robson M, Faller B, Ogilvie R, Rapaport A, and DeVeber GA: Continuous ambulatory peritoneal dialysis. A new era in the treatment of chronic renal failure. Clin Nephrol 11: 125, 1979
8. Pyle KW, Moncrief JW, and Popovich RP: Peritoneal transport evaluation in CAPD. In Moncrief JW, and Popovich RP (Eds), CAPD Update. New York and Paris: Masson Publishing, 1981, p 35
9. Henderson IS, Couper I, and Lumsden A: Potentially irritant glucose metabolites in unused CAPD fluid. Peritoneal Dial Bull 4(Suppl): 530, 1984
10. Williams P, Marliss EB, Anderson GH, Oren A, Stein A, Khanna R, Pettit J, Brandes L, Rodella H, Mupas L, Dombros N, and Oreopoulos DG: Amino acid absorption following intraperitoneal administration in CAPD patients. Peritoneal Dial Bull 2: 124, 1982
11. Heaton, A, Johnston DG, Ward MK, Alberti KGMM, and Kerr DNA: Glycerol instead of glucose as an osmotic agent in CAPD. Peritoneal Dial Bull 4(Suppl): S30, 1984
12. Twardowski ZJ, Nolph KD, McGary TJ, and Moore HL: Polyanions and glucose as osmotic agents in simulated peritoneal dialysis. Artif Organs 7: 420, 1983
13. Twardowski ZJ, Hain H, McGary TJ, Moore HL, and Keller RS: Sustained ultrafiltration with gelatin dialysis fluid during long dwell dialysis exchange in rats. Peritoneal Dial Bull 4(Suppl): S67, 1984
14. Bazzato G, Coli U, Landini S, Fracasso A, Moraciello P, Righetto F, and Scanferla F: Xylitol and low dosages of insulin: New perspectives for diabetic uremic patients on CAPD. Peritoneal Dial Bull 2: 161, 1981
15. Berlyne GM, Brewis RAL, Boath EM, and Mallick NP: A soluble glucose polymer for use in renal failure and calorie deprivation state. Lancet 1: 689, 1969
16. Andersen DW, Filer LJ Jr, Wu-Rideout MYC, White LB, and Stegink LD. Utilization of intravenously administered glucose-oligosaccharides in growing miniature pigs. Pediatr Res 16: 304, 1982
17. Nolph KD, Twardowski ZJ, Popovich RP, and Rubin J: Equilibration of peritoneal dialysis solutions during long dwell exchanges. J Lab Clin Med 93: 246, 1979
18. Silverman M: Brush disorder disaccharides in dog kidney and their spatial relationship to glucose transport receptors. J Clin Invest 52: 2486, 1973
19. Young JM, and Weser E: The metabolism of circulating maltose in man. J Clin Invest 501: 246, 1979
20. Van Handle E: Trehalase and maltase in the serum of vertebrates. Comp Biochem Physiol 26: 561, 1968
21. Ohneda AS, Yamagata S, Tsutsumi K, and Fujiwara H: Distribution of maltose intravenously administered to rabbits and its metabolism in the kidney. Tohoku J Exp Med 112: 141, 1974
22. Young EA, Drummond A, Cool DA, Cioletti LA, Crain M, Taylor JB, and Weser E: The effect of insulin on the metabolism of parenteral maltose in man. J Clin Endocrinol Metab 50: 764, 1980

C.D. Mistry, R. Gokal, and N.P. Mallick

44

Glucose Polymer As an Osmotic Agent in CAPD

SUMMARY

As an alternative osmotic agent for peritoneal dialysis, 5% and 10% glucose polymer solutions were studied in five patients and compared to 1.36% and 3.86% anhydrous dextrose. The ultrafiltration rate was higher with the polymer with a 6 h dwell compared to dextrose dialysis, and the equilibration rate for small solutes was faster despite the higher volume. A lower fraction of the polymer was absorbed from dialysate compared to dextrose but by weight more polymer was absorbed. The polymer was degraded to maltose and maltotriose, which were eliminated slowly in the absence of normal renal function.

INTRODUCTION

Presently available CAPD solutions, using dextrose as an osmotic agent, are safe, effective, and economical but are associated with the disadvantage of rapid dextrose absorption.[1] This results in short duration of ultrafiltration[2] and metabolic complications such as obesity[3] and hyperlipidemia.[4] Glucose polymers, isolated by fractionation of hydrolysed corn starch, have been widely used to provide a palatable high energy source in dietary management of patients with renal[5] and hepatic failure. They are a mixture of oligosaccharides of variable chain length, ranging from one to more than twelve glucose units

---

From the Manchester Royal Infirmary, Manchester, United Kingdom.

linked by α-1,4 glucosidic bonds with some α-1,6 linkages; the average length is between five and six units with average molecular weight of approximately 960 daltons. They may be potentially useful alternatives to dextrose on theoretic grounds; their large size should limit the rate of absorption from the peritoneal cavity, and intraperitoneal metabolism should generate smaller osmotically active particles, thus providing more sustained ultrafiltration. The aim of the present study was to compare glucose polymers (5 and 10%) with commercially available anhydrous dextrose solutions (1.36 and 3.86%) with respect to ultrafiltration and solute clearances.

SUBJECTS AND METHODS

We studied 5 nondiabetic patients (3 male, 2 female) aged 22–53 years who had been on CAPD for a mean period of 17.1 months (range 3.5–32 months), on four exchanges/day, and who had been free of peritonitis for at least 3 months prior to study. Each patient underwent four separate 6 hour exchanges, in a random order, using 2 L dialysis fluid containing either 1.36 or 3.86% dextrose (G) or glucose polymer (GP) 5 or 10%. The electrolyte composition was identical in all solutions. The 1.36% G and 5% GP are referred to as isotonic, whereas 3.86% G and 10% GP were known as hypertonic solutions.

After an overnight fast (10–12 hours), subjects were admitted to the hospital metabolic procedure room overnight, dialysate was drained and 2 L fresh dialysis fluid were infused by gravity over 10 minutes. Blood and dialysate samples were taken ¡mul-

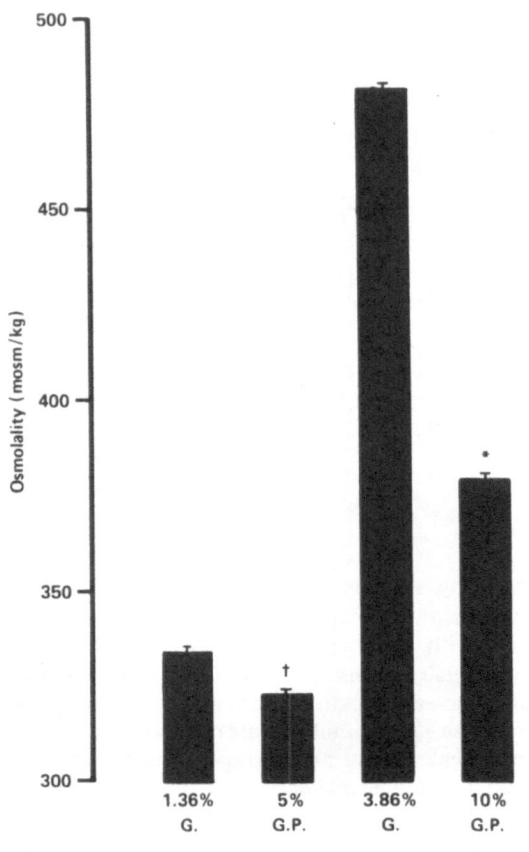

Fig. 1. Initial osmolality of the dialysis fluid. G: dextrose; GP: glucose polymer.

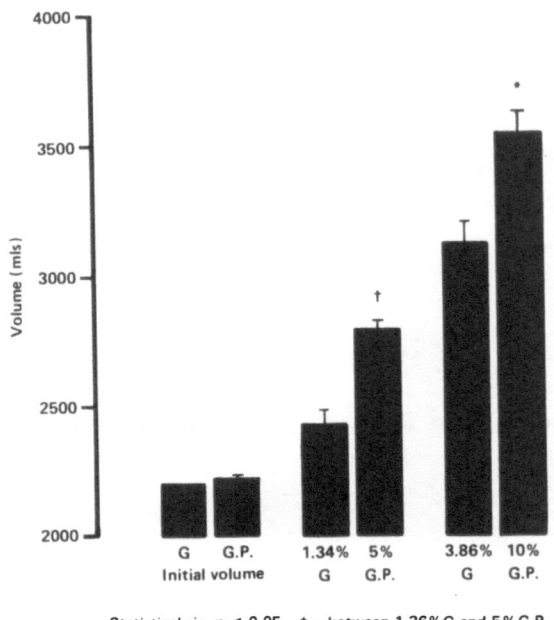

Fig. 2. Total dialysate (drained) volume after 6 hours dwell.

taneously before and at 0, 15, 30, 60, 90, 120, 180, 240 and 360 minutes, time zero being the end of the infusion. Subjects remained fasting throughout the 6 hours exchange period, drinking water freely. At the end of each study, the fluid was drained and volume recorded. Normal dialysis schedule resumed, except after the use of GP, when the dialysis was discontinued for 24 hours and additional blood samples were taken at 3, 14, and 24 hours. Each study was separated by a 48 to 72 hours interval.

Assay Methods

The serum and dialysate biochemistry was determined by the Vickers M300 multichannel autoanalyser, glucose by glucose oxidase method, osmolality by the freezing point depression method, and glucose polymer by gel-permeation chromatography, on Bio-gel P_2, using modified Jelco 6AH automatic carbohydrate analyser with orcinol-sulphuric acid detection system.[6] Statistical analysis was by Student's paired t tests. All values are expressed as mean ± standard error of mean (SEM).

RESULTS

The initial dialysate osmolality of GP solutions was significantly lower as compared to G, for both isotonic (323 ± 0.86 versus 334 ± 1.5 mOsm/kg; $p < 0.05$) and hypertonic (378 ± 2.3 versus 482 ± 1.6 mOsm/kg; $p < 0.05$) solutions (Fig. 1); yet the net ultrafiltration achieved was 2.5 and 1.4 times greater respectively (Fig. 2). This appears to be related to a slower rate of dissipation of the osmotic gradient compared to G (Fig. 3).

Dialysate/plasma ratios were obtained for urea, creatinine, uric acid, and phosphate in relation to dwell time (Figs. 4–7). Urea (60 daltons) diffused rapidly and equilibrated within 6 hours, with both GP and G solutions; however the rate of equilibration was much faster with polymers. Creatinine, uric acid and phosphate attained faster equilibration with

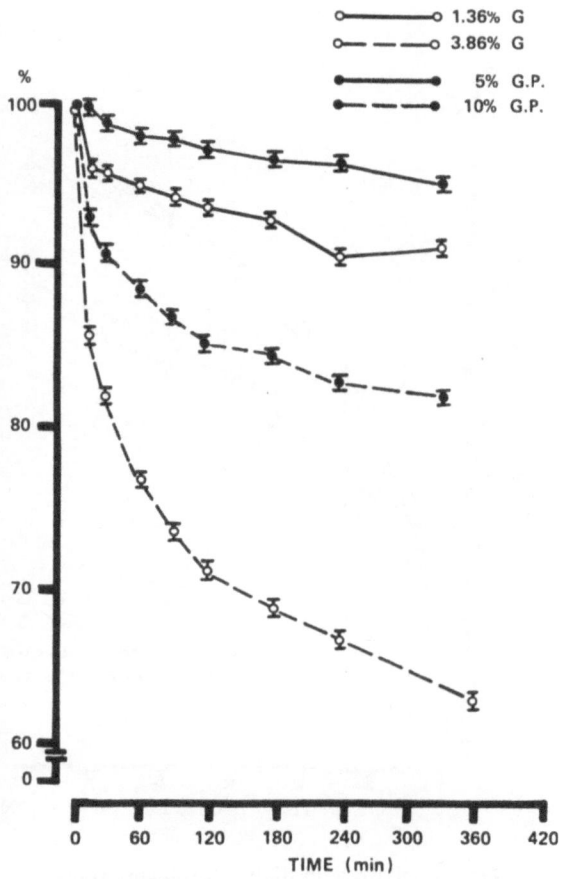

Osmolality expressed as % of initial value.

Fig. 3. Dialysate osmolality in relation to dwell time; osmolality expressed as percent of initial value.

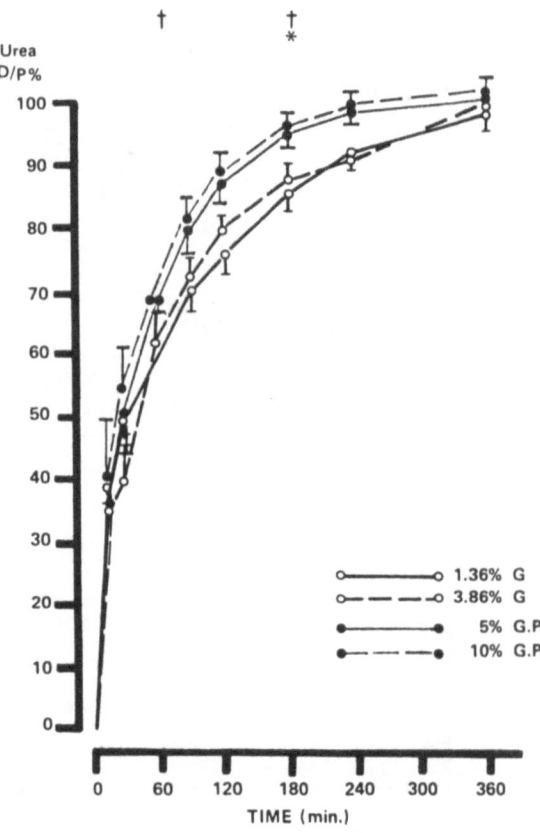

Fig. 4. Urea dialysate/plasma ratio, expressed as percentages.

GP at both concentrations. Significant differences occurred as early as 60 minutes after the onset of dialysis and progressively increased throughout the cycle, so that at 6 hours, 14.8, 19, and 21 percent greater equilibration was achieved for creatinine, uric acid and phosphate respectively.

Similarly, average clearances of solutes (Table 1) were also significantly greater with GP solutions at both concentrations ($p < 0.03$) and appear to be particularly marked for higher molecular weight solutes. Hypertonic solutions resulted in overall increase in clearances values by 25% as compared to their respective isotonic fluids, but the percentage increase was similar for all solutes, irrespective of their molecular size. Furthermore, when hypertonic

dextrose G (3.86%) was compared with isotonic GP (5%) solution, glucose solution failed to achieve comparable solute clearances, with exception of urea, in spite of augmentation in ultrafiltration of 325 ml.

Blood glucose, peaked (6.7 ± 0.3 mmol/L) at 30 minutes after the onset of hypertonic dextrose dialysis and fell thereafter to fasting level within 6 hours. No appreciable change in blood glucose occurs with any of the other solutions (Fig. 8). Analysis of glucose polymers concentrations in the serum and dialysate were available in three patients.

The data indicate (Table 2) that the percentage absorption of the total glucose polymer infused from the peritoneal cavity was lower as compared to dextrose (42.5 to 59% versus 65.5 to 68.9%); however the total amount of carbohydrate absorbed was greater, providing a caloric load 1.7 to 4.3 times greater than with dextrose dialysis.

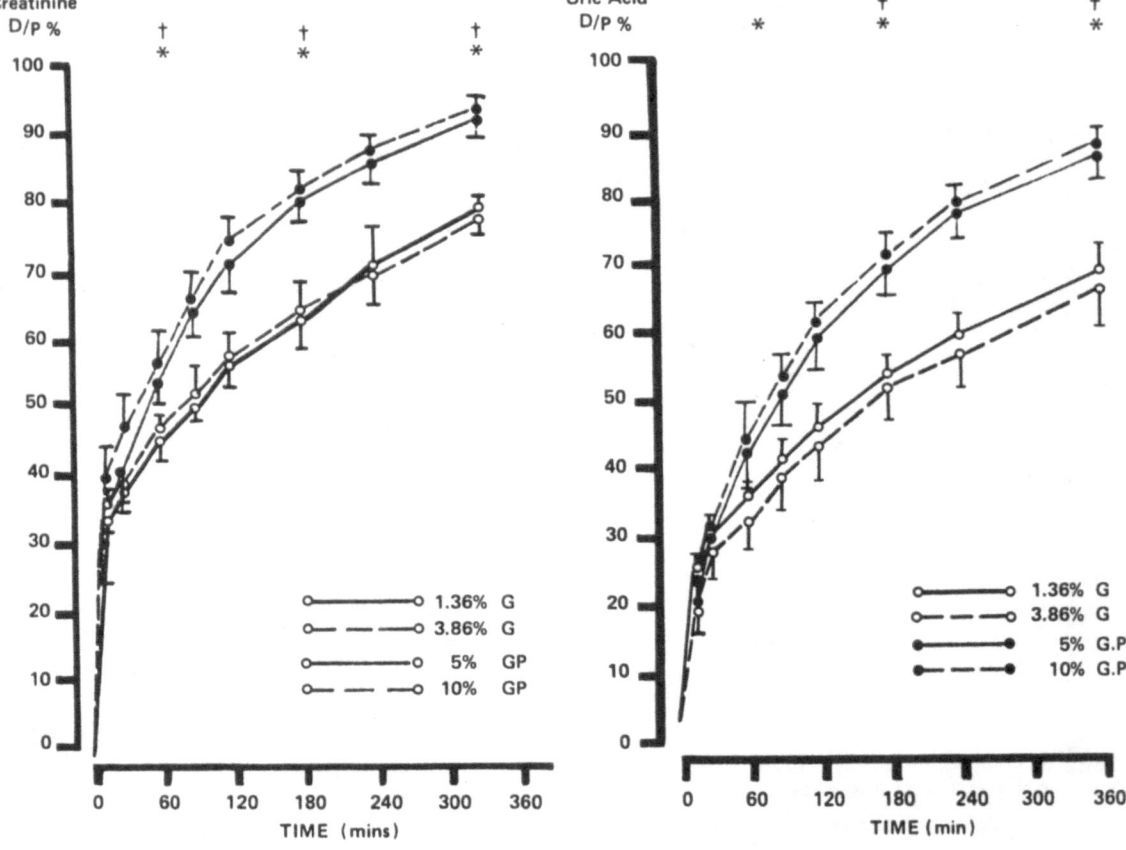

Fig. 5. Creatinine dialysate/plasma ratio.   **Fig. 6.** Uric acid dialysate/plasma ratio.

The loss of individual polymer fraction from the peritoneal cavity varied considerably, depending on molecular size. Generally, up to 75% loss occurred for small fractions (2 to 12 glucose units), but only 13 to 37% for larger fractions (12 glucose units). After a 6 hour dwell, the serum profile (Fig. 9) showed predominant elevation of maltose and maltotriose (2 and 3 glucose units), accounting for 60 to 70% of the total polymer rise; with only minimal rise in the fraction above 5 glucose units. Serum maltose (G_2) and maltotriose (G_3) (Fig. 10) rose rapidly, reaching 80% of their peak values 2 hours after the onset of dialysis. The peak values of the above fractions, however, occurred at different times with two concentrations of polymer; 10% solution produced a peak at the end of the dialysis, whereas it was delayed with 5% solution, to 14 hours post dialysis. The clearances from plasma were slow; up to 80 to 90% maltose and 55 to 75% of maltotriose persisting

24 hours after stopping the dialysis. No adverse effect was noted, in any patients using GP solutions.

DISCUSSION

This study shows that glucose polymers achieve a superior rate of ultrafiltration and clearances of low molecular weight solutes (urea, creatinine, uric acid, phosphate). On a weight basis, GP exhibits an osmotic pressure about one fifth that of dextrose. The current GP solutions (5 and 10%) were only 3.7 and 2.7 greater in weight than dextrose solutions (1.36 and 3.86%); the resulting osmolalities were correspondingly lower. However, the net ultrafiltration rate achieved by GP solutions were significantly superior. This important function of polymer appears to reflect the higher average molecular weight, within the peritoneal cavity, and concomitant de-

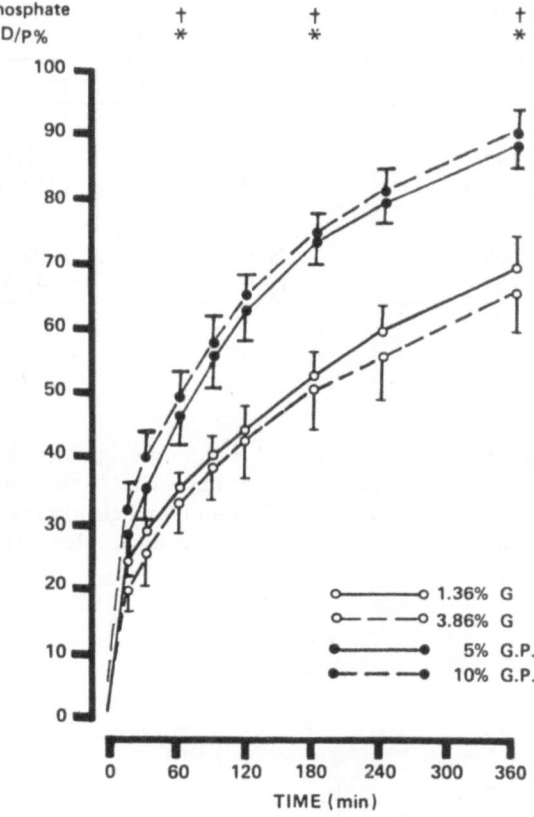

Fig. 7. Phosphate dialysate/plasma ratio.

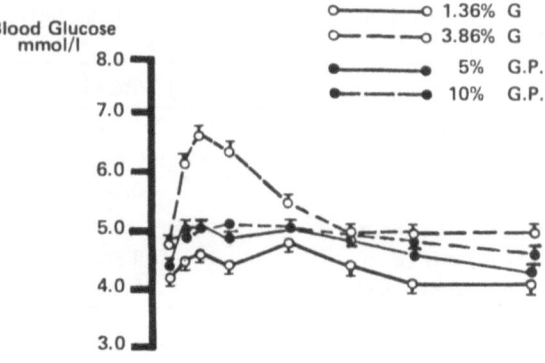

Fig. 8. Blood glucose profile during 6 hours dwell.

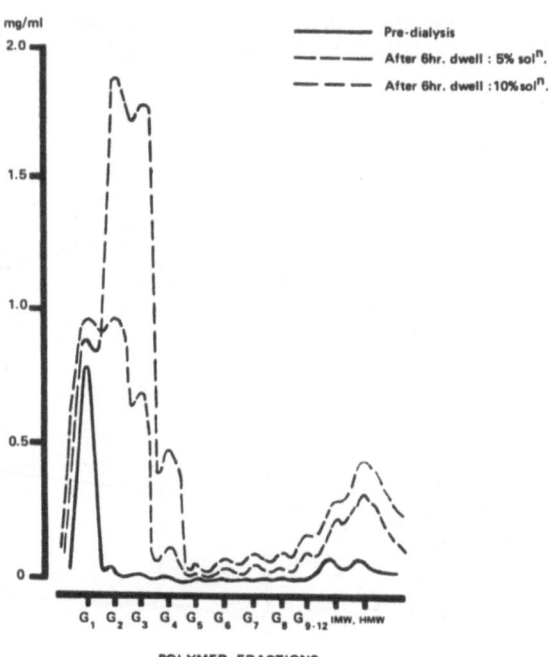

crease in percentage loss to the circulation. Fractions with 5 to 9 glucose units show the highest intraperitoneal fall in concentration (about 75%) without concomitant rise in serum levels, whereas, maltose and maltotriose with a slightly lower fall (60 to 65%) produce a substantial rise in serum levels, suggesting considerable breakdown of intermediate molecules to smaller units.

This effect may augment GP-induced ultrafiltration by contributing towards maintenance of intra-

Table 1. Solute Clearances (C, ml/min) (mean ± SEM).

	1.36% G	5% GP	3.86% G	10% GP
C. Urea	6.7 ± 0.14	7.9 ± 0.14	8.7 ± 0.23	10.0 ± 0.32
C. Creatinine	5.3 ± 0.27	7.2 ± 0.09	6.7 ± 0.18	9.2 ± 0.32
C. Uric acid	4.6 ± 0.27	6.7 ± 0.18	5.7 ± 0.27	8.5 ± 0.36
C. Phosphate	4.7 ± 0.36	6.9 ± 0.18	5.7 ± 0.27	8.8 ± 0.41

Comparing 1.36% G with 5% GP and 3.86% G with 10% GP, the differences between the values are all statistically significant ($p < 0.03$).

Table 2. Carbohydrate (CHO) Content Predialysis and After 6 Hour Dwell for Glucose and Polymer (GP) Solutions.

	1.36% G	5% GP	3.86% G	10% GP
Total CHO (g)				
predialysis	29.4	140.3	82.14	225.1
at 6 hour	10.14	57.33	25.52	129.46
Total CHO absorbed				
at 6 hour (g)	19.26	82.97	56.62	95.64
% of initial CHO	65.5	59.0	68.9	42.5

G = Glucose (n = 5).
GP = Glucose polymer (n = 3).

peritoneal osmolality, as smaller osmotically active particles are generated. Overall, although the percentage of total polymers lost from the peritoneum is relatively small, the total amount absorbed has a potential caloric load 1.7 to 4.3 times greater than glucose. Polymer solutions appear to have a profound effect on the equilibration and clearances of various solutes, particularly for molecules larger

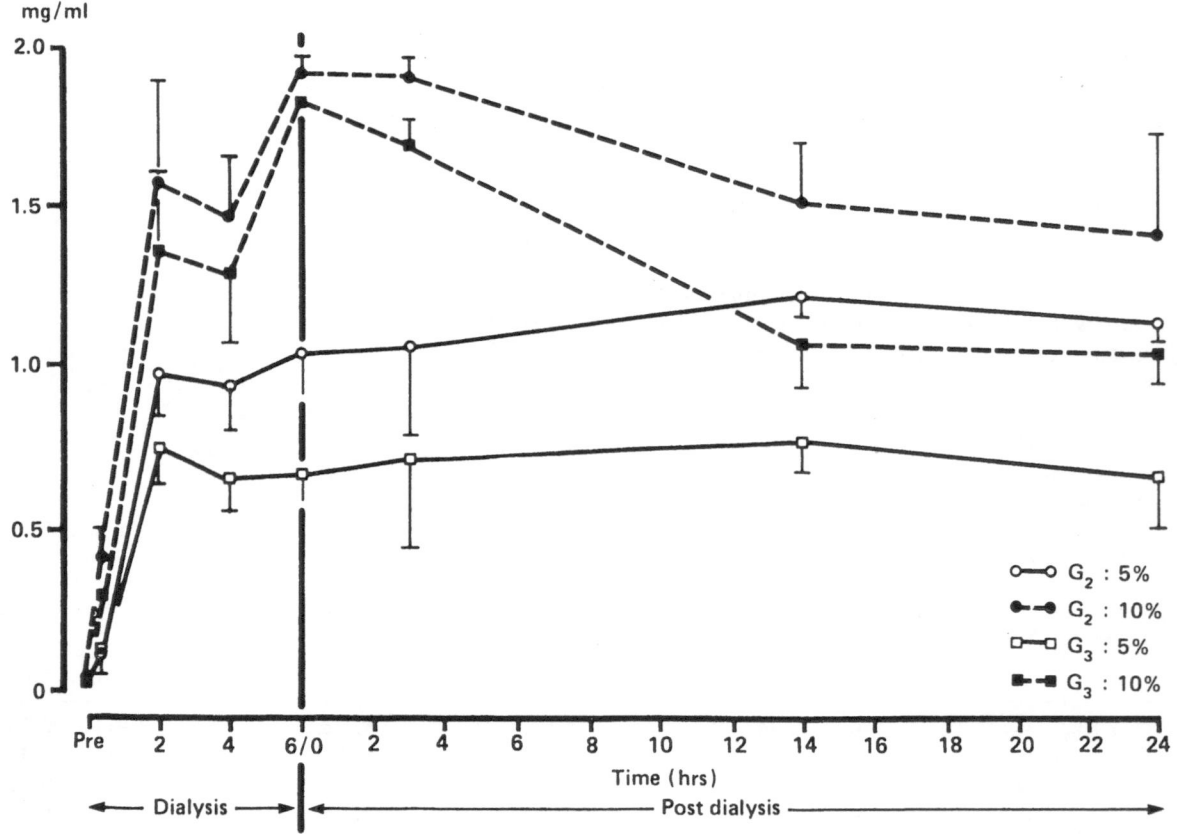

Fig. 10. Serum glucose polymer (G$_2$ ± G$_3$) profile.

than urea. It could be argued that the observed effect may be the result of an increased ultrafiltration rate. However, two important observations are noteworthy. Firstly the hypertonic solutions, G and GP, both produced a similar increase in ultrafiltration and overall solute clearances, compared to their respective isotonic solutions, without significant effect on equilibration or selective increase in clearances of larger molecules. Secondly, although ultrafiltration was lower with isotonic GP (5%) than hypertonic G (3.86%) by 325 ml, resulting solute clearances were greater, except for urea. These observations suggest that polymer solutions may alter the permeability of the peritoneum to molecules larger than urea. Assessment of mass transfer area coefficient (MTAC) of the above solutes will answer this question more specifically. Recent study in dogs has not confirmed this speculation.[6]

Maltose and maltotriose are the end products of the degradation of glucose polymer by serum and various tissue amylases. Maltase activity is virtually absent in the circulating blood of man,[7,8] but it has been demonstrated in a variety of extraintestinal tissues,[9] particularly kidney. Kidney tissue exhibits relatively high maltase activity,[10,11] which has been associated with the brush border and apical membrane of proximal renal tubules.[12,13] Ohneda et al.[14] reported that infused maltose was rapidly cleared from the plasma of intact rabbits, but was cleared only slowly by nephrectomized animals, suggesting that renal handling of this disaccharide is an important factor in its metabolism. This may explain the slow clearance of maltose and maltotriose in our patients, in whom mean residual creatinine clearance was only 1.7 ml/min. The long-term effects of high maltose and maltotriose are unknown, although from animal studies there is evidence that suggests that maltose can enter cells by diffusion and could subsequently be hydrolysed.[15] Alternatively, a portion of cellular maltose may be converted to higher polymers of glucose without prior hydrolysis to glucose.[16] The above mechanisms may account for essentially unaltered blood glucose levels during GP dialysis in our study. Similar findings were reported when dextrin[17] and maltose[16] were infused intravenously in normal human subjects.

In conclusion, glucose polymers appear to be well tolerated with superior ultrafiltration and solute clearance characteristics. The use of present formulation is limited by slow metabolism of the rapidly absorbed maltose and maltotriose. Further modification of the polymer profile may reduce this to acceptable levels.

ACKNOWLEDGMENTS

CDM is in receipt of a grant from the Manchester and North West Kidney Research Association. The G.P. was supplied by Milner Scientific Co. and prepared for infusion by Boots Co. G.P. assays were undertaken by Dr. J. Fox. To all those we extend our thanks.

REFERENCES

1. Nolph KD, Twardowski ZJ, Popovich R.P., and Rubin J: Equilibration of peritoneal dialysis solution during long dwell exchange. J Lab Clin Med 93: 246, 1979
2. Pyle KW, Moncreif JW, and Popovich RP: Peritoneal transport evaluation in CAPD. In Moncreif JW, and Popovich RP (Eds), CAPD update. New York and Paris: Masson Publishing, 1981, p 35
3. Ramos JM, Gokal R, Siamopolous K, Ward MK, Wilkinson R, and Kerr DNS: Continuous ambulatory dialysis: Three years experience. Q J Med 52: 165, 1983
4. Gokal R, Ramos JM, McGurk JC, Ward MK, and Kerr DNS: Hyperlipidaemia in patients on continuous ambulatory peritoneal dialysis. In Gahl GM, Kessel M, and Nolph KD (Eds), Advances in peritoneal dialysis: Proceedings of the 2nd international symposium on peritoneal dialysis. Amsterdam: Excerpta Medica, 1981, p 430
5. Berlyne GM, Brewis RAL, Boath EM, and Mallick NP: A soluble glucose polymer for use in renal failure and calorie deprivation states. Lancet 1: 689, 1969
6. Kennedy JF, and Fox JE: Fully automatic gel-permeation chromatographic analysis of neutral oligosaccharides. In Whistler RL, and BeMiller JN (Eds), Methods in carbohydrate chemistry, Vol 8. New York: Academic Press, 1980, p 13
7. Young JM, and Weser E: The metabolism of circulating maltose in man. J Clin Invest 50: 246, 1979
8. Van Handle E: Trehalase and maltase in the serum of vertebrates. Com Biochem Physiol 26: 561, 1968
9. Dreyfus JC, and Alexandre Y. Electrophoretic characterization of acid and neutral amylo 1–4 glucosidase (acid maltase) in human tissues and evidence for two electrophoretic variants in acid maltase deficiency. Biochem Biophys Res Comm 48: 914, 1972
10. Bittencourt HMH, Sleisenger M, Weser E: Studies of serum and tissue maltase in the rat. Gastroenterology 57: 410, 1969
11. Silverman M: Brush border disaccharides in dog kidney and their spatial relationship to glucose transport receptors. J Clin Invest 52: 2486, 1973
12. Berger SJ, and Sackfor B: Preparation and biochemical characterization of brush border from rabbit kidney. J Cell Biol 47: 637, 1970

13.   Stevenson FK: Studies on the surface maltase of the rabbit renal cortex. Biochem Biophys Acta 311: 409, 1973

14.   Ohneda AS, Yamagata S, Tsutsumi K, and Fujiwara H: Distribution of maltose intravenously administered to rabbits and its metabolism in the kidney. Tohoku J Exp Med 112: 141, 1974

15.   Young EA, and Weser E: Uptake of maltose and other sugars by rat diaphragm. J Clin Invest 53: 87a, 1974

16.   Young EA, Drummond A, Cool DA, Cioletti LA, Crain M, Taylor JB, and Weser E: The effect of insulin on the metabolism of parenteral maltose in man. J Clin Endocrinol Metab 50: 764, 1980

17.   Bibby RJ, Davies D, Mallick MP, Atherton ST, Wright DM, Rickett CR, and Milner J: Intravenous infusion of a dextrin, Caloreen, in human subjects. Metabolic Studies. Br J Nutr 38: 341, 1977

Z.J. Twardowski, H. Hain, T.J. McGary,
H.L. Moore, and R.S. Keller

45

Sustained UF with Gelatin Dialysis Solution during Long Dwell Dialysis Exchanges in Rats

SUMMARY

Two Haemaccel solutions (5.5% and 10%) were developed to contain electrolyte concentrations similar to rat serum. Twenty ml of each solution was studied during long dwell exchanges in nonuremic rats. Commercial Dianeal solutions served as controls.

Whereas the typical ultrafiltration pattern of an absorbable osmotic agent was seen with Dianeal, Haemaccel yielded sustained ultrafiltration. The rate of ultrafiltration with 4.25% Dianeal solution after a 6 hour dwell time was similar to that of 5.5% Haemaccel and markedly lower than that of 10% Haemaccel. There were no untoward effects of Haemaccel, no electrolyte disturbances and the peritoneal membrane looked normal on light and scanning electron microscopy.

It is therefore concluded that Haemaccel or other gelatin derivatives may be valuable as alternate osmotic agents for peritoneal dialysis.

INTRODUCTION

Commercially available peritoneal dialysis solutions contain dextrose as the osmotic agent to obtain ultrafiltration. However, dextrose has several disadvantages. Some patients cannot achieve adequate ultrafiltration even with the most hypertonic exchanges, due to rapid absorption of dextrose from the peritoneal cavity.[1] The continuous absorption of dextrose from the dialysate may be responsible for obesity and hypertriglyceridema.[2] Thus, a slowly absorbable osmotic agent might be useful, especially in patients with poor ultrafiltration. The larger the size of the osmotic agent, the longer ultrafiltration lasts, because solute absorption through the peritoneal membrane is slower for larger molecules.

The osmotic driving force depends on the osmolality, which is a measure of the total number of osmotically active molecules in solution. It is directly related to the molar concentration of a solute, i.e., the number of moles per kilogram of solute. Larger molecular weight solutes must be dissolved at higher percentage concentrations to obtain the same osmolality. Therefore, it is difficult to achieve a high ultrafiltration with uncharged molecules even though the rate of ultrafiltration may be sustained longer.

The properties of charged molecules used as osmotic agents are different. The osmotic driving force in such solutions depends mainly on the concentration of ionized electrolytes that cannot cross the membrane because they must balance the opposite charge of the polyion.[3] Polymer molecules *per se* contribute little to the total osmotic driving force.[4] Solutions containing polyacrylate and dextran sulfate have been showed to yield high and sustained ultrafiltration in an *in vitro* simulation of perito-

From the Division of Nephrology, Department of Medicine, Harry S. Truman Memorial Veterans Administration Hospital, and from the University of Missouri Health Sciences Center, Columbia, Missouri.

neal dialysis.[5] However, several synthetic polymers tested in both rats and rabbits induced intraperitoneal bleeding, cardiovascular instability,[6] and damaged the peritoneal membrane.

Preliminary studies in rats with gelatin solutions demonstrated desirable ultrafiltration rates. There were no untoward effects of gelatin on rats and the peritoneal membrane looked normal on light and scanning electronmicroscopy.[6] However, crude gelatin solutions were difficult to work with because of viscosity and gelation.

The present study had three major purposes: to prepare a solution of Haemaccel, a gelatin derivative, with the desired concentration of the electrolytes; to assess ultrafiltration patterns during long dwell exchanges in rats using two concentrations of Haemaccel compared to commercially available peritoneal dialysis solutions; and to test whether Haemaccel would induce electrolyte disturbances and/or acute toxic effects.

MATERIALS AND METHODS

Haemaccel Solution Preparation

The method of polymer solution preparation to obtain the desired concentration of diffusible electrolytes has been previously described.[5] In brief, 3.5% Haemaccel (Beringwerke, Marburg, Germany) solution with an average molecular weight of 35,000 daltons was dialyzed in a Travenol 1512 hollow fiber dialyser against an electrolyte solution containing (mEq/L); potassium—4.0; sodium—138.8; chloride—110; magnesium—0.48; calcium—3.50; and lactate—35.0. The mean transmembrane pressure of 30 mm Hg was maintained throughout the dialysis to prevent excessive polymer dilution. When electrolyte concentrations in inflowing and outflowing dialysates were equal, dialysis was discontinued and a higher transmembrane pressure was applied on the perfusate side to obtain a Haemaccel concentration of 10%. The concentration of electrolytes in the ultrafiltrate equal to those in the dialysates were considered as proof of equilibration. A portion of the 10% solution was diluted with dialysate to obtain a solution of 5.5% Haemaccel. All solutions were heat sterilized at 60°C for 10 hours in a Thelco Laboratory Oven (Model 18, Precision Scientific, Chicago, IL).

Glucose Solution Preparation

Glucose solution was commercially available Dianeal (Baxter-Travenol Laboratories, Deerfield, IL) with added potassium of 4.0 mEq/L.

Dialysis Technique

All dialysis exchanges were performed in non-uremic Sprague-Dawley rats weighing 310–390 g.

Table 1. Composition of Haemaccel and Electrolyte Solutions at the Completion of Polymer Preparation.

	Na^+ mEq–L	K^+ mEq–L	Mg^{++} mEq–L	Ca^{++} mEq–L	Cl^- mEq–L	Osmolality mOsm/kg	pH
Haemaccel 3.5%							
Beringwerke	139.3	4.9	0.3	12.69	142		
Inflowing dialysate	138.8	4.0	0.48	3.50	110	272	5.9
Outflowing dialysate	138.7	4.0	0.48	3.52	110	273	5.9
Ultrafiltrate	141.1	4.1	0.46	3.54	111	272	6.2
Haemaccel 5.5%	147.6	4.3	0.59	4.79	108	290	6.0
Total/diffusible cation ratio	1.05	1.05	1.28	1.35			
Gibbs-Donnan distribution ratio					0.97		
Haemaccel 10%	149.3	4.5	.64	5.23	105	298	6.0
Total/diffusible cation ratio	1.06	1.10	1.39	1.48			
Gibbs-Donnan distribution ratio					0.95		

The rats were anesthetized with a subcutaneous injection of pentobarbital sodium and a silicone catheter without cuffs was inserted into the peritoneal cavity through a small incision in the midline of the abdomen below the sternum. The catheter tip was positioned in the right inferior quadrant.

Arterial and venous cannulae were inserted into femoral artery and jugular vein respectively for monitoring of vital signs and fluid replacement. Fluid losses were replaced with lactated Ringers solution.

The dialysis solution was prewarmed to 30°C and a 20 ml volume was introduced into the peritoneal cavity over one minute. The solution was immediately drained and the volume measured to estimate the undrainable volume retained in the peritoneal cavity. The same solution was then reinfused immediately after the volume measurements. The measurements of drainage volumes were repeated at 1, 2, 3, 4, and 5 hours. At the 6th hour the solution was drained, tissue samples taken, and the rat sacrificed.

Ultrafiltration volumes were calculated by adding the undrainable volume retained in the peritoneal cavity to the apparent ultrafiltration volumes at the particular dwell times.

Chemical Determinations

Sodium and potassium concentrations were determined by flame photometry (model 143; Instrumentation Laboratories, Inc., Lexington, MA). Chloride was measured by a chloridometer (Buchler Instruments, Inc., Fort Lee, NJ). Calcium and

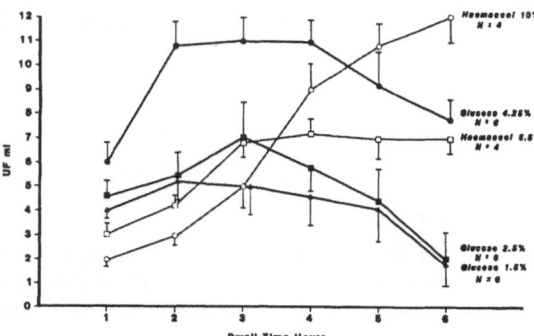

Fig. 1. Mean ultrafiltration (UF) ± SEM related to dwell time with gelatin isocyanate (Haemaccel), and glucose (Dianeal). Symbols: open circles, 10% Haemaccel; open squares, 5.5% Haemaccel; closed circles, 4.25% Dianeal; closed squares, 2.5% Dianeal; closed triangles, 1.5% Dianeal. Note sustained ultrafiltration with poorly absorbable gelatin isocyanate molecules.

magnesium were determined by atomic absorption spectrophotometry (Atomic Absorption Spectrophotometer, Model 403; Perkin-Elmer, Norwalk, CT). Osmolality was measured by freezing point depression (Osmette Automatic Osmometer; Precision Systems, Inc., Waltham, MA).

Pathologic Studies

The specimens of the peritoneum were taken immediately after the completion of dialysis, and stained with silver nitrate for an *en face* light

Table 2. Mean ± SEM Rat Serum Electrolyte Concentrations at the End of Dialysis.

Dialysis Solution	N	Na^+ mEq/L	K^+ mEq/L	Mg^{++} mEq/L	Ca^{++} mEq/L	Cl^- mEq/L
Dianeal 1.5%	6	135.9 ±1.0	4.7 0.14	2.27 0.14	4.57 0.19	104.7 1.6
Dianeal 2.5%	6	148.3 ±2.4	5.4 0.20	1.69 0.04	4.24 0.16	104.0 0.7
Dianeal 4.25%	6	145.4 ±1.8	5.5 0.13	1.70 0.09	4.07 0.06	104.5 1.7
Haemaccel 5.5%	3	139.9 ±1.6	5.4 0.22	2.31 0.11	4.46 0.30	106.7 0.7
Haemaccel 10%	4	141.7 ±1.6	5.4 0.18	2.28 0.15	4.66 0.15	112.8 2.2

microscopy examination. The technique has been previously described.[7]

RESULTS

Haemaccel Solutions

Table 1 shows compositions of Haemaccel electrolyte solutions at the completion of the preparation. The concentrations of electrolytes in inflowing and outflowing dialysates were similar to each other and also were similar to the concentrations of electrolytes in the ultrafiltrate indicating complete equilibration. Concentrations of the cations were higher in Haemaccel solutions due to binding to the negatively charged polymer residues.

Rat Vital Signs

Blood pressures, heart and respiration rates were essentially stable throughout the dialysis in all rats. Slight decreases in blood pressure, observed during most hypertonic exchanges of both solutions, were easily corrected with fluid replacement.

Ultrafiltration

Figure 1 shows total net ultrafiltration with Haemaccel and Dianeal solutions. Whereas, typical ultrafiltration patterns for diffusible osmotic agents were obtained with Dianeal, a sustained ultrafiltration with Haemaccel was achieved up to a 6 hour cycle time.

Serum Electrolytes

Table 2 presents serum concentration of electrolytes upon completion of dialysis. No electrolyte derangements were observed with either Dianeal or Haemaccel solutions.

Dialysate Electrolytes

Table 3 shows concentrations of electrolytes in dialysates drained after 6 hours. Cation concentrations in the Haemaccel dialysate were higher than in the serum although lower than in the dialysis solutions prior to infusion indicating that a substantial amount of Haemaccel molecules were retained in the dialysate.

Peritoneal Membrane Morphology

The peritoneal membrane after dialysis with 10% Haemaccel solution looked essentially normal on light microscopy, only cell boundaries seemed less pleated (Figs. 2 and 3).

DISCUSSION

Gelatin is obtained from collagen, which constitutes 30% of the total body protein. The collagen molecule consists of three polypeptide chains with a total molecular mass of approximately 300,000 to 320,000 daltons with the chemical structure being similar in all species.[8] The immunogenicity of collagen is weak due to this similarity of primary structure as well as the absence of tryptophan and deficiency of tyrosine.[9]

Table 3. Mean ± SEM Drained Dialysate Electrolyte Concentrations.

Dialysate	N	Na+ mEq/L	K+ mEq/L	Mg++ mEq/L	Ca++ mEq/L	CC- mEq/L	Osmolality mOsm/kg
Dianeal 1.5%	6	131.6 ±4.8	4.0 0.17	0.90 0.05	1.81 0.24	98.5 4.9	268.3 11.7
Dianeal 2.5%	6	141.2 ±0.9	4.4 0.08	0.67 0.04	1.53 0.22	104.0 1.2	282.7 2.7
Dianeal 4.25%	6	136.8 ±1.8	4.2 0.11	0.66 0.03	1.52 0.18	101.3 1.5	275.2 3.5
Haemaccel 5.5%	4	143.2 ±1.0	5.0 0.32	1.48 0.13	4.03 0.05	102.5 0.9	294.8 2.6
Haemaccel 10%	4	145.3 ±0.2	5.1 0.06	1.48 0.05	4.42 0.09	103.0 0.9	304.5 2.9

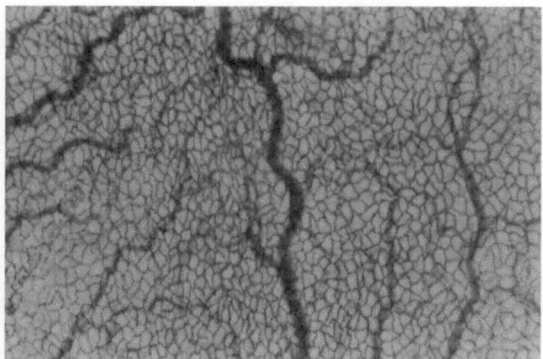

Fig. 2. Normal peritoneal membrane on rat mesentery by light microscopy using an *en face* silver stain. Note pleated cell boundaries and occasional intercellular gaps (× 80).

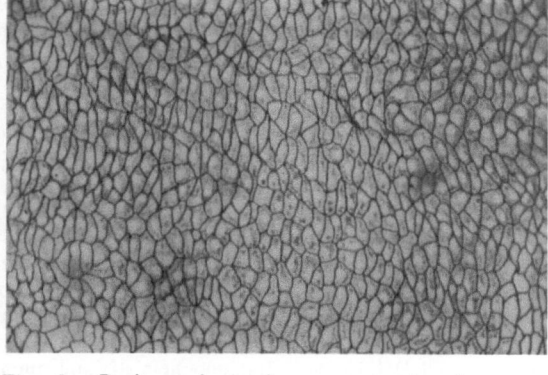

Fig. 3. Peritoneal membrane on gut by the same technique as in Figure 2 after 10% Haemaccel dialysis. Note less pleated cell boundaries, otherwise the membrane looks normal.

Historically, gelatin solutions were used by Hogan in 1915 as plasma substitutes in the treatment of shock patients.[10] Problems with viscosity and sterilization as well as the development of blood transfusions decreased the interest in gelatin as a plasma substitute. Approximately 40 years ago Frank, Seligman, and Fine used gelatin as an osmotic agent in acute peritoneal dialysis.[11] In recent years there have been no further reports of gelatin solutions used in peritoneal dialysis.

A revival of gelatin as a plasma substitute occurred in the early 1950s due to the fact that the point of gel formation could be lowered to less than 10°C by chemical modification.[12]

One of these derivatives is Haemaccel, a gelatin isocyanate, currently used in Europe as a plasma expander. Haemaccel is easily metabolized in the body with a mean half life of 22 hours in hemodialysis patients.[13]

Our preliminary studies suggest that solutions containing Haemaccel as the osmotic agent yield sustained ultrafiltration in rats. The ultrafiltration rate with 4.25% Dianeal solution after a 6 hour cycle time is comparable to that of a 5.5% Haemaccel solution and markedly lower than that of a 10% Haemaccel solution. Also no electrolyte disturbances were observed with the Haemaccel solutions.

Less pleated mesothelial cell boundaries (Fig. 3) may reflect a slight shrinkage of cells exposed to a high colloid osmotic pressure solution.

These studies suggest that Haemaccel is a very promising alternative osmotic agent for CAPD especially in patients who require high dextrose concentrations to achieve ultrafiltration. However, long term studies are needed to establish the rates of absorption, chronic toxicity, possible immunogenicity, and metabolism of these solutions in continuous ambulatory peritoneal dialysis.

ACKNOWLEDGMENTS

Supported in part by Nephrology Research Funds and Travenol Laboratories, Inc. The authors thank Dr. Oswald Zwisler of Beringwerke AG for generous supply of Haemaccel, and Cindy Franklin for secretarial assistance.

REFERENCES

1. Nolph KD: Factors affecting ultrafiltration in continuous ambulatory peritoneal dialysis; first report of an international cooperative study. Peritoneal Dial Bull 4: 14, 1984
2. Oreopoulos DG, Robson M, Faller B, Ogilvie R, Rapport A, and de Veber GA: Continuous ambulatory peritoneal dialysis: A new era in the treatment of chronic renal failure. Clin Nephrol 11: 125, 1979
3. Twardowski ZJ, Nolph KD, Popovich R, and Hopkins C: Comparison of polymer, glucose, and hydrostatic pressure induced ultrafiltration in a hollow fiber dialyzer; effects on convective solute transport. J Lab Clin Med 92: 619, 1978
4. Morawetz H: Macromolecules in solution (2nd Ed). New York, Wiley-Interscience, 1975

5. Twardowski ZJ, Nolph KD, McGary TJ, and Moore HL: Polyanions and glucose as osmotic agents in simulated peritoneal dialysis. Artif Organs 7: 420, 1983

6. Twardowski ZJ, Moore HL, McGary TJ, Poskuta M, Hirszel P, and Stathakis C: Polymers as osmotic agents for peritoneal dialysis. Peritoneal Dial Bull 3(Suppl 4): 125, 1984

7. Verger C, Luger A, Moore HL, and Nolph KD: Acute changes in peritoneal morphology and transport properties with infectious peritonitis and mechanical injury. Kidney Int 23: 823, 1983

8. Veis A: The macromolecular chemistry of gelatin. New York and London, Academic Press, 1964

9. Schwick HG, Heide K: Immunochemistry and immunology of collagen and gelatin. In Lundsgaard-Hansen P, Hassig A, and Nitschman HS (Eds), Modified gelatins as plasma substitutes. Basel/New York: Karger, 1969 p 111

10. Hogan JJ: The intravenous use of colloidal (gelatin) solutions in shock. JAMA 64: 721, 1915

11. Frank HA, Seligman AM, and Fine J: Further experiences with peritoneal irrigation for acute renal failure. Ann Surg 128: 561, 1948

12. Lundsgaard-Hansen P, Hassig A, and Nitschman HS (Eds); Modified gelatins as plasma substitutes. Basel/New York: Karger, 1969

13. Schutterle G, Dieker P, Knopp K: Plasma substitutes and the artificial kidney. In Lundsgaard-Hansen P, Hassig A and Nitschman HS (Eds), Modified gelatins as plasma substitutes. Basel/New York: Karger, 1969, p 581

A. Heaton, D.G. Johnston, M.K. Ward, K.G.M.M. Alberti,
and D.N.S. Kerr

46

Glycerol Instead of Dextrose As an Osmotic Agent in CAPD

SUMMARY

Glycerol replaced dextrose as the osmotic agent in dialysis fluid for six patients undergoing CAPD. This resulted in lower plasma glucose concentrations and insulin levels. No toxicity was detected from glycerol absorption, even in one patient so exposed for 6 months. On a molar basis, however, glycerol induced less ultrafiltration than dextrose did. Because of the lower dialysate volume, clearances were less with glycerol than with dextrose.

INTRODUCTION

Numerous metabolic problems have been described in patients with chronic renal failure. Impaired glucose tolerance was noted many years ago and occurs with both oral and intravenous glucose,[1] while fasting hyperglycemia is less common.[2] The occurrence of hyperinsulinemia in association with impaired glucose tolerance has been attributed to peripheral insulin resistance.[3] Recent studies have shown normal binding of insulin to surface receptors and the site of resistance is therefore probably in the postreceptor actions of insulin.[4] Other abnormalities include innappropriately raised levels of circulating glucagon,[5] and growth hormone,[6] but they do not appear to cause glucose intolerance and have no evident clinical significance. Lipid metabolism is also deranged in uremia. Hypertriglyceridemia is the predominant abnormality,[7] but hypercholesterolemia is found in a minority of patients.[8] Raised circulating very low density lipoprotein (VLDL) triglyceride levels are due to a combination of increased production and reduced clearance.[9]

Dialysis may modify these abnormalities. Partial reversal of glucose intolerance has been reported following efficient hemodialysis[10] but this is not invariable. Hemodialysis does not improve hyperlipidemia and it may make it worse.[11] Intermittent peritoneal dialysis may also improve oral glucose tolerance,[12] but has also been reported to induce hyperglycemia and hyperosmolality[13] as a result of glucose absorption from the dialysis fluid. CAPD provides good biochemical control in uremic patients, which may improve some of these metabolic abnormalities. The control of fluid balance in CAPD patients is achieved by varying the osmolality of the dialysis fluid and absorption of the osmotic agent may further modify any metabolic derangement.

Various osmotic agents have been tried in dialysis fluids but the only osmotic agent in common use is dextrose. Dextrose is safe, effective, and cheap, and when absorbed is rapidly metabolized and provides useful calories in malnourished patients.[14] There are, however, significant disadvantages with the use of dialysis fluid dextrose. The obligatory caloric load can induce excessive weight gain and hypertriglyceridemia and the insulin requirements

---

From the Royal Victoria Infirmary, Newcastle upon Tyne, United Kingdom.

Table 1. Composition of the Various Dialysis Fluids Used.

Solute	Concentration (mmol/L)		
	Low	Medium	High
Dextrose	76	126	215
Glycerol	92	152	272
Na^+	132	132	132
Cl^-	102	102	102
Ca^{2+}	1.75	1.75	1.75
Mg^{2+}	0.75	0.75	0.75
Lactate	35	35	35

of diabetic patients on CAPD may be increased. Dextrose based solutions require acidification to prevent caramelization during sterilization and the low pH of the solution may cause abdominal pain and inhibit leucocyte phagocytosis.[15]

The ideal osmotic agent would not be absorbed, but would be safe and effective. Molecules smaller than glucose would exert a higher osmotic effect at equal weight concentration, but would be more rapidly absorbed and need to be readily metabolized. Larger molecules would have to be present in high concentrations to have adequate osmotic effect, but would have the advantage of being more slowly absorbed. However, most larger molecules under consideration are nonphysiologic with unknown toxicity. The agents currently under study are amino acids, xylitol, and polyanions.[16] Although amino acids are promising as osmotic agents,[17] they are relatively expensive and the ideal combination and concentration has yet to be found. Xylitol may cause hyperuricemia,[18] and the polyanions studied have proven to be too toxic to justify use in humans.

Glycerol is a three-carbon sugar alcohol that has been used therapeutically for many years in the treatment of cerebral edema and glaucoma. It has a lower molecular weight (92 daltons) than glucose and is produced naturally in human metabolism during glycolysis. It has a calorific value approximately half that of glucose. It is a potent gluconeogenic precursor and is metabolized rapidly in the liver. Glycerol-based dialysis fluids should therefore be able to provide adequate osmotic effect with a lower total caloric load, even allowing for the more rapid absorption of glycerol during dialysis. We have examined the metabolic effects of dextrose over a single dialysis cycle, compared this with the effects of glycerol, and assessed the use of glycerol-based dialysis fluid in a patient over a 6 month period.

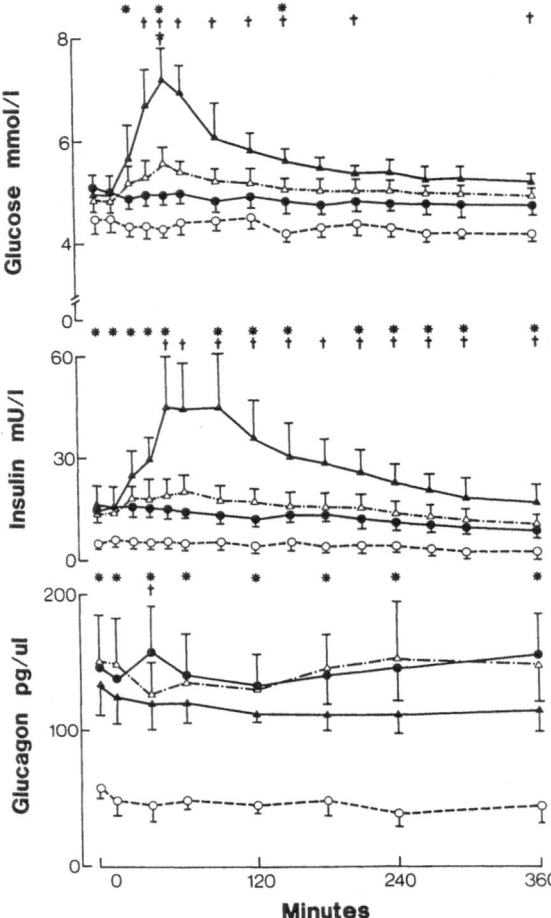

Fig. 1. Blood glucose, serum insulin and plasma glucagon concentrations over 6 hours in normal subjects (○·········○) and in CAPD patients undialysed (●———●), during isotonic (76 mmol dextrose/L) dialysis (Δ·—·—·Δ) and during hypertonic (215 mmol dextrose/L) dialysis (▲———▲). Values are expressed as mean ± SEM. Points of differences (p < 0.05 or less) are shown: (*) between normal and undialysed CAPD patients,(†) between undialysed and hypertonic dialysis, and (‡) between undialysed and isotonic dialysis.

PATIENTS AND METHODS

Study 1

Six patients, aged 30 to 65 years, established on CAPD, were studied to determine the effect of a single dialysis cycle, using dextrose-based dialysis fluid, on hormone and intermediary metabolite status. Results were compared with seven normal controls aged 22 to 61 years.

Study 2

Six further patients, aged 33 to 63 years, were studied to compare the effects of dextrose- and glycerol-based dialysis fluids (Table 1) over a 6 hour dialysis cycle and to assess glycerol as a possible therapeutic agent in CAPD.

Study 3

One patient, a 43-year-old man who had been on CAPD for 12 months, was followed for 6 months using glycerol-based dialysis fluid only and then for a further 6 months using conventional dextrose-based fluid to assess the long-term effects of glycerol-based dialysis fluids in CAPD.

ANALYTIC METHODS

Glucose, glycerol, lactate, pyruvate, alanine, and 3-hydroxybutyrate were assayed by an automated fluorometric enzyme method,[19] and acetoacetate by a manual spectrophotometric assay.[20] Insulin was assayed by double antibody radioimmunoassay[21] and glucagon by C-terminal specific radioimmunoassay.[22] Intraperitoneal volume was assessed by a hemoglobin dilution method.[23]

RESULTS

Study 1

Glucose, insulin, and glucagon levels over a 6 hour dialysis cycle are shown in Figure 1. Basal glucose levels in CAPD patients were 0.5 mmol/L higher than in normal controls. Mean blood glucose levels peaked 45 minutes following the onset of dialysis and fell slowly thereafter. Insulin concentrations followed a similar pattern, with fasting hyperinsulinemia in CAPD patients and a rapid rise during dialysis, particularly with the use of high dextrose concentration dialysis fluid. Glucagon levels were high throughout the dialysis cycle when compared to fasting normal controls.

Blood lactate and alanine levels were elevated in CAPD patients throughout the three studies but levels were highest during hypertonic dialysis. Total ketone concentrations (3-hydroxybutyrate + acetoacetate) were decreased in CAPD, especially during the use of high dextrose concentration dialysis fluid.

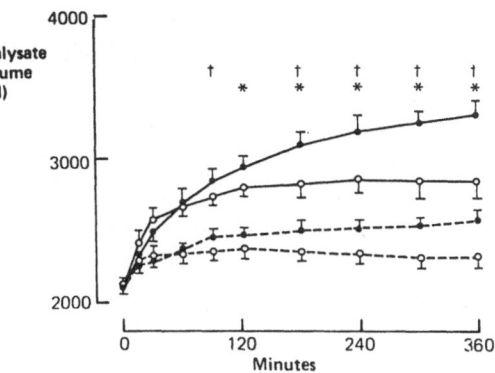

Fig. 2. Intraperitoneal volumes estimated by the hemoglobin dilution method over 6 hours in CAPD patients with dextrose (76 mmol ●--------● and 215 mmol/L ●———●) and glycerol (92 mmol/L ○--------○ and 272 mmol/L ○———○) as osmotic agents. Values are expressed as mean ± SEM. Points of difference ($p < 0.05$ or less) between isotonic dextrose and isotonic glycerol (†) and hypertonic dextrose and hypertonic glycerol (*) are shown at the top of each graph.

Study 2

Glycerol-based dialysis fluid was well tolerated in this short-term study. Intraperitoneal volumes using the four different solutions are shown in Figure 2. Volumes were lower than anticipated using glycerol-based dialysis fluid, despite the higher initial osmolality. This is confirmed when net ultrafiltration (volume drained-volume instilled) after 6 hours is compared. The dialysis fluid containing 215 mmol/L dextrose resulted in a mean net loss of 965 ml, compared to 500 ml using fluid containing 272 mmol/L glycerol ($p < 0.01$).

A mean of 72% of dialysis solution dextrose was absorbed over 6 hours compared to 84% of glycerol. This resulted in a net saving of about 20% of the calorific value of the absorbed osmotic agent when glycerol was used in place of dextrose.

The equilibration of creatinine, urea, and K^+ in the dialysate was similar in all four solutions, but 6 hour creatinine clearance was less using glycerol due to the smaller dialysate volumes.

Blood glycerol levels rose rapidly, reaching a peak of 4.3 ± 0.8 mmol/L at 150 minutes with glycerol 272 mmol/L solution and fell slowly. Using the lowest strength glycerol solution, the peak was 0.42 ± 0.08 mmol/L but this value was still ten times

Table 2. Mean Blood Hormone and Metabolite Levels Over a
Single 6 Hour Dialysis Cycle Using Dialysis Fluid Containing
Dextrose or Glycerol.

Blood Hormone/ Metabolite	Osmotic Agent		Significance
	Dextrose (215 mmol/L)	Glycerol (272 mmol/L)	
Glucose (mmol/L)	6.71 ± 0.50	5.10 ± 0.05	$p < 0.01$
Lactate (mmol/L)	1.23 ± 0.22	1.11 ± 0.07	NS
Pyruvate (mmol/L)	0.074 ± 0.004	0.070 ± 0.004	NS
Alanine (mmol/L)	0.40 ± 0.03	0.38 ± 0.03	NS
Insulin (mU/l)	18.8 ± 3.5	6.3 ± 0.4	$p < 0.001$
Glucagon (pg/μl)	111 ± 20	163 ± 18	$p < 0.05$

NS = Not significant.

greater than the levels during dialysis with dextrose
based solutions.

Mean levels of the gluconeogenic precursors
lactate, pyruvate and alanine were similar with
dextrose and glycerol. Glycerol, in contrast to dextrose, did not induce a glycemic or insulin response
(Table 2).

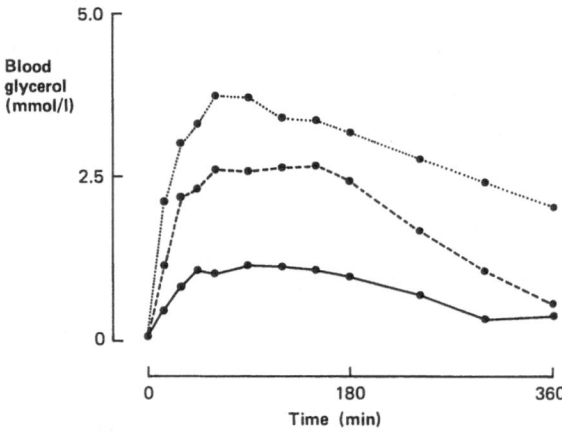

Fig. 3. Blood glycerol levels over 6 hours in a single CAPD patient using dialysis fluid containing 272
mmol/L of glycerol at start of treatment (●———●),
after 1 month of treatment (●·······●) and after 3
months treatment (●---------●) with dialysis fluid
containing glycerol.

Study 3

The patient tolerated long-term dialysis with
glycerol-based fluid well. He felt no different and
had no toxic effects using glycerol. There was no
evidence of progressive accumulation of glycerol in
this patient (Fig. 3).

Fluid balance, blood pressure and plasma creatinine and urea concentrations were maintained
over the study period. His weight, which had been
steadily increasing on CAPD, stabilized, although he
remained obese. Triglyceride concentrations were
marginally higher with glycerol than with dextrose,
but cholesterol levels were unchanged (Table 3).
There was no change in serum bilirubin, haptoglobin, alkaline phosphatase, glutamic oxaloacetic
transaminase, or urate throughout the study period.

DISCUSSION

Patients on CAPD constantly absorb the osmotic substrate dextrose from their peritoneal cavities. This process causes and exacerbates some of
the abnormalities described in CAPD patients. The
most obvious effect is hyperglycemia, which we observed in fasted CAPD patients, and during dialysis,
which leads to persistently high ambient insulin levels. Hyperinsulinemia in turn may stimulate glycolysis and inhibit gluconeogenesis and thus explain the

Table 3. Clinical Details of a Single Patient Using Glycerol-Based Dialysis Fluid.

Dialysis Fluid	Dextrose	Glycerol			Dextrose		
Months	0	1	3	6	1	3	6
Weight (kg)	97.7	95.7	95.8	95.9	95.8	95.9	95.9
Blood pressure (mm Hg)	160/105	140/90	160/90	150/90	120/70	160/105	160/100
Exchanges per day*	3L 1H	3L 1H	3L 1H	3L 1H	3L 1H	3L 1H	3L 1H
Creatinine (μmol/L)	790	876	908	1026	1116	1139	1104
Urea (mmol/L)	20.9	24.7	21.0	22.4	23.1	21.8	21.7
Triglyceride (mmol/L)	2.40	4.12	4.80	4.50	2.71	4.65	3.57
Cholesterol (mmol/L)	6.35	7.44	7.08	8.35	9.19	7.87	9.11

* = Low concentration, M = Medium concentration, H = High concentration.

elevated levels of the circulating gluconeogenic precursors lactate and alanine. Decreased circulating levels of the ketone bodies may also be explained by insulin mediated reduction in nonesterified fatty acid substrate supply.

There is therefore good reason to study alternative osmotic agents. Glycerol was well tolerated and free of side-effects in the short-term studies and in one patient in the long-term. As expected, glycerol was more rapidly absorbed than dextrose, but the calorific value of the absorbed glycerol was nevertheless significantly lower than that of the absorbed glucose and this would be a worthwhile saving, particularly in obese patients. However, ultrafiltration with glycerol-based fluids was substantially less than with dextrose-based fluids, despite an adequate osmotic gradient, possibly due to an alteration in the characteristics in the peritoneal membrane by either agent. The concentration of glycerol in dialysis fluid would therefore have to be increased to improve ultrafiltration and the resulting increase in glycerol would probably offset the calorific advantage.

The main advantage of glycerol observed in these studies was that it was associated with substantially lower plasma glucose levels and consequently reduced circulating insulin concentrations. Despite this, we observed no immediate alteration in intermediate metabolite concentrations. Studies on the use of glycerol in diabetic patients on CAPD would be justified as glycerol metabolism occurs in the absence of an insulin response.

The high glycerol levels observed during dialysis with glycerol-based dialysis fluid caused no apparent toxic effect. No accumulation of glycerol was observed over 6 months continuous use of glycerol-based fluids in one patient.

That glycerol could be successfully used as an osmotic agent in CAPD was demonstrated over 6 months in one patient. There were no problems with fluid balance and he remained well dialysed. However, no advantage of glycerol over glucose emerged in this study, despite reduced insulin levels, indeed triglyceride concentrations were increased rather than decreased in our patient and it seems justified to study the use of glycerol in several more patients to establish whether or not glycerol has any clinical advantages.

ACKNOWLEDGMENTS

Figure 1 reprinted by permission from Clinical Science 65:539, copyright © 1983, The Biochemical Society, London. Figure 2 reprinted by permission from Clinical Science 67 in press, copyright © 1984, The Biochemical Society, London. A. Heaton is supported by MRC Project Grant No. 412203. D.G. Johnston is a Wellcome Senior Research Fellow. Financial aid from the British Diabetic Association and Travenol Laboratories is also acknowledged.

REFERENCES

1. Spitz IM, Rubenstein AH, Bersohn I, Abrahams C, and Lowry C: Carbohydrate metabolism in renal disease. QJ Med 39: 201, 1970
2. Cerletty JM, and Engbring NH: Azotemia and glucose intolerance. Ann Intern Med 66: 1097, 1967
3. Westervelt FB: Insulin effect in uremia. J Lab Clin Med 74: 79, 1969
4. Smith D, and Defronzo RA: Insulin resistance in uremia mediated by postbinding defects. Kidney Int 22: 54, 1982
5. Jaspan JB, and Rubenstein AH: Circulating glucagon: Plasma profiles and metabolism in health and disease. Diabetes 26: 887, 1977
6. Samaan NA, and Freeman RM: Growth hormone levels in severe renal failure. Metabolism 19: 102, 1970
7. Bagdade JD, Porte D Jr, and Bierman EL: Hypertriglyceridemia, a metabolic consequence of chronic renal failure. N Engl J Med 279: 181, 1968
8. Norbeck HE, and Carlson LA: The uremic dyslipoproteinaemia: Its characteristics and relations to clinical factors. Acta Med Scand 209: 489, 1981
9. Chan MK, Varghese Z, Persaud JW, Baillod RA, and Moorhead JF: Hyperlipidaemia in patients on maintenance haemo- and peritoneal dialysis: The relative pathogenetic roles of triglyceride production and triglyceride removal. Clin Nephrol 17: 183, 1982
10. Hampers CL, Soeldner JS, Doak PB, and Merrill JP: Effect of chronic renal failure and hemodialysis on carbohydrate metabolism. J Clin Invest 45: 1719, 1966
11. McCosh EJ, Solangi K, Rivers JM, and Goodman A: Hypertriglyceridemia in patients with chronic renal failure insufficiency. Am J Clin Nutr 28: 1036, 1975
12. Spitz I, Rubenstein AH, Bersohn I, Lawrence AM, and Kirsteins L: The effect of dialysis on the carbohydrate intolerance of chronic renal failure. Hormone Metab Res 2: 86, 1970
13. Boyer J, Gill GN, and Epstein FH: Hyperglycemia and hyperosmolality complicating peritoneal dialysis. Ann Intern Med 67: 568, 1967
14. Desanto NG, Capodicasa G, Senatore R, Cicchetti T, Cirillo D, Damiano M, Torella R, Giugliano D, Improta L, and Giordano C: Glucose utilization from dialysate in patients on continuous ambulatory peritoneal dialysis (CAPD). Int J Artif Organs 2: 119, 1979
15. Vas SI, Duwe A, and Weatherhead J: Natural defence mechanisms of the peritoneum: The effect of peritoneal dialysis fluid on polymorphonuclear cells. In Atkins RC, Thompson NM, and Farrell PC (Eds), Peritoneal dialysis. Edinburgh: Churchill Livingstone, 1981, p 41
16. McGary TJ, Nolph KD, and Kartinos NJ: Polyanions as osmotic agents in a simulated in vitro model of peritoneal dialysis. Trans Am Soc Artif Intern Organs 27: 314, 1981
17. Williams P, Marliss EB, Anderson GH, Oren A, Stein A, Khanna R, Pettit J, Brandes L, Rodella H, Mupas L, Dombros N, and Oreopoulos DG: Amino acid absorption following intraperitoneal administration in CAPD patients. Peritoneal Dial Bull 2: 124, 1982
18. Bazzato G, Coli U, Landini S, Fracasso A, Moraciello P, Righetto F, and Scanferla F: Xylitol and low dosages of insulin: New perspectives for diabetic uremic patients on CAPD. Peritoneal Dial Bull 2: 161, 1981
19. Lloyd B, Burrin JM, Smythe P, and Alberti KGMM; Enzymatic fluorometric continuous flow assay for blood glucose, lactate, pyruvate, alanine, glycerol and 3-hydroxybutyrate. Clin Chem 24: 1724, 1978
20. Price CP, Lloyd B, and Alberti KGMM: A kinetic spectrophotometric assay for rapid determination of acetoacetate in blood. Clin Chem 23: 1893, 1977
21. Soeldner JS, and Slone D: Critical variables in the radioimmunoassay of serum insulin using the double antibody technic. Diabetes 14: 771, 1965
22. Orskov H, Thomsen HG, and Yde H: Wick chromatography for rapid and reliable immunoassay of insulin, glucagon and growth hormone. Nature (London) 219: 193, 1968
23. Canaud B, Liendo-Liendo C, Claret G, Mion H, and Mion C: Etude in situ de la cinetique de l'ultrafiltration en cours de dialyse peritoneale avec periodes de diffusion prolongee. Nephrologie 1: 126, 1980

I.S. Henderson, I.A. Couper, and A. Lumsden

47

Potentially Irritant Glucose Metabolites in Unused CAPD Fluid

SUMMARY

Many CAPD patients experience discomfort on infusion of hypertonic peritoneal dialysis fluid which can be relieved by the addition of 8.4% sodium bicarbonate prior to use. The irritant effect has been attributed to low pH or the presence of glucose metabolites including 5-hydroxymethylfurfural (5-HMF). In a study designed to evaluate this problem we demonstrated that the relief of pain induced by bicarbonate was not completely due to pH neutralization; pH decreased and the concentration of 5-HMF increased with age of fluid as did the clinical experience of pain. There was a qualitative change in the wavelength of peak absorbance on UV spectrometry indicating formation of species other than 5-HMF. Peritoneal dialysis fluid should be used as quickly as possible after manufacture, and statutory limits for pH and 5-HMF should be defined.

INTRODUCTION

Pain that occurs during inflow of dialysate has been variously attributed to excessively hot or cold fluid[1] or, in the case of hypertonic dextrose dialysis fluid, to low pH, often necessitating neutralization with sodium hydroxide[2] or sodium bicarbonate[3] for pain relief.

The low pH of dextrose-containing dialysis fluid results from the need to adjust the pH to ap-

proximately 5.0 prior to autoclaving. This limits the caramelization of glucose to colored products[4] and reduces the formation of glucose metabolites, of which 5-hydroxymethylfurfural (5-HMF) is the commonest and most readily detectable.[5] Prolonged storage of hypertonic dextrose dialysis fluid might also be expected to result in glucose degradation along the same pathway with accumulation of 5-HMF and some of its acidic metabolites[6] (Fig. 1).

Approximately 10% of our CAPD patient population experienced "hypertonic infusion pain" (HIP) requiring prior injection of sodium bicarbonate into the dialysate for its relief. We set out to investigate the clinical and chemical effects of the use of hypertonic dialysis solutions of varying ages.

PATIENTS AND METHODS

Ten of 70 patients on our CAPD program experienced HIP and were included in the study. The group comprised six males and four females. As there might conceivably have been other etiologies for pain, patients established on CAPD for less than 3 months were not considered as suffering from HIP. The diagnosis of HIP was confirmed by relief of pain with 8.4% sodium bicarbonate, usually at a dose of 4 ml/L of dialysis solution. Prior to the initiation of treatment with 8.4% sodium bicarbonate, the incidence of bacterial peritonitis was comparable in both HIP and non-HIP patients. The degree of pain was gauged with a bar chart graded from 0 (no pain) to 10 (extreme pain) which the patients were asked to score during an attack of pain.

From the Renal Unit and Pharmacy, Glasgow Royal Infirmary, Glasgow, Scotland.

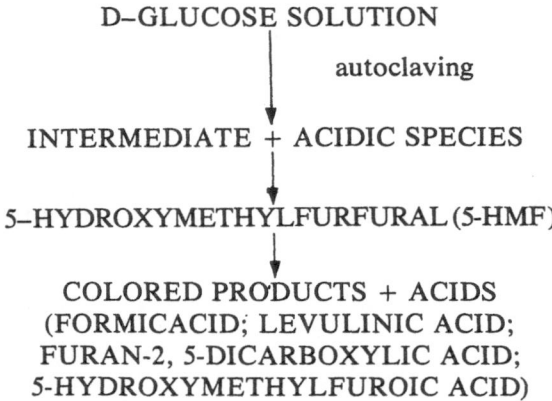

Fig. 1. Postulated pathway for degradation of D-glucose aqueous solutions.

Dialysis solution pH was measured by standard methods and the approximate levels of glucose metabolites (principally 5-HMF) by UV absorbance at about 284 nm using a Pye Unicam SP8-400 spectrophotometer.[7] Results are expressed as mean ± one standard deviation. The hypertonic dialysis fluid used in these studies was Peritoflex 4.25% (Fresenius, Bad Homburg).

RESULTS

Clinical Studies

Effect of age of dialysis fluid on HIP (Fig. 2). There was a significant correlation between the clinical experience of pain and age of the dialysis fluid, the severest pain being caused by dialysis solution more than 18 months old.

Amount of 8.4% bicarbonate required to reduce HIP due to dialysis fluid 24 months old (Fig. 3). When 2 ml/L 8.4% sodium bicarbonate was added to 24-month-old hypertonic dialysis fluid prior to infusion, there was little alleviation of pain. By contrast, 4 ml/L 8.4% sodium bicarbonate almost completely abolished HIP.

Incidence of bacterial peritonitis during bicarbonate therapy. During 6 months of regular bicarbonate injections, the incidence of bacterial

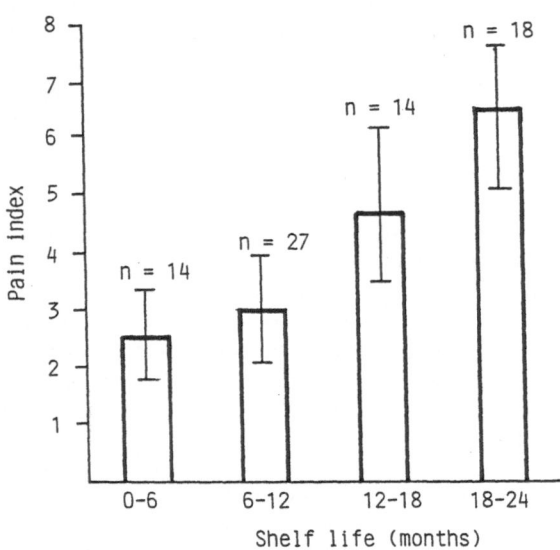

Fig. 2. Relationship between HIP to shelf life of hypertonic CAPD fluid (mo)—10 patients; 73 occasions.

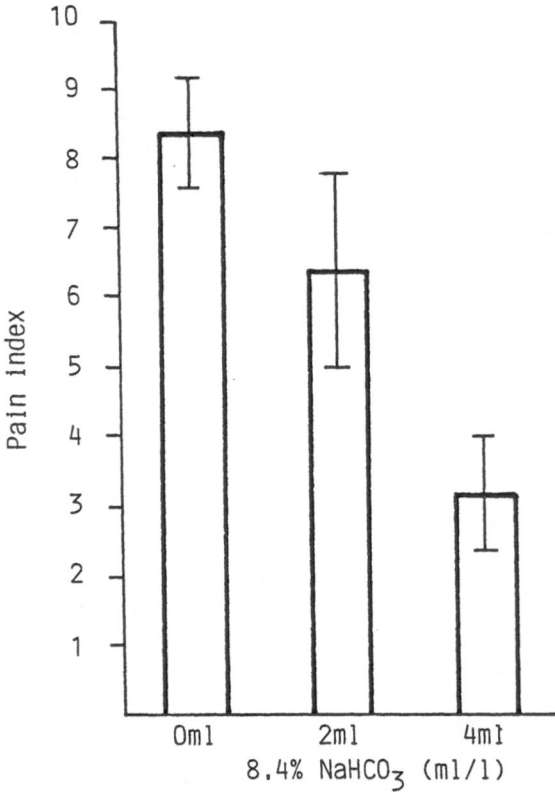

Fig. 3. Dose of 8.4% $NaHCO_3$ (ml/L) required to counter HIP induced by 24 mo old hypertonic dialysis solution (10 episodes for each dose).

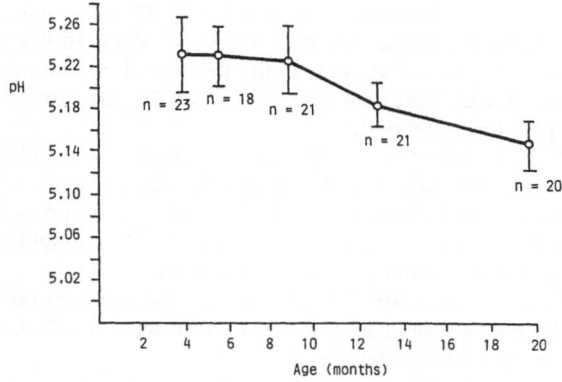

Fig. 4. Effect of age of hypertonic dialysis solution on pH.

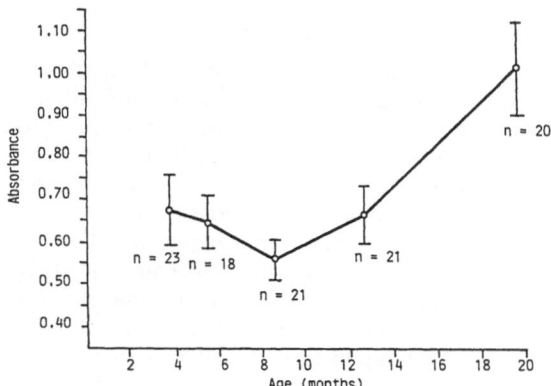

Fig. 6. Change in UV absorbance at 284 nm related to age of dialysis fluid.

peritonitis in the 10 patients studied was 1 episode/4 patient months. In a similar period following bicarbonate therapy, the incidence was 1 episode/9 patient months.

Chemical Studies

Effect of age of hypertonic dialysis fluid on pH (Fig. 4). During the process of 20 months storage in the manufacturers recommended conditions, the pH of hypertonic dialysate fell considerably.

Effect of titration of 8.4% sodium bicarbonate on pH of old and new isotonic and hypertonic dialysis fluid (Fig. 5). pH values of both "new" (3 months old) and "old" (24 months old) hypertonic and isotonic dialysis solutions were situated within a

narrow range, although that of old hypertonic fluid was the lowest. On titration with 8.4% sodium bicarbonate, approximately 2.5 ml/L was required to raise the pH of old hypertonic fluid to the same level as new dialysis fluid. This is significantly less than the 4 ml/L sodium bicarbonate required to abolish HIP. Even after addition of 5.5 ml sodium bicarbonate, hypertonic dialysis fluid remained more acidic than isotonic.

Effect of age of hypertonic dialysate on UV absorbance of 284 nm (Fig. 6). There was significant accumulation of 5-HMF and related substances after storage for 20 months. There were also changes in the wavelength of peak absorbance indicating degradation of 5-HMF into other chemical species.

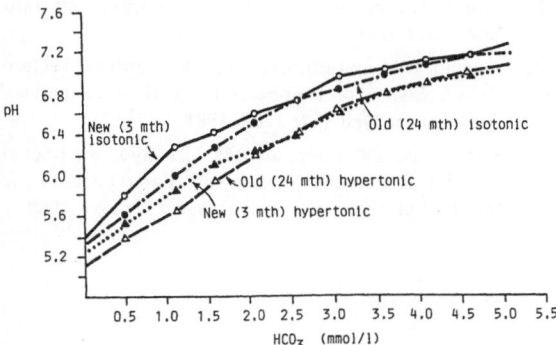

Fig. 5. Effect of addition of 8.4% sodium bicarbonate on old (24 mo old) and new (3 mo old) isotonic and hypertonic dialysis solutions.

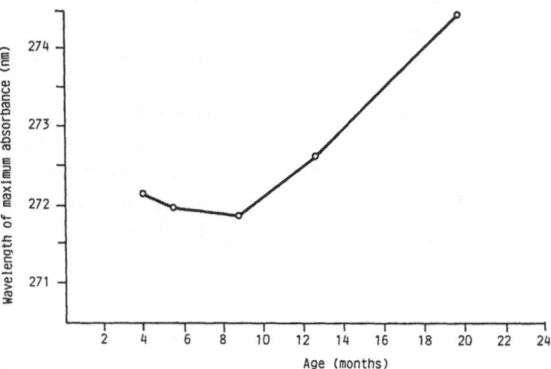

Fig. 7. Effect of age of hypertonic dialysis fluid on wavelength of maximum absorbance of 5-HMF and related substances.

264

Henderson, et al.

DISCUSSION

Our results indicate that the clinical experience of hypertonic infusion pain (HIP) correlates with the length of time the dialysis fluid was stored prior to use. In the past, HIP has been attributed solely to low pH[8] on the basis of its abolition by the addition of alkaline solutions, but as less bicarbonate is needed to raise the pH of old hypertonic fluid to reasonable levels than to abolish the pain, it is likely that the accumulation of other glucose metabolites may also play a role. With age of the solution there is certainly a build-up of 5-HMF and probably also of some of its metabolites (Fig.1) as indicated by the change in wavelength of peak UV absorbance. Chemical studies have suggested that furan acids may be implicated.[6]

Which of the various chemical species thus formed is responsible for HIP and whether in the long term damage to the peritoneum results, has not yet been evaluated. In the absence of data on the peritoneum, it is interesting to note the study by Fonkalsrud et al.[9] on postinfusion thrombophlebitis with 5% dextrose. The incidence of this complication was reduced by 50% on prior neutralization of the dextrose, but was not completely abolished. Moreover, different manufacturers' solutions neutralized to the same pH produced different incidences of thrombophlebitis, again probably implicating other chemicals.

At the present time, there are no statutory limits for pH or for glucose degradation products in peritoneal dialysis solutions. The only available guidelines are those laid down for 5% dextrose for parenteral use in the British and U.S. Pharmacopoeias[7] ("5-HMF and related substances: The UV absorbance of a solution containing 1 g of dextrose diluted to 250 ml with water at about 284 nm is not more than 0.25"). Even 24 month old hypertonic dialysis solution conformed to these limits in our study. However, statutory limits must be defined for peritoneal dialysis solutions to which patients may be exposed over many years as opposed to much shorter periods in the case of 5% dextrose for intravenous use.

Further chemical studies using more sophisticated analytical techniques including high perform-ance liquid chromatography (HPLC)[6] will be needed to characterize glucose degradation products in PD fluid and animal studies on the peritoneal irritation induced by these substances will enable statutory limits to be defined.

As there was a lower incidence of HIP using dialysis solutions less then 18 months old, we recommend a rapid turnover of fluid stocks and reconsideration of the current 2 year shelf life. This should reduce the experience of a troublesome complication and eliminate the extra procedure involved in the addition of bicarbonate with the attendant risk of bacterial contamination.

REFERENCES

1. Mion CM: Practical use of peritoneal dialysis. In Drukker W, Parsons FM, and Maher JF (Eds), Replacement of renal function by dialysis. The Hague: Martinus Nijhoff, 1983, p 457
2. Tenckhoff H: Chronic Peritoneal Dialysis Manual. Seattle, University of Washington School of Medicine, 1974, p 57
3. Robson M, Pinto T, Kao E, and Oren A: The metabolism of lactate and bicarbonate in CAPD. In Atkins RC, Thomson NM, and Farrell PC (Eds), Peritoneal dialysis. Edinburgh: Churchill Livingstone, 1981, p 211
4. Jurgens RW, Lacz JP, and Welco AD: Color analysis of dextrose solutions using color difference meter. J Pharm Sci 67: 1485, 1978
5. Shpak RS: Determination of glucose stability in a concentrated plasma substituting Ringers solution. Khim Pharm Zh 6: 50, 1972
6. Hung CT, Selkirk AB, and Taylor RB: Chromatographic QC procedure based on HPLC for 5-HMF in autoclaved D-glucose infusion fluids. J Clin Hosp Pharm 7: 17, 1982
7. British Pharmacopoeia. Dextrose intravenous infusion. 1980, p 601
8. Schmidt RW, and Blumenkrantz M: Peritoneal sclerosis—A Sword of Democles for peritoneal dialysis? Arch Intern Med 141: 1265, 1981
9. Fonkalsrud EW, Pederson BM, Murray J, and Beckerman JH: Reduction of infusion thrombophlebitis with buffered glucose solutions. Surgery 63: 280, 1968

J.J. Frifelt and F. Bangsgaard Pedersen

48

CAPD Using a High Calcium Concentration

SUMMARY

The daily calcium transfer was studied in two groups of CAPD patients using two different dialysis fluids containing 2.25 and 1.75 mmol/L of calcium, respectively. In the first group 4.43 mmol per day of calcium was taken up from the fluid and in the second group 1.89 mmol, which was significantly lower.

Furthermore the long term effects were studied in eight patients treated with dialysis fluid containing 2.25 mmol/L of calcium and in 18 patients treated with fluid containing 1.75 mmol/L of calcium. After 10 months a significant rise of serum calcium and phosphate and a fall in serum PTH was demonstrated in the first group. In the second group no significant changes took place.

The present studies indicate that CAPD using a calcium concentration of 2.25 mmol/L might be advantageous in comparison to one of 1.75 mmol/L with respect of reducing serum PTH.

INTRODUCTION

This study was undertaken to investigate calcium transfer in CAPD at two different concentrations of calcium in the dialysis fluid. Furthermore over 10 months we investigated two groups of CAPD patients using different concentrations of calcium in the dialysis fluid to examine long-term effects on parathyroid and bone metabolism.

From the Nephrology Department of Odense University Hospital, Denmark.

MATERIAL AND METHODS

Transfer Studies

Two groups of end stage renal disease (ESRD) patients treated with CAPD were investigated. All patients were on CAPD with four exchanges/day. The bag volume in both groups was 2.0 L and the calcium concentration in the dialysis fluid used in group I was 1.75 mmol/L and in group II 2.25 mmol/L. There were five patients in each group. During four consecutive cycles, dialysis fluid was sampled before instillation and after outflow, for determination of calcium. Serum calcium and albumin were analyzed and the weight of the bag before instillation and after outflow was registered for determination of the ultrafiltration volume. Hence the net calcium flux could be determined.

Blood and dialysate analyses were performed by routine methods at our laboratory. The statistical method used was Student's unpaired t-test.

Longitudinal Study

Two groups of patients with ESRD were included in the study. Eight patients dialyzed with a fluid concentration of calcium of 2.25 mmol/L (group I), and 18 patients dialyzed with a fluid concentration of 1.75 mmol/L (group II). All patients dialyzed in their homes with four daily exchanges with bag sizes varying from 1 to 2 L. All were given a free daily diet containing about 1 g of calcium. Group I comprised four men and four women with a mean age of 46.3 years. Group II comprised 10 men and

Table 1. The Total Net Transport of Calcium per Day (Mean ± SD).

	Group I*	Group II†	Significance
Net flow of calcium (mmol/day)	1.89 ± 0.94	4.43 ± 1.19	$p < 0.005$
Ultrafiltration (g/day)	592 ± 351	473 ± 443	n.s.‡
Total serum calcium (mmol/L)	2.38 ± 0.21	2.38 ± 0.23	n.s.
Serum albumin (g/L)	39	37	n.s.

* Concentration of calcium in dialysis fluid 1.75 mmol/L.
† Concentration of calcium in dialysis fluid 2.25 mmol/L.
‡ n.s. = not significant.

eight women with a mean age of 48.2 years. Each month blood samples were drawn to analyze the serum values of calcium, phosphate, albumin, and alkaline phosphatase by routine methods. Every 3 months serum parathormone (PTH) was analyzed by radioimmunoassay for C-terminal PTH while bone densitometry was performed by photoabsorptiometry using ^{121}I as the radioactive isotope. The administration of vitamin D analogues and phosphate binders were recorded.

The statistical method used was Student's paired and unpaired t-tests. In the description of the results, all values are given as means (± 1 SD) after 1 and 2 months (start) and after 9 and 10 months (end).

RESULTS

Transfer Studies

The results are shown in Table 1. In both groups there was a positive mean net transfer of calcium into the patients. Comparing the transfer of calcium in the two groups, there was a significantly greater net input in group II with the higher calcium concentration in the dialysis fluid. There was no significant difference between the serum concentration of total calcium and the ultrafiltration volume between the two groups.

Table 2. Serum Values in Group I* at Start and End of the Study Period (Mean ± SD).

	Start	End	Significance
Serum calcium (mmol/L)	2.40 ± 0.17	2.55 ± 0.18	$p < 0.05$
Serum phosphate (mmol/L)	1.71 ± 0.48	2.34 ± 0.72	$p < 0.025$
Alkaline phosphatase (U/L)	160 ± 68	146 ± 44	n.s.†
Albumin (g/L)	33 ± 4	34 ± 3	n.s.
PTH (μg/L)	4.88 ± 2.36	2.20 ± 0.69	$p < 0.01$

* Calcium concentration in dialysis fluid 2.25 mmol/L.
† n.s. = not significant.

Table 3. Serum Values in Group II* at Start and End of the Study Period (Mean ± SD).

	Start	End	Significance
Serum calcium (mmol/L)	2.35 ± 0.22	2.38 ± 0.16	n.s.†
Serum phosphate (mmol/L)	1.66 ± 0.37	1.77 ± 0.46	n.s.
Alkaline phosphatase (U/L)	155 ± 52	138 ± 56	n.s.
Serum albumin (g/L)	36 ± 4	37 ± 3	n.s.
PTH (μg/L)	4.20 ± 3.18	3.30 ± 3.59	n.s.

* Calcium concentration in dialysis fluid 1.75 mmol/L.
n.s. = not significant.

Longitudinal Studies

Serum total calcium. In group I (Table 2) mean serum calcium at the start of the period under study was 2.40 ± 0.17 mmol/L, rising significantly to 2.55 ± 0.18 mmol/L by the end ($p < 0.05$). In group II (Table 3) mean serum calcium rose, but not significantly, from 2.35 ± 0.22 mmol/L at the start, to 2.38 ± 0.16 mmol/L at the end of the study period. The rise in serum calcium during the period under study in group I was significantly greater than that of group II ($p < 0.0125$) (Table 4). The range of reference values for calcium was 2.29–2.67 mmol/L.

Serum phosphate. The initial value of phosphate in group I (Table 2) was 1.71 ± 0.48 mmol/L, rising significantly during the study period to 2.34 ± 0.72 mmol/L ($p < 0.025$). In group II no significant rise took place; the initial value was 1.66 ± 0.37 mmol/L and the final value was 1.77 ± 0.46 mmol/L (Table 3). The rise in serum phosphate was significantly greater in group I than in group II ($p < 0.0125$) (Table 4). The range of reference value for phosphate was 0.79–1.56 mmol/L.

Serum albumin. In group I the initial value of albumin was 33 ± 4 g/L, which rose to 34 ± 3 g/L (Table 2). This was not significant, nor was the rise in group II from a value of 36 ± 4 g/L to 37 ± 3 g/L (Table 3).

Mean albumin concentration was significantly higher in group II than in group I. The range of reference for albumin was 36–46 g/L.

Table 4. Serum Values in Group I and II (Mean ± SD).

		Group I	Group II	Significance
Total serum calcium (mmol/L)	start	2.40 ± 0.17	2.35 ± 0.22	n.s.*
	end	2.55 ± 0.18	2.38 ± 0.16	$p < 0.0125$
Serum phosphate (mmol/L)	start	1.71 ± 0.48	1.66 ± 0.37	n.s.
	end	2.34 ± 0.72	1.77 ± 0.46	$p < 0.0125$
Serum alkaline phosphatases (U/L)	start	169 ± 67	155 ± 52	n.s.
	end	146 ± 44	138 ± 56	n.s.
Albumin (g/L)	start	33 ± 4	36 ± 4	$p < 0.05$
	end	34 ± 3	37 ± 3	$p < 0.025$
PTH (μg/L)	start	4.88 ± 2.36	4.20 ± 3.18	n.s.
	end	2.20 ± 0.69	3.30 ± 3.59	n.s.

* n.s. = not significant.

Serum alkaline phosphatase. At the start of the study, the value in group I was 160 ± 68 U/L, and during the observation period it fell to an end value of 146 ± 44 U/L (Table 2). In group II the value declined from 155 ± 52 U/L to 138 ± 56 U/L (Table 3). None of these changes were significant, nor was there a difference between the values in group I and II (Table 4). The range of reference for alkaline phosphatase was 80–275 U/L.

Parathormone (PTH). In group I there was a significant fall from an initial value of 4.88 ± 2.36 μg/L to a final value of 2.20 ± 0.69 μg/L ($p < 0.01$) (Table 2). In group II the fall from 4.20 ± 3.18 μg/L to 3.30 ± 3.59 μg/L was not significant (Table 3). There were no significant differences between the initial or final values between the two groups (Table 4). The range of reference for PTH is 0.22–0.50 μg/L.

Bone densitometry. The initial values for bone densitometry in groups I and II were not significantly different (0.68 ± 0.20 and 0.58 ± 0.20 U respectively), and no significant changes took place within the groups during the observation period. In group I the initial value was 0.68 ± 0.20 and the final value was 0.69 ± 0.19 U. In group II the initial value was 0.58 ± 0.20 and the final value 0.57 ± 0.19 U.

Medical administration. One patient in group I and three patients in group II received 1α-hydroxy-cholecalciferol. The doses given varied between 0.25 μg and 1 μg daily. Phosphate binders were given as a liquid solution of aluminum aminoacetate in a daily dose of 2.5–7.5 g. Four patients in group I and 17 patients in group II received phosphate binders.

DISCUSSION

In our transport study, we found that, with a calcium concentration of 2.25 mmol/L in the dialysis fluid, an average of 4.43 mmol was taken up, which equals 173 mg/day of calcium. With a calcium concentration of 1.75 mmol/L, the daily uptake was 1.89 mmol, which equals 75.6 mg/day.

The long term effect of using a concentration of 2.25 mmol/L of calcium in the dialysis fluid was a fall in serum PTH and alkaline phosphatase, although the latter was not statistically significant, and a rise in serum calcium and phosphate. These findings indicate that better control of renal osteodystrophy might have been obtained, although we were unable to demonstrate a rise in bone density during 10 months observation. The rising serum phosphate may be explained by inadequate dosage of phosphate binders in these patients.

In the group of patients using a calcium concentration of 1.75 mmol/L in the fluid, no significant changes took place. In these patients there were no significant signs of a better control of the hyperparathyroidism.

Similar studies have been made by others. Tielemans et al.[1] found that an average of 2.4 ± 13.9 mg calcium/day was taken up from dialysis fluid containing 1.75 mmol/L calcium with some patients having negative calcium balance. Furthermore, they found that when using a calcium concentration of 1.75 mmol/L in the fluid, without vitamin D analogues or oral calcium supplements, that serum calcium decreased and alkaline phosphatase increased. On the other hand, when supplying 3 g calcium carbonate/day, a rise in serum calcium and a fall in serum PTH could be demonstrated after 4 to 6 months.[1] Kurtz et al.[2] found a mean calcium uptake of 16 ± 28 mg/24 hours using a calcium concentration of 1.75 mmol/L in the dialysis fluid. On the background of a long-term study of CAPD patients during 6 to 12 months, they recommended that the serum calcium should be maintained high (2.25–2.73 mmol/L) either by vitamin D analogues and calcium supplements, or by increasing the calcium concentration in the dialysis fluid to 1.88 or 2.0 mmol/L.

Delmez et al.[3] also studied CAPD patients using dialysis fluids with calcium concentrations of 1.75 mmol/L. The daily uptake of calcium in these patients was found to be only 9.9 mg. They recommended that an increased concentration of calcium should be used in the dialysis fluids.

Thus, several authors have suggested that a calcium concentration higher than 1.75 mmol/L should be used in the dialysis fluid, to establish better control of the dialysis-related osteodystrophy. This is the first report of a long-term study with CAPD patients using a calcium concentration of 2.25 mmol/L in the fluid, and our results indicate that this concentration might be advantageous in comparison with a concentration of 1.75 mmol/L. Whether a calcium concentration of 2.25 mmol/L is too high, remains to be established.

REFERENCES

1. Tielemans C, Aubry C, and Dratwa M: The effects of continuous peritoneal dialysis (CAPD) on renal osteodystrophy. In Gahl GM, Kessel M, and Nolph KD

(Eds), Advances in peritoneal dialysis: Proceedings of the 2nd international symposium on peritoneal dialysis. Amsterdam: Exerpta Medica, 1981, p 455

2. Kurtz SB, McCarthy JT, and Kumar R: Hypercalcemia in continuous ambulatory peritoneal dialysis (CAPD) patients: Observations on parameters of calcium metabolism. In Gahl GM, Kessel M, and Nolph KD (Eds), Advances in peritoneal dialysis: Proceedings of the 2nd international symposium on peritoneal dialysis. Amsterdam: Excerpta Medica, 1981, p 467

3. Delmez JA, Slatopolsky E, Martin KJ, Gearing BN, and Harter HR: Minerals, vitamin D, and parathyroid hormone in continuous ambulatory peritoneal dialysis. Kidney Int 21: 862, 1982

A. Katirtzoglou, G.E. Digenis, P. Kontesis,
B. Karamanos, and A. Symvoulidis

49

Is Peritoneal Ultrafiltration Influenced by Acetate or Lactate Buffers?

SUMMARY

Loss of net ultrafiltration (UF) of the peritoneum is a serious complication in patients undergoing CAPD, and acetate has been considered as one of the possible causes. Three different peritoneal solutions (Brand A: acetate (A) or lactate (L_1); Brand B: lactate (L_2)) produced by two different firms were used in six patients treated by CAPD. Net UF and absolute glucose absorption (GA) from the peritoneum as well as plasma glucose (PG) and insulin levels (PI) were measured before and during the experiment. There was no difference in net UF and PG levels with the three peritoneal solutions used, but GA was significantly lower with solution L_2 in comparison to L_1 and A. Concerning the changes in PI levels and the insulinogenic index $\left(\dfrac{PI}{PE}\right)$ there was a trend for higher levels with both lactates compared to acetate, but the differences were not statistically significant. These findings do not support the hypothesis that acetate or lactate can be incriminated in the decrease of peritoneal UF.

INTRODUCTION

The peritoneal dialysis (PD) system can be considered to be based on the ultrafiltration (UF) capacity of the peritoneal membrane.

From the Second Department of Internal Medicine, Athens University Medical School, Hippokration Hospital, Athens, Greece.

Reduction of the peritoneal UF has been reported as a complication in a few patients treated with intermittent PD,[1,2] but it has been more frequently noted among CAPD patients.[3]

The severity of this complication is emphasized by the fact that patients with severe reduction of peritoneal UF have to be transferred to another type of dialysis (i.e., hemodialysis). The etiology of this impairment of peritoneal functional capacity remains unknown, although various factors have been incriminated. Acetate has been considered as one of the possible causative factors.

In the present study we have tried to elucidate the role of acetate as a possible cause of loss of UF by comparing the net UF produced by solutions containing either acetate or lactate, in the same group of patients. In addition, in an effort to explain possible differences we have studied the changes in plasma insulin levels occurring during the infusion of acetate or lactate solutions.

MATERIAL AND METHODS

Six patients with end stage renal failure treated by CAPD were studied (2 male, 4 female aged 38 to 67 years, average 55 years).

All patients were transferred from hemodialysis and the duration of treatment with CAPD was 9 to 310 days, with an average stay of 164 days. None was diabetic or had vascular disease. The primary renal disease was chronic glomerulonephritis in five patients and pyelonephritis in one. Their residual renal function (endogenous creatinine clearance)

Table 1. Net Ultrafiltration and Glucose Absorption with the
Three Different Solutions.

	Net UF (mL)	Amount of Glucose Absorbed (g)	Significance
Brand A, A	841 ± 247	65.9 ± 1.6	net UF n.s. GA*
Brand A, L$_1$	783 ± 238	67.1 ± 1.1	net UF n.s. GA†
Brand B, L$_2$	770 ± 226	63.5 ± 1.5	net UF n.s. GA†

* $p < 0.05$.
† $p < 0.01$.
n.s. = not significant.

was zero. Four patients had never had peritonitis. The remaining two had each had one episode of peritonitis, but the study was performed not less than one month after each episode of peritonitis. CAPD was performed through a peritoneal catheter (TWH type) that had been implanted surgically under general anesthesia. All patients were dialysed with four, 2 L exchanges/day with peritoneal solutions containing acetate. The study was carried out with informed patient consent.

For the purpose of the study three kinds of dialysis solutions from two different manufacturers were used. The first brand contained acetate (A) or lactate (L$_1$), while the second brand contained lactate (L$_2$).

Every patient had one bag exchange of each dialysate on 3 different days according to the following protocol. The patient fasted in the morning and was permitted to drink only water up to the end of the experiment. After draining the peritoneal cavity from the regular dialysate (1.5% acetate type), which had been infused the previous midnight, 2 L of the peritoneal solution under study (concentration of anhydrous glucose 3.86 g/dL) was instilled.

The dwell time (from the end of the infusion to the beginning of drainage was 4 hours. The difference between the weight of the bag before the infusion and after drainage was considered net UF. Blood samples for plasma glucose (PG) and insulin (PI) levels, which were measured by an enzymatic technique and a RIA method[4] respectively, were taken at the beginning of the experiment and at the end of the first, second, third, and fourth hours. The dialysate glucose concentration was measured, in order to calculate the amount of glucose absorbed (GA) through the peritoneal membrane.

For better estimation of the insulin–glucose interactions, the insulinogenic index (plasma insulin/plasma glucose) was used. In order to compare the changes in insulin and glucose levels during the experiment, the absolute values of these parameters before the infusion were taken as 100, and the subsequent values were expressed as a percentage of the primary one.[5]

The statistical analysis of the results was performed using the Student's paired t-test.

RESULTS

Table 1 shows the net UF produced by each peritoneal solution and the amount of glucose absorbed. There was no difference in net UF with the three peritoneal solutions used, but glucose absorption was significantly lower with L$_2$ solution in comparison to L$_1$ ($p < 0.01$) and solution A ($p < 0.05$) (Fig. 1).

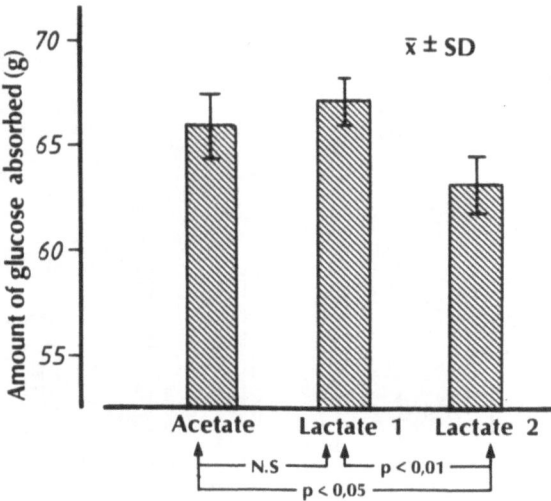

Fig. 1. Glucose absorption with the three different peritoneal solutions.

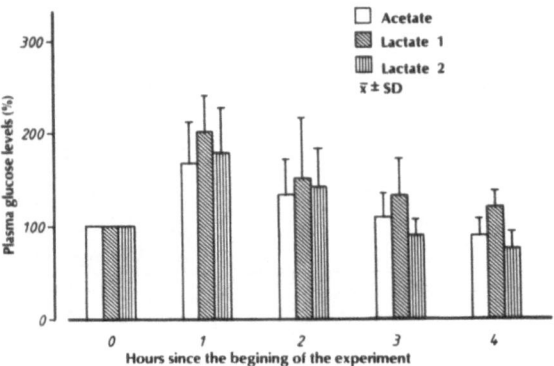

Fig. 2. Plasma glucose levels during the experiment with the three different peritoneal solutions.

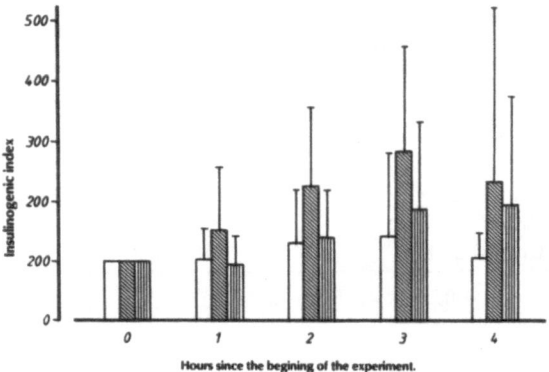

Fig. 4. Insulinogenic index during the experiment with the three different peritoneal solutions.

Figures 2 and 3 demonstrate the changes in plasma glucose and plasma insulin levels, respectively, during the experiment. The differences in plasma glucose levels were not statistically significant. As for the plasma insulin levels, both lactates (L_1 and L_2) were associated with a trend toward higher levels compared to acetate, which, however, was not statistically significant, except between the L_1 and A solutions at the end of the 3rd hour ($p < 0.05$).

The changes in the insulinogenic index are shown in Figure 4. I also showed a trend to be higher with both lactates, but the differences were not statistically significant.

CONCLUSIONS

The more experience we gain with the use of CAPD in the treatment of end stage renal failure, the more we are faced with new complications. Loss of peritoneal UF was known as a complication of intermittent PD, but it has also been described in CAPD patients, especially in Europe.[6,7]

The severity of this complication becomes clear from the fact that it can cause the dynamic failure of CAPD because of inability to maintain fluid balance.

The cause remains obscure and the incidence varies widely among the different CAPD centers. In fact, an incidence of 2.8% has been described in Toronto, Canada,[8] and 1.6% in the USA,[9] while in Europe, the situation is quite different. In one French center, a partial loss of peritoneal UF of 10% during the first, and 20% during the second year of CAPD treatment has been reported and 24% of these patients finally had to change their dialysis method.[6] Similar results were reported from another center in France.[3]

Little is known concerning the factors implicated in this complication. Regarding age, the incidence of loss of peritoneal UF was higher in older patients in Toronto, while in France there was no difference between young and old. The duration of CAPD seems to be an important factor, although there are cases that have presented loss of UF soon after the initiation of CAPD.[8]

The number of episodes of peritonitis before the loss of UF does not seem to be a stable factor, as conflicting data are reported from different CAPD centers.[3,8]

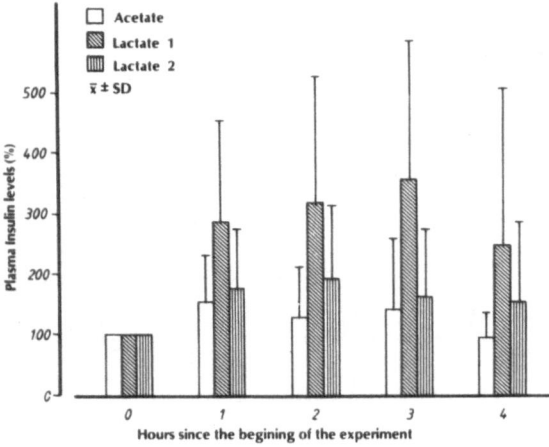

Fig. 3. Plasma insulin levels during the experiment with the three different peritoneal solutions.

The composition of the peritoneal solution has been considered as a possible source of peritoneal toxicity by several authors. As the solutions used in America and France differ in their base equivalent (lactate in America and acetate in France), acetate has been incriminated as the causative agent.[6,9]

In the present study, the peritoneal membrane of each patient was exposed to three different peritoneal solutions (acetate and two different brands of lactate). In the polycentric study designed by Nolph and collaborators,[9] however, the evaluation was based only on one bag exchange with the dialysate used by the patient.

In our study there was no difference in net UF produced with the three different peritoneal solutions. Also the stimulation of insulin secretion was not different with the dialysis fluids used. In fact, experimental data concerning the influence of acetate or lactate on insulin secretion are contradictory.[10,11] The peritoneal glucose absorption was similar with the acetate and lactate solutions of one brand, but significantly lower with the lactate solution of the second brand.

Therefore, based on these data, it does not seem that acetate or lactate is the causative factor of peritoneal UF loss, and further investigations should be carried on to elucidate whether factors other than the base equivalent and related to the brand itself are to be considered.

REFERENCES

1. Mion C, Slingeneyer A, Canaud B, and Elie M: A review of 7 year's home peritoneal dialysis. Proc Eur Dial Transplant Assoc 18: 91, 1981

2. Oreopoulos DG, Gotloib L, Calderaro V, and Khanna R: How long can peritoneal dialysis be continued? Can Med Assoc J 124: 12, 1981

3. Faller B, and Marichal JF: Loss of ultrafiltration in continuous ambulatory peritoneal dialysis: Clinical data. In Gahl GM, Kessel M, and Nolph KD (Eds), Advances in peritoneal dialysis: Proceedings of the 2nd international symposium on peritoneal dialysis. Amsterdam: Excerpta Medica, 1981, p 227

4. Midgley AR, Rebar RW, and Niswender GD: Radioimmunoassays employing double antibody techniques. Acta Endocrinol [Suppl] (Copenh) 142: 247, 1969

5. Perley M, and Wipnis DM: Plasma insulin responses to oral and I.V. infused glucose. J Clin Invest 46: 1954, 1967

6. Slingeneyer A, Canaud B, and Mion C: Permanent loss of ultrafiltration capacity of the peritoneum in long-term peritoneal dialysis: An epidemiological study. Nephron 33: 133, 1983

7. Faller B, and Marichal JF: Loss of ultrafiltration in continuous ambulatory peritoneal dialysis: A role for acetate. Peritoneal Dial Bull 4: 10, 1984

8. Manuel MA, and the University of Toronto Collaborative Dialysis Group: Failure of ultrafiltration in patient in patients on CAPD. Peritoneal Dial Bull [Suppl] 3: S38, 1983

9. Nolph KD, Ryan L, Moore H, Legrain M, Mion C, Oreopoulos DG, and Participants of the International Cooperative Study: Factors effecting ultrafiltration in continuous ambulatory peritoneal dialysis. Peritoneal Dial Bull 4: 14, 1984

10. Wathen RI, Ward RA, Harding GB, and Meyer LC: Acidbase and metabolic responses to anion infusion in the anesthetized dog. Kidney Int 21: 592, 1982

11. Federspil G, Zaccaria M, Pedrazzoli S, Zago E, DePalo C, and Scandellari C: Effects of sodium DC-lactate on insulin secretion in anesthetized dogs. Diabetes 29: 33, 1980

B. Faller and J.F. Marichal

50

Evolution of Ultrafiltration in CAPD According to the Dialysis Fluid Buffer

SUMMARY

The evolution of the peritoneal ultrafiltration rate as dialysis was continued for 30 mo in nine patients treated with CAPD using acetate buffer was compared to that in seven patients using dialysis fluid containing lactate. A 4 h dwell of 2 L of lactated hypertonic dialysis solution induced about 900 ml of ultrafiltration and this rate persisted for 30 mo. Dialysis with acetate solution yielded less ultrafiltrate and the ultrafiltration rate decreased progressively with time. When patients switched from acetate to lactate dialysis the ultrafiltrate volume increased significantly from 340 ml to 585 ml over the course of 11 mo.

INTRODUCTION

The ultrafiltration (UF) capacity of the peritoneal membrane enables water balance in chronic renal patients treated with continuous ambulatory peritoneal dialysis (CAPD) to be maintained. UF is achieved with dialysis solutions that contain high dextrose concentrations (1.50–4.33 g/dL) that are hyperosmolar to body fluids.[1] Since 1981, inability to maintain adequate UF has been described mainly in patients using acetate buffered peritoneal fluids.[2-4] This is an attempt to demonstrate the role of the acetate buffered solutions in the loss of UF.

From the Service de Néphrologie of the Hôpital Pasteur, Colmar, France.

PATIENTS AND METHODS

From May 1978 to May 1984, 77 patients entered our CAPD program. The study concerns the evolution of UF in 16 patients treated with this technique for more than 2 years. There were 7 males and 9 females, with a mean age 45.2 ± 14 years. The cumulative duration of CAPD was 49 years and the average duration per patient was 42.9 ± 7.3 months.

Dialysis Devices

Two types of CAPD devices have been used. The characteristics of both systems are summarized in Tables 1 and 2. The main difference concerns the buffer: acetate or lactate. Since May 1983, lactate buffered solutions made by Aguettant Labs have also been available. Dextrose concentration in hypertonic acetate peritoneal dialysis (PD) fluids is slightly higher than in lactate PD fluids: 4.33 g/dL versus 4.12 g/dL. In certain conditions (surgery, peritonitis), we use a PD machine and fluids available in 10 L containers (Dubernard Laboratory, Bordeaux, France). These solutions were buffered with acetate until September 1983; since then, they have contained lactate.

Patient Groups

The 16 patients included in the study were divided into 2 groups. Group A had 9 patients (3 male, 6 female, aged 44.2 ± 13 years) who had been using acetate- then lactate-containing solutions. From

Table 1. Characteristics of the Two Types of CAPD Solutions, Bags, and Delivery Sets.

	Aguettant	Travenol
Dialysate—Buffer	Acetate	Lactate
—pH	6.5	5.5
Container	PVC	PVC
Heat sterilization	110°C/60 minute	121°C/minute
Tubing set	Silicone	PVC
Connection site	Heat welding polycarbonate	Heat welding polyester

May 1978 to May 1983, the patients had used solutions buffered with acetate for an average duration per patient of 32.3 ± 9 months. Since June 1983, CAPD was performed with Aguettant lactate solutions during an average of 7 months/patient; then with Travenol lactate solutions during an average of 5 months. Group B had 7 patients (4 male, 3 female, aged 46.2 ± 15 years) who had exclusively been using lactate-containing solutions and CAPD devices from Travenol Laboratories during an average time per patient of 42.3 ± 5 months.

CAPD Technique

All patients performed daily CAPD with 2 L exchanges. CAPD was not stopped during the night; 87% of the patients exchanged four times/day, 6.5% three times/day, and 6.5% five times/day.

Peritonitis

The peritonitis rate in group A was 1.1 episodes/patient/year and in group B it was 0.84 episode/patient/year. The treatment of each episode was always done on an in-center basis with acetate buffered solutions in 10 L containers or 2 L bags containing antibiotics. From 1978 to 1981, treatment consisted of continuous lavage with a machine until negative dialysate cultures were obtained on three consecutive days. From 1981 to 1983, the lavage time was reduced to 12 hours, followed by CAPD with six daily exchanges. Since January 1983, we have used the technique described by Williams et al.[5]

Measurement of UF and Dextrose Absorption

Measurements of UF were done with a hypertonic (4.33 or 4.12 g/dl dextrose) 2 L, 4 hour dwell exchange. The fresh bag was weighed before instillation, and the effluent bag weighed following drainage.[6] The difference was reported as net UF. After weighing, a sample of the peritoneal effluent was drawn and dextrose concentration was measured by the hexokinase technique. Dextrose absorption during an exchange corresponded to the difference in dextrose concentration between dialysate before instillation and after drainage.

Statistical Analysis

For most variables, the mean values were compared by the Student's t-test. When the difference of the variances between two values were high, the Mann-Whitney and Wilcoxon test was used.

Table 2. Dialysate Composition (mmole/L).

	Aguettant		Travenol	
Sodium	130		132	
Calcium	1.75		1.75	
Magnesium	0.75		0.75	
Acetate	35		—	
Lactate	—		35	
Chloride	97.25		102	
Glucose	83	238	82.5	226

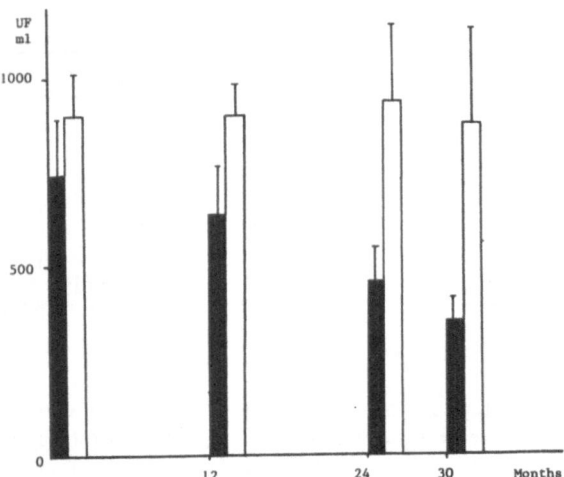

Fig. 1. Ultrafiltration rate according to dialysis fluid buffer (■ acetate, □ lactate).

RESULTS

Patients from group A underwent two periods of treatment: a first period of CAPD with acetate-containing solutions and a second period with lactate-containing solutions. During the same time, patients from group B can be considered as the reference group. We report the evolution of UF during both periods in both groups, and dextrose absorption in both groups, but only after replacing acetate by lactate-containing solutions.

Evolution of UF Volumes

UF volumes in group A during the acetate period versus UF volumes in group B are shown in Figure 1 as the mean drainage volumes obtained with hypertonic PD fluids according to the buffer and the duration of CAPD.

In group A at the initiation of CAPD, 2 L hypertonic dialysate removed 736 ± 150 ml (mean $\pm$ SD) of body water; after one year, 645 ± 119 ml; after 2 years, 460 ± 97 ml; and at 30 months, 340 ± 65 ml. In these patients, the UF volumes from the initiation of CAPD to 30 months decreased significantly ($p < 0.01$). In group B UF remained stable from the beginning of CAPD to 30 months: at the initiation, UF volumes reached 905 ± 113 ml; at one year, 902 ± 83 ml; at 2 years, 936 ± 193 ml; and at 30 months, 892 ± 295 ml. The difference between UF volumes from the initiation of CAPD to 30 months is not statistically significant. At each measurement, even at the initiation of CAPD, UF in group A was always significantly lower ($p < 0.01$) than in group B.

UF volumes in group A during the lactate period versus UF volumes in group B are shown in Figure 2. In group A at the beginning of the lactate period (June 1983), mean UF with an hypertonic, 4 hour exchange reached only 340 ± 65 ml. In May 1984, UF increased significantly to 585 ± 204 ml ($p < 0.01$). In group B during the same time, we did not observe any significant changes in UF volumes obtained in patients from group B: 907 ± 120 ml in June 1983 versus 907 ± 272 ml in May 1984.

Evolution of Dextrose Absorption

In group A (Fig. 3), the amount of dextrose absorbed from hypertonic solution during a 4 hour exchange was 3650 ± 890 mg/dl in June 1983. One year later, it decreased significantly to 3350 ± 1240 mg/dl ($p < 0.001$).

In group B, as we observed with UF volumes, dextrose absorption did not change from June 1983 to May 1984: it was respectively 3230 ± 1060 mg/dl and 3130 ± 1720 mg/dl (not significant).

Finally, dextrose absorption in June 1983 in group A and group B are statistically different ($p < 0.01$). The difference remains significant ($p < 0.01$) between both groups in May 1984.

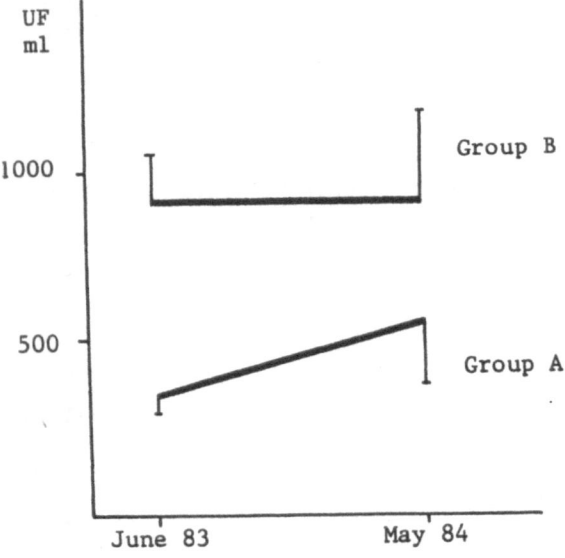

Fig. 2. Evolution of ultrafiltration after changing dialysis fluid buffer.

DISCUSSION

Loss of UF can be defined as a progressive reduction of water removal with a certain dialysis solution and for the same dwell-time.[7] The methodology of the evaluation of the peritoneal permeability has been critically analysed by Nolph et al.[8] Weighing the effluent bags and measuring dextrose concentration in the effluent fluid after a 4 hour dwell time of hypertonic solution represents the protocol used in the International Cooperative Study concerning factors affecting UF in CAPD.[8]

Maintaining water balance in patients treated with peritoneal dialysis appeared to be difficult in certain conditions. The reduction of UF capacity of the peritoneal membrane without impairment of biochemical results was first mentioned in a few patients treated with intermittent peritoneal dialysis.[9,10] This problem became particularly severe in CAPD patients; we reported a decrease in drainage volumes over the years in 73% of the patients[2] and Verger et al.[3] mentioned the same complication in 3 of 13 patients. Slingeneyer et al.[4] reported that 10% and 30% of patients lost UF at 1 and 2 years respectively. All these reports came from French Units. In contrast, in North America, loss of UF has been described in only occasional cases: 1.6% of 4838 patients from the USA CAPD Registry[8] and 2.7% of 508 patients from Toronto, Canada.[11]

We have explored possible explanations for these differences. It appeared that most patients who had experienced severe loss of UF had been using acetate solutions, while patients using lactate-containing solutions maintained their UF capacities. In North America, lactate solutions have been almost exclusively used. In two retrospective clinical studies, we confirmed the role of acetate: in the first,[7] UF obtained with hypertonic acetate solutions in 31 patients (average time on CAPD was 15.1 months) was significantly lower than in 14 patients using lactate solutions. In the second evaluation of UF reported here, the longitudinal study compares two groups of patients treated for more than 2 years: a significant decrease of UF occurred in the patients using acetate buffered fluids, whereas over the same time UF did not change in patients using lactate fluid.

In both groups using acetate, there was an inverse relationship of net UF to time. The duration of the peritoneum's exposure to acetate-containing solutions seems to play an important role in loss of UF. Though acetate dialysis solutions have been used in all patients after implantation of the catheter and in

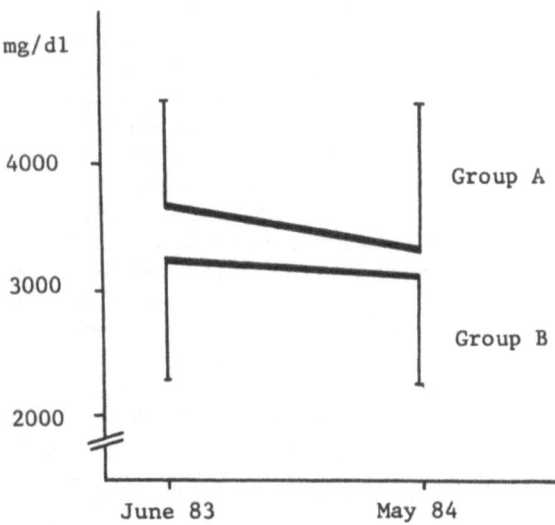

Fig. 3. Evolution of dextrose absorption after changing dialysis fluid buffer.

all peritonitis episodes, a severe reduction of UF has been observed only when CAPD was carried on with acetate solutions. Rubin et al.[12] showed no significant differences in transport features of acetate versus lactate buffered solutions in acute studies. The chronic use of acetate solutions seems to damage the UF capacities of the peritoneal membrane.

To explore more thoroughly the geographic differences in UF, an International Cooperative Study was begun in March 1983. However, in Europe, different brands of CAPD solutions have been used. The first report of the study[8] gives the results of 210 patients. The conclusion is that "the chronic use of acetate solutions appeared to be associated with more rapid decreases in dialysate glucose and low UF."

It has now been admitted that the reduction of the peritoneal membrane area is unusual[8] and that peritonitis does not influence UF over the long term. The mechanism behind loss of UF is a rapid dissipation of the osmotic gradient between plasma and peritoneal fluid.[1] Glucose may be rapidly absorbed if the peritoneal membrane becomes hyperpermeable, and the glucose concentration in the peritoneal effluent will rapidly become low. Dextrose absorption in patients from group S using acetate solutions was higher than in patients from group B using lactate solutions. The difference in glucose absorption is even more striking because the initial glucose concentration is higher in the acetate solutions than in the lactate solutions.

On the basis of these results, even if we assumed that acetate alone is not involved in loss of UF, we replaced it by lactate. During 7 months only the buffer was changed, bags were still manufactured by the same company. In December 1983, we had to stop using the French CAPD solutions. Nevertheless, one year after using exclusively lactate solutions in both groups of patients, we observed a significant increase in drainage volumes associated with a decrease in glucose absorption. Both changes were statistically significant. This means that the hyperpermeability of the peritoneum decreases and that the UF capacity partially recovered, even after a long (average 32.2 ± 9 months) exposure to acetate. Patients also mentioned less discomfort during the infusion of the lactate dialysate compared with the acetate solutions.

In patients with low UF and hyperpermeable peritoneum, Verger et al.[3] observed a patchy or total destruction of the mesothelial layer of the peritoneal membrane. It would be particularly important to see if histologic changes occur in the same way as functional changes in cases of recovery of UF. We need also to know more about peritoneal pathophysiology and mesothelial cells, and to find out the factors that would prevent structural changes in the cells or would allow their complete regeneration.[13] These factors might consist of a "rest" of the peritoneum, or in changes in the peritoneal fluid composition. The moment and the duration of the "rest" have still to be defined, and the "toxic" components of any peritoneal dialysis solution need to be identified.

REFERENCES

1. Nolph KD, Miller FN, Pyle WK, Popovich RP, and Sorkin MI: An hypothesis to explain the ultrafiltration characteristics of peritoneal dialysis. Kidney Int 20: 543, 1981
2. Faller B, and Marichal JF: Loss of ultrafiltration in CAPD: Clinical data. In Gahl GM, Kessel M, and Nolph KD (Eds), Advances in peritoneal dialysis: Proceeding of the 2nd international symposium on peritoneal dialysis. Amsterdam: Excerpta Medica, 1981, p 227
3. Verger C, Brunschvieg O, LeCharpentier Y, Lavergne A, and Vantelon J: Structural peritoneal membrane changes and permeability alterations during continuous ambulatory peritoneal dialysis. Proc Eur Dial Transplant Assoc 18: 199, 1981
4. Slingeneyer A, Canaud B, and Mion C: Permanent loss of ultrafiltration capacity of the peritoneum in long-term peritoneal dialysis: An epidemiological study. Nephron 33: 133, 1983
5. Williams P, Khanna R, and Oreopoulos DG: Treatment of peritonitis in patients on CAPD: No longer a controversy. Dial Transplant 10: 272, 1981
6. Rubin J, Nolph KD, Popovich RP, Moncrief JW, and Prowant B: Drainage volumes during continuous ambulatory peritoneal dialysis. asaio J 2: 54, 1979
7. Faller B, and Marichal JF: Loss of ultrafiltration in continuous ambulatory peritoneal dialysis: A role for acetate. Peritoneal Dial Bull 4: 10, 1984
8. Nolph KD, Legrain M, Mion C, and Oreopoulos DG: First report of an International Cooperative Study on factors affecting ultrafiltration in continuous ambulatory peritoneal dialysis. Peritoneal Dial Bull 4: 14, 1984
9. Tenckhoff H: Advantages and shortcomings of peritoneal dialysis in the management of chronic renal failure. In Kuss R, and Legrain M (Eds), Seminars in Uro-Néphrologie de la Pitié-Salpètrière. Paris: Masson 1977, p 107
10. Oreopoulos DG, Gotloib L, Calderaro V, and Khanna R: How long can peritoneal dialysis be continued? Can Med Assoc J 124: 12, 1981
11. Williams CC, and the University of Toronto Collaborative Dialysis Group: CAPD in Toronto—An overview. Peritoneal Dial Bull [Suppl] 3: S6, 1983
12. Rubin J, Nolph KD, Arfania D, Wiegman DL, Miller FH, and Harris PD: Comparison of the effects of lactate and acetate on clinical peritoneal clearances. Clin Nephrol 12: 145, 1979
13. Verger C, Luger A, Moore HL, and Nolph KD: Acute changes in peritoneal morphology and transport properties with infectious peritonitis and mechanical injury. Kidney Int 23: 823, 1983

M. DePaepe, J. Kips, F. Belpaire, and N. Lameire

51

Comparison of Different Volume Markers in Peritoneal Dialysis

SUMMARY

To assess intraperitoneal volume repeatedly during the course of peritoneal dialysis the indicator dilution technique has been used. This study compared different volume markers, both in rabbits and in man. Recoveries of ^{14}C dextran and ^{125}I albumin were less than recovery of blue dextran. When corrected for diffusion, calculated volumes were comparable with either marker, but uncorrected calculations gave spuriously high values beginning at 60 min of intraperitoneal dwell. In patients recovery of ^{131}I albumin was 82% and that of hemoglobin 81% after intraperitoneal instillation. When corrected for diffusion, calculated volumes with either marker were nearly identical to measured volumes. Because of availability and safety hemoglobin is recommended as an indicator dilution marker, but with this technique a correction for diffusion should be made.

INTRODUCTION

During peritoneal dialysis, the intraperitoneal volume changes with time. Measurement of the intraperitoneal volume during the dwell could help in optimizing the peritoneal dialysis regimen for a given patient. From these measurements one could define the optimal dwell-time, whereby maximal ultrafiltration, for example, is achieved for a given

---

From the Renal Division and Heymans Institute of Pharmacology (J.K. and F.B.) of the State University of Gent, Gent, Belgium.

solution. It is also necessary, in order to study the membrane properties of the peritoneum, to know the intraperitoneal volume at any time during the dwell. The measurement is most accurately performed *in situ* according to the indicator dilution technique. An indicator, or in this setting, a volume marker should possess the following properties: it should not diffuse, or it should minimally diffuse across the peritoneal membrane; it should be nontoxic; and preferably it should be inexpensive. Different substances have been used as volume markers. Pyle et al.[1] used radioisotopically-labeled ^{14}C dextran (mean mol wt 70,000 daltons). Others used radioactive albumin[2] (mol wt 64,000 daltons), or recently, hemoglobin[3] (mol wt 68,000 daltons). Blue dextran (mean mol wt 5×10^6 daltons) has been used in rats.[4] In this study, different volume markers were compared both in rabbits and in man.

METHODS

In six rabbits (group I), blue dextran (0.1 g/dl) was compared to ^{14}C dextran (25 μCi/L over a dwell time of 4 hours, using a dialysis solution containing 3.86% anhydrous dextrose (Dianeal®). In another six rabbits (Group II), blue dextran was compared to ^{125}I albumin (50 μCi/L) using the same protocol.

Rabbits were anesthetized with urethane, and a catheter was implanted in the left abdominal fossa through a midline incision and 75 ml/kg dialysis fluid instilled. Blood and dialysate samples (± 3 ml) were taken at 0 (immediately postinfusion), 5, 10, 15, 30, 60, 120, and 240 minutes. The peritoneum was then

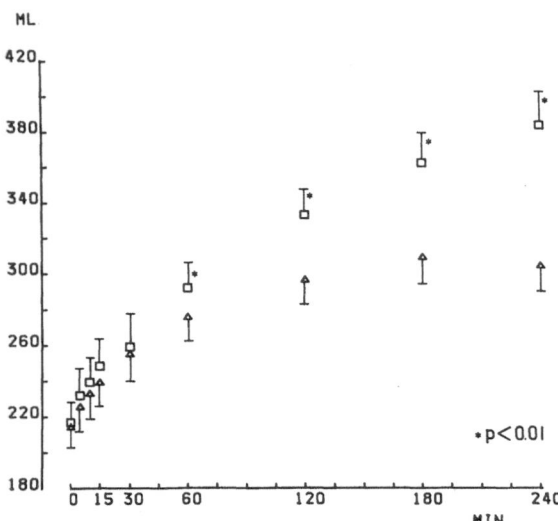

Fig. 1. Volume-time profile, non corrected, ^{14}C dextran (□) vs blue dextran (Δ), (rabbits, n = 6).

drained and rinsed twice with 100 ml saline and the recovery of the markers was calculated.

In eight patients, hemoglobin and ^{131}I albumin as volume markers were studied during a 6 hour dwell time essentially using the same protocol as in the rabbits, but taking two additional samples at 300 and 360 minutes. Sample size of dialysate in the patients was approximately 10 ml. Approximately

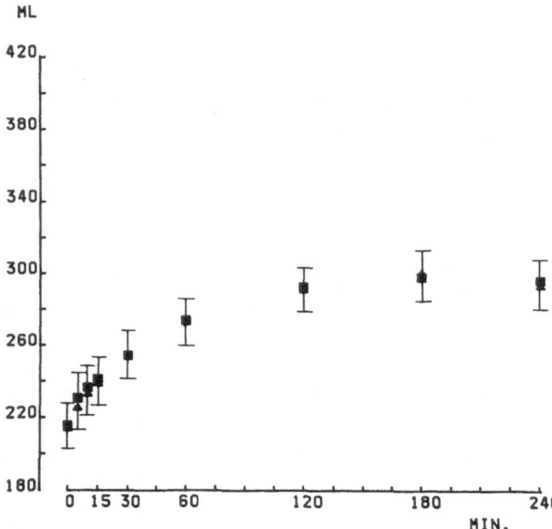

Fig. 2. Volume-time profile, corrected, ^{14}C dextran (■) vs blue dextran (▲) (rabbits, n = 6).

400 mg hemoglobin and 1 μCi ^{131}I albumin were injected into the 2 L bag.

After drainage, the peritoneal cavity was rinsed twice with 1 L saline (recovery study). The free hemoglobin was prepared as described by Canaud et al.[2] Radioactive iodine and ^{14}C levels were determined by standard liquid scintillation counting. Absorbance readings were obtained at 630 nm for blue dextran and 540 nm for hemoglobin using a Zeiss spectrophotometer. The volumes obtained by the dilution technique were corrected for both the diffusion of the markers across the peritoneal membrane and the quantity of marker removed during the sampling procedure.

The correction was made from the recovery studies assuming first order kinetics for the diffusion process. Statistical analysis was performed using three way analysis of variance (ANOVA) and Student's t test for paired observations.

RESULTS

In group I rabbits, recovery of ^{14}C dextran was 71 ± 3% compared to 92 ± 1% for blue dextran, ($p < 0.001$). In group II, the recovery of ^{125}I albumin was 78 ± 4% compared to blue dextran, 85 ± 2%; ($p > 0.05$).

The volume curves (not corrected for diffusion of the marker) obtained with ^{14}C dextran and blue dextran (Group I) are shown in Figure 1. The two curves are different (ANOVA). The volume obtained with ^{14}C dextran was higher ($p < 0.02$) after 60 minutes (Student's t test). The uncorrected volumes obtained with ^{125}I albumin and blue dextran (Group II) are also different from 60 minutes on, the

Table 1. Comparison of Measured and Calculated (Mean ± SEM) End Volumes in Rabbits.

	Measured Volume* (ml)	Calculated Volume (ml)
Group I (n = 6)		
Blue dextran	246 ± 21	259 ± 25
^{125}I albumin	250 ± 22	257 ± 23
Group II (n = 6)		
Blue dextran	283 ± 17	280 ± 15
^{14}C dextran	283 ± 17	289 ± 17

* Residual volume calculated.

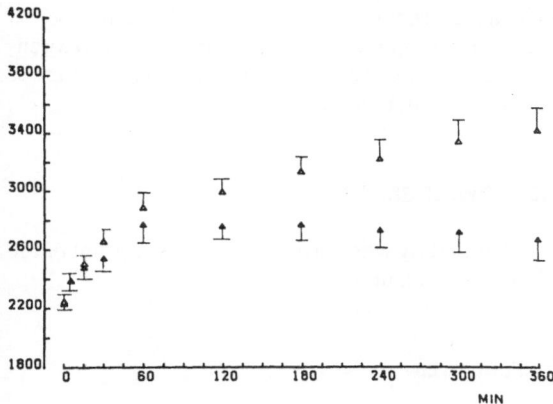

Fig. 3. Volume-time profile, hemoglobin, corrected (▲) vs non corrected (△), (patients, n = 8).

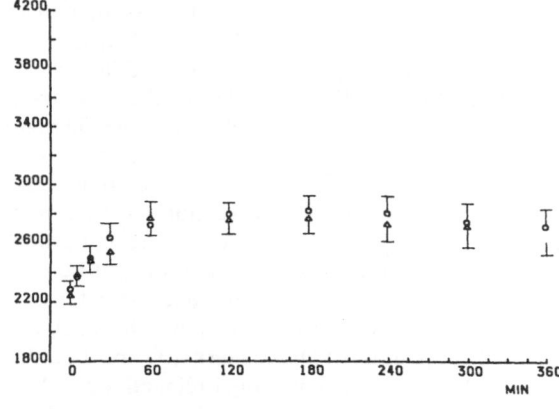

Fig. 4. Volume-time profile, corrective, hemoglobin (△) vs ^{131}I albumin (○), (patients, n = 8).

use of ^{125}I albumin resulting in larger volumes (not shown). The corrected volume profiles obtained with ^{14}C dextran and blue dextran (Group I) are shown in Figure 2. After correction, both curves show a similar profile. Also, the corrected volumes obtained with ^{125}I albumin and blue dextran are not different (not shown). It appears therefore that the noncorrected volume profile curves in both groups overestimate the intraperitoneal volume, e.g., by 4% at 60 minutes, 10% at 120 minutes, and 30% at 240 minutes for ^{125}I albumin, and by 3% at 120 minutes and 15% at 240 minutes for blue dextran.

These results show that correction for diffusion is necessary when using volume markers. Without correction, larger volumes are calculated and reabsorption in the second half of the dwell is not observed. It is also worthy of note that the corrected volume curves with different markers give the same results.

The end volumes measured with the three different dilution techniques were compared to the volumes drained (Table 1).

No difference was obtained between the calculated (and corrected) volumes and the measured volumes at the end of the dwell. These results suggest that the correction for diffusion was necessary and also adequate.

In patients, the recovery of ^{131}I albumin was 82 ± 1% and of hemoglobin was 81 ± 3%, data which were not statistically significantly different. The corrected and noncorrected volume profile curves obtained with hemoglobin are shown in Figure 3. Again as expected, a higher volume was obtained when no

correction was made (+5% at 60 minutes, +10% at 120 minutes, +30% at 360 minutes).

Corrected and noncorrected volume profile curves obtained with ^{131}I albumin show an overestimation in the same order of magnitude as with hemoglobin. The corrected volume profiles curves for both markers are identical (Fig. 4). The measured end volumes and those calculated from the dilution technique in the patient group showed comparable values (Table 2).

DISCUSSION

Different volume markers can be used in peritoneal dialysis, provided the dilution curves are corrected for the diffusion of the markers. In previous studies,[2,3] this correction was not performed and the results obtained were regarded as satisfactory. However, for estimating membrane parameters more accurate measurements are necessary. Pyle et

Table 2. Comparison of Measured and Calculated End Volumes (Mean ± SEM) in Eight Patients.

	Measured Volume* (ml)	Calculated Volume (ml)
^{131}I albumin	2691 ± 116	2695 ± 126
Hemoglobin	2641 ± 119	2607 ± 116

* Residual volume calculated.

al.[1] corrected for the diffusion of ^{14}C dextran with a mass balance using serum levels of ^{14}C dextran and distribution volumes of dextran reported in the literature. In Pyle et al.[1] calculation of the mass balance may not be correct, since it is conceivable that dextrans with lower molecular weight may diffuse preferentially across the peritoneal membrane. A simpler way to perform this correction is to measure the recovery of the marker and to assume first order kinetics for the diffusion process. As might be expected, only minimal correction is necessary for the marker with the largest molecular weight, such as blue dextran, but this volume marker is not suitable in clinical practice. When using radioactive labeled markers, albumin compared to dextran is a better choice, since it has a relatively short half life ($t_{\frac{1}{2}} = 8$ days).

Based on our results, hemoglobin behaves like albumin as far as diffusion and volume profiles are concerned, which is not surprising in view of the similarity in their molecular weights. Hemoglobin however, has, several advantages; it is nonradioactive; it is always available, and is easy to prepare; and it gives comparable results to radioactive albumin.

In conclusion, different volume markers can be used in peritoneal dialysis, with similar results as long as correction for diffusion of the marker is made. In our opinion, the least harmful, least expensive, and clinically most practical volume marker seems to be hemoglobin.

ACKNOWLEDGMENT

This study was partially funded by a grant of the NFWGO, Belgium.

REFERENCES

1. Pyle W, Moncrief JW, and Popovich RP: Peritoneal transport evaluation in CAPD. In Moncrief JW, and Popovich RP (Eds), CAPD update. New York: Masson, 1981, p 35
2. Shear L, Swartz C, Shinaberger JA, and Barry KG: Kinetics of peritoneal fluid absorption in adult man. N Engl J Med 272: 123, 1965
3. Canaud B, Liendo-Liendo C, Claret G, Mion H, and Mion C: Etude 'in situ' de la cinétique de l'ultrafiltration en cours de dialyse péritonéale avec périodes de diffusion prolongée. Nephrologie 1: 126, 1980
4. Daniels FH, Leonard EF, and Cortell S: Glucose and glycerol compared as osmotic agents for peritoneal dialysis. Kidney Int 25: 20, 1984

J. Rottembourg, A. Crayon, D. Benoliel, F. Peluso, and P. Ozanne

52

Critical Evaluation of the Injection Site for Insulin in CAPD for Diabetic Patients

SUMMARY

Diabetic patients with renal failure treated by CAPD seem ideal candidates for intra-peritoneal insulin administration. This investigation evaluated the injection port of three different commercial bags in order to study: 1) the insulin retention in the injection site 2) the amount of insulin contained in the first 50 ml of dialysis fluid entering the peritoneal cavity, and 3) the amount of insulin in the last 1950 ml. The bags used for the investigation were Dianeal Travenol bag, the Aguettant bag with an injection port on the connecting tube of the bag, and a new device designed by Travenol with an injection port on the connecting tube of the bag in a form of a reverse Y. The insulins used were: ^{125}I labelled insulin and regular insulin. The injection ports of the new Travenol and Aguettant bags allow a bolus of insulin in the peritoneal cavity, with no retention of insulin at the injection site. The use of old Travenol bags is associated with important retention of insulin in the plastic bag, and does not give a bolus of insulin into the peritoneal cavity.

INTRODUCTION

An increasing number of patients with diabetic nephropathy have recently entered dialysis programs.[1,2] Recently, continuous ambulatory perito-

From the Departments of Nephrology (JR) and Biochemistry (AC and DB) of the Hopital de la Pitie, Paris, France, and from Travenol Laboratories Nivelles Belgique (FP and PO), Plaisir, France.

neal dialysis (CAPD) has been proposed as the first dialysis choice for a large number of insulin dependent diabetic patients.[2] These patients seem ideal candidates for intraperitoneal insulin administration as proposed first by Flynn and Nanson.[3] Other similar indications were described by Stephen et al.[4] and Mirouze et al.[5] Studies in diabetic patients have demonstrated that approximately one-half of the insulin delivered intraperitoneally by bolus injection appears in the systemic circulation.[6] Since insulin is absorbed from the peritoneal cavity via the hepatic portal system and the portal vein, it seems likely that this would be a physiologic delivery route.[7] Higher insulin requirements might be the result of adsorption on the plastic bag.[8]

The aim of this experimental investigation was to evaluate the injection site of different bags. Two types of insulin were tested: ^{125}I labeled insulin in order to learn the exact distribution of the hormone, and regular insulin in to order to reproduce *ex vivo* the human regimen.

MATERIALS AND METHODS

Materials

Three different available commercial bags were used. Syringes and needles were common for all procedures: 40 U syringes and needles, gauge 25, and length 15 mm. All experiments were carried out at an ambient temperature of 22°C to 24°C. The Travenol "T" Dianeal Bag is from Travenol Laboratories in Deerfield, IL, Figure 1. The injection port is connected directly to the bag, located laterally to the

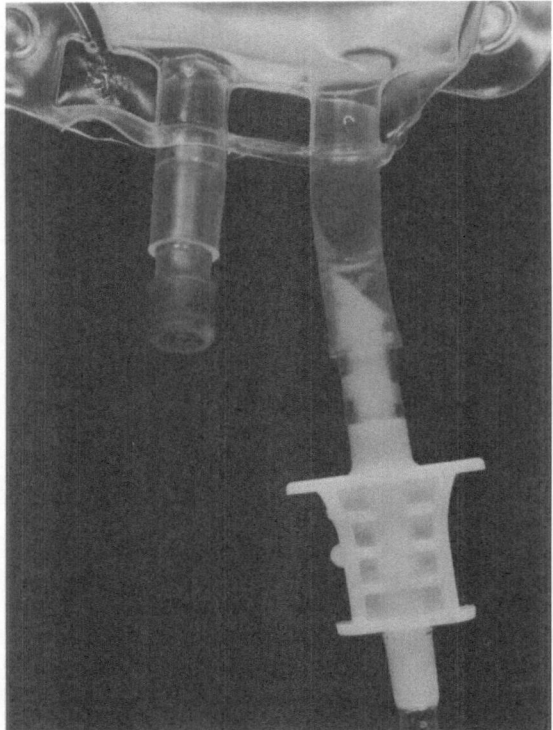

Fig. 1. Injection port of bag T (Dianeal Travenol, Deerfield, IL).

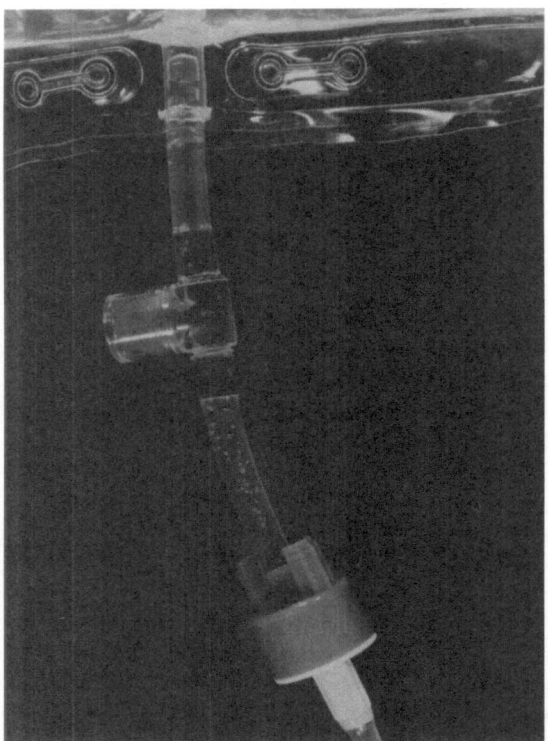

Fig. 2. Injection port of bag A (Aguettant, Lyon, France).

tubing line. The insulin is injected in a narrow channel, mixed with dialysis fluid, before entering with the fluid through the tubing into the peritoneal cavity.

The Aguettant "A" Bag (Lyon France) appears in Figure 2. The injection port is located on the connecting tube of each bag. The insulin is injected directly in the tubing line while the upper part of the tubing between the port and the bag is clamped. With this device, the insulin penetrates directly as a bolus into peritoneal cavity.

The new Travenol "N" Dianeal Bag (Nivelles, Belgium) is shown in Figure 3. The injection port is located on the connecting tube of each bag. It is designed to facilitate the injection when the bag is hung. The insulin is injected directly in the tubing line, while the upper part of the tubing between the port and the bag is clamped. The insulin penetrates directly as a bolus into the peritoneal cavity.

Experimental Design

The experimental procedure was performed in a laboratory with the usual material distributed to the patients. The material was tested with three goals: to measure insulin retention in the injection port of each bag, to measure the amount of insulin contained in the first 50 ml of dialysis fluid drained out of the bag; and to measure the amount of insulin contained in the last 1950 ml of dialysis fluid instilled. Each complete procedure was performed twice; once with radioactive insulin (three different bags of each brand were tested). The second part of the study was performed with regular insulin (six different bags of each brand were tested).

To measure insulin retention in the injection port after injection of insulin and drainage of the fluid, the residual amount of insulin remaining in the syringe and the port was counted (^{125}I insulin) or measured (regular insulin).

To measure the amount of insulin in the first 50 ml of dialysis fluid, after injection of insulin in the port, the tubing line was opened and the first 50 ml of dialysate drained collected in a precise graduated cylinder. Samples were taken for measurement of insulin. Finally, to measure the amount of insulin in the last 1950 ml of dialysis fluid, after the previous procedure, the bag was emptied into a cylinder that was weighed to find the exact remaining volume of fluid. Samples were taken for insulin measurement.

Type of Insulin

Two types of insulin were used successively for this experimental procedure. [125]I labeled porcine insulin (400 μCi/mg) was diluted in 0.5 ml of dialysis fluid to give 1.8×10^6 cpm. After injection, the insulin remaining in the syringe was counted in order to determine the amount injected. Each measurement was made three times. The radioactivity was counted with an automatic gamma counting system (Packard 5110). The results were expressed as percent of total radioactivity injected.

Normal regular Actrapid Novo® insulin was used at a dosage of 20 IU diluted in 0.5 ml. After each procedure samples were taken and measured using a radioimmunoassay technique with reference to a standard scale.[7] Results were expressed as percent of the total injected dose.

RESULTS

Radioactive Insulin

Three bags of each brand were tested. The results are shown in Table 1. The amount injected was high (between 84.7% and 90.3%) and a small amount of insulin remained in the syringes. Very little insulin remained in the injection ports of bag "A" (Fig. 2)

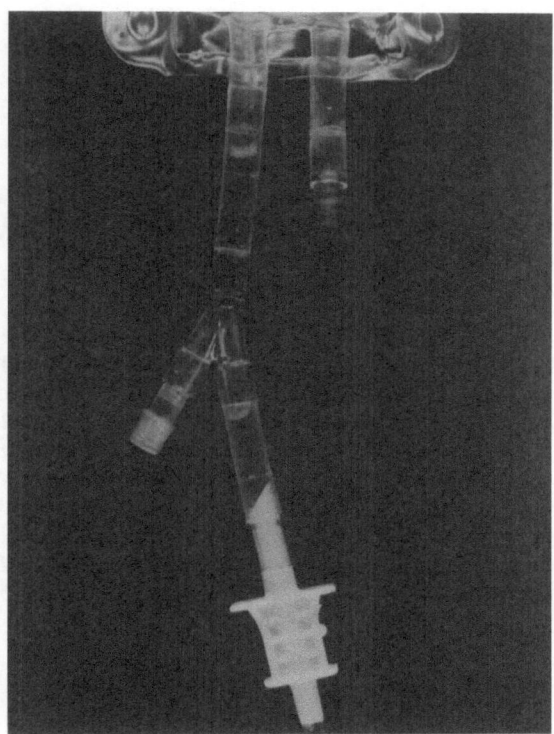

Fig. 3. Injection port of new bag N (Travenol, Nivelles, Belgium).

$1.5 \pm 0.17\%$ and bag "N" (Fig. 3) $3.5 \pm 4\%$, while there was an important retention of radioactive insulin in the injection port of bag "T" (Fig. 1) $22.7 \pm 19\%$; 73.3% to 75.7% of the radioactivity was counted in the first 50 ml of bags A and N. However, the radioactivity of the first 50 ml in bag T was only

Table 1. Results of the Experimental Procedure.

Insulin	Procedure*		Bag T	Bag A	Bag N
Injection Product		%	86.2 ± 3.3	90.3 ± 1.6	84.7 ± 1.4
[125]I-labeled	I	%	22.7 ± 19	0.15 ± 0.17	3.5 ± 4
radioactive insulin	II	%	38.1 ± 8.1	73.3 ± 11.9	75.7 ± 4.4
	III	%	26.9 ± 12.9	2.6 ± 1.8	4.3 ± 2.7
(400 μCi/mg)	II + III	%	65.1 ± 16.6	75.9 ± 10.1	80.1 ± 2
Actrapid novo© insulin	I	%	8.5 ± 3.4	0.47 ± 0.32	1.4 ± 0.9
	II	%	23.2 ± 25.4	99.3 ± 0.5	97.6 ± 1.4
	III	%	68.2 ± 23.4	0.19 ± 0.14	0.9 ± 0.8
(20 IU)	II + III	%	91.4 ± 3.4	99.5 ± 0.41	98.5 ± 0.9
Total amount of insulin found in the dialysis fluid (IU)			5 ± 5?	25 ± 5	25 ± 5

* Procedure I = retention of insulin in the port; II = first 50 mL; III = last 1950 mL.

38%. An important ratio of radioactivity is obtained with bag T in the last 1950 ml. The total radioactive insulin delivered was 65% of the initial dose with bag T, 76% with bag A, and 80% with bag N.

Actrapid Insulin Novo R

Six bags of each brand were used. The results are similar to those obtained with radioactive insulin. They are listed in Table 1. There was no insulin retention at the injection port of bag A and bag N, but there was $8.5 \pm 3.4\%$ with bag T. Most of the injected insulin was contained in the first 50 ml dialysis fluid drained from bag A ($99.3 \pm 0.5\%$) or bag N ($97.7 \pm 1.4\%$). However, there was only $23.2 \pm 25.4\%$ of injected insulin in the first 50 ml from bag T. The most important quantity of insulin is delivered with the last 1950 ml. With bag T this was only 68.2 ± 23.2, while there was more insulin delivered with bags A and N (see above). The total amount of insulin found in the dialysis fluid was around 25 ± 5 U for bags A and N and only 5 ± 5 U for bag T.

CONCLUSIONS

Intraperitoneal administration of insulin in insulin-dependent diabetic patients treated by CAPD is currently reported as a satisfactory method to obtain good blood glucose control.[9] Wide variation in insulin binding to the dialysate containers has been reported.[8, 10–13] No study has been reported on the influence of the injection port, and very few studies have used the same protocol with radioactive insulin and regular insulin. The use of radioactive insulin allows more precise measurement, but the physicochemical properties of radioactive insulin are not exactly the same as that of the insulin used in clinical practice.

The radioactivity measurements at the injection ports gave negligible residual insulin in bags A and N, but there was a significant amount of insulin in bag T. In bags A and N, 73 to 76% of the insulin was contained in the first 50 ml and 2.6 to 4.3% in the remaining dialysis fluid. In bag T, the same amount of insulin was contained in the first 50 ml or in the last 1950 ml sample. These differences are explained by the different location of the injection port: directly connected to the bag for bag T, on the tubing line for bags A and N. The use of bag T does not allow a bolus of insulin to be delivered intraperitoneally.

The use of regular insulin gave similar results to that with radioactive insulin. The amount of insulin measured in the dialysis fluid after completion of the protocol was similar in bags A and N (around 25 ± 5 IU), and allows good mixing between the two ports. But the small amount of insulin found in the drained dialysis fluid of bag T suggests important adsorption on the bag material.

With regular insulin Amidon et al.[10] and more recently, Wideroe et al.[13] found large insulin binding to the bags. Twardowski and colleagues,[11, 12] using ^{125}I insulin, found insulin binding around 4%. These differences prove the different affinities of radioactive and regular insulin to the plastic bags. Despite these facts, with regular insulin, large differences exist in the distribution of the injected doses, 23% in the first 50 ml from bag T, compared to 99.3% from bag A and 97% from bag N. In clinical practice there are also many differences in the reported doses. The mean daily doses of insulin used by the 28 Canadian patients reported recently by Amair et al.[14] is 138 ± 36 IU using bag T, while the mean daily doses used in 38 patients in Paris using bag A is 83 ± 16 IU.[15] With bag T, patients need more insulin to obtain a comparable stable blood glucose levels than with bag A.

In conclusion, the clinical implications of this experimental study are important. If one wishes to deliver a bolus of insulin into the peritoneal cavity and obtain a large and rapid peritoneal transfer, the injection ports of bags A and N should be used. The use of bag T is associated with important binding of insulin to plastic and does not allow a bolus of insulin to be delivered into the peritoneal cavity.

REFERENCES

1. Jacobs C, Brunner FP, Brynger H, Challah S, Kramer P, Selwood NH, and Wing AJ: The changing scene in the treatment of diabetic patients with terminal uraemia in Europe. In Legrain M, and Kean H (Eds), Prevention and treatment of diabetic nephropathy. London: MTP Press, 1983, p 21
2. Legrain M. Diabetics with end stage renal disease. The best buy. Diabetic Nephropathy 23: 1, 1983
3. Flynn CT, and Nanson JA: Intraperitoneal insulin with CAPD: An artificial pancreas. Trans Am Soc Artif Intern Organs 25: 114, 1979
4. Stephen RL, Jacobsen SC, Maxwell JG, Kablitz C, Maddock RK, and Tyler FH. Long-term intraperitoneal insulin treatment. Preliminary studies in 12 diabetic patients. In Friedman EA, and L'Esperance F (Eds), Diabetic renal retinal syndrome II. New York: Grune & Stratton, 1982, p 447
5. Mirouze J, Selam JL, Slingeneyer A, Chaptal PA, Franetzki M, Prestele K, and Mion C: One year continuous run with a totally implantable insulin infusion

pump in a human diabetic. Trans Am Soc Artif Intern Organs 29: 709, 1983

6. Schade DS, and Eaton RP: The peritoneum—a potential insulin delivery route for a mechanical pancreas. Diabetes Care 3: 229, 1980

7. Balducci A, Slama G, Rottembourg J, Baumelou A, and DeLage A: Intraperitoneal insulin in uraemic diabetics undergoing continuous ambulatory peritoneal dialysis. Br Med J 283: 1021, 1981

8. Hirsh JL, Fratkin MJ, and Wood JH: Clinical significance of the insulin adsorption by polyvinyl chloride infusion systems. Am J Hosp Pharm 34: 583, 1977

9. Shade DS, Eaton RP, Friedman N, and Spencer W: The intravenous intraperitoneal and subcutaneous routes of insulin delivery in diabetic man. Diabetes 28: 1069, 1979

10. Amidon G, Reicher J, Curtis MS, and Johnson A: Absorption of insulin to the surface of polyvinyl chloride CAPD solution containers. Clin Dial Transplant Forum 10: 296, 1980

11. Twardowski ZJ: Insulin absorption to peritoneal dialysis bags. Peritoneal Dial Bull 3: 113, 1983

12. Twardowski ZJ, Nolph KD, MacGary TJ, Moore HL, Collin P, Ausman RK, and Slimac WS: Insulin binding to plastic bags. Methodological study. Am J Hosp Pharm 40: 575, 1983

13. Wideroe TE, Smeby LC, Berg KJ, Jorstad S, and Svartas TM: Intraperitoneal (I 125) insulin absorption during intermittent and continuous peritoneal dialysis. Kidney Int 23: 22, 1983

14. Amair P, Khanna R, Leibel B, Pierratos A, Vas S, Meema E, Blair G, Chisholm L, Vas M, Zingg W, Digenis G, and Oreopoulos DG: Continuous ambulatory peritoneal dialysis in diabetics with end stage renal disease. N Engl J Med 306: 625, 1982

15. Rottembourg J, Issad B, Poignet JL, Strippoli P, Balducci A, Slama G, and Gahl GM: Residual renal function and control of blood glucose levels in insulin dependent diabetic patients treated by CAPD. In Legrain M, and Keen H (Eds), Prevention and treatment of diabetic nephropathy. London: MTP Press, 1983, p 339

SECTION III

Clinical Experiences

S.J. Cutler, S.M. Steinberg, K.D. Nolph, and J.W. Novak

53

Overview of Three Year Experience of the National CAPD Registry of the National Institutes of Health

SUMMARY

Since its inception in January 1981, 9008 patients have been registered in the NIH-CAPD registry. Other forms of ESRD therapy had not been used in 3670 of the patients. CAPD and CCPD were used respectively by 56% and 54% males and 78% and 74% white patients, while 5% and 18% were younger than 21 years. Approximately 66.9% remained on CAPD at one year and 45.4% at two years. Peritonitis is likely to develop in 25% of patients within the first three months, and in 66% of patients within the first 12 mo of initiating CAPD.

INTRODUCTION

The National continuous ambulatory peritoneal dialysis (CAPD) Registry is sponsored by the National Institute of Arthritis, Diabetes, and Digestive and Kidney Diseases of the National Institutes of Health. The Registry Program was initiated in January 1981 on a pilot basis and became fully operational in October of that year. As of April 5, 1984, 9008 patients had been registered by 270 treatment centers in the United States; follow-up information was available on 7701 patients (CAPD—7404, CCPD or continuous cyclical peritoneal dialysis—297).

CAPD or CCPD was initiated for 67% of the 7701 patients at the time they were first followed by the Registry Program. The balance (2520 patients) had been on CAPD/CCPD for varying lengths of time when the centers at which they were being treated joined the Registry Program. Of the 5181 patients who have been followed by the Registry since they started on CAPD or CCPD, 1878 (36%) had not received prior therapy for end-stage renal disease (ESRD).

The sex distributions for the two forms of peritoneal dialysis were similar—56% males for CAPD, 54% for CCPD. The race distributions were also similar—78% white for CAPD, 74% for CCPD. However, the age distributions were different—5% of the CAPD patients were 20 years of age or younger compared to 18% of CCPD patients.

Three types of primary renal disease accounted for 59% of all the patients in the program—diabetic glomerulosclerosis (22%), chronic glomerulonephritis (21%), hypertensive renal disease (16%).

CAPD promises to be a therapy that patients can maintain for reasonably long periods of time. Using standard life table methods for determining survival probabilities, it was found that approximately two thirds of patients (66.9%) were continuing on CAPD at one year, and 45.4% were receiving CAPD by the second anniversary of that treatment. In that analysis, patients who transferred to another form of therapy, who left dialysis without return of

From the National Institutes of Health CAPD Registry and from the EMES Corporation, Rockville, Maryland.

Note: The information contained in this paper is a brief summary of the data collected. More complete analyses appear in the *Report of the National CAPD Registry of the National Institutes of Health.*

kidney function, or who died while on CAPD were considered failures; patients whose kidney function returned or who received a transplant were considered withdrawn from follow-up. There are differences in the probability of remaining on CAPD between diabetics and nondiabetics. For example, at 12 months, the probability that a diabetic will still be on CAPD is 63%; for a nondiabetic it is 73%. Age also makes a difference; the 12-month rate for a patient 60 years of age or older is 63% compared to 75% for patients between 20 and 60 years of age.

Among those patients who have been followed by the Registry since they started on CAPD, 369 (7.5%) were transferred to hemodialysis within 6 months, and an additional 396 (8.1%) were transferred during the next 18 months. The reasons reported for the transfer were: non-dialysis-related medical reasons—39%; noncompliance with technique/excessive peritonitis—27%; patient/family choice—15%; poor fluid/chemical control—10%; socioeconomic factors—1%; and other reasons—8%.

The three complications associated with CAPD that are reported to the Registry are: peritonitis, exit site/tunnel infections, and catheter replacements. Occurrence rates were computed by relating the number of occurrences reported to the number of patient-years of observations. Among the patients who were first followed by the Registry Program at the time they started on CAPD, the occurrence rates were 1.6 incidents/patient-year for peritonitis, 0.9 incidents/patient-year for exit site/tunnel infection, and 0.3 incidents/year for replacements. While the time between successive complications may not be constant, these rates indicate that in an "average" patient, peritonitis occurred every 7.5 months, an exit site/tunnel infection occurred every 15.1 months, and a catheter replacement was performed every 41.5 months.

Analysis of patient experience with complications by means of the life table method indicates that in patients starting on CAPD, 25% may be expected to develop peritonitis within 3 months, and 66% within 12 months. The corresponding figures for exit site/tunnel infection are 18% within 3 months and 41% within 12 months. For catheter replacements the figures are 8% within 3 months and 20% within 12 months.

The corresponding figures for hospitalization due to CAPD-related complications are 23% by 3 months and 57% by 12 months. No difference was observed in hospitalization rates between diabetics and nondiabetics, or between patients under 60 years of age and those 60 years and over.

R. Gokal, C. Lloyd, R. Baillod, F. Marsh, C. Ogg,
D. Oliver, M. Ward, and R. Wilkinson

54

Multi-center Study on the Outcome of Patients on CAPD and Hemodialysis

SUMMARY

Seven renal units in England entered 361 patients into a multicenter study of CAPD. After one year 92 patients on CAPD were compared to 42 on hemodialysis. CAPD was preferentially used for patients with diabetes mellitus or cardiac problems. Actuarial patient survival and technique survival did not differ with the two treatments. The hospitalization rate for vascular access problems complicating hemodialysis therapy was nearly as high as that for peritonitis and catheter problems in CAPD patients. The peritonitis rate was 2.4 episodes/patient yr.

INTRODUCTION

Since its first introduction into the United Kingdom in late 1978, CAPD has become an accepted form of dialysis therapy for patients with end stage renal failure.[1] However, early reports on the outcome of this treatment suggested inferior patient and technique survival rates and higher morbidity, compared to hemodialysis patients.[2,3] Data from the European Dialysis and Transplant (EDTA) Registry showed a CAPD technique survival of only 46% at 2 years, and that only 30% were on CAPD at the end of that period, if deaths were included.[3]

There may be several reasons for the differences in the two treatment modalities. These include

_____

From the Royal Infirmary, Manchester, Guys, Royal Free, and London Hospitals, London, Royal Victoria Infirmary, and Freeman Road Hospital, Newcastle, and the Churchill Hospital, Oxford, England.

patient selection, whereby those who are elderly, suffering from cardiocerebrovascular diseases and diabetes mellitus may be preferentially placed on CAPD. The selection policy may be biased by inadequate hemodialysis facilities, and the high 'drop-out' rate on CAPD may reflect early experience as centers acquired the expertise and developed adequate facilities and staff to conduct CAPD. Intercenter differences in policy, and even differences in diagnostic reporting techniques might make pooled data (such as EDTA) difficult to interpret.

In order to study these questions, a prospective study was started in January 1983 in seven large and established renal units in England, involving all new patients taken on for dialysis treatment. This report is based on the analysis of the first year of the study.

METHODS

Aims of the Study

The study aimed to determine patient and technique survival for both groups of patients (CAPD and HD) and to relate these to reasons for choice of therapy and complicating disease and social factors as defined at the commencement of dialysis treatment. Also, it aimed to ascertain hospitalization and reasons for this; to determine the incidence of specific CAPD related problems of peritonitis and catheters and relate them to possible causative influences; and to determine outcome of patients on various dialysis treatments and causes for failure.

Table 1. Details of Patients in Study
(U = 139).

	HD	CAPD
Number (male/female)	47 (35/12)	92 (64/28)
Age (mean ± SD) (years)	43 ± 15	47 ± 14
Median duration of treatment (days)	151 (2–365)	204 (2–365)
Number on therapy for 12 months	12	27

Table 2. Primary Renal Disease
(% of Patients) in the Hemodialysis
and CAPD Groups.

Renal Disease	HD n = 42	CAPD n = 92
Glomerulonephritis	30	26
Unknown	17	19
Pyelonephritis	11	9
Polycystic kidneys	13	9
Diabetes mellitus	2	15
Other	27	22

Patients and Definitions

All new patients coming on to dialysis therapy for the first time were entered into the study. One person (CL) collated the data from each centre, using a defined protocol. There were set definitions for such factors as peritonitis, relapse of peritonitis,[4] temporary modality change, hospitalization, and catheter related problems. The choice of therapy was determined by the policy of individual units and there was no attempt to randomize patients into treatment groups.

End Point of the Study. The patients left the study when there was a permanent change in dialysis therapy, death, return of renal function, or transfer to another renal unit. Those patients who had completed 12 months on the initial therapy were deemed to have reached the "end point."

Statistics. Student's t-test, χ^2, and actuarial life table analysis were utilized.

RESULTS

Over the first 15 months of the study, 361 new patients were entered into the study; of these 123 started on hemodialysis and 238 on CAPD. However, the current report is based on those reaching end point or who had been on dialysis for 12 months; 139 patients (47 HD, 92 CAPD) (Table 1).

Primary renal diseases. Diseases leading to end stage renal failure, based on the EDTA coding, did not differ significantly in incidence in the two groups other than for diabetes mellitus (Table 2).

Reasons governing choice of therapy and complicating factors. From a list of 37 medical, social, and other factors, the main reasons that determined whether a patient was treated by HD or CAPD were

recorded (Table 3). Often there were multiple determinants in an individual patient. Similar factors present at start of treatment, but not necessarily determining it are given in Table 3.

Outcome. The details of outcome in the two groups are shown in Table 4, which also lists the cause of death and reasons for change to another dialysis modality in the CAPD group. A major cause of discontinuation of dialysis therapy in both groups was successful transplantation.

Hospitalization. The various reasons leading to hospitalization after the patient was discharged home following initial admission or completion of training are given in Table 5, expressed as days/patient year of therapy. The hospitalization rate for vascular access in HD patients almost equalled that for CAPD related problems in the other groups. Surgical reasons refer to causes other than vascular access or catheter problems.

Peritonitis. The overall peritonitis rate was 2.4 episodes/patient year of treatment. A total of 126 episodes were recorded in 52.2 patient years of therapy. Of these 27% were culture negative and 2% eosinophilic. The relapse rate (defined as recurrence of peritonitis with the same organism within one month of stopping antibiotics) was 17% while 4% of episodes necessitated catheter removal with an additional 4% following a relapse. Twenty-nine percent of the patients had not experienced any peritonitis whereas another 53% had 1–2 episodes. The proportion of peritonitis episodes involving admission to the hospital for either the primary infection or a subsequent relapse was 35%. The rest were managed entirely at home.

Catheter problems. A total of 31 catheter removals were undertaken in 92 patients for reasons other than peritonitis or post transplantation.

Table 3. Complicating Factors and Reasons Governing Choice of Therapy in Patients under Study.

	HD	CAPD	$p\,(\chi^2)$
Complicating factors at start of therapy (% of patients)			
Cardiac			
Angina	2	13	NS
Heart failure	6	19	NS
Myocardial infarction	2	12	NS
Diabetes mellitus	2	15	0.005
Cerebrovascular accidents	0	8	NS
Steroid/Cytotoxic therapy	26	5	0.002
Reasons governing choice of therapy			
Cardiac			
Angina	0	12	0.033
Heart failure	0	19	0.004
Myocardial infarction	0	12	0.033
Inadequate HD facilities	0	9	NS
Awaiting early transplant	21	20	NS
Age	9	15	NS
Patient preference	21	15	NS
Renal unit policy	0	17	0.006

Twenty-seven of these were related to outflow/inflow obstruction of peritoneal dialysis fluid and two to fluid leaks.

DISCUSSION

The use of CAPD in the United Kingdom has risen so dramatically that between 25 to 30% of all dialysis patients are on this therapy.[3,5] This study reveals that in seven large centers in England, CAPD is used twice as often as HD in managing patients with terminal renal failure. Whether this reflects a definitive change to accepting CAPD as a primary choice of therapy or a move to accommodate the increasing number of patients in the face of limited HD facilities is difficult to ascertain; a few units have reported a decline in the use of HD as it

Table 4. Outcome of Patients under Study.

	HD (n = 47)	CAPD (n = 92)
Continue original therapy	12 (26%)	27 (29%)
Transplanted	23 (49%)	39 (42%
Death	5 (11%)	9 (10%)
Changed dialysis therapy	4 (9%)	15 (16%)
	all to CAPD	5 to Home HD
		9 to Hosp HD
		1 to IPD
Reasons for change in CAPD patients	Peritonitis	4
	Other CAPD problems	6
	Patient preference	2
Cause of death (No. of patients)		
Cardiac	1	4
Cerebrovascular accident	1	—
Hemorrhage	1	1
Pulmonary infection tuberculosis	—	2
Others	2	2

Table 5. Reasons for Hospitalization
in Patients under Study.

Reasons	HD	CAPD
	(days/patient year of therapy)	
Overall	16.0	18.0
Medical	7.1	7.0
Surgical	2.7	2.1
Vascular access	6.2	0.4
Peritonitis	—	6.0
Catheter	—	2.0

has become unit policy to place most patients on CAPD as the initial therapy (Table 3).

In spite of the short duration of follow-up and the small numbers, several aspects of the study results are interesting. Firstly, all centers utilized CAPD preferentially in patients with known cardiovascular problems and for the management of diabetic end stage renal disease. It was not possible to correlate the outcome on CAPD or HD with either reason for choice of therapy or complicating factors at the start of dialysis because of small numbers and the short follow-up. However, the tendency for patients with cardiac disease to be treated with CAPD rather than HD suggests that cardiac mortality may be higher in the former group, as noted in other predictions and survival studies in patients with end stage renal disease.[6,7]

A significant cause of "drop-out" from both groups was successful transplantation, which has always been regarded as the treatment of choice in most centers in the UK. A common impression that CAPD is preferred to HD as a "holding" therapy prior to a planned or early transplantation has not been confirmed so far in this study.

The actuarial patient and technique survival was almost identical in the two groups, although the follow-up is short. In view of previous pessimism over the prospects of CAPD, it is relevant that such results were obtained despite a bias to the inclusion of high risk patients in the group treated with CAPD. Nevertheless, the results are comparable to single unit reports[8] and more recent EDTA statistics[9] and may reflect acquisition of the requisite expertise with CAPD practiced with the appropriate facilities.

Hospitalization was fairly high in the two groups but did not differ significantly between them. The rate for CAPD related factors was only slightly greater than for vascular access on HD—a some-

what surprising finding. It would be interesting to see if this trend persists with longer follow-up. A disquieting feature in CAPD patients was the high peritonitis rate of 2.4 episodes/patient year and an equally high relapse rate. No obvious reasons came to light from this study but points to greater needs to minimize the factors contributing to peritonitis.

Overall, the study shows that the use of CAPD is twice as high as HD. Over the 12 months of follow-up, CAPD compared favorably with HD in terms of patient and technique survival as well as hospitalization. Peritonitis remains a major problem.

ACKNOWLEDGMENTS

The study was made possible through a research grant from the National Federation of Kidney Patients Association and Travenol Laboratories. Our thanks to Linda Hunt for her help with the statistics and computerizing the data.

REFERENCES

1. Gokal R: Continuous ambulatory peritoneal dialysis (CAPD)—current state in the United Kingdom. In Parsons FM, and Ogg CS (Eds]), Renal failure—who cares? Lancaster: MPT Press, 1982, p 137
2. Jacobs C, Broyer M, Brunner FB, Brynger H, Donckerwolcke RA, Kramer P, Selwood NH, Wing AJ, and Blake PH: Combined report on regular dialysis and transplantation in Europe XI, 1980. Proc Eur Dial Transplant Assoc 18: 2, 1981
3. Broyer M, Brunner FP, Brynger H, Donckerwolcke RA, Jacobs C, Kramer P, Selwood NH, and Wing AJ: Combined report on regular dialysis and transplantation in Europe XII, 1981. Proc Eur Dial Transplant Assoc 19: 2, 1982
4. Oreopoulos DG: Let us all speak the same language. Peritoneal Dial Bull 4: 1, 1984
5. Gokal R: Chapter 19. In Saunders KB (Ed), Continuous ambulatory peritoneal dialysis in advanced medicine. London: Pitman Publishing, 1983, p 38
6. Hutchinson TA, Thomas DE, and MacGribbon B: Predicting survival in adults with end stage renal disease: An age equivalent index. Ann Intern Med 96: 417, 1982
7. Wu G: Cardiovascular deaths among CAPD patients. Peritoneal Dial Bull (Suppl)3: 523, 1983
8. Ramos JM, Gokal R, Siamopolous K, Ward MK, Wilkinson R, and Kerr DNS: CAPD: Three years experience. Q J Med 52: 165, 1983
9. Wing AJ, Broyer M, Brunner FP, Brynger H, Challah S, Donckerwolcke RA, Gretz N, Jacobs C, Kramer P, Selwood NH, and Wing AJ: Combined report on regular dialysis and transplantation in Europe XIII, 1982. Proc Eur Dial Transplant Assoc 20: 2, 1983

G. Piccoli, G.P. Segoloni, F. Quarello,
and A. Vercellone

55

CAPD in Italy: A Multicenter Study

SUMMARY

Experience of the first 4 years of the Italian Multicenter Study on CAPD were reviewed. Twenty-one centers had 460 patients being treated by CAPD. For more than 50% of them this was the first type of dialysis used and there was a preponderance of elderly patients. One year patient survival was 83.9%, comparable to that of hospital hemodialysis. Survival was much higher in "standard" patients, i.e. young uncomplicated adults. After 18 months 75% of patients remained on CAPD. Peritonitis was the main reason for dropouts.

INTRODUCTION

In Italy we admit to dialysis on average 65 new patients per year per million inhabitants, but in many regions the acceptance rate is 70 or more, and in only a few areas is there a serious limitation of hemodialysis facilities. This satisfactory situation, and the good results in terms of survival and rehabilitation achieved by hemodialysis,[1-4] initially were obstacles to widespread use of CAPD in our country. In September 1979, to facilitate an exchange of infor-

Representing the Italian Multicenter Study Group on CAPD, San Giovani Hospital, Turin, Italy. Other members are G. D'Amico, L. Minetti, C. Ponticelli, A. Giangrande, R. Maiorca, L. Scarpioni, P. Zucchelli, M. Fusaroli, G. LaGreca, S. Lamperi, A. Vercellone, G. Piccoli, S. Zini, A. Ramello, R. Cavagna, F. Pecchini, G. Maschio, G. Mioni, R. Gusmano, G. Mecca, A. Passione.

mation and opinion about this treatment, 16 Italian centers decided to join in a collaborative study on CAPD. A registry was then set up to analyze the demographic characteristics of patients treated by CAPD, and to keep a constant record of their condition.[5]

A sufficient amount of information for an overall view of CAPD in Italy is now provided by the data of this registry and those of the annual census[6] of the Italian Association of Patients on Dialysis (ANED). Additional information to compare CAPD with hemodialysis has been obtained from the Dialysis and Transplantation Registry of Piedmont.

METHODS

The Registry of the Italian Multicenter Study on CAPD was started at the end of 1979 by 16 centers. Up to date (December 31, 1983) 21 centers from several Italian regions were taking part; there are now 861 patients on file (data of 20 patients, accepted to CAPD after Dec. 1, 1983 have not been processed for survival percentages) and 460 patients on treatment (Table 1).

The Piedmont Region Dialysis and Transplantation Registry was started on January 1, 1981; data are processed by the Local Government Data Processing Center. Every 6 months it gathers data from all of the 19 centers operating in Piedmont, North Italian Region with 4,600,000 inhabitants. Information is supplied on 100% of patients treated. On December 31, 1983, there were 2218 patients on file: 1467 patients on treatment, 150 of whom were on

Table 1. Patients in the Registries.

	Italian Multicenter Study on CAPD	Piedmont Region Dialysis Registry (RPDR)*	ANED Registry*
1983†			
Centers	21	19	363
Patients on file	861	2218	
Patients on treatment†			
1980	163		12,759
1981	306	1339	14,515
1982	391	1432	16,051
1983	460	1467	17,360

* All modes of dialysis.

† December 31st.

CAPD from a pool of 306 CAPD patients on file. Three centers of Piedmont are taking part of the Italian Multicenter Study on CAPD. Two hundred and one patients are included in both registries, 23% of the cases on file in the Multicenter Study.

The ANED (Italian Association of Patients on Dialysis) annual census gathers the demographic characteristics of nearly 100% of Italian patients on dialysis. Data from Piedmont Regional Registry were organized into a SAS (Statistical Analysis System)[7] data set. Data from the CAPD Italian Registry were kept on a BMDP (Biomedical Computer Program P-series).[8] Survival curves were analyzed by means of a Hitachi OH-5560 Computer (IBM compatible). Differences between the curves were calculated according to the methods of Breslow[9] and Mantel.[10] All data were processed by applying the BMDP-1L procedure, and life tables and survival functions were derived by BMDP statistical software.[8]

RESULTS AND DISCUSSION

On December 31, 1983, 1067 of 17,360 patients on dialysis in Italy (6%) were being treated by CAPD. On the same date, in the collaborating centers of the CAPD Registry, this treatment was being used in 460 cases: 18% of their overall dialysis population, and about 50% of all Italian CAPD patients (Table 2). In these units, during the past years the number of patients treated by CAPD has continued to increase and in five of them this was the first mode of therapy for more than 50% of all new patients admitted to dialysis. However the attitude to the use of CAPD differed widely and, at the end of the year, in the Registry, the ratio of CAPD patients to all patients in treatment was only slightly higher than the year before.

In Italian centers as elsewhere, older patients are more likely to be treated by peritoneal dialysis: 66% of the patients on file in the Registry are over 50

Table 2. Development of CAPD in the Italian Multicenter Study.

Year*	Centers	New patients		Patients		
		Total Number	CAPD 1st Treatment	Starting CAPD	On CAPD	On Dialysis*
1980	16	402	101 (25%)	168	143 (8.8%)	1625
1981	20	502	172 (34%)	237	308 (14.7%)	2090
1982	22	559	162 (29%)	220	391 (15.5%)	2526
1983	21	612	153 (25%)	194	460 (17.8%)	2584

* At December 31, 1983.

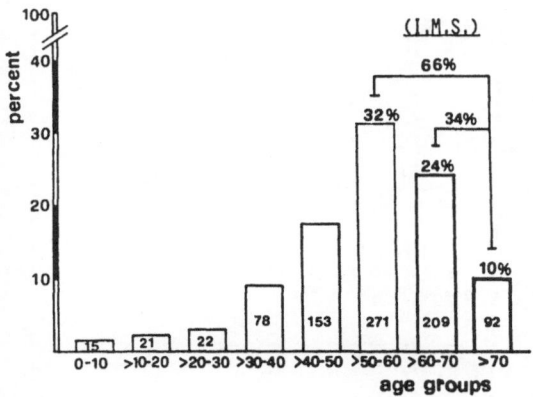

Fig. 1. Age distribution of all CAPD patients in the registry (I.M.S. = Italian Multicenter Study).

Table 3. Primary Renal Disease (Italian Multicenter Study).

	Patients	%
Chronic glomerulonephritis	201	23
Interstitial	169	20
Diabetes	97	11
Nephroangiosclerosis	87	10
Polycystic kidney diseases	77	9
Systemic diseases	23	3
Other	27	3
Unknown	180	21

years old; 10% are over 70 years of age (Fig. 1). In the Piedmont Dialysis and Transplantation Registry, 74% of the patients accepted on CAPD (1st choice) from January 1981 to December 1983 are over 50 years old and 24% over 70 Years old.

In the CAPD Centers of Piedmont (11/19) this treatment was the initiating modality of therapy for 40% of 157 patients over 70 years old (versus 24% for all patients). A large number of new patients over 60 years old is now being admitted to dialysis (Fig. 2); probably this is due both to a new attitude towards elderly people, and to increased use of CAPD treat-

ment, often very well tolerated by these patients. The influence of risk factors on the choice of CAPD is analogous: at least one major risk factor was present in 57% of the patients on file in the Registry and in 64% of 190 patients treated by CAPD as first therapy in Piedmont; 53% of the 960 new patients admitted to dialysis in this Region, during the last three years, presented with at least one major risk factor.

The causes of uremia in CAPD patients of the Italian Collaborative Group correspond to those reported by other groups[11]; a large number of diabetics has been treated by CAPD (Table 3). In the Italian Multicenter Study, the actuarial survival rate of the CAPD population as a whole is 83.9% at 12 months, 70.2% at 24 months, and 55% at 36 months (death on CAPD—or on another treatment—was defined as death occurring while the patient was being maintained on that particular treatment, or within the first month of leaving it) (Fig. 3).

Survival figures concerning CAPD and hospital hemodialysis patients entered on dialysis in Pied-

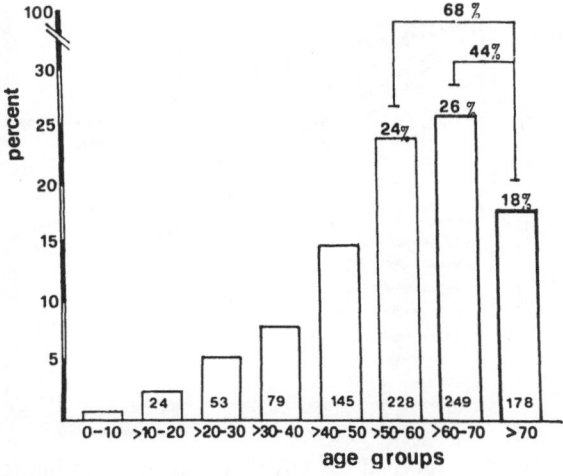

Fig. 2. Age distribution among 960 new patients accepted on dialysis from Jan. 1, 1981 to Dec. 31, 1983 in Piedmont (R.P.D.R. = Piedmont Region Dialysis and Transplantation Registry).

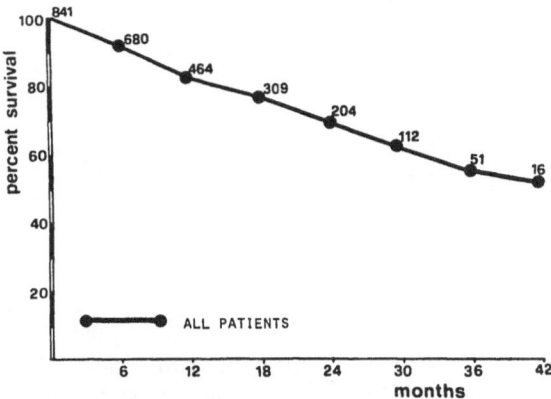

Fig. 3. Italian Multicenter Study on CAPD, all patients. Percent survival.

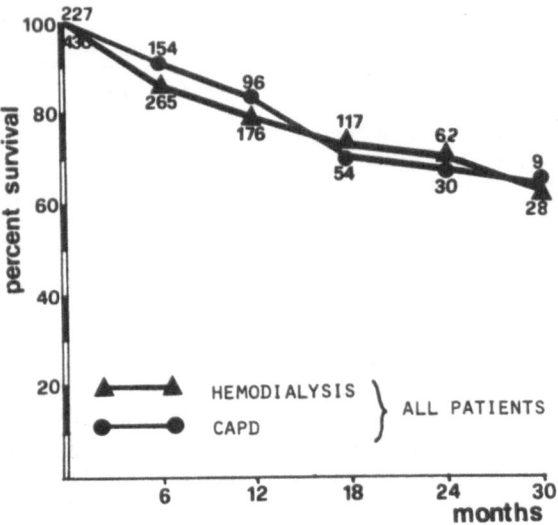

Fig. 4. Cumulative survival in CAPD and hospital hemodialysis patients admitted to dialysis since Jan. 1, 1981.

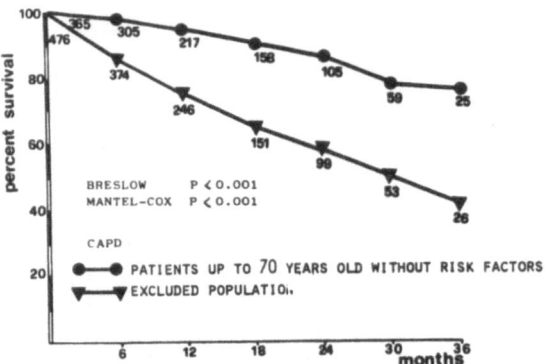

Fig. 6. Patient survival according to the presence of risk factors (I.M.S.).

mont since January 1, 1981, are very similar (Fig. 4). In the standard population—as defined by Kjellstrand[12] the survival rates are 96.6% at 12 months, 94% at 24 months, and 85.6 at 36 months. For the CAPD and hospital hemodialysis standard population in Piedmont, the data are again identical: 98% at 12 months and 94.9% at 24 months (Fig. 5).

In agreement with other reports, survival rates for the various groups vary widely according to presence of major risk factors (Fig. 6) and age groups (Figs. 7 & 8). For patients over 70 years old, the survival data were 70.3% at 12 months and 41.7% at 24 months. Once more the figures from the Piedmont Registry confirm that CAPD and hemodialysis give comparable results (Fig. 9).

A study on peritonitis, with a special questionnaire, is now in progress. The data so far available indicate that the frequency of peritonitis is on average still high: one every 13.6% patient-months in 1983. Nearly 50% of the patients had their first epi-

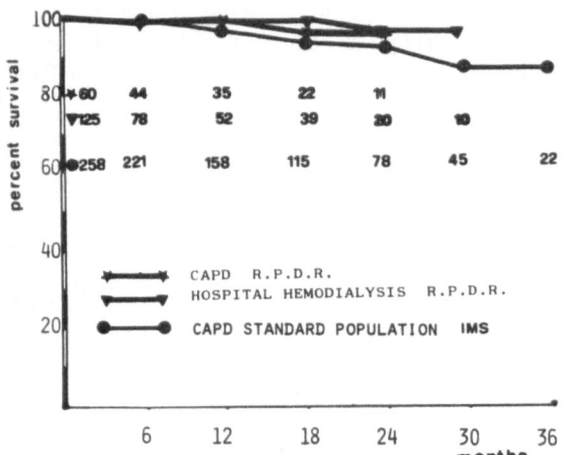

Fig. 5. Survival in CAPD standard patients (Italian Multicenter Study and Piedmont Region Dialysis Registry) and in hospital hemodialysis standard patients.

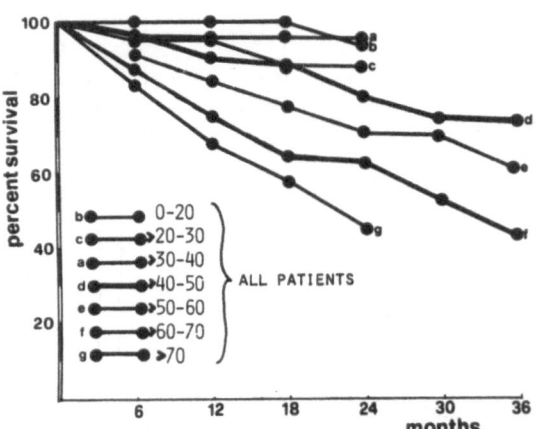

Fig. 7. Survival for CAPD patients according to age (complete period of observation). For patients transferred to another treatment: all subsequent treatment modes. Survival data computed only for the CAPD period of treatment are strictly similar.

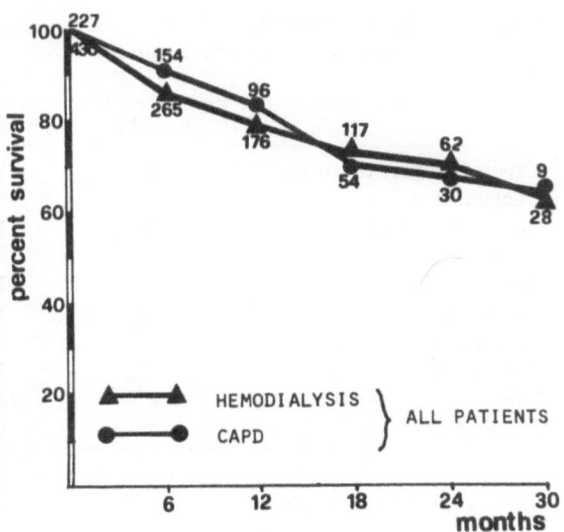

Fig. 8. Survival for CAPD patients aged 20 to 40/40 to 50/50 to 60 years without risk factors (standard population).

sode of peritonitis during the first 6 months of treatment.[13] After 15 months 26% were still free from peritonitis. However, after 3 years, almost all patients had experienced peritonitis (Fig. 10). After 15 months on CAPD, over half of the patients had had two episodes of peritonitis.

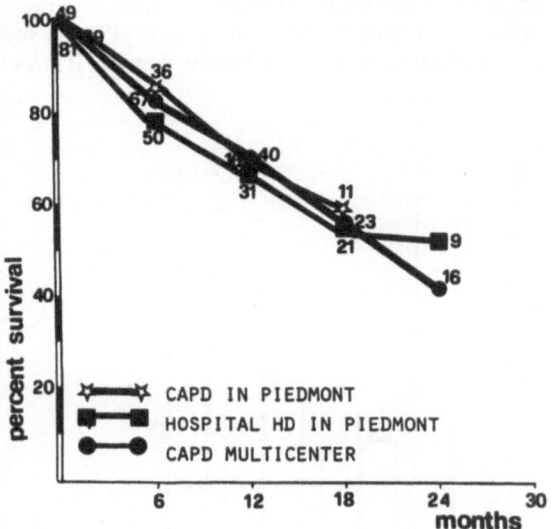

Fig. 9. Survival for CAPD and hospital hemodialysis patients over 70 years old.

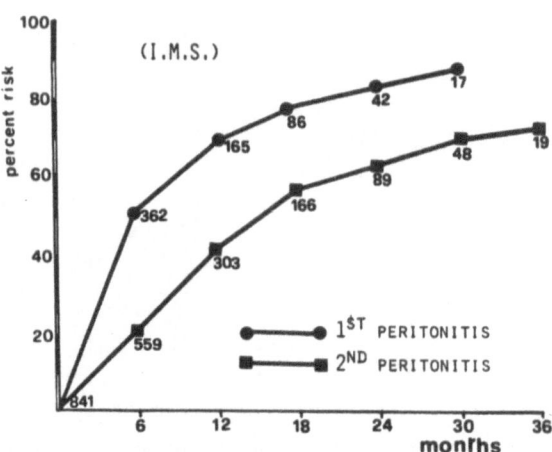

Fig. 10. First and second peritonitis in all patients.

However there are large differences within the group; the situation is now improving mostly because of the adoption of the Ẏ connector in many centers.[14, 15] Drop-outs are still very frequent; the percentage of patients requiring dialysis who remain on CAPD is 75% at 18 months, and 52% at 42 months (death, recovery of renal function, or kidney transplantation are considered as a loss to risk) (Fig. 11). At 36 months the percentage of patients still on CAPD was down to 30% (Fig. 12). Among the reasons for leaving CAPD for other dialysis therapies, peritonitis accounts for 42% of drop-outs; noncompliance accounts for another 8% (Table 4). In our program we still cannot distinguish between "loss of ultrafiltration capacity" and "inability to control

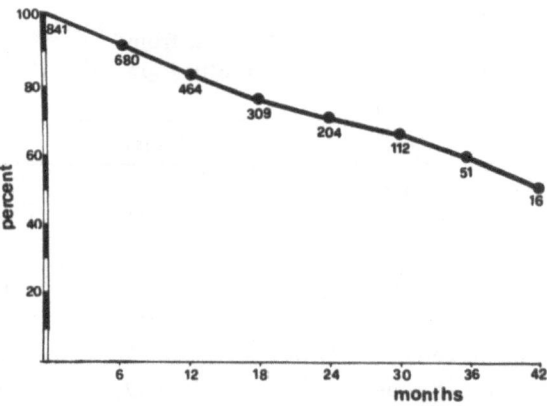

Fig. 11. Cumulative percentages of patients not transferring to hemodialysis, hemofiltration or IPD (I.M.S.).

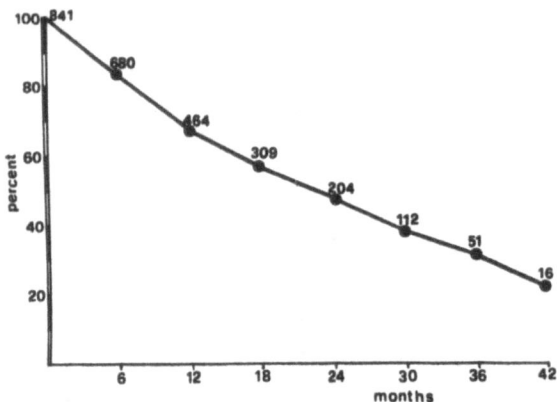

Fig. 12. Percentages of patients not leaving CAPD for any reason.

Table 5. Causes of Death in Patients on CAPD (Italian Multicenter Study on CAPD).

	Patients	%
Cardiovascular diseases	63	35
Cachexia	30	16
Myocardial infarction	20	11
Peritonitis	12	7
Sepsis	4	2
Neoplasia	5	3
Chronic liver disease	3	2
Pancreatitis	2	1
Other	27	15
Uncertain	15	8

chemistry," but at least in our experience, the loss of ultrafiltration capacity is a quite infrequent event (2 of 152 patients treated by CAPD in the S. Giovanni Hospital of Turin).

Cardiovascular diseases are the major causes of death (Table 5). Peritonitis accounts for 7% of deaths (12 patients of this group). The analysis of the rehabilitation rate of CAPD patients, according to EDTA, is not, in the whole group, particularly outstanding (Fig. 13), but in the "standard population" the results are quite satisfactory.

Unfortunately it is very difficult to state what quality of life these patients have. Direct experience shows that often patients on CAPD are feeling very well and have fewer problems than the hospital hemodialysis patients with similar physical conditions.

The transfer from CAPD to an alternative treatment modality does not affect patient survival (79% at 12 months for 131 cases examined) in the experience of the Multicenter Study (Fig. 14).

CONCLUSIONS

Even in Italy, where hemodialysis is widely used and carried out with satisfactory results, CAPD has quickly and outstandingly achieved diffusion. Only in some areas this wide application provides an immediate answer to patients who otherwise would not have received any treatment at all, and this might indeed be an element for support of CAPD. Its success is often to be attributed to the fact that it is well

Table 4. Reasons for Drop-out from CAPD (Italian Multicenter Study on CAPD).

	Patients	%
Excessive peritonitis	67	42
Medical reasons	29	18
CAPD not able to control fluid or chemistry	20	13
Catheter dysfunction	11	7
Patient choice	12	8
Unable to cope	12	8
Others	6	4
Total	157	100

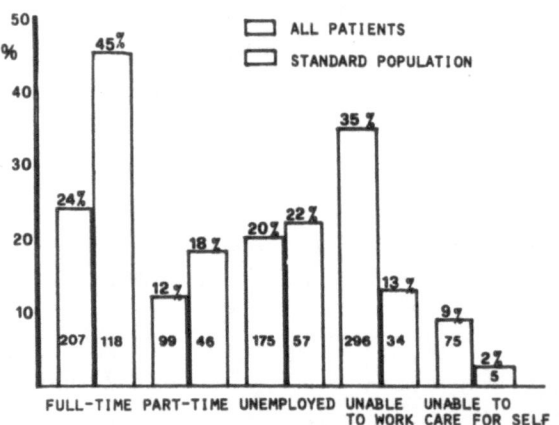

Fig. 13. Rehabilitation in CAPD patients (I.M.S.).

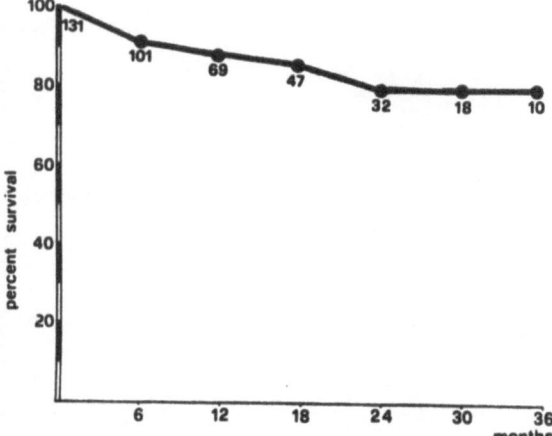

Fig. 14. Survival after transfer from CAPD to hemodialysis, hemofiltration or IPD (Italian Multicenter Study on CAPD).

tolerated by elderly people and by those with various clinical problems; more generally, CAPD fits very well into the lifestyle of a large number of patients of different backgrounds.

When properly applied, CAPD seems to give analogous results in terms of survival to hemodialysis, at least for the first years. The saving of resources and the increase in home treatments are other points of considerable importance. The high drop-out figures and the rate of peritonitis, reduced but not to the rate we would wish, still constitute the most negative aspects of this technique. In the Italian experience hemodialysis still remains the standard treatment, but CAPD has established itself as an alternative technique for a considerable percentage of patients.

ACKNOWLEDGMENTS

The authors would like to aknowledge Dr. L. Pia and Dr. G. Romano (C.S.I. Institute of Turin), A. Jayme (S. Giovanni Hospital of Turin) for their work in data processing and invaluable assistance; A. Mirone (Health Dept. of Piedmont) for her constant help; P. Belardi M.D., F. Bonello, M.D., C. Guarena, M.D., G. Salamone, M.D., A. Pacitti, M.D. and D. Pelizza, M.D. for their skilled assistance in data collection and in preparation of this manuscript. Members of the Piedmont Region Nephrology and Dialysis Centers included A. Vercellone, G. Piccoli, F. Linari, R. Triolo, G. Riva, A. Ramello, A. Arnaud, A. Tafuri, G. Verzetti, C. Peona, P. Bajardi, G. Boccardo, P.L. Cavalli, M. Ventura, M. Gonella, L. Fiorina, R. Ragni, R. Cardelli, and P.M. Ghezzi.

REFERENCES

1. Vercellone A, Segoloni GG, Giacchino F, Canavese C, Messina M, Pozzato M, Rotunno M, Squiccimarro G, Thea A, and Camussi G: Immune responsiveness versus dialytic age. In Giordano C, and Friedman EA (Eds), Uremia. Milano: Wichtig, 1981, p 274
2. Piccoli G, Giachino G, Jeantet A, Quarello F, Bossi P, Squiccimarro G, Zatteri R, Rossi P, and Vercellone A: Bone disease in hemodialyzed patients treated for ten years or more. In Giordano C, and Friedman EA (Eds), Uremia. Milano: Wichtig, 1981, p 90
3. Vercellone A, and Segoloni GP: Dialysis without choice. In proc. IV uremia conference, Capri 1983 (in press)
4. Cambi V, Garini G, Savazzi G, Arisi L, David S, Zanelli P, Bon F, and Gardini F: Short dialysis. Proc Eur Dial Transplant Assoc 20: 111, 1983
5. Segoloni GP: Up to date on CAPD in Italy, In LaGreca G, Biasioli S, Ronco C (Eds), Peritoneal dialysis proc 1st int course on peritoneal dial. Vicenza, Italy, Wichtig Editore, Milano, 1982, p 527
6. Censimento dei Servizi di dialisi e trapianto italiani al 31 dicembre '80–'81–'82–'83 ANED, Associazione Italiana Emodializzati, Milano
7. SAS Institute Inc. Version 1982. Cary, North Carolina
8. WJ Dixon (Ed): BMDP Statistical Software, Los Angeles, University of California Press, Oct, 1983
9. Breslow A: A generalized Kruskal-Wallis test for comparing k samples subject to unequal patterns of censorship. Biometrika 57: 579, 1970
10. Mantel N: Evaluation of survival data and two rank order statistics arising in its consideration. Cancer Chemother Rep 50: 163, 1966
11. Khanna R, Wu G, Vas S, and Oreopoulos D: Mortality and morbidity on CAPD. asaio J 6: 197, 1983
12. Kjellstrand CM: Introduction to workshop on morbidity and mortality in hemodialysis, hemofiltration and CAPD. asaio J 6: 167, 1983
13. Pierratos A, Amair P, Corey P, Vas S, Khanna R, and Oreopoulos D: Statistical analysis of the incidence of peritonitis on CAPD. Peritoneal Dial Bull 2: 32, 1982
14. Maiorca R, Cancarini GC, Broccoli R, Brasa S, Cantaluppi A, Scalamogna A, Graziani G, and Ponticelli C: Prospective controlled trial of a Y connector and disinfectant to prevent peritonitis in CAPD. Lancet 2: 642, 1983
15. Buoncristiani U, Bianchi P, and Cozzari M: A new safe simple connection system for CAPD. Int J Nephrol Urol Androl 1: 50, 1980

S. Shaldon

56

Is CAPD a Second Class Treatment?

SUMMARY

The origin of the term "second class" is described. Because CAPD has a shorter duration of technique life than other treatment modalities for ESRD and it is associated with sclerosing peritonitis, a lethal complication attributed to continuous stimulation of peritoneal macrophages, it is deemed second class. The widespread proliferation of this therapy is called into question.

INTRODUCTION

Second-class is an adjective that was introduced into the English language in 1837[1] to describe railway carriages of a design that were cheaper to construct because of less luxurious seating accommodation, and an anticipated life span of less than the first class carriages (Fig. 1). Thus, the term is defined as of or belonging to the class next to first. Its pejorative connotation arose by association with second-rate, an adjective describing ships of an inferior condition with a higher insurance liability: this term came into use in 1689 with the beginning of marine insurance at Lloyd's. These terms were eventually associated in the following manner: of the second-class in quality or excellence; not first rate, of only moderate quality. However, the historical implications of "second-class" imply less durable and more hazardous; and it is essentially in these senses that one may consider CAPD in relationship to other forms of ESRD therapy.

Let me first dispense with the obvious. Where no reasonable alternative form of therapy exists, it is conceded that CAPD is an acceptable alternative to death, and thus the use of CAPD in those situations, where the authors have made this point clear, seems a correct ethical use of this treatment.[2,3] It is with the less selective and more widespread use of CAPD that I take exception.[4] The remarkable achievement of "the medical-industrial complex"[5] to launch CAPD on a dead paradigm[6] and thereafter to obtain government endorsement for the therapy as "the preferred method of treatment"[7] demonstrates the clear superiority of marketing intelligence compared to that of present day metanephrologic judgement. The recent estimates of over 16,000 patients receiving CAPD suggest that this cannot be due to lack of alternative facilities entirely. In U.S.A., CAPD is clearly being offered in preference to hemodialysis, rather than as a treatment without available alternative as in UK or Canada. This state of affairs persists in spite of repeated questioning of the advisability of continued expansion of CAPD in the light of the recent NIH Registry report[8] showing 56% mortality or drop out rate and 84% prevalence of at least one hospitalization in the first year of therapy. EDTA statistics[9] had previously shown very similar figures. Indeed, as will be discussed later, the true morbidity and mortality figures associated with CAPD may be higher, as the hazards associated with this type of therapy may be lethal even many months after a change from CAPD to hemodialysis.

From the Department of Nephrology, University Hospital, Nimes, France.

Sclerosing encapsulating peritonitis is a particularly disturbing complication of CAPD that has been identified recently.[10, 11] Forty cases have been recognized in Europe in the past year, with an 80% mortality in patients whose mean age was under 45 years. The disease may present months or years after cessation of peritoneal dialysis. Its pathogenesis is unknown. The clinical features include wasting, intractable ascites, loss of peritoneal transport function (with consequence of under dialysis of those continuing on peritoneal dialysis), and bowel obstruction. Post mortem studies reveal obliteration of the peritoneal cavity by fibrous adhesions, sacs with high protein fluid, and extreme thickening of the peritoneal membrane, which comes to resemble a fibrous band rather than an ultrathin membrane. The disease is not restricted to CAPD because it was previously described in patients on intermittent peritoneal dialysis.[12] The pathology resembles practolol peritonitis.[13] Analysis of the risk factors in CAPD indicate a mean exposure of treatment of at least 2 years of CAPD in patients below age 60 years, often with a history of recurrent bacterial peritonitis. The incidence has been higher in patients dialyzed with acetate in the fluid rather than lactate. Recently it has been suggested that the use of a bacterial filter to reduce the risk of peritonitis may increase the probability of developing sclerosing peritonitis. The detection of Interleukin-1 in the drain fluid of patients on CAPD and the observation that this monocyte hormone can stimulate fibroblast proliferation suggests that substances stimulating peritoneal macrophages to produce IL-1 are responsible for starting the process towards sclerosing peritonitis. The presence of a bacterial filter can explain an increased pyrogen load entering the peritoneal cavity, secondary to presumed bacterial multiplication on the upstream surface of the filter.[14] Other examples of increased stimulation of peritoneal macrophages with undesirable results such as loss of ultrafiltration may be explained by the production of prostacyclin in the prostaglandin cascade secondary to arachidonic acid synthesis by the macrophage.[15, 16] Interference with phagocytosis (a macrophage dependent function) in the peritoneal cavity has also been reported.[17] It seems probable that these macrophage stimulants (eg, pyrogen) do not induce fever when introduced into the peritoneal cavity[18] and thus the warning signs of inflammatory response to pyrogen introduction into the peritoneal cavity may be reduced or absent, leaving the patient and clinician in a state of ill advised complacency. The only sign of value may be the loss of ultrafiltration capacity due to increased absorption of glucose and hence re-

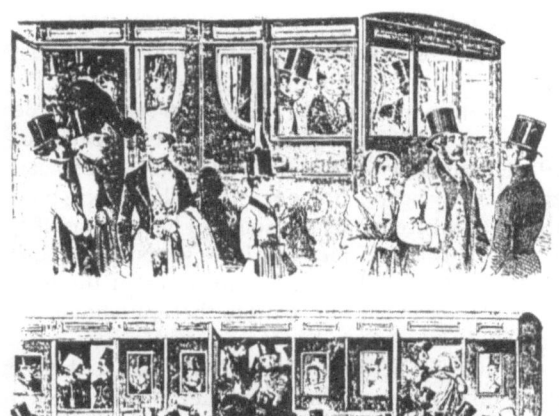

Fig. 1.   CAPD is a second class treatment. (From Illustrated London News. May 14, 1982.) "Snobbery and class prejudice is exemplified in these cameos of the classes going off to the Derby in 1842; the second-class passengers are given faces more befitting to Neanderthal Man. The first class carriage has a coupé compartment at the end; these were locked when next to the engine."

duced osmotic force to move water into the peritoneal cavity. The increase in peritoneal blood flow secondary to macrophage production of prostacylin might link loss of UF as a forerunner of sclerosing peritonitis, as Interleukin-1 is a potent stimulator of prostacylin production by macrophages.[16]

The consequence of repeated stimulation of peritoneal macrophages remains uncertain. Moreover the possibility that stimulants other than exogenous pyrogen may also stimulate macrophages cannot be excluded, such as silicone particles from the catheter and plasticizers leaching from the sacs and tubing sets.

However, a fundamental question that remains unanswered and is yet extremely relevant to the hypothesis, is why do only 10% of patients repeatedly stimulated develop sclerosing peritonitis, if the mechanism is operative in all patients? The presumption is that multiple factors are responsible, not least being the reason why fibroblast proliferation continues after the cessation of CAPD therapy. The possibility that the lesion becomes irreversible because of the development of autonomous fibroblast production remains an intriguing suggestion.

The true incidence of the disease remains to be evaluated. It is of interest that at a recent meeting of 59 internationally known nephrologists whose mean age was 47 years, not one would have accepted CAPD as the treatment of choice for her or himself.[19] This confirms the plea made 5 years ago about CAPD,[20] that until more is known about the long term results expansion of this therapy should be limited.

Thus, by accepting that CAPD has a shorter duration of technique life than other forms of ESRD therapy and that the use of it implies a greater risk for the patient due to the continuous stimulation of the peritoneal macrophage, one may conclude that the treatment is indeed second-class.

REFERENCES

1. The Shorter Oxford English on Historical Principles, Vol 2 (3rd ed). Oxford, Oxford University Press, 1973, p 1924
2. Clark RD: Peritonitis prevented in continuous ambulatory peritoneal dialysis by using the Hong Kong connection. Br Med J 228: 353, 1984
3. Gabriel R: Continuous ambulatory peritoneal dialysis in patients aged over 60. Br Med J 288: 407, 1984
4. Stragier A: CAPD after 5 years—the amazing growth of a new therapy. Eur Dial Transplant Nursing Assoc J 2: 3, 1983
5. Relman AS: The new medical-industrial complex. N Engl J Med 303: 963, 1980
6. Shaldon S, Koch KM: Are standards and checklists needed in uremia therapy? Kidney Int (in press)
7. Fisher AB: Washington reins in the dialysis business. Fortune Int July 25: 66, 1983
8. CAPD Patient Registry. Report No. 83-1. April 15th 1983. The National Institute of Health. Bethesda, MD, 1983
9. Kramer P, Broyer M, Brunner FP, Brynger H, Donckerwolcke RA, Jacobs C, Selwood NH, and Wing AJ: Combined report on regular dialysis and transplantation in Europe, XII, 1981. Proc Eur Dial Transplant Assoc 19: 4, 1982
10. Slingeneyer A, Mion C, Mourad G, Canaud B, Faller B, and Beraud JJ: Progressive sclerosing peritonitis: A late and severe complication of maintenance peritoneal dialysis. Trans Am Soc Artif Intern Organs 29: 633, 1983
11. Rottembourg J, Gahl GM, Poignet JL, Mertani E, Strippoli S, Langlois P, Tranbaloc P, and Legrain M: Severe abdominal complications in patients undergoing continuous ambulatory dialysis. Proc Eur Dial Transplant Assoc 20: 236, 1983
12. Gandhi VC, Humayum H, Ing TS, Daugirdas JT, Jablokow VR, Iwatsuki S, Geis P, and Hano JE: Scerotic thickening of the peritoneal membrane in maintenance peritoneal dialysis patients. Arch Intern Med 140: 1201, 1980
13. Marshall AJ, Baddeley H, Barritt DW, Davies JD, Lee REJ, Low-Beer TS, and Read AE: Practolol peritonitis: A study of 16 cases and a survey of small bowel function in patients taking beta adrenergic blockers. Q J Med 46: 145, 1977
14. Shaldon S, Koch KM, Quellhorst E, and Dinarello CA: Pathogenesis of sclerosing peritonitis in CAPD. Trans Am Soc Artif Intern Organs (in press)
15. Foegh F, Maddox YT, Winchester J, Rakowski T, Schreiner G, and Ramwell PW: Prostacyclin and thromboxane release from human peritoneal macrophages. In Samuelsson B, Paoletti R, and Ramwell P (Eds), Advances in prostaglandin, thromboxane, and leukotriene research, Vol 12. New York: Raven Press, 1983, p 45
16. Dinarello CA, Marnoy SO, and Rosenwasser LJ: Role of arachidonate metabolism in the immunoregulatory function of human leucocytic pyrogen/lymphocyte-activating factor/interleukin 1. J Immunol 130: 890, 1983
17. Keane FW, Comty CM, Verbrugh HA, and Peterson PK: Opsonic deficiency of peritoneal dialysis effluent in continuous ambulatory peritoneal dialysis. Kidney Int 25: 539, 1984
18. Bennett IL: Studies on the pathogenesis of fever. V. The fever accompanying pneumococcal infection in the rabbit. Bull John Hopkins Hosp 98: 216, 1956
19. 4th Capri Uremia Meeting. September 1983 (in press)
20. Shaldon S: A cynical critique of continuous ambulatory peritoneal dialysis. In Legrain M (Ed), Continuous ambulatory peritoneal dialysis. Amsterdam: Excerpta Medica, 1980, p 137

A. Saito, H. Ogawa, T.G. Chung, K. Maeda

57

CAPD and Protein-Permeating Hemodialysis: A Clinical Comparison

SUMMARY

Blood laboratory data were compared .before and after one year's treatment, respectively, from 12 patients on continuous ambulatory peritoneal dialysis (CAPD) and 12 patients on protein-permeating-hemodialysis (P-P-HD), the latter with a protein loss in one week the equivalent of those on CAPD. In CAPD patients, Dianeal (Travenol) was continuously exchanged four times/day (4.25% dextrose solution, once and, 1.5% dextrose solution, three exchanges) Kuraray KF-101-12C dialyzer was used in the P-P-HD patients thrice weekly (5 hours/treatment). Weekly albumin removal in CAPD was 18673.2 ± 3654.3 mg, against 22365.0 ± 3759.6 mg in P-P-HD after one year of treatment. Both forms of therapy resulted in significantly higher erythrocyte count, hemoglobin, transferrin, and β-lipoprotein levels. P-P-HD patients showed a significant increase in total cholesterol, triglyceride and HDL-cholesterol, whereas CAPD patients had a similar increasing trend. Serum β_2 microglobulin levels were lowered significantly in P-P-HD patients and a decrease was also apparent in CAPD patients. P-P-HD patients had a significant decrease in total protein and albumin levels, but in CAPD patients these remained unchanged. Although seven other low molecular weight proteins were removed by both CAPD and P-P-HD treatments, their serum levels did not fall, whereas α_1-acidic glycoprotein, β_2-glycoprotein I and α_1-antitrypsin increased moderately.

From the Bio-dynamics Research Institute and Nagoya University Branch Hospital, Nagoya, Japan.

INTRODUCTION

Compared to hemodialysis, removal of low molecular weight substances by CAPD is inferior, but it offers outstanding advantages in removal of medium molecular weight and large molecular weight substances.[1,2] These features can presumably be used effectively for clinical improvement, but at the same time CAPD results in some loss of needed nutritional and immunological substances such as albumin, IgG, IgA, IgM, and complement components C_3 and C_4.[3,4] Also, the transfer into blood of dextrose from a high concentration in the dialysis fluid is considered to have a major effect on both carbohydrate and lipid metabolisms.[5,6] It is as yet unclear what contribution CAPD makes at the clinical level.

In the present study, hemodialysis was performed using a hemodialyzer with a higher molecular weight cut-off point than a conventional hemodialyzer, which had better middle molecular weight range removal and weekly protein loss comparable to that of CAPD. A comparison was made with clinical CAPD data.

MATERIALS AND METHODS

Comparison of laboratory data was made between 12 patients on CAPD for more than one year, and 12 patients on protein-permeating hemodialysis (P-P-HD). The CAPD group consisted of eight middle-aged males and four females, mean age 48.8 years. Ten of the 12 had changed from long-term hemodialysis to CAPD therapy, while two were on CAPD from the very start. Creatinine clearance in all 12 was under 4 ml/minute, protein intake was 1.4 g/kg/day and caloric intake was 2000–2200 cal/day. For the CAPD solution, all 12 used 4.25% dextrose Dianeal (Travenol) at 2 L once daily and 1.5% dextrose Dianeal 2 L three times/day for a total of four exchanges/day on a continuous basis. Four of the 12 patients on CAPD developed peritonitis a total of eight times during their first year on CAPD.

Of the 12 patients on P-P-HD, nine were males and three were females, mean age 53.4 years, with an average of 6.8 years on artificial kidney treatment. During conventional hemodialysis therapy using a cuprophan dialyzer, various complications had developed, prompting the change to P-P-HD. The dialyzer was a Kuraray KF-101-12C with a membrane surface area of 1.2 m², a cut-off point of 80,000 daltons, and an ultrafiltration rate of 6.0 ml/mm Hg/hour. Hemodialysis was done three times per week (5 hours each) with a blood flow of 200 ml/minute and dialysate flow of 500 ml/minute. All 12 patients had a creatinine clearance less than 4 ml/minute. Protein intake with meals was 1.4 g/kg/day, and caloric intake was 2200–2400/day. Blood laboratory data were checked before initiation of treatment and after one year of both CAPD and P-P-HD treatment regimens, and a comparison was made.

The used dialysate from 10 of the 12 patients in each group was collected for one week, and the protein removal was measured. The amount of fluid removed per day was measured for each patient, the hemodialysate was concentrated 100-fold and the peritoneal dialysate was concentrated 10-fold before proteins were measured by radial immunodiffusion.[7] Measured proteins were as follows: β_2-microglobu-

lin, retinol-binding protein, α_1-acidic glycoprotein, β_2-glycoprotein I, α_2-HS-glycoprotein, α_1-antitrypsin, prealbumin, hemopexin, albumin, and transferrin. The same method was employed to measure the protein concentrations in the blood of the 12 patients in each group both before and one year after being put on CAPD and P-P-HD, respectively.

RESULTS

Table 1 presents the one-week removal rates by CAPD and P-P-HD for 10 different kinds of proteins. P-P-HD treatment tended to remove more proteins than CAPD with the exception of α_1-acidic glycoprotein. Table 2 and 3 show the pretreatment and one-year blood levels for each of the 12 CAPD and P-P-HD patients. Table 4 gives the blood concentrations of small molecular weight serum proteins in the two groups, before, and one year following initiation of the respective treatment. Erythrocyte count, hemoglobin, transferrin and β-lipoprotein significantly increased over a year in both P-P-HD and CAPD patients. CAPD patients had a significant decrease in serum uric acid, and the trend was similar in P-P-HD patients. β_2-microglobulin fell significantly in the P-P-HD group, and also decreased somewhat in the CAPD group. Total protein and albumin decreased significantly in the P-P-HD group, but was unchanged in the CAPD group. Serum potassium decreased significantly in the CAPD patients and serum magnesium increased significantly, but there was no change in any P-P-HD patient. Inorganic phosphate significantly increased in P-P-HD but tended to decrease with CAPD.

Table 1. Weekly Removal of Plasma Proteins During CAPD and P-P-HD.

Protein	M.W. (daltons)	CAPD (n = 10) mg/week	P-P-HD (n = 10) mg/week
β_2-microglobulin	(11,800)	229.5 ± 31.4	246.7 ± 26.1
Retinol-binding protein	(21,000)	180.2 ± 30.6	232.5 ± 42.1
α_1-acidic glycoprotein	(40,000)	896.4 ± 206.4	855.9 ± 189.4
β_2-glycoprotein I	(40,000)	147.3 ± 29.4	152.4 ± 40.8
α_2-HS-glycoprotein	(49,000)	259.6 ± 164.5	368.7 ± 162.2
α_1-antitrypsin	(54,000)	1766.1 ± 351.4	1896.2 ± 412.7
Prealbumin	(55,000)	192.6 ± 54.8	248.4 ± 50.8
Hemopexin	(57,000)	390.9 ± 67.2	478.2 ± 86.6
Albumin	(67,000)	18673.2 ± 3654.3	22365.0 ± 3759.6
Transferrin	(76,000)	1252.8 ± 368.4	1430.4 ± 540.9

Table 2. Blood Laboratory Data Before and One Year After CAPD and P-P-HD Treatment (I).

	CAPD (n = 12)		P-P-HD (n = 12)	
	Before	After One Year	Before	After One Year
Erythrocyte count ($\times 10^4/mm^3$)	250.4 ± 61.2	307.6 ± 64.2*	286.0 ± 65.8	311.3 ± 64.1*
Hematocrit (%)	22.5 ± 4.9	28.6 ± 6.2	25.1 ± 5.0	27.8 ± 4.7
Hemoglobin (g/dl)	7.4 ± 1.6	9.5 ± 2.1*	8.6 ± 1.6	9.5 ± 2.1*
Urea nitrogen (mg/dl)	80.2 ± 23.5	62.3 ± 16.7	80.4 ± 19.6	75.3 ± 18.6
Creatinine (mg/dl)	10.9 ± 1.8	10.7 ± 1.4	13.7 ± 2.9	14.4 ± 3.1
Uric acid (mg/dl)	9.0 ± 1.0	7.4 ± 0.6†	9.0 ± 1.5	8.4 ± 1.0
Total protein (g/dl)	6.6 ± 0.8	6.9 ± 0.8	6.8 ± 0.5	6.2 ± 0.6*
Albumin (g/dl)	3.5 ± 0.4	3.7 ± 0.5	4.2 ± 0.5	3.6 ± 0.6*
Transferrin (mg/dl)	191.1 ± 57.1	247.9 ± 67.4†	202.8 ± 51.9	242.3 ± 56.8*
β_2-microglobulin (mg/dl)	5.1 ± 2.0	3.7 ± 1.5	6.0 ± 1.6	4.8 ± 1.5*
C-PTH (ng/ml)	2.6 ± 1.5	3.2 ± 2.7	2.4 ± 1.5	3.1 ± 2.0

* $p < 0.05$, † $p < 0.01$.

As to the change in small-molecule protein levels, aside from β_2-microglobulin and transferrin, there was no change of significant nature, either increase or decrease, in either group. Despite their removal by both forms of treatment, α_1-antitrypsin showed an increasing trend.

Clinical conditions were as follows. Of two CAPD patients with pruritis, one improved. Recovery was seen in four patients on P-P-HD with painful osteodystrophy, three of four with uremic peripheral neuropathy and one patient with pruritus.

DISCUSSION

The present study compares laboratory data between CAPD patients and those on hemodialysis. One-week protein removal by P-P-HD was comparable to that of CAPD, and effective removal of middle and large molecules exceeded that by conventional hemodialysis. With these two different forms of therapy, in which there are similarities in solute removal, there should have been common changes in the laboratory data from patients on

Table 3. Blood Laboratory Data Before and One Year After CAPD and P-P-HD Treatment (II).

	CAPD (n = 12)		P-P-HD (n = 12)	
	Before	After One Year	Before	After One Year
Total cholesterol (mg/dl)	177.5 ± 32.6	191.2 ± 38.0	151.3 ± 55.5	219.8 ± 72.6†
Triglyceride (mg/dl)	155.3 ± 53.5	167.8 ± 73.5	149.2 ± 82.4	176.1 ± 84.4*
HDL-cholesterol (mg/dl)	26.5 ± 11.8	29.8 ± 12.7	30.1 ± 7.9	36.8 ± 11.0*
β-lipoprotein (mg/dl)	556.9 ± 147.0	709.1 ± 92.0*	496.3 ± 110.2	697.2 ± 72.1†
Na (mEq/l)	136.8 ± 3.2	135.5 ± 1.6	138.1 ± 2.8	138.0 ± 2.8
K (mEq/l)	4.5 ± 0.2	3.9 ± 0.7*	5.0 ± 0.6	5.1 ± 0.8
Cl (mEq/l)	103.4 ± 6.2	101.3 ± 2.2	103.0 ± 4.3	105.1 ± 4.2
Ca (mg/dl)	8.4 ± 1.0	9.2 ± 0.8	9.3 ± 1.1	8.7 ± 1.0
Mg (mg/dl)	2.4 ± 0.5	3.3 ± 0.4†	2.8 ± 1.0	2.6 ± 0.6
Inorganic P (mg/dl)	6.9 ± 2.6	6.4 ± 2.6	6.6 ± 2.2	7.6 ± 1.9*

* $p < 0.05$, † $p < 0.01$.

Table 4. Serum Concentrations of Low Molecular Weight Proteins Before and After CAPD and P-P-HD Treatment.

	CAPD (mg/dl)		P-P-HD (mg/dl)		
	Before (n = 12)	After One Year (n = 12)	Before (n = 12)	After One Year (n = 12)	Normal Range (mg/dl)
β_2-microglobulin	5.1 ± 2.0	3.7 ± 1.5	6.0 ± 1.6	4.8 ± 1.5†	0.08–0.24
Retinol-binding protein	23.8 ± 3.7	23.6 ± 6.3	31.8 ± 5.6	27.5 ± 8.2	3–6
α_1-acidic glycoprotein	127.6 ± 44.4	148.6 ± 49.6	94.1 ± 36.6	103.7 ± 40.8	40–80
β_2-glyco-protein I	32.3 ± 2.5	38.1 ± 8.5	29.6 ± 5.1	31.6 ± 6.0	10–20
α_2-HS-glycoprotein	64.2 ± 13.1	78.1 ± 18.8	57.5 ± 5.0	50.8 ± 5.4	30–70
α_1-antitrypsin	149.3 ± 28.8	156.4 ± 48.6	133.8 ± 30.6	150.0 ± 40.1	170–360
Prealbumin	40.1 ± 5.0	42.2 ± 11.7	43.3 ± 7.6	39.2 ± 6.8	12–28
Hemopexin	73.1 ± 6.0	70.0 ± 13.8	76.3 ± 10.6	68.5 ± 12.1	40–60
Albumin	3500 ± 410	3720 ± 508	4220 ± 521	3601 ± 597*	3500–5000
Transferrin	191.1 ± 57.1	247.9 ± 67.4†	202.8 ± 51.9	242.3 ± 56.8*	210–290

* $p < 0.05$, † $p < 0.01$.

each. Common changes in laboratory data with the two methods were increases in hemoglobin and erythrocyte count, and either an increase or an increasing trend in β-lipoprotein, total cholesterol, triglyceride, and HDL-cholesterol. Also, transferrin significantly increased, while β_2-microglobulin either fell or tended to decrease.

Many investigators have reported recovery from uremic anemia by CAPD treatment,[8–10] but the reason has not been elucidated to date. The anemia of chronic renal failure is characterized by erythropoietin deficiency, inhibition of erythropoiesis, and shortened red cell life span, among others. CAPD has a lower clearance of small molecular weight substances than conventional hemodialysis does, but that of middle molecules is higher.[1,2] It is thought that there may be some substance among the middle molecules which triggers inhibition of erythropoiesis. The recovery from anemia seen in CAPD patients, together with the increase in red cell mass, also may accompany plasma volume reduction, according to certain reports.[11] The common feature of both methods under investigation here was improved removal of middle and large molecular substances not eliminated well by conventional hemodialysis. This could explain the recovery from anemia.

McGonigle et al.[12] reported that, in both regular dialysis treatment as well as CAPD therapy, there was no correlation between erythropoietin concentration and hematocrit, but there was a direct relationship between inhibition of erythroid colony (CFU-E) formation and hematocrit. Brunner et al.[13] found that a fraction from a uremic ultrafiltrate with a molecular mass exceeding 10,000 daltons markedly inhibited ^{3}H-thymidine incorporation in rat bone marrow cell culture. Freedman et al.[14] reported that a fraction from uremic serum of more than 47,000 daltons molecular weight, acted as an erythropoietic inhibitor. From these studies it seems possible that there is a correlation between the recovery from anemia and the marked increase in the removal of inhibitors of erythropoiesis, in both forms of therapy under study here.

As to the increase in β-lipoprotein, total cholesterol, triglyceride and HDL-cholesterol, both methods of treatment showed common variations. Only P-P-HD was associated with significant increase in total cholesterol, triglyceride and HDL-cholesterol, although with CAPD there was also some increase. The increase in lipids with CAPD can be attributed to the role played by continuous glucose absorption from the dialysate in addition to dietary caloric intake. However, in P-P-HD, in which the glucose level of dialysis fluid is 150 mg/dl, the glucose load cannot be of much importance. Thus, the presence or absence of increased dietary caloric intake in P-P-HD treatment deserves study, but from the similarities evident with both treatments the occurrence of hyperlipidemia suggests some connection with protein loss. The enzyme taking part in lipid metabolism may have been eliminated by one or both methods; this hypothesis requires further study.

As to the protein loss, P-P-HD appears to remove more protein than CAPD, but by and large they have a similar effect. Among the plasma proteins studied in the present cases, only β_2-microglobulin was lowered by the two treatments. Although more than 1000 mg of transferrin was removed in one week, it significantly increased in the blood of patients on either P-P-HD or CAPD, attaining normal levels. Other small molecular weight plasma proteins did not show any major change. However, despite the removal of α_1-acidic glycoprotein, β_2-glycoprotein I and α_1-antitrypsin, with both forms of treatment the proteins increased after one year of therapy. Serum albumin decreased significantly with P-P-HD, but was unchanged with CAPD. Among the proteins eliminated by both treatments, were those which decreased, remained the same or increased. Close study of the metabolism each of these proteins is required but at this juncture it is clear that at least transferrin synthesis is promoted by P-P-HD and CAPD. Substances inhibiting transferrin synthesis in renal failure accumulate, and perhaps CAPD and P-P-HD both serve to remove them. Whether the difference in serum albumin is attributable to the difference in removal in CAPD and P-P-HD, or depends on overall nutritional status, is a subject for future investigation.

REFERENCES

1. Popovich RP, and Moncrief JW: Kinetic modeling of peritoneal transport. Contrib Nephrol 17: 59, 1979
2. Saito A, Chung TG, Niwa T, Maeda K, and Kobayashi K: Middle molecular substances in peritoneal dialysis fluid of uremic patients. In Gahl GM, Kessel M, and Nolph KD (Eds), Advances in peritoneal dialysis: Proceedings of the 2nd international symposium on peritoneal dialysis. Amsterdam: Excerpta Medica, 1981, p 54
3. Twardowski Z, Ksiazek A, Majdan M, Janicka L, Bocheńska-Nowacka E, Sokolowska G, Gutka A, and Żbikowska A: Kinetics of continuous ambulatory peritoneal dialysis (CAPD) with four exchanges per day. Clin Nephrol 15: 119, 1981
4. Blumenkrantz MJ, Gahl GH, Kopple JD, Kamdar AV, Jones MR, Kessel M, and Coburn JW: Protein losses during peritoneal dialysis. Kidney Int 19: 593, 1981
5. Norbeck HE: Lipid abnormalities in continuous ambulatory peritoneal dialysis patients. In Legrain M (Ed), Continuous ambulatory peritoneal dialysis. Amsterdam: Excerpta Medica, 1979, p 298
6. Keusch G, Bommatter F, Mordasini R, and Binswanger U: Serum lipoprotein concentrations during continuous ambulatory peritoneal dialysis: In Gahl GM, Kessel M, and Nolph KD (Eds), Advances in peritoneal dialysis: Proceedings of the 2nd international symposium on peritoneal dialysis. Amsterdam: Excerpta Medica, 1981, p 427
7. Mancini G, Carbonara AO, and Heremans JF: Immunochemical quantitation of antigens by single radial immunodiffusion. Immunochemistry 2: 235, 1965
8. Popovich RP, Moncrief JW, Nolph KD, Ghods AJ, Twardowski ZJ, and Pyle WK: Continuous ambulatory peritoneal dialysis. Ann Intern Med 88: 449, 1978
9. Oreopoulos DG, Robson M, Faller B, Ogilvie R, Rapoport A, and DeVeber GA: Continuous ambulatory peritoneal dialysis: A new era in the treatment of chronic renal failure. Clin Nephrol 11: 125, 1979
10. Zappacosta AR, Caro J, and Erslev A: Normalization of hematocrit in patients with end-stage renal disease on continuous ambulatory peritoneal dialysis. Am J Med 72: 53, 1982
11. DePaepe MBJ, Schelstraete KHG, Ringoir SMG, and Lameire NH: Influence of continuous ambulatory peritoneal dialysis on the anemia of endstage renal disease. Kidney Int 23: 744, 1983
12. McGonigle RJS, Husserl F, Wallin JD, and Fisher JW: Hemodialysis and continuous ambulatory peritoneal dialysis effects on erythropoiesis in renal failure. Kidney Int 25: 430, 1984
13. Brunner H, Mann H, Essers U, and Byrne T: Large-scale isolation of middle and higher molecular weight uremic toxins. Artif Organs 4(Suppl); 41, 1980
14. Freedman MH, Grunberger T, and Saunders EF: Erythropoietic inhibitors in uremic serum. Clin Invest Med 5: 237, 1982

A.R. Nissenson, D.E. Gentile, R. Soderblom, and C. Brax

58

CAPD in the Elderly—Regional Experience

SUMMARY

Experience with 775 patients over age 60 years treated by CAPD is reported. After 11.6 months 78% were alive and 32% were still on CAPD. Death was attributed to vascular disease in 62%. By the end of one year, 55% had their first episode of peritonitis, but 88% still had their original catheter. CAPD is a reasonable treatment for elderly patients with ESRD. Except for the expected increased mortality in this age group, the elderly compared favorably with younger patients treated by CAPD.

INTRODUCTION

Most investigators agree that CAPD is an equivalent form of treatment to hemodialysis for "standard" patients (ages 21–60 years nondiabetic, no associated medical problems).[1-3] In addition, most pediatric nephrologists consider CAPD or CCPD the dialysis modality of choice for children awaiting renal transplantation.[4] Though the outcome of CAPD in the elderly seems favorable,[5,6] no large experience with such individuals has been reported.

PATIENTS AND METHODS

Between early 1979 and December 31, 1983, 775 patients have started on CAPD and entered in the CAPD study in NCC #4, which includes Southern California and Southern Nevada. A total experience of 204.25 patient years has accumulated in the 183 patients (23.6% of the total CAPD population) over 60 years of age at the time of initiation of CAPD. For this elderly group, mean time on CAPD is 11.6 months (range 0.5–46 months). Patients entered the study when they completed CAPD training and initiated CAPD as their only treatment modality. A registration form was completed initially to collect basic demographic data and quarterly patient status update forms were completed to provide outcome data.

Demographic data was tabulated and where appropriate, percent prevalence was calculated. Life-table analyses were then performed, using standard methods[7] for selected outcome variables.

RESULTS

Demographic Analysis

The group was 59.2% male and 40.8% female, comparable to the overall CAPD patient sex distribution. There were 74.3% white, 13.1% Mexican-American, and 7.9% black patients, compared with 65.8%, 16.5%, and 11% for the same racial groups respectively in the overall CAPD population. ESRD was caused by chronic glomerulonephritis in 25.1%, nephrosclerosis in 22%, polycystic kidney disease in 14.1%, and diabetes mellitus in 12.6%, similar to the overall CAPD population.

Patient Outcome (Table 1)

At the end of the study 32% of the patients were still on CAPD, 39% had transferred to hemodialysis, and 22% had died.

From the Department of Medicine, Division of Nephrology, UCLA School of Medicine and NCC #4 Los Angeles, California; and the Medical Review Board, National Coordinating Council No. 4.

Table 1. Patient Outcome.

Still on CAPD	32%
Transferred to hemodialysis	39%
Died	22%
Recovered renal function	2%
Lost-to-follow-up	4%
Unknown	1%

Table 2. Reasons for Changing Dialysis Mode.

Peritonitis	37%
Other medical	23%
Patient or family choice	18%
Tunnel infection	13%
Inadequate clearances	7%
Socioeconomic	2%

Reasons for Changing Dialysis Mode (Table 2)

Of the patients who switched to hemodialysis 37% did so because of recurrent peritonitis, and 13% because of tunnel infection. Only 18% switched because of patient or family preference and 7% because of inadequate clearances.

Cause of Death (Table 3)

Death was attributed to vascular causes (MI, other cardiac or cerebrovascular) in 62% while 12% died of septicemia. The remainder of deaths resulted from a wide variety of causes.

Life-Table Analyses (Figs. 1–6).

Patient survival. Patient survival was 79% at 1 year, 63% at 2 years, and 52% at 2 1/2 years. Survival was significantly lower, as expected, in the elderly compared to the younger patients.

Patients remaining on CAPD. Overall, 53% of patients were still on CAPD at 1 year, 24% at 2 years, and 15% at 2 1/2 years. Significantly fewer elderly patients remained on CAPD at these time periods compared to younger patients.

Technique survival. Excluding death and transplantation, 67% of patients were still on CAPD at 1 year, 37% at 2 years, and 29% at 2 1/2 years. Technique survival was significantly less in the elderly compared to the 0–20-year-old patients, but not different from that seen in the 21–60-year-old patients.

Hospitalizations. By the end of 1 year, 62% of patients had been hospitalized at least once, 76% by the end of two years, and 79% by 2 1/2 years. There were no differences in time to first hospitalization between the elderly and the other two age groups.

Peritonitis. By the end of 1 year, 55% of patients had their first episode of peritonitis, 65% by the end of 2 years, and 70% by the end of 2 1/2 years. There were no differences in time to first peritonitis episode among the three age groups.

Catheter replacement. By the end of 1 year, 88% of patients still had their original catheter, 86% at the end of 2 years, and 81% at the end of 3 1/2 years. Elderly patients had significantly better catheter longevity than did patients age 0–20 years.

Hospitalizations (Table 4)

Elderly patients spent an average of 19.1 days/patient-year in the hospital compared to 17.8 days/patient-year for the overall CAPD population. CAPD related problems including peritonitis accounted for 60% of all hospital days.

DISCUSSION

In the 5 years since the widespread application of CAPD, many data have been published on outcome of large heterogenous populations.[1–3,8,9] Lit-

Table 3. Cause of Death.

Acute myocardial infarction	33%
Cardiac (excluding MI and pericarditis)	21%
Septicemia	12%
Unknown	10%
Cerebrovascular	8%
GI hemorrhage	6%
Other	6%
Pulmonary infection	2%
Withdrawal from dialysis	2%

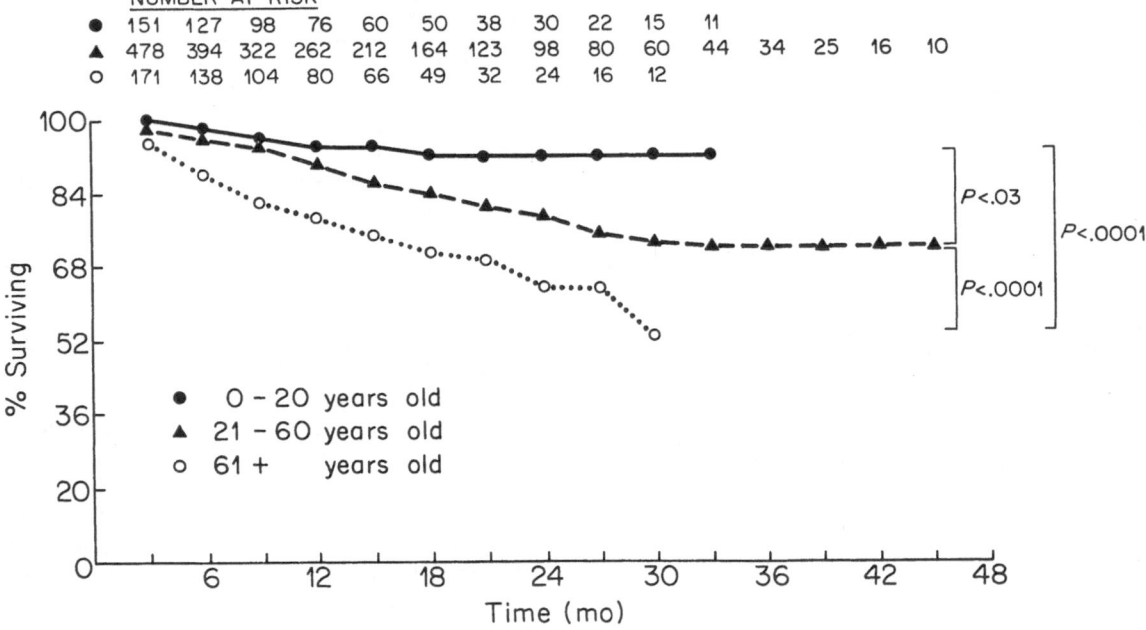

Fig. 1. Patient survival for each age group on CAPD.

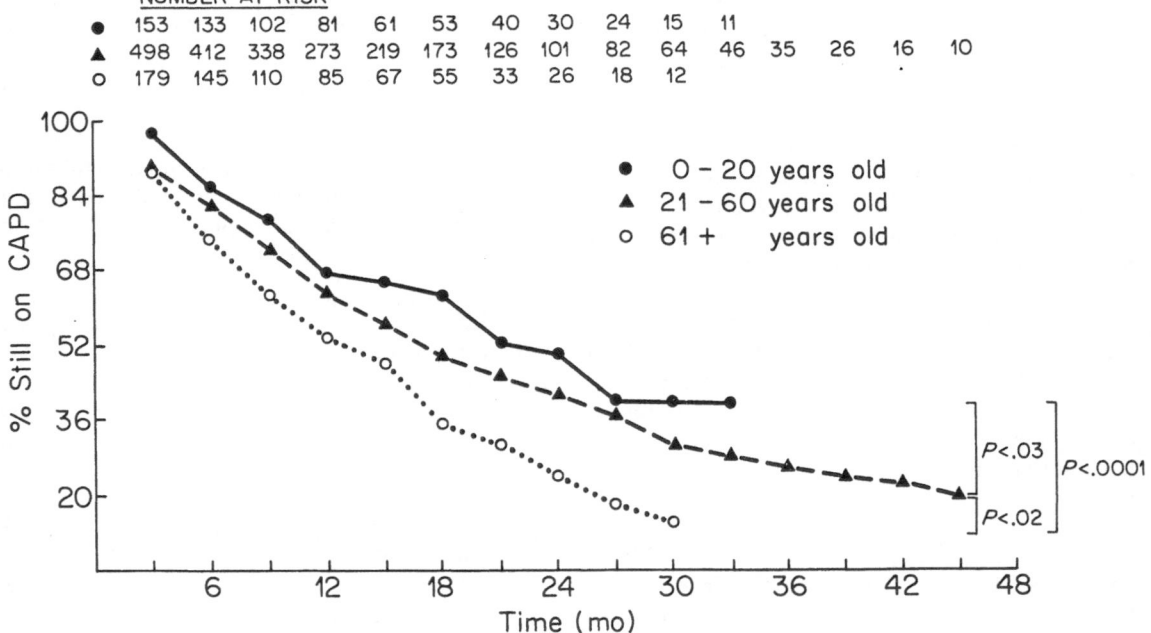

Fig. 2. Percent of patients remaining on CAPD by age group.

NUMBER AT RISK
● 152 127 98 76 60 52 40 30 23 15 11
▲ 491 406 331 266 214 171 123 99 80 62 45 35 26 16 10
○ 172 140 107 83 65 55 33 25 18 11
% Not Changing Dialysis Modality
100
84
68
52
36
20
0
6
12
18
24
30
36
42
48
Time (mo)
● 0 - 20 years old
▲ 21 - 60 years old
○ 61 + years old
P<.0001
P<.0001

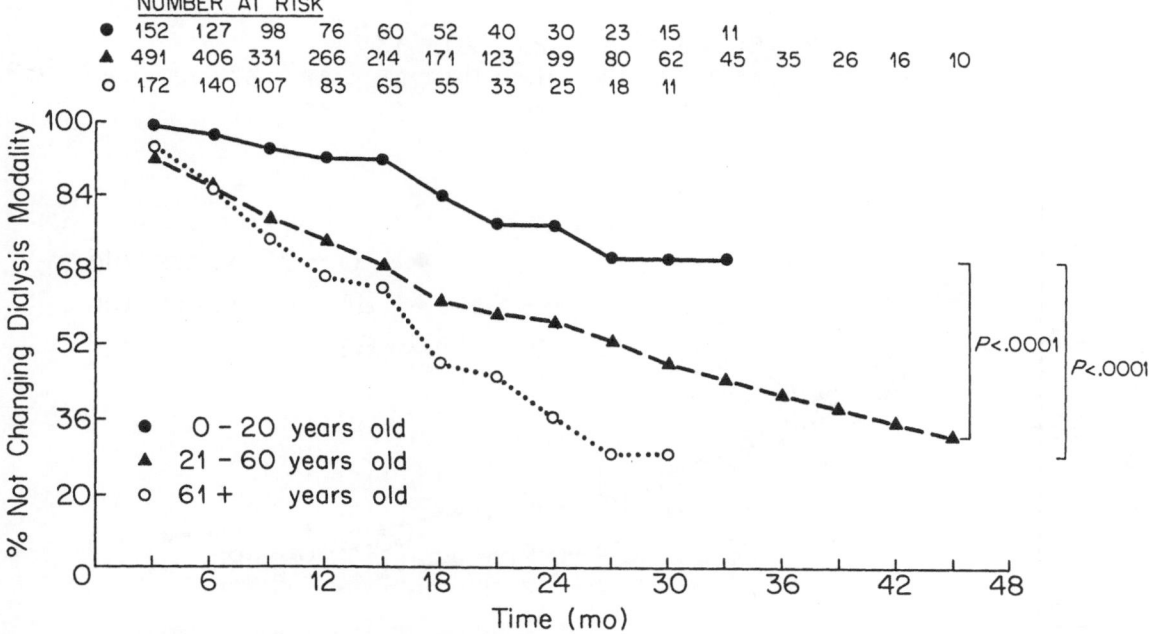

Fig. 3. Technique survival on CAPD (death and transplantation are considered "lost-to-follow-up").

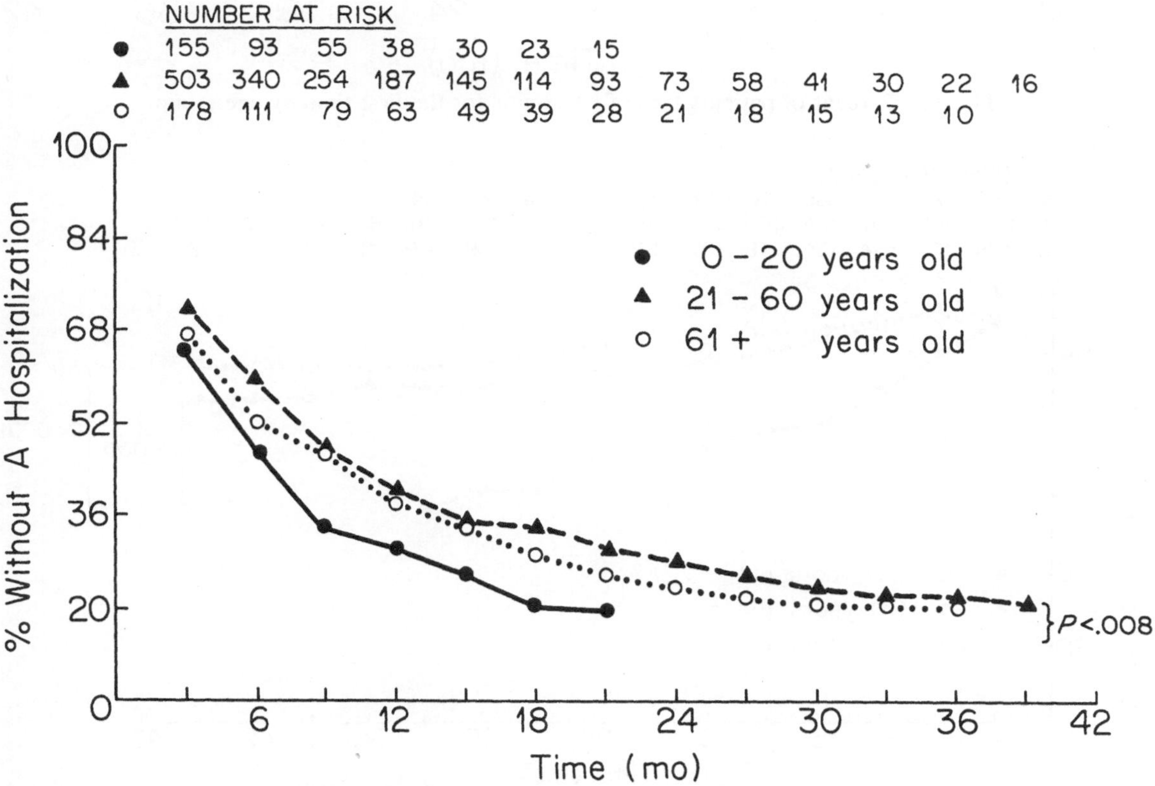

NUMBER AT RISK
● 155 93 55 38 30 23 15
▲ 503 340 254 187 145 114 93 73 58 41 30 22 16
○ 178 111 79 63 49 39 28 21 18 15 13 10
% Without A Hospitalization
100
84
68
52
36
20
0
6
12
18
24
30
36
42
Time (mo)
● 0 - 20 years old
▲ 21 - 60 years old
○ 61 + years old
P<.008

Fig. 4. Percent of patients hospitalized for the first time by age group

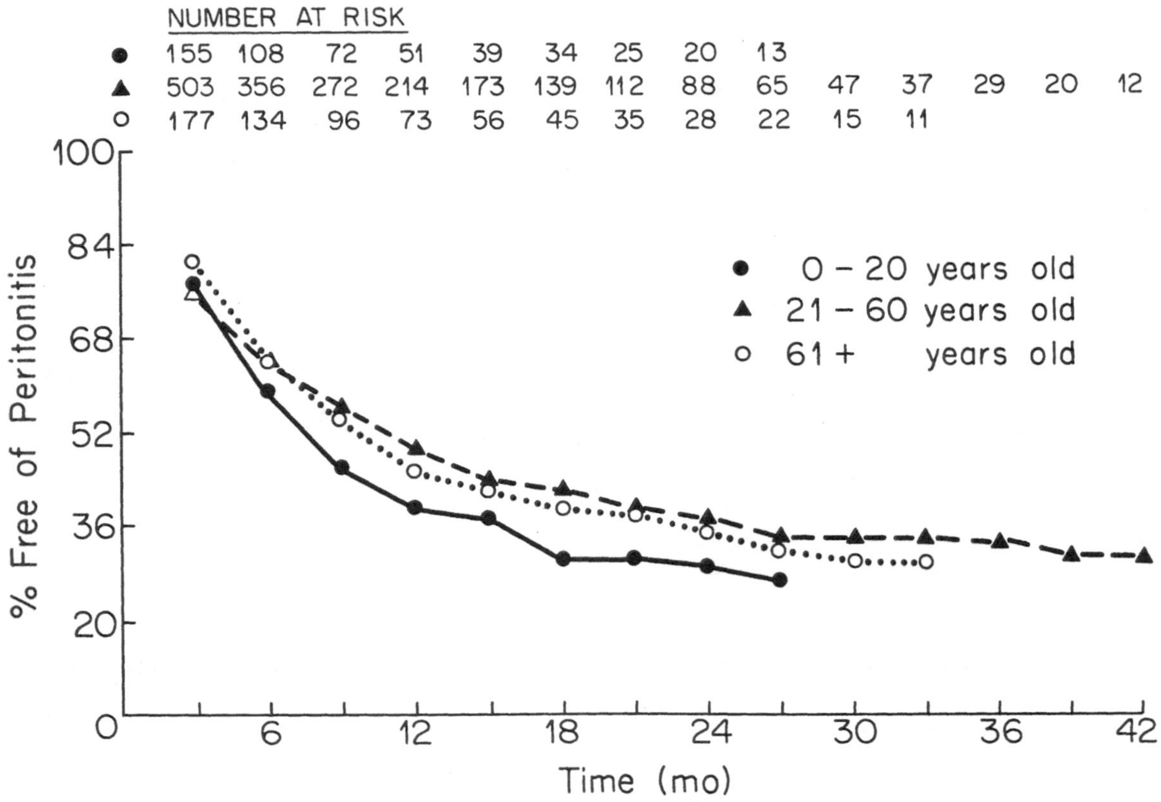

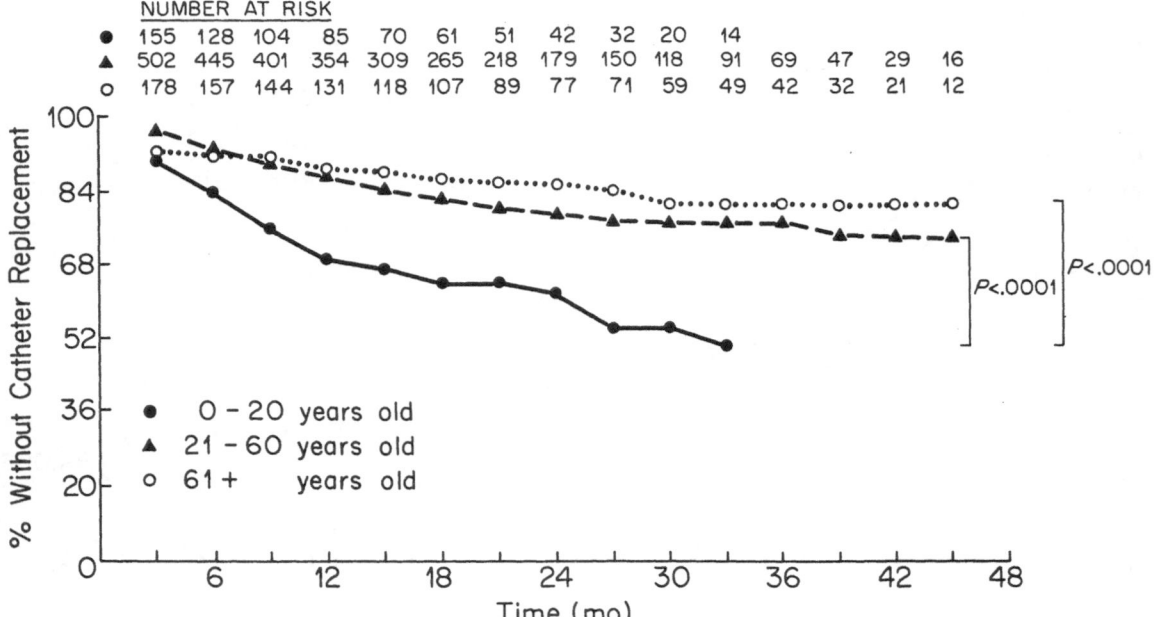

Fig. 5. Percent of patients free of peritonitis for the first time by age group.

Fig. 6. Percent of patients without a catheter replacement by age group.

Table 4. Hospitalizations.

Reasons for Hospitalization	Total Number of Hospital		
	Admissions	Days	Days/ Patient-year
Peritonitis	142	1317	6.5
CAPD related problems other than peritonitis	130	957	4.7
Vascular problems	68	630	3.1
Other problems	97	989	4.8
All reasons	437	3893	19.1

tle has been written, however, on the elderly patient, a rapidly growing segment of the ESRD population. This type of data is particularly cogent since age is a major factor excluding patients from dialysis in some countries.[10]

Kaye et al.[5] reported on 18 patients age 65 years or older on CAPD in Montreal, and compared them to 26 younger CAPD patients. They found that in most respects (biochemical control, complications, failure rate) elderly patients were comparable to younger ones. Though more elderly patients died than younger ones during the period of observation, the difference was not statistically significant.

Nicholls et al.[6] described 38 patients aged over 60 years treated with CAPD. Most of these patients were considered unsuitable for hemodialysis by criteria that were applied in the United Kingdom prior to the availability of CAPD. Two patients subsequently transferred to hemodialysis while the remainder stayed on CAPD. Patient survival was 72% at 1 year and 61% at two years, and 21% of the 23 survivors were "fully rehabilitated."

The present report is the largest series of elderly CAPD patients yet described. The demographic features of this group, other than age, were similar to those of the overall NCC #4 CAPD population. Overall patient and technique survival were comparable to the previous reports, but survival was significantly lower compared to the overall NCC #4 CAPD population. Technique survival, hospitalization rate, peritonitis rate and catheter survival rates were similar in our young and older patients, though the latter was somewhat better in the elderly.

In conclusion, CAPD is a reasonable alternative treatment for the elderly patient with ESRD. Except for the expected increase in death in this group, the elderly compared favorably in other aspects of morbidity to younger patients receiving this modality of therapy.

REFERENCES

1. Khanna R, Wu G, Vas S, and Oreopoulos DG: Mortality and morbidity on CAPD. asaio J 6: 197, 1983
2. Mion CM, Mourad G, Canaud B, Chong G, Polito C, Oules R, Branger B, Granolleras C, Issautier R, Slingeneyer A, Ramperez P, Flavier J, Deschodt G, Emond C, Cozette P, Florence P, Chouzenoox R, Huchard G, Fitte H, Marty L, Grolleau-Raoux R, and Shaldon S: Maintenance dialysis: A survey of 17 years' experience in Languedoc-Roussillon with a comparison of methods in a "standard population." asaio J 6: 205, 1983
3. Wing AJ, Broyer M, Brunner FP, Brynger H, Donckerwolcke RA, Jacobs C, Kramer P, Selwood NH, and Challah S: The contribution of CAPD in Europe. asaio J 6: 214, 1983
4. Baum M, Powell D, Calvin S, McDaid T, McHenry K, Mar H, and Potter D: CAPD in children. N Engl J Med 307: 1537, 1982
5. Kaye M, Pajel PA, and Somerville PJ: Four years' experience with CAPD in the elderly. Peritoneal Dial Bull 3: 17, 1983
6. Nicholls AJ, Waldek S, Platts MM, Moorhead PJ, and Brown CB: Impact of CAPD on treatment of renal failure in patients aged over 60. Br Med J 288: 18, 1984
7. Cutler SJ, and Ederer F: Maximum utilization of the life table method in analyzing survival. J Chron Dis 8: 699, 1958
8. Nissenson AR, Gentile DE, Soderblom R, and Brax C: Long-term outcome of CAPD—regional experience. Dial Transplant 13: 34, 1984
9. Diaz-Buxo J: Intermittent, continuous ambulatory and continuous cycling peritoneal dialysis. In Nissenson AR, Fine RN, and Gentile DE (Eds), Clinical dialysis. Norwalk, CN, Appleton-Century-Crofts, 1984, p 263
10. Challah S, Wing AJ, Bauer R, Morris RW, and Schroeder SA: Negative selection of patients for dialysis and transplantation in the United Kingdom. Br Med J 288: 1119, 1984

G. Triolo, A. Cantaluppi, S. Bellocchi, S. Carozzi,
A. Jayme, M. Remondino, and G.P. Segoloni

59

Italian Multicentric Study on Diabetic Uremic Patients Treated by CAPD

SUMMARY

A multicenter evaluation of diabetic patients undergoing CAPD has compared results to those of nondiabetic patients treated by CAPD and of diabetic patients treated by hemodialysis. The study involved 22 Italian dialysis centers and evaluated 97 diabetic patients and 764 nondiabetic patients who were comparable in age. The mortality rate was higher in the diabetic group, but the peritonitis rate was similar. The technique survival rate was lower in the diabetic patients. The patient survival rate was no different when diabetic patients treated by CAPD were compared to the diabetic group treated by hemodialysis. Moreover, when high risk nondiabetic patients were compared to the diabetic group, CAPD patient survival rates were comparable. CAPD is a useful treatment for diabetic uremic patients.

INTRODUCTION

The relatively few diabetic ESRD patients treated in our country with hemodialysis and with CAPD, even in those centers committed to such treatments limit the objective evaluation of the advantages and disadvantages of such techniques. To assess the value of CAPD, which from the very beginning seemed to have some advantages in the treatment of diabetics, a study, which is part of a greater multicentric national registry on CAPD[1] involving 861 patients (40.3% of the total national pool for 1982) in 22 centers of 17 provinces, was under-

taken. The aims of our study were to compare the clinical picture of uremic diabetic patients with that of our other patients, the survival rates, and technique failure rates of diabetics on CAPD with nondiabetics and diabetics undergoing hemodialysis, and the incidence of peritonitis in diabetic and nondiabetic patients.

PATIENTS AND METHODS

Our study involved 97 diabetic and 764 nondiabetic patients, the characteristics of whom are summarized in Table 1. Data from 32 diabetic patients starting treatment with hemodialysis were also recorded. To obtain our data we asked the centers to fill in a questionnaire with 39 items. All data were processed at the Computer Center of Ospedale San Giovanni, Turin, in collaboration with the Piemonte CSI, by applying the BMDP-1L procedure: "Life tables and survival functions" from BMDP statistical software,[2] developed at the Health Science Computing Facility, UCLA (NIH Special Research Resources, grant RR—3), (Program revised October 1983). Survival curves were analyzed following the method of Kaplan and Meier.[3] Differences between the curves were calculated by the methods of Breslow[4] and Mantel,[5] and, between single points by a two-sided test of significance for normal distributions. In our study the male/female ratio of the diabetic group was 2.03, and their average age was 53.6 ± 11.8 years, 36% being under 50 years. In the patients 83% had previously undergone conservative treatment; CAPD was chosen as pri-

Table 1. Case Series of the Italian CAPD Multicenter Study (1980–1983).

Diabetic	Group	Nondiabetic
97	Number of patients	764
65/32 (2.03)	Males/females	422/341 (1.2)
100%	High risk (%)	51%
53.6 ± 11.8 (27–79)	Average age at beginning CAPD (years) (range)	54.06 ± 15.3 (1–83)
35 (36%)	<50 years	251 (32.8%)
62 (64%)	>50 years	513 (67.1%)
	Reasons for CAPD	
41 (42.2%)	Policy of the center	241 (31.5%)
23 (23.7%)	Patient's wish	173 (31.5%)
6 (6.1%)	Difficult vascular access	93 (12.1%)
6 (6.1%)	Poor hemodialysis tolerance	56 (7.3%)
21 (21.6%)	Other	201 (26.3%)
	Previous Treatment	
81 (83.5%)	Conservative	543 (71.0%)
8 (8.2%)	Hemodialysis	156 (20.4%)
3 (3.0%)	Hemofiltration	9 (1.1%)
5 (5.1%)	IPD	46 (6.1%)
	Period Under CAPD	
11.7 ± 8.3 (1–33)	Observation (months) (range)	15.3 ± 11.4 (1–53)

Table 2. Causes of Drop-Out (%).

Diabetics	Group	Nondiabetics
28 (58.3%)	Died	153 (46.9%)
5 (10.4%)	Peritonitis	62 (19.0%)
3 (6.3%)	Other clinical complications	26 (7.9%)
4 (8.3%)	Incapability of the patient	8 (2.6%)
2 (4.2%)	Dialytic ineffectiveness	18 (5.5%)
—	Wish of patient to discontinue	12 (3.9%)
2 (4.2%)	Catheter complications	9 (2.9%)
3 (6.2%)	Functional recovery	11 (3.2%)
1 (2.0%)	Transplant	21 (6.5%)
—	Other	6 (1.6%)

Table 3. Number of Patients Free from First Peritonitis at
Time Intervals.

| | Patients | | | |
| | Diabetic | | Nondiabetic | |
Months	At Risk (n)	Survival Rate (%)	At Risk (n)	Survival Rate (%)
1	97	90.5 ± 3	746	88.7 ± 1.1
3	67	64.4 ± 5.0	507	67.6 ± 1.7
6	37	46.1 ± 5.4	325	48.8 ± 1.9
12	15	30.6 ± 5.4	150	30.5 ± 1.9
24	5	20.3 ± 6.1	38	17.5 ± 1.9

p = N.S.

mary treatment by the center in 50% of cases, by the patient in 28%, and in 22% for other various reasons.

In the remaining 17% of cases, CAPD was usually chosen as secondary treatment to overcome difficulties deriving from previous treatment. The same data were calculated for nondiabetic patients (Table 1).

RESULTS

Treatment was interrupted by 49% of diabetic and 42.6% of nondiabetic patients for the following reasons: death (58% and 47% respectively), peritonitis (10% and 19%), other clinical complications (6% and 7%) (Table 2).

The number of patients free from the first episode of peritonitis was surprisingly similar in both groups (46% and 48% at the sixth mo 30.6% and 30.5% at the twelfth mo) (Table 3). While 61 patients had suffered one episode of peritonitis, 42 had two episodes, with an incidence of 1 episode/every 6.4

patient-month. Among the causes of death, vascular complications were responsible in 12 diabetic and 22 nondiabetic patients; infection was responsible for respectively 3 and 17 cases; cachexia for respectively 5 and 25 cases (Table 4). Patient survival rates during treatment were 89.6 ± 3.2%, 74.2 ± 5.3%, 49.5 ± 8.6% at 6, 12, and 24 months (Table 5). Whereas for nondiabetic patients survival rate at the same time intervals were 92.6, 85, and 72%, diabetic patients seemed to be at greater risk but approximately at the same risk when compared to nondiabetic patients at "high risk" (patient survivals 89, 74, 49% compared to 87, 75, and 58% respectively sixth, twelfth, and twenty-fourth months) (Table 6).

Overall survival rate of diabetic patients on CAPD from the beginning, compared to diabetics undergoing hemodialysis, revealed no significant differences (Table 7).

Diabetic patients encountered a higher number of CAPD failures[6] compared to nondiabetics (76, 61, 33% versus 86, 71, and 52% of technique survival respectively sixth, twelfth, and twenty-fourth) (Table 8).

The survival rate of diabetic drop-outs calculated from the thirtieth day after interrupting treatment, was not significantly different when compared to the nondiabetic drop-out survival rate (Table 9). One must bear in mind in interpreting these results the different treatments given after drop-out in the two groups (Table 10).

In conclusion, even if survival rates are obviously lower than in nondiabetic patients, our results show that the survival rates of diabetic patients on CAPD are similar to those of high risk nondiabetics, who constitute over 50% of the population undergo-

Table 4. Causes of Death.

Diabetic	Patients	Nondiabetic
8 (28.5%)	Cardiac	56 (36.6%)
4 (14.2%)	Cerebral	16 (10.5%)
3 (10.7%)	Infectious	17 (11.1%)
(2)	(peritonitis)	(10)
(1)	(pulmonary)	(7)
5 (17.8%)	Cachexia	25 (16.3%)
8 (28.5%)	Other	39 (25.4%)

Table 5. Survival Rate during CAPD (%).

	Patients				
	Diabetic			Nondiabetic	
Months	At Risk	Survival Rate		At Risk	Survival Rate
1	97	98.9 ± 1		746	99.6 ± 0.2
3	91	96.7 ± 1.8		706	96.6 ± 0.6
6	74	89.6 ± 3.2		606	92.6 ± 1.0
12	41	74.1 ± 5.3		423	85.0 ± 1.4
24	13	49.5 ± 8.6		191	72.3 ± 2.1

$p = 0.0076$ (BRESLOW); $p = 0.0027$ (MANTEL–COX).

Table 6. Patient Survival Rate during CAPD in Diabetics and High Risk Nondiabetics (%).

	Patients				
	Diabetic			"High Risk"	
Months	At Risk	Survival Rate		At Risk	Survival Rate
1	97	98.8 ± 1.1		388	99.4 ± 0.3
3	84	96.4 ± 1.8		368	94.6 ± 1.1
6	67	89.6 ± 3.2		308	87.5 ± 1.7
12	37	74.2 ± 5.3		210	75.4 ± 2.6
24	12	49.5 ± 8.6		87	58.4 ± 3.3

p = N.S.

ing CAPD, and are similar to the results obtained in patients treated with hemodialysis. From our experience CAPD is a useful additional means of treating uremic diabetic patients not only for the clinical results obtained, but also for its easy application and operation. Over the last years the percentage of patients undergoing hemodialysis has not changed whereas the percentage of diabetics in treatment has grown from 4.2% in 1979 to 8.4% of new admissions in 1983, leading us to believe that finally an adequate policy for the full treatment of all diabetic patients will be achieved.

ACKNOWLEDGMENTS

We thank M. Mostert, M.D., M. Salomone, M.D., and D. Pelizza, M.D. for their collaboration and helpful criticism.

STUDY CENTERS

Torino: Molinette (A. Vercellone), Nuova Astanteria Martini (G. Piccoli); Pinerolo: E. Agnelli (A. Ramello); Milano: Maggiore-Policlinico (C.

Table 7. Overall Survival of Diabetic Patients.

	Treatment	
Months	CAPD Survival Rate (%)	Hemodialysis Survival Rate (%)
1	97 ± 1.6	92.9 ± 4.8
3	97 ± 1.6	92.9 ± 4.8
6	91.2 ± 3.2	92.9 ± 4.8
12	87.1 ± 3.8	85.6 ± 6.9
24	65.1 ± 6.5	64.7 ± 11

Table 8. Technique Survival Rate.

Months	Patients			
	Diabetic		Nondiabetic	
1	97	98.9 ± 1.0	746	99.4 ± 0.2
2	91	92.5 ± 2.7	706	93.3 ± 0.9
6	74	76.3 ± 4.4	606	86.3 ± 1.3
12	41	61.7 ± 5.4	423	71.3 ± 1.7
24	13	33.7 ± 6.8	191	52.4 ± 2.2

$p = 0.0173$ (BRESLOW); $p = 0.0094$ (MANTEL–COX).

Table 9. Patient Survival Rate after Drop-out (%).

Months	Patients			
	Diabetic		Nondiabetic	
1	16	93.7 ± 6	115	100 ± 0
3	13	93.7 ± 6	109	94.3 ± 2.2
6	11	85.9 ± 9.3	90	91.3 ± 2.7
12	6	85.9 ± 9.3	63	88.7 ± 3.2
24		—	30	80.9 ± 4.8

p = N.S.

Table 10. Post-CAPD Drop-Out Treatment.

Diabetic	Patients	Nondiabetic
11 (61.1%)	HD acetate	116 (71.6%)
1 (55%)	HD bicarbonate	12 (7.4%)
4 (22.2%)	Hemofiltration	3 (1.9%)
1 (5.5%)	IPD	10 (6.1%)
—	Cadaver transplant	17 (10.4%)
1 (5.5%)	Living donor transplant	4 (2.4%)

Ponticelli); S. Carlo Borromeo (G. D'Amico), Niguarda-Ca' Granda (L. Minetti); Bergamo: Rinuiti (G. Mecca); Brescia: Spedali Civili (R. Maiorca); Cremona: Istituti Ospitalieri (F. Pecchini); Busto Arsizio: Provinciale (A. Giangrande); Verona: Istituti Ospitalieri (G. Maschio); Vicenza: S. Bortolo (G. LaGreca); Udine: Regionale (G. Mioni); Genova: S. Martino (S. Lamperi), Gaslini (R. Gusmano); Bologna: M. Malpighi (P. Zucchelli); Piacenza: Provinciale (L. Scarpioni); Ravenna: S. Maria Delle Croci (M. Fusaroli); Reggio Emilia: S. Maria Nuova (S. Zini); Ancona: Umberto I (L. Mioli); Ascoli Piceno: G. Mazzoni (M. Ragaiolo); Foggia: Riuniti (A. Passione).

REFERENCES

1. Segoloni GP: Evaluation of the clinical and organizational impact of CAPD in the three year period from 1980–1983; the experience of 21 Italian Centers. J Artif Organs (in press)
2. Dixon WJ (Ed): BMDP statistical software, October Edition. Los Angeles, University of California Press, 1983
3. Kaplan EL, and Meier P: Nonparametric estimation from incomplete observations. J Am Statist Assoc 53: 457, 1958
4. Breslow N: A generalized Kruskal-Wallis test for comparing k samples subject to unequal patterns of censorship. Biometrika 57: 579, 1970
5. Mantel N: Evaluation of survival data and two rank order statistics arising in its consideration. Cancer Chemother Rep 50: 163, 1966
6. Pierratos A: Peritoneal dialysis glossary. Peritoneal Dial Bull 4: 1, 1984

N.M. Thomson, R.W. Simpson, R.C. Atkins, and N. Boyce

60

CAPD in the Diabetic; Comparison with Nondiabetics on CAPD

SUMMARY

Twenty-five patients with endstage renal failure due to diabetic nephropathy have received CAPD for a mean time of more than 1 year. Their capacity to learn self dialysis, adequacy of dialysis, patient and technique survival, complications of CAPD and quality of life have been assessed and compared to those of a group of 135 nondiabetic patients on CAPD over the same period. All diabetic patients were successfully trained for home CAPD (with aid of a relative if blind). Adequacy of dialysis was comparable for the two groups as was the survival of the technique of CAPD. Patient survival at 1 year was 78% for diabetic and 93% for nondiabetic patients, the principal cause of death in the diabetic group being complications of degenerative vascular disease. The incidence of peritonitis was similar in both groups and hypertriglyceridemia was significantly less in the diabetic group.

The use of intraperitoneal insulin resulted in better control of blood sugar than with subcutaneous insulin. Deterioration of diabetic retinopathy was uncommon in patients on CAPD as opposed to those on hemodialysis. It is concluded that CAPD is the preferable type of dialysis for the diabetic with end-stage renal failure, with results similar to that for CAPD in the nondiabetic.

From the Department of Nephrology and Medical Research Centre, Prince Henry's Hospital, Melbourne, Australia.

INTRODUCTION

The management of the diabetic with end-stage renal failure by dialysis and transplantation has undoubtedly improved over the last 15 to 20 years with 1 year survival increasing from 20 to 60% in the early 1970s[1-3] to 60 to 90% in the late 1970s.[4-7] However, survival is still less than in the nondiabetic patients, largely due to the cardiovascular, cerebrovascular, and peripheral vascular complications of diabetes. Improved mortality for the diabetic with end-stage renal failure is probably related to better control of hypertension and earlier dialysis. With improved survival more and more diabetics are being offered dialysis and transplantation and in some centers diabetics comprise up to 20% of all patients.

Controversy still surrounds whether renal transplantation or dialysis is the better treatment for the diabetic patient. However, most diabetics will receive dialysis at least initially and the decision must be made as to hemodialysis (HD) or peritoneal dialysis (PD). Studies reported in the late 1970s[8-12] showed that intermittent PD had several advantages over HD, notably, better control of retinopathy and vascular instability although control of blood glucose was often difficult. With the introduction of CAPD in 1976[13] and its refinement[14] a number of groups including ourselves[15-17] reported preliminary studies of the use of CAPD in diabetic patients and found CAPD to be an effective treatment with many advantages over HD and IPD.

In this paper we report our experience of CAPD in 25 patients with diabetic renal failure and compare results to those of 135 nondiabetics treated by CAPD in the same period.

METHODS

Patients

Since 1978, 25 insulin-dependent diabetic patients (19 males, 6 females; mean age 41 years, range 22 to 69 years) with end-stage renal failure due to diabetic nephropathy have been accepted into our CAPD program. In the same period 135 nondiabetic patients (mean age 43.8 years, range 5 to 73 years) have commenced CAPD. All diabetics had diabetic retinopathy (seven blind), 11 (44%) had diabetic peripheral neuropathy, five (20%) had clinically obvious peripheral vascular disease, six (24%) had clinical or ECG evidence of ischemic heart disease and five (20%) had clinical features of autonomic neuropathy. Three diabetic patients (12%) had suffered a minor cerebrovascular accident prior to dialysis. By comparison the incidence of ischemic heart disease in the nondiabetics was (22%) while that of peripheral vascular disease was only (4%) and prior stroke had occurred in no patient.

Technique of CAPD and Diet

All patients were trained for home CAPD using three, four or five exchanges per day as previously described.[18, 19] Diabetic patients were prescribed a diet to provide 30 to 35 Kcal/kg lean body weight/ day of which protein comprised 18% (predominantly lean red or white meat), fat (ratio of polyunsaturated: saturated = one) 32%, and carbohydrate (unrefined carbohydrate rich foods) 50%. Control of blood glucose with insulin is described below.

Clinical and Laboratory Observations

The following observations and comparisons were made between the diabetic and nondiabetic groups. Patient survival and outcome of CAPD; The cumulative survival of diabetic and nondiabetic patients on CAPD and the survival of the technique of CAPD in the two groups was determined using the life table method of Cutler and Ederer. The patient groups were compared using the log rank test. Capacity to learn CAPD and perform home dialysis; adequacy of dialysis as assessed by general health, biochemical parameters and, control of hypertension and salt and water balance were as-

sessed. Complications of CAPD, particularly peritonitis, hyperlipidemia and complications related to diabetic vascular disease, and control of blood glucose in the diabetic were watched. Adequacy of glucose control with intraperitoneal (IP) insulin administration was formally compared to control with subcutaneous (SC) insulin. In all diabetics blood glucose was initially controlled with twice daily SC administration of a mixture of short-acting (Actrapid) and long-acting (Monotard) insulin. Home capillary blood glucose was monitored by glucose oxidase strips (and reflectance meter) aiming to achieve a postprandial blood glucose concentration between 4 and 8 mmol/L. After stable control for at least 6 weeks, a formal 24 hour assessment of blood glucose concentration was obtained using free-flowing hourly samples from an indwelling Teflon cannula (eight patients). Eighteen patients were then changed to a regime of IP insulin using soluble insulin (Actrapid). Again when adequate control of blood glucose was obtained with home monitoring for at least 6 weeks a formal 24 hours assessment was obtained (seven patients). In addition glycosylated hemoglobin (Hb a1c) levels were compared for the two regimes of insulin administration. Progress of retinopathy was assessed by monitoring visual acuity, fundoscopy and fluorescein angiography at 6 month intervals. An assessment of quality of life in the diabetics was made using the parameters of capacity to work, and general sense of wellbeing.

RESULTS

Patient Survival and Outcome

The mean time diabetics spent on CAPD was 13.4 months (range 2 to 35 months) compared to 15.3 months (range 3 to 66 months) for nondiabetics. Seven diabetics are still on CAPD, nine have had successful renal transplants (12 renal transplants have been performed overall), four were transferred to HD (recurrent peritonitis) and five died while on CAPD (myocardial infarction, suicide, fungal peritonitis/meningitis, and dialysis was withdrawn from two patients with very poor quality of life) (Table 1). Survival at 1 and 2 years for diabetics was 78% and 70% respectively compared to 93% and 86% for nondiabetics $(0.1> p> 0.05)$ (Fig. 1). Survival of the technique of CAPD was 71% and 49% for diabetics at 1 and 2 years respectively and 78% and 58% for nondiabetics $[p> 0.1]$ (Fig. 2).

Table 1. Reasons for Cessation of CAPD.

| | Group | |
	Diabetic (n = 25)	Nondiabetic (n = 135)
Still on CAPD	7	53
Ceased CAPD	18	82
Renal transplantation	9	27
Transfer to another unit	—	2
Temporary CAPD	—	4
Transfer to HD	4	31
recurrent peritonitis	4	23
poor dialysis	—	4
abdominal pain	—	1
hydrothorax	—	3
Died	5	18
cardiovascular	1	11
suicide	1	—
peritonitis	1	6
dialysis withdrawn	2	1

Home Dialysis

All diabetic and nondiabetic patients were successfully trained for home dialysis. However six (24%) of diabetics (all blind) required the aid of a relative. Only one blind diabetic was self-sufficient.

In the blind diabetics home dialysis was associated with considerable family stress and disruption.

Adequacy of Dialysis

Adequacy of dialysis as assessed by serum creatinine and urea concentrations was similar for both

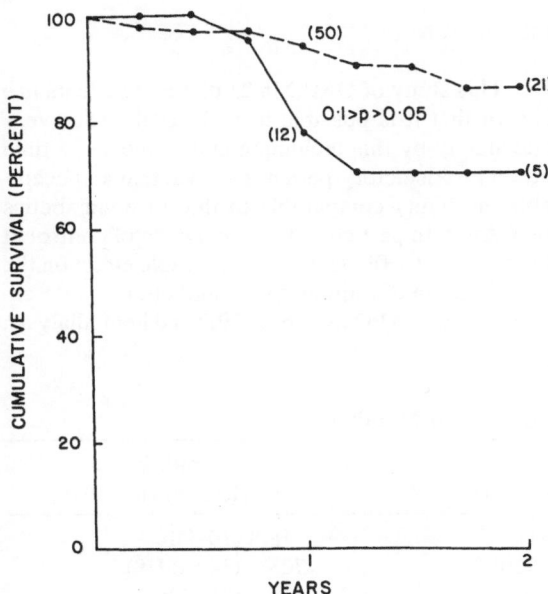

Fig. 1. Cumulative patient survival for 25 diabetic (——) and 135 nondiabetic (----) patients on CAPD.

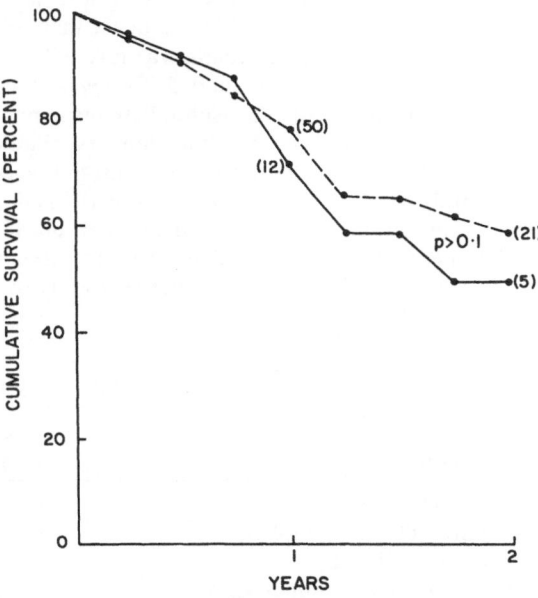

Fig. 2. Cumulative CAPD technique survival for diabetic (——) and nondiabetic (----) patients.

groups (Table 2). Nerve conduction velocity improved in ten diabetics, remained stable in six and deteriorated in one. Sustained hypertension was seen in two diabetics (8%) compared to 7% of nondiabetics, while persistent saline retention due to poor peritoneal ultrafiltration was seen in one diabetic (4%) and in 3% of nondiabetic patients.

Complications

Peritonitis occurred at a rate of one episode every 6.2 patient months in diabetic patients and one episode every 5.3 patient months in nondiabetics ($p > 0.1$). Death related to peritonitis occurred in 4% of both patient groups. The causative organisms were similar in both groups being predominantly *Staphylococcus epidermidis* and *aureus*. Fungal peritonitis developed in two (8%) diabetics and 12 (8%) nondiabetic patients.

Serum triglyceride and cholesterol concentrations were elevated in both groups although serum triglyceride concentrations were significantly less in diabetics than in nondiabetics ($p > 0.05$) (Table 2). Other diabetic complications included depression (in six blind patients), limb amputation (two patients) and deterioration in retinopathy (four patients, see below).

Control of Blood Glucose

IP insulin administration was associated with significantly better control of blood glucose than SC insulin ($p < 0.05$). Hypoglycemia was rare with IP insulin. Postprandial rise of blood glucose was however not normalized with SC insulin. Patients appreciated the freedom from SC injection associated with IP insulin. Hemoglobin a1c concentration was significantly less ($p < 0.05$) in diabetics on IP insulin (mean 11.6%, range 8.3 to 14.6) than when on SC insulin (mean 14.1%, range 11.8 to 15.9%) although results were rarely in the normal range (<9%). However, nondiabetics on CAPD also had elevated concentrations (mean 11.1%, range 8.0 to 14.2%).

Retinopathy

Of the 18 diabetic patients with useful vision at the commencement of CAPD deterioration in retinopathy was seen in only four. Each of these patients had one or more episodes of vitreous hemorrhage (eight episodes in all) but in only two did a significant decline in visual acuity occur. The incidence of vitreous hemorrhage was once every 30.3 patient months which compared to one episode every 3.4 patient months in five diabetics on recurrent hemodialysis.

Quality of Life

Eleven diabetics (44%) had a good quality of life in that they were able to work or perform household duties and felt well. Six (24%) had a moderately impaired quality of life as a consequence of poor vision, repeated episodes of peritonitis, peripheral vascular disease or cardiac disease. Quality of life was judged to be poor in eight diabetics (32%) principally as a result of blindness resulting in depression although severe peripheral vascular disease was a factor in two of the patients.

DISCUSSION

This study of CAPD in 25 diabetic patients has shown that it is possible to dialyse diabetics very adequately by this technique and at the same time attain a satisfactory patient survival and an acceptable morbidity comparable to that of nondiabetics on CAPD. In particular the excellence of control of blood sugar by IP insulin and favorable effect on the deterioration of retinopathy, stand out as major advantages of CAPD over both IPD and hemodialysis.

Table 2. Biochemical Parameters of Adequacy of Dialysis (at 6 Months).

Serum (Normal)	Diabetics (Range) (n = 21)	Nondiabetics (Range) (n = 94)
Urea (1.7–6.7 mmol/L)	20.2 (11–31)	18.8 (10–28)
Creatinine (60–120 μmol/L)	708 (569–980)	725 (340–1410)
Albumin (33–48 g/L)	33 (28–40)	32 (25–40)
Triglycerides (<1.1 mmol/L)	2.9 (0.9–5.9)	4.1 (0.7–12.3) [$p < 0.05$]
Cholesterol (<6.5 mmol/L)	5.8 (3.9–7.8)	6.9 (4.3–11.0)
Hemoglobin (11–17 g/dl)	10.2 (7.7–14.0)	9.6 (6.2–14.0)

Moreover, the continuous gentle nature of CAPD is not associated with the sudden hemodynamic changes seen with hemodialysis and has allowed excellent control of blood pressure and salt and water retention, factors that are thought to be associated with the often rapidly accelerating retinopathy seen in diabetics on hemodialysis.

Adequacy of dialysis in our diabetics on CAPD has been as satisfactory as in nondiabetics on CAPD. It is recognized that the mean time patients have been on CAPD is short and the possibility remains of peritoneal membrane failure (either for dialysis or ultrafiltration) with long term CAPD especially if diabetic microvascular disease should involve peritoneal vessels. The improvement and stability of peripheral neuropathy in our diabetics also attests to the adequacy of dialysis. Other studies have shown that hemodialysis in the diabetic patient is often associated with deterioration of neuropathy.[2]

The incidence of peritonitis in diabetics on CAPD was equal to that for nondiabetics despite the theoretic reasons for a greater incidence with diabetes. Similar results have been reported for IPD[4, 8, 10] and for CAPD.[20] Hyperlipidemia, although of concern, was significantly less for diabetics than for nondiabetics on CAPD. This may be related to the greater attention to diet paid by diabetic patients, particularly the use of white meat and polyunsaturated fats. Deterioration in peripheral vascular disease leading to limb amputation remained a problem in the diabetic on CAPD but was not a problem in the nondiabetic. Intraperitoneal insulin has resulted in better control of blood glucose in diabetics on CAPD than with SC insulin, and better control than that reported for diabetics on IPD.[4, 10–12, 21] However, the postprandial and prebreakfast rises in blood glucose were still seen even with IP insulin. IP administration also has the ooher advantages of more direct delivery of insulin into the portal vascular system and thus into the liver, the principle site of insulin action.

Accelerated retinopathy in association with hemodialysis in the diabetic has been one of the major causes of morbidity in the diabetic on dialysis. This may be related to the sudden hemodynamic changes associated with hemodialysis, poorer control of hypertension and the use of heparin. In our patients, deterioration in retinopathy was documented in only four patients. Moreover in the five diabetic patients on hemodialysis, the incidence of vitreous hemorrhage was markedly greater than with CAPD although the number of patients was small and time on hemodialysis was short.

Survival for our diabetics on CAPD (78% at one year) was less (but not significantly less) than for nondiabetics on CAPD (93%). However, survival for our diabetics compares favorably with the best reports from other centers. In a collaborative study from Toronto,[22] of 64 diabetics and 345 nondiabetics on CAPD, patient survival at one year was 90% and 93% respectively although at 7 years there was a 10% difference (although not significant) in survival (72% and 82%). There must be a limit to the degree that either dialysis or transplantation can be expected to improve survival of the diabetic in that the severity of diabetic complications present prior to commencing dialysis will limit survival. The trend to earlier commencement of dialysis in diabetics rather than to await ESRD will hopefully prevent or delay some of these irreversible complications of the diabetic state. The success of the technique of CAPD in the diabetics has been equal to that in nondiabetics.

Perhaps the most distressing problem in the treatment of diabetics with ESRF is that of the blind patient. Of the seven blind diabetics we treated with CAPD, six had a very poor quality of life largely related to the restrictions imposed by their loss of vision coupled with the new demands of a life of dialysis. Transplantation for the blind diabetic does offer the possibility of a life style equal to other blind people but the interim period of dialysis, be it CAPD or hemodialysis, can be very distressing to all concerned. Again the early institution of CAPD before the acceleration of retinopathy associated with the last few months before ESRF, should reduce the incidence of blindness.

Following this study our approach to the diabetic with chronic renal failure is to consider all diabetics for the dialysis transplant program. If it is judged that they are likely to have an acceptable quality of life with dialysis or transplantation, they commence CAPD once the serum creatinine has reached 500–600 μ mol/L, especially if hypertension or retinopathy are problems. Once on CAPD, we recommend IP insulin administration for control of blood glucose. If the patient is less than 50 years old, does not have severe ischemic heart disease or severe microvascular disease we would recommend renal transplantation as this treatment modality probably still offers the best chance of long-term survival for the diabetic patient.

REFERENCES

1. Blagg CR, Eschbach JW, Sawyer TK, and Casaretto AA: Dialysis for endstage diabetic nephropathy. Proc Dial Transplant Forum 1: 133, 1971

2. Ghavamian M, Gutch CF, Kopp KF, and Kolff WJ: The sad truth about hemodialysis in diabetic nephropathy. JAMA 222: 1386, 1972

3. White N, Snowden SA, Parsons U, Sheidon J, and Berwick M: The management of terminal renal failure in diabetic patients by regular dialysis therapy. Nephron 11: 261, 1973

4. Mitchell JC: Endstage renal failure in juvenile diabetes mellitus; A 5 year follow-up of treatment. Mayo Clinic Proc 52: 281, 1977

5. Jacobs C, Rottembourg J, Frantz P, Slama G, and Legrain NM: Treatment of endstage renal failure in the insulin-dependent diabetic patient. Adv Nephrol 8: 101, 1979

6. Goetz FC, and Kjellstrand CM: The treatment of diabetic kidney disease. Diabetologia 17: 267, 1979

7. Najarian JC, Sutherland DER, Simmons RL, Howard RJ, Kjellstrand GM, Mauer SM, Kennedy W, Ramsay R, Barbosa J, and Goetz FC: Kidney transplantation for uremic diabetic patients. Surg Gynecol Obstet 144: 682, 1977

8. Blumenkrantz MJ, Kamdar AK, and Coburn JW: Peritoneal dialysis for diabetic patients with endstage nephropathy. Dial Tranplant 6: 47, 1977

9. Finkelstein FD, Kliger AS, Bastl C, Yap P, and Goffinet J: Chronic peritoneal dialysis in diabetic patients with endstage renal failure. Proc Clin Dial Transplant Forum 5: 141, 1975

10. Rubin JE, Oreopoulos DG, Blair RDG, Chisholm LDJ, Meema HE, and deVeber GA: Chronic peritoneal dialysis in the management of diabetics with terminal renal failure. Nephron 19: 265, 1977

11. Mitchell JC, Frohnert PO, Kurtz SB, and Anderson CF: Chronic peritoneal dialysis in juvenile-onset diabetes mellitus: A comparison with hemodialysis. Mayo Clin Proc 53: 775, 1978

12. Quellhorst E, Schuenemann B, Mietzsch G, and Jacob I: Haemo- and peritoneal dialysis treatment of patients with diabetic nephropathy: A comparative study. Proc Eur Dial Transplant Assoc 15: 205, 1978

13. Popovich RP, Moncreif JW, Decherd JF, Bomar JB, and Pyle WK: The definition of a novel portable/wearable equilibrium peritoneal dialysis technique. Abst Am Soc Artif Intern Organs 5: 64, 1976

14. Oreopoulos DG, Robson N, Izatt S, Clayton S, and deVeber GA: A simple and safe technique for continuous ambulatory peritoneal dialysis. Trans Am Soc Artif Intern Organs 25: 484, 1978

15. Moncrief JW, Popovich RP, Nolph KD, Rubin J, Robson M, Dombros N, de Veber GA, and Oreopoulos DG: Clinical experience with continuous ambulatory peritoneal dialysis. 2: 114, 1979

16. Flynn CT, Hibbard J, and Dohrman B: Advantages of continuous ambulatory peritoneal dialysis to the diabetic with renal failure. Proc Eur Dial Transplant Assoc 16: 184, 1980

17. Thomson NM, Simpson RW, Hooke DH, and Atkins RC: Peritoneal dialysis in the treatment of diabetic endstage renal failure. In Atkins RC, Thomson NM, and Farrell PC (Eds), Peritoneal dialysis. Edinburgh: Churchill Livingstone, 1981, p 345

18. Thomson NM, Atkins RC, Hooke DH, Maydom B, and Scott DF: Efficacy and clinical experience of continuous ambulatory peritoneal dialysis. Long term clinical experience in Australia. In Atkins RC, Thomson NM, and Farrell PC (Eds), Peritoneal dialysis. Edinburgh: Churchill Livingstone, 1981, p 93

19. Thomson NM, Atkins RC, Humphrey TJ, Agar JMcD, and Scott DR: Continuous ambulatory peritoneal dialysis (CAPD); An established treatment for endstage renal failure. Aust NZ J Med 13: 489, 1983

20. Amair P, Khanna R, Leibel B, Pierratos A, Vas S, Meema E, Blair G, Chisholm L, Vas M, Zingg W, Digenis G, and Oreopoulos D: Continuous ambulatory peritoneal dialysis in diabetics with endstage renal disease. N Engl J Med 306: 625, 1982

21. Crossley K, and Kjellstrand CM: Intraperitoneal insulin for control of blood sugar in diabetics patients during peritoneal dialysis. Br Med J 1: 269, 1971

22. Williams C, Belvedere D, Cattran D, Clayton S, Cole E, Fenton S, Gutman K, Khanna R, Knight S, Manuel A, Oreopoulos D, Pierratos A, Roscoe J, Saiphoo C, and Vas S: Experience with CAPD in diabetic patients in Toronto. Peritoneal Dial Bull 2: S12, 1982

E.C. Kohaut, and D. Appell

61

CAPD in Infants

SUMMARY

Continuous ambulatory peritoneal dialysis is possible in the very young infant with renal insufficiency. Whether it will prevent growth retardation is speculative. Our eight patients did not grow normally, but they did grow better than the conservatively managed patients. Whether mental retardation that is associated with renal insufficiency, seen in the first year of life, will be prevented is uncertain but the neurological data presented suggest its prevention.

INTRODUCTION

In 1949, Swan and Gordon[1] reported the use of peritoneal lavage in five children with anuria. In the early 1960s reports by Segar et al[2] and Etteldorf et al.[6] popularized this form of therapy in children. In 1967 Levin and Winklestein[4] reported the use of intermittent peritoneal dialysis in the treatment of a pediatric patient with chronic renal failure. However, due to the lack of peritoneal access, repeated punctures were required and dialysis was only done monthly in conjunction with vigorous dietary management which was the main mode of therapy. The development of a chronic peritoneal access device by Palmer, which was refined by Tenckhoff,[5] coupled with the development of automated cycling ma-

chines by Boen,[6] provided the capability to treat patients with chronic renal failure with intermittent peritoneal dialysis (IPD). In 1968 Counts et al.[7] initiated an IPD program in children, and since then other authors[8-10] have described similar programs.

Intermittent peritoneal dialysis was never used extensively in the treatment of children with chronic renal failure. Of the 823 children under the age of 15 years who are alive on dialysis in the member countries of the European Dialysis and Transplant Association on December 31, 1979, only 38 (4.6%) were being treated with peritoneal dialysis.[11] In 1976 Popovich et al.[12] first described a new form of peritoneal dialysis called continuous ambulatory peritoneal dialysis (CAPD). The authors recognized that the peritoneal membrane was inefficient, but demonstrated that if dialysis was done continuously, adequate dialysis could be obtained. They then designed a system that was wearable and portable so that convenient, continuous dialysis could be provided. This form of dialysis reached prominence in 1978 after the publication of the combined clinical experiences of Moncrief and Nolph.[13] In 1980 the first preliminary reports of the use of CAPD in children appeared.[14] In 1981 more extensive experience was reported,[15, 16] and the following year Baum et al.[17] presented definitive data demonstrating that CAPD was an attractive alternative to hemodialysis in the pediatric population. The possibilities that CAPD could be used in very small infants has been suggested by a number of authors.[14-16] In this paper we will describe our experiences in the treatment of eight infants started on CAPD at less than 3 months of age.

From the Department of Pediatric Nephrology, The Children's Hospital, The University of Alabama in Birmingham, Birmingham, Alabama.

Table 1. Status of Eight Patients Started on CAPD Prior to Age 3 Months.

Died on CAPD	2/8
Transplanted	4/8
Alive on CAPD	2/8

PATIENT POPULATION

Eight patients were started on CAPD at less than 3 months of age. Three had renal failure secondary to dysplasia, three had obstructive uropathy, one had acute renal failure without recovery, and one patient had renal aplasia. Six of the patients were started on therapy in the first month of life, one at age 6 weeks, and one at age 10 weeks. All of the patients had endogenous creatinine clearances less than 5 ml/m²/minute. Six of the patients were started on CAPD because of inability to control fluid and electrolyte status with vigorous medical management. Two patients were started on CAPD due to failure to thrive despite vigorous medical management which included nutritional supplementation.

METHODS

Therapy was initiated after placement of a Tenckhoff catheter utilizing the procedure described by Alexander and Tank.[18] Initially double-cuff catheters were used, however, the last six patients had catheters with only a peritoneal cuff implanted. Originally the catheter was placed in the midline, however, as experience was gained we

Table 2. Complications/Patient-Months in Neonates and Older Children.

	<3 Months	>3 Months
Total months experience	78	371
Mortality	1/39	1/185 $p < 0.01$
Peritonitis	1/4	1/7 N.S.
Significant hypotension	1/6	1/92 $p < 0.01$
Catheter loss*	1/3	1/11 $p < 0.01$
Hyponatremia	1/3	1/80 $p < 0.01$

* Does not include catheters removed post transplant or because of changes in therapy not related to catheter problems or peritonitis.

found that a catheter placed at the lateral edge of the rectus muscle was more effective.

Dialysate volume used in this group of patients varied anywhere from 600 ml/m² to 1200 ml/m². As we previously reported,[19] dialysate volume is a major determinant of ultrafiltration. Six patients had residual urine output and the need for a large amount of ultrafiltration was not only unnecessary but undesirable, therefore, lower dialysate volumes could be used. However, in two anuric patients dialysate volumes approaching 1200 ml/m² were required before adequate ultrafiltration was obtained. The majority of our patients were treated utilizing a dialysate containing 2.5% dextrose. Higher glucose concentrations were used in the anuric patients where increased ultrafiltration was critical. Early in our experience Dianeal® 137 was used, however, as soon as Dianeal® PD-2 became available, it was used and provided better control of both serum magnesium concentration and improved acid–base balance.[20] All patients underwent at least five CAPD cycles a day. At times the number of cycles was increased if required for better control of metabolic parameters. One patient was treated with CCPD for a short time during this study period.

RESULTS

A total of 78 patient-months of experience with this group of patients has been gained. The status of these patients is outlined in Table 1. Two patients died while on CAPD. One patient died secondary to entrapment of a piece of bowel in a column-disk catheter, which led to necrosis of that segment of bowel and sepsis. The second patient died due to an inability to ever effect adequate dialysis because of multiple mechanical problems. Four patients had received transplants, and two are alive on CAPD. Some of the complications seen in this group of patients are shown in Table 2 and compared to our older patient population. The mortality rate in the neonates was 1/39 patient-months of therapy. This was significantly higher than that seen in our older patient group, where the mortality rate was 1/185 patient-months of therapy. Peritonitis was seen once every 4 patient-months in the neonatal population, whereas in our older patient group the rate is 1/7 patient-months of therapy. This difference is not significant. Significant hypotension is defined as having symptomatic changes in blood pressure, which required the patient to receive intravenous fluid support. This was seen in the neonatal population at a rate of 1/6 patient-months but only 1/92 patient-months in our older patients. Catheter loss is defined as those catheters that are lost because of nonfunction, or those catheters that had to be removed because of chronic peritonitis. This figure does not include catheters removed after a successful transplant, or catheters that were removed due to a change in therapy not related to catheter problems or peritonitis. The neonates had a significantly higher rate of catheter loss than the older patients. Hyponatremia was a problem that was seen commonly in this population, at a rate of one episode every 3 patient-months, while in our older population this was only seen once every 80 patient-months. Hyponatremia was defined as a serum sodium less than 130 mEq/L.

Many of our patients were not able to maintain adequate nutritional intake. It was our goal that these patients take in at least 100% of the recommended dietary allowance for calories and at least 4 g/kg/day of protein. When this patient population developed peritonitis or even minor viral infections their intake dropped dramatically. Early in our experience we noted that if the patients developed anorexia due to an intercurrent illness it took a long time for this to recover. We, therefore, have adopted a policy where we set a minimum amount of nutrient intake that a patient must take per day. If the patient does not take this, the patient is gavage fed. This patient population required gavage feeding an average of 5.3 days/month. Two of the patients developed prolonged anorexia, coupled with intermittent vomiting, and were placed on chronic transpyloric feedings for a period of 1 and 3 months respectively (Table 3).

Growth was not as good in this population as it was in our patients who were started on CAPD at greater than 3 months of age. Our older children had a height that was 1.62 SD average below the normal mean at the onset of therapy, and this improved to 1.38 SD average below mean normal at the end of therapy. However, in the infant population, their length at the beginning of therapy was 0.72 SD below the normal mean, and at the end of therapy declined to 1.95 SD below the normal mean.

Table 4 gives the patients' neurologic status at the end of the treatment period. We were able to study five of the six surviving patients. Neurologic exams were performed by a pediatric neurologist who had no knowledge of the patients' treatment course. He felt that two of the patients were normal developmentally for age, two were normal except for a 1 to 2 month delay in gross motor function, and one had a 3 month delay in developmental parameters. Three of the five patients had normal CAT scans. On one of the five we could not obtain a CAT

scan, but had a normal sonogram of the head. One patient had mild cerebral atrophy as demonstrated on CAT scan.

Table 3. Forced Feeding.

Patients were gavage fed an average of 5.3 days/month.

Two patients required constant transpyloric feedings.

RECOMMENDATIONS

Gavage feed during periods of stress.

Constant feedings when patient intake remains inadequate.

DISCUSSION

The aggressive treatment of young infants with renal failure brings to the surface as many social and moral questions, as it does questions pertinent to the therapy. Previously the approach to such patients was to provide aggressive medical management, and if they survived the first few years of life provide dialysis and then ultimately transplant. However, this approach has resulted in some significant complications. Betts and McGrath[21] demonstrated that those patients born with renal insufficiency have very poor growth in the first year or two of life and that it is nearly impossible to regain the growth lost during that period. It is extremely difficult to produce catch-up growth either with dialysis or transplantation.[22] Therefore, if patients are left untreated during this period of time, even if they do survive, they will almost certainly be dwarfed. Of possible more importance, Rotundo et al.[23] followed 23 patients with renal insufficiency in the first year of life and found that 20 had serious and permanent neurologic dysfunction in follow-up. These data suggest that if normal growth and neurologic function is to be

Table 4. Neurological Assessment.

5/6—Surviving patients studied

2/5—Normal

2/5—Normal except for 1 and 2 month delays in gross motor function

1/5—Three month delay in all areas

3/5—Normal CAT scan

1/5—Normal sonogram

1/5—Mild cerebral atrophy

obtained, therapy for renal insufficiency should be early and aggressive.

When we decided to treat young infants with CAPD we adopted the following criteria for treatment: those patients with renal insufficiency would first be treated with aggressive medical management, which would include correction of their acid-base status, control of metabolic parameters, and aggressive nutritional support. Only after failure to thrive on this therapy would the patient be placed on CAPD. Those patients whose creatinine clearances exceeded 5 ml/m²/minute have done relatively well without CAPD, while those with lower clearances failed to thrive and required dialysis.

Therapy for the infant on CAPD differs somewhat from that of the older child and adult. Since the infant cannot reach a fluid source unaided, his thirst mechanism is not operational and fluid intake must be controlled. We have had more problems with low intake than with excessive intake. Hypotension is a significant problem. Therefore, we prescribe a minimum daily amount of fluids. When not imbibed, it must be given by gavage feeding. The minimum intake is calculated by adding insensible losses, residual urine output, and dialysis ultrafiltration. In those patients where residual urine output is small, we would rather increase ultrafiltration and, thus, preserve caloric intake rather than limiting fluids. As previously reported,[19] adequate ultrafiltration often depends on providing a dialysate volume of 1200 ml/m². In some infants we are unable to do this because of the patient's limited respiratory capacity and, therefore, short dwell times and/or a more hypertonic dialysate is required to achieve ultrafiltration.

Nutritional support is essential in these young infants. The formula we have used in this patient population is outlined in Table 5. The amount of Propac, a protein supplement, given daily is altered dependent upon the volume of formula delivered, the patient's BUN and serum albumin concentration. One of our older patients on CAPD developed clinical signs of zinc deficiency. Since that time our

Table 5. Infant Formula.

Base:	Similac 20	20 cal/oz
Additives:	Polycose, one teaspoon/oz	10 cal/tsp
	Propac, 2–3 tablespoons/day	4 g/tbs
	Final caloric content, 32–36 cal/oz	

patients receive a daily trace element supplement similar to that given with total parenteral nutrition. The daily intake of this formula is strictly monitored by the caretaker. Should the patient not ingest the minimum amount required for adequate nutrition and salt and water balance, gavage feedings are done during the evening to supplement the oral intake. In two of our patients this form of therapy did not work. One patient required gavage feedings almost twice a day, and the other would vomit the gavage feeding. These patients were placed on transpyloric, constant feedings at an amount required to maintain nutritional and fluid balance. With this approach, their average intake exceeded the RDA for calories. In our older patients, growth has been associated with a protein intake of greater than 2 g/kg/day.[24] However, we found that many of our patients were taking 4 to 6 g/kg/day of protein. This is very similar to the elective intake of the healthy infant.

Hyponatremia was seen almost exclusively in this group of young patients. The formula provided has relatively little sodium in it. In those patients that required much ultrafiltration, dialysate sodium losses well exceeded sodium intake. Those patients required oral sodium chloride supplements to maintain a normal serum sodium concentration. When hyponatremia was seen despite minimal ultrafiltration, most such patients had obstructive uropathy and excessive urinary salt losses. These patients also required oral sodium chloride supplements. Occasionally hyponatremia was seen due to inadequate ultrafiltration of water.

The maintenance of normal bone metabolism is important to the growth of the patient on CAPD.[24] Our aim is to maintain serum parathormone levels at a level that is less than twice the upper limits of normal. To accomplish this, these patients require rather large doses of 1,25 dihydroxycholecalciferol (Rocaltrol, 0.5–2 μg/day). We have also used calcium supplementation, first in the form of calcium gluconate and later in the form of calcium carbonate. With peritoneal dialysis and calcium supplements, we have not had to use a great deal of aluminum hydroxide phosphate binders. The average intake of elemental aluminum in this population has been approximately 60 mg/day. This is fortunate since aluminum intoxication has been associated with significant bone disease.[25]

Previous experiences with forms of constant peritoneal dialysis in the treatment of the very young infant have been limited. Conley et al.[26] treated three infants under 6 months of age with chronic peritoneal dialysis. They did not use traditional CAPD, but rather designed a system using a Y-tubing that allowed multiple (7–10) exchanges per day while entering the system only once. This allows for the use of lower dialysate volumes and should reduce the incidence of peritonitis. Conley et al.[26] provided aggressive nutritional support with constant nasogastric feedings. Two of these patients have been successfully transplanted after reaching appropriate size. The third died. Alexander[27] initiated CAPD at less than 6 months of age in two patients. One is alive on CAPD. The other died. He also advocates constant gavage feedings to maintain adequate intake. Adding our series to the above experience, the mortality for the treatment of young infants with forms of constant peritoneal dialysis is 29%, much higher than seen in older patients. Unfortunately, no control data are available, however, the mortality rate in a similar group of patients left untreated should be higher.

The experiences of all three centers emphasize the importance of nutritional management in the care of the young infant with renal failure. Gavage feedings, either constant or intermittent, were universal, as was the use of caloric supplements. The patients treated by Conley et al.[26] received 3.5–4.5 g/kg/day of protein, similar to the amount our patients received.

REFERENCES

1. Swan H, and Gordon H: Peritoneal lavage in the treatment of anuria in children. Pediatrics 4: 586, 1949
2. Segar WE, Gibson RK, and Rhomy R: Peritoneal dialysis in infants and small children. Pediatrics 27: 603, 1961
3. Etteldorf JN, Dobbin WT, Sweeney MJ, Smith JD, Whittington GL, Sheffield JA, and Meadowsn RW: Intermittent peritoneal dialysis in the management of acute renal failure in children. J Pediatr 60: 327, 1962
4. Levin S, and Winklestein JA: Diet and infrequent peritoneal dialysis in chronic anuric uremia. N Engl J Med 277: 619, 1961
5. Tenckhoff H, and Schechter H: A bacteriologically safe peritoneal access device. Trans Am Soc Artif Intern Organs 14: 181, 1968
6. Boen ST, Mion C, Curtis PK, and Shilipetar G: Periodic peritoneal dialysis using the repeated puncture technique and automated cycling machine. Trans Am Soc Artif Intern Organs 10: 409, 1964
7. Counts S, Hickman R, Garbaccio A, and Tenckhoff H: Chronic home peritoneal dialysis in children. Trans Am Soc Artif Intern Organs 19: 157, 1973
8. Brouhand BM, Berger M, and Cunningham RJ: Home peritoneal dialysis in children. Trans Am Soc Artif Intern Organs 25: 90, 1979
9. Feldman W, Balisk T, and Drummond K: Intermittent peritoneal dialysis in the management of chronic renal failure in children. Am J Dis Child 16: 30, 1968
10. Day RE, and White RHR: Peritoneal dialysis in children. Arch Dis Child 62: 56, 1977
11. Donckerwolcke RA, Chantler C, Broyer M, Brunner FP, Brynger H, Jacobs C, Kramer P, Selwood NH, and Wing AJ: Combined report on regular dialysis and transplantation of children in Europe. Proc Eur Dial Transplant Assoc 17: 89, 1979
12. Popovich RP, Moncrief JW, Decherd JF, Bomar JB, and Pyle WK: The definition of a novel portable, wearable equilibrium peritoneal dialysis technique. Abst Am Soc Artif Intern Organs 5: 64, 1976
13. Popovich RP, Moncrief JW, Nolph KD, Ghods AJ, Twardowski ZJ, and Pyle WK: Continuous ambulatory peritoneal dialysis. Ann Intern Med 88: 449, 1968
14. Alexander SR, Tseng CH, Maksym KA, and Talwalker YB: Early clinical experience with continuous ambulatory peritoneal dialysis (CAPD) in infants and children. Clin Res 28: 131A, 1980
15. Kohaut EC: Continuous ambulatory peritoneal dialysis, a preliminary pediatric experience. Am J Dis Child 135: 270, 1981
16. Balfe JW, Vigneux A, Willumsen J, and Hardy BE: The use of CAPD in the treatment of children with end stage renal disease. Peritoneal Dial Bull 1: 35, 1981
17. Baum M, Powell D, and Calvin S: Continuous ambulatory peritoneal dialysis in children. N Engl J Med 307: 1537, 1982
18. Alexander SR, and Tank ES: Surgical aspects of continuous ambulatory peritoneal dialysis in infants, children and adolescents. J Urol 127: 501, 1982
19. Kohaut EC: Effect of dialysate volume on ultrafiltration in young children. Eur J Pediatr 140: 179A, 1983
20. Kohaut EC, Balfe JW, Potter D, Alexander SR, and Lum G: Hypermagnesemia and mild hypocarbia in pediatric patients on continuous ambulatory peritoneal dialysis. Peritoneal Dial Bull 3: 42, 1983
21. Betts PR, and McGrath G: Growth pattern and dietary intake of children with chronic renal insufficiency. Br Med J 2: 189, 1974
22. West CD, and Smith WC: An attempt to elucidate the cause of growth retardation in renal disease. Am J Dis Child 91: 460, 1956
23. Rotundo A, Nevins TE, Lipton M, Lockman LA, Mauer SM, and Michael AF. Progressive encephalopathy in children with chronic renal insufficiency in infancy. Kidney Int 21: 686, 1982
24. Kohaut EC: Growth in children treated with continuous ambulatory peritoneal dialysis. Int J Pediatr Nephrol 4: 93, 1983
25. Andreoli SP, Bergstein JM, and Sheppard DJ: Aluminum intoxication from aluminum containing phosphate binders in children with azotemia not undergoing dialysis. N Engl J Med 310: 1079, 1984
26. Conley SB, Brewer ED, Grady S, and Payne W: Normal growth in very small children on peritoneal dialysis. Abst National Kidney Foundation, 1982, p 8
27. Alexander SR: Personal communication, 1984

J. Manos, N.P. Mallick, and R. Gokal

62

Outcome of High Risk Patients on CAPD

SUMMARY

High risk (HR) patients treated by CAPD were followed for a minimum of 6 months. Patient survival was significantly inferior to other patients but technique survival was better. Both groups had similar rates of peritonitis, but hospitalization was more frequent in the high risk group and their rehabilitation rate was somewhat lower. The higher morbidity and mortality in high risk patients related to the complicating disease, rather than to CAPD related problems.

INTRODUCTION

Over the past 5 years the introduction of CAPD led to an increase in the total number of patients with terminal renal failure accepted for renal replacement therapy. CAPD has enabled nephrologists to offer treatment to patients who previously might have been denied it either due to lack of hemodialysis facilities or because they were felt unsuitable for this form of therapy on medical grounds. In Britain, a similar pattern prevails and such high risk (HR) patients (those suffering from cardio/cerebrovascular disease, diabetes mellitus, the elderly,[1] and social and psychiatric problems) have been increasingly accepted for replacement therapy and managed predominantly[2,3] on CAPD. CAPD is a simple and efficacious form of therapy and several studies[4,5] have

From the Manchester Royal Infirmary, Manchester, United Kingdom.

shown acceptable results in this group of patients. We analyze here the outcome of 29 patients, deemed "high risk," in our CAPD program over the last 3 years.

PATIENTS AND METHODS

Between September 1980 and August 1983, 97 patients began CAPD; in 87 this was the initial form of therapy, and 29 of 97 were characterized as being "high risk" (HR). These comprised diabetes mellitus (10), severe cardio/cerebrovascular disease (19), and a helper performing exchanges (8). A quarter of these patients had up to three of the above factors (Table 1).

A minimum 6 months follow-up was available for all patients. The outcome in this group of 29 was compared to that of the remaining CAPD population comprising 68 patients. The two groups were compared for actuarial and technique survival, peritonitis, and hospitalization rates and rehabilitation. Kaplan-Meier curves[6] for the actuarial patient survival and the classification for rehabilitation according to the EDTA registry were used.[7]

RESULTS

Demographic data were not significantly different in the two groups of patients (Table 2).

Actuarial patient and technique survival. Actuarial patient survival rate in the HR group was significantly inferior to the rest (Fig. 1). Seven patients (three diabetics and four with severe ischemic heart disease) died in the HR group. The cause of death was cardiac in five and in the remaining two, treatment was discontinued at patient's or relatives' request. However, CAPD technique survival showed the opposite result, with a higher technique survival in the HR group (Fig. 2). Only two patients were required to change to hemodialysis (HD) because of peritonitis. In the other groups, 17 of the 68 patients (25%) changed to hemodialysis within the 3 year period (in 76% of the cases, due to peritonitis).

Peritonitis and Hospitalization. Although both groups had similar peritonitis rates, the overall hospitalization was greater in the HR group of patients (Table 3). Hospitalization was significantly higher for non-CAPD related reasons, and was due mainly to diabetic and cardiac complications (Table 3).

Rehabilitation. At the end of the study period or at the time of death 16 of the 29 high risk patients were working or able to work, nine were not fit for work, but able to look after themselves and five patients required daily care by spouse or other relatives. In comparison, the rehabilitation in 68 remaining patients in the CAPD program for the above three respective groups was 51, 17, and 0 patients. These differences between the HR and the remaining patients was not significant.

DISCUSSION

In the United Kingdom, because of the lack of hemodialysis facilities and, to some extent, lack of referral to Renal Units, the acceptance rates for patients taken on for renal replacement therapy has been particularly low compared to other European countries.[2,7] The patients discriminated against, are the elderly, those with diabetes mellitus and cardiovascular problems. However, CAPD has enabled

Table 1. Risk Factors and Patients Distribution.

Factor	No. of Patients
Diabetes mellitus (DM)	10
Cardiovascular disease (CVD)	19
Helper performing exchanges (HPE)	8
DM + CVD	1
DM + CVD + HPE	1
CVD + HPE	2
DM + HPE	3

many units to manage these patients and our data show that other than having a higher mortality rate, which is not too surprising, they do not differ in outcome in relation to other parameters studied. Of interest is the superior technique survival in the higher risk group as compared to the rest. This could relate to the desire to maintain these patients on CAPD as other treatments may well be inappropriate or unsuitable for them, whereas in the remaining group, the switch to hemodialysis would have been readily undertaken for complications of peritonitis.

Our findings are consistent with recent reports[2,5] on the outcome of 'elderly' and diabetic patients on CAPD; these subjects show results comparable to other treatment groups on CAPD. In our study we did not consider the older age groups as an independent risk factor. Of the few patients who were over 60 years old and did not have concurrent cardiovascular problems or disabilities the outcome was extremely good.

The morbidity of patients in the high-risk group is related to the complicating disease rather than CAPD related problems. This is reflected in the high hospitalization rate for this group, predominantly related to diabetic and cardiac complications. There was no difference in the peritonitis or hospitalization rates related to CAPD technique.

Table 2. Demographics.

Group	No.	m/f	Mean Age (years) (Range)	Training Time (days)
HR	29	25/4	47.2 ± 12.4 (20–61)	11.6 ± 4.5
Rest	68	41/27	37.4 ± 15.4 (16–71)	10.5 ± 5.2

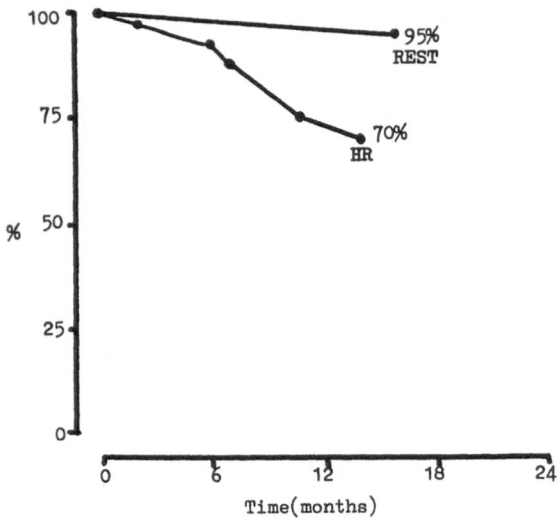

Fig. 1. Patients' survival.

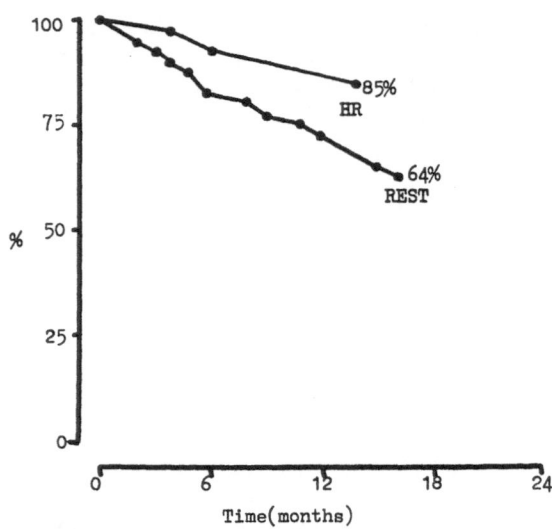

Fig. 2. Technique survival.

Table 3. Peritonitis and Hospitalization.

Group	Follow-up (months)	Peritonitis (episodes/ patient-year)	Hospital Days CAPD Related	Hospital Days Non-CAPD
HR	11.1 ± 5.7	2.2	30 ± 37	7.5 ± 21
				$p < 0.005$
Rest	10.3 ± 7.7	2	16 ± 21	1.6 ± 5

Although long term results are unknown in this group of HR patients, our results show that many achieve acceptable rehabilitation and need not be denied treatment. In the future detailed consideration will be needed in each individual to assess the risk factors present, for these will determine the eventual outcome.

REFERENCES

1. Berlyne GM: Over 50 and uraemic death. Nephron 31: 189, 1982
2. Wing AJ, Broyer M, Brunner FP, Brynger H, Challah S, Donckerwolcke RA, Gretz N, Jacobs C, Kramer P, and Selwood NH: Combined report on regular dialysis and transplantation in Europe XIII 1982. Proc Eur Dial Transplant Assoc 20: 5, 1983
3. Lancet Editorial: Long-term survival on dialysis. 2: 889, 1983
4. Taube DH, Winder EA, Ogg CS, Bewick M, Cameron JS, Rudge CJ, and Williams DG: Successful treatment of middle-aged and elderly patients with end-stage renal disease. Br Med J 286: 2018, 1983
5. Nicholls AD, Waldek S, Platts MM, Moorhead PJ, and Brown CB: Impact of CAPD on treatment of renal failure on patients aged over 60. Br Med J 288: 18, 1984 over 60. Br Med J 288: 18, 1984
6. Peto R, Pike MC, Armitage P, Breslow NE, Cox DR, Howard SV, Mantel N, McPherson K, Peto J, and Smith PG: Design and analysis of randomized clinical trials requiring prolonged observation of each patient. Br J Cancer 35: 1, 1977
7. Broyer M, Brunner FP, Brynger H, Donckerwolcke RA, Jacobs S, Kramer P, Selwood NH, and Wing AJ: Combined report on regular dialysis and transplantation in Europe XIII 1981. Proc Eur Dial Transplant Assoc 19: 2, 1982

A. Locatelli, L. DeBenedetti, M. Fuentes, E. Chaya,
C. Marelli, E. Castiglioni, N. Marchetta, A. Heilbron,
L. Lef, and R. Valtuille

63

Four Year Experience in CAPD

SUMMARY

CAPD provides a viable alternative to hemodialysis for ESRD, because of the serum chemistry and clinic results obtained and the independence and quality of life that patients can achieve. Nineteen patients treated by CAPD for an average of 19.4 mo demonstrate the adequacy of this treatment.

INTRODUCTION

CAPD can be considered an optional treatment for the end stage renal disease (ESRD). First described by Popovich, Moncrief et al.[1] as a therapeutic alternative for ESRD, it was then largely developed by Oreopoulos et al. at Toronto Western Hospital, using collapsible plastic bags.[2]

MATERIAL AND METHODS

From December 1979 to December 1983, 19 patients were trained for CAPD (12 females and 7 males average age 40.3 years [26–56 years]). The average duration on CAPD was 19.4 patient-months, giving a total experience of 369 patient-months. The causes of renal failure and duration of CAPD are listed in Tables 1 and 2 respectively. Priority to be included was given to insulin-dependent diabetic (IDD) patients, to those living 100 km

From the Policlinico Metalúrgico Central, Buenos Aires, Argentina.

away from the dialysis unit and those who, having chosen the method, showed no contraindication. Dianeal 137 in 2000 ml bags with 1.5, 2.5, or 4.5% dextrose concentration were used. Dialysis techniques have been described elsewhere.[3] Intraperitoneal administration of insulin was adopted for IDD patients, doses being from 50 to 100% higher than those used before initiating CAPD.[4]

RESULTS

A sense of well-being, as well as acceptable plasma concentrations of urea, creatinine, and potassium were observed in patients on CAPD (Table 3). The relation of hemoglobin and albumin concentrations to the duration of treatment are shown in Table 4. Table 5 shows the motor nerve conduction velocity (MNCV) results, which were decreased in most patients on starting CAPD. Four diabetics presented inexcitability of the peripheral nerves of the lower extremities. During treatment MNCV remained stable or became slightly increased. Nondiabetics showed no clinical peripheral neuropathy. Table 6 shows data pertinent to phosphorus and calcium metabolism. The dose of aluminum hydroxide required to keep normal levels of phosphorus was in general lower than that in patients on hemodialysis. The decreasing number of peritonitis episodes can be seen in Table 7. Other infectious complications are discussed elsewhere.[5] Good control of blood pressure, especially in IDD patients was achieved since, dry weight was attained by means of adequate dextrose concentration in the dialysis fluid. Noninfectious complications are

Table 1. Etiology of Renal Disease in Study Group (n = 19).

Diabetes mellitus type I	6
Chronic glomerulonephritis	4
Systemic lupus	3
Polycystic disease	2
Chronic pyelonephritis	1
Diabetes mellitus type II	1

Table 2. Duration of CAPD.

Months	Patients
6–12	8
12–24	3
24–36	7
>36	1

Table 3. Serum Chemistry Values (mg/dl).

Urea	136 ± 38
Creatinine	9.7 ± 2.5
Potassium	4.4 ± 0.4

Table 4. Hemoglobin (g/dl) and Albumin (g/dl) Evolution.

Predialysis	6.65 ± 1.5	3.14 ± 0.4
6th month	9.30 ± 1.9	3.46 ± 0.4
12th month	10.30 ± 2.2	3.95 ± 0.6
18th month	10.00 ± 2.8	3.40 ± 0.3
24th month	10.30 ± 2.4	3.86 ± 0.5

Table 5. Evolution of MNCV (m/sec).

Predialysis	39.2 ± 2.7
6th month	40.2 ± 2.8
12th month	39.7 ± 2.7
24th month	41.4 ± 2.4

Table 6. Phosphorus and Calcium Data.

Patients	M.B.C.	Ca	P	A.P.	PTH
2	100%	N	N	N	N/<4000
3	>90%	N	N/↑	N/↑	3000/9000
3	>80%	N	N	N/↑	6000/9000
1	>60	N	↑	↑	>9000

M.B.C.: Mineral Bone Content.
Ca: Calcium.
P: Phosphorus.
AP: Alkaline Phosphatase.
PTH: Immunoreactive Parathyroid Hormone (units).

shown on Table 8. Two patients developed obesity despite low-caloric diets (20–25 kcal/kg/day). Six episodes of pericatheter dialysate leak in the immediate post-operative period were resolved by reducing number and volume of exchanges. Two patients died during treatment, both of them being IDD after 32 and 8 months of treatment respectively. The former died of sepsis due to peritonitis and the latter, who presented severe autonomic neuropathy together with gastroparesis and severe malnutrition, died after complications following thrombosis of the femoral artery. Table 9 shows the causes of drop-out on CAPD. Table 10 shows the rehabilitation according to European Dialysis and Transplant Association Registry criteria[6] of the nine patients who are still on the program.

Adequate control of blood glucose was obtained on IDD patients. On beginning treatment three-eyes were blind, three suffered from severe proliferative retinopathy with blurred vision and six maintained visual acuity satisfactory enough to begin CAPD. The three eyes with blurred vision worsened to blindness and the remaining six had unvarying visual acuity during an average of 22 patient-months. Figure 1 shows the survival curve of the patients and the dialytic therapy. At the end of the first year there was a 6% mortality and an 11% drop-out. After 2 years mortality remained stable and the technique survival was 60%.

DISCUSSION

Our experience proves that CAPD is a useful alternative therapy for ESRD. Patients report a more steady-state, have less dietary restrictions and need less aluminum hydroxide and antihypertensive drugs. There still exist problems as regards to access to the peritoneum, as the device to prevent the exit-site or tunnel infections has not yet been found.

Table 7. Peritonitis Episodes.

Period	Experience/ Months	Peritonitis	Average (episode/ patient-months)
1-12-79 to 31-7-81	112	24	4.6
1- 8-81 to 31-7-82	104	14	7.4
1- 8-82 to 31-7-83	106	14	7.5
1-12-79 to 31-7-83	332	52	6.2

Table 8. Complications (except Peritonitis).

I Salt/water balance	Overhydration	7
	Orthostatic hypotension	9
II Others	Obesity	2
	Hemorragic effluent	4
	Cuff extrusion	2
	Pericatheter leakage	6
	Umbilical hernia	2
	Eventration	1
	Vaginal dialysate leak	1
	Severe malnutrition	1

Table 9. Causes of Drop-Out.

No adaptation	2
Loss of UF	2
Peritonitis TBC	1
Recurrent peritonitis	1
Eventration	1
Transplantation	1

Table 10. Rehabilitation.*

Fit for work	Full time	3
	Part time	6
	Unemployed	—
	Retired	—
Unable to work	Living at home	—
	Requiring hospital care	—

* According to the European Dialysis and Transplant Association.

There are important factors that must be taken into account, as they bear on the amount of drop-out after two years on CAPD.[7] Dietary control of protein and calorie intake is a factor to be controlled continuously in order to prevent protein malnutrition as well as obesity. Another aspect to be considered is the efficiency of the peritoneal membrane with time and the influence of dextrose and other components of the dialysate. In the Argentine Republic, the inclusion of patients in a CAPD program remains difficult because of problems in obtaining bags and tubes, due to the lack of adequate national technology. Despite the necessity to use imported bags, CAPD is 15% cheaper than hemodialysis. At present, 3000 patients are in dialytic programs, about 100 million population while only 1% are trained in CAPD.

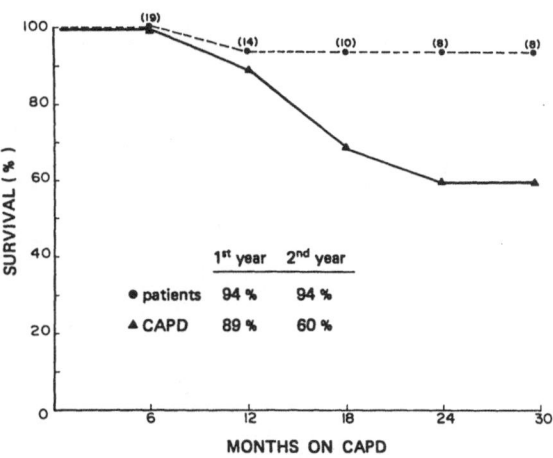

Fig. 1. Four year experience of continuous ambulatory peritoneal dialysis (CAPD).

REFERENCES

1. Popovich RP, Moncrief J, Decherd JF, Bomar JB, and Pyle WK: The definition of a novel portable/wearable equilibrium peritoneal dialysis. Abst Am Soc Artif Intern Organs 5: 64, 1976
2. Oreopoulos DG, Robson M, Izatti S, Clayton S, and deVeber GA: A simple and safe technique for continuous ambulatory peritoneal dialysis. Trans Am Soc Artif Intern Organs 24: 484, 1978
3. Locatelli AJ, Nesse A, Arrizurieta E, DeBenedetti L, Chaya E, Marelli C, and Paparone R: Middle and low molecular weight (MLMW) substances in patients treated with continuous ambulatory peritoneal dialysis (CAPD). In Gahl G, Kessel M, and Nolph K (Eds), Advances in peritoneal dialysis. Proceedings of the 2nd international symposium on peritoneal dialysis. Amsterdam: Excerpta Medica, 1981, p 220
4. Flynn C, and Navson J: Intraperitoneal insulin with CAPD. An artificial pancreas. Trans Am Soc Artif Intern Organs 25: 114, 1979
5. Locatelli AJ: The peritoneal access. In LaGreca G, Biasoli S, and Ronco C (Eds), Peritoneal dialysis. Milano: Wichtig, 1982, p 151
6. Jacobs C, Brunner FP, Chantler C, Donckerwolcke RA, Gurland HJ, Hathway RA, Selwood JH, and Wing AJ: Combined report on regular dialysis and transplantation in Europe. Proc Eur Dial Transplant Assoc 1977, p 4
7. Oreopoulos DG: Why the high drop-out rate in CAPD. Peritoneal Dial Bull 2: 57, 1982

R.C. Mackow, W.P. Argy, T.A. Rakowski,
J.F. Winchester, A.C. Chester, A.S. Siemsen,
S. Jenkins, and G.E. Schreiner

64

Prognostic Correlates in Ambulatory Peritoneal Dialysis Versus Hemodialysis

SUMMARY

The importance of race and geographic location have been described as variables in comparing hemodialysis populations. We have extended our investigations into our CAPD population. Survival in our ambulatory peritoneal dialysis patients is better than that of hemodialysis patients in two geographic areas. To interpret data from diverse dialysis populations, many considerations must be evaluated for adequate interpretation.

INTRODUCTION

We have previously demonstrated the importance of race and geographic distribution as variables in evaluating diverse hemodialysis populations and we have also shown the need for using multi-variant analysis in comparing varied hemodialysis populations.[1] There is, however, little information relating these and other variables to prognosis in ambulatory peritoneal dialysis.

MATERIALS AND METHODS

To predict the prognosis for patients receiving ambulatory peritoneal dialysis (APD) we compared a group of 81 APD patients in Washington, DC to two diverse hemodialysis (HD) populations. Sev-

From the Division of Nephrology, Department of Medicine, Georgetown University Medical Center, Washington, D.C. and Institute for Kidney Diseases, St. Francis Hospital, University of Hawaii, Honolulu, Hawaii.

enty-nine HD patients from Washington, D.C. and 71 HD patients from Hawaii were compared to the APD group with respect to factors that might influence morbidity and mortality.

All HD patients were dialyzed three days a week 4 to 4 ½ hours/day with various dialysis membranes. All APD patients were dialyzed using four 2 L exchanges/day of Dianeal® (Travenol Laboratories, Deerfield, IL), 7 days a week. Dextrose concentrations in the dialysis fluid were 1.5, 2.5, and 4.25%. The fluids were varied depending on each patient's fluid balance.

Blood pressures were measured in the semi-recumbent position before hemodialysis or on a visit to the outpatient clinic in the case of peritoneal dialysis patients. Dialysis to dry weight was attempted in all patients.

The two different hemodialysis populations were located in Metropolitan Washington, D.C. (79 patients) and dialysis centers serviced by the Institute for Kidney Diseases, St. Francis Hospital, University of Hawaii, Honolulu, HI (71 patients). The peritoneal dialysis patients were located at Georgetown University Medical Center, Washington, D.C. (81 patients).

All blood pressure determinations and laboratory values represent the mean ± SE of 10 random readings throughout each patient's course on dialysis.

RESULTS

The demographics of the three separate dialysis populations are listed in Table 1. The Hawaii population was older than the other two populations and

341

Table 1. Demographics of Three Separate Dialysis Populations.

	APD	HD-W	HD-H
No.	81	79	71
Age ± SEM	48.0 ± 1.4	45.3 ± 1.9	52.0 ± 1.6
Total months on dialysis	50.1 ± 3.9*	24.1 ± 2.4	36.6 ± 2.4
Male	39	41	40
Female	42	38	31
Black	36	38	0
White	45	41	11
Asian or ethnic Hawaiian	0	0	60
Percent hypertensive	28	53	20

* 19.5 ± 1.3 mos. on APD.
APD—ambulatory peritoneal dialysis.
HD-W—hemodialysis Washington.
HD-H—hemodialysis Hawaii.

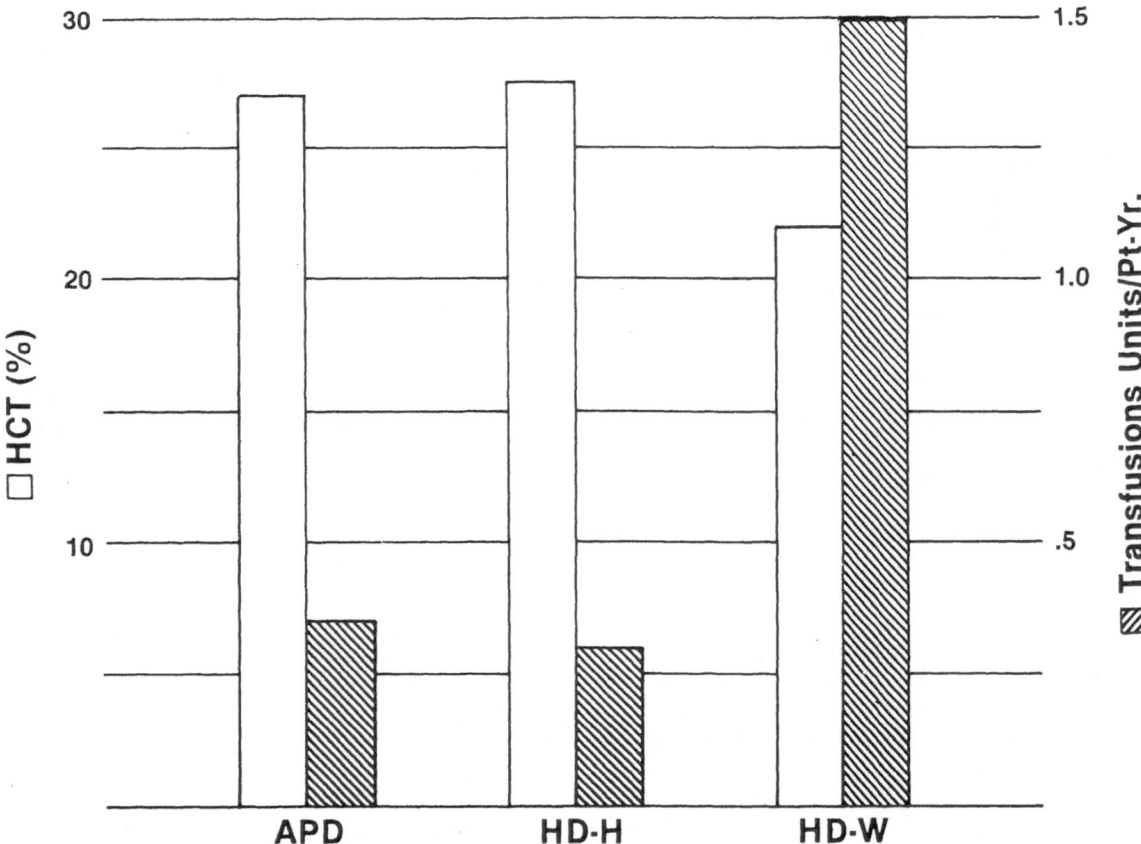

Fig. 1. Hematocrit and transfusion requirements differ in three dialysis populations.

Table 2. Diagnostic Categories of ESRD of the Three Populations (%).

	APD	HD-W	HD-H
Glomerulonephritis	17*	28	39
Diabetic nephropathy	15*	11†	35
Tubulointerstitial disease	10	16†	3
Nephrosclerosis hypertensive	28*	22†	4
PCKD	10	9	5
Other	20	14	14

* Difference APD and HD-H, $p < .05$.
† Difference HD-W and HD-H, $p < .05$.

had been dialyzed for approximately 1 year longer than the Washington populations. The APD patients had been on dialysis for a total of 50.1 patient months, however, with only 19.5 months spent on APD, previously being treated with hemodialysis prior to starting APD. The hemodialysis Washington population had a larger number of hypertensive patients (53%) compared to 20% for HD Hawaii and 27% for APD.

Hematocrit and transfusion requirements also differed dramatically. In APD in Washington and HD Hawaii, patients had similar transfusion requirements at 0.37 and 0.27 U/patient/year. Transfusion requirements in the Washington group were 1.5

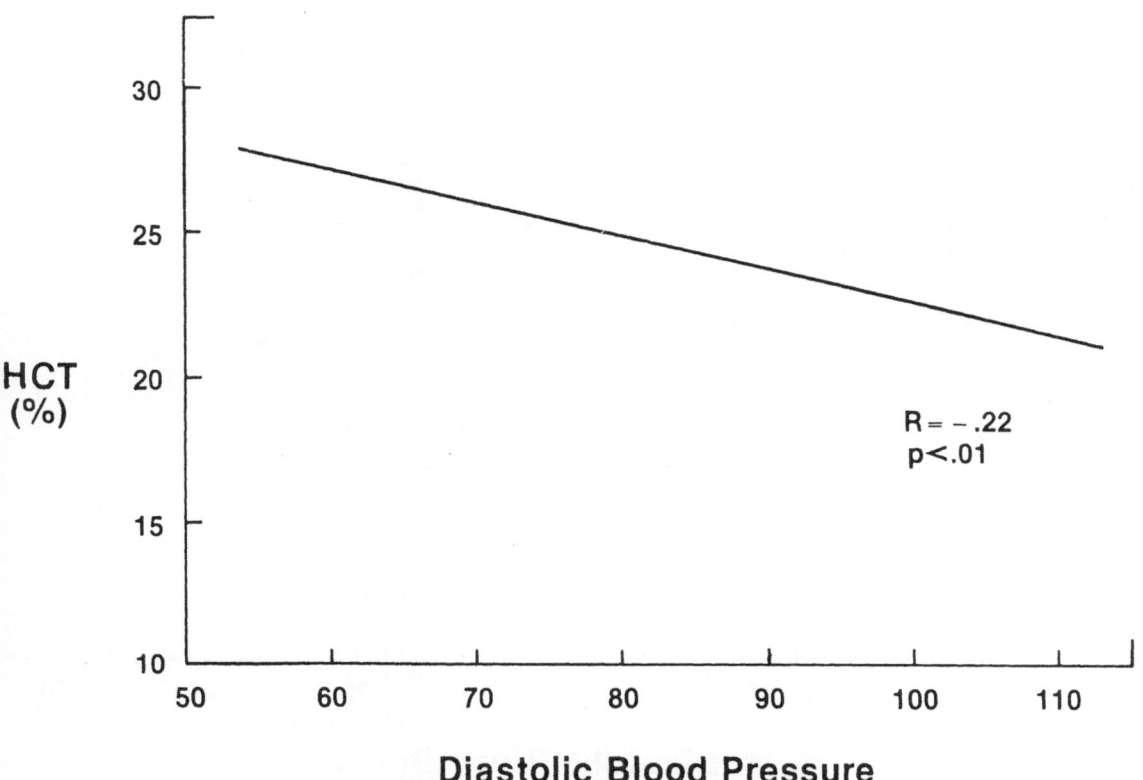

Fig. 2. The correlation of diastolic blood pressure and hematocrit is shown for hemodialysis patients. No significant correlation was shown for APD patients, $r = -0.036$.

U/patient/year (Fig. 1.). The hematocrit (HCT) in APD was 27 ± 0.7%, in HD-Hawaii 27.5 ± 0.07%, and in HD Washington 21.7 ± 0.5%. The HCT in APD and HD-Hawaii were statistically significantly higher than in HD-Washington.

The diagnostic categories for end-stage renal disease in the three populations were compared (Table 2). The APD group had a lower incidence of glomerulonephritis, 17%, than either of the two hemodialysis populations, 28% and 39% for HD-Washington and HD-Hawaii, respectively.

APD and HD-Washington had a higher incidence of nephrosclerosis than HD-Hawaii with the APD population having the highest incidence at 26%. Diastolic blood pressure correlated inversely with HCT in the pooled HD population. No such

correlation was found in the APD group (Fig. 2). Diastolic blood pressure also correlated inversely with age in the pooled HD population and again there was no such correlation in the APD patients (Fig. 3).

The higher incidence of nephrosclerosis in the APD and HD-Washington populations may reflect racial composition since the APD and HD-Washington population has a large percentage of black patients as compared to HD-Hawaii population where the HD population was Asian American, ethnic Hawaiian and Caucasian.

Actuarial survival in the three dialysis populations was compared (Fig. 4). Actuarial survival for the APD group at 1, 2, and 3 years was 91, 82, and 82% respectively. This more closely parallelled HD-

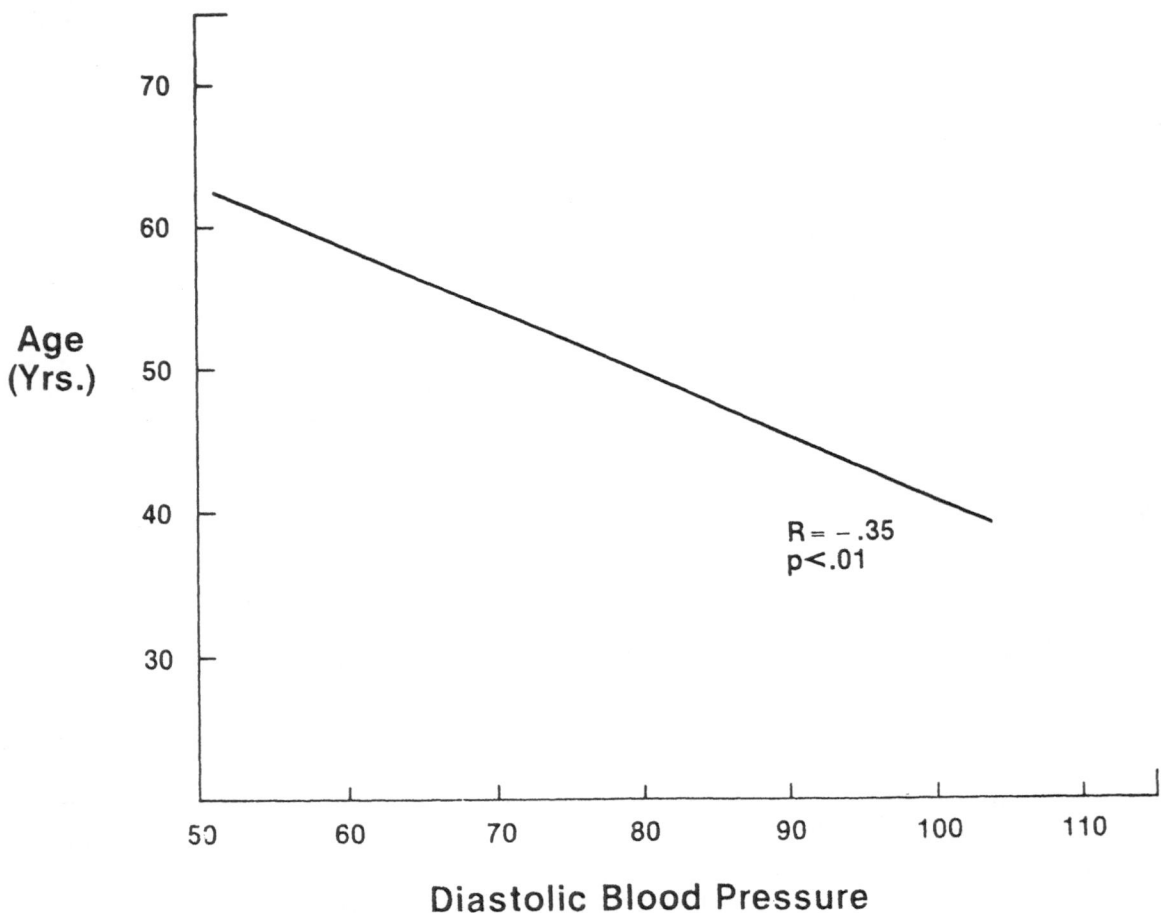

Fig. 3. The correlation of diastolic blood pressure and age is shown for hemodialysis patients. No significant correlation was shown for APD patients, r = −0.11.

Hawaii at 82, 70, 63%, than it did HD-Washington at 70, 55, 51%.

DISCUSSION

We have examined an urban APD population and compared it to an urban HD population located in the same geographical area and having similar racial composition, and to an HD population of white, Asian American, and ethnic Hawaiian patients. Both HD centers had liberal standards for acceptance of patients. Patients were rarely rejected except for terminal nonrenal disease. Similar HD equipment was used in both centers for dialysis procedures. The APD population differed from the incenter HD population in that it was somewhat selected; that is, the patient must be able to be trained in the technique of APD. In this way it more closely resembled a home HD population. The number of patients in each group was comparable.

We have previously described a strong negative correlation between diastolic blood pressure and hematocrit,[2] shown in this pooled HD population.[2] This correlation, however, did not hold in the APD population. The reason for this lack of correlation between hematocrit and blood pressure in the APD population might be secondary to the different factors controlling erythropoiesis, which may be operating in the different populations. For instance, it has been shown that erythropoiesis might be increased in patients on APD as compared to those

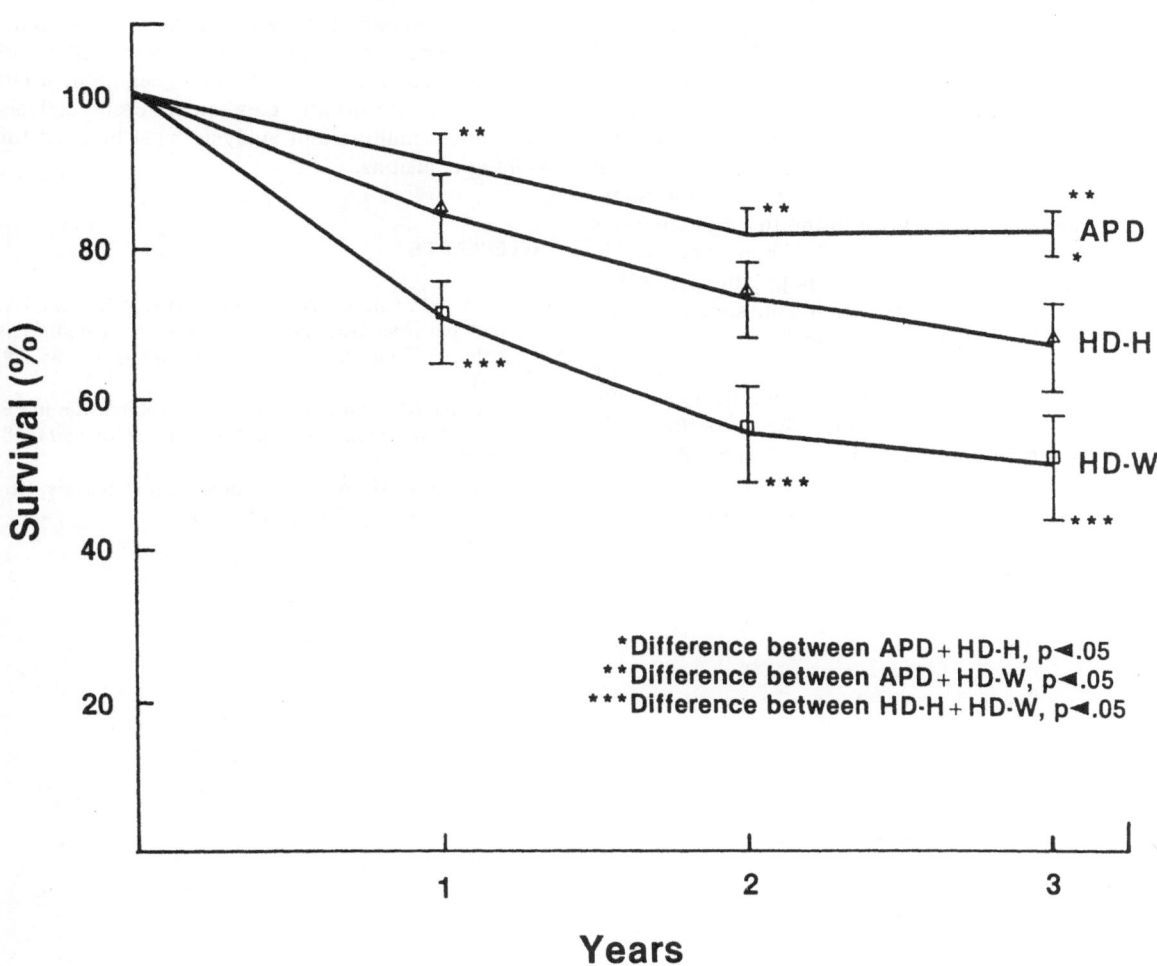

Fig. 4. Actuarial patient survival.

patients on HD.[3] A higher HCT was found in our APD population, when compared with the HD-Washington population. However, the HD-Hawaii population and the APD population were almost identical with respect to hematocrit and transfusion requirement. This highlights the necessity for taking into account multiple variables when comparing different modalities of therapy for end-stage renal disease.

Despite the high incidence of arteriolar nephrosclerosis as a diagnosis in the end-stage renal disease population of HD-Washington, and APD Washington, the APD population had a low incidence of hypertension. The APD population had much lower incidence of hypertension than HD-Washington and this was comparable to the low incidence of hypertension in the HD-Hawaii group. This might reflect better fluid balance achieved by APD as compared to HD in a heavily hypertensive black population in Washington, DC. The incidence of hypertension and nephrosclerosis was much lower in the HD-Hawaii population. It must be noted that the diagnosis of hypertensive nephrosclerosis in these populations was essentially a clinical one and most diagnoses were made without renal biopsy. These clinical judgments are subject to interpretative limitations.

The actuarial survival in the three populations differed, with the highest survival being achieved in the APD group. Of the two HD populations, the HD-Hawaii subgroup most resembled the survival statistics found in APD. This could be due to the low icidence of hypertension in these two groups, as we have previously documented the significance of diastolic hypertension as a mortality risk factor in patients undergoing hemodialysis.[2] The APD population was a somewhat more selected population than either of the HD populations, as we have pre-viously noted. For our actuarial curves we have calculated only the time on APD with respect to survival and as noted in Table 1 the patients on APD had a total of 50.1 months on dialysis, 19.5 of that spent on APD. This is a further selection bias since these patients obviously had survived quite well on hemodialysis, perhaps because of the benefit of other good prognostic indicators of which we are not aware.

In conclusion, we can state that survival for our population of APD patients seems better than for HD patients in the two diverse geographic areas and that various characteristics of the HD-Washington population are quite different from the APD population despite a similar end-stage renal disease pool found in Washington, D.C. We have again shown that interpretation of data from different dialysis populations has many risks. There are substantial differences between populations in different racial, ethnic, and geographic areas and there are substantial differences between populations of APD and hemodialysis patients in the same geographic area. Clearly, in interpreting data on different dialysis modalities, multivariant analysis must be used for valid conclusions.

REFERENCES

1. Argy WP, Chester AC, Siemsen AS, Rakowski TA, and Schreiner GE: Hypertension in two hemodialysis cohorts. Trans Am Soc Artif Intern Organs 28: 329, 1982
2. Chester AC, and Schreiner GE: Hypertension in hemodialysis. Trans Am Soc Artif Intern Organs 24: 38, 1978
3. Winchester JF: Anemia, androgens and dialysis. Perspect Peritoneal Dial 2: 10, 1984

"P." A.J. Sorrels-Akar, M. Bobbitt, F. Aguirre,
J.W. Moncrief, and R.P. Popovich

65

Peritoneal Dialysis for In-Hospital Patients

SUMMARY

To facilitate peritoneal dialysis for acute renal failure a procedure of continuous peritoneal dialysis using the Lasker cycler has been evaluated for 4 years in 140 patients. There were only five episodes of peritonitis. Individualized dialysis prescriptions were achieved and a closed system was maintained. The system, however, was bulky. Dialysis personnel and hospital staff shared responsibility for the conduct of the dialysis.

INTRODUCTION

By 1975, manual or automated peritoneal dialysis (PD) for acute renal failure had become standard practice in many hospitals. Peritonitis, though more prominent with manual exchanges, occurred in more than 50% of all patients undergoing PD for acute renal failure. The advent of continuous ambulatory peritoneal dialysis (CAPD) in the late 1970s further increased the in-hospital use of PD by adding end stage renal disease (ESRD) patients to the potential population. However, the high incidence of hospital acquired peritonitis dictated the necessity for a safe PD system for in-hospital use.

Historically, this institution's hospital affiliation contract made no provision for peritoneal dialysis, and it was therfore performed (upon physi-

cian order) by nondialysis hospital staff. Efforts at utilizing CAPD staff for in-hospital PD eliminated peritonitis as a complication but created a myriad of other problems. Assembling and connecting the Lasker cycler proved satisfactory, but hospital staff relied on dialysis personnel for the slightest malfunction of the system. Thus on-call personnel spent many expensive and wasteful hours at the hospital. The same waste, accompanied by staff burn-out, resulted when dialysis staff performed the CAPD technique on hospitalized patients.

In August 1983, Moncrief and colleagues developed a procedure for in-hospital manual continuous peritoneal dialysis (CPD). Adapting the multipronged manifolds developed for use with the Lasker cycler and techniques developed for CAPD, a safe, relatively simple process resulted.

PROCEDURES

The CPD system adjusts quite easily to CAPD procedures. The "spike" of the CAPD solution transfer set connects directly into the patient adapter of the multipronged manifold (Fig. 1). Adapting the CAPD exchange procedure (Table 1), the connection becomes a safe means with which to initiate PD, and a Betadine Connection Shield℗ fits snugly in place at the connection site.

Also using CAPD exchange technique, multipronged "spikes" may be inserted into plastic dialysis solution containers. Because of the configuration of the finger guards on the manifold "spikes" it is impossible to utilize Betadine Connection Shields℗,

From the Acorn Research Laboratory, the Austin Diagnostic Clinic, and the University of Texas at Austin, Austin, Texas.

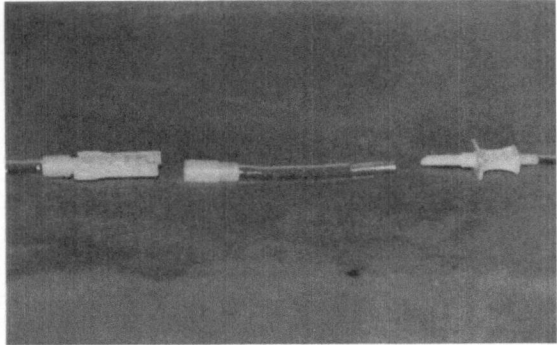

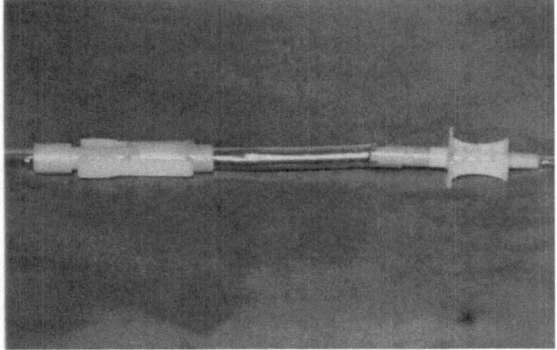

Fig. 1. Using CAPD technique, patient is attached to CPD system by inserting "spike" of transfer set into patient adapter of manifold.

thus making it necessary to revert to the traditional betadine "wrap" dressings at the connection sites.

A titanium adapter and a solution transfer set should be attached during the Tenckhoff catheter placement procedure. The occlusive clamp must be closed and the transfer set taped securely to the patient's abdomen in order to prevent contamination (Fig. 2). Therefore, the "closed system" of CAPD is established in a sterile environment and need not be violated when connecting the patient to the CPD system.

According to physician order, solution containers are prepared and aligned in the order that exchanges will occur (Fig. 3). After closing all occlusive clamps and using the CAPD exchange technique, each "spike" of the manifold should be inserted into a solution container and the connection dressed in the appropriate manner. The system can then be hung to allow for the purging of air by alternately opening two sets of tubing at a time in order to maintain the "closed system." Aseptically, and again using the CAPD technique, the patient adapter

is attached, and the solution transfer "spike" is inserted into the system (Fig. 4). The patient is now connected to the CPD manifold, and dialysis may commence via gravity.

Solution containers are numbered according to an exchange schedule dictated by the physician. Dialysis staff then prepare a dialysis flow sheet (Fig. 5) which indicates a specific time for inflow and outflow as well as the infusion and drained volumes. If specific drained volume measurements are required, a gram scale may be used to weigh the solution container prior to infusion and after drainage to determine ultrafiltration without contaminating the system. After proper inservice, hospital staff may then perform the dialysis by simply opening and closing occlusive clamps and weighing the containers if necessary.

Solution containers are exchanged by dialysis staff upon depletion of supplies or physician's order changes. All betadine dressings must be changed daily to ensure the presence of moisture at the connections. The multipronged manifold should be changed whenever the system is disconnected from the patient, or biweekly. In addition, a procedure for emergency disconnection of the system allows hospital staff to detach the manifold for surgical, diagnostic, or lifesaving measures.

PERITONITIS

Since August 1980, 140 acute and chronic patients have undergone in-hospital CPD. Time on dialysis has ranged from 6 hours to 90 days. Five patients contracted peritonitis while undergoing CPD during that time.

Patient #1, a chronic hemodialysis patient for 5 years, had been performing CAPD for 3 months. He entered the hospital for bilateral femoral popliteal bypass, which proved unsuccessful and resulted in a right below-knee amputation. During this traumatic period, the patient underwent CPD in order to alleviate any additional stress. After a month on CPD the patient developed diverticulitis and died within 4 days of the diagnosis.

Patient #2 was admitted to hospital with a diagnosis of acute renal failure, etiology unknown. Diagnostic evaluation proved inconclusive, although renal function failed to return. Peritoneal access was obtained, and CPD was initiated and progressed well for 20 days, when turbidity appeared, accompanied by an elevated white blood count and no growth seen in the dialysate cultures. Hemodialysis, the patient's choice of chronic treatment, was instituted and the

Table 1. Procedure for In-Hospital Continuous Peritoneal Dialysis (Acute or Chronic).

Equipment
1. Masks (2)
2. Plastic hemostats "gizmos" (1)
3. Multipronged PD tubing (1)
4. Bags of peritoneal dialysis solution (8)
5. Packages of 4 × 4 Betadine gauze pads (7)
6. Packages of 3 × 9 Betadine gauze pads (10)
7. Roll of one inch tape
8. "C" clamps for multipronged tubing
9. Heating pad

Procedure
1. The titanium adapter and solution transfer set should be attached during the Tenckhoff catheter placement. The occlusive clamp must be closed, then taped securely to the dressing.
2. Gather supplies.
3. Mask (all persons in room).
4. Open outer wrap of all peritoneal dialysis bags. Check bags for leaks.
5. Wash hands thoroughly with soap and water.
6. Open outer wrap of multi-pronged connector.
7. Close occlusive clamps on each prong completely. Clamp "gizmo" on patient end of multipronged tubing.
8. Add medications to bags at this time according to "Procedure for Adding Medications."
9. Each bag must be attached using sterile procedure to one prong of the multi-pronged connector then dressed in accordance with the "CAPD Exchange Instructions."
10. Hangs bags in infusion position.
11. Maintaining a closed system, purge tubing of air. (In order to clear each prong, two occlusive clamps should be opened alternately until each prong is filled with fluid.) Attach and close "C" clamps to each of the tubes.
12. Remove protective cover from patient end of multipronged connector, being careful to avoid contamination of sterile tip.
13. Remove protective cover from distal end (spike end) of transfer set.
14. Insert spike into sterile tip of multipronged connector set, making sure the sterile ends meet at the shoulder of the spike.
15. Dress the connection in accordance with the "CAPD Exchange Instructions."
16. To purge the transfer set of air, one bag should be placed below the level of the abdomen, both clamps opened, and the fluid allowed to flow via gravity from the peritoneal cavity into the bag. If no residual fluid is present in peritoneal and air remains in the transfer set, proceed with fluid installation.
17. Fill out a room flow sheet and number the dialysis bags.
18. Bags may be warmed using a "K-pad" or heating pad, but never by immersing in warm water.

---

peritoneal catheter removed without further investigation of the turbid effluent.

Patient #3 was a very stable chronic dialysis patient who had been performing CAPD for two years. He was admitted to the hospital after a cerebrovascular accident that produced dysphasia and some dysfunction of motor skills. CPD was initiated, but numerous disconnections and connections were required to allow for multiple diagnostic evaluations. Peritonitis was diagnosed within 7 days, and the causative organism was *Staphylococcus aureus*. The episode was attributed to contamination; the

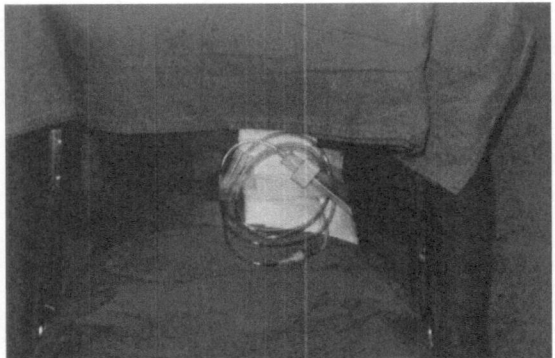

Fig. 2. "Closed system" should be established in sterile atmosphere with titanium adapter and solution transfer set attached in the operating room.

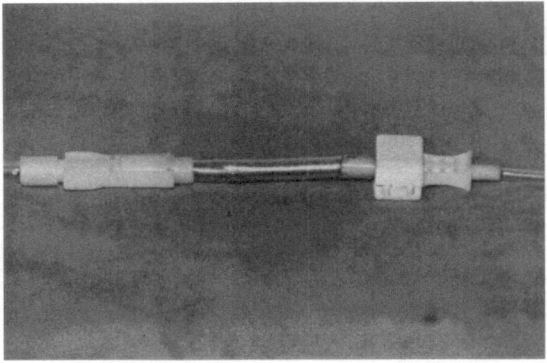

Fig. 4. Patient is attached to "closed system" by which dialysis can be accomplished with minimal risk of external contamination.

patient treated with appropriate antibiotics, and CPD continued for another week at which time the patient was again able to perform CAPD.

Patient #4, a historically noncompliant hemodialysis patient for 5 years, had been a marginally compliant CAPD patient for 10 months. The patient's major problems were fluid abuse, which caused persistent hypertension, and poor dietary habits, resulting in malnutrition. The patient suffered an acute myocardial infarction, and was immediately placed on CPD in the coronary care unit. Within 3 days, the patient developed a rigid, tender abdomen, accompanied by bloody, turbid dialysate. White blood cell and red blood cell counts were extremely high, and the surgeon diagnosed an acute abdomen. Emergency laparotomy revealed an infarcted bowel, which was repaired.

The catheter was removed, and the patient returned to hemodialysis.

Patient #5 was hospitalized for cholecystectomy and developed acute renal failure postoperatively. During the course of CPD, cardiac tamponade occurred, and an emergency cardiac window was performed at the bedside. In the midst of the surgical procedure, the hospital staff improperly disconnected the PD system and contaminated the patient. The patient did not receive prophylactic antibiotics, however, because two broad spectrum antibiotics were already in use. Effluent turbidity occurred within 48 hours, and *Pseudomonas aeruginosa* was the causative organism. Tobramycin protocols were initiated upon physician order, and the dialysate cleared within 96 hours. CPD was continued until the patient regained renal function after 90 days of dialysis therapy.

RESULTS

Of the 140 patients treated with in-hospital continuous peritoneal dialysis, only in the five cases above did turbidity or a suspicion of contamination occur. Of the 135 patients who had no peritonitis, success of treatment was very encouraging. As with any process, there are advantages and disadvantages; however for the hospital setting, CPD has proven to be the most feasible,

Advantages. CPD provides an individualized, flexible dialysis with easy observation and evaluation of problems. The dialysis prescription can be changed quickly and changes initiated by draining

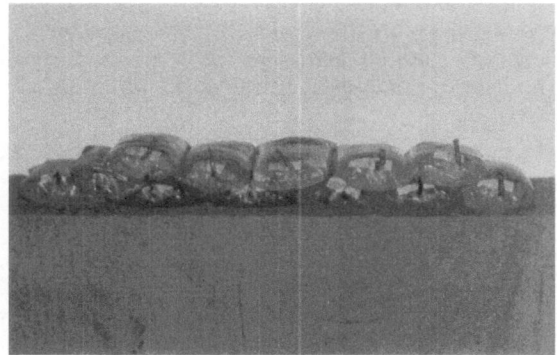

Fig. 3. Solution containers should be aligned in order of prescription to make "spiking" easier when preparing the system.

Continuous Peritoneal Dialysis
Room Flow Sheet

Patient Name: _____ Room #: _____ Date: _____

The CAPD staff has initiated peritoneal dialysis on this patient. The following table is provided for recording ten (10) complete exchanges.

#1 _____ Infuse _____ Volume _____ Drain _____ Volume _____

#2 _____ Infuse _____ Volume _____ Drain _____ Volume _____

#3 _____ Infuse _____ Volume _____ Drain _____ Volume _____

#4 _____ Infuse _____ Volume _____ Drain _____ Volume _____

#5 _____ Infuse _____ Volume _____ Drain _____ Volume _____

#6 _____ Infuse _____ Volume _____ Drain _____ Volume _____

#7 _____ Infuse _____ Volume _____ Drain _____ Volume _____

#8 _____ Infuse _____ Volume _____ Drain _____ Volume _____

#9 _____ Infuse _____ Volume _____ Drain _____ Volume _____

#10 _____ Infuse _____ Volume _____ Drain _____ Volume _____

Make sure the occlusive roller clamp on the transfer tubing remains closed during dwell times. For any leakage noted around the catheter exit site or any type of bag or tubing leakage or disconnection, please contact the CAPD unit STAT. *Do not violate the closed system by changing bags or adding medications.* A nurse can be reached 24 hours daily via the medical exchange.

Fig. 5. Flow sheet for continuous peritoneal dialysis.

the peritoneal cavity and instilling fresh solution. Dialysis of uremic toxins and/or ultrafiltration can be determined with each exchange and altered by changing dwell times and solution tonicity.

Because it is peritoneal dialysis and less efficient, CPD is more gentle and therefore less traumatic to other systems of the body. In addition, electrolyte balance is achieved and maintained with much less stress to the patient by the addition or deletion of medications to the solution containers.

The third, and possibly most important advantage, is that CPD eliminates much of the dialysis related stress for hospital and dialysis staff alike. Dialysis staff establish and maintain the "closed system." which virtually eliminates external contamination as a peritonitis risk factor. On the other hand, hospital staff are not made responsible for the major tasks of dialysis, but for the simple procedures of infusing solution and draining effluent for the patient. Thus, dialysis tasks are shared, and wasteful, time consuming procedures, which often lead to burn-out are not the burden of either staff.

Disadvantages. Although it can be made as convenient as possible, CPD is an extremely bulky, cumbersome system. Because at least eight solution containers are attached and at the bedside, patient care is often hindered, and hospital staff do not appreciate the necessity of maintaining an orderly

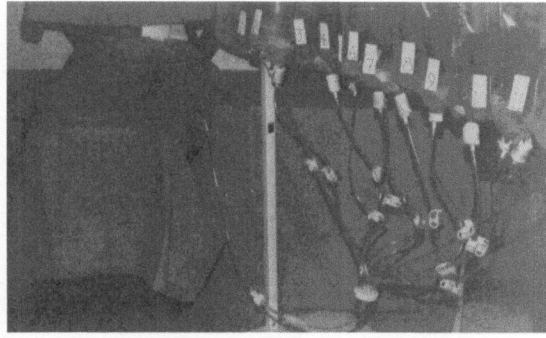

Fig. 6. Maintaining an orderly system is necessary to allow hospital staff to give adequate bedside care without hindrance.

system (Fig. 6). In addition, bulkiness prevents the patient from ambulating alone; someone must be responsible for the CPD system as the patient moves about. This often creates a burden for busy hospital staff and may prevent the patient from ambulating because no one is available for assistance.

Since peritoneal dialysis is less efficient than hemodialysis, CPD is not the treatment of choice in some situations. Primarily, these are conditions that require rapid removal of toxins, such as drug overdose, and/or rapid ultrafiltration, such as pulmonary edema or congestive heart failure. Although CPD has been successful in treating such conditions when hemodialysis was contraindicated, the more efficient modality is preferred at this institution.

CONCLUSIONS

During the 4 year experience with in-hospital continuous peritoneal dialysis at this institution, the system has evolved into a convenient, highly efficient means with which to deliver hospital dialysis to patients with either acute or chronic renal failure. However, there are some principles that must be rigidly applied to ensure the success of CPD.

Procedures must be precise with strict adherence to established CAPD techniques. Therefore, PD staff should be responsible for maintaining the "closed system," which entails having an on-call rotation. On-call can still be quite time consuming when several patients are undergoing CPD simultaneously; however, the flexibility of the system allows the dialysis staff member to arrange CPD schedules such that container changes are performed at convenient intervals.

In addition, hospital staff must be properly educated in emergency actions and problem solving techniques. They must also be taught what "violation of the closed system" means and how to avoid it at all costs. They need to be aware of the dangers of performing procedures for which they have not been trained as well as the potential hazards to the patient.

The physician must be well educated in the theoretical and practical implications of CAPD and must be able to apply these to the acute as well as chronic in-hospital patient. The physician must also be willing to support dialysis staff by evaluating and writing orders on CPD patients consistently to allow dialysis staff to be informed of patient regimens.

Proper education and sharing of responsibilities between dialysis and hospital staff can make CPD a most beneficial dialytic therapy. It can also foster shared concern for the patient's quality of care in addition to a well organized means of treating hospitalized renal failure patients.

C.J. Wood, N.M. Thomson, D.F. Scott, S.R. Holdsworth,
N. Boyce, and R.C. Atkins

66

Renal Transplantation in Patients on CAPD

SUMMARY

Graft and patient survival in 37 patients receiving a renal allograft while on CAPD have been compared to that in 102 hemodialysis patients transplanted in the same period. Graft and patient survival was similar in both groups. Blood transfusion prior to transplantation was associated with better graft survival in both CAPD and hemodialysis patients. Although peritonitis occurred in 6 of 30 patients in whom the peritoneal catheter was left *in situ* at transplantation, the peritonitis rapidly subsided with antibiotics without sequelae. Thus renal transplantation may be safely and effectively performed in patients on CAPD and the catheter left *in situ* and used if necessary for postoperative dialysis.

INTRODUCTION

Since the introduction in 1978 of continuous ambulatory peritoneal dialysis (CAPD) into our program of care for patients with endstage renal failure, 148 patients have received CAPD for periods from 3–52 months.[1–3] Adequacy of dialysis, quality of life and patient survival have been comparable to that for our patients on hemodialysis (HD). With the increasing popularity of CAPD as a treatment for end stage renal failure, an increasing number of pa-

tients are likely to be using this form of therapy at the time of renal transplantation. There has previously been some concern expressed that transplantation in patients on CAPD is associated with poor graft survival and increased morbidity due to infection in relation to the presence of the peritoneal dialysis catheter. In addition, the value of blood transfusion in improving graft survival has not been adequately determined for patient transplanted while on CAPD.

This study is a retrospective analysis of graft and patient survival for patients on CAPD who have undergone renal transplantation, comparing these results to those of a comparable group of patients transplanted while on hemodialysis; the benefit of pretransplantation blood transfusions on graft survival for patients on CAPD, and infective complications due directly to the *in situ* peritoneal catheter.

METHODS

During the 5 year period 1978 to 1983, 38 renal allografts were performed in 37 patients on CAPD (22 female, 15 male). Thirty four were from cadaveric donors and four from living related donors. In the same period 102 cadaveric renal allografts were performed in patients on hemodialysis. The mean age of the transplanted CAPD patients (39.3 years: range 13 to 55 years) was not significantly different from that of hemodialysis patients (37.2 years: range 6 to 61 years). The etiology of endstage renal failure was similar between groups except that diabetic nephropathy was more frequent in CAPD patients (Table 1).

From the Departments of Nephrology and Surgery, Monash University, Prince Henry's Hospital, Melbourne, Australia.

Table 1. Causes of End-Stage Renal Failure—Cadaveric Transplants.

Disease	CAPD Group (n = 33)	HD Group (n = 102)
Glomerulonephritis	9 (27%)	43 (42%)
Diabetes mellitus	9 (27%)	2 (2%)
Reflux nephropathy	5 (15%)	18 (17%)
Polycystic kidneys	3 (9%)	12 (12%)
Analgesic nephropathy	3 (9%)	14 (14%)
Hypertension	2 (6%)	5 (5%)
Others	2 (6%)	8 (8%)

Initially patients in both groups did or did not receive a course (3 to 4 U) of pretransplantation blood transfusion as part of a controlled trial of blood transfusion in transplantation. However, on cessation of the trial all patients were transfused prior to transplantation. Immunosuppression was identical in the CAPD and hemodialysis groups (low dose prednisolone 30 mg/day initially) and azathioprine (2–2.5 mg/kg/day). The treatment of rejection in both groups was with IV methylprednisolone, plus more recently antithymocyte globulin (ATGAM).

At transplantation the peritoneal dialysis catheter (Tenckhoff) was left *in situ* unless there was or had been evidence of chronic infection in the catheter tract. In the latter situation the catheter was removed and the patient given parenteral antibiotics for 5 to 10 days. Peritoneal dialysis (usually as a CAPD regime) was recommended immediately post transplantation if diuresis did not occur. CAPD was

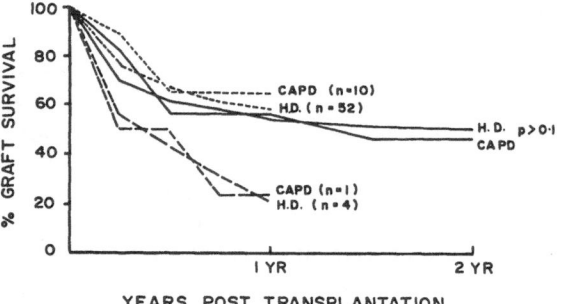

Fig. 1. Cadaveric graft survival for 33 recipients on CAPD and 102 recipients on hemodialysis (HD). All patients (——), transfused recipients (- - - -) and non-transfused recipients (– – –).

also used during episodes of renal failure resulting from severe rejection.

RESULTS

Graft and Patient Survival

Actuarial cadaveric graft survival at 1 year was 56 and 54% for the CAPD and hemodialysis group respectively ($p > 0.1$) (Fig. 1). Eighty percent of CAPD patients and 82% of hemodialysis patients had received one or more blood transfusions prior to transplantation. Graft survival for transfused patients was 65 and 58% for the CAPD and hemodialysis patients respectively compared to only 23 and 21% for untransfused CAPD and hemodialysis patients (insufficient numbers of untransfused CAPD patients to allow meaningful statistical analysis).

Patient survival at 1 year was 96% for CAPD patients and 87% for HD patients (N.S.). Death due to a transplant related problem occurred in only one CAPD patient; the cause of death being CMV colitis with perforation of the colon and subsequent fecal peritonitis.

Postoperative Abdominal Wall and Peritoneal Infection

The intraperitoneal catheter was removed perioperatively in seven patients, left *in situ* in 30 and subsequently removed 1–10 weeks later in 23 patients. CAPD was continued in the postoperative period in 14 patients. Eight infective episodes occurred posttransplantation in six patients (seven peritonitis, one catheter tract infection). One episode of peritonitis was associated with septicemia but this and all other episodes responded rapidly to parenteral and intraperitoneal antibiotics. The intraperitoneal catheter was subsequently removed within 2–5 days in five of these patients. One patient, with a poorly functioning allograft associated with severe rejection, suffered three episodes of peritonitis within 4 months after transplantation. This patient was noted to have a high incidence of peritonitis both prior to transplantation and following graft failure and withdrawal of immunosuppression.

Four of the six patients developing peritonitis were receiving peritoneal dialysis in the post-transplant period. In the other two patients the catheter had been capped at transplantation and peritonitis developed 12 and 21 days postoperatively. In patients not requiring postoperative dialysis routine

Table 2. Infective Episodes in CAPD Patients after Transplantation.

Patient	Primary Disease	Onset Transplant	CAPD in Use	Organism	Catheter Removed	Response to Treatment
1	reflux	3 episodes in 4 months	yes	*Staph. epiderm. I* *Staph. epiderm. II*	no	yes
2	reflux	10 days	yes	*E. coli*	yes	yes
3	polycystic	10 weeks	no	*Staph. aureus*	yes	yes
4	GN	4 weeks	yes	*Staph. epiderm.*	yes	yes
5	diabetes	2 weeks (catheter tract infection)	no	*E. coli*	yes	yes
6	diabetes	4 weeks	no	*Staph. aureus*	yes	yes

GN = glomerulonephritis.

lavage and culture of peritoneal fluid was not performed unless the possibility of peritonitis was raised.

The most frequent organism in patients with peritonitis was *Staphylococcus*. These infective episodes are summarized in Table 2.

Transplant wound infection was seen in two patients (6%) on CAPD and in five patients (5%) on hemodialysis. The peritoneal catheter tract healed rapidly in all patients following removal of the catheter including patients in whom the catheter was removed at the transplant operation because of tract infection.

DISCUSSION

This study has shown that cadaveric renal allograft survival in patients transplanted when on CAPD is equal to that of hemodialysis patients and supports the findings of two other studies of smaller groups of patients.[4,5] Similarly patient survival was equal for both groups with no CAPD patient dying as a result of complications of CAPD.

The beneficial effect of blood transfusion for patients transplanted when on hemodialysis has been well documented[6] but until now not reported for CAPD patients. Our study has shown a marked improvement in graft survival in CAPD patients receiving pretransplantation transfusions and we now insist on two or more transfusions before transplant-

ing CAPD patients. We cannot comment as yet on the incidence and severity of sensitization to HLA antigens following routine transfusion in patients on CAPD, compared to hemodialysis patients.

Although we have found a significant incidence of peritonitis in CAPD patients posttransplantation, significant morbidity has not been seen and we believe the risk of peritonitis is acceptable. Other studies[7-10] of smaller groups of adult or pediatric patients have also found a low or zero incidence of posttransplant CAPD-related infective complications. We would however advocate the immediate removal of any peritoneal catheter that shows evidence of acute or chronic tract infection at the time of transplantation. If not infected the catheter can be safely left *in situ*, used if dialysis is necessary and then removed when graft function is stable. Should peritonitis develop, routine treatment with the appropriate antibiotic (and in some patients subsequent removal of the catheter) is successful without compromising the patient or graft function.

REFERENCES

1. Thomson NM, Walker R, Whiteside GM, Scott D, and Atkins RC: Continuous ambulatory peritoneal dialysis (CAPD) in the treatment of end-stage renal failure. Proc Eur Dial Transplant Assoc 16: 171, 1979
2. Thomson NM, Atkins RC, Hooke D, Maydom B, and Scott DF: Long term clinical experience in Australia with continuous ambulatory peritoneal dialysis. In

Atkins RC, Thomson NM, and Farrell PC (Eds), Peritoneal dialysis. Edinburgh: Churchill Livingstone, 1981, p 93

3. Thomson NM, Atkins RC, Humphrey TJ, Agar JMcD, and Scott DF: Continuous ambulatory peritoneal dialysis (CAPD): An established treatment for endstage renal failure. Aust NZ J Med 13: 489, 1983

4. Gokal R, Ramos JM, Veitch P, Proud G, Talor RMR, Ward MK, Wilkinson R, and Kerr DNS: Renal transplantation in patients on continuous ambulatory peritoneal dialysis. Proc Eur Dial Transplant Assoc 18: 222, 1981

5. Evans DH, Sorkin MI, Nolph KD, and Whittier FC: Continuous ambulatory peritoneal dialysis and transplantation. Trans Am Soc Artif Intern Organs 27: 320, 1981

6. Opelz G, and Terasaki P: Dominant effect of transfusions on kidney graft survival. Transplantation 29: 153, 1980

7. Cardella CJ: Renal transplantation in patients on peritoneal dialysis. Peritoneal Dial Bull 1: 12, 1980

8. Gokal R, Ramos JM, and Veitch P: Renal transplantation in patients on CAPD. Dial Transplant 2: 125, 1982

9. Stephanidis GJ, Balfe JW, Arbus GS, Hardy BE, Churchill BM, and Rance CP: Renal transplantation in children treated with CAPD. Peritoneal Dial Bull 3: 5, 1983

10. Ryckelynch JP, Verger C, Pierre D, Sabatier JC, Faller B, and Beaud JM. Early post transplant infection in CAPD patients. Peritoneal Dial Bull 4: 1, 1984

B. Prowant

67

Hemodialysis Requirements of CAPD Patients

SUMMARY

A restrospective review of the need for hemodialysis among 97 patients treated by CAPD was undertaken. After 1 year, 36% had required hemodialysis, after 2 years 52%, and after 3 years 76%, 25% permanently transferring to hemodialysis. Older and Black patients required hemodialysis more often than others. The most frequent reasons for instituting hemodialysis were peritonitis, catheter tunnel infections, technical catheter problems and dialysate leaks. Vascular access was usually achieved by percutaneous catheters but it is recommended that patients who require two or more periods of acute hemodialysis should have a permanent angioaccess.

INTRODUCTION

It has been recognized that a significant number of continuous ambulatory peritoneal dialysis (CAPD) patients transfer to chronic hemodialysis therapy.[1,2] The purposes of this study were to document the acute, as well as chronic, hemodialysis requirements of CAPD patients and to evaluate the need for permanent arteriovenous access in the CAPD population.

From the University of Missouri-Columbia School of Medicine.

METHODS

Chart review of 97 CAPD patients followed at the University of Missouri Hospital and Clinics and Dialysis Clinics, Inc. from May 1977 through December 1983 was undertaken. All patients with outpatient dialysis charts were included in the study. Time on CAPD ranged from 0.5 to 79.5 months with a mean of 20.0 months/patient and a total of 162 patient-years. All patients had had the opportunity to remain on CAPD for at least 6 months. All hemodialysis treatments which took place after the successful initiation of CAPD were included in the study data.

RESULTS

Life table analysis of the time on CAPD until first hemodialysis showed that 36, 52, and 76% of the patient population had required hemodialysis at 1, 2, and 3 years respectively (Fig. 1). The average duration of acute hemodialysis was 8.0 treatments. Twenty-five percent of the population had permanently transferred to hemodialysis during the study period.

Figure 2 indicates the percentage of CAPD patients requiring acute and chronic hemodialysis in relation to the year of CAPD therapy. The requirement for acute hemodialysis was consistent irrespective of the length of time on CAPD. However,

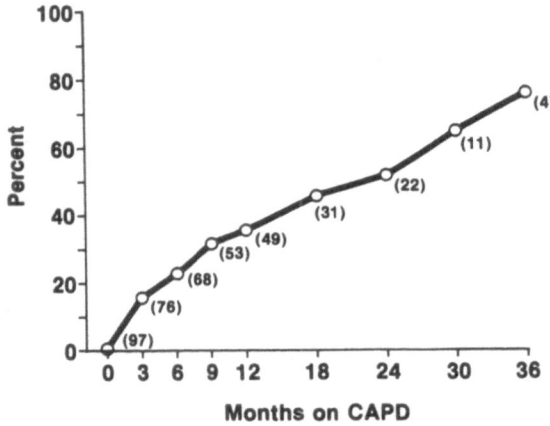

Fig. 1. Probability of first hemodialysis.

Table 1. Patient Characteristics.

	Required HD	No HD
Male (%)	59.6	57.8
Black (%)	9.6	2.2
Mean age (years)	52.4	45.5*
Over 55 years (%)	51.9	35.5
Diabetics (%)	23.1	20.5
Permanent HD access (%)	21.2	31.5
Functioning HD access (%)	15.4	Unknown

* $p = 0.024$.

the percentage of patients who transferred to chronic hemodialysis therapy gradually declined with each year of therapy.

Table 1 compares characteristics of patients who required hemodialysis and those who did not. Th mean age of patients requiring hemodialysis was significantly higher ($p = 0.024$) than of those who did not need hemodialysis. Black patients (the only nonwhite group in our population) also tended to be more likely to require hemodialysis treatment. Diabetic CAPD patients were no more likely to undergo hemodialysis than their nondiabetic counterparts. The presence of a preexisting permanent blood access did not correlate with the use of hemodialysis therapy.

The reasons CAPD patients received hemodialysis therapy are shown in Figure 3. CAPD complications comprised the indication for hemodialysis therapy in 73% of the cases. Peritonitis most frequently resulted in hemodialysis, followed by infections of the subcutaneous tunnel, dialysate leaks, and technical catheter problems. Dialysate leaks included exit site leaks, fluid leaks into herniae, and leaks into the subcutaneous tissue. Other catheter problems included poorly functioning catheters, malposition, a broken catheter, and chronic irritation at the catheter tip. Hemodialysis was also used to manage patients with superimposed medical problems, after surgical procedures, to manage fluid overload and electrolyte abnormalities, and for patients with unacceptably high serum urea and creatinine levels. Hemodialysis was occasionally required in malnourished patients and those unable to continue self-care and home dialysis.

The type of hemodialysis access used for acute dialysis is shown in Figure 4. Only 21% of the patients who required hemodialysis had a preexisting permanent arteriovenous access. Seventy-three

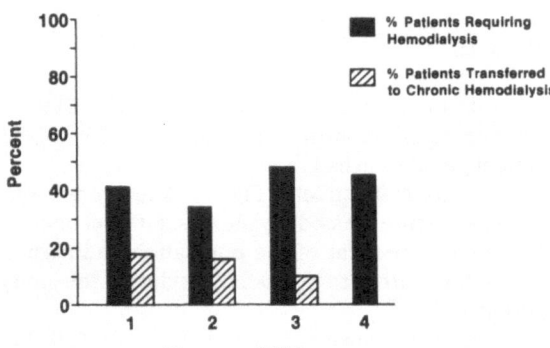

Fig. 2. Percent of CAPD population requiring acute and chronic hemodialysis in relation to year of therapy.

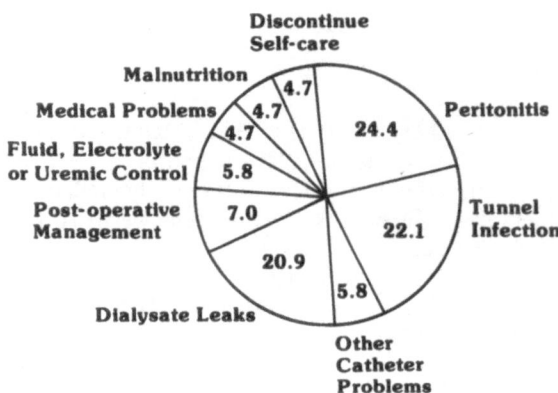

Fig. 3. Reasons for hemodialysis.

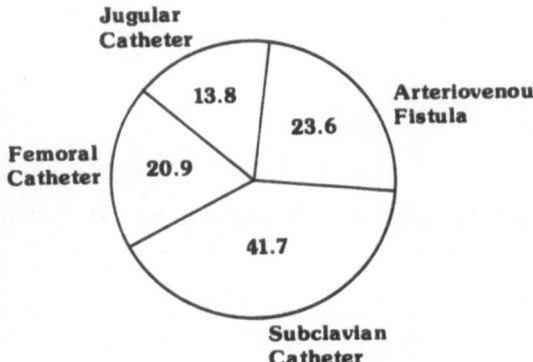

Fig. 4.   Type of hemodialysis access.

percent of these functioned adequately for hemodialysis and permanent access was used for 23% of the acute treatments. Subclavian catheters were used most frequently for acute access (41.7% of treatments) followed by femoral (20.9%) and jugular catheters (13.8%).

DISCUSSION

Although 76% of the patients on CAPD at 36 months had required hemodialysis, only 15% had an adequate preexisting vascular access. Thirty-two percent of all CAPD patients required three or more periods of hemodialysis and a permanent vascular access would be avantageous. However, it remains difficult to identify these individuals prospectively. At present it seems that all CAPD patients who require two or more periods of acute hemodialysis should have a permanent vascular access and that a prudent approach would be to place a chronic arteriovenous access in all patients prior to or early after the commencement of CAPD. Studies that determine the long-term patency of permanent vascular access in CAPD patients, document the complication rates and morbidity associated with both acute and chronic access and compare costs are required to support this recommendation.

REFERENCES

1. Pyle WK, Hiatt MP, and Nolph KD: The Registry pilot project, patent population demographics and selected outcome measures for the period January 1, 1981 through December 31, 1981. The National Institutes of Health CAPD Patient Registry, 1982, p 12
2. Kramer P, Broyer M, Brunner FP, Brynger H, Donckerwolcke RA, Jacobs C, Selwood NH, and Wing AJ: Combined report on regular dialysis and transplantation in Europe, XII, 1981. Proc Eur Dial Transplant Assoc 20: 32, 1983

J. Moon, L. Uttley, J. Manos, N.P. Mallick, and R. Gokal

68

Home CAPD Nurse—An Asset to a CAPD Program

SUMMARY

In the Manchester region the home care nurse provided a valuable service for the patients by maintaining the vital link between home and hospital and achieving a significant reduction in the number of hospital visits. Her role made the out patient treatment of peritonitis more practicable and furnished immediate and close contact during times of difficulty for the patient. Her unique position allows insight into the patient's family and social situation, giving the ability to envisage and resolve problems sooner than a hospital based team would be able. Patient reaction consistently indicated, particularly from the more vulnerable patients, that the provision of a home nurse was a welcome facility. We feel that the home CAPD nurse is an invaluable member of the CAPD team in any CAPD program but more so in a large one undertaking care of all types of patients but in particular those deemed high risk.

INTRODUCTION

CAPD has now become an accepted form of dialysis therapy for end stage renal failure (ESRF) patients. It is a treatment that allows patients to be managed readily at home, with a very short training time in hospital as compared to home hemodialysis patients. An adequate number of nursing staff is a necessary prerequisite of any successful CAPD pro-

gram, so that the CAPD team can train patients efficiently and manage them during readmissions.[1,2] In most renal centers, the Unit advises the patient after discharge predominantly at out-patient visits. However, since its inception our CAPD program has had a home CAPD nurse (now two) as part of the team. The nurse aims to help manage patients in the home, so as to reduce morbidity, increase support, and help in achieving rehabilitation. This report relates to the experience of the CAPD nurse and her role in the program.

CAPD PROGRAM AT MANCHESTER ROYAL INFIRMARY

CAPD was commenced at the Manchester Royal Infirmary in 1980 as part of an already well established and integrated program for ESRF offering transplantation, maintenance, and home hemodialysis. The CAPD team comprised of consultants, medical registrars, social workers, a dietitian, and nursing staff. Initially, training of the patients was carried out by the nursing staff of the medical wards to which patients were readmitted for any subsequent problems, but a full-time nurse for CAPD was soon appointed.

At the commencement of the program a home visiting nurse was appointed to aid continuity of care between hospital and home, as had always been the practice with our home hemodialysis program. During the 3 year period from October 1, 1980 to September 30, 1983, a total of 104 patients were trained for CAPD. Of these, 53 continue on CAPD, 26 were

From the Manchester Royal Infirmary, Manchester, England.

successfully transplanted, 19 transferred to hemodialysis and there were 13 deaths. The average time of CAPD was 10.75 months. Included in these 104 patients were 37 who were classed as being high risk (defined as those with cerebrovascular or cardiovascular disease, diabetes mellitus, age greater than 65 years, spouse performing exchanges, and those with social/psychiatric problems). These were patients who were unlikely to have received treatment on hemodialysis because of the shortage of hemodialysis facilities.[3] Although these enjoyed reasonable quality of life, they were likely to provide greater problems in care and follow up.

The catchment area for our unit covers the North West region of England, stretching as far as 150 miles from the hospital. It was felt that the home nurse should minimize visits to hospital for those living a distance away.

AIMS OF HOME CAPD NURSE

The aims of the home nurse were seen as promoting the general well being of the patients by preventing peritonitis, reducing hospital visits/stays to a minimum, continuing and reinforcing the learning process, encouraging return to previous or improved social status, nurturing a close link between home and hospital, and giving moral support to the patient and family.

ROLE

The above aims of the home CAPD nurse were achieved by performing the following roles.

Assessing the Patient's Home (Pre-Home Dialysis)

When a patient is approaching ESRF a report on his social and work conditions is usually prepared by the social worker. This alerts the team to problems the patient is likely to face on CAPD. A home visit is undertaken at this stage and is even more important for patients who are admitted for the first time, already in ESRF. While the patient is undergoing CAPD training in hospital a further home assessment is undertaken before discharge. This is carried out in the presence of the patient and his family, preferably after he has undergone some exchanges, making it easier for him to assimilate the recommendations for his home care. This is always done in the

presence of the home CAPD nurse. This visit enables both the patient and his family to question the nurse away from the strange and often restrictive environment of the hospital. It also affords the opportunity to assess the patient's own standards of hygiene and the family's interest in his well being and future care. It has proven to be the first essential step in nurturing a mutually trusting and supportive relationship.

Discharge from the Hospital

The home nurse has always been present for the first exchange at home, thus giving the reassurance and practical advice for the adaptation from hospital to home environment. Immediately thereafter, close telephone contact is maintained with further home visits planned according to the individual needs of each patient.

Record Keeping

In our program all patients are requested to keep records of each exchange showing the strength of solution used, clarity of effluent, and drainage volume. In addition, weight, state of exit site, drugs used and any other relevant comments are recorded on a daily basis. Accurate record keeping is essential to help resolve problems and the home nurse has played an important role in ensuring that these were adequately maintained. If a patient takes the time to record these data accurately, neatly and with attention to detail, he or she is far more likely to be treating the rest of his or her obligations with the same diligence. These records are checked at outpatient visits in the hospital at which the home CAPD nurse is also present.

Observations of Exchange Procedure

It is quite common for the patient to deviate inadvertently from the accepted routine, becoming more prone to infection. Awareness that the nurse will be checking the exchange procedure at regular intervals reinforces the importance of scrupulous adherence to the correct exchange procedure.

Set Changes

Set changes performed in the home resulted in a reduction in the number of hospital visits for the patient, particularly important for those with full time employment or limited mobility. This procedure also gives, where necessary, the opportunity to separate the patient from family and allows plenty of time for discussion.

Routine Visits

Every home visit furnishes the nurse with the opportunity to assess the patient's knowledge regarding both the illness and treatment and to update this as necessary. It is essential to ensure that there is sufficient visiting time to give physical and moral support to both the patient and family. Each patient must feel he or she is "the only patient" during a home visit.

Peritonitis Protocol

On occasions treatment for peritonitis has been initiated at home and dialysate specimens have been collected and taken to the hospital for culture and sensitivity. During the training period, patients are taught injection procedures for intraperitoneal antibiotic therapy but many, through lack of practice, have lost confidence and dexterity when they are actually required to do this. Satisfactory fluid balance suddenly becomes more difficult to maintain and understand, particularly if they feel unwell; there is usually a temporary loss of ultrafiltration caused by the peritonitis and fluid balance becomes even more important. Frequent visits, procedure observation and telephone contact are essential to ensure satisfactory recovery. During peritonitis the patient is likely to be more receptive than usual to reeducation. The home CAPD nurse has always used this opportunity to reinforce the exchange procedure hygiene and proper self-care.

Employment

We regard it as important to attempt to return the patient to his or her previous social status. A life revolving around CAPD exchanges alone is unmotivating, and it is essential to encourage the patient to return to useful employment. In our program, the home nurse has been the most suitable person to do this, for she or he develops an intimate knowledge of the patient's medical condition and family background and so can liaise with the employer. The nurse is able to inform the patient's employer of the expected physical state of the employee, and any physical restrictions that may affect working capacity. The amount of time to be spent on hospital visits and future prognosis with regard to the employment

is also explained. The home nurse visits the place of work, assesses its suitability for performing exchanges and, if necessary, checks on an exchange done at work. Occupational health personnel are briefed. All this extends further the care and support of the patient.

Other Health Disciplines

The home nurse has turned out to be the key person in providing the link between home and hospital, involving general practitioners, social workers and other community resources as necessary, therefore encouraging a mutual rapport for the benefit of the patient.

Bereavement Visits

When death occurs, whether expected or not, there will be many questions the family wish to ask. They have been closely and intimately involved with the hospital and gentle severence from this union aids the mourning process.

High Risk Patients

A special role played by the home nurse has been in the management of a group of patients deemed high risk. The group comprised the following patients.

BLIND

Although blind patients adapt well to the CAPD exchange procedure, it is a difficult process for them initially. The anomaly of performing a "no-touch" technique by touch is difficult to grasp at first and frequent observations of their technique is essential, both for their physical protection and to maintain their confidence. The nurse has been able to monitor this in the usual home setting giving the best reassurance to the patient about his or her ability. The use of manual devices to aid the blind has helped considerably in their training and rehabilitation.

DIABETICS

Although CAPD is a more successful form of treatment than hemodialysis for this group of patients, the presence of a home nurse has made it possible to achieve better blood sugar and blood pressure control by careful monitoring. There has also been a reduction in the number of hospital out patient visits for a group of patients who often find traveling long distances irksome.

SEVERE CARDIOVASCULAR DISEASE

A reduction in the number of hospital out-patient appointments has been a real bonus to this group, as CAPD does not necessarily result in physical improvement for those patients severely crippled by cardiac or cerebral conditions and simply adds a further "disability," often leading to depression. The home nurse has been able to provide an essential service in maintaining good fluid balance control, helping to motivate the patient and liaising with other community resources.

POORLY MOTIVATED PATIENTS

Lack of both patient selection and hospital dialysis facilities has led to patients psychologically unsuited to CAPD therapy managed by this treatment. Frequent home visits for this group are essential to obtain a satisfactory degree of motivation and commitment.

HELP IN PERFORMING EXCHANGES

Helpers were involved in the care of seven patients (four diabetics, blind and with peripheral neuropathy, two previous severe cardiovascular accidents with poor motor recovery and one manic depressive). Patients classed in this category were usually severely physically debilitated with poor prognosis or had psychosocial problems, such that the patient was unable to perform the exchanges himself or herself. This group has proved to be the most difficult for the home nurse. Lack of physical improvement and further dependence on the spouse resulted in severe depression for the patient. Extra responsibility and further physical involvement in aiding the patient proved difficult for the helper to cope with. This resulted in "helper fatigue" and necessitated patient admission to the wards to give the helper a break. Ironically, CAPD problems tended to be few and peritonitis rates low in this group. Visiting priorities were high for this group with the home nurse acting as friend and mentor and liaising with other community health resources. Our experience shows that this form of helper in CAPD is not desirable and should be avoided whenever possible.

Visiting Priorities

In a large CAPD program, as ours is, with a current total of over 60 patients, it is difficult to cover all the patient's needs. A visiting priorities list has been formulated to try and work on those issues that are of prime importance.

Newly discharged patients, with their subsequent vulnerability are first in the list of visiting priorities, with the high risk and poorly motivated patients falling naturally into place. While the elderly are not necessarily deemed to be at greater risk, they do require more support than the younger, more physically able patients, particularly if living alone.

With the Manchester experience, the large percentage of high risk patients greatly affected the balance of care, resulting in a large proportion of the home visits being expended on a group of poor achievers, with subsequent gaps in the care of the "better" patients.

The Home-Hospital Link

This is important. The home nurse visited and discussed CAPD treatment and adjustment to home while the patient was still training in hospital. In addition each out patient session was attended by the home nurse, as were weekly meetings of the CAPD team, held to discuss the medical, social, and other concerns of each CAPD patient.

Necessary Prerequisites of a Home Nurse

It is vital that the nurse is able to work at odd hours and at evenings, to accommodate patient lifestyles and work schedules. The nurse needs to be enthusiastic, and able to drive long distances. It is our estimate that one CAPD nurse working full-time may well be required for up to 40 patients.

REFERENCES

1. Gokal R: Continuous ambulatory peritoneal dialysis. In Parsons FM, and Ogg CS (Eds), Renal failure—who cares? Lancaster: MTP Press, 1982, p 137
2. Oreopoulos DG: Requirements for the organization of a CAPD program. Nephron 24: 261, 1979
3. Pryor JS: Comparison of facilities in United Kingdom and in Europe for dialysis and transplantation. In Parsons FM, and Ogg CS (Eds), Renal failure—who cares? Lancaster: MTP Press, 1982, p 17

W.F. Barnard, N. Kloberdanz, W.P. Argy, T.A. Rakowski,
and J.F. Winchester

69

The Telephone—An Underestimated Resource for CAPD Nursing Management

SUMMARY

Telephone communication between CAPD nursing staff and patients, avoids unnecessary delays in dealing with simple problems, giving support to patients, and judging whether patients have serious problems necessitating acute nursing/medical management. The telephone serves as a vital link between patient and nursing personnel.

INTRODUCTION

Patients treated at home for any major disease must remain in contact with nursing personnel for continued management. Many diseases do not require contact except at regular clinic visits (e.g., review of blood glucose recordings at diabetic clinics and blood pressure values at hypertension clinics). After a period of home dialysis training patients often feel the need for support, to discuss machine dysfunction and symptoms. We have always felt that the telephone was a vital link to patient management, even in the relatively proximate vicinity of the Washington Metropolitan area (none of our patients lives more than 40 miles from our center), and could be of even greater value for patients at great distance from the hospital. Since we have always maintained a daily log of patient calls, with reasons for the call, and a resolution of problems, we retrospectively

From Georgetown University Hospital, Washington, D.C.

364

analyzed the calls to determine the major reasons for such calls.

METHODS

Over a 3 month period, when following a total pool of 55 patients, we examined our telephone log of reasons for call, time of call, patient name, nurse accepting call, and resolution of call. Since we have a 24 hour 7 day on-call system, we examined the frequency of calls, by day and by nursing shift (three 8 hour shifts/day). In addition nurse initiated calls were also recorded.

RESULTS

Over a 3 month period, 338 calls were received. As expected most calls were received on Monday, and most calls (on all days) were received on the first nursing shift of the day (Table 1). The most frequent reason for patient initiated calls were problems with fluid balance (dehydration, edema, hypotension, hypertension), while nurse-initiated calls were related to resolution of this problem or for peritonitis. Peritonitis (diagnosis and therapy) was the most frequent CAPD related problem prompting the patient to call. Table 2 gives the breakdown of the reasons for telephone contact.

The calls were divided into categories as to the reason for the call; questions about fluid balance were the most frequent, 27.2%. Nurse-initiated calls were the next largest block of time spent, on the

Table 1. Frequency of Calls by Day (338 Calls Received Over a 3 Month Period).

Day	%
Monday	24.3
Tuesday	20.0
Wednesday	17.8
Thursday	11.2
Friday	18.3
Saturday	4.7
Sunday	3.6

Most calls occurred: first morning shift. Time spent on each call: average 5–10 minutes.

Table 2. Reasons for Telephone Contact Between CAPD Patient and CAPD Nurse.

Reason for Call	%
Fluid Balance	27.2
Nurse initiated follow-up	19.5
CAPD-related	17.8
Non-CAPD-related	13.6
Drug prescriptions	7.4
Lab test results	7.1
Logistics (Billing/clinic)	5.0
Reassurance	2.7

telephone at 19.5%. These were calls by the nurses to check on patients who had problems or who had called in previously. It is worth noting that time is also spent by the nurses giving reassurance during all the other calls, while they are sorting out other problems.

DISCUSSION

We started our telephone log originally as an aid to better communication among the nursing staff, as the nurses were not in the office at the same time, but were on various units in the hospital giving inservice to nursing staff regarding our renal patients. There was no way to communicate the calls coming in and the action taken without written records. This also proved to be a valuable means of communication between the day time and evening nurses.

We found the telephone to be a vital link for patients. It has provided them with a confidence base; informed them as to current self-care expectations; helped to minimize complications, as minor problems are handled before they become monumental complications, and helped the patients learn to problem solve. We aided them in looking at a problem such as fluid status and helping them decide how to solve their problem.

We also found we had saved the physicians valuable time, as we have screened the calls and have only involved the physician when it has been absolutely necessary. Few calls have ever had to be direct, between patient and physician. We have managed patient fluid balance and all other aspects of their dialysis requirements. We have provided accurate, detailed, and up-to-date written records of the status of each patient, and the entire program from a nursing level under the guidance of our nephrologists. We have provided the physician with an up-to-date status report of all patients with current problems, so that if the patient does need to contact our physicians, he or she will have ready knowledge of the problem.

After keeping our detailed log and examining it closely, we have determined that the telephone is a vital, absolutely essential part of a CAPD program. We feel strongly that the CAPD related as well as the non-CAPD related calls, provide the patient with a confidence base necessary for successful self-care management. By utilizing the telephone as a positive element, the nurses have saved the physicians valuable time and have provided essential program management.

G. Omotosho

70

Psychological and Economic Assessment of Peritoneal Dialysis Patients in Nigeria

SUMMARY

Psychological and social problems accompany treatment of end stage renal disease by peritoneal dialysis. This paper reviews the varied problems encountered in six patients from Nigeria. It is recommended that psychological intervention and rehabilitative physical therapy be used regularly.

INTRODUCTION

It is well known that patients in end-stage renal failure have psychological and social difficulties. Acceptance of the disease and change in their socioeconomic life style are loathed by a good percentage especially at the initiation of treatment. To assess the psychosocioeconomic status of peritoneal dialysis patients, 22 patients were studied over 2 years on intermittent peritoneal dialysis for 24 hours three times weekly using an automated peritoneal dialyzer with 1.36 to 3.86% Dianeal 137. This reports six patients who were closely studied.

Nigeria is situated in West Africa with a population of over eighty million. There are many teaching and local hospitals in all the 19 states of the Federation of Nigeria. Peritoneal dialysis had been the treatment of choice for few patients in various hospitals over 10 years until September 1981 when the Lagos University Teaching Hospital, Lagos, decided to have a dialysis center for hemodialysis and peritoneal dialysis.

From Lagos University Teaching Hospital, Nigeria, West Africa.

CASE REPORTS

The first patient is a 36-year-old executive of an oil company with a good marital relationship and job satisfaction. He was edematous from heart failure. Water was removed from the patient by dialysing with 3.86% Dianeal 137. Blood pressure and pulse were monitored carefully to avoid hypotension and shock. He would always ask his wife to find out about his electrolyte results. The wife was always delighted to be around at each exchange of the dialysate asking questions about turbidity of fluid if it occurred. She looked forward to their twenty-first wedding anniversary and how they would jointly manage the affairs of their new company, which they were planning. She was very optimistic about the maintenance of her husband's chronic illness on automated peritoneal dialysis. He was maintained for 2 years on peritoneal dialysis without any complication, but on the 4th of February, 1984, a shunt and fistula was created and he is now being maintained on hemodialysis.

The second patient, anticipated her 20 and 18-year-old daughters' ambition to achieve their life goals. She would always talk about the children. On one occasion, the returning fluid was bloodstained. She was very upset and asked many questions about peritonitis. She would recall that her first daughter would take another 3 years to graduate as a law student and get married. Although she knew she had a chronic illness, she believed and relied on the fact that she could live on peritoneal dialysis for many more years in order to see her girls achieve their life goals. Peritoneal dialysis was stopped for a few days and conservative treatment was given. She later agreed to hemodialysis and had a shunt and fistula created. Her access routes created a lot of problems. A graft that was inserted became nonfunctional when she knocked her hand against the wall. She is now being dialysed via subclavian and femoral routes.

Loneliness and boredom led to a suicidal attempt by the third patient who is a 36-year-old trained nurse with chronic glomerulonephritis. All members of staff are, at some time, the target of aggressive feelings, and the medical social worker expressed these negative feelings secretly. We accept and understand this. It was discovered that this patient lacked affection and did not receive emotional support from her husband. She is married and blessed with four children including a set of twins. She realized that the husband had been staying very long in the office and did not bother to ask about her peritoneal dialysis treatment. She cut off her peritoneal catheter twice with her teeth and removed the catheter once. She said that she would prefer to die. At each suicidal attempt, she was caught by the nurses. This vigilance increased her animosity toward the nurses, who spend a lot of time telling her that she has reasons to be alive. The medical social worker and occupational therapist kept her busy. She loves talking and sharing views with everybody, but decided not to look after her appearance and lost interest in her surrounding. After all the long counseling, she improved socially, She started changing her apparel and taking care of her hair. She decided that she would like to reapply for her job. A fistula was created and she is now on hemodialysis. She has since resumed her duty and is doing well on hemodialysis twice weekly on a 6 hour basis.

A 26-year-old teacher was admitted with high blood pressure. He complained of constant severe headaches coupled with blurred vision. He looked very ill and worried. Serum chemistry determinations show a very high creatinine, potassium and blood urea. The renal condition was discussed with the family and initial deposit was paid. It was discovered from the discussion with a nurse that the patient's family borrowed money to pay for the initial deposit. The medical social worker and psychologist were consulted. The patient asked the nephrologist to remove the peritoneal catheter as he would like to be treated by a spiritualist. He had no money to pay for the renal treatment.

A 25-year-old accounts clerk was admitted following a post abortal sepsis from a private hospital. She was in severe pain and had a fever. Blood specimens and culture were sent and she was treated accordingly. Peritoneal dialysis was started with a broad spectrum antibiotic added to the dialysate. She sometimes complained of shoulder pain. She improved after five (24 hour) exchanges spread over 10 days. She became worried about the loss of the pregnancy especially as it was the first after her marriage. She was afraid of the peritoneal catheter despite the fact that everything about dialysis was explained to her. Her septicemic state was treated and she felt better. She requested that she would like to stop peritoneal dialysis and that she would prefer conservative treatment at the out-patient medical clinic. She defaulted after her in-patient discharge.

A 43-year-old business tycoon was being treated for chronic renal failure. She had the chronic peritoneal catheter inserted. She had ascites and congestive cardiac failure. After 9 months on peritoneal dialysis, the omentum wrapped round the catheter. The patient was told of an operation that would be performed on her. She took her discharge. Her husband reported that she was flown to India for kidney transplantation.

Finally, looking at the problem on a larger scale, psychiatric and psychological consultations should continue. Rehabilitative physical therapy should be encouraged to alleviate boredom.

A. Treviño-Becerra and A.G. Valencia

71

CAPD on Alternate Days

SUMMARY

Four patients, (previously on CAPD for a mean of 16 months during a patient experience of 36 months ($\overline{X}$9), were treated with CAPD-A that consist of four exchanges in 24 hours and for the next day only one exchange in 24 hours. Comparison of average results obtained: Glucose: CAPD, 82.5 ± 6.0 mg/dl; CAPD-A 65.0 ± 2.0 mg/dl; Albumin: CAPD 3.3 ± 0.31 g/dl; CAPD-A 3.9 ± 0.36 g/dl; CO_2: CAPD, 29.6 ± 1.5 mEq/l, CAPD-A 25.7 ± 1.03 mEq/L. With CAPD, the peritonitis rate was 3.25 per patient, one infection every 4 months. With CAPD-A only one patient had peritonitis twice in 7.7 months and two patients remained infection free. Infection rate decreased 0.6 infections/patient/year. Levels of urea, Cr., uric acid, Hb., HCT., Na., K., Cl., Ca. and blood pressure were similar with both methods. There was 1.0 g protein increase with CAPD-A.

CAPD-A is a useful procedure to correct CAPD complications. Fewer exchanges leave the patient free for 24 hours every third day and there is a reduction in the amount of dialysis solution by one third.

INTRODUCTION

With the advent of continuous ambulatory peritoneal dialysis (CAPD) by Popovich and colleagues in 1977,[1] this method has become more and more popular due to its beneficial effects in maintaining end-stage chronic renal failure patients in acceptable condition.[2,3] Other variations have been suggested to reduce the incidence of complications particularly peritonitis.[4,5] Modifications in the number of exchanges, the volume of solution and the dwell time have been suggested alternatives.[6-8]

The objectives of these modifications have been to reduce the incidence of peritonitis and other infections, reduce the cost of treatment, and make the patient feel more free. Mass transfer that takes place during four exchanges of dialysis solution in CAPD or continuous cyclic peritoneal dialysis,[9] demonstrate that when exchanges are very rapid, equilibrium is not reached. Some authors claim that the basis for the effectiveness of CAPD (4 to 6 hour exchanges) and its hallmark, i.e., a more physiologic dialysis may be complicated by increased passage of glucose into the patient,[1] higher protein excretion, and lactate or acetate transfer from dialysis fluid into plasma resulting in extreme metabolic alkalosis.[10]

Another concern is that with time the constant instillation into and removal of fluid from the peritoneal cavity may cause loss of peritoneal ultrafiltration.[11]

This study was carried out in four patients on CAPD who were changed to continuous peritoneal dialysis on alternate days (CAPD-A) so as to assess their clinical and biochemical status, reduce complications and the previously mentioned undesirable effects and make the patient feel freer.

MATERIAL AND METHODS

Four chronic renal failure patients were studied (3 females, 1 male) ages ranging from 35 to 40 years (mean 37.5 years). Patients were selected from the

From the Nephrology Department, Specialties Hospital, "La Raza" Medical Center, IMSS, Mexico.

Table 1. General Data of Four Patients Included in the Peritoneal Dialysis on Alternate Days Program (CAPD-A).

Patient	Age (years)	Sex	Diagnosis	Creatinine Clearance (ml/minute)	
				Initial	Current
1	37	M	Glomerulonephritis	1.0	0.1
2	40	F	Glomerulonephritis	1.5	0.03
3	35	F	Pyelonephritis	2.4	6.0
4	38	F	Glomerulonephritis	1.2	—

CAPD group according to their compliance and follow-up in their therapeutic and dietary regimens. Evolution on CAPD varied from 5 to 37 months (mean 16 months) with a peritonitis rate of 4.5 months/patient. Patients were in good general condition and the daily diet consisted of 30 to 40 Kcal/Kg of ideal BW, 1 to 1.5 g/Kg of protein/70 to 100 mEq K; 60 to 100 mEq Na and liberal fluid intake.

Patients were on propranolol and hydralazine, dose adjusted according to blood pressure. Their creatinine clearance was 4 ml/minute or less (Table 1).

In the CAPD program there were four daily exchanges of 2 L dialysis solution (1.5% dextrose) and occasionally one exchange of 4.25% dextrose at night depending on fluid retention. In CAPD-A, four 1.5% dextrose exchanges were performed, and the following day only one exchange with 2 L of solution (1.5% or 4.25% dextrose depending on fluid status) leaving this exchange inside the peritoneal cavity for 24 hours and continuing this protocol on alternate days. The number of connections was reduced from 28 to 16 to 19/week and the volume of dialysis solution from 56 L to 32 L to 38 L weekly. Up to now patients have been followed from 6–20 months (mean 14.5 months). Biochemical control investigated during CAPD-A included Hb, HCT, glucose, urea, creatinine, uric acid, Na, K, Cl, CO_2, Ca, P, cholesterol, protein, and albumin concentrations.

Patient 1 had symptoms of uremia on the days when only one exchange was made, so he was changed to three and two exchanges on alternate days, maintaining five exchanges every 2 days as in the other patients.

RESULTS

Table 2 shows the duration of different treatments, a mean of 15.8 months with CAPD (range 5 to 37 months) and in CAPD-A, mean 14.5 months (range 6 to 37 months.) It is important to observe that patients 1, 2, and 3 were on CAPD-A over a year. This table also shows peritonitis incidence with both procedures. With CAPD, 13 episodes of peritonitis,

Table 2. Time and Peritonitis Episodes in Four Patients on CAPD and CAPD-A.

Patient	Time (Months)		Peritonitis Episodes		Peritonitis Rate (Months/Patient)	
	CAPD	CAPD-A	CAPD	CAPD-A	CAPD	CAPD-A
1	37	15	4	0	9.2	—
2	11	20	3	0	3.7	—
3	10	17	4	2	2.5	6.0
4	5	6	2	0	2.5	—
Total	63	58	13	2		
$\bar{x}$	15.8	14.5	3.25	0.5	4.47	
$S\bar{x}$	14.4	6.0	0.95	1.0	3.2	

a mean of 3.25 infections/patient and an interval of 4.5 months/patient between infections; this figure is consistent with previous finding from our group.

When treatment was changed to CAPD-A, patient 3 had two episodes of peritonitis at the beginning of the dialysis program, but this has never recurred. The other three patients were infection free. Two patients have been without an infection for 15 to 20 months, a lower incidence than on CAPD, so peritonitis decreased with a decrease in the number of exchanges. With CAPD (7560 connections) 13 episodes of peritonitis occurred, yielding an average of one infection per 581 connections while with CAPD-A (4265 exchanges) there were two cases of peritonitis, giving an average of only one per 2132.5.

The biochemical findings showed that the average urea concentration was similar in both, (CAPD 113 ± 33 mg/dl versus CAPD-A 127 ± 12 mg/dl; p, N.S. Serum creatinine values were also very similar in both treatments, (CAPD 9.22 ± 3.5 mg/dl and CAPD-A 9.25 + 1.8 mg/dl; p, N.S.) Uric acid levels, were also not significantly different, 6.1 versus 6.3 mg/dl. A remarkable finding was the HCT increase from 30.5 ± 3% with CAPD to 34 ± 6% with CAPD-A. In two patients it was very similar with both procedures, but it increased considerably 6 and 10%, in patients 3 and 4. These patients were those that had undergone dialysis for a shorter time (Table 3).

Serum electrolyte values are shown in Table 4. There was no difference in serum sodium or potassium concentrations with the two treatments. A moderate metabolic alkalosis was found in patients 1, 3, 4, on CAPD, but CO_2 returned to normal when these patients were changed to CAPD-A.

There was a slight decrease in serum calcium with CAPD-A when compared to CAPD. In three patients levels were normal, but patient 2 had hypo-calcemia that became worse on CAPD-A. Concerning phosphorus, the mean value on CAPD was 4.8 ± 2.6, changing to 3.7 ± 1.3 mg/dl with CAPD-A, although this was not statistically significant (Table 4).

Table 5 shows biochemical parameters related to nutrition. Average serum protein values increased from 6.7 ± 0.9 to 7.4 ± 0.8 g/dl, mainly due to a rise in albumin; in three patients initial hypoalbuminemia increased from 3.2 to 3.9 g/dl.

All patients had normal plasma glucose levels. The mean value decreased significantly from 82.5 ± 12–65.2 ± 4 in parallel to a decrease in the glucose load. Finally, plasma cholesterol increased in two patients and decreased in the other two.

Average values per patient of systolic and diastolic blood pressures show negligible differences: 167/102 mm Hg with CAPD and 162/104 mm Hg in the CAPD-A group.

DISCUSSION

There have been several modifications of the original CAPD technique in order to reduce complications such as peritonitis, as well as reducing the number of daily exchanges. Another objective is to try to control metabolic alterations because of uremia and the treatment itself. A significant reduction in the incidence of peritonitis was observed in our patients; in three this complication never occurred and one patient had two episodes during the initial phase but has remained infection free for the last 13 months. We consider that the main factor for infection reduction has been less connections. We infer that patient fatigue is involved in the process of contamination and with CAPD-A this factor is significantly reduced. We found that uremic serum chemical values did not change appreciably when

Table 3.   Serum Chemistry and Hematocrit Values on CAPD and CAPD-A.

Patient	Urea (mg/dl)		Creatinine (mg/dl)		Uric Acid (mg/dl)		Hematocrit (%)	
	CAPD	CAPD-A	CAPD	CAPD-A	CAPD	CAPD-A	CAPD	CAPD-A
1	91	123	9.7	9.7	6.8	7.5	28	27
2	133	113	12.0	11.2	7.25	6.6	32	31
3	80	130	4.1	6.9	4.14	4.3	34	40
4	148	141	11.1	9.2	6.2	6.7	28	38
Mean	113	126.7	9.22	9.25	6.1	6.27	30.5	34
p	NS		NS		NS		NS	

patients were changed to CAPD-A, and clinically only one patient had symptoms of uremia making necessary a regimen of three and two exchanges on alternate days, a total of five in two days as in the rest of the patients.

Improvement in hemoglobin and hematocrit in two patients after some time on CAPD-A is typical of patients who have been on CAPD. It has been established that the longer they are on CAPD the greater the improvement of hemoglobin and hematocrit levels. Patients that changed from CAPD to CAPD-A improved their alkalosis and low albumin values probably due to less protein loss. Levels of glycemia decreased.

On correction of all these alterations, more favorable conditions are present to maintain patients in better physical condition with CAPD-A. We consider that CAPD-A is useful to maintain chronic renal failure patients in acceptable condition. This work is preliminary and should be extended to larger numbers of cases. The patients are completely free to carry out daily life activities every 48, hours there is less use of solutions and certain metabolic complications are blunted. These important points support the concept of CAPD-A.

CONCLUSIONS

Changing patients from CAPD to CAPD-A gave the following results. There was a reduction in the incidence of peritonitis. Moderate elevation of uremic solutes was not significantly higher and did not have clinical effects with the exception of one patient who was changed to three and two exchanges on alternate days. Hematocrit remained stable and in some it even increased. Electrolyte balance remained stable when changing from one type of dialysis to another. CO_2 was normalized. Improvement of total proteins and albumin occurred. Glycemia decreased, and hypocalcemia remained stable. Finally, arterial blood pressure was not changed on CAPD-A.

REFERENCES

1. Popovich RP, Moncrif JW, Nolph KD, Ghods AJ, Twardowski ZJ, and Pyle WK: Continuous ambulatory peritoneal dialysis. Ann Intern Med 88: 449, 1978
2. Robson MD, Oreopoulos DG, Clayton S, Izett S, Rapoport A, and deVeber GA: Comparison of intermittent with continuous perioneal dialysis. Proc Eur Dial Transplant Assoc 15: 197, 1978

Table 4. Serum Electrolytes on CAPD and CAPD-A.

Patient	Sodium (mEq/L)		Potassium (mEq/L)		CO_2 (mEq/L)		Calcium (mg/dl)		Phosphorus (mg/dl)	
	CAPD	CAPD-A	CAPD	CAPD-A	CAPD	CAPD-A	CAPD	CAPD-A	CAPD	CAPD-A
1	137	140	5.7	4.2	33.0	27	11.5	8.0	4.5	3.8
2	143	141	5.5	5.8	25.0	27.5	8.1	6.4	2.2	2.4
3	143	143	3.8	4.8	31.1	25.2	10	9.9	4.1	31
4	138	141	4.3	5.4	27.0	23.0	10	9.5	8.5	5.4
Mean	140.2	141.2	4.8	5.0	29.0	25.7	9.9	9.3	4.8	3.7
Standard Deviation	3.2	1.2	0.9	0.7	3.6	2.0	1.4	2.8	2.6	1.3
p	NS		NS		NS		NS		NS	

Table 5. Nutritional Biochemical Parameters Comparing CAPD with CAPD-A.

Patient	Total Proteins (g/dl)		Albumin (g/dl)		Glucose (mg/dl)		Cholesterol (mg/dl)	
	CAPD	CAPD-A	CAPD	CAPD-A	CAPD	CAPD-A	CAPD	CAPD-A
1	8.0	8.3	5.1	4.7	83	64	312	235
2	6.4	7.3	2.6	4.2	68	62	258	203
3	6.1	6.4	2.5	3.0	97	64	232	308
4	6.3	7.7	2.7	2.8	82	71	341	415
Mean	6.7	7.42	3.2	3.9	82.5	65.2	285	290
Standard Deviation	0.9	0.9	1.2	0.7	11.8	3.9	49	99
p	NS		NS		0.01		NS	

3. Prowant B, Ryan L, and Nolph KD: Six years of experience with perionitis in a CAPD Program. Peritoneal Dial Bull 3: 199, 1983

4. Prowant B, and Nolph KD: Five years' experience with peritonitis in CAPD program. Peritoneal Dial Bull 2: 169, 1982

5. Wu G: A review of peritonitis episodes that caused interruption of CAPD. Peritoneal Dial Bull (Suppl 3): S11, 1983

6. Cantarovich F, Perez LJ, Chena C, Wilberg R, Vernetti J, Correa C, and Tizado J: CAPD-3 daily exchanges, In Moncrief JW, and Popovich RP (Eds), CAPD update. New York, Paris: Masson Publishing, 1981, p 117

7. Forbes AM, Reed V, and Goldsmith HJ: CAPD-A Scheme to allow reduction of daily bag exchange. Clin Nephrol 15: 264, 1981

8. Twardowski ZJ, Prowant BF, Nolph KD, Martínez AJ, and Lamoton LM: High volume low frequency continuous ambulatory peritoneal dialysis. Kidney Int 23: 64, 1983

9. Díaz-Buxo JA, Farmer CD, Walker PJ, Chandler JT, and Holt KL: Continuous cyclic peritoneal dialysis: A preliminary report. Artif Organs 5: 157, 1981

10. Slingeneyer A, Mion C, and Selem JL: Home intermittent (IPD) and continuous ambulatory peritoneal dialysis (CAPD) as a long term treatment of end-stage renal failure in diabetics. In Gahl GM, Kessel M, and Nolph KD, (Eds), Advances in peritoneal dialysis: Proceeding of the 2nd international symposium on peritoneal dialysis. Amsterdam: Excerpta Medica, 1981, p 378

11. Faller B, and Marichal JF: Loss of ultrafiltration in continuous ambulatory peritoneal dialysis: A role for acetate. Peritoneal Dial Bull 4: 10, 1984

R.C. Mackow, W.P. Argy, T.A. Rakowski, J.F. Winchester,
S. Jenkins, J.I. Shapiro, and G.E. Schreiner

72

Low BUN: A Negative Prognostic Indicator Early in CAPD

SUMMARY

A low mean value for predialysis BUN has been associated with decreased survival and decreased parameters of well-being in hemodialysis patients. We sought to extend our investigations into our CAPD population. Early in CAPD a population exists with a low mean BUN who will fail to thrive. Postulates as to mechanisms of disease are discussed.

INTRODUCTION

The exact role that nitrogenous wastes play in the pathogenesis of the uremic syndrome is a subject of interest and remains controversial. The use of blood urea nitrogen (BUN) as a marker for dialysis adequacy has been proposed.[1]

In prior work with two groups of hemodialysis patients we have shown that a low mean value for predialysis BUN is associated with decreased survival on hemodialysis.[2] A high BUN on the other hand is associated with decreased morbidity in terms of annual frequency of hospitalizations. Indeed, patients with a higher BUN in this hemodialysis population have a significantly higher hematocrit. We sought, therefore, to analyze survival and morbidity as well as indices of well-being in our population of CAPD patients when subdivided into low and high BUN groups.

From the Division of Nephrology, Department of Medicine, Georgetown University Medical Center, Washington, D.C.

METHODS

The CAPD population at Georgetown University Medical Center was analyzed for the period July, 1979, to December, 1982. Of 86 patients trained on CAPD, 81 had adequate follow-up data. The CAPD regimen consisted of four, 2 L exchanges/day with 1.5, 2.5, or 4.25% dextrose dialysis solution as required to maintain target weight. All patients initiated CAPD on 1.5 g/kg protein diets with *ad libitum* sodium, potassium, and water intake. Biochemical values, procedures and clinical data were obtained over the total course of CAPD. All laboratory values are expressed as the mean ± SEM of 10 randomly selected values.

Two subgroups were arbitrarily created by dividing patients into two populations by mean BUN: BUN < 60 mg/dl designated group I, and BUN > 80 mg/dl designated group II. Data analysis was performed by Student's t-test, chi square analysis, Fisher exact test, and life table analysis where appropriate.[3] Life table analysis included CAPD patients who eventually changed their therapy to hemodialysis or renal transplantation, or who died.

Morbidity was analyzed by life table as the cumulative probability of remaining unhospitalized versus time after initiation of CAPD. Only hospitalizations for acute or subacute illnesses were included in the analysis. Admissions, for example, for minor vascular access problems were excluded.

RESULTS

The status of the 81 patients entered into the study is given in Table 1. Forty-seven continue CAPD, whereas 17 patients have returned to hemo-

373

Table.1. CAPD Population
Characteristics.

86 patients were initiated on CAPD from 7/79 to 12/82	
81 patients had adequate follow-up Status as of 12/82 was:	
CAPD	47
Hemodialysis	17
Transplanted	8
Dead	9

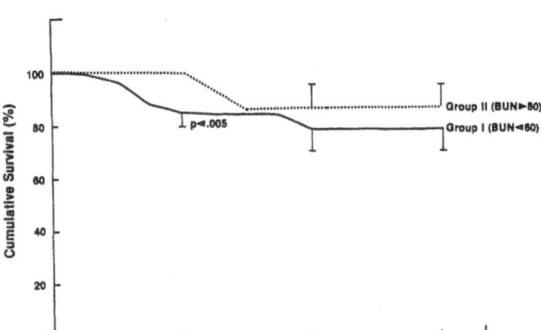

Fig. 1. Actuarial survival on CAPD of a patient group with high BUN Contrasted to a group with low BUN.

dialysis for renal replacement therapy. Of note, about half of these 17 patients returned to hemodialysis for reasons of personal preference. The other major reason was recurrent peritonitis. Eight patients trained for CAPD were transplanted and nine died.

Demographics of the two groups are compared in Table 2. Thirty-seven patients are included in group I and 23 in group II. The average BUN for group I was 50 ± 1.4 mg/dl and for group II was 90 ± 1.6 mg/dl. A significantly different sex distribution existed in the two groups $p < 0.001$. Racial distribution on the other hand was not significantly different. The low BUN (group I) patients were slightly younger than the high BUN (group II) patients: 45.2 ± 2.7 years versus 48.9 ± 2.1 years. Average months of CAPD treatment was not different between the two groups, but prior time on hemodialysis, hence total duration of dialytic therapy was shorter in group I versus group II. The average body weights of group I, 77.7 ± 13 kg and group II, 78.1 ± 3.1 kg were not different. Approximately an equal percentage of patients in each BUN group carry a diagnosis of hypertension, 24% in group I and 35% in group II.

Group I and group II patients were analyzed in terms of cause of end-stage renal disease. The etiology of ESRD was largely made on clinical grounds

as renal biopsy had not been performed in most patients. In Table 3 the frequency of various diseases is given for group I versus group II. None of these differences in disease distribution reached statistical significance. Notable, however, was the apparent uneven distribution and increased proportion of patients with diabetes mellitus in group I, 6/37 (16%) versus group II, 1/23 (4.3%). By Fisher exact test, this difference was not significantly different.

The groups did not differ in mean hematocrit or systolic and diastolic blood pressure. Serum calcium, on the other hand, was slightly higher in group I patients and serum phosphorus was higher in group II (Table 4). Morbidity, including episodes of peritotis and hospitalizations per year were higher in the low BUN (group I) patients.

Cumulative survival at 10 months was better for group II (100%) than for group I (86%), ($p < 0.001$). There were no differences in survival after 20 or 30 months of CAPD. At 10 months morbidity, defined by avoiding hospitalizations for acute illness, was

Table 2. Comparison of Population Subgroups.

	Group I (BUN < 60 mg/dl)	Group II (BUN > 80 mg/dl)	
Number	37	23	
Sex F/M	27/10	4/19	$p < 0.001$
Race B/W	20/17	6/17	ns
Age (years)	45.2 ± 2.7	48.9 ± 2.1	$p < 0.001$
Months on CAPD	17.5 ± 1.2	17.0 ± 2.1	ns
Total months on dialysis	29 ± 4.8	33 ± 8.0	$p < 0.05$

significantly less in the high BUN (group II) patients, 79% than in the low BUN group (49%) ($p < 0.02$). No difference in this measure of cumulative morbidity was seen at 20 or 30 months.

No association between diabetes mellitus and early mortality in the first 12 months of CAPD could be demonstrated. Despite more males in group II and more female patients in group I, no association between sex and early mortality could be demonstrated. Tables 5 and 6 show data for group I and group II patients combined. No relationship between diabetes mellitus and early morbid events during the first 12 months or between sex and early morbid events was demonstrated.

DISCUSSION

BUN alone is a poor indicator of adequacy of dialysis unless associated with nutritional considerations. A dialysis regimen based on BUN alone could be dangerous. Both in hemodialysis patients and in our CAPD population, we have shown that patients with a low BUN are at significantly greater risk of morbidity and mortality.[2]

The assessment of dialysis adequacy and patient prognosis is a complex interplay of many factors. Total solute clearance (peritoneal residual renal clearance), nutrition, presence of hyperten-

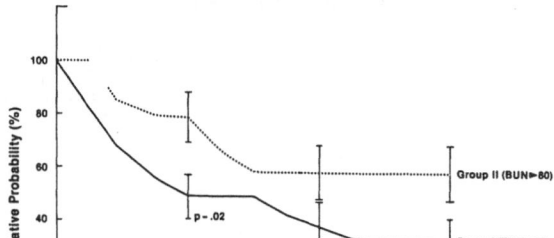

Fig. 2. A comparison of the probability of remaining free of a morbid event in two groups of patients on CAPD.

sion, and other underlying diseases are but a few. As a whole, survival of the CAPD patient group reported here is similar to other series.[4] Our patients were adequately dialyzed. They had initiation of a high protein diet, during CAPD training, which has been shown to be adequate to maintain nitrogen balance.[5]

Several factors may have played a role in the urea nitrogen values of the low BUN group. It is well

Table 3. Causes of ESRD in the BUN Subgroups.

	Group I (%)	Group II (%)	
GN	9 (24)	2 (9)	ns
DM	6 (17)	1 (4)	ns
NS	9 (24)	8 (35)	ns
TIN	2 (5)	4 (17)	ns
PCKD	3 (8)	3 (13)	ns
Other	8 (22)	5 (22)	ns

Table 4. Comparison of Population Subgroups.

	Group I (BUN < 60 mg/dl)	Group II (BUN > 80 mg/dl)	
HCT	$27.6 \pm .88$	27.6 ± 1.4	ns
BP systolic/diastolic	$141 \pm 3.4/83 \pm 1.7$	$139 \pm 4.4/85 \pm 2.2$	ns
Calcium	$9.3 \pm .11$	$9.2 \pm .15$	$p < .01$
Phosphorus	$5.6 \pm .21$	$6.2 \pm .24$	$p < .001$
Episodes of peritonitis/year	$3.2 \pm .59$	$2.1 \pm .48$	$p < .0005$
Hospitalizations/year	$2.2 \pm .033$	$0.9 \pm .20$	$p < .001$

Table 5. Morbid Events in Diabetic Versus Nondiabetic Patients during First 12 Months of CAPD.

	Patients Having Early Morbid Events	Patients Having No Early Morbid Events	
Diabetic	3	4	ns
Nondiabetic	19	34	ns

Table 6. Early Morbid Events in Male Versus Female Patients during First 12 Months of CAPD.

	Patients Having Early Morbid Events	Patients Having No Early Morbid Events	
Male	8	22	ns
Female	14	16	ns

known that in acute peritonitis, increased peritoneal protein losses occur and although these losses may be massive they are usually transient and return to baseline in a few days. Since group I (low BUN) patients had a higher incidence of peritonitis, peritoneal protein loss may partly explain their lower BUN. On the other hand, continued dietary adequacy is difficult to assess. The lower serum phosphorus in the low BUN patients supports lower protein intake in this group, however, sufficient dietary follow-up or nitrogen output measurements were not available for us to determine for certain whether group I patients were simply undernourished. In similarly dialyzed patients, all other parameters being equal, BUN itself directly correlates with protein intake.[5,6] This supports low dietary protein intake as the cause of the low BUN in group I patients.

We have shown then that patients with a low BUN have increased morbidity and mortality early in the course of CAPD. The low BUN in these patients is most likely related to nutritional factors. Similar findings of excess morbidity and mortality have previously been related to low BUN in some hemodialysis populations.[1,7] Our results, therefore, are compatible. These differences in early morbidity and mortality in our CAPD patients could not be correlated with the cause of ESRD or sex. A potential factor could be the disproportionate number of diabetics, although this was not statistically significantly different, in the low BUN group. For this reason, however, we looked more closely for relationships between diabetes mellitus and early mor-

bidity and mortality and although our numbers are small, found none. Later in the course of CAPD, after 10 months, BUN was not a prognostic indicator positively or negatively in our CAPD population.

Early in CAPD a population exists with a low BUN who will fail to thrive. Undernutrition is a likely cause of the low BUN seen in this population. the finding of a low BUN over time in a CAPD patient should stimulate diligent attention to dietary adequacy.

ACKNOWLEGEMENT

Supported in part by Georgetown University Nephritis Research Fund.

REFERENCES

1. Lowrie EG, Laird NM, Parker TF, and Sargent JA: Effect of hemodialysis prescription on patient morbidity. N Engl J Med 305: 1176, 1981
2. Shapiro JI, Argy WP, Rakowski TA, Chester A, Siemsen AS, and Schreiner GE: The unsuitability of BUN as a criterion for prescription dialysis. Trans Am Soc Artif Intern Organs 29: 129, 1983
3. Cutler SJ, and Ederer F: Maximum utilization of the life table method in analyzing survival. J Chronic Dis 8: 699, 1958
4. Williams D, Cattran C, Clayton S, Cole E, Fenton S, Gutman K, Khanna R, Knight S, Manuel A, Roscoe J, Saiphoo C, Tattersall S, Vas S, and Oreopoulos D:

CAPD in Toronto. The first five years. Abst Am Soc Nephrol 16: 125A, 1983

5. Blumenkrantz MJ:Studies of protein and nitrogen metabolism during continuous ambulatory peritoneal dialysis. In Gahl GM, Kessel M, and Nolph KD (Eds), Advances in peritoneal dialysis: Proceedings of the 2nd international symposium on peritoneal dialysis. Amsterdam: Excerpta Medica, 1981, p 391

6. Nolph KD, Sorkin MJ, Prowant B, and Moore H: Protein intake can be estimated from BUN with CAPD. In Gahl GM, Kessel M, and Nolph KD (Eds), Advances in peritoneal dialysis: Proceedings of the 2nd international symposium on peritoneal dialysis. Amsterdam: Excerpta Medica 1981, p 405

7. Degoulet P, Legrain M, Reach I, Aime F, Devries C, Rojas P, and Jacobs C: Mortality risk factors in patients treated with chronic hemodialysis. Nephron 31: 103, 1982

Z.J. Twardowski, R. Khanna, L.M. Burrows, L.M. Schmidt,
L.P. Ryan, and R.J. Satalowich

73

Two Years Experience with High Volume Low Frequency CAPD

SUMMARY

Thirty-nine stable CAPD patients were challenged with 3 L volume exchanges. Long term tolerance to this high volume dialysis was observed in 30% of patients. Taller and heavier patients tolerated large volumes better. Dialysate flow increased 13 to 50% when patients were switched from low to high volume dialysis.

After an initial decrease, BUN and serum creatinine levels later rose, concomitantly with a gradual decline in residual renal function. Hematocrit increased significantly on high volume dialysis, which might indicate better control of uremia.

Unexpectedly, the peritonitis rate tended to be higher in high volume dialysis patients compared to our remaining low volume population, probably related to an unusually high incidence of catheter tunnel infections in the former group.

It is concluded that high volume dialysis is a convenient and effective method for some CAPD patients, and increases the flexibility of the recommended dialysis schedule.

INTRODUCTION

During continuous ambulatory peritoneal dialysis (CAPD), similar daily peritoneal clearances are achieved with higher volume exchanges performed less frequently compared to more frequent, lower volume exchanges, provided that dialysate flow re-

---

From the Division of Nephrology, Department of Medicine, University of Missouri, and Dialysis Clinics, Inc., Columbia, Missouri.

mains the same, i.e., the total drainage volume per day is similar with both methods.[1] Larger volume exchanges yield higher daily clearances of small and middle molecules with essentially unchanged protein losses compared to lower volume exchanges.[1]

Preliminary results of CAPD, using three 2.5 L exchanges/day were first reported at the Second International Symposium on Peritoneal Dialysis in Berlin in 1981.[2] More than 80% of patients in Poland[2,3] tolerated these 2.5 L exchanges during 1 to 13 months of CAPD. Short term experience at the University of Missouri indicated that up to 50% of the patients could tolerate 3 L volumes.[4] The major objective determinant of high volume tolerance was adequate pulmonary function,[4] but the ultimate criterion was the patient's subjective assessment.[5] Review of long term tolerance of high volume dialysis, complications, blood chemistries, and rates of peritonitis are the subjects of the present study.

MATERIAL AND METHODS

Patients

At the University of Missouri-Columbia, between October 1981 and April 1984, 110 patients were treated by CAPD. The patients who tolerated 2 L volume exchanges during CAPD without any discomfort were offered the option of using 3 L volume exchanges.

High Volume Exchange Implementation

During a regular clinic visit, after obtaining informed consent, the patients were infused with 3 L of dialysis fluid. On the initial challenge if they felt

Table 1. Symptoms and Signs in Patients Challenged with 3 L Volume.

Group	Dyspnea	Discomfort	Leak	Hernia	Body Image	Total
I Intolerant	3	9	1		2	15
II Short-Term Tolerant		7	2	1		10
III Long-Term Tolerant						14
Total	3	15	3	1	2	39

little or no discomfort they were maintained on 3 L volume exchanges for a trial period of one week. Patients were advised to continue 3 L exchanges indefinitely if the one week trial with use of this volume was uneventful.

Treatment of Complications

Peritonitis was treated according to our established protocol without changing the volume of exchanges.[5] The amount of antibiotics added to 3 L volume of peritoneal dialysis solution was adjusted to maintain essentially the same concentration as for 2 L volume with minor deviations to avoid cumbersome calculation. Dialysate leaks and hernias were treated surgically but high volume exchanges were discontinued after surgical operation.

RESULTS

Tolerance

Of the 110 patients, 39 were challenged with a 3 L volume exchange (Table 1). Of the 39 patients challenged with 3 L volume 15 were intolerant to this high volume because of discomfort, dyspnea, dialysate leak, or concern for change of body image due to increased abdominal girth. Ten patients tolerated 3 L volume for more than a week but eventually discontinued the use of this high volume because of discomfort, leak, or hernia. Fourteen patients have never returned to low volume exchanges, two were transplanted, two died, and ten were still using 3 L volume exchanges at the end of April 1984. Ten patients used three exchanges and four patients used four exchanges/day.

Technique survival of patients while on high volume exchanges computed by life table analysis is shown in Figure 1. Long-term tolerance to high volume is seen in almost 30 percent of patients who were challenged with the high volume exchanges.

In Table 2 are presented the height, weight, and body surface area of the 39 patients who were challenged with 3 L volume exchanges. The patients

were divided into tolerant and intolerant groups. Taller and heavier patients appeared to tolerate high volume dialysis better. The differences are significant (all $p = 0.05$) between intolerant and long term tolerant patients.

Blood Chemistries

Figure 2 shows the serial mean values of BUN, serum creatinine, hematocrit, and serum albumin as a percent of the last value obtained before 3 L volume implementation in 19 patients. Body weight and urine output are also shown in Figure 2. There was a tendency for hematocrit to rise during high volume dialysis. Both creatinine and BUN after an initial fall, increased concomitant with gradual decline in urine output with time on dialysis. Serum albumin did not change. The mean body weight for the group increased. Dialysate flow increased 13 to 50% in all patients.

Peritonitis

Twenty-four patients who were on 3 L volume exchanges for more than a week experienced 25 peritonitis episodes during 195 months of treatment, for a peritonitis rate of one episode/7.8 patient-

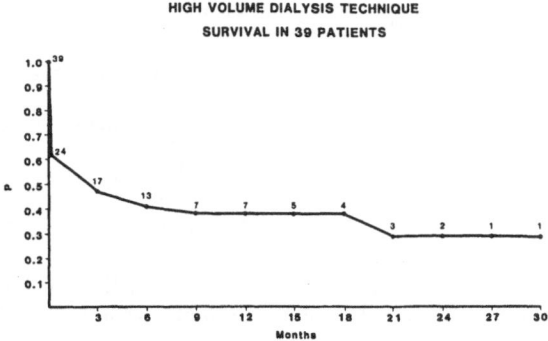

Fig. 1. High volume dialysis technique survival in 39 patients. Number of patients still under treatment are given at each period.

Table 2. Height, Weight, and Body Surface Area (BSA) in Relation to Tolerance of 3 L Volume.

Group	N	Height	Weight	BSA
I Intolerant	9	166 ± 12	70 ± 12	1.79 ± 0.17
II Short-Term Tolerant	9	170 ± 11	86 ± 17	1.99 ± 0.20
III Long-Term Tolerant	10	174 ± 11	85 ± 16	1.99 ± 0.20

Table 3. Peritonitis.

	Patients on 2 L Exchanges October 1981– April 1984	Patients on 2 L Exchanges Prior to 3 L Implementation	Patients on 3 L Exchanges For More Than a Week
Population	86	24	24
Treatment Time (Months)	1140	359	194
Peritonitis Episodes	78	27	25
Patient Months Per Episode	14.6	13.3	7.8

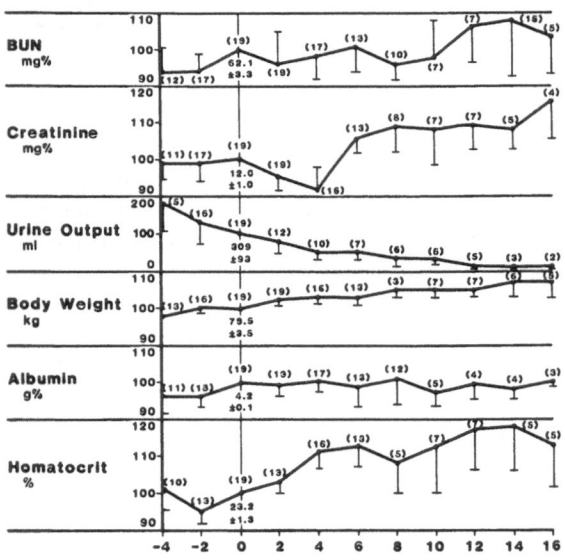

Fig. 2. Mean percentages (+ or − SEM) of last value before 3 L volume implementation for 19 patients who were on high volume dialysis for more than 2 months. Numbers in parentheses = N. Actual means ± SEM of 100% values are also shown at time 0.

months. Fifteen episodes occurred in three patients due to catheter tunnel infection. The same 24 patients had 27 peritonitis episodes during the preceeding 359 months of 2 L volume exchanges, for a peritonitis rate of one episode/13.3 patient-months. In the period between October 1981 and April 1984 in 86 patients who were on 2 L volume there were 78 peritonitis episodes during 1140 months of treatment, i.e., one peritonitis episode/14.6 patient-months (Table 3).

DISCUSSION

Our original intention of high volume implementation was to decrease the number of daily exchanges from four to three. Although in the majority of patients the exchange frequency was reduced to three during high volume dialysis, four patients retained four exchanges/day because of symptoms and signs of underdialysis due to gradually decreasing residual renal function. Six such patients were offered an option of five daily exchanges of 2 L volume or four exchanges of 3 L volume. Four of these patients chose four high volume daily exchanges, one switched to hemodialysis, and one is contemplating CCPD while on five exchanges of 2 L volume.

Dialysate flow increased 13 to 50% in all patients. Albumin levels did not change (Fig. 2) on high

Table 4.   High Volume Exchange.

Advantages	Disadvantages
Lower Exchange Number 　↑ Schedule Flexibility 　↓ Connections 　　↓ Risk of Contamination 　↓ Cost Same Exchange Number 　↑ Dialysate Flow 　↑ Small Solute Mass 　　Transfer	↑ Discomfort ↓ Appetite ↑ Intraabdominal Pressure ↓ Pulmonary Functions ↓ Cardiac Performance ↑ Abdominal Girth ↑ Risk of Leakage ↑ Risk of Hernias ↑ Risk of Back Pain?

volume dialysis, indicating satisfactory protein balance. After the initial decrease, BUN and serum creatinine levels rose later probably due to the gradual decline of residual renal function. Increased body weight, which partly might be related to increased muscle mass may also contribute to the rise in serum creatinine (Fig. 2).

An interesting finding was the significant increase in the hematocrit during the high volume dialysis. This increase might be partly related to the increased amount of dialysis with better removal of inhibitory substances claimed to be responsible for bone marrow suppression in uremia.[6] Hypoxemia due to compromised pulmonary functions, certainly could be an additional factor causing the observed change. However, the latter explanation seems less likely as the patients tolerant to high volume dialysis did not show significant decrease in vital capacity with intraperitoneal fluid volume up to 5 L.[5] Further studies are needed to explain this phenomenon.

The peritonitis rate in our patients on high volume dialysis was higher compared to their rate during their 2 L exchange period. This rate was also higher compared to the other patients who during the same period were on 2 L volume exchanges. This observation is not only surprising but is in contrast to the findings of Kim et al.[7] who found a significantly lower rate of peritonitis in patients on 3 L compared to the 2 L volumes patients. The higher rate of peritonitis in our patients was associated with an unusually high incidence of catheter tunnel infections negating the beneficial effect of reduced chances of external contamination due to the lower number of connection/disconnection procedures during higher volume lower frequency exchanges. This high rate of peritonitis episodes associated with catheter tunnel infections may explain the difference between our findings and that of Kim and associates.[7]

Table 4 summarizes the advantages and disadvantages of high volume dialysis. Only the patients can judge whether advantages or disadvantages prevail and which volume and schedule they prefer for routine dialysis.

Dialysis solutions in 2.5 L volume bags are commercially not available in the U.S.A. In view of the tolerance of 2.5 L volume by a high percentage of patients,[3] marketing a dialysis solution containing 2.5 L is highly desirable.

REFERENCES

1. Twardowski ZJ, Nolph KD, Prowant BF, and Moore HL: Efficiency of high volume, low frequency continuous ambulatory peritoneal dialysis. Trans Am Soc Artif Intern Organs 29: 53, 1981
2. Twardowski ZJ, Janicka L, Majdan M, Bochenska-Nowacka E, and Pawlin W: Efficiency of continuous ambulatory peritoneal dialysis with three 2.5 liter exchanges per day. In Gahl GM, Kessel M, and Nolph KD (Eds), Advances in peritoneal dialysis: Proceedings of the 2nd international symposium on peritoneal dialysis. Amsterdam, Excerpta Medica, 1981, p 111
3. Twardowski ZJ, and Janicka L: Three exchanges with a 2.5 liter volume for continuous ambulatory peritoneal dialysis. Kidney Int 20: 281, 1981
4. Twardowski ZJ, Prowant BF, Nolph KD, Martinez AJ, and Lampton LM. High volume, low frequency continuous ambulatory peritoneal dialysis. Kidney Int 23:64, 1983
5. Twardowski ZJ, and Nolph KD: Optimal exchange volume for continuous ambulatory peritoneal dialysis (CAPD) (Editorial review). Peritoneal Dial Bull 2: 154, 1982
6. Lamperi S, Carozzi S, and Icardi A: Hematological aspects of peritoneal dialysis. In La Greca G, Biasoli S, and Ronco C (Eds), Peritoneal dialysis: Proceedings of 1st international course on peritoneal dialysis. Milano: Wichtig Editore, 1982, p 431
7. Kim D, Khanna R, Wu D, Vas S, and Oreopoulos DG: Continuous ambulatory peritoneal dialysis with three 3 L exchanges per day. Peritoneal Dial Bull 4: S32, 1984

D. Kim, R. Khanna, G. Wu, P. Fountas, M. Druck,
and D.G. Oreopoulos

74

Successful Use of CAPD in Refractory Heart Failure

SUMMARY

Four patients with end-stage heart failure, massive ascites refractory to medical intervention, and a variable degree of renal failure were treated successfully with CAPD for 8 to 24 months. The New York Heart Association functional class improved in all four. In two patients, who presented initially with signs and symptoms mainly of right-sided heart failure, ejection fraction improved. Each day dialysis achieved a significant degree of ultrafiltration and a negative sodium balance. We propose that CAPD is an alternative therapeutic modality in patients with severe heart failure refractory to conventional medical treatment.

INTRODUCTION

The advent of potent diuretics and preload and afterload reducing agents has had a major impact in the treatment of refractory congestive heart failure. Recently, captopril, an angiotensin-converting enzyme inhibitor, has been used with major benefit in some patients.[1] However, some patients still do not respond to these treatments and their management presents a major therapeutic challenge. Furthermore, overzealous therapy with diuretics may lead to intravascular volume depletion resulting in hypotension, azotemia, and electrolyte disturbances, which further complicate management.

In the past, intermittent peritoneal dialysis (IPD) or hemodialysis (HD) has been used to remove

From the Divisions of Nephrology and Cardiology, Toronto Western Hospital and the Department of Medicine, University of Toronto.

fluid from patients with intractable edema due to heart failure.[2-7] But the benefit is only transient and fluid accumulates again, requiring repeated sessions of acute dialysis. However, hypotension is a frequent complication during either form of acute dialysis especially in hemodynamically unstable patients due to rapid removal of large amounts of fluid from the intravascular space.

Continuous ambulatory peritoneal dialysis (CAPD), whose main characteristic is the slow continuous removal of sodium and water, offers obvious advantages in patients with intractable heart failure.

This paper describes our experience with four patients with intractable heart failure who have been treated with CAPD for 8 to 24 months.

PATIENTS AND METHODS

Tables 1 and 2 show the clinical features of these four patients. All had severe underlying cardiac pathology with left ventricular ejection fractions ranging from 0.19 to 0.36. In addition, each patient had a variable degree of renal failure.

At the initial presentation (Table 2) two patients were New York Heart Association (NYHA) functional class IV, and the other two were class III. All had significant electrolyte disturbances. Their response to therapy is shown in Figure 1. Patients #3 and #4 had signs and symptoms consistent with predominant right ventricular failure. All had massive ascites refractory to medical intervention.

In patients #1 and #2, assessment of the efficacy of various preload and afterload reducing agents with Swan-Ganz catheterization was carried out. Patient #1 was treated with hydralazine, prazosine, nitrates (Isordil) and large doses of furosemide

Table 1. Clinical Profile.

	Patient #1	Patient #2	Patient #3	Patient #4
Age	50	28	56	59
Sex	Male	Male	Male	Male
Cardiac Dx	Ischemic heart disease	Aortic insufficiency	Idiopathic congestive cardiomyopathy	Idiopathic congestive cardiomyopathy
Renal dx	Nephrosclerosis	Goodpasture's syndrome	unknown	Diabetic nephropathy

and spironolactone without improvement (Table 2). Patient #2, who had no urine output, did not improve on optimal medical therapy. Patients #3 and #4 did not respond to maximum doses of furosemide in combination with spironolactone. Both could not tolerate afterload reducing agents due to symptomatic hypotension. We did not try captopril in these patients because it was not available at the beginning of our study.

Peritoneal dialysis was the initial mode of dialysis rather than HD in three of four patients (patients #1, #3, #4) because of very unstable cardiovascular status and severe ascites. Patient #4 was also diabetic. Patient #2 had been on HD for 7 years before he developed recurrent episodes of congestive heart failure and ascites, and was transferred to the PD service.

Initially acute intermittent peritoneal dialysis (IPD) was used to remove fluid and to correct electrolyte imbalances. Patient #3 had several sessions of IPD over a period of one month during which he lost 50 kg. To avoid hypotension due to excessive ascitic fluid removal, it was removed at a rate of 500 ml during each hourly exchange, emptying the abdomen completely over several days. Subsequently, all four patients were started on CAPD. Patient one, who had only a moderate degree of renal failure, was dialysed with 1 L exchanges rather than the conventional 2 L regimen.

Three of four patients achieved a significant degree of ultrafiltration and sodium removal through peritoneal dialysis. Patient #4 did not require large ultrafiltration by PD because of an adequate urinary excretion of sodium and water once he became stable on CAPD (Table 3). Although all patients had significant ascites before PD was started, the average daily protein loss through CAPD (11.4 g) was only slightly higher than the average value, 8–10 g/24 hours, seen in other CAPD patients.[11]

The left ventricular ejection fraction (LVEF) was measured by radionuclide angiography (RNA),

when patients became stable after several sessions of acute peritoneal dialysis and when they were stable on CAPD 6 to 12 months later (Fig. 2). In two of the four patients (#3, #4), who manifested signs and symptoms of predominant right ventricular failure, LVEF increased significantly after 8 and 9 months on CAPD, respectively. (Standard error of ejection fraction measured by RNA at our lab is about 5%, when compared to that measured by cardiac catheterization.)

All the patients described in this paper had remarkable clinical improvement in terms of general well being and relief from symptoms of CHF. New York Heart Association functional class improved in all of them (Fig. 1). Patient #1 no longer experienced orthopnea or paroxysmal nocturnal dyspnea and, while on vacation, was able to swim. However, after being on CAPD for one and one-half years, he suffered a severe decline in renal function to total anuria. He was not able to tolerate a dialysis volume greater than 1 L and hence suffered from underdialysis (hemodialysis was not feasible because of cardiovascular instability). He died of renal failure. Patients #2 and #3 are stable on CAPD after 8 and 24 months, respectively; each has a minimal degree of dyspnea on exertion. Patient #4 has had recurrent episodes of peritonitis which have impaired ultrafiltration; in addition to CAPD he requires large doses of furosemide to control his heart and renal failure.

DISCUSSION

Schneison et al.[2] first described the treatment of intractable cardiac edema by continuous peritoneal irrigation 34 years ago. Since then several authors [2-4] have reported the use of acute peritoneal dialysis to treat refractory CHF that is not amenable to conventional medical therapy. Peritoneal dialysis has also been used to treat CHF, which follows of acute myocardial infarction, or to prepare patients for cardiac surgery.[5-7] Hemodynamic studies in these pa-

Table 2. Clinical Features on Admission.

NYHA Functional Class	Patient #1	Patient #2	Patient #3	Patient #4
	IV	IV	III	III
Medications on Admission	Digoxin 0.125 mg OD	Digoxin 0.125 mg 4×/wk	Digoxin 0.125 mg 3×/wk	Digoxin 0.125 mg 3×/wk
	Hydralazine 50 mg qid	Hydralazine 50 mg qid	Isordil 30 mg qid	Lasix 500 mg OD
	Minipress 5 mg qid	Isordil 15 mg qid	Aldactone 25 mg tid	Aldactone 25 mg tid
	Isordil 15 mg qid	Nitropaste 2 mg qid		
	Lasix 250 mg OD			
	Aldactone 25 mg tid			
Supine B.P. (mm Hg)	100/60	150/100	85/56	100/50
Ascites	marked	marked	marked	marked
Serum				
Na	129	132	125	130
K	3.7	3.7	3.0	3.2
Cl	80	88	82	86
HCO$_3$ (meq/l)	31	27	30	28
Serum Creatinine (mg/dl)	3.9	7.5	7.5	4.4
BUN (mg/dl)	157	90	75	74
Weight Loss Following IPD	5.1 kg	8.3 kg	50 kg	15 kg
RNA Findings	LVEF = 0.19. Enlarged LV with generalized hypokinesis; inferior & anterior akinesis.	LVEF = 0.36. Severe global LV hypokinesis; RV enlargement.	LVEF = 0.19. Biventricular enlargement with global hypokinesis.	LVEF = 0.24. Biventricular enlargement with global hypokinesis.

tients show a decrease in venous pressure and blood volume. Cairns et al.[8] found that, after acute PD, the cardiac index (CI) rose in six of eight patients; all six entered a period of remission. On the other hand, Mailloux, et al.[3] found that cardiac output increased in only one of five patients.

Invariably acute intermittent PD ameliorates the symptoms of CHF but the improvement is temporary and the long-term results disappointing.[9] Edema and ascites return between dialyses, and the interval between dialyses progressively shortens. Other drawbacks of IPD in these patients include hypotension due to rapid intravascular-volume depletion, hyperglycemia due to large glucose load, and aggravation of pulmonary edema due to interdialytic weight gain. Hemodialysis also is particularly hazardous in these patients. The presence of an AV fistula can further stress an already compromised cardiac function. Development of hypotension and pulmonary edema, for the same reasons as IPD, is a

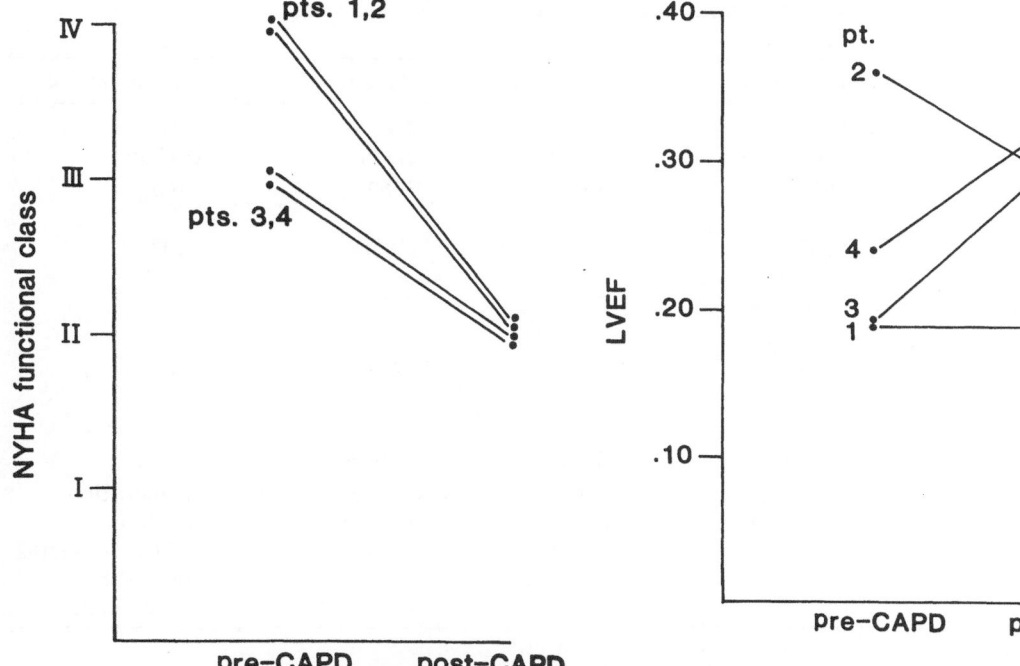

Fig. 1.   NY Heart Association functional class.

Fig. 2.   Left ventricular ejection fraction by radio-nuclide angiography.

further drawback to hemodialysis. CAPD, with its characteristics, gradual removal of sodium and water, might prevent these complications and hence offer better therapy. CAPD has an added advantage of improving hematocrit, which especially benefits these patients. Robson et al.[10] employed CAPD in three patients with refractory CHF, but their results were discouraging because of frequent peritonitis. Although their stort-term results were satisfactory, they had to discontinue CAPD at 3, 5, and 6 months. Each patient died within 2 weeks of stopping dialysis. Our patients maintained their initial clinical improvement over a long follow-up period. The high degree of ultrafiltration and the net sodium balance allowed our patients to eat a more liberal diet. Our initial concern about excessive protein loss through CAPD in these patients with massive ascites proved groundless.[11]

The clinical improvement observed with our patients could be due to two factors. First, continuous removal of fluid, by itself, could have improved the patients' overall functional status without improvement in cardiac function. Secondly, the improvement in LVEF as observed in two of our patients may have played some role. The improvement in LVEF after being on CAPD for 6 to 12 months might be explained in three ways: First, because the left and right ventricles share a common septum, chronic right ventricular overload, which displaces the septum into the left ventricular wall, may interfere with left ventricular filling and emptying.[12] Second, the shape of the left ventricular diastolic pressure–volume curve to sustain volume overload can be significantly modified by the pericardium. The pericardium is more resistant than the myocardium to stretch. Thus the dilated heart is restrained by the pericardium.[13] Third, there is a theoretical possibility that the left ventricles of these patients might be operating on the down-slope portion of Starling's curve. Thus, CAPD, by continuously reducing preload on a long-term basis, may facilitate left ventricular emptying by modifying these factors. Although all our patients had concomitant moderate to severe renal failure, some patients with minimal renal impairment may benefit from CAPD simply for continuous fluid removal.

In summary, we have presented four patients with refractory heart failure who were successfully treated with CAPD for 1 to 2 years. CAPD slowly and continuously removes sodium and water. Thus CAPD prevents a rapid shift of fluid across body compartments and a large interdialytic weight gain

Table 3. CAPD Schedule, Ultrafiltration, Sodium Balance, and Protein Loss thru CAPD, and Clinical Outcome.

	Patient #1	Patient #2	Patient #3	Patient #4
Daily CAPD Schedule	1 L × 4 exchanges	2 L × 4 exchanges	2 L × 4 exchanges	2 L × 3 exchanges
Daily ultrafiltration	1690	2240	3060	140
urine output (ml/day)	900	0	0	1200
Total Na$^+$ removal (PD + urine) (mEq/day)	165	144	294	88
Protein loss (PD + urine) (g/day)	14.6	11.2	10.6	9.2
Outcome	died after 18 months	stable on CAPD for 2 years	stable on CAPD for 10 months	malnutrition stable on IPD × 6 months, on CAPD × 10 months

as seen with IPD or HD. We believe that CAPD will be recognized as an adjunct to the medical treatment of refractory congestive heart failure.

ACKNOWLEDGMENT

This work was supported by the Peritoneal Research Fund of the Toronto Western Hospital.

REFERENCES

1. Dzau VJ, Colucci WS, Williams GH, Curfman G, Meggs L, and Hollenberg NK: Sustained effectiveness of converting enzyme inhibition in patients with severe congestive heart failure. N Engl J Med 25: 1373, 1980
2. Schneison SJ: Continuous peritoneal irrigation in the treatment of intractable edema of cardiac origin. Am J Med Sci 218: 76, 1949
3. Mailloux LU, Swartz CD, Onesti G, Heider C, Ramirez O, and Brest AN: Peritoneal dialysis for refractory congestive heart failure. JAMA 199: 873, 1967
4. Raja RM, Krasnoff SO, Moros JH, Kramer MS, and Rosenbaum JL: Repeated peritoneal dialysis in treatment of heart failure. JAMA 213: 2268, 1970
5. Chopra MP, Galati RB, Portal RW, and Aber CP: Peritoneal dialysis for pulmonary edema after acute myocardial infarction. Br Med J 3: 77, 1970
6. Malach M: Peritoneal dialysis for intractable heart failure in acute myocardial infarction. Am J Cardiol 29: 61, 1972
7. Lund HG, and Hughes RK: Peritoneal dialysis before cardiac surgery. Thorac Surg 4: 470, 1967
8. Cairns KB, Porter GA, Kloster FE, Bristow JD, and Griswold HE: Clinical and hemodynamic results of peritoneal dialysis for severe cardiac failure. Am Heart J 76: 227, 1968
9. Shapira J, Lang R, Jutrin I, Robson M, and Ravid M: Peritoneal dialysis in refractory congestive heart failure. Intermittent peritoneal dialysis. Peritoneal Dial Bull 3: 130, 1983
10. Robson M, Biro A, Knobel B, Schai G, and Ravid M: Peritoneal dialysis in refractory congestive heart failure. II. Continuous ambulatory peritoneal dialysis. Peritoneal Dial Bull 3: 133, 1983
11. Katirtzoglou A, Oreopoulos DG, Husdan H, Leung M, Ogilvie R, and Dombros N: Reappraisal of protein losses in patients undergoing continuous ambulatory peritoneal dialysis. Nephron 26: 230, 1980
12. Ludbrook PA, Byrne JD, and McNight RC: Influence of right ventricular hemodynamics on left ventricular diastolic pressure–volume relations in man. Circulation 59: 21, 1979
13. Bhargava V, Shabetal R, Ross JJ, Shirato K, Parelec RS, and Mason PA: Influence of the pericardium on left ventricular diastolic pressure–volume curves in dogs with sustained volume overload. Am Heart J 6: 995, 1983

Nutritional, Metabolic, and Physiological Effects

J.D. Kopple

75

Nutritional Requirements with CAPD

SUMMARY

Based on balance studies and other investigations, nutrient allowances are recommended for adult patients undergoing CAPD. The daily protein allowance should be 1.2 to 1.3 g/kg/day. Dietary carbohydrates should be complex predominantly and should provide about 35% of ingested calories, the remainder provided by dietary fat, preferably with a polyunsaturated : saturated fatty acid ratio of unity. Energy intake should be 35 to 42 kcal/kg/day. Mineral requirements in CAPD include phosphorus restriction, calcium supplementation and a liberal sodium and water intake. Water soluble vitamins and vitamin D should be supplemented, but vitamins A and E should not.

INTRODUCTION

Despite much interest in the nutritional status and requirements of patients undergoing CAPD, many of these patients continue to suffer from wasting, malnutrition, or impaired growth. On the one hand, adults frequently gain weight and body fat during CAPD.[1] In children undergoing CAPD, the Z-scores for height and weight, although low initially, do not decrease further.[2] (The Z-score is a patient's anthropometric measurement expressed in terms of the number of standard deviations above or below the mean normal value.) Indeed, in prepubertal children undergoing CAPD, the Z-scores for mid-arm

---

From the Division of Nephrology and Hypertension, Department of Medicine, Harbor-UCLA Medical Center, Los Angeles, California.

muscle circumference, when compared to normal children of the same height-age, may increase.[2]

On the other hand, depletion of somatic and visceral proteins may be found in CAPD patients,[1-5] and vitamin and mineral depletion or mineral excess may occur (see below). Serum total protein, albumin, transferrin, and C3 are, on average, subnormal, but usually do not decrease further during treatment.[1] In one report, extravascular albumin and total exchangeable albumin were reduced in CAPD patients,[3] while in another study, body albumin pools were normal.[6] In a large series of adult CAPD patients, there was no increase in arm muscle circumference.[7] Williams et al.[4] monitored total body potassium and nitrogen in patients undergoing CAPD: total body potassium remained unchanged or increased, but total body nitrogen fell significantly. Others reported a reduction in total body potassium in CAPD patients who sustained multiple episodes of peritonitis.[5] Lindholm and Bergström[8] performed muscle biopsies in 24 CAPD patients and described increased muscle intracellular and extracellular water and increased muscle potassium when expressed per unit of fat free solids but not when expressed per liter of intracellular water.

PREVIOUS RESEARCH CONCERNING DIETARY REQUIREMENTS IN ADULT CAPD PATIENTS

Protein

Blumenkrantz et al.[9] assessed nutritional requirements in adults undergoing CAPD by studying protein and mineral balances in eight clinically stable men. Patients were evaluated in a clinical research center during 13 metabolic balance studies of 14–33 days duration. Age was 43.8 ± 3.4 (SEM) years, and duration of treatment with all types of maintenance dialysis was 49.3 ± 14 months. The glomerular filtration rate was 1.0–3.0 ml/min in three patients; the others were anuric. Total urea clearance from dialysate and urine combined was 10.7 ± 0.3 L/day. Body weight was 77.9 ± 2.2 kg (relative body weight, 104 ± 3.9%). They were fed diets that provided an average of 0.98 g protein/kg/day or 1.44 g protein/kg/day. Over 50% of the protein was of high biological value. Five patients received both diets; two were fed the lower protein diet first. No patient was fed the same diet twice. Total energy intake (diet plus dialysis solution) was 41.3 ± 1.9 and 42.1 ± 1.2 kcal/kg/day with the low and high protein diets, respectively. Patients were given supplemental multivitamins and, to control serum phosphorus levels, varying amounts of aluminum hydroxide. Most patients received five dialysate exchanges per day; those with more residual renal function received less. Two liter bags (Dianeal®, Travenol Laboratories, Deerfield, IL) were used for each exchange.

The balance studies for nitrogen and minerals are shown in Table 1 and Figure 1. The nitrogen and mineral balance data are calculated for the entire 14–33 days of study in each patient but are not adjusted for unmeasured losses from skin, sweat, blood sampling, hair and nail growth, and (for nitrogen balances) losses from respiration and flatus. The nitrogen balances are corrected for changes in body urea nitrogen and were +0.35 ± 0.83 g/day with the low protein diet and +2.94 ± 0.54 g/day with the 1.44 g/kg/day protein intake. These values did not differ significantly ($p = 0.06$ by paired t test among the five patients fed both diets), but only the high protein diet was significantly different from zero. If nitrogen balances are adjusted by about 1.0 g/day for the unmeasured losses through skin, respiration, flatus, and blood sampling,[10] balances still would be not different from zero with the 1.0 g/kg protein diet, but would remain significantly positive with the higher protein intake. There was a curvilinear relationship between dietary protein intake and nitrogen balance in the 13 studies (Fig. 1). Nitrogen balance rose as protein intake increased until protein intake was 1.09 g/kg/day. At this level, balance was positive. As dietary protein increased above this level, there was little or no further increment in nitrogen balance.

The results of other workers, in general, are consistent with these data. Giordano et al.[11] re-

Table 1. Nitrogen and Mineral Balances and Serum Chemistries in Eight Patients Undergoing CAPD.[a]

Balances

	0.98 g/kg/day					1.44 g/kg/day				
	Diet	Dialysate[b]	Urine[c]	Feces	Balance	Diet	Dialysate[b]	Urine[c]	Feces	Balance
Nitrogen g/day	12.06 ± 0.51(7)[d]	−9.80 ± 0.65	0.97–1.72	1.61 ± 0.09	+0.35 ± 0.83	18.32 ± 0.27(6)[h]	−12.67 ± 0.93	2.61	1.80 ± 0.08[f]	+2.94 ± 0.54[c,g]
Potassium mEq/day	64 ± 4.1(7)	−36.6 ± 2.6	2.7–11.6	16.9 ± 1.1	+6.8 ± 4.6	84.1 ± 5.0(6)[a]	−44.5 ± 3.5	8.7	20.4 ± 2.1	+17.8 ± 4.0
Phosphorus mg/day	1047 ± 37(7)	−324 ± 23	16–103	468 ± 53	+227 ± 77	1915 ± 117(6)[a]	−332 ± 36	223	839 ± 67[a]	+708 ± 152
Calcium mg/day	769 ± 74(6)	+100 ± 30	2–17	753 ± 110	+112 ± 51	1356 ± 108(6)[h]	+67 ± 18	33	1220 ± 213	+198 ± 194[e,g]
Magnesium mg/day	259 ± 25(6)	−48 ± 10	12–31	158 ± 23	+46 ± 10	320 ± 11(6)[a]	−44 ± 12	40	203 ± 30	+66 ± 28[f]

Serum Chemistries

	0.98 g/kg/day	1.44 g/kg/day
Urea Nitrogen mg/dl	67 ± 5.5	91 ± 7.0
Potassium mEq/l	4.0 ± 0.19	4.6 ± 0.31
Phosphorus mg/dl	4.5 ± 0.27	4.8 ± 0.43
Magnesium mg/dl	3.1 ± 0.10	3.1 ± 0.15
Calcium mg/dl	8.9 ± 0.46	9.2 ± 0.26

[a] Data represent mean ± standard error of data collected during the 14–33 days of study. Adapted from reference 9.
[b] Minus sign indicates net loss from patient into dialysate; positive sign indicates net uptake from dialysate into patient.
[c] Indicates values in the three patients studied with the 0.98 g/protein/kg/day diet and the one patient with the 1.44 g/protein/kg/day diet who had urine output.
[d] Parentheses indicate the number of men studied with each diet; no patient was studied twice with the same diet.
[e] Nitrogen balance is adjusted for changes in body urea nitrogen content but not for losses from cutaneous structures, respiration, flatus or blood drawing.
Significantly different from corresponding values obtained with the 0.98 g/kg/day protein diet: [f] $p < 0.05$, [g] $p < 0.01$, [h] $p < 0.001$. Statistics were calculated either by nonpaired t tests of all the data or by paired t tests of values from the five patients studied with both diets.
One patient received 0.25 μg/day of 1,25-dihydroxycholecalciferol during the last 12 days of study.

ported neutral or positive nitrogen balance in seven of eight CAPD patients who were fed about 1.2 g protein/kg/day. Gahl et al.[12] reported neutral or positive nitrogen balance in five CAPD patients ingesting diets that provided 0.71–0.96 g protein/kg/day. Interpretation of these data is difficult, however, because the subjects were studied as outpatients and feces were not collected. If our values for fecal nitrogen output and unmeasured losses are applied to their data, then two of their patients probably would be in negative nitrogen balance. Lindholm et al.[13] carried out short term (10–14 day) balance studies in ten patients undergoing CAPD who were fed diets containing 0.76–2.07 g protein/kg/day. Total energy intake was 120–122 kJ/kg/day. Nitrogen balance, adjusted for unmeasured losses, was positive in all. However, nitrogen balance correlated positively with both protein intake and energy intake in these patients. Mihindukulasuriya et al.[14] studied six CAPD patients who underwent nitrogen balances for two 4-day periods following nine days of equilibration on the same diet, seven at home and two during the study. Protein intake varied from 1.1–1.7 g/kg/day. Nitrogen balance was negative in one patient fed about 1.2 g protein/kg/day; if nitrogen balance is adjusted for unmeasured losses, balance would probably be catalogued as negative in one other patient fed about 1.2 g protein/kg/day.

The serum urea nitrogen levels with the diets providing 0.98 and 1.44 g protein/kg/day were not greater than predialysis values commonly found in maintenance hemodialysis patients (Table 1). The serum urea nitrogen, obtained serially during the entire 14–33 day period of study with each diet, averaged 67 ± 5.5 and 91 ± 7.0 mg/dl with the low and high protein diets, respectively.

The anthropometric data also indicated that patients were anabolic with the diet providing 1.44 g protein/kg/day. Body weight increased in all, mid-arm muscle circumference increased in five of six, and the sum of the triceps and subscapular skinfold thickness increased in four of six patients. In contrast, with the 0.98 g protein/kg/day diet, anthropometric measurements did not improve. Serum total protein, albumin, and transferrin concentrations did not change with either diet.

These observations suggest that the protein intake that will promote neutral or positive nitrogen balance in most clinically stable CAPD patients is about 1.1–1.2 g/kg/day. To allow for individual variability, 1.2–1.3 g protein/kg/day is considered safe. For malnourished clinically stable CAPD patients, there may be value in offering 1.5 g protein/kg/day.

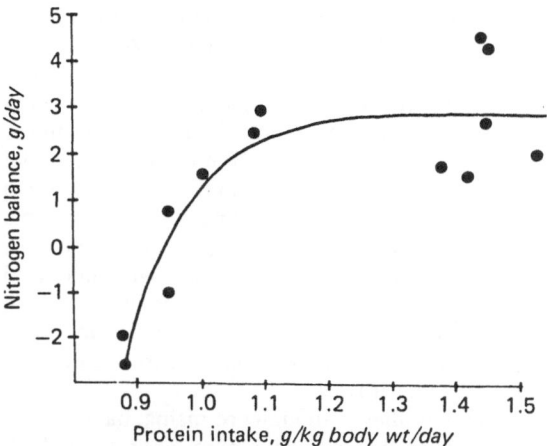

Fig. 1. Relationship between protein intake and nitrogen balance during 13 studies in eight men undergoing CAPD. Each circle represents the mean of data collected in an individual study of 14–33 days duration. Nitrogen balance was adjusted for changes in body urea nitrogen but not for unmeasured losses. The curved line depicts the calculated relationship between protein intake and nitrogen balance. Reproduced with permission from reference 9.

Amino Acids

Patients undergoing CAPD lose into dialysate each day about 1.7–3.4 g of amino acids and about 9 g of protein.[15–18] Several investigators advocate adding amino acids to peritoneal dialysis fluid to increase the total daily amino acid intake. By modifying the proportions of the amino acids in dialysate, it may also be possible to normalize plasma and intracellular concentrations of many amino acids. There is the unproven possibility that normalizing such pools may promote anabolism. Also, by substituting amino acids for glucose in dialysate, it may be possible to decrease the daily intake of purified sugars, the production of triglycerides, and in patients with diabetes mellitus, the requirement for insulin.

Williams et al.[19] and Oren et al.[20] investigated the addition of amino acids to dialysis fluid in CAPD patients. A dialysis solution containing 2 g/dl of amino acids without glucose has an osmolality and promotes a volume of ultrafiltrate comparable to the same dialysis solution without amino acids and containing 4.25 g/dl dextrose. In a dialysis solution containing a 2% mixture of essential and nonessential amino acids and no glucose, 80–90% of the amino acids were absorbed by six hours. The mean plasma amino acid concentration increased approximately two to three times at one hour after instillation of the dialysis fluid and fell to preinstillation values by six hours. Plasma levels of several amino acids were still slightly elevated at six hours. These investigators studied nutritional status for four weeks in six CAPD patients receiving a 1% mixture of essential and nonessential amino acids and no glucose in two of their four daily 2 L exchanges.[20] The patients continued to ingest their usual diet. After four weeks, the patients' serum urea nitrogen increased from 64–102 mg/dl, total body nitrogen (excluding body urea nitrogen) from 1333–1350 g, serum transferrin from 175–222 mg/dl, and the serum anion gap from 15.1–17.3 mEq/L.

These studies, although promising, have not yet demonstrated that adding amino acids to dialysis fluid is preferable to the less expensive alternatives of prescribing protein or amino acid supplements or simply increasing the intake of protein-containing foods. The use of amino acids in dialysis fluid may be of particular value for patients who will not eat food or nutritional supplements. Also, it appears that the addition of amino acids to dialysis fluid reduces modestly the daily total sugar load (diet plus dialysis fluid) and may not have a major effect on serum triglyceride levels. As shown by Baeyer et al.[21] and Salusky et al.,[22] the mean values for serum triglyceride levels, although often elevated in CAPD patients, do not change after patients commence CAPD. In those who begin CAPD with high serum triglyceride levels, they tend to remain high. Those with low serum triglycerides at the onset of CAPD tend to maintain low concentrations.

Peritoneal dialysis has also been suggested as a method for providing total parenteral nutrition.[23] Theoretically, it could provide the daily requirements for amino acids, water soluble vitamins, and minerals including trace elements. The problem is to provide sufficient calories. It is difficult to accomplish this with glucose because of the hypertonic nature of concentrated dextrose solutions. The degree to which lipids can be absorbed from the peritoneal cavity has not been adequately evaluated. If fat or larger carbohydrate molecules can be demonstrated to be readily absorbed from the peritoneal cavity, rapidly metabolized and safe, and if fat soluble vitamins can be administered safely through the peritoneal cavity, then total peritoneal nutrition may become feasible.

Energy

Energy requirements in CAPD patients have never been systematically evaluated. Several surveys indicate that total energy intake (diet plus dialysis fluid) averages about 30 kcal/kg/day in CAPD patients, which is below that recommended for normal people with typical daily activities. Our current policy is to maintain total energy intake between 35–42 kcal/kg/day in nonobese patients (i.e., body weight equal to or less than 120% of the mean body weight of normal individuals of the same age, height, and sex). This is based on the following considerations: First, CAPD patients may be protein depleted (see above). Second, our data in clinically stable nondialyzed patients with chronic renal failure and patients undergoing maintenance hemodialysis indicates that energy expenditure is normal.[24] The energy requirements for stable nondialyzed patients with chronic renal failure is close to 35 kcal/kg/day.[24]

Contribution of Glucose

In our experience, there is a close correlation between the amount of glucose absorbed from the peritoneum each day (y) and the quantity instilled into the peritoneal cavity (x): $y(g/day) = 0.89x$ $(g/day) - 43$, $r = 0.91$.[25] Our patients, who usually underwent five dialysate exchanges each day, had a mean intraperitoneal instillation of dextrose of 252 ± 62 g/day (range 185–395 g/day); 182 ± 61 g/day glucose were absorbed, which provided 8.4 ± 2.7 kcal/kg/day. These calculations are based upon the quantity of anhydrous dextrose in dialysis fluid (1.30 ± 0.11 g anhydrous dextrose in the 1.5% solution and 3.76 ± 0.12 g in the 4.25% solution) and the yield of 3.74 kcal/g of anhydrous glucose.[25]

Minerals

There are few data concerning mineral requirements in CAPD patients. In the studies of Blumenkrantz et al.,[9] the independent variable was the protein intake, and the mineral balances were dependent variables. Dietary potassium, phosphorus, calcium, and magnesium each correlated directly with the nitrogen intake. Hence, it is possible that the balances for a given mineral were influenced by the intake and balance of nitrogen or other minerals as well as by the intake of the mineral in question. Nonetheless, the relationships between the mineral intakes and balances should have some relevance for determining dietary requirements.

Potassium intake averaged 64 mEq/day with the lower protein diet and was significantly greater, 84 mEq/day, with the higher protein diet (Table 1). Dialysate losses accounted for approximately 70% of potassium output, and fecal losses contributed about 30%. Potassium balance did not differ from zero with the low protein diet and was significantly positive, 17.8 ± 4.0 mEq/day, with the higher intake. Potassium balance (y) correlated directly with potassium intake (x): y(mEq/day) = 0.64x (mEq/day) − 35, r = 0.80, $p < 0.01$. When potassium intake was 67 mEq/day or greater, potassium balance was invariably positive. Serum potassium concentration did not differ with the low and high protein diets and was usually within normal limits, 4.0 ± 0.19 and 4.6 ± 0.31 mEq/L, respectively. The SUN and serum electrolytes referred to in these studies are the average of the values obtained periodically throughout the entire 14–33 days of study with the two diets.

Phosphorus intake averaged 1047 and 1915 mg/day, respectively, with the low and high protein diets. Dietary and fecal phosphorus were each greater with the 1.44 g/kg protein diet, and phosphorus balance was significantly positive with both diets (Table 1). Serum phosphorus, measured periodically during the studies, averaged 4.5 ± 0.27 and 4.8 ± 0.43 mg/dl with the low and high protein diets, respectively. Serum phosphorus was slightly increased in several patients despite 7.8 ± 1.0 g/day of aluminum hydroxide gel during the 13 studies. Despite the phosphate binders, net intestinal absorption of phosphorus (dietary minus fecal phosphorus) correlated directly with phosphorus intake (r = 0.87). The serum phosphorus level was always 5.1 mg/dl or less when phosphorus intake was 1200 mg/day or lower.

Dietary magnesium averaged 259 and 320 mg/day, respectively, with the low and high protein diets. The intake and balance for magnesium were greater with the higher protein diet, and magnesium balance was significantly positive with both diets. Mean serum magnesium concentrations were abnormally high, 3.1 ± 0.10 and 3.1 ± 0.15 mg/dl, respectively, with the low and high protein diets. Net intestinal magnesium absorption ranged from 74–200 mg/day except for one patient who had a net intestinal magnesium loss of 49 mg/day. This patient also had large fecal phosphorus and calcium losses. The positive magnesium balance and high serum magnesium levels were related to the rather small magnesium losses into dialysate, which averaged 48 and 44 mg/day with the low and high protein diets, respectively. This low removal rate was related to the high magnesium concentrations in the dialysis solution, 1.85 mg/dl. With the lower dialysis fluid magnesium concentrations now available, patients should tolerate these magnesium intakes better.

Dietary calcium averaged 769 and 1356 mg/day, respectively, with the low and high protein diets. The intake and balance were significantly greater with the high protein diet (Table 1). Feces were the major source of calcium loss. Calcium balance was not significantly positive with the high protein diet because of the large fecal calcium losses in the patient with the large fecal phosphorus and magnesium output. Except for this patient, calcium balance was always neutral or positive when dietary intake was 720 mg/day or greater in the 13 studies. There was a net uptake of calcium from dialysate which averaged 84 mg/day. The dialysis fluid calcium concentration was 3.5 mEq/L, and net calcium absorption from dialysate correlated inversely with the serum calcium concentration.

Delmez et al.[26] and Kurtz et al.[27] found that calcium uptake in CAPD patients was affected by both the serum ionized calcium and the dialysis fluid concentration of glucose, which is a determinant of the ultrafiltrate volume. Delmez et al.[26] also used a dialysis fluid calcium concentration of 3.5 mEq/L. They studied ten CAPD patients who had a mean serum ionized calcium of 4.9 mg/dl. In those who had a serum ionized calcium above normal (5.0 mg/dl), there was a net calcium loss into dialysate of 77 mg/day. A serum ionized calcium below normal (less than 4.4 mg/dl) was associated with a net calcium uptake from dialysate of 44 mg/day. With a single 1.5% dextrose exchange, net calcium uptake was 9.8 mg per exchange, and with a 4.25% dextrose exchange, there was a net calcium loss into dialysate of 21 mg per exchange.

With the calcium concentrations currently employed in peritoneal dialysis fluids, calcium uptake and losses from dialysate will be small. Most calcium taken into the body will come from the diet. Excluding the patient with large fecal losses in our studies, the calcium intake necessary for neutral or positive calcium balance was 720 mg/day. This quantity of dietary calcium is greater than many people will eat, and dietary noncompliance will be accentuated if a margin of safety of several hundred mg per day is added to the recommended calcium intake to allow for individual variability among patients. Thus, to ensure neutral or positive calcium balance in CAPD patients, it seems necessary to either prescribe a calcium supplement or to increase the dialysis fluid calcium concentration.

Vitamins

Blumberg et al.[28] evaluated blood vitamin levels in ten CAPD patients who were eating normally and not receiving vitamin supplements. They reported low or borderline normal vitamin levels of thiamine (vitamin B_1) in five patients, pyridoxine (vitamin B_6) in eight patients, folic acid in six patients, and vitamin C in four patients. Riboflavin (vitamin B_2) and vitamin B_{12} were normal. Serum levels of vitamins A and E and retinol binding protein were elevated. Dietary intake of vitamin A, vitamin B_1, vitamin B_6, vitamin B_{12}, and nicotinamide were often reduced below the recommended daily allowances for normal adults. These observations are consistent with previous reports of low dietary intakes for many vitamins in nondialyzed patients with chronic renal failure and in patients undergoing maintenance hemodialysis.[29]

These authors then prescribed a daily supplement that provided 16 mg each of thiamine hydrochloride, riboflavin, and pyridoxine hydrochloride (quantities of the free thiamine and pyridoxine were lower), 200 mg of vitamin C and 4 mg of folic acid, and they reevaluated vitamin status in nine of the patients.[28] After receiving these vitamin supplements for seven weeks, vitamins A and E and retinol binding protein were still elevated. Thiamine levels were still low in five of nine patients when assessed by erythrocyte transketolase activity. However, thiamine levels were normal in all patients tested when evaluated by the erythrocyte transketolase activity index. This latter test is considered to be a more sensitive index of vitamin B_1 status.[30] Hence, it could be argued that 16 mg/day of thiamine hydrochloride corrected the vitamin depletion in all of the patients, and that an even lower dose might be sufficient to prevent or treat vitamin B_1 deficiency. Indeed, we have observed no evidence for thiamine deficiency in nondialyzed chronically uremic patients and in hemodialysis patients, many of whom received a daily vitamin supplement that provided only one to several mg per day of thiamine hydrochloride.[31] Since dialysis of thiamine should not be substantially greater with CAPD than with hemodialysis, it is not clear why the dietary requirement should be greater with CAPD.

The activity and the activity index of erythrocyte aspartate-amino-transferase, indicators of vitamin B_6 status, were normal in all nine patients studied after supplementation, although low pyridoxal phosphate levels persisted in one patient.[28] Vitamin B_2 (riboflavin) and vitamin B_{12} remained normal; patients were not given vitamin B_{12} supplements, and vitamin B_{12} levels decreased slightly during the study. Folic acid levels were sometimes normal and usually markedly elevated after supplementation with 4 mg/day of this vitamin.

Several investigators have evaluated vitamin D nutrition in CAPD patients. Since vitamin D is protein bound, there is a concern that CAPD patients may be particularly susceptible to vitamin D deficiency. Aloni et al.[32] reported decreased serum-25-hydroxyvitamin D concentrations and 25-hydroxyvitamin D binding capacity in CAPD patients. The patients had a mean daily loss of 25-hydroxyvitamin D in peritoneal fluid of 1491 ± 260 ng/day and a loss of 25-hydroxyvitamin D binding capacity into dialysate of 153 ± 28 nmol/day. The serum 25-hydroxyvitamin D levels were also lower than in maintenance hemodialysis patients. Kurtz et al.[27] found very low levels of serum 1,25-dihydroxyvitamin D levels and 24,25-dihydroxyvitamin D concentrations in CAPD patients. Serum 25-hydroxyvitamin D was only slightly decreased and did not change with 6–12 months of treatment with CAPD. However, Gokal et al.[33] observed that serum 25-hydroxyvitamin D levels fell with time in CAPD patients. In contrast, Delmez et al.[26] reported that patients treated with CAPD for six months had normal serum concentrations of 25-hydroxyvitamin D, 21 ± 3 ng/ml; these values did not differ from those of maintenance hemodialysis patients (28 ± 6 ng/ml). Serum 25-hydroxyvitamin D did not change in five CAPD patients in whom levels were measured serially. The CAPD patients lost an average of 6.2 ± 2.2 mg of vitamin D binding protein with each 1.5% dextrose exchange. Despite these losses, serum vitamin D binding protein levels were normal in their CAPD patients, 610 ± 21 μg/ml (normal range 400–650 μg/ml), and were significantly higher than those of maintenance hemodialysis patients.

These conflicting data suggest that 25-hydroxyvitamin D levels may or may not be decreased in CAPD patients; serum 1,25-dihydroxyvitamin D and 24,25-dihydroxyvitamin D appear to be reduced in these individuals as they are in patients undergoing maintenance hemodialysis. At present, indications for administering 1,25-dihydroxycholecalciferol to CAPD patients probably should be considered similar to those for hemodialysis patients and include osteomalacia not due to aluminum toxicity, osteoporosis, and hypocalcemia.

Trace Elements

Thompson et al.[34] describe normal plasma zinc, copper, and manganese; increased plasma aluminum; decreased red cell zinc and copper; normal red cell lead; increased whole blood chromium; and normal whole blood cadmium in CAPD patients. Wallaeys et al.[35] found normal serum and red cell cesium, copper, iron, and manganese; increased serum chromium and cobalt; low serum and red cell bromide; and low serum selenium and zinc in five CAPD patients. Rubidium was normal in serum and low in red cells. Zinc was increased, while cobalt and selenium were normal in red cells. The increased chromium levels may be related to the uptake of this element from dialysate. The findings of elevated serum cobalt levels in CAPD patients may indicate that CAPD patients should not receive vitamin preparations that contain cobalt supplements.

Several researchers have also found increased serum aluminum levels in CAPD patients.[34, 36, 37] Serum aluminum is elevated in CAPD patients who have not received oral aluminum binders of phosphate, but serum aluminum levels also correlate with the total intake of aluminum phosphate binders.[37] Hercz et al.[37] reported that daily losses of aluminum into dialysate averaged 206 ± 23 μg. Aluminum-related osteomalacia has been described in CAPD patients. Some have been treated with desferrioxamine to remove aluminum; in one CAPD patient who was given 6 g of desferrioxamine IV, the aluminum losses into peritoneal dialysate increased by 3.5–4.7 mg/24 h.[37]

Lipids and Carnitine.

As indicated above, CAPD was originally thought to accelerate or worsen serum cholesterol and triglyceride levels. However, several studies now indicate that in most patients CAPD does not substantially increase the frequency or severity of these lipid abnormalities. Nonetheless, elevated serum total cholesterol, triglycerides, LDL and VLDL cholesterol and low HDL cholesterol are aften observed in these patients.[38–41] The hypertriglyceridemia may be severe. There are multiple causes of elevated serum cholesterol and triglyceride levels in patients with chronic renal failure, including those undergoing CAPD.[42, 43] Hypertriglyceridemia is primarily caused by impaired clearance of triglycerides, but the high glucose intake from dialysis fluid may also stimulate triglyceride synthesis. Carnitine deficiency can cause hypertriglyceridemia, and low carnitine levels have been reported in serum and sometimes in muscle in patients with chronic renal failure.[44–46] Whether CAPD patients should be given carnitine routinely has not been established.

RECOMMENDED NUTRIENT ALLOWANCES FOR ADULT PATIENTS UNDERGOING CAPD

A tentative proposal for daily nutrient allowances for clinically stable adult CAPD patients is proposed based on the foregoing consideration (Table 2). These recommendations should be considered a first approximation and a basis for further

inquiry. Additional research will undoubtedly modify these recommended allowances. Since excessive and insufficient intakes may each be hazardous to the CAPD patient, it would be desirable to indicate both the upper and lower ranges of safe nutritional allowances. Malnourished patients may have greater requirements than well-nourished patients for protein, energy, and other nutrients. Also, patients with moderate or severe obesity may require less energy. Patients with abnormal serum lipid and lipoprotein concentrations may require changes in the fat and carbohydrate composition of the diet. Changes in the dialysis regimen or in dialysis solution composition may also alter dietary allowances; thus, the dietary requirement for patients undergoing continuous cyclic peritoneal dialysis may be somewhat altered. In addition, CAPD patients with superimposed catabolic illnesses may have different nutritional needs. Finally, the nutrient intake should always be adjusted according to the clinical and metabolic response of the individual patient.

The recommended daily protein intake is based upon the observation that nitrogen balance became more positive as protein intake was increased to 1.09 g/kg/day and greater protein intakes did not cause more positive nitrogen balance. Allowing for individual variation, we propose a daily protein allowance of 1.2–1.3 g/kg/day (Table 2). Serum urea nitrogen concentrations should not be excessive with this protein intake (Table 1). If the dietary requirements for essential amino acids in CAPD patients resemble those of normal individuals, then allowing 50% of the daily protein intake to be of high biological value should provide a surfeit of these amino acids. Patients who are given amino acids in dialysis fluid may have a lower dietary protein requirement. If patients are not obese or hypertriglyceridemic, it is recommended that attempts should be made to maintain total energy intake (diet plus dialysis fluid) at 42 kcal/kg/day; unfortunately, such a high energy intake will be difficult to attain for many CAPD patients.

Dietary carbohydrate should be composed primarily of complex carbohydrates and should provide about 35% of ingested calories. Dietary fat should provide the remainder of the ingested nonprotein calories. The polyunsaturated to saturated fatty acid ratio should be about 1.0 : 1.0. These recommendations are based on the observations of Sanfelippo et al.[48, 49] in nondialyzed chronically uremic and maintenance hemodialysis patients that such types of dietary modifications may reduce serum triglyceride levels. The glucose absorbed from the dialysate will increase the proportion of calories

Table 2. Daily Dietary Allowances for CAPD Patients—
A Tentative Proposal.[a]

Protein	1.2–1.3 g/kg normalized body weight[b]
Energy (oral and dialysate)	35–42 kcal/kg normalized body weight[b]
Carbohydrate (oral)	35% of ingested calories[c]
Fat	Remainder of ingested nonprotein calories[c]
Polyunsaturated : saturated fatty acid ratio	1.0 : 1.0[c]
Total fiber	20–25 g[c]
Calcium	1000–1400 mg[d]
Phosphorus	800–1200 mg[e]
Magnesium	200–300 mg
Potassium	70–80 mEq
Sodium and water	As tolerated by water balances and serum sodium
Supplemental vitamins[f]	
Ascorbic acid	100 mg
Pyridoxine hydrochloride (B$_6$)	10 mg
Thiamine hydrochloride (B$_1$)	2.0 mg
Folic acid	1 mg
Other water soluble vitamins	Recommended daily allowances for normal adults[51]
Vitamins A, E and K	None
Vitamin D	See text
Trace elements	See text

[a] See text for discussion of recommendations, adapted from reference 47.
[b] A patient's normalized body weight is the average body weight of normal persons of the same age, height, and sex as the patient.
[c] These dietary recommendations may increase the arduousness of the diet and may not be as critical for health as many of the other recommended intakes. Therefore we do not urge compliance with the same intensity as is used for the proteins, energy, minerals, and vitamins.
[d] As an alternative to this high intake, patients may be given a vitamin D preparation such as 1,25-dihydroxycholecalciferol, or the dialysate calcium concentration may be increased.
[e] Phosphate binders are often needed in addition.
[f] Refers to vitamin intake in addition to vitamins present in food.

derived from carbohydrates above 35% of total energy intake (diet plus dialysis fluid). However, further reductions in dietary carbohydrate to below 35% of ingested calories would make dietary compliance too difficult for most patients. Currently, carnitine is not routinely prescribed, but if there is hypertriglyceridemia or unexplained weakness, particularly of the proximal muscles, serum, and possibly muscle carnitine should be measured. If carnitine levels are low, a therapeutic trial of L-carnitine, 0.5–1.0 g/day orally, may be tried.

Dietary fiber may enhance health in several ways. These include improved glucose tolerance, reduced serum lipids, more normal bowel function, and possibly reduced risk of certain malignancies.[50] However, foods containing fiber are often high in minerals, particularly magnesium and phosphorus. We recommend a dietary total fiber intake of 20–25

g/day. This is lower than the high fiber intakes often recommended for health-enhancing diets, but exceeds the total fiber intake of a typical American diet. Unfortunately, the foregoing modifications in dietary lipids and carbohydrates and even this quantity of total fiber often make the diet less palatable and more arduous. These proposed dietary modifications may not be as critical for health as many of the other recommended nutrient intakes. Therefore, although patients are encouraged to adhere to these dietary recommendations, we do not urge compliance with the same intensity that is used for the protein, energy, mineral, and vitamin intake.

The daily recommended dietary phosphorus intake is 800–1200 mg. Phosphorus intakes closer to 800 mg/day may decrease the risk of severe hyperparathyroidism and the need for aluminum binders of phosphate. On the other hand, a diet that provides only about 800 mg/day of phosphorus may be unpalatable and difficult to ingest, particularly with a daily protein intake of 1.2–1.3 g/kg. We therefore recommend a dietary phosphorus intake as close to 800 mg/day as the patient can comfortably tolerate, but do not prescribe more than 1200 mg/day. Aluminum binders of phosphate are prescribed as necessary to maintain normal serum phosphorus concentrations. These binders may increase the serum levels and body burden of aluminum.[37,51] Increased serum aluminum concentrations and aluminum related osteomalacia have been reported in CAPD patients, and it is therefore considered important to restrict the aluminum intake. Currently, new phosphate binders are being developed that do not contain aluminum. If these agents can be shown to be safe and effective, they may markedly diminish the problem of aluminum toxicity in patients with renal failure.

The recommended magnesium intake of 200–300 mg/day is based upon the use of a dialysis solution with magnesium concentrations of 0.05–0.75 mEq/L. The proposed dietary calcium intake of 1000–1400 mg/day is most easily attained with the use of calcium supplements. Conversely, a higher dialysis fluid calcium concentration could be employed to increase the net calcium intake. If vitamin D analogues (e.g., 1,25-dihydroxycholecalciferol) or a high dialysis fluid calcium are used, the dietary calcium intake may be decreased. Vitamin D analogues or calcium supplements should not be prescribed to CAPD patients unless the serum phosphorus is normal.

Since sodium and water can be removed easily with CAPD, a liberal salt and water intake is usually allowed. If the patient maintains a high dietary sodium and water intake, the quantity of fluid removed from the patient and, hence, the daily dialysate volume can be increased. This may be beneficial, since with CAPD the clearance of small and middle-sized molecules correlates directly with the dialysate volume. Thus, a higher sodium and water intake (e.g., 6–8 g/day of sodium and 3 L/day of water) will enable some patients to use more hypertonic glucose exchanges to increase their dialysate volume; this, in turn, should lead to higher clearances and more glucose and energy uptake from dialysate. This technique may be less desirable for obese, hypertriglyceridemic, or diabetic patients because of the greater need for hypertonic glucose exchanges. Also, some patients may become habituated to high salt and water intakes. If they change to hemodialysis therapy, they may have difficulty in curtailing their sodium and water intake.

Dietary requirements for trace elements are not established. At the present time, trace element supplements are not recommended unless there is both (1) a low serum or tissue concentration of a trace element and (2) clinical manifestations of deficiency of this element. The exception is iron. CAPD patients are routinely given iron, usually 300 mg ferrous sulfate three times a day approximately one-half hour after meals, unless the patient has evidence for normal serum iron or iron overload. If oral iron therapy causes gastrointestinal symptoms, changing to another oral iron compound sometimes may alleviate the problem. Otherwise, iron dextran may be given parenterally on an intermittent basis.

Supplemental vitamin A and E are not recommended because serum levels are increased in CAPD patients. Supplemental vitamin K is not considered necessary unless the patient is not eating and is receiving antibiotics which may suppress intestinal bacteria that synthesize vitamin K. Vitamin D analogues are given as with hemodialysis patients, although there may be a greater need for supplementation.[26,27,33]

The recommendations for the water soluble vitamins are based on studies conducted primarily in nondialyzed chronically uremic patients and patients undergoing maintenance hemodialysis. The work of Blumberg et al.[28] does not seem to have defined the minimum safe allowance for the water soluble vitamins, since essentially every patient had evidence for normal vitamin nutritional status after receiving their supplements. It is recommended that CAPD patients should receive as a supplement the recommended dietary allowances[52] for normal nonpregnant nonlactating adults for each of the water soluble vitamins with the following modifications: pyridoxine hydrochloride, 10 mg/day (8.12 mg/day of pyridoxine); thiamine hydrochloride, 2 mg/day; ascorbic acid, 100 mg/day; folic acid, 1.0 mg/day. Further studies will be necessary to ascertain whether a greater daily intake of thiamine is necessary.

REFERENCES

1. Heide B, Pierratos A, Khanna R, Pettit J, Ogilvie R, Harrison J, McNeil K, and Oreopoulos DG: Nutritional status of patients undergoing continuous ambulatory peritoneal dialysis (CAPD). Peritoneal Dial Bull 3: 138, 1983

2. Salusky IB, Fine RN, Nelson P, and Kopple JD: Factors affecting growth and nutritional status in children undergoing CAPD. Kidney Int (Abstract) 25: 260, 1984

3. Jones MR, Blumenkrantz MJ, and Kopple JD: Albumin metabolism in patients with chronic renal failure. Fed Proc (Abstract) 39: 561, 1980

4. Williams P, Kay R, Harrison J, McNeil K, Pettit J, Kelman B, Mendez M, Klein M, Ogilvie R, Khanna R, Carmichael D, and Oreopoulos D: Nutritional and anthropometric assessment of patients on CAPD over one year: Contrasting changes in total body nitrogen and potassium. Peritoneal Dial Bull 1: 82, 1981

5. Rubin J, Flynn MA, and Nolph KD: Total body potassium—a guide to nutritional health in patients undergoing continuous ambulatory peritoneal dialysis. Am J Clin Nutr 34: 94, 1981

6. Kaysen G, and Schoenfeld P: Albumin homeostasis during CAPD. Kidney Int 23: 153, 1983

7. Bodnar D, Schreiber M, and Vidt D: Protein status of patients during the first year on CAPD. Kidney Int (Abstract) (in press)

8. Lindholm B, and Bergström J: Personal communication

9. Blumenkrantz MJ, Kopple JD, Moran JK, and Coburn JW: Metabolic balance studies and dietary protein requirements in patients undergoing continuous ambulatory peritoneal dialysis. Kidney Int 21: 849, 1982

10. Calloway DH, Odell ACF, and Margen S: Sweat and miscellaneous nitrogen losses in human balance studies. J Nutr 101: 775, 1971

11. Giordano C, DeSanto NG, Pluvio M, DiLeo VA, Capodicasa G, Cirillo D, Esposito R, and Damiano M: Protein requirement of patients on CAPD: a study on nitrogen balance. Int J Artif Organs 3: 11, 1980

12. Gahl GM, Baeyer HU, Averdunk R, Reidinger H, Borowzak B, Schurig R, Becker H, and Kessel M: Outpatient evaluation of dietary intake and nitrogen removal in continuous ambulatory peritoneal dialysis. Ann Intern Med 94: 643, 1981

13. Lindholm B, Alvestrand A, Fürst P, Karlander SG, Norbeck HE, Ahlberg M, Tranaeus A, and Bergström J: Metabolic effects of continuous ambulatory peritoneal dialysis. Proc Eur Dial Transplant Assoc 17: 283, 1980

14. Mihindukulasuriya MB, Talbot S, Rowlands A, and Lee HA: Protein requirements of patients on chronic ambulatory peritoneal dialysis (CAPD). J Int Biomed Inf Data 3: 37, 1982

15. Giordano C, DeSanto NG, Capodicasa G, DiLeo VA, DiSerafino A, Cirillo D, Esposito R, Fiore R, Damiano M, Buonadonna L, Cocco F, and DiIorio B: Amino acid losses during CAPD. Clin Nephrol 14: 230, 1980

16. Randerson DH, Chapman GV, and Farrell PC: Amino acid and dietary status in CAPD patients. In Atkins RC, Thomson NM, and Farrell PC (Eds), Continuous ambulatory peritoneal dialysis. London: Churchill-Livingstone, 1981, p 179

17. Kopple JD, Blumenkrantz MJ, Jones MR, Moran JK, and Coburn JW: Plasma amino acid levels and amino acid losses during continuous ambulatory peritoneal dialysis. Am J Clin Nutr 36: 395, 1982

18. Dombros N, Oren A, Marliss EB, Anderson GH, Stein AN, Khanna R, Pettit J, Brandes L, Rodella H, Libel BS, and Oreopoulos DG: Plasma amino acid profiles and amino acid losses in patients undergoing CAPD. Peritoneal Dial Bull 2: 27, 1982

19. Williams PF, Marliss E, Anderson GH, Oren A, Stein A, Khanna R, Pettit J, Brandes L, Rodella H, Mupas L, Dombros, N, and Oreopoulos DG: Amino acid absorption following intraperitoneal administration in CAPD patients. Peritoneal Dial Bull 2: 124, 1982

20. Oren A, Wu G, Anderson GH, Marliss E, Khanna R, Pettit J, Mupas L, Rhodella H, Brandes L, Roncari DL, Kakis G, Harrison J, McNeil K, and Oreopoulos DG: Effective use of amino acid dialysate over four weeks in CAPD patients. Peritoneal Dial Bull 3: 66, 1983

21. Baeyer HV, Gahl GM, Riedinger H, Borowzak R, Averdunk R, Schurig R, and Kessel M: Adaptation of CAPD patients to the continuous peritoneal energy uptake. Kidney Int 23: 29, 1983

22. Salusky IB, Kopple JD, and Fine RN: Continuous ambulatory peritoneal dialysis in pediatric patients: A 20 month experience. Kidney Int 24(Suppl 15): S101, 1983

23. Leleiko NS, Bronstein AD, Murphy J, Fox J, and Lieberman K: Studies in the use of the intraperitoneal route for parenteral nutrition in the rat. J Parenteral Ent Nutr 7: 381, 1983

24. Kopple JD, Shaib JK, and Monteon F: Energy expenditure in chronic renal failure and hemodialysis patients. Kidney Int (Abstract) 25: 187, 1984

25. Grodstein GP, Blumenkrantz MJ, Kopple JD, Moran JK, and Coburn JW: Glucose absorption during continuous ambulatory peritoneal dialysis. Kidney Int 19: 564, 1981

26. Delmez JA, Slatopolsky E, Martin KJ, Gearing BN, and Harter HR: Minerals, vitamin D, and parathyroid hormone in continuous ambulatory peritoneal dialysis. Kidney Int 21: 862, 1982

27. Kurtz SB, McCarthy JT, and Kumar R: Hypercalcemia in continuous ambulatory peritoneal dialysis (CAPD) patients: Observations on parameters of calcium metabolism. In Gahl GM, Kessel M, and Nolph KD (Eds), Advances in peritoneal dialysis: Proceedings of the 2nd international symposium on peritoneal dialysis. Amsterdam: Excerpta Medica, 1981, p 467

28. Blumberg, Hanck A, and Sander G: Vitamin nutrition in patients on continuous ambulatory peritoneal dialysis (CAPD). Clin Nephrol 20: 244, 1983

29. Kopple JD, and Swendseid ME: Vitamin nutrition in patients undergoing maintenance hemodialysis. Kidney Int 7: S79, 1975

30. Sauberlich HE, Skala JH, and Dowdy RP: Laboratory tests for the assessment of nutritional status. Thiamine (Vitamin B_1). Ohio: CRC Press, 1974, p 30

31. Kopple JD, Dirige OV, Jacob M, Wang M, and Swendseid ME: Transketolase activity in red blood

cells in chronic uremia. Trans Am Soc Artif Intern Organs 18: 250, 1972

32. Aloni Y, Shany S, and Chaimovitz C: Losses of 25-hydroxyvitamin D in peritoneal fluid: Possible mechanism for bone disease in uremia patients treated with chronic ambulatory peritoneal dialysis. Mineral Electrolyte Metab 9: 82, 1983

33. Gokal R, Ellis HA, Ramos JM, Dewar J, Sweeting V, Ward MK, and Kerr DNS: Improvement in secondary hyperparathyroidism in patients on continuous ambulatory peritoneal dialysis. In Gahl GM, Kessel M, and Nolph KD (Eds), Advances in peritoneal dialysis: Proceedings of the 2nd international symposium on peritoneal dialysis. Amsterdam: Excerpta Medica, 1981, p 461

34. Thompson N, Stevens B, Humphery T, and Atkins R: Comparison of trace elements in peritoneal dialysis, hemodialysis and uremia. Kidney Int 23: 9, 1983

35. Wallaeys B, Cornelis R, and Lameire N: The trace elements Br, Co, Cr, Cs, Cu Fe, Mn, Rb, Se and Zn in serum, packed cells and dialysate of CAPD patients. Peritoneal Dial Bull 4: S70, 1984

36. Gokal R, Parkinson IS, Ramos M, Ward MK, and Kerr DNS: Elevated serum aluminum levels in patients on continuous ambulatory peritoneal dialysis. In Gahl GM, Kessel M, and Nolph KD (Eds), Advances in peritoneal dialysis: Proceedings of the 2nd international symposium on peritoneal dialysis. Amsterdam: Excerpta Medica, 1981, p 478

37. Hercz G, Milliner D, Shinaberger J, Nissenson AR, Cutler RE, Goodman WG, Gentile DE, Kraus AP, and Coburn JW: Aluminum metabolism and removal during CAPD. Kidney Int (Abstract) 25: 257, 1984

38. Khanna R, Breckenridge C, Roncari D, Digenis G, and Oreopoulos DG: Lipid abnormalities in patients undergoing CAPD. In endocrine and metabolic implications of CAPD. Peritoneal Dial Bull 3(Suppl): S13, 1983

39. Lindholm B, Karlander SG, Norbeck HE, and Bergström J: Glucose and lipid metabolism in peritoneal dialysis. In LaGreca G, Biasoli S, and Ronco C (Eds), Peritoneal dialysis. Milano: Wichtig Editore, 1982, p 219

40. Monteón F, Treviño A, González D, Toledo M, Aviles C, Navarro A, Aragón L, Acuña F, and Scott O: Hypertriglyceridemia in patients on CAPD. In Gahl GM, Kessel M, and Nolph KD (Eds), Advances in peritoneal dialysis: Proceedings of the 2nd international symposium on peritoneal dialysis. Amsterdam: Excerpta Medica, 1981, p 437

41. Cattran DC: The significance of lipid abnormalities in patients receiving dialysis therapy. Peritoneal Dial Bull 3: 529, 1983

42. Heuck CC, Ritz E, Liersch M, and Mehls O: Serum lipids in renal insufficiency. Am J Clin Nutr 31: 1547, 1978

43. Chan MK, Varghese Z, and Persaud JW: Hyperlipidemia in patients on maintenance hemo- and peritoneal dialysis: The relative pathogenetic roles of triglyceride production and triglyceride removal. Clin Nephrol 17: 183, 1982

44. Buoncristiani U, DiPaolo N, Carobi C, Cozzari M, Quintaliani G, and Bracaglia R: Carnitine depletion with CAPD. In Gahl GM, Kessel M, and Nolph KD (Eds), Advances in peritoneal dialysis: Proceedings of the 2nd international symposium on peritoneal dialysis. Amsterdam: Excerpta Medica, 1981, p 441

45. Albright RK, Kram BW, and White RP: Carnitine status of CAPD patients. Lancet 2: 218, 1982

46. Bartel LL, Hussey JL, and Shrago E: Effect of dialysis on serum carnitine, free fatty acids, and triglyceride levels in man and the rat. Metabolism 31: 944, 1982

47. Kopple JD, and Blumenkrantz MJ: Nutritional requirements for patients undergoing continuous ambulatory peritoneal dialysis. Kidney Int 24(Suppl 16): S295, 1983

48. Sanfelippo ML, Swenson RS, and Relen GM: Reduction of plasma triglycerides by diet in subjects with chronic renal failure. Kidney Int 11: 54, 1977

49. Sanfelippo ML, Swenson RS, and Reaven GM: Response of plasma triglycerides to dietary change in patients on hemodialysis. Kidney Int 14: 180, 1978

50. Nutrition Coordinating Committee of the National Institutes of Health: Symposium on role of dietary fiber in health. Am J Clin Nutr 31: S1, 1978

51. Lam M: Influence of aluminum-containing antacids on plasma aluminum. Kidney Int (Abstract) 23: 129, 1983

52. Recommended dietary allowances. 9th Revised Edition. Washington, D.C.: National Academy of Sciences, 1980

B. Lindholm, A. Alvestrand, and J. Bergström

76

Muscle Free Amino Acids in Patients Treated with CAPD

SUMMARY

Plasma and muscle intracellular free amino acid concentrations were quantified in 15 patients on continuous ambulatory peritoneal dialysis (CAPD) and 36 healthy control subjects. Most essential and some nonessential amino acids were decreased in plasma. These changes probably reflect metabolic and nutritional derangements of uremia rather than the modest losses into peritoneal dialysate. A few nonessential amino acids are increased in plasma and muscle. The distribution of several amino acids between plasma and intracellular fluid was abnormal in these patients. Taurine concentration in muscle was markedly reduced indicating depletion of this amino acid.

INTRODUCTION

Patients with advanced renal failure have deranged metabolism of amino acids, most obviously reflected in an abnormal pattern of plasma amino acids, with low concentrations of most essential amino acids, including tyrosine and histidine, and increased concentrations of several nonessential amino acids.[1,2] Some of these alterations appear to be typical for uremia *per se*, whereas others may reflect the commonly present protein-energy malnutrition in uremic patients.

From the Department of Renal Medicine, Karolinska Institute, Huddinge University Hospital, Stockholm, Sweden.

A more specific and a partly different uremic amino acid pattern is found in intracellular amino acids in skeletal muscle, which contains the largest pool of free amino acids in the body. The typical muscle free amino acid abnormalities in untreated uremic patients include decreased concentrations of threonine, valine, tyrosine, lysine, and sometimes histidine, whereas leucine and isoleucine concentrations usually are normal. As in plasma, the concentrations of several nonessential amino acids are increased in muscle.[1,2] Many of these abnormalities persist in uremic patients in spite of treatment with hemodialysis (HD) or intermittent peritoneal dialysis (IPD), nor are amino acid abnormalities fully normalized by supplementation of essential amino acids in conventional proportions.[1-3]

CAPD may lead to a better control of various uremic symptoms than other forms of therapy.[4] Several signs, including increasing body weights and positive nitrogen balance during the first months of the treatment, indicate that CAPD may induce an anabolic state. These positive effects have been attributed to the continuous dialytic process and to effective removal of uremic middle molecules. The long-term results are more uncertain, however. CAPD patients continuously lose proteins (5–15 g/24 h) and amino acids (2–4 g/24 h) into the dialysate.[4] Both protein and energy seem to decrease over time, and the nutritional intakes may be inadequate in some patients. These changes may possibly result in long-term negative nitrogen balance in CAPD patients.

Since deficient amino acid pools may limit protein synthesis, it is of interest to investigate the amino acid status of CAPD patients. Previous studies have shown abnormal plasma amino acid concentrations in CAPD patients.[5-12] In this study, which comprises a larger number of patients (15 males) than in earlier studies, we confirm these findings. Furthermore, we describe here for the first time the presence of an abnormal pattern of muscle intracellular free amino acids in CAPD patients. Our results show that most patients have markedly reduced intracellular concentrations of taurine, and several patients also show decreased concentrations of tyrosine in muscle. On the other hand, none of the essential amino acids were significantly decreased in muscle.

MATERIAL AND METHODS

Fifteen male nondiabetic uremic patients, aged 27–76 years (mean 58 years), were studied. They had been treated with CAPD according to the technique of Oreopoulos et al.[13] for 2–21 months (mean 10 months) before the study. Patients exchanged 2 L dialysis fluid (Dianeal®, Travenol Laboratories; manufactured either in Deerfield, IL, or Halden, Norway) three to five times in 24 hours. The dialysis solutions contained dextrose (anhydrous) at concentrations of either 1.36, 2.27, or 3.86 g/dl, and Na 132 mmol/L, Cl 102 mmol/L, Ca 1.75 mmol/L, Mg 0.75 mmol/L, and lactate 35 mmol/L. Glomerular filtration rate was less than 5 ml/min in all patients when they started CAPD. All patients had been recommended a high protein intake (1.2 g/kg/day, or more). Metabolic studies[8] in seven of the patients at the time of amino acid investigations showed daily protein intakes between 0.76–2.09 g/kg (1.47 ± 0.41 g/kg; mean + SD) and total energy intakes per 24 hours (including absorption of glucose from dialysis fluid) between 153–213 kJ/kg (186 ± 18 kJ/kg). Their body weights ranged between 57–84 kg (67.6 ± 6.4 kg); Broca's index ranged between 0.70–1.07 (0.88 ± 0.09). Mean serum concentrations were: urea 24.4 ± 5.3 mmol/L; creatinine 854 ± 475 μmol/L; albumin 33 ± 10 g/L.

The patients were studied at about eight hours after a ten-hour overnight fast. Since CAPD is associated with a continuous absorption of glucose from the dialysate, the patients were, strictly speaking, never in a completely fasted state. To standardize fasting conditions, all patients therefore used 1.36% dialysis fluid for 10 hours overnight without exchanging the fluid before the investigations.

Percutaneous muscle biopsies for determinations of muscle intracellular free amino acids were taken from the quadriceps femoris according to the technique of Bergström.[14] Venous blood samples for determinations of plasma free amino acids, serum total protein, and serum electrolytes were obtained at the time of each muscle biopsy. The methods for determination of free amino acids in muscle and plasma have been described earlier,[15] as has also the calculation of intracellular amino acid concentrations based on the chloride method.[16, 17]

The results were compared with data from 36 male apparently healthy control subjects of similar age to the patients. The investigations were approved by the Ethical Committee of the Karolinska Institute after informed consent was obtained from patients and control subjects. The t test for comparison of two independent means was used to evaluate the results.

Table 1. Plasma and Muscle Intracellular Free Amino Acids in 15 Male CAPD Patients as Compared to Data from 36 Healthy, Age-Matched Male Control Subjects.

	Percentage of Normal (Mean Values)[a]	
Essential	Plasma	Muscle
Tyrosine[b]	58%***	62%**
Threonine	58%***	90%
Histidine[b]	59%***	90%
Valine	61%***	83%
Lysine	63%***	126%*
Leucine	65%***	92%
Phenylalanine	89%	125%
Isoleucine	90%	98%
Methionine	97%	—
Nonessential	Plasma	Muscle
Serine	44%***	84%
Taurine	63%**	68%***
Ornithine	65%***	98%
Glutamine	66%***	98%
Glycine	81%**	97%
Alanine	85%*	105%
Proline	105%	99%
Asparagine	120%*	310%***
Glutamic acid	130%*	117%*
Citrulline	221%***	142%
Aspartic acid	307%***	133%***
3-methylhistidine	914%***	189%*

[a] Significant changes versus healthy controls are marked: * = p < 0.05, ** = p < 0.01 and *** = p < 0.001.
[b] Considered as an essential amino acid in uremia.

RESULTS

Plasma Amino Acids

The mean concentrations of most essential amino acids were decreased in the patients as compared to the control subjects; however, the differences were not statistically significant for isoleucine, methionine, and phenylalanine (Table 1). Several nonessential amino acids had decreased plasma concentrations, and some were increased.

Muscle Intracellular Concentrations

In contrast to the findings in plasma, only tyrosine of the essential amino acids had a significantly decreased mean concentration in the muscle intracellular compartment, but lysine was significantly increased (Table 1). However, the taurine concentration was significantly decreased in muscle ($p < 0.001$). Several of the nonessential amino acids were significantly increased in muscle.

DISCUSSION

Plasma amino acid concentrations are abnormal in nondiabetic CAPD patients, as shown in this study and in previous investigations.[5–12] Thus, we and most of the other authors report significantly reduced plasma concentrations of the essential amino acids leucine, lysine, threonine and valine; decreased tyrosine (considered as essential in uremia) and serine levels, and increased plasma concentrations of several nonessential amino acids. Low plasma histidine concentrations in CAPD patients has previously been reported in only one study in females undergoing CAPD.[10] Low plasma taurine concentrations in CAPD has previously been reported in one study,[6] whereas increased concentrations of taurine were found in another study.[11]

The plasma amino acid abnormalities in CAPD patients are similar to those observed in untreated uremic patients, and therefore probably reflect the metabolic and nutritional derangements of uremia rather than depletion due to amino acid losses into the dialysate. Furthermore, these losses are relatively small: on average 1.2–3.4 g/24 h of free amino acids are lost into the dialysate during CAPD.[5–7,9–11,18] In addition, the reduced plasma amino acid concentrations may to some extent reflect the commonly observed hyperinsulinemia in uremic patients, especially since hyperinsulinemia is accentuated during CAPD due to the continuous

absorption of glucose from the dialysate. On the other hand insulin resistance in uremia does not appear to involve an insulin effect on amino acids.[19]

Differences in the published results may reflect methodological differences, as well as variations in age and sex distribution and protein intake between different patient groups. Furthermore, interpretation of the results will depend on whether the control group is matched with regard to age and sex, since these factors influence the concentration of free amino acids in plasma as well as in muscle. In our study, the number of control subjects was relatively large; patients and control subjects were all men and of similar age.

The distribution of several amino acids between the extra- and intracellular compartments are altered in uremia.[1] Thus, plasma amino acid levels may not correlate well with intracellular amino acid composition. Direct measurement of muscle free intracellular amino acids, which comprise the largest free amino acid pool in the body, may therefore give more relevant information in the assessment of the total free amino acid pool in uremic patients. The results of these measurements may allow conclusions concerning possible deficiencies of amino acids.

Our results show that CAPD patients have an abnormal intracellular amino acid pattern. In accordance with the above-mentioned observations, the intracellular pattern differed from the amino acid pattern in plasma. Thus, except for tyrosine, the essential amino acids were significantly reduced in muscle, whereas most essential amino acids were decreased in plasma. The intracellular muscle concentration of valine is markedly reduced in untreated uremic patients.[2] In CAPD patients, muscle free valine tended to be low, but was not significantly reduced in comparison to controls, suggesting that this feature of uremia is relatively well controlled by CAPD. Furthermore, the mean intracellular concentration of tyrosine was reduced to 62% of normal. This finding suggests depletion of tyrosine in CAPD patients and a need for supplementation with this amino acid.

In addition, the markedly reduced intracellular concentration of taurine indicates depletion of this amino acid. Taurine has become increasingly acknowledged as a factor involved in the functional regulation of the cardiovascular and nervous system.[20] Taurine metabolism in man is largely unknown and it cannot be excluded that uremia and CAPD may negatively affect its synthesis. Thus, it is possible that CAPD patients might benefit from supplementation with taurine.

Increased concentration of lysine in muscle has previously been described in patients undergoing intermittent peritoneal dialysis (IPD),[1] whereas untreated uremic patients have decreased intracellular lysine levels.[2] The cause of high free lysine in muscle in peritoneal dialysis patients is not known, High intracellular concentrations of basic amino acids have been observed in patients with severe potassium depletion[17]; however, muscle potassium has not been found to be low in IPD patients[16] or in CAPD patients (unpublished observations).

During long-term treatment with CAPD, many patients appear to have inadequate intakes of both protein and energy.[4] A major concern is that the inadequate nutritional intakes and the continuous losses of proteins and amino acids into the dialysate may lead to long-term negative nitrogen balance in CAPD patients.[21] To improve the nutritional status of CAPD patients, attempts have been made to substitute amino acids for glucose as osmotic agents in peritoneal dialysis solutions; however, the effects on plasma amino acid profiles were marginal.[12,22] It remains to be further investigated how the amino acid composition should be optimized for a solution intended for peritoneal use in order to obtain both an efficient osmotic effect and the best possible nutritive effect with improvement or normaliztion of plasma and muscle aminograms.

ACKNOWLEDGMENTS

This study was supported by National Institutes of Health, Grant No. RO1-AM-27519.

REFERENCES

1. Bergström J, Fürst P, Noree LO, and Vinnars E: Intracellular free amino acids in muscle tissue of patients with chronic uraemia: Effect of peritoneal dialysis and infusion of essential amino acids. Clin Sci Mol Med 54: 51, 1978
2. Alvestrand A, Fürst P, and Bergström J: Plasma and muscle free amino acids in uremia: Influence of nutrition with amino acids. Clin Nephrol 18: 297, 1982
3. Fürst P, Alvestrand A, and Bergström J: Effects of nutrition and catabolic stress on intracellular amino acid pools in uremia. Am J Clin Nutr 33: 1387, 1980
4. Lindholm B, Alvestrand A, Norbeck HE, Tranaues A, and Bergström J: Long-term metabolic consequences of continuous ambulatory peritoneal dialysis (CAPD). In Robinson RR (Ed), Proceedings of the 1984 international congress of nephrology. New York: Springer Verlag, in press
5. Armstrong VW, Buschmann U, Ebert R, Fuchs C, Rieger J, and Scheler F: Biochemical investigations of CAPD: Plasma levels of trace elements and amino acids and impaired glucose tolerance during the course of treatment. Int J Artif Organs 3: 237, 1980
6. Giordano C, De Santo NG, Capodicasa G, Di Leo VA, Di Serafino A, Cirillo D, Espositio R, Fiore R, Damiano M, Buonadonna L, Cocco F, and Di Iorio B: Amino acid losses during CAPD. Clin Nephrol 14: 230, 1980
7. Fürst P, Bergström J, and Lindholm B: Studies of amino-acid metabolism in continuous ambulatory peritoneal dialysis patients—preliminary results. In Legrain M (Ed), Continuous ambulatory peritoneal dialysis. Amsterdam: Excerpta Medica, 1980, p 292
8. Lindholm B, Alvestrand A, Fürst P, Tranaeus A, and Bergström J: Efficacy and clinical experience of CAPD—Stockholm, Sweden. In Atkins RC, Thomson NM, and Farrell PC (Eds), Peritoneal dialysis. Edinburgh: Churchill Livingstone, 1981, p 147
9. Randerson DH, Chapman GV, and Farrell P: Amino acid and dietary status in CAPD patients. In Atkins RC, Thomson NM, and Farrell PC (Eds), Peritoneal dialysis. Edinburgh: Churchill Livingstone, 1981, p 179
10. Dombros N, Oren A, Marliss EB, Anderson GH, Stein AN, Khanna R, Petit J, Brandes L, Rodella H, Leibel BS, and Oreopoulos D: Plasma amino acid profiles and amino acid losses in patients undergoing CAPD. Peritoneal Dial Bull 2: 27, 1982
11. Kopple JD, Blumenkrantz MJ, Jones MR, Moran JK, and Coburn JW: Plasma amino acid levels and amino acid losses during continuous ambulatory peritoneal dialysis. Am J Clin Nutr 36: 395, 1982
12. Oren A, Wu G, Anderson GH, Marliss E, Khanna R, Pettit J, Mupas L, Rodella H, Brandes L, Roncari DA, Kakis G, Harrison J, McNeil K, and Oreopoulos DG: Effective use of amino acid dialysate over four weeks in CAPD patients. Peritoneal Dial Bull 3: 66, 1983
13. Oreopoulos DG, Robson M, Izatt S, Clayton S, and DeVeber GA: A simple and safe technique for continuous ambulatory peritoneal dialysis (CAPD). Am Soc Artif Intern Organs J 24: 484, 1978
14. Bergström J: Muscle electrolytes in man. Determined by neutron activation analysis in needle biopsy specimens. A study on normal subjects, kidney patients, and patients with chronic diarrhoea. Scand J Clin Lab Invest 14: Suppl 68, 1962
15. Bergström J, Fürst P, Noree LO, and Vinnars E: Intracellular free amino acid concentration in human muscle tissue. J Appl Physiol 36: 693, 1974
16. Bergström J, and Hultman E: Water, electrolyte and glycogen content of muscle tissue in patients undergoing regular dialysis therapy. Clin Nephrol 2: 24, 1974
17. Bergström J, Alvestrand A, Fürst P, Hultman E, Sahlin K, Vinnars E, and Widström A: Influence of severe potassium depletion and subsequent repletion

with potassium on muscle electrolytes, metabolites and amino acids in man. Clin Sci Mol Med 51: 589, 1976

18. von Baeyer H, Gahl GM, Riedinger H, Borowzak B, and Kessel M: Nutritional behaviour of patients on continuous ambulatory peritoneal dialysis. Proc Eur Dial Transplant Assoc 18: 193, 1981

19. DeFronzo RA, Smith D, and Alvestrand A: Insulin action in uremia. Kidney Int 24: S102, 1982

20. Hayes KC: Taurine in metabolism. Ann Rev Nutr 1: 401, 1981

21. Heide B, Pierratos A, Khanna R, Pettit J, Ogilvie R, Harrison J, McNeil K, Siccion Z, and Oreopoulos DG: Nutritional status of patients undergoing continuous ambulatory peritoneal dialysis (CAPD). Peritoneal Dial Bull 3: 138, 1983

22. Williams PF, Marliss EB, Anderson GH, Oren A, Stein AN, Khanna R, Pettit J, Brandes L, Rodella H, Mupas L, Dombros N, and Oreopoulos JDG: Amino acid absorption following intraperitoneal administration in CAPD patients. Peritoneal Dial Bull 2: 124, 1982

T.H.J. Goodship, B. Clayton, D. Rodham, M.K. Ward, and D.N.S. Kerr

77

Total Body Potassium and Fat Free Mass in CAPD

SUMMARY

Total body potassium and fat free mass were measured in 52 CAPD patients and 52 age-matched controls. Hand-grip strength and anthropometric measurements were also made in order to measure nutritional status in the two groups. Total body potassium correlated less well with free fat mass (and quantitatively was less) in CAPD patients than in normal controls. Anthropometric measurements, however, were not different in the two groups, suggesting that total body potassium measurements in CAPD patients do not specifically reflect protein stores. Protein-calorie malnutrition was no more common in CAPD patients than in normal controls.

INTRODUCTION

Protein-calorie malnutrition is one of the complications associated with CAPD. Persisting uremia, loss of appetite, and loss of protein and amino acids in the peritoneal dialysate may be important in its etiology.[1] The diagnosis of malnutrition, both clinically and in research, relies on the use of indicators of nutritional status that are accurate, precise, sensitive and specific.[2,3] Total body potassium (TBK) and anthropometric assessment of fat free mass (FFM) are two measurements that are commonly used. In this study we have looked at the relationship between TBK and FFM in normal subjects and

From the Departments of Medicine and Medical Physics, University of Newcastle upon Tyne, England.

patients with chronic renal failure treated by CAPD. At the same time we have compared nutritional status in the two groups using anthropometric data.

METHODS

Subjects

Fifty-two patients on CAPD and 52 age- and sex-matched volunteers were studied. There were 28 male and 24 female subjects in each group. The mean ($\pm$ SD) age of the CAPD patients was 46.3 $\pm$ 1.9 years, and of the normal volunteers was 45.1 $\pm$ 2.0 years. The mean time on dialysis of the CAPD patients was 18.1 $\pm$ 1.7 months. The volunteers were all in good health and taking no medication known to affect the measurement of TBK or nutritional status. Approval for the study and the use of the radioisotope ^{42}K in a subgroup of both patients and normal volunteers was given by the ethical committee of the Newcastle Area Health Authority.

Measurement of Total Body Potassium

TBK was measured using a shadow shield whole body counter to detect the naturally occurring radioisotope ^{40}K, which constitutes approximately 0.012% of all potassium. In order to derive TBK from the counts obtained from the gamma emission of ^{40}K it is necessary to apply a calibration factor to the ratio of the counts obtained from the subject and a phantom containing a known amount of potassium.[4]

Table 1. Anthropometric Measurements.

	CAPD	Normal	
Weight (kg)	67.8 ± 1.8	67.9 ± 1.7	NS
Height (m)	1.67 ± 0.01	1.68 ± 0.01	NS
BMI (wt/ht²)	24.3 ± 0.5	24.0 ± 0.5*	NS
% Fat	25.6 ± 1.3	26.9 ± 1.1	NS
FFM (kg)	50.2 ± 1.4	49.6 ± 1.4	NS
AMA (mm²)	4474 ± 158	4540 ± 170	NS

* Acceptable range = 20.1–25.0.

$$TBK \ (g) \ = \ \frac{(subject \ ^{40}K \ CPM) \times F}{(phantom \ ^{40}K \ CPM/g \ K)}$$

F depends upon the physical characteristics of the subject, notably the height and weight. F was determined by giving an oral dose of 10 μCi of the radioisotope ^{42}K to 29 CAPD patients and 28 normal volunteers. Urine and dialysis effluent were collected for the 24-hour period between administration of the ^{42}K and whole body counting to determine the interim loss of radioactivity. F was then determined from Equation (1):

$$F \ = \ \frac{CPM/\ \mu Ci^{42}K \ phantom}{CPM/\ \mu Ci^{42}K \ subject} \qquad (1)$$

A regression equation was computed by the least squares method, relating F and the weight (W)

Table 2. Hand-grip in the Dominant and Nondominant Hand.

	CAPD	Normal	
Dominant	33.7 ± 1.3	41.1 ± 1.9	p < 0.01
Nondominant	32.9 ± 1.5	37.2 ± 1.7	NS

and height (H) of the subject. For volunteers and patients combined:

$$F \ = \ 0.26 + 0.0075 \ W + 0.00017 \ H \qquad (2)$$

No significant difference was found between the regression equations for each individual group, and the above equation was therefore used in all the studies.

Anthropometric Measurements

The subjects weight and height were measured in light indoor clothing without shoes. Skin-fold thicknesses were measured using Harpenden calipers at the triceps, biceps, suprailiac, and subscapular sites on the left side. If the patient had a fistula on that side, the other arm was used. Mid-arm circumference was measured on the same side. The mean of five measurements at each site was used. Hand-grip was measured for both hands using a Harpenden hand-grip dynamometer, and the greatest of three readings for each hand was taken. Per-

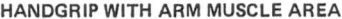

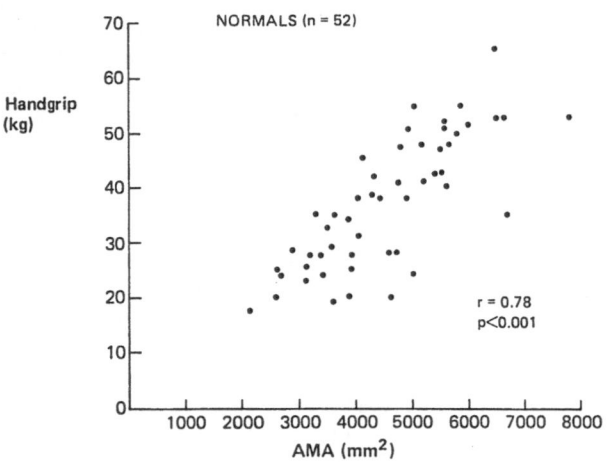

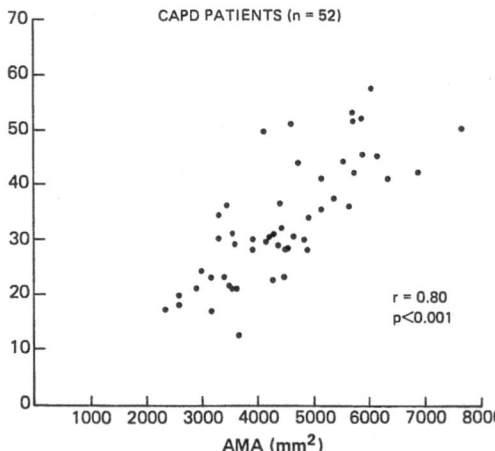

Fig. 1. Relationship between hand-grip and arm muscle area in normal subjects and CAPD patients.

centage fat was calculated using the regression equations from Durnin and Womersley.[5] Arm muscle area (AMA) was calculated according to the method of Frisancho.[6] Body mass index (BMI) was calculated from weight/(height × height).

RESULTS

The results of the anthropometric assessment (Table 1) showed no significant difference in the weight, height, % fat, FFM, or AMA of the two groups. BMI provides a crude index of obesity[7]; there was no significant difference between the two groups, and both lie within what is quoted to be an acceptable range.

Hand-grip was weaker in the CAPD patients in both the dominant and nondominant hand, significantly so in the former (Table 2). There was a good correlation in both groups between hand-grip and arm muscle area (Fig. 1). The total body potassium results have been expressed both corrected and uncorrected for weight and fat free mass (Table 3). In all three ways, TBK was significantly lower in the CAPD patients. In both groups there was a good correlation between TBK and FFM (Fig. 2). It is

Table 3. TBK Corrected and Uncorrected for FFM.

	CAPD	Normal	
TBK (g)	106 ± 3	116 ± 4	p < 0.05
g/kg weight	1.59 ± 0.04	1.71 ± 0.04	p < 0.05
g/kg FFM	2.12 ± 0.04	2.33 ± 0.03	p < 0.001

noticeable, however, that the scatter was greater and the correlation weaker in the CAPD patients.

DISCUSSION

The interpretation of anthropometric measurements and TBK in patients on CAPD is difficult. The major problem associated with the measurement of skinfold thickness is that the regression equations used are drawn from a different population from the one to which they are applied. Moreover the extent to which tissue turgor and edema affect the measurement of skinfold thickness in CAPD patients is not certain.

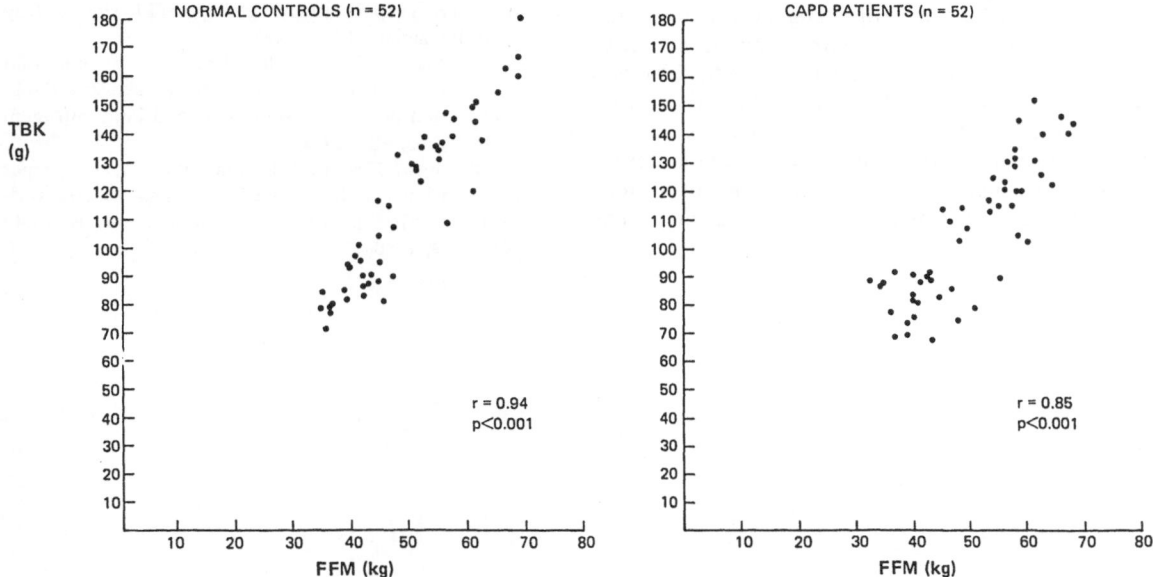

Fig. 2. Relationship between total body potassium and fat free mass in normal subjects and CAPD patients.

The use of TBK as an accurate indicator of protein status in CAPD patients has been questioned. Heide et al.[1] in a longitudinal survey of nutritional status found that total body nitrogen decreased with time on CAPD whilst TBK increased. In normal volunteers a close correlation between total body nitrogen and TBK has been found.[8] This suggests that other factors apart from protein status may be affecting the measurement of TBK in CAPD patients. Our finding that TBK correlated less well with fat free mass in CAPD patients than normal volunteers supports this hypothesis. Likewise, the finding that total body potassium was lower in CAPD patients whilst anthropometric assessment of protein stores showed no difference suggests loss of specificity. The way to determine which more accurately reflects protein stores would be to measure total body nitrogen as well. Studies comparing fat free mass, TBK, and total body nitrogen in normal volunteers have shown a good correlation amongst all three patients.[8]

The measurement of hand-grip has been proposed as an accurate indicator of functional nutritional status. In surgical patients it has been found to be of prognostic value for postoperative complications.[9] Its measurement in CAPD patients may be limited by other factors affecting muscle power. Although none of our patients had clinical evidence of a neuropathy, without electromyography it is impossible to say that the lower hand-grip strength we observed was not due to peripheral neuropathy.

In conclusion, this study suggests that protein calorie malnutrition is no more common in CAPD patients than normal volunteers, as judged by anthropometric assessment. Although TBK correlates well with FFM in CAPD patients, the observation that it does not do so as well as in normal volunteers, suggests that use of TBK as in indicator of protein status may not have as much "power" as in normal subjects.

ACKNOWLEDGMENT

Supported by MRC Project Grant No. G8115291SB.

REFERENCES

1. Heide B, Pierratos A, Khanna R, Pettit J, Ogilvie R, Harrison J, McNeil K, and Oreopoulos DG: Nutritional status of patients undergoing CAPD. Peritoneal Dial Bull 3: 138, 1983
2. Haas JD, and Flegal KM: Anthropometric measurements. In Newell GR, and Ellison NM (Eds), Nutrition and cancer: Etiology and treatment. New York: Raven Press, 1981, p 123
3. Katch FI, and Katch VL: Measurement and prediction errors in body composition assessment and the search for the perfect prediction equation. Res Exercise Sport 51: 249, 1980
4. Boddy K, King PC, Tothill P, and Strong JA: Measurement of total body potassium with a Shadow Shield whole-body counter: Calibration and errors. Phys Med Biol 16: 275, 1971
5. Durnin JVGA, and Womersley J: Body fat assessed from total body density and its estimation from skinfold thicknesses; measurements on 481 men and women aged from 16 to 72 years. Br J Nutr 32: 77, 1974
6. Frisancho AR: Triceps skinfold and upper arm size norms for assessment of nutritional status. Am J Clin Nutr 27: 1052, 1974
7. Obesity. A report of Royal College of Physicians. Roy Coll Physicians 17: 5, 1983
8. Morgan DB, and Burkinshaw L: Estimation of non-fat body tissues from measurements of skinfold thickness, total body potassium and total body nitrogen. Clin Sci 65: 407, 1983
9. Klidjian AM, Foster KJ, Kammerling RM, and Cooper A: Relation of anthropometric and dynamometric variables to serious postoperative complications. Br Med J 281: 899, 1980

A. Oren, R. Bernhard, L.J. Riley, Jr., P. Mojaverian,
and R.K. Ferguson

78

Effect of Increased Insulin Secretion during CAPD on Potassium Metabolism

SUMMARY

The explanation for control of plasma potassium in patients undergoing CAPD despite low removal rates was studied in Sprague-Dawley rats. Decrements in serum potassium concentrations correlated with absorption of glucose from dialysate and the insulin response to it. In a group that also received somatostatin, the rise in insulin was blunted and there was less of a fall in serum potassium. A reactivation of the inhibited cell membrane Na-K-ATPase may promote the cellular uptake of potassium.

INTRODUCTION

In 1982, Oreopoulos and Khanna,[1] summarizing the five-year experience with CAPD, noted that a major medical advantage over hemodialysis, along with better control of anemia and control of hypertension, was control of serum potassium. "While CAPD removes a relatively small amount of potassium (30 to 35 mEq/day), for reasons that are not well explained, serum potassium remains low or normal even though these patients enjoy a diet without potassium restriction."[1] Blumenkrantz et al.[2] reported a lower mean clearance of potassium with CAPD of 65 ± 2.5 L/week, compared to calculated

values of 80 to 90 L/week for potassium dialysance during hemodialysis. In view of these circumstances, the normal or low serum potassium of CAPD patients is most likely associated with either potassium retention in the body or high fecal potassium losses, or both.[2-4] Williams et al.[5] measured changes in total body potassium in 13 CAPD patients and observed that, concurrent with the decrease in total body nitrogen, probably reflecting protein and amino acid losses with dialysate, these patients had sustained elevations in total body potassium (TBK) with time. Since serum potassium levels remained within normal range or sometimes even lower, it is conceivable that intracellular potassium accumulates during CAPD.

To determine the mechanism of such transcellular potassium redistribution, the secretion of insulin, stimulated by continuous glucose absorption from dialysate with each exchange on CAPD was studied. The effect of insulin on enhancing the cellular uptake of potassium is well known.[6-7] This ability of insulin to accelerate transcellular shifts of potassium is used clinically in the treatment of acute hyperkalemia.[8] The purpose of this work was to elucidate the role of insulin on potassium distribution in a rat model of CAPD.

MATERIALS AND METHODS

All experiments were performed on 18 male Sprague-Dawley rats, 250–300 g, (Charles River Breeding Lakes, Wilmington, DE). Renal dysfunc-

From the Division of Clinical Pharmacology, Department of Medicine, Jefferson Medical College, Philadelphia, Pennsylvania.

tion was produced by a single intravenous injection of uranyl nitrate, 5 mg/kg[9] as a 5 mg/ml solution via a permanent jugular vein cannula. On the sixth day following uranyl nitrate injection, 7 ml of peritoneal dialysis solution containing 4.25% dextrose was injected IP in each of six rats, while three other rats were given IP injections of an equal volume of normal saline. Blood samples were collected before IP injection (time 0) and at 0.5, 2, 4, 6, and 24 hours thereafter. Nine additional rats were similarly cannulated and injected with uranyl nitrate and were studied in a second experiment. Three rats received an intravenous injection of somatostatin (Wyeth Laboratories), 250 mg/kg, a small polypeptide that has been shown to inhibit glucose-induced synthesis and secretion of insulin.[10] In six other rats, an equal volume of normal saline was administered by IV injection. Peritoneal dialysis fluid was instilled in all nine rats immediately after the IV infusion. Blood samples were taken prior to IV infusion (time 0) and at 0.5, 1, 2, 4, and 6 hours after injection of peritoneal dialysis solution. In the six rats that did not receive somatostatin, another peritoneal dialysis fluid infusion was begun at the completion of the six-hour dwell time. Blood samples were collected from these rats 30 minutes after this second peritoneal infusion.

The blood samples were analyzed for concentration of serum potassium by Digital Flame Photometer (Instrumentation Laboratory, Inc.), insulin by the radioimmunoassay technique (Micromedic system), and glucose by the colorimetric method at 520 nm (Sigma Diagnostic Kit). Student's paired t test was used for intragroup and unpaired-for intergroup comparison.

RESULTS

On the sixth day after uranyl nitrate injection, all rats demonstrated deterioration of kidney function as evidenced by serum creatinine concentrations ranging from 4.8–7.0 mg/dl and BUN levels of 142–209 mg/dl. Mean serum potassium before uranyl nitrate injection was 4.1 ± 0.3 mEq/L and increased on the sixth day to 5.2 ± 0.6 mEq/L.

Within 30 minutes after IP administration of dialysis fluid in six rats, mean serum potassium decreased from 5.2 ± 0.6 to 4.6 ± 0.6 mEq/L ($p < 0.05$) and remained at this level for the following six hours (Fig. 1). Serum potassium subsequently increased in these rats toward baseline at 24 hours after the start of the peritoneal infusion. In the group of rats that received normal saline IP, no changes in serum potassium concentration were observed throughout

the experiment (Fig. 1). The mean changes in serum concentrations of glucose, insulin, and potassium in six rats are illustrated in Figure 2. The fall in serum potassium after the first administration of peritoneal dialysate corresponds to the peak levels of serum glucose and insulin concentrations. The second peritoneal infusion, six hours later, resulted in a similar increase in serum glucose and insulin concentration, but without the change in serum potassium concentration.

In the three rats that received the somatostatin infusion, an increase in serum glucose at 30 minutes was similar to that observed in the six rats that received IV normal saline (from 126 ± 13 to 226 ± 14 mg/dl and from 188 ± 23 to 261 ± 37 mg/dl, respectively). However, the rats administered somatostatin had a smaller rise in serum insulin (from 10.6 ± 1.6 to 24.4 ± 13.6 μU/ml versus from 10.8 ± 2.4 to 37.7 ± 13.1 μU/ml in the control group), and a correspondingly small decrease in serum potassium concentration (from 5.2 ± 0.6 to 4.9 ± 0.4 mEq/L) ($p < 0.01$ and < 0.05, respectively). Figure 3 illustrates the mean changes in serum glucose, insulin, and potassium concentrations of these two groups of rats 30 minutes after instillation of peritoneal dialysate.

DISCUSSION

While patients with ESRD may exhibit high or normal serum potassium levels, most of them are TBK deficient.[11] The skeletal muscles of uremic patients have revealed significant decreases in intracellular potassium and increases in intracellular sodium.[12,13] Although this abnormality can be temporarily corrected by hemodialysis,[12,13] the majority of chronic hemodialysis patients still have significant deficits in TBK stores.[14,15]

In 1964, Welt et al.[16] described an electrolyte abnormality in red blood cells of uremic patients and presented evidence that activity of the Na-K pump responsible for potassium influx was diminished in uremics as compared with normals. They suggested that uremia produces inhibition of some alkali-metal sensitive component of adenosine-triphosphatase (Na-K-ATPase) that determines active transport of sodium from the cells and accumulation of potassium in the cell interior.[17,18] Many subsequent investigations confirmed this theory; activity of Na-K-ATPase appeared to be reduced in advanced renal failure.[19–23] Whether this inhibition is due to a circulating natriuretic factor[24] or to other uremic toxins or conditions remains to be determined.

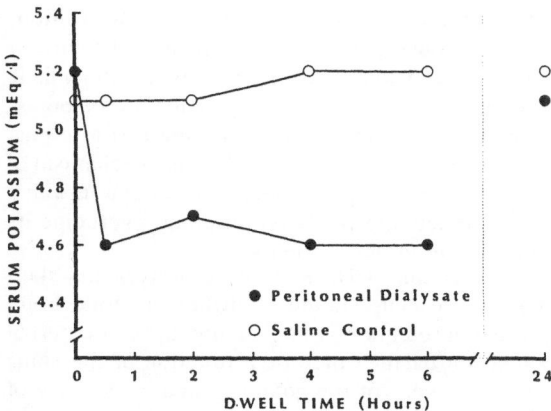

Fig. 1. Mean serum potassium concentration of rats that received intraperitoneal dialysate (n = 6) and rats that received intraperitoneally normal saline (n = 3).

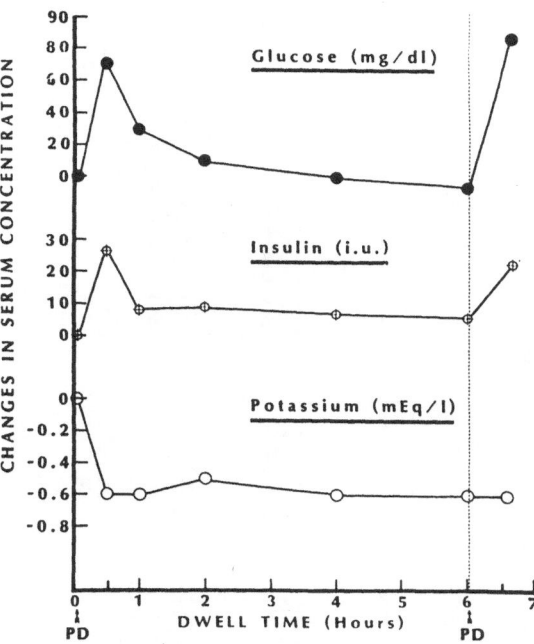

Fig. 2. Mean changes in serum glucose, insulin and potassium concentrations (n = 6). Peritoneal dialysate was instilled immediately after blood sampling at time 0 and 6 hours.

With an impaired sodium-potassium pump, the role of insulin as stimulator of cellular potassium uptake may become more important. Lack of insulin in uremic diabetics probably contributes to their tendency to develop hyperkalemia.[11] It is also possible that insulin resistance or inhibition of insulin activity in uremia[25] created a relative insulinopenic condition where more insulin is necessary to provide an adequate potassium influx into cells.[26] Westervelt[27] found that the rate of potassium uptake by skeletal muscle was abnormal in uremic patients. However, during insulin infusion in these patients, response of potassium uptake was quite similar to that of normal subjects. Early studies by Zierler[28] provided evidence that insulin-mediated potassium transfer in muscle occurs independently of glucose. He suggested that insulin hyperpolarizes the muscle membrane by some unexplained mechanism, thereby enhancing potassium transport into muscle cells. Analysis of this mechanism of insulin action was also undertaken by Moore.[29] His experiments on frog skeletal muscle indicated that insulin, in some way, increases the activity of the Na-K pump. Later observations confirmed that insulin, in fact, stimulates the activity of Na-K-ATPase.[30] When Na-K-ATPase was inhibited by ouabain, large concentrations of insulin were shown to overcome this inhibition and stimulate potassium influx. On the other hand, when activity of the pump was maximally stimulated, insulin had no additional effect.

In the present study, intravenous infusion or uranyl nitrate produced advanced renal failure with a rise in serum creatinine up to 7.0 mg/dl within six days. An increase in serum potassium from 4.1–5.2 mEq/L was assumed to be a function of renal failure and at least partially due to compromised activity of Na-K-ATPase. Following the intraperitoneal administration of glucose-containing dialysate, plasma insulin concentrations began to rise, reaching peak levels within the first 30 minutes. Simultaneously, serum potassium concentrations dropped significantly in all rats. A transcellular shift of potassium from serum to cells, perhaps reflecting enhanced activation of Na-K-ATPase, was a likely explanation for this rapid change in serum potassium. Although glucose absorption from dialysate continued and insulin levels remained stimulated for the subsequent hours, no additional changes in potassium concentration were observed. Furthermore, serum potassium remained stable when a second peritoneal exchange was administered six hours later, despite similar elevations in plasma glucose and insulin. This could indicate that maximal activation of Na-K-ATPase in these rats was achieved during the first exchange. This self-limiting mechanism seems to be very important and may explain why marked hypo-

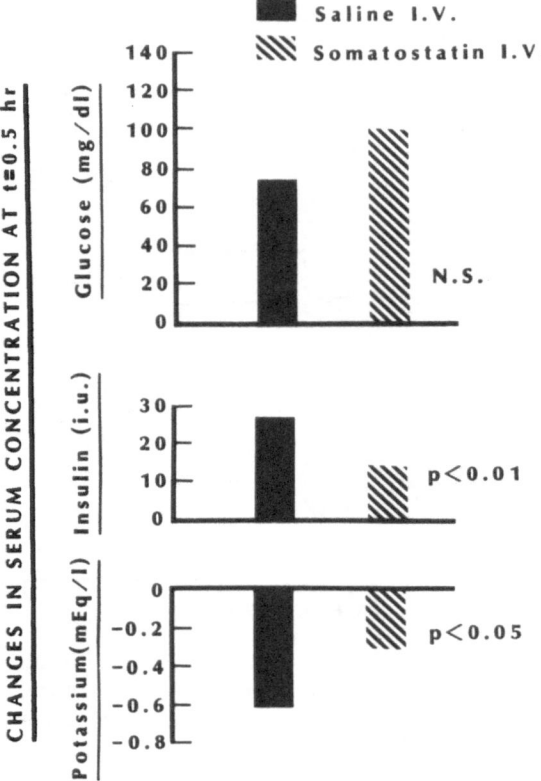

CHANGES IN SERUM CONCENTRATION AT t=0.5 hr

■ Saline I.V.

▨ Somatostatin I.V.

Fig. 3. Mean changes in serum glucose, insulin and potassium concentrations within 30 minutes of instillation of peritoneal dialysate in rats that received IV normal saline (n = 6) and rats that received IV somatostatin (n = 3).

kalemia is rare in CAPD patients, even though enhanced insulin secretion occurred with each exchange. When somatostatin was administered, insulin hypersecretion in response to glucose absorption was partially blocked. Activation of Na-K-ATPase at this insulin level was probably incomplete, and consequently, smaller decreases in serum potassium were observed.

Recent data show that, during CAPD, continuous absorption of glucose induces an increased production of proinsulin and results in hyperinsulinemia, which persists for a longer period of time than that which occurs after an oral load of the same amount of glucose.[31] The repeated challenges with a high peritoneal glucose load per exchange (approximately every 6 hours) exaggerates insulin production, which becomes essentially permanent in CAPD patients. In diabetic patients, the same state is

achieved due to exogenous insulin administration, which is adjusted to the glucose load.[32] The current study suggests that this chronic hyperinsulinemia is responsible for returning cellular uptake of potassium toward normal and decreasing serum potassium levels in patients on CAPD. The mechanism of this action may well be mediated through insulin's ability to activate Na-K-ATPase and overcome its inhibition in uremic patients.

Activation of Na-K-ATPase in liver and skeletal muscle cells should contribute to total body potassium retention, while maintenance of external potassium balance may be a function of the same process in cells of the colonic mucosa. Activity of Na-K-ATPase in these cells is stimulated in normal individuals with increased potassium intake, augmenting fecal potassium output,[33] which was proposed as an important pathway for maintenance of potassium balance in severely uremic patients.[34] Increased potassium excretion and sodium absorption in the colon of rats with renal insufficiency, fed high potassium diets, were found to be accompanied by increased activity of Na-K-ATPase in colonic mucosal cells.[35] One could assume that the net effect of uremic inhibition and insulin stimulation of Na-K-ATPase during CAPD is a further activation of the colonic mucosal Na-K-ATPase, which allows these patients to increase their fecal potassium. Indeed, Blumenkrantz et al.[2] reported that fecal potassium losses of patients on CAPD correlated significantly with dietary potassium intake.

In addition to control of serum potassium, other notable features of CAPD, such as control of anemia and hypertension, might also be explained on the basis of insulin-stimulated Na-K-ATPase activity. With depressed erythropoiesis, the minimal hemolysis observed in patients with chronic renal failure becomes a major cause of anemia.[36–39] Early studies on red blood cells from uremic patients revealed that the shortened survival of these cells was accompanied by a decrease in their potassium concentration.[36,40] High sodium, low potassium red blood cells have been described in a wide variety of states as a cause of hemolysis probably due to osmotic fragility.[41] Thus, uremic inhibition of Na-K-ATPase appeared to be responsible for hemolysis and, coupled with deficiency of erythropoietin, for anemia in chronic renal failure.[38] The dramatic increase in hemoglobin after initiation of CAPD[42–44] may be a consequence of reactivation of Na-K-ATPase by insulin and restoration of a normal red blood cell electrolyte concentration with prolongation of their survival time. It was recently reported that red cell survival of patients on CAPD was significantly

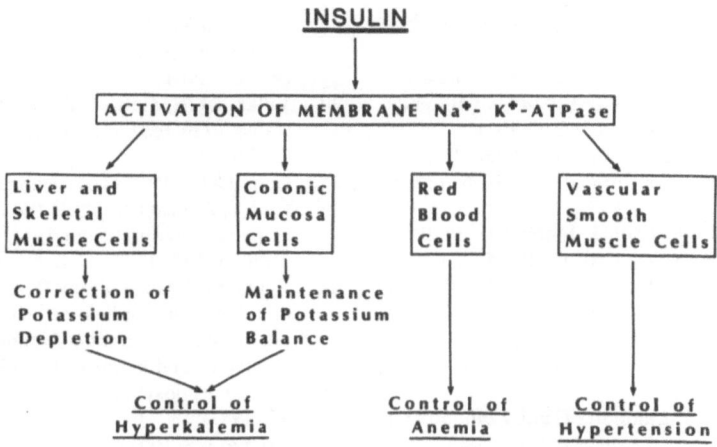

Fig. 4. Hypothetical scheme of benefits provided by insulin hypersecretion during CAPD.

longer than that of patient on hemodialysis, and that it increased with time on CAPD.[45,46]

Inhibition of Na-K-ATPase in vascular smooth muscle cells may be an important factor in the pathogenesis of hypertension.[47] Whether this defect is a result of putative inherited factors as in essential hypertension,[48] or acquired as in secondary hypertension,[49-51] it causes accumulation of intracellular sodium and free calcium in vascular smooth muscle,[52,53] which increases vascular tone and elevates arterial pressure.[54] It might be that counteracting this mechanism by reactivation of Na-K-ATPase is responsible for reducing the CAPD patient's need for antihypertensive medications. Consequently, the only requirement for maintenance of normotension becomes controlled balance of body fluid.[55]

In conclusion, increased secretion of insulin following glucose absorption via the peritoneal route appears to be responsible for the decrease in serum potassium concentration in uranyl nitrate induced uremic rats. A possible explanation for this phenomenon is reactivation of the inhibited cell membrane Na-K-ATPase by hyperinsulinemia and promotion of cellular potassium uptake.

We suggest that such stimulation of Na-K-ATPase (Fig. 4) may be a common mechanism operating in patients on CAPD to produce the following favorable effects:

1. Total body potassium depletion is corrected mainly due to Na-K pump stimulation in skeletal muscle cells.
2. Further activation of Na-K-ATPase in colonic mucosal cells may enhance the ability to excrete fecal potassium in larger amounts in response to dietary potassium intake, possibly representing a major mechanism for maintenance of potassium balance on CAPD. Together, these two events can explain the observed control of hyperkalemia in patients on CAPD.
3. Reactivation of Na-K-ATPase restores normal Na/K ratio in red blood cells, possibly contributing to prolongation of their survival with consequent control of anemia in CAPD patients.
4. In vascular smooth muscle cells, activation of Na-K-ATPase can be expected to release intracellular sodium and free calcium, providing an important factor in the control of hypertension.

We believe that this unifying theory of CAPD benefits needs to be tested and compels further investigation.

ACKNOWLEDGMENT

We thank Dr. Erick L. Lien, Wyeth Laboratories, Radnor, Pennsylvania, for providing somatostatin for this study.

REFERENCES

1. Oreopoulos DG, and Khanna R: The present and future role of continuous ambulatory peritoneal dialysis (CAPD). Am J Kidney Dis 2: 381, 1982
2. Blumenkrantz MJ, Kopple JD, Moran JK, and Coburn JW: Metabolic balance studies and dietary protein requirements in patients undergoing continu-

ous ambulatory peritoneal dialysis. Kidney Int 21: 849, 1982

3. Moncrief JW: Continuous ambulatory peritoneal dialysis: Impact on management of patients with end-stage renal disease. Nephron 27: 226, 1981

4. Oreopoulos DG, Khanna R, Williams P, and Vas SI: Continuous ambulatory peritoneal dialysis. Nephron 30: 293, 1982

5. Williams P, Kay R, Harrison J, McNeil K. Pettit J, Kelman B, Mendez M, Klein M, Ogilvie R, Khanna R, Carmichael D, and Oreopoulos DG: Nutritional and anthropometric assessment of patients on CAPD over one year: Contrasting changes in total body nitrogen and potassium. Peritoneal Dial Bull 1: 82, 1981

6. Kestens PJ, Haxhe JJ, Lambotte I, and Lambotte C: The effect of insulin on the uptake of potassium and phosphate by the isolated perfused canine liver. Metabolism 12: 941, 1963

7. DeFronzo R, Felig P, Ferrannini E, and Wahren J; Effect of graded doses of insulin on splanchnic and peripheral potassium metabolism in man. Am J Physiol 238: 421, 1980

8. Bricker NS: Acute renal failure. In Beeson P, and McDermott N (Eds), Textbook of medicine. Philadelphia: WB Saunders Company, 1975, p 1107

9. Giacomini KM, Roberts SM, and Levy G: Evaluation of methods for producing renal dysfunction in rats. J Pharm Sci 70: 117, 1981

10. Bent-Hansen L, Capito K, and Hedeskov CJ: The effect of calcium on somatostatin inhibition of insulin release and cyclic AMP production in mouse pancreatic islets. Biochim Biophys Acta 585: 240, 1979

11. van Ypersele de Strihou C: Potassium homeostasis in renal failure. Kidney Int 11: 491, 1977

12. Bilbrey GL, Carber NW, White MG, Schilling JF, and Knochel JP: Potassium deficiency in chronic renal failure. Kidney Int 4: 423, 1973

13. Cotton JR, Woodard T, Carter NW, and Knochel JP: Resting skeletal muscle membrane potential as an index of uremic toxicity. J Clin Invest 63: 501, 1979

14. Seedat YK: Exchangeable potassium study in patients undergoing chronic hemodialysis. Br Med J 2: 344, 1969

15. Butkus DE, Alfrey AC, and Miller NL: Tissue potassium in chronic dialysis patients. Nephron 13: 314, 1974

16. Welt LG, Sachs JR, and McManus TJ: An ion transport defect in erythrocytes from uremic subjects. Trans Assoc Am Phys 77: 169, 1964

17. Whittam R: Potassium movements and ATP in human red cells. J Physiol 140: 479, 1958

18. Post RL, Merritt CR, Kinsolving CR, and Albright CD: Membrane adenosine triphosphatase as a participant in the active transport of sodium and potassium in the human erythrocyte. J Biol Chem 235: 1796, 1960

19. Kuroyanagi T, Kurisu A, Sugiyama H, and Saito M: The ADP and ATP levels and the phosphorylating

activity of erythrocytes in patients with uremia associated with chronic renal failure. Tohoku J Exp Med 84: 105, 1964

20. Villamil MF, Rettori V, and Kleeman CR: Sodium transport by red blood cells in uremia. J Lab Clin Med 72: 308, 1968

21. Cole CH: Decreased ouabain-sensitive adenosine triphosphatase activity in the erythrocyte membrane of patients with chronic renal disease. Clin Sci Mol Med 45: 775, 1973

22. Kramer HJ, Gospodinov D, and Kruck F: Functional and metabolic studies on red blood cell sodium transport in chronic uremia. Nephron 16: 344, 1976

23. Walter U, and Becht E: Red blood cell sodium transport and phosphate release in uremia. Nephron 34: 35, 1983

24. Bricker NS, Bourgoignie JJ, and Klahr A: A humoral inhibitor of sodium transport in uremic serum. Arch Intern Med 126: 860, 1970

25. Mondon CE, Dolkas CB, and Reaven GM: The site of insulin resistance in acute uremia. Diabetes 27: 571, 1978

26. Knochel JP: Role of glucoregulatory hormones in potassium homeostasis. Kidney Int 11: 443, 1977

27. Westervelt FB: Insulin effect in uremia. J Lab Clin Med 74: 79, 1969

28. Zierler KL: Hyperpolarization of muscle by insulin in a glucose-free environment. Am J Physiol 197: 524, 1959

29. Moore RD: Effect of insulin upon the sodium pump in frog skeletal muscle. J Physiol 232: 23, 1973

30. Gaveryck WA, Moore RD, and Thompson RC: Effect of insulin upon membrane-bound (Na$^+$-K$^+$)-ATPase extracted from frog skeletal muscle. J Physiol 252: 43, 1975

31. Wideroe T-E, Smeby LC, and Myking OL: Plasma concentrations and transperitoneal transport of native insulin and C-peptide in patients on continuous ambulatory peritoneal dialysis. Kidney Int 25: 82, 1984

32. Wideroe T-E, Smeby LC, Berg KJ, Jorstad S, and Svartas TM: Intraperitoneal (^{125}I) insulin absorption during intermittent and continuous peritoneal dialysis. Kidney Int 23: 22, 1983

33. Silva P, Charney AN, and Epstein FH: Potassium adaptation and Na-K-ATPase activity in mucosa of colon. Am J Physiol 229: 1576, 1975

34. Hayes Jr CP, McLeod MI, and Robinson R: An extrarenal mechanism for the maintenance of potassium balance in severe chronic renal failure. Trans Assoc Am Phys 80: 207, 1967

35. Bastl C, Hayslett JP, and Binder HJ: Increased large intestinal secretion of potassium in renal insufficiency. Kidney Int 12: 9, 1977

36. Giovannetti S, Balestri PL, and Cioni L: Spontaneous in vitro autohaemolysis of blood from chronic uraemic patients. Clin Sci 29: 407, 1965

37. Shaw AB: Haemolysis in chronic renal failure. Br Med J 2: 213, 1967

38. Cohen BD: Uremia and blood cell dysfunction. Adv Intern Med 19: 27, 1974

39. Hocken AG: Haemolysis in chronic renal failure. Nephron 32: 28, 1982

40. Rees SB, Scheitlin WG, Pond JC, McManus TJ, Guild WR, and Merrill JR: Effect of dialysis and purine ribosides upon the anemia of uremia. J Clin Invest 36: 923, 1957

41. Parker JC, and Welt LG: Pathological alterations of cation movements in red blood cells. Arch Intern Med 129: 320, 1972

42. Oreopoulos DG, Dombros, N, Robson M, and Pierratos A: First year's experience with continuous ambulatory peritoneal dialysis (CAPD). Trans Am Soc Artif Intern Organs 8: 242, 1978

43. Moncrief JW, Nolph KD, Rubin J, and Popovich RP: Additional experience with continuous ambulatory peritoneal dialysis (CAPD). Trans Am Soc Artif Intern Organs 24: 476, 1978

44. Gokal R, McHugh M, Fryer R, Ward MK, and Kerr DNS: One year's experience in a UK dialysis unit. Br Med J 281: 494, 1980

45. Summerfield GP, Gyde OHB, Forbes AMW, Goldsmith HJ, and Bellingham AJ: Haemoglobin concentration in patients on continuous ambulatory peritoneal dialysis (CAPD). Br J Haematol 51: 331, 1983

46. Salahudeen AK, Hawkins T, Keavey PM, and Wilkinson R: Is anaemia during continuous ambulatory peritoneal dialysis really better than during haemodialysis? Lancet 2: 1046, 1983

47. DeWardener HE, and MacGregor GA: The relation of a circulating sodium transport inhibitor (the natriuretic hormone?) to hypertension. Medicine 62: 310, 1983

48. Garay RP, Dagher G, Pernollet MG, Devynck MA, and Meyer P: Inherited defect in Na$^+$, K$^+$ co-transport system in erythrocytes from essential hypertensive patients. Nature 284: 281, 1980

49. Bricker NS: The control of sodium excretion with normal and reduced nephron populations: The pre-eminence of third factor. Am J Med 43: 313, 1967

50. Haddy FJ, and Overbeck HW: The role of humoral agents in volume expanded hypertension. Life Sci 19: 935, 1976

51. Huot S, Pamnani M, Clough D, and Haddy F: The role of sodium intake, the Na$^+$-K$^+$ pump and ouabain-like humoral agent in the genesis of reduced renal mass hypertension. Am J Nephrol 3: 92, 1983

52. Blaustein MP: Sodium ions, calcium ions, blood pressure regulation and hypertension: A reassessment and a hypothesis. Am J Physiol 232: C165, 1977

53. Haddy FJ: What is the link between vascular smooth muscle, sodium pump and hypertension? Clin Exp Hypertension 3: 179, 1981

54. Johansson B: Process involved in vascular smooth muscle contraction and relaxation. Circ Res 43(Suppl 1): 1, 1978

55. Khanna R, and Oreopoulos DG: Peritoneal dialysis. In Levine DZ (Ed), Care of the renal patient. Philadelphia: WB Saunders Company, 1983, p 322

J.W. Balfe, R.M. Hanning, and S.H. Zlotkin

79

Amino Acid Versus Glucose Dialysis in Children on CAPD

SUMMARY

Nineteen children on CAPD have undergone short-term trials wherein amino acids have substituted for dextrose as osmotic agents in peritoneal dialysis fluid. Amino acid concentrations of 1.1% and 2.0% had osmolal concentrations comparable to 2.5% and 4.25% dextrose. Maximal absorption of amino acids and dextrose occurred within 1 hour after instillation. Fluid, urea, and creatinine removal were satisfactory with the modified dialysis solution and no adverse effects were noted. Long-term trials are recommended.

INTRODUCTION

It is well recognized that children with chronic renal failure (CRF) grow poorly and are frequently malnourished. Inadequate dietary intake is only one of several factors that have been implicated in the etiology of the growth failure,[1-3] yet its importance must not be underestimated. Nutritional management of CRF usually involves the restriction of protein, phosphate, sodium, and potassium, which severely limits food selection for these often anorexic patients. With the introduction of dialysis, especially CAPD, more liberal diets may be prescribed.

From the University of Toronto and the Research Institute, The Hospital for Sick Children, Toronto, Ontario, Canada.

Pediatric CAPD has become increasingly popular since it was first introduced at The Hospital for Sick Children, Toronto, in 1978. Currently, over 40% of Canadian dialysis patients under 15 years of age are managed by CAPD.[4] Despite its popularity and a more permissive diet, CAPD has failed to normalize growth[1] and reverse the malnutrition of CRF.[5] Indeed, a number of nutrition-related problems have been identified in infants and children undergoing CAPD.

Traditionally, dextrose has been used as the osmotic agent in peritoneal dialysis solutions. Approximately 77% of the dextrose is absorbed during the course of a dialysis exchange,[6,7] with absorption being relatively greater on a per kilogram body weight basis in younger versus older children and children versus adult dialysis patients.[7] While dextrose absorbed from dialysate provides up to 21% of a child's caloric intake,[8] resultant episodes of elevated blood glucose may contribute to the decreased appetite[6] and the hypertriglyceridemia characteristically observed in CAPD patients.[9]

In addition, protein and amino acids are lost in effluent dialysis fluid. These losses amount to 8–10 g/day of protein[10-12] and 2–3.5 g/day of amino acids[13,10] in adult CAPD patients, and are relatively greater on a per kilogram body weight basis in infants and children.[7,14] Considering also the increased protein and amino acid requirements for growth, the losses in the young and often anorexic CAPD patients may be critical. It is unlikely that they may be easily replaced by increased dietary intake, as has been suggested in adults.[15]

Dombros et al.[12] found that amino acid losses in effluent dialysate are in proportion to their plasma concentrations. It therefore seems that CAPD neither improves nor worsens the abnormal plasma amino acid profile of uremia.

Alternative dialysis fluid osmotic agents have been sought. It appears that dextrose may not be the ideal dialysis fluid osmotic agent, especially for infants and children, and thus the use of alternatives such as xylitol and sorbitol have been investigated.[16] More recently, the use of amino acids has been proposed.[17, 18]

When we began our studies of the efficacy and short-term metabolic consequences of amino acid dialysis in children in 1982, amino acid dialysis was a very new concept. As early as 1968, Gjessing[20] demonstrated that amino acids could be absorbed across the peritoneum. In 1979, Kobayashi et al.[21] and Jackson et al.[22] reported that amino acids could be given via the peritoneal cavity and counteract dialy-

sis amino acid losses. Oreopoulos et at.[23] formulated amino acid solutions with comparable osmolalities to the traditional dextrose dialysis solutions used for CAPD patients. Trials of amino acid dialysis in rabbits and one adult patient by Oreopoulos et al.[24] and our own experience with one infant, indicated that

Table 1. Dialysis Solutions.*

2.5% dextrose	
1.1% amino acid (Travasol® based)	osmolality
1.3% amino acid (Vamin® based)	384
4.25% dextrose	
2.0% amino acid (Travasol® based)	osmolality
2.3% amino acid (Vamin® based)	463

* All dialysis fluids and Travasol® from Baxter Travenol (Deerfield, Michigan).
Vamin® from Pharmacia.

Table 2. Composition of Dialysis Solutions.

Dialysis Fluid (Composition/L)		4.25% dextrose (Baxter-Travenol)	2% Amino Acid (Travasol®-based)	2% Amino Acid (Vamin®-based)
dextrose, hydrous g		42.5	—	—
Na	mEq/L	132	132	132
Ca	mEq/L	3	3	4
Mg	mEq/L	1.5	1.5	2
Cl	mEq/L	102	113	108
Lactate		35	26	29
Acetate			13	
Na bisulfate			1	
L Leucine	mg		1238	1511
L Phenylalanine	mg		1238	1568
L Methionine	mg		1158	542
L Lysine	mg		1158	1112
L Isoleucine	mg		957	1112
L Valine	mg		917	1226
L Histidine	mg		877	684
L Threonine	mg		837	855
L Tryptophan	mg		360	285
L Alanine	gm		4.15	0.8555
Amino acetic acid	gm		4.15	—
L Arginine	mg		2075	941
L Proline	mg		837	2309
L Tyrosine	mg		80	143
L Cysteine/Cystine	mg			399
L Aspartic Acid	mg			1169
L Glutamic Acid	mg			2565
L Glycine	mg			599
L Serine	mg			2138

amino acids were effective dialysis osmotic agents, and showed promise in the reversal of hypoproteinemia and hypertriglyceridemia.

These early studies suggested that amino acid dialysis solutions would be as effective as dextrose-containing solutions, removing excess fluid and metabolic waste products, and yet would prevent the transient hyperglycemia and reverse the net loss of amino acids associated with dextrose dialysis.

As amino acids appear to be absorbed by diffusion,[25] it might also be possible to normalize the plasma and/or intracellular amino acid profile by altering the dialysis solution amino acid composition and thereby improve nitrogen balance[26] and growth.[27]

METHODS

Between February 1982 and June 1983, 19 patients with chronic renal failure (age 0.5–19 years) participated in a short-term trial of amino acid versus dextrose dialysis. Patients were studied over the course of four single fasted morning dialysis exchanges using each of four dialysis solutions in a randomly selected order. These comprised dextrose solutions at two concentrations, 2.5% and 4.25% (Dianeal®, Baxter-Travenol), and amino acid solutions at approximately 1.1 and 2.0% concentrations, the osmolal concentrations of which were comparable to the dextrose solutions (Table 1). In this way, each patient was able to act as his or her own control.

Blood and peritoneal fluid aliquots were samples over the course of the five-hour dialysis exchange. The blood glucose, amino acid, electrolyte, urea, creatinine, and insulin responses to the amino acid and glucose solutions were compared. Amino acid and glucose absorption from the respective dialysis solutions and losses in effluent dialysate were assessed. Changes in peritoneal fluid osmolality, urea, and creatinine concentrations were monitored and total protein, amino acid, albumin, and insulin losses were quantified.

The first nine patients were studied using amino acid solutions based on Travasol® (Baxter-Travenol), and solutions based on Vamin® (Pharmacia) were used on the latter group of children as described in Table 2. The plasma amino acid response to different amino acid concentrations and profiles could then be assessed.

Follow-up studies were made in a subsample of patients, using a similar protocol at a three-month follow-up period. The response to an amino acid dialysis exchange was also studied in the fed state. The blood glucose and amino acid levels at the time of peak absorbance from both the gastrointestinal tract and the peritoneal cavity could then be determined and potential amino acid toxicities and imbalances identified (Fig. 1).

RESULTS

We have found that maximal glucose and amino acid absorption from dialysate occurs within one hour after instillation. Gastrointestinal absorption

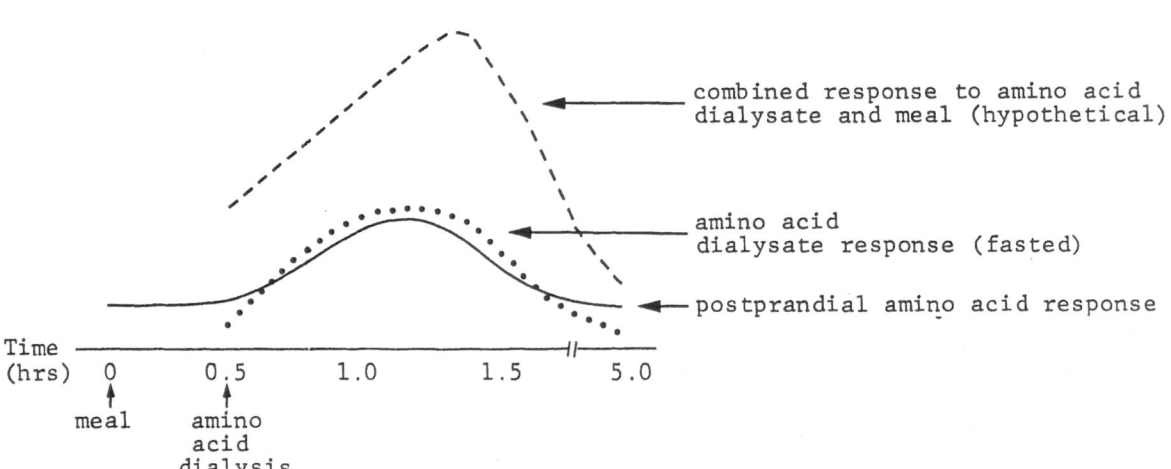

Fig. 1. Hypothetical plasma response to amino acid dialysate in the fed state.

rates for nutrients are variable, depending on the age of the child and the nutrient density and composition of the meal. In order to maintain uniform nutrient density and composition, a nutritionally complete food supplement (Ensure®, Ross Laboratories) was used in a fixed volume per kilogram body weight to each subject. A short pilot study showed that maximal plasma glucose and amino acid levels occur about 1.5 hours after the ingestion of this liquid meal.

DISCUSSION

The results of these studies have been reported in abstract form.[18,19] In general, our studies support the findings of Oreopoulos et al.[17] in adults. Amino acids appear to be effective osmotic agents in a dialysis solution and provide satisfactory fluid, urea, and creatinine removal. Amino acid dialysis solutions maintain normal blood glucose levels and result in net amino acid absorption.

The elevation of certain plasma amino acids at the end of a five-hour dialysis exchange with either Travasol® or Vamin® based solutions suggested that modification of the dialysate amino acid profiles used in these studies was needed. It is appreciated, however, that the abnormalities in plasma amino acids in uremia do not always reflect the larger intracellular amino acid pool.[28] The findings of Alvestrand et al.[26,29] that oral amino acid supplements can correct plasma and muscle amino acid abnormalities, and appear to improve nitrogen utilization in untreated uremic patients, is encouraging.

The success of the short-term studies has led us to consider the long-term use of amino acid dialysis in infants and children on CAPD. Using a new amino acid solution, we are currently assessing the daily use of one amino acid dialysis exchange versus exclusive dextrose dialysis in a three-month randomized crossover design trial. Amino acid administered via the peritoneal dialysis solution may provide the needed nutritional support for infants and children on CAPD and ultimately enhance growth.

ACKNOWLEDGMENTS

Supported in part by a grant from Baxter Travenol Canada.

REFERENCES

1. Stefanidis CJ, Hewitt IK, and Balfe JW: Growth in children receiving continuous ambulatory peritoneal dialysis. J Pediatr 102: 681, 1983
2. Hsu AC, Kooh SW, Fraser D, Cumming WA, and Fornasier VL: Renal osteodystrophy in children with chronic renal failure: An unexpectedly common and incapacitating complication. Pediatrics 70: 742, 1982
3. Holliday MA, and Chantler C: Metabolic and nutritional factors in children with renal insufficiency. Kidney Int 14: 306, 1978
4. Canadian Renal Failure Register: 1982 Report. Kidney Foundation of Canada.
5. Salusky IB, Fine RN, Nelson P, Blumenkrantz MJ, and Kopple JD: Nutritional status of children undergoing continuous ambulatory peritoneal dialysis. Am J Clin Nutr 38: 599, 1983
6. Grodstein GP, Blumenkrantz MJ, Kopple JD, Moran JK, and Coburn JW: Glucose absorption during continuous ambulatory peritoneal dialysis. Kidney Int 19: 564, 1981
7. Balfe JW, Vigneux A, Willumsen J, and Hardy BE: The use of CAPD in the treatment of children with end stage renal disease. Peritoneal Dial Bull 1: 35, 1981
8. Potter DE, McDaid TK, McHenry K, and Mar H: Continuous ambulatory peritoneal dialysis (CAPD) in children. Trans Am Soc Artif Intern Organs 27: 64, 1981
9. Moncrief J, Pyle W, Simon P, and Popovich R: Hypertriglyceridemia, diabetes mellitus and insulin administration in patients undergoing CAPD. In Moncrief JW, and Popovich (Eds), CAPD update. New York: Masson Publishing, 1981, p 143
10. Kopple JD, and Blumenkrantz MJ: Nutritional requirements for patients undergoing continuous ambulatory peritoneal dialysis. Kidney Int 24(Suppl 16): S295, 1983
11. Katirzoglou A, Oreopoulos DG, Husdan H, Leung M, Ogilvie R, and Dombros N: Reappraisal of protein losses in patients undergoing CAPD. Nephron 26: 230, 1980
12. Rubin J, Nolph KD, Arfania D, Prowant B, Fruto L, Brown P, and Moore H: Protein losses in continuous ambulatory peritoneal dialysis. Nephron 28: 218, 1981
13. Dombros N, Oren A, Marliss EB, Anderson GH, Stein AN, Khanna R, Petit J, Brandes L, Rodella H, Leibel BS, and Oreopoulos DE: Plasma amino acid profiles and amino acid losses in patients undergoing CAPD. Peritoneal Dial Bull 2: 27, 1982
14. Giordano C, DeSanto NG, Capodicasa G, DiLeo VA, Diserafi A, Cirillo D, Esposito R, Damiano M, and Buonadon L: Amino acid losses during CAPD in children. Int J Pediatr Nephrol 2: 85, 1981
15. Kopple JD, Blumenkrantz MJ, Jones MR, Moran JK, and Coburn JW: Plasma amino acid levels and amino acid losses during continuous ambulatory peritoneal dialysis. Am J Clin Nutr 36: 395, 1982
16. Wu G: Osmotic agents for peritoneal dialysis solutions. Peritoneal Dial Bull 2: 151, 1982
17. Oreopoulos DG, Marliss E, and Anderson GH: Nutritional aspects of CAPD and the potential use of amino

acid containing dialysis solutions. Peritoneal Dial Bull 3(Suppl): S10, 1983

18. Hanning RM, Balfe JW, and Zlotkin SH. The efficacy of amino acid vs glucose dialysis in children on continuous ambulatory peritoneal dialysis Pediatr Res (Abstract) 17: 1590, 1983

19. Balfe JW, Zlotkin SH, and Hanning RM: Amino acid vs glucose dialysis in children on continuous ambulatory peritoneal dialysis. Peritoneal Dial Bull 4(Suppl): S3, 1984

20. Gjessing J: Addition of acids to peritoneal dialysis fluid. Lancet 2: 812, 1968

21. Kobayashi K, Manji T, Hiramatsu S, Maeda K, and Uemura J: Nitrogen metabolism in patients on peritoneal dialysis. Contrib Nephrol 17: 93, 1979

22. Jackson M, Thomas D, Talbot S, and Lee H: Prevention of amino acid losses during peritoneal dialysis. Postgrad Med J 55: 533, 1979

23. Oreopoulos DG, Crassweller P, Katirtzoglou A, Ogilvie R, Zellerman G, Rodella H, and Vas SI: Amino acids as an osmotic agent (instead of glucose) in continuous ambulatory peritoneal dialysis. In Legrain M (Ed), Continuous ambulatory peritoneal dialysis: Proceedings of an international symposium, Paris, 1979. Amsterdam: Excerpta Medica, 1980, p 335

24. Oreopoulos DG, Balfe JW, Khanna R, Crassweller P, Gotloib L, Rodella H, Zellerman G, Brandes L, McReady W, Ogilvie R, and Husdan H: Further experience with the use of amino acid containing dialysate (amino-dianeal) in peritoneal dialysis. In Moncrief JW, and Popovich RP (Eds), CAPD update: continuous ambulatory peritoneal dialysis. New York: Masson Publishing, 1981, p 109

25. Williams PF, Marliss EB, Anderson GH, Oren A, Stein AN, Khanna R, Petitt J, Brandes L, Rodella H, Mupas L, Dombros N, and Oreopoulos DG: Amino acid absorption following intraperitoneal administration in CAPD patients. Peritoneal Dial Bull 2: 124, 1982

26. Alvestrand A, Fürst P, and Bergström J: Plasma and muscle free amino acids in uremia: Influence of nutrition with amino acids. Clin Nephrol 18: 297, 1982

27. Broyer M, Jean G, Dartois AM, and Kleinknecht C: Plasma and muscle free amino acids in children at the early stages of renal failure. Am J Clin Nutr 33:1396, 1980

28. Alvestrand A, Fürst P, and Bergström J: Intracellular amino acids in uremia. Kidney Int 24(Suppl 16): 9, 1983

29. Alvestrand A, Ahlberg M, Fürst P, and Bergström J: Clinical results of long-term treatment with a low protein diet and a new amino acid preparation in patients with chronic uremia. Clin Nephrol 19: 67, 1983

K.E. Bonzel, K. Bonatz, C. Senghaas, D.E. Mueller-Wiefel,
R. Wartha, N. Gretz, E. Moeller, and O. Mehls

80

Nutritional Aspects in Children on CAPD

SUMMARY

Eight children on CAPD and nine treated by hemodialysis were surveyed with regard to nutritional intake and were studied by IV glucose tolerance test. Children on CAPD adapt to the glucose absorption from dialysis fluid by spontaneously decreasing their carbohydrate intake in favor of fats. The energy intake is maintained, but the spontaneous protein intake is low. Protein losses into dialysate averaged 10% of protein intake. The diet should be modified to provide a high protein intake and should be monitored.

INTRODUCTION

CAPD has become an alternative to hemodialysis (HD) in children with end-stage renal disease (ESRD).[1-4] Because most of the technical and infectious problems with CAPD have been minimized during the past five years, the metabolic consequences of long-term CAPD have become of primary interest.[2,4]

It has been claimed that growth in children on HD can be increased by oral calorie supplementation.[5] In this regard, glucose uptake from dialysate should act as an important source of calories in children on CAPD. Recent studies do not support the concept that growth in ESRD patients can be improved by calorie supplementation.[6] Further-

more, a potential disadvantage of the high glucose intake with CAPD is hypertriglyceridemia.[4,7,8] The aim of this study was to assess the spontaneous nutritional intake of children on CAPD and HD and to determine the extent to which the nutritional intake and the metabolic consequences were influenced by the type of dialysis procedure.

METHODS

Eight children on CAPD (5 males, 3 females), and nine children on HD (5 males, 4 females) of similar age and weight were studied (Table 1). All tests were performed at least three months after initiation of dialysis. Median time on both CAPD and HD was 8.5 months. HD was performed three times a week for four hours each dialysis. CAPD was performed with a commercial dialysis fluid with a dextrose content of 2.3%. Each patient received four exchanges daily, which provided 35 ml/kg of body weight of dialysis fluid/exchange. Five CAPD and five HD patients were anuric.

All children were on self-selected diets. No prescription for energy and protein intake was given for at least three months prior to the study. The nutritional survey was done by the exact weighing method with a seven-day record recorded at home.[9] Protein, cabohydrate, and fat intake were calculated according to standard tables of food analysis.[10,11] Since German[12-14] and American[15] standards of nutritional intake do not differ widely, the data were calculated and expressed as percent of the recommended daily allowance (RDA). Glucose was ana-

From the University Children's Hospital, Division of Pediatric Nephrology, Heidelberg, FRG.

Table 1. Nutritional Survey, List of Patients.

	Hemodialysis					CAPD			
#	True Age (yrs)	Height Age (yrs)	Body Weight (kg)	Body Height (cm)	#	True Age (yrs)	Height Age (yrs)	Body Weight (kg)	Body Height (cm)
1	5.0	3.5	14	96	1	5.0	3.0	15	92
2	8.6	5.7	17	111	2	5.5	2.5	15	91
3	8.1	5.4	20	118	3	6.0	6.0	20	115
4	7.8	7.0	20	120	4	9.8	7.3	21	118
5	9.5	8.0	24	123	5	13.3	10.3	25	140
6	14.5	10.0	28	138	6	15.2	9.5	29	133
7	12.6	7.5	30	130	7	13.3	8.5	30	133
8	10.0	8.8	31	135	8	10.3	11.0	40	148
9	13.9	10.0	32	140	—				
Median:					Median:				
	9.5	7.5	24	123		10.0	7.9	23	125

lyzed by the hexokinase method. The protein content of serum and dialysate was determined by the Biuret method, and the albumin content by electrophoretic methods. Amino acids (AA) were measured by ion exchange chromatography (LKB 4400, automatic program for physiologic AA with lithium buffer system). Intravenous (IV) glucose tolerance tests (IV GTT)[16] were performed after an overnight fast; in CAPD patients the last exchange was completed 12 hours prior to the test and the abdominal cavity was not empty during the test period. Glucose in an amount of 0.5 g/kg body weight was injected IV within three minutes. Samples for glucose determination were taken at 0, 15, 30, 40, 50, and 60 minutes. The glucose slope after the IV GTT was described by the glucose assimilation coefficient K[17], which is the drop of glucose concentration in %/min expressed on a logarithmic scale. Blood samples for radioimmunoassay analysis of insulin and C-peptide were taken at 0, 30, and 60 minutes. Statistical analysis were performed by Wilcoxon test for random samples and by students t test.

RESULTS

The daily glucose absorption from the dialysate of children on CAPD is shown in Figure 1. The median uptake in children with a body weight between 15–40 kg was 9.5 cal/kg/day. It was higher in the very young children with a body weight below 15 kg. The oral energy intake accounted for 75% of the RDA and was equal in the children undergoing CAPD and HD (Table 2); however, the total energy intake, i.e., the oral intake plus the dextrose supplement from dialysis fluid, was slightly higher in children on CAPD. The spontaneous oral carbohydrate intake was lower in the patients undergoing CAPD than in HD patients. This was compensated for by a higher intake of fat in CAPD patients.

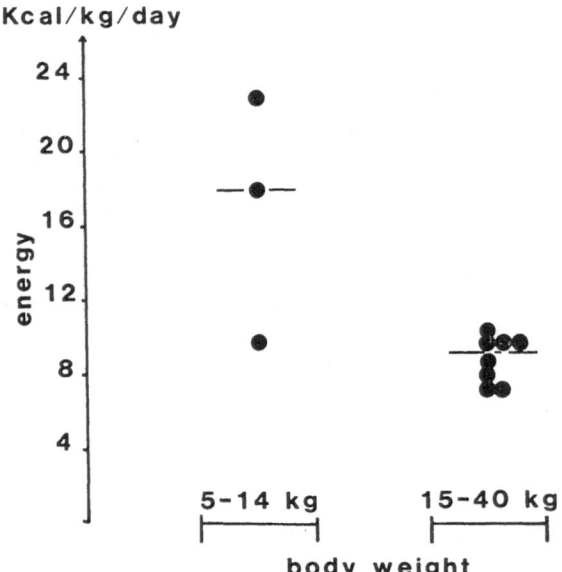

Fig. 1. Energy from glucose by peritoneal fluid; 5–14 kg: glucose 2.3% and 4.25%, 15–40 kg body weight: glucose 2.3% only, — median values.

Table 2. Energy Intake of Pediatric Dialysis Patients.

	Hemodialysis			CAPD			
				Oral Intake		Total Intake	
#	(kcal/kg/day)	(% RDA)	#	(kcal/kg/day)	(% RDA)	(kcal/kg/day)	(% RDA)
1	45	52	1	46	53	55	63
2	72	99	2	60	69	70	81
3	70	84	3	78	103	86	118
4	55	69	4	53	72	61	82
5	57	81	5	52	76	62	91
6	43	54	6	45	66	54	79
7	54	87	7	60	88	68	100
8	48	71	8	43	63	51	75
9	52	75	—				
mean ± SD	55 ± 10	75 ± 15	mean ± SD	51 ± 14	72 ± 16	60 ± 15	84 ± 17
carbohydrate % total energy		53			46		51
fat % total energy		35			42		37

IV GTT were normal in both CAPD and HD (Figs. 2 & 3) and glucose assimilation coefficients (K) did not differ significantly. Basal serum insulin levels were within the normal range in CAPD and HD patients, with the exception of one CAPD patient (Fig. 4). The late insulin response after 30 minutes was abnormal in four of four children on HD and in four of seven on CAPD. Two children of each group showed markedly elevated insulin values. In those children, the insulin levels were still elevated after 60 minutes. The serum levels for C-peptide were elevated under basal conditions in both groups and raised slightly after the IV GTT (Fig. 4).

The spontaneous protein intake (Table 3) was found to be significantly higher in HD than in CAPD patients ($P < 0.05$). This difference was more significant ($P < 0.01$) when the net intake (oral intake minus peritoneal loss) of CAPD patients was used for comparison.

The protein loss into the dialysate of CAPD patients is shown in Table 4. The mean value of 0.15 g/kg/day is confined to children of a body of 15–40 kg and who did not have peritonitis for at least three months. The protein losses during peritonitis (Table 4) varied widely depending on the severity of inflammation. Under proper treatment, the dialysate became clear after the fourth day. At this time, the protein loss was dramatically reduced, although a slight elevation could be noted one month after peritonitis.

The overall loss of AA was lower in CAPD than in HD children (Table 5). The amount of AA lost across the peritoneal membrane correlated with the respective serum values. The quotient between substrate concentration in dialysate and substrate concentration in blood (S_D/S_B) was within the same range for most AA with increasing dwell time (middle curve of Fig. 5). The lower curve of Figure 5 is representative for taurine, threonine, glutamine, arginine, valine, lysine, ornithine, and 1,3 methylhistidine, which have a S_D/S_B ratio below 0.4 after 4 hours dwell time. Only proline and tyrosine showed significantly higher S_D/S_B ratios amounting to 0.74 after four hours.

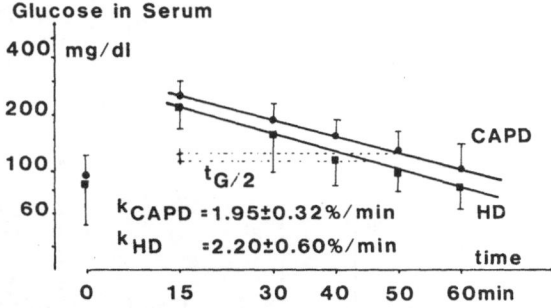

Fig. 2. IV glucose tolerance test in children on HD (■, n = 9) and CAPD (●, n = 6); k = glucose assimilation coefficient, mean ± SD.

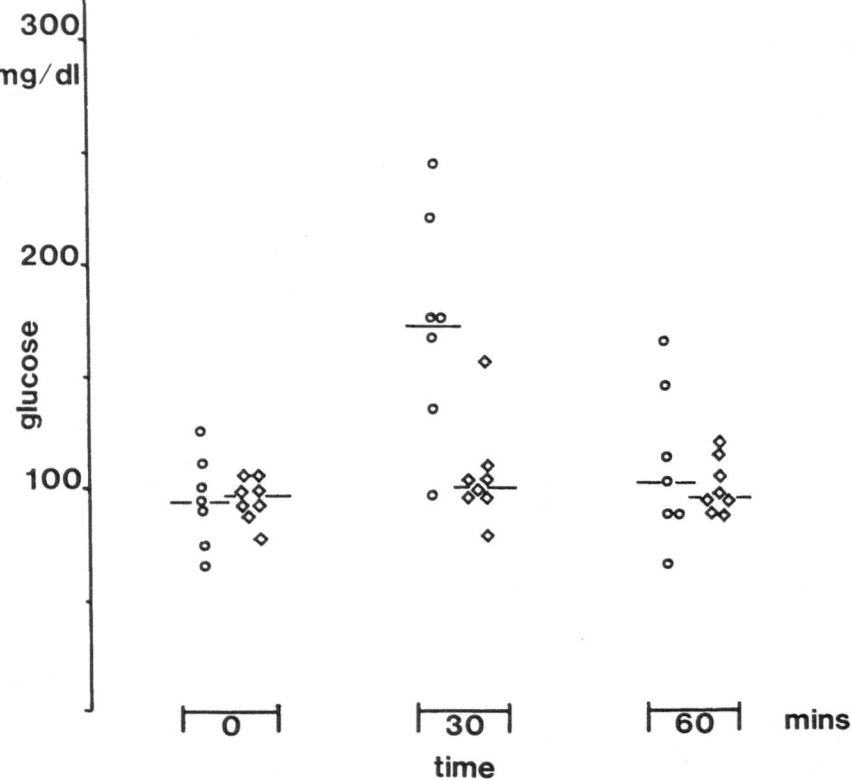

Fig. 3. Glucose in blood of CAPD patients after IV glucose injection of 0.5 g/kg/3 min (○, n = 7) and during continuous peritoneal glucose uptake (0.5 g/kg/4 h) following a bag exchange (◇, n = 8), glucose content of dialysis fluid: 2.3%, — median values.

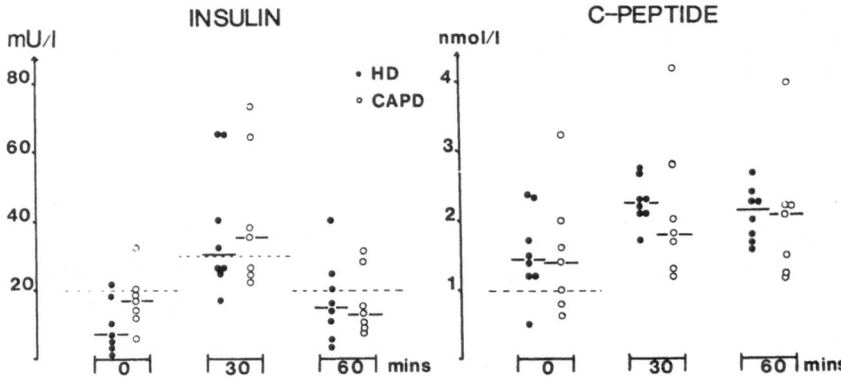

Fig. 4. Insulin and C-peptide after IV glucose 0.5 g/kg body weight in HD (●) and in CAPD (○), — median values, --- upper normal range.

Table 3. Protein Intake in Pediatric Dialysis Patients.

| | Hemodialysis | | | CAPD | | | |
| | | | | Oral Intake | | Total Intake | |
#	(g/kg/day)	(% RDA)	#	(g/kg/day)	(% RDA)	(g/kg/day)	(% RDA)
1	2.4	104	1	1.6	70	1.5	63
2	2.2	114	2	1.4	61	1.2	54
3	2.4	124	3	1.9	90	1.7	88
4	2.4	85	4	1.2	60	1.1	53
5	1.7	85	5	1.4	78	1.2	69
6	1.0	52	6	1.3	68	1.2	61
7	1.1	59	7	2.1	110	1.9	102
8	1.5	58	8	1.2	70	1.1	62
9	1.1	75					
mean ± SD	1.75 ± 0.60	87 ± 28		1.51 ± 0.33	76 ± 16	13.6 ± 0.30	69 ± 17

DISCUSSION

Glucose intolerance and insulin resistance are common in adults[18] and children[19] with chronic renal failure. These abnormalities in carbohydrate metabolism are potentially of importance in children with chronic renal failure because defective glucose utilization may result in abnormal protein metabolism, inadequate anabolism, and poor growth. Abnormal carbohydrate metabolism may also be associated with hyperlipidemia,[20] which carries the potential risk of premature arteriosclerosis. This potential risk is theoretically aggravated in children on CAPD because of the continuous load of glucose absorbed from the dialysate.

Our children on CAPD had a self-selected, spontaneous dietary energy intake of 60% of the RDA. The total energy intake, including the glucose absorbed from the dialysate, was 84% RDA. This value is slightly above the spontaneous energy intake of HD children. It is of interest, however, that CAPD children adapted to the continuous peritoneal uptake of glucose by eating more fat instead of glucose. A similar adaptation has been observed in adults by Von Baeyer et al.[21]

Under the conditions of free and spontaneous oral energy and protein intake, IV GTT were normal (K values) in CAPD and HD children. Normal GTT does not exclude abnormal carbohydrate metabolism, since accurate, quantitative measurement can only be obtained by the glucose clamp technique.[22] Elevated insulin and C-peptide levels in many of our patients point to insulin resistance in both HD and

CAPD patients. These results are in agreement with the results of other authors who studied adults[23-26] and children on HD.[16,19,27] In contrast, DeSanto et al.[28] and Mak et al.[29] did not find hyperinsulinemia and insulin resistance in children undergoing CAPD.

It is important to determine if the spontaneous energy intake of our children on HD and CAPD was

Table 4. Protein Loss with and without Peritonitis (N = 6, Mean ± SD).

Time	Ultra-filtration	Protein Loss (g/kg/day)
Without peritonitis	normal	0.15 ± 0.04
With peritonitis		
day 1–3	reduced	up to 1.0
day 4–7	reduced	0.18 − 0.56
week 2	reduced	0.22 ± 0.08
week 3	normalized	0.2 ± 0.10
week 4–8	normalized	0.17 ± 0.08

Table 5. Amino Acid Loss into the Dialysate (Mean ± SD).

	Hemodialysis	CAPD
Number of patients	23	10
AA (mg/kg/day)	57 ± 20	34 ± 8
(nM/kg/day)	(366 ± 160)	(272 ± 64)

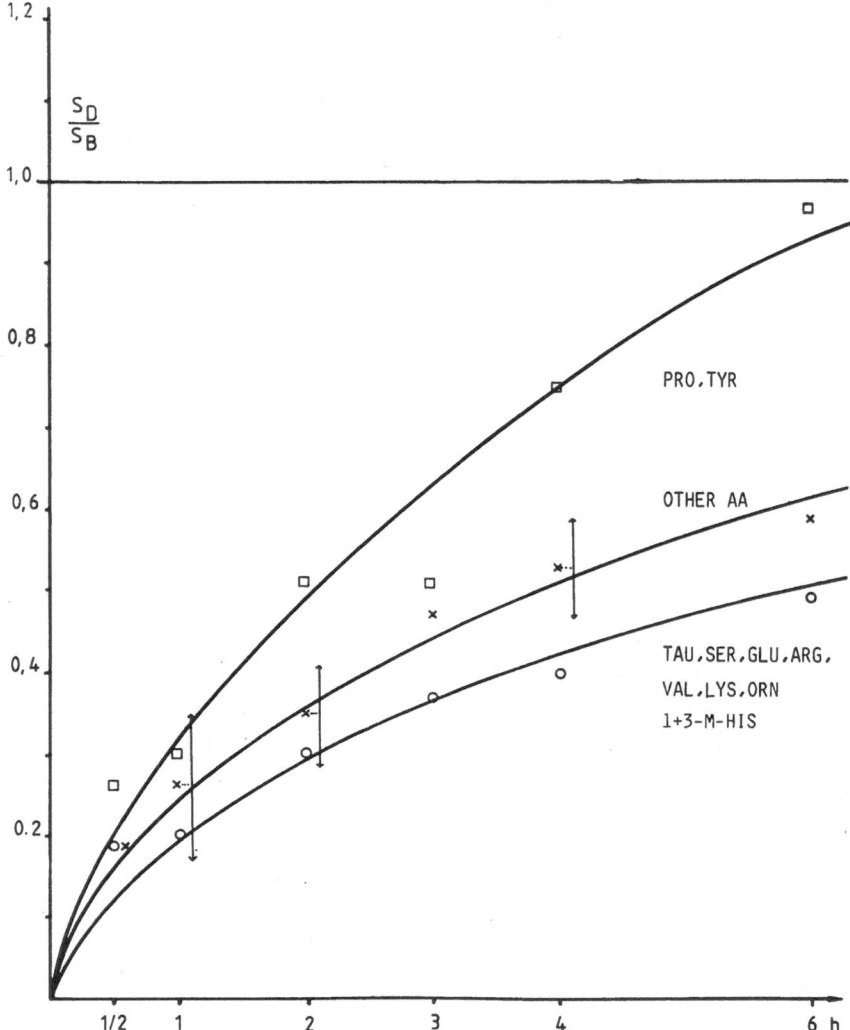

Fig. 5. Kinetics of peritoneal amino acid transfer in children on CAPD. S_D/S_B = transfer ratio substrate concentration in dialysate divided by substrate concentration in blood; groups of AA with different 4 h S_D/S_B ratios of <0.4, 0.4 to 0.5 and >0.5 (mean $\pm$ SD).

sufficient for optimal growth. There is no question that undernutrition interferes with growth. Contrary to expectations, force feeding ($>70\%$ of RDA) does not improve the growth velocity in dialyzed children in our experience[6] and that of others[30] during the last decade. We believe that the slightly reduced energy intake is a consequence of, and not the reason for, a reduced growth velocity rate of children with ESRD.

The protein losses into the dialysate of our children on CAPD with a body weight >15 kg amounted to 10% of their total protein intake. This is in agreement with the reported observations in children[31,32] and adults.[33] The amino acid losses into the dialysate appear to be negligible. The amount was about 3% of oral intake, which is in agreement with the results obtained by Giordano et al.[34] This is less than in patients undergoing HD or hemofiltration.[35] Only proline and tyrosine were lost in greater amounts (higher S_D/S_B ratio) in the dialysate. Measurement of proline is associated with well-known technical problems and artifacts cannot be excluded. Whether

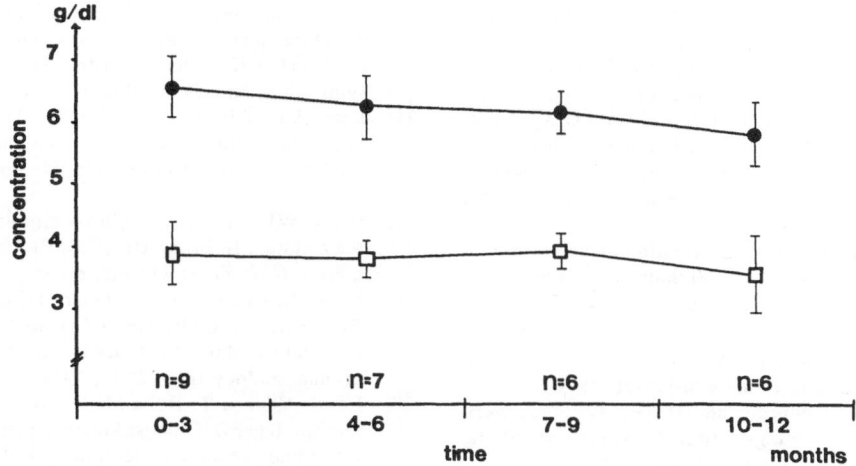

Fig. 6. Serum protein (●) and albumin (□) concentrations in relationship to time on CAPD, mean ± SD.

tyrosine losses are of clinical importance is unknown at this time.

Children on CAPD do not appear to adapt to the protein losses of the dialysis procedure, since the net protein intake was less than in children undergoing HD. Although the protein intake of about 1.36 g/kg/day has not been shown to be too low, we and others[31] have found a slight reduction of the serum albumin level with increasing time on CAPD. Therefore, it seems prudent not to rely on the spontaneous protein intake of children on CAPD but to prescribe an oral intake of at least 2 g/kg/day and to check the oral protein intake regularly.

CONCLUSION

Children on CAPD adapt to glucose absorption from the dialysis is fluid by eating more fat instead of carbohydrate. The overall spontaneous energy intake seems to be sufficient. In contrast, the spontaneous protein intake is low. It is prudent to prescribe a high protein intake and to measure regularly the intake using dietary records.

ACKNOWLEDGMENTS

We thank Dr. Schmidt-Gayk for insulin and C-peptide analysis; Dr. Harms for amino acid analysis; and Mrs. Meye and Ms. Karen Varma for their secretarial work.

REFERENCES

1. Balfe JW, Vigneux A, Willumsen J, and Hardy BE: The use of CAPD in the treatment of children with end-stage renal disease. Peritoneal Dial Bull 1: 35, 1981
2. Guillot M, Clermont MJ, Gagnadoux MF, and Broyer M: Nineteen months' experience with continuous ambulatory peritoneal dialysis in children: Main clinical and biological results. In Gahl GM, Kessel M, and Nolph KD (Eds), Advances in peritoneal dialysis: Proceedings of the 2nd international symposium on peritoneal dialysis. Amsterdam: Excerpta Medica, 1981, p 203
3. Salusky IB, Kopple JD, and Fine RN: Continuous ambulatory peritoneal dialysis in children—A 20 months' experience. Kidney Int 24(Suppl 15): S101, 1983
4. Salusky IB, Fine RN, Nelson P, Blumenkrantz MJ, and Kopple JD: Nutritional status of children undergoing continuous ambulatory peritoneal dialysis. J Clin Nutr 38: 599, 1983
5. Simmons JM, Wilson CJ, Potter DE, and Holliday MA: Relation of calorie deficiency to growth failure in children on hemodialysis and the growth response to calorie supplementation. N Engl J Med 285: 653, 1971
6. Mehls O, Gilli G, and Schaerer K: Analysis of growth and food intake in uremic children. Kidney Int 24(Suppl 16): S344(A), 1983
7. Lindholm B, Bergström J, and Norbeck HE: Lipoprotein metabolism in patients on continuous ambulatory peritoneal dialysis. In Gahl GM, Kessel M, and Nolph KD (Eds), Advances in peritoneal dialysis: Proceedings of the 2nd international symposium on

peritoneal dialysis. Amsterdam: Excerpta Medica, 1981, p 434

8. Gokal R, Ramos JM, McGurk JG, Ward MK, and Kerr DNS: Hyperlipidemia in patients on continuous ambulatory peritoneal dialysis. In Gahl GM, Kessel M, and Nolph KD (Eds), Advances in peritoneal dialysis: Proceedings of the 2nd international symposium on peritoneal dialysis. Amsterdam: Excerpta Medica, 1981, p 430

9. Stolley H, Droese W, and Kersting M: Energie- und Nahrstoffversorung im Verlauf der Kindheit. I. Nahrungsmenge und Energie. Mon Schr Kinderheilk 125: 80, 1977

10. Cremer HD, and Aign W: Die grosse Naehrwerttabelle. Munchen: Grafe und Unzer, 1984

11. Stolley H, Kersting M, and Droese W: Naehrwerttabelle des Forschungsinstituts fur Kinderernahrung. Hans Munchen: Marseille Verlag, 1980

12. Droese W, Stolley H, and Kersting M: Energie- und Nahrstoffversorung im Verlauf der Kindheit. II. Protein, Mon Schr Kinderheilk 126: 524, 1978

13. Stolley H, Droese W, and Kersting M: Energie-und Nagrstoffversorumg im Verlauf der Kindheit. III. Fett, Linolsaure, Cholesterin. Mon Schr Kinderheilk 127: 80, 1979

14. Droe W, Stolley H, and Kersting M: Energie- und Nahrstoffversorung im Verlauf der Kindheit. IV. Khlenhydrate, Rohfaser. Mon Schr Kinderheilk 127: 405, 1979

15. Recommended dietary allowances. Food and Nutritional Board, National Research Council, USA, revised, 1980

16. El-Bishti MM, Counahan R, Bloom SR, and Chantler C: Hormonal and metabolic responses to intravenous glucose in children on regular hemodialysis. Am J Clin Nutr 31: 1865, 1978

17. Rescigno A, and Segre G: Drug and tracer kinetics. Toronto: Waltham, Blaisdell Publishing Company, 1966, p 7

18. DeFronzo RA, Andres R, Edgar P, and Walker GW: Carbohydrate metabolism in uremia: A review. Medicine (Baltimore) 52: 469, 1973

19. Mak RH, Haycock GB, and Chantler C: Glucose intolerance in children with chronic renal failure. Kidney Int 24: S22, 1983

20. Chantler C: Hyperlipidaemia in children on regular haemodialysis. Arch Dis Child 52: 932, 1977

21. VonBaeyer H, Gahl GM, Riedinger H, Borowzak R, Averdunk R, Schurig R, and Kessel M: Adaptation of CAPD patients to the continuous peritoneal energy uptake. Kidney Int 23: 29, 1983

22. DeFronzo RA, Tobin JD, and Andres R: Glucose clamp technique. A method for quantifying insulin secretion and resistance. Am J Physiol 237: E214, 1979

23. Armstrong VW, Fuchs C, and Scheler F: Effect of dialysate glucose load on plasma glucose and insulin levels in CAPD patients. Abstracts, 2nd international symposium on peritoneal dialysis. Berlin, 1981, p 2

24. Ferrani E, Pilo A, and Tuoni M: The response to intravenous glucose of patients on maintenance hemodialysis: Effects of dialysis. Metabolism 28: 125, 1979

25. Brech WJ: Uraemische Glukoseintoleranz—Diabetes mellitus. In Franz HE (Ed), Blutreiningingsverfahren. New York: Thieme, p 168

26. Fiasci E, Companacci L, Guarnieri GF, Faccini L, Bellini G, Caretta R, and D'Angelo A: Glucose content and hexokinase activity in patients with chronic uremia. Kidney Int 7: S341, 1975

27. Ronda-Vildosa T, Bulla M, Herkenrath P, Roth B, and Hubinger D: Glucose kinetics, plasma insulin and C-peptide in children undergoing chronic hemodialysis treatment. Eur J Pediatr 40: 164, 1983

28. DeSanto NG, Capodicasa G, Gilli G, DiLeo VA, Capasso G, and Giordano C: Metabolic aspects of continuous ambulatory peritoneal dialysis with reference to energy-protein input and growth. Int J Pediatr Nephrol 3: 279, 1982

29. Mak R, Turner C, Rigden S, Woods C, Haycock G, and Chantler C: Glucose metabolism in uremia: Effect of haemodialysis and CAPD. Abstracts, 1st international congress on continuous ambulatory peritoneal dialysis (CAPD) in children. Heidelberg, 1984, p 4

30. Arnold WC, Danford D, and Holliday MA: Effects of caloric supplementation on growth in children with uremia. Kidney Int 24: 205, 1983

31. Broyer M, Niaudet P, Champion G, Jean G, Chopin N, and Chernichow P: Nutritional and metabolic studies in children on continuous ambulatory peritoneal dialysis. Kidney Int 24: S106, 1983

32. Drachman R, Niaudet P, and Broyer M: Protein losses during peritoneal dialysis in children. Abstracts, 1st international congress on continuous ambulatory peritoneal dialysis (CAPD) in children. Heidelberg, 1984, p 19

33. Heide B, Pihatos A, Khanna R, Pettit J, Olgivie R, Harrison J, McNeil K, Siccion Z, and Oreopoulos DG: Nutritional status of patients undergoing continuous ambulatory peritoneal dialysis (CAPD). Peritoneal Dial Bull 3: 138, 1983

34. Giordano C, DeSanto NG, and Capodicasa G: Amino acid loss during CAPD in children. Int J Ped Nephrol 2: 85, 1981

35. Bonzel KE, Muller-Wiefel DE, Rauh W, Grobe H, Harms E, Diekmann L, and Mehls O: Serum amino acids (AA) and AA losses in uremic children treated with hemodialysis (HD), hemofiltration (HF) and continuous ambulatory peritoneal dialysis (CAPD). Eur J Pediatr 140: 174, 1983

J.J. Sanchez, R. Schurig, A. Mahiout, A. Pustelnik,
C. Haase, H. Becker, G.M. Gahl, and M. Kessel.

81

Intraperitoneal Versus Oral Glucose Load in CAPD Patients

SUMMARY

A comparison of the response of plasma glucose concentrations in patients with end-stage renal disease was made between oral glucose loading and intraperitoneal instillation. On CAPD plasma glucose was a function of the dialysis fluid dextrose concentration, but at all loads fractional absorption was comparable and peak plasma levels were below those attained by oral loading. Because intestinal absorption is faster then diffusion across the peritoneum an active transport process is suggested.

INTRODUCTION

CAPD is routinely used to dialyze patients with end-stage renal disease (ESRD).[1] Glucose intolerance and hyperglycemia in uremic patients have been postulated since the 1900s[2,3] and many mechanisms have been proposed to explain this problem.[4-6] In the treatment of ESRD patients with peritoneal dialysis, it is now customary to use solutions containing dextrose as the major osmotic agent. The usual dextrose (monohydrate) concentrations are 15 g/L, 22.7 g/L, and 42.5 g/L. Therefore, patients on CAPD are subject to a glucose load due to absorption from the dialysate during each exchange. Therefore, we studied the effects of different dialysis solution-dextrose concentrations on plasma glucose levels in CAPD patients, and compared them to an oral glucose tolerance test in ESRD patients not on peritoneal dialysis.

MATERIALS AND METHODS

Twenty ESRD patients were divided in two groups: group 1 (n = 10) received an oral glucose load of 1 g/kg body weight and group 2 (n = 10) received 0.5 g/kg. The CAPD patients were divided into three groups, each patient receiving 2 L of dialysis solution for the purposes of the study. Group 3 (n = 7) received dialysis fluid containing dextrose 42.5 g/L; group 4 (n = 6) received 22.7 g/L solutions, and group 5 (n = 5 received 15.0 g/L solutions. All patients had no personal or family history of diabetes mellitus. The patients fasted during the four-hour study and clinically were stable during the study. The composition of the dialysis solutions were Na 134 mmol/L, Ca 1.75 mmol/L, Mg 0.5 mmol/L, Cl 103 mmol/L, lactate 35.0 mmol/L and the dialysis fluid dextrose concentrations were 15.0 g/L, 22.7 g/L, and 42.25 g/L glucose, respectively (Fresenius AG, Bad Homburg, FRG). At the end of the study the remaining dextrose concentration in the dialysate was measured and the amount absorbed was calculated.

Plasma glucose levels were measured continuously using a glucose monitor (Miles, Life Science Instruments, Indiana) designed for clinical application requiring continuous blood assays. The monitoring period had a response time of less than 90 seconds from blood withdrawal to glucose read-out. The measurement principle is based on an electro-

From the Department of Nephrology, Universitätsklinikum Charlottenburg, Freie Universität Berlin, F.R.G.

Table 1. Clinical Data of Patients.

Groups	Sex	Age, Range (years)	Basic Disease		Duration of Dialysis, Range (years)
1	6 f, 4 m	46–72	CGN CPN CN	7 2 1	0.6–12
2	2 f, 8 m	52–74	CGN CPN CN	3 6 1	0.8–8
3	2 f, 5 m	41–73	CGN CPN	2 5	0.1–1.6
4	3 f, 3 m	61–79	CGN CPN	2 4	0.2–1.3
5	2 f, 3 m	42–72	CGN CPN	2 3	0.1–0.9

CGN = chronic glomerulonephritis; CPN = chronic pyelonephritis; CN = cystic disease.

chemical glucose sensor, which polarographically measures hydrogen peroxide generated by the reaction between the blood glucose and membrane coupled glucose oxidase enzyme.

RESULTS

Table 1 gives a general description of the patients in each group. Figure 1 and Table 2 show the time course of the blood glucose concentrations after the oral or intraperitoneal glucose application. Table 2 depicts also the glucose load in each group as mean ± SD. In all groups the highest blood glucose concentrations were reached in similar times be-

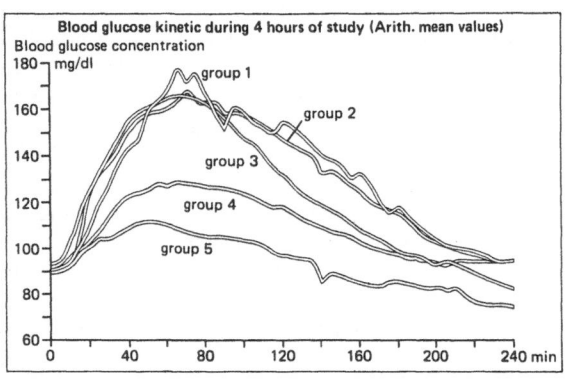

Fig. 1. Time course of blood glucose level during four hours (Arithmetic mean values).

Table 2. Blood Glucose Levels During the Study Values are Expressed as Mean ± SD.

Groups	Glucose Load (g)	Blood Glucose Concentration (mg/dl)								
		0 min	30 min	60 min	90 min	120 min	150 min	180 min	210 min	240 min
1	62 ± 14	90 ± 10	136 ± 24	166 ± 51	171 ± 57	152 ± 67	136 ± 52	118 ± 37	98 ± 28	94 ± 18
2	34 ± 6	90 ± 19	128 ± 33	162 ± 46	156 ± 44	131 ± 43	114 ± 39	99 ± 33	92 ± 33	83 ± 40
3	69 ± 8	94 ± 12	140 ± 21	164 ± 25	163 ± 25	148 ± 25	131 ± 20	115 ± 21	100 ± 18	97 ± 11
4	28 ± 3	84 ± 13	115 ± 11	127 ± 15	126 ± 19	116 ± 16	106 ± 18	98 ± 18	96 ± 21	96 ± 19
5	20 ± 3	91 ± 16	104 ± 20	110 ± 25	105 ± 21	96 ± 18	87 ± 24	80 ± 21	80 ± 22	78 ± 23

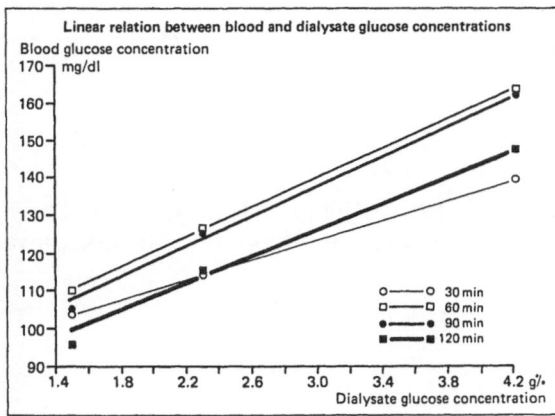

Fig. 2. Linear relationship between blood glucose levels and dialysis fluid dextrose concentration.

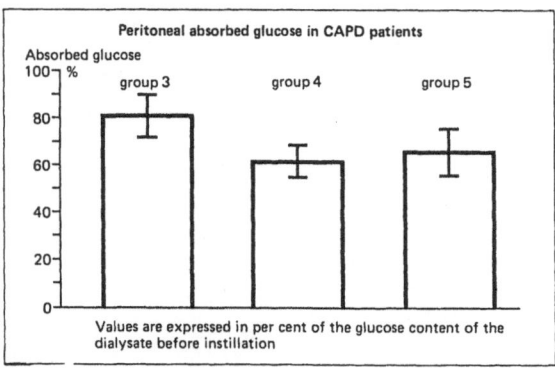

Fig. 3. Peritoneal absorbed glucose in CAPD patients (values are expressed in percentage of the dextrose content of the bags before instillation).

tween 40–100 minutes. With oral glucose (group 1 and 2), identical peak blood concentrations were obtained. In contrast with IP dextrose, blood glucose levels were lower and dose dependent. Only with the 42.5 g/L dextrose solutions were rises in blood glucose concentrations obtained comparable to those with the oral doses. Furthermore, in the CAPD patients, a linear relationship existed between blood concentration and the dialysis fluid dextrose concentration (Fig. 2).

In all CAPD groups the mean glucose load absorbed was 75% of the total dextrose instilled; group 3 absorbed 69 ± 8 g, group 4 absorbed 28 ± 3 g, and group 5 absorbed 20 ± 3 g glucose, respectively. A high degree of variation in glucose absorption in all the patients was observed (Fig. 3).

CONCLUSIONS

The blood glucose levels in CAPD patients were dose dependent, as was the absorbed glucose load. However, the absorption of glucose by the peritoneum appears to be slower than by the intestine; this results in lower blood glucose concentrations after peritoneal dextrose instillation compared with the same glucose load orally. This could be explained in part by the existence of an active transport in the bowel, in contrast to diffusive transport in the peritoneum.

REFERENCES

1. Popovich RP, Moncrief J, Nolph KD, Ghods AO, Twardowski ZJ, and Pyle WK: Continuous ambulatory peritoneal dialysis. Ann Intern Med 88: 449, 1978

2. Lindner GC, Hiller A, and Van Slyke DD: Carbohydrate metabolism in nephritis. J Clin Invest 1: 247, 1925

3. Horton ES, Johnson C, and Lebovitz HE: Carbohydrate metabolism in uremia. Ann Intern Med 68: 63, 1968

4. Delmez JA, Rutherford WE, Klahr S, and Blondin J: Studies on the role of the liver and splanchnic tissues in the production of carbohydrate intolerance in uremia. Metabolism 30: 7, 1981

5. Schauder P, Matthaei D, Hennig HV, Scheler F, and Langenbeck U: Blood levels of branched chain alfa-keto acids in uremia: Effect of an oral glucose test. Klin Woschr 59: 845, 1981

6. Balducci A, Slama G, Rottembourg J, and Baumelou A: Intraperitoneal insulin in uraemic diabetics undergoing continuous ambulatory peritoneal dialysis. Br Med J 283: 1021, 1981

7. DeFronzo RA, Reubin A, Edgar P, and Gordon W: Carbohydrate metabolism in uremia: A review. Medicine 52: 469, 1973

8. Lauristen KB, and Moody AJ: The association between plasma GIP and insulin after oral glucose. Scand J Gastroenterol 15: 953, 1980

9. Briggs JD, Buchanan KD, Luke RG, and McKiddie MT: Role of insulin in glucose intolerance in uremia. Lancet 1: 462, 1967

10. Quintanilla A, Shambaugh GE III, Gibson TP, and Craig R: Glucose metabolism in uremia. Am J Clin Nutr 33: 1446, 1980

11. Boyer J, Gill GN, and Epstein FH: Hyperglycemia and hyperosmolality complicating peritoneal dialysis. Ann Intern Med 67: 3, 1967

K. Ozawa, K. Goto, Y. Kijima, I. Nakayama, T. Shoji,
T. Sasaoka, T. Akiba, and S. Nakagawa

82

The Effect of CAPD on Lipid Abnormalities Detected by Apoproteins and Ultracentrifugal Lipid Subfractions

SUMMARY

The hyperlipidemic tendency of CAPD patients (CAPD) has been described elsewhere without detailed data on apoproteins and ultracentrifugal lipid subfractions. In order to understand the details of hyperlipidemia, especially in light of the protective role of apoproteins, we compared the total cholesterol (TC), free cholesterol (FC), phospholipid (PL), triglyceride (TG), their ultracentrifugal subfractions, and apoproteins A-I, A-II, C-II, and E present in the uremic serum of CAPD with those in hemodialysis patients (HD) and in healthy normal controls (N).

TC, FC, PL, and TG were elevated in CAPD, whereas only the elevation of TG was noted in HD. Hypercholesterolemia was due to an increase in the VLDL and LDL fractions. HDL cholesterol, and especially HDL$_2$ cholesterol, in CAPD were significantly lower than in N. Apo A-I and A-IC were within normal limits in CAPD. Apo C-II and E levels were higher in CAPD than in N. Accordingly, the HDL cholesterol/apo A-I ratio was lower in CAPD than in N. But the VLDL-TG/apo C-II ratio was higher in CAPD than in N.

It is suggested that apoproteins do not perform their protective role against atherogenesis in CAPD.

From the Dialysis Unit, Department of Medicine, Yokosuka Kyosai Hospital, Yokosuka, Kanagawa, and the Second Department of Medicine, Tokyo Medical and Dental University, Tokyo, Japan.

INTRODUCTION

Since the advent of continuous ambulatory peritoneal dialysis (CAPD), it has been claimed that patients tend to develop lipid abnormalities mainly in the pattern of hypertriglyceridemia and hypo-HDL-cholesterolemia.[1,2] This abnormality is a feature common to uremic patients,[3] and one that neither hemodialysis[4] nor transplantation[5] improves. CAPD may even aggravate this abnormality.[2] Although accelerated atherosclerosis is multifactorial in origin, the literature to date has suggested a major role for lipid abnormalities. In this regard, it is questioned whether or not CAPD has a beneficial influence on the cardiovascular system over a long-term period. On the other hand, detailed analyses of lipid abnormalities with respect to apoproteins and ultracentrifugal lipid subfractions have been lacking. The present study was undertaken to obtain more information about the role of protective apoproteins in association with ultracentrifugal lipid subfractions in the genesis of lipid abnormalities in CAPD.

MATERIALS AND METHODS

Eighteen uremic patients (12 males and 6 females age range 19 to 61 years, average 45.2 years) maintained on CAPD were studied. Duration on CAPD therapy averaged 17.8 months and ranged from 3 to 42 months. Prior to CAPD, 14 of 18 patients had been treated by hemodialysis. Their original

Table 1. Fractional Concentration of Total Cholesterol (mg/dl).

Group	Whole* Serum	VLDL	LDL	HDL$_2$	HDL$_3$
Control	165 ± 25	11 ± 6	106 ± 22	32 ± 9	18 ± 4
HD	168 ± 26	19 ± 15*	107 ± 25	27 ± 2*	15 ± 4*
CAPD	229 ± 55!	49 ± 39!	142 ± 51!	22 ± 8!	17 ± 4

* : $p < 0.01$ (HD or CAPD vs Control).
! : $p < 0.01$ (CAPD vs HD).

diseases were chronic glomerulonephritis in 15, renal tuberculosis in one, polycystic kidneys in one and chronic pyelonephritis in one. Diabetics were excluded from the study. The data obtained from CAPD were compared with those from healthy normal controls (N)—11 males and 11 females with a mean age of 36 years—and hemodialysis patients (HD)—11 males and 7 females with a mean age of 42.5 years. Hemodialysis averaged 91 months in duration.CAPD was performed using the Travenol system and Dianeal solution. With four 2 L exchanges, including one volume of solution with 4.25% dextrose and 3 volumes of solutions with 1.5% dextrose as a rule, the average drainage volume per day was 2.3 L.

Blood samples were collected after a 12-hour overnight fast without interruption of dialysis. The last exchange was done at least 10 hours prior to the collection of blood samples. Patients whose blood glucose exceeded 130 mg/dl were excluded from the study, even though diabetes was not among their original diseases. Blood samples were collected in EDTA tubes, separated, and stored at 4°C. The fractionation of lipid was completed within four days. Plasma (175 μl) was ultracentrifuged for the fractionation of HDL with LDL. For the fractionation of HDL or HDL$_3$, a 90 μl sample of plasma adjusted in gravity was overlaid with an equal volume of prepared KBr solution. The ultracentrifuging was done for four hours in an LP-42 Ti angle rotor at 42,000 rpm at 4°C in a Beckman L5-65 ultracentrifuge system. Total cholesterol (TC), free cholesterol (FC), phospholipid (PL), and triglyceride (TG) were determined by an enzyme method. The lipid subfractions in HDL, HDL$_3$, and HDL with LDL were also determined by this method. The concentration of each lipid in VLDL, LDL, or HDL$_2$ was mathematically calculated. Apoproteins A-I, A-II, C-II, and E were measured by a single radial immunodiffusion assay using an Apoprotein plate from Daiichi Kagaku Laboratory (Tokyo, Japan). Statistical anal-

yses were performed by Student's t test. If variance in two groups were not equal by Fisher's test, the data were reanalyzed by Welch's test.

RESULTS

Cholesterol

The total cholesterol level of whole serum in CAPD was significantly higher than in N and HD (Table 1). This finding is attributable to an increase

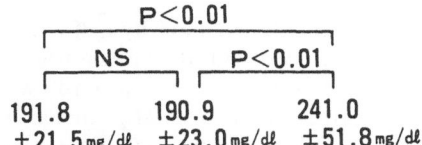

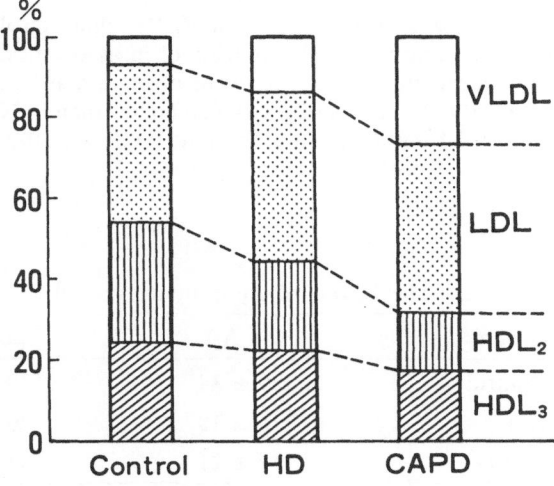

Fig. 1. Serum phospholipid levels and their fractional percentage.

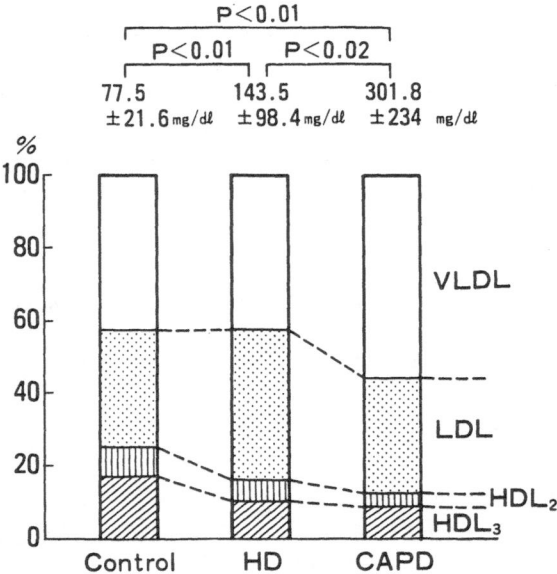

Fig. 2. Serum triglyceride levels and their fractional percentages.

Phospholipid

PL was also elevated in CAPD (Fig. 1). The range of abnormal distribution in PL presented a pattern very similar to that of TC.

Triglyceride

The most striking abnormality was observed in TG concentration and distribution. CAPD had TG levels four times higher than N and twice that of HD (Fig. 2). Although the percentage of HDL-TG was decreased, a consideration of the absolute contents showed a greater increase in CAPD than in N and HD.

Apoproteins

Apo A-I and A-II did not yield statistical differences among the three groups. The apo C-II in HD and CAPD was more elevated than in N. Between HD and CAPD there was no significant difference. The apo E in CAPD was double that in N and HD (Table 2). The HDL cholesterol/apo A-I ratio in uremic groups was signficantly lower than that in N (Fig. 3). The VLDL-TG/apo C-II ratio of CAPD was higher than that of N and HD (Fig. 4).

in VLDL and LDL fractions by half-and-half distribution. In contrast with the increase of VLDL and LDL cholesterol, HDL_2 cholesterol was significantly decreased. The HDL_2 cholesterol/HDL_3 cholesterol ratio was lower in CAPD than in N (1.36 $\pm$ 0.56 vs 1.89 $\pm$ 0.67, p < 0.02).

In HD, a slight increase of VLDL cholesterol and a decrease of HLD cholesterol in association with normocholesterolemia were observed. FC in CAPD (76.9 $\pm$ 21 mg/dl) was also higher than in N (45.6 $\pm$ 7.8 mg/dl, p < 0.01) and in HD (54.6 $\pm$ 10.8 mg/dl, p < 0.01).

DISCUSSION

In this study, CAPD was complicated by hypercholesterolemia in association with hypertriglyceridemia. Hypo-HDL-cholesterolemia was also observed in CAPD as well as in HD. Previous papers[2,6] describe the hypercholesterolemia in CAPD as caused by an increase of VLDL cholesterol. In this study, the increase was observed in both LDL and VLDL fractions. As to the cause of hypertriglyceridemia, a decrease in clearance due to the presence of the inhibitor[7] of lipoprotein lipase (LPL) in the uremic serum, and a reduction in apo C-II,[8]

Table 2. The Levels of Apoproteins (mg/dl).

Group	Apo A-I	Apo A-II	Apo C-II	Apo E
Control	120 ± 14	30 ± 4	3.0 ± 0.8	3.2 ± 0.7
HD	116 ± 19	30 ± 5	4.8 ± 2.0*	3.3 ± 1.0*
CAPD	115 ± 21	31 ± 5	5.8 ± 3.8*	6.4 ± 3.4!*

* : p < 0.01 (HD or CAPD vs Control).
! : p < 0.01 (CAPD vs HD).

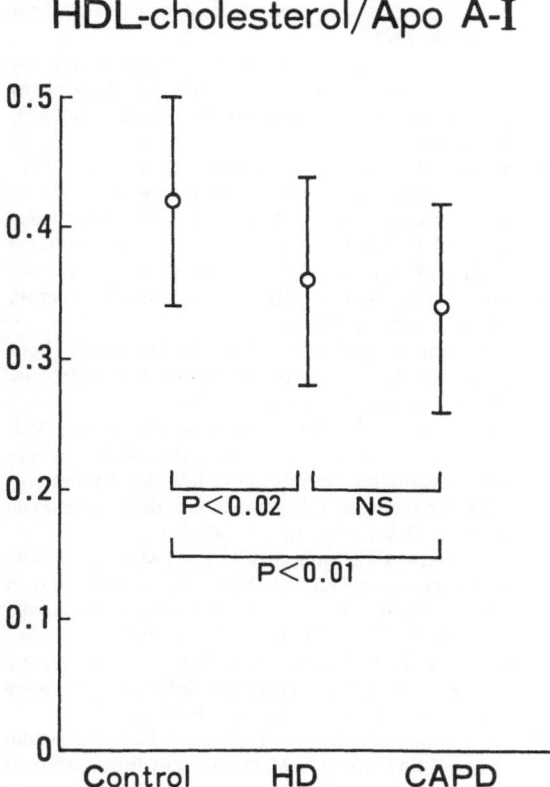

Fig. 3. The ratio of HDL cholesterol/Apo A-I.

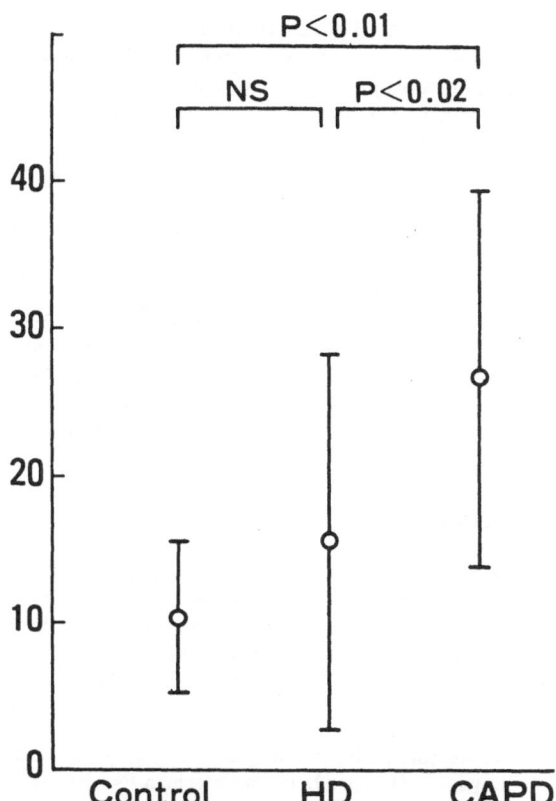

Fig. 4. The ratio of VLDL triglyceride/Apo C-II.

which is an activator of LPL, have been considered. In addition, in CAPD, a persistent and continuous peritoneal absorption of glucose leads to hyperinsulinemia,[9] which may result in the hepatic overproduction of VLDL. However, under the conditions of a delayed process from VLDL to LDL, the hepatic overproducion of VLDL may not cause hyper-LDL-cholesterolemia, if clearance of LDL is not disturbed. In the present study, LDL cholesterol was also increased to the same degree as that of VLDL cholesterol. Therefore, a disturbance in clearance of LDL via the LDL pathway is suggested.[10]

The mechanism causing this abnormality in clearance of LDL can be hypothesized as follows. Apoprotein B in the native LDL is modified by acetylation,[11] carbamylation,[12] glycosylation,[13] or reaction with malondialdehyde,[14] producing denatured LDL. Denatured LDL decreases the ability of LDL to bind to high-affinity receptor sites on human skin fibroblasts. Moreover, the clearance of glyco-

sylated LDL is decreased, as Sasaki and Cottam[15] have demonstrated in the plasma of rabbits. With respect to CAPD, glycosylation and carbamylation seem to be most important modifications when we consider the fact that the hemoglobin A_{1c} concentration is elevated in CAPD.[9] In uremia, carbamylated hemoglobin is produced[16] by the condensation of urea-derived cyanate with the N-terminal aminogroup. In CAPD, apoprotein B as well as hemoglobin may be susceptible to glycosylation and carbamylation. It seems likely that the unfavorable capacity of glycosylation and carbamylation could result in hypercholesterolemia as a result of denatured LDL production.

Apoproteins A-I and A-II did not differ among three groups, nor was apo A-I/A-II ratio changed. Apo A-I is a co-factor in the activation of lecithin-cholesterol acyl transferase (LCAT). Apo A-I was reported to be an available marker of angiographically assessed coronary artery disease.[17] On the other hand, apo C-II is a co-factor in LPL activation. In view of these protective functions, the findings in which normal apo A-I and increased apo C-II were observed in CAPD can be interpreted as playing a preventive role in atherogenesis, provided these apoproteins are qualitatively normal. However, in the present study, HDL-cholesterol/apo A-I or VLDL-TG/apo C-II ratios were abnormal in spite of normal or increased apoprotein levels in CAPD. The low HDL_2 cholesterol/HDL_3 cholesterol ratio suggests the delayed maturation of HDL probably caused by a reduction in LCAT activity. The abnormal composition of lipoprotein particles may in part result from the decreased function of protective apoprotein modified by glycosylation or carbamylation.

REFERENCES

1. Oreopoulos DG, Clayton S, Dombros N, Zellerman G, and Katirtzoglou A: Nineteen months experience with continuous ambulatory peritoneal dialysis. Proc Eur Dial Transplant Assoc 16: 178, 1979

2. Ramos JM, Heaton A, McGurk JG, Ward MK, and Kerr DNS: Sequential change in serum lipids and their subfractions in patients receiving continuous ambulatory peritoneal dialysis. Nephron 35: 20, 1983

3. Bagdade JD, Porte D Jr, and Bierman EL: Hypertriglyceridemia. A metabolic consequence of chronic renal failure. N Engl J Med 279, 181, 1968

4. McCosh EJ, Solangi K, Rivers JM, and Goodman A: Hypertriglyceridemia in patients with chronic renal insufficiency. Am J Clin Nutr 28: 1036, 1975

5. Savdie ES, Gibson JC, Crawford GA, Simons LA, and Mahony JF: Impaired plasma triglyceride clearance as a feature of both uremic and posttransplant triglyceridemia. Kidney Int 18, 774, 1980

6. Roncari DAK, Breckenridge WC, Khanna R, and Oreopoulos DG: Rise in high-density lipoprotein cholesterol in some patients treated with CAPD. Peritoneal Dial Bull 1: 136, 1981

7. Murase T, Cattran DC, Rubenstein B, and Steiner G: Inhibition of lipoprotein lipase by uremic plasma. A possible cause of hypertriglyceridemia. Metabolism 24: 1279, 1975

8. Rapoport J, Aviram M, Chaimovitz C, and Brook JG: Defective high-density lipoprotein composition in patients on chronic hemodialysis. N Engl J Med 299: 1326, 1978

9. Lindholm B, Bergström J, and Karlamder SG: Glucose metabolism in patients on continuous ambulatory peritonial dialysis (CAPD). In Gahl GM, Kessel M, and Nolph KD (Eds), Advances in peritoneal dialysis. Proceedings of the 2nd international symposium on peritoneal dialysis. Amsterdam: Excerpta Medica, 1981, p 413

10. Goldstein JL, and Brown MS: The low density lipoprotein pathway and its relation to atherosclerosis. Annu Rev Biochem 46: 897, 1977

11. Goldstein JL, Ho YK, Basu SK, and Brown MS: Binding site on macrophages that mediates uptake and degradation of acetylated low density lipoprotein, producing massive cholesterol deposition. Proc Natl Acad Sci USA 76: 333, 1979

12. Weisgraber KH, Innerarity TL, and Mahley W: Role of the lysine residues of plasma lipoproteins in high affinity binding to cell surface receptors on human fibroblasts. J Biol Chem 253:9053, 1978

13. Gonen B, Baenziger J, Schonfeld G, Jacobson D, and Farrar P: Non enzymatic glycosylation of low density lipoproteins in vitro. Diabetes 30: 875, 1981

14. Fogelman AM, Shechter I, Seager J, Hokon M, Child JS, and Edwards PA: Malondialdehyde alteration of low density lipoproteins leads to cholesterol ester accumulation in human monocyte-macrophages. Proc Natl Acad Sci USA 77: 2214, 1980

15. Sasaki J, and Cottam GL: Glycosylation of LDL decreases its ability to interact with high-affinity receptors of human fibroblasts in vitro and decreases its clearance from rabbit plasma in vivo. Biochim Biophys Acta 713: 199, 1982

16. Flückiges R, Harmon W, Meier W, Loo S, and Gabby KH: Hemoglobin carbamylation in uremia. N Engl J Med 304: 823, 1981

17. Maciejko JJ, Holmes DR, Kottke BA, Zinsmeister AR, Dinh DM, and Mao SJT: Apolipoprotein A-I as a marker of angiographically assessed coronary-artery disease. N Engl J Med 309: 385, 1983

M.K. Chan, J.W. Persaud, Z. Varghese, R.A. Baillod,
and J.F. Moorhead

83

Post-Heparin Lipolytic Enzymes in Patients on CAPD

SUMMARY

Serum TC, TG and HDL-C concentrations as well as post-heparin hepatic lipase and lipoprotein lipase activities were studied in CAPD patients and compared to those obtained in normal subjects and HD patients. Female CAPD patients had higher serum TC concentrations than did normal subjects or HD patients. Their mean HDL-C concentration was no different from that of normal subjects, but higher than the corresponding value in HD patients. Male CAPD patients, like their HD counterparts, had markedly reduced HDL-C concentrations. Both male and female CAPD patients had reduced hepatic lipase and lipoprotein lipase activities, but the mean lipoprotein lipase activity of female CAPD patients was higher than that of female HD patients. An inverse correlation between lipoprotein lipase activity and log-TG concentrations and a positive correlation between lipoprotein lipase activity and HDL-C concentrations were established in normal subjects and HD patients, but could not be demonstrated in CAPD patients. Hepatic lipase activity did not correlate with any of the other parameters of lipid metabolism. Reduced lipoprotein lipase activity, which would cause defective triglyceride metabolism, cannot adequately explain the hyperlipidemia in CAPD patients.

From the Department of Nephrology and Transplantation, The Royal Free Hospital, London, and the Department of Medicine, University of Hong Kong, Queen Mary Hospital, Hong Kong.

INTRODUCTION

Hyperlipidemia is common in CAPD patients.[1,2] Its pathogenesis remains unclear. The hyperlipidemia is of the combined type, but hypertriglyceridemia is usually more prominent than hypercholesterolemia. In the present study we have measured the activities of lipoprotein lipase and hepatic lipase in the post-heparin plasma of CAPD patients. Lipoprotein lipase is a key enzyme in the catabolism of triglyceride-rich lipoproteins.

PATIENTS AND METHODS

Forty-two CAPD patients (25 males, 17 females) were included in the study. The male patients had a mean age of 50.3 years and the females 42.9 years. They had been on CAPD from 6–36 months, with a mean of 14.4 months. Five patients received antihpertensives in the form of atenolol from 50–100 mg daily. All except two patients carried out 2 L exchanges daily using 1.36% (anhydrous) dextrose solutions. Hypertonic solutions were not regularly used. All studies were performed in the fasting state, when there was no dialysis solution in the abdominal cavity. Blood samples were taken for the determination of serum cholesterol (TC), triglyceride (TG), and high-density lipoprotein cholesterol (HDL-C) concentrations by enzymatic methods as described elsewhere.[3] Post-heparin plasma was collected 15 minutes after an intravenous injection (100 U/kg of heparin from 27 patients for the measurement of hepatic lipase and lipoprotein lipase activities by a

Table 1. Parameters of Lipid Metabolism in Normal Subjects, CAPD, and Hemodialysis Patients (Mean ± SD), Statistical Significance Evaluated by Mann-Whitney Test.

		A Normal Male N = 10 Female N = 12	Difference A & B	B CAPD Male N = 17 Female N = 25	Difference B & C	C HD N = 23	Difference C & A
Age (yrs)	Male	38.70 ± 10.10	ns	42.90 ± 14.00	ns	41.50 ± 10.10	ns
	Female	49.70 ± 10.40	ns	50.30 ± 13.70	ns	46.40 ± 9.70	ns
TC μM/L	Male	5.93 ± 1.39	p = 0.03	7.46 ± 2.24	p = 0.02	5.94 ± 1.34	ns
	Female	6.13 ± 1.07	ns	6.30 ± 2.09	ns	5.61 ± 1.12	ns
TG μM/L	Male	1.14 ± 0.57	p = 0.01	3.06 ± 2.66	ns	3.41 ± 3.89	p < 0.01
	Female	1.88 ± 0.95	ns	2.47 ± 1.63	ns	3.29 ± 2.74	p = 0.02
HDL-C μM/L	Male	1.20 ± 0.23	ns	1.11 ± 0.25	p < 0.05	0.83 ± 0.23	p = 0.008
	Female	1.03 ± 0.29	p = 0.01	0.78 ± 0.21†	ns	0.70 ± 0.17	p = 0.003
HL μM/FFA/ml/h	Male	14.28 ± 4.30	p = 0.01	9.31 ± 4.56§	ns	11.89 ± 4.82††	ns
	Female	22.40 ± 6.26*	p = 0.007	14.08 ± 5.56**	ns	14.84 ± 6.06§§	p = 0.005
LPL μM/FFA/ml/h	Male	6.75 ± 0.97	p = 0.0001	3.70 ± 1.53§	p = 0.04	2.54 ± 1.30††	p = 0.0001
	Female	5.86 ± 1.72*	p = 0.004	3.02 ± 1.36**	ns	2.68 ± 1.11§§	p = 0.001

* n = 11; † n = 22; §n = 12; **n = 15; ††n = 20; §§n = 21.

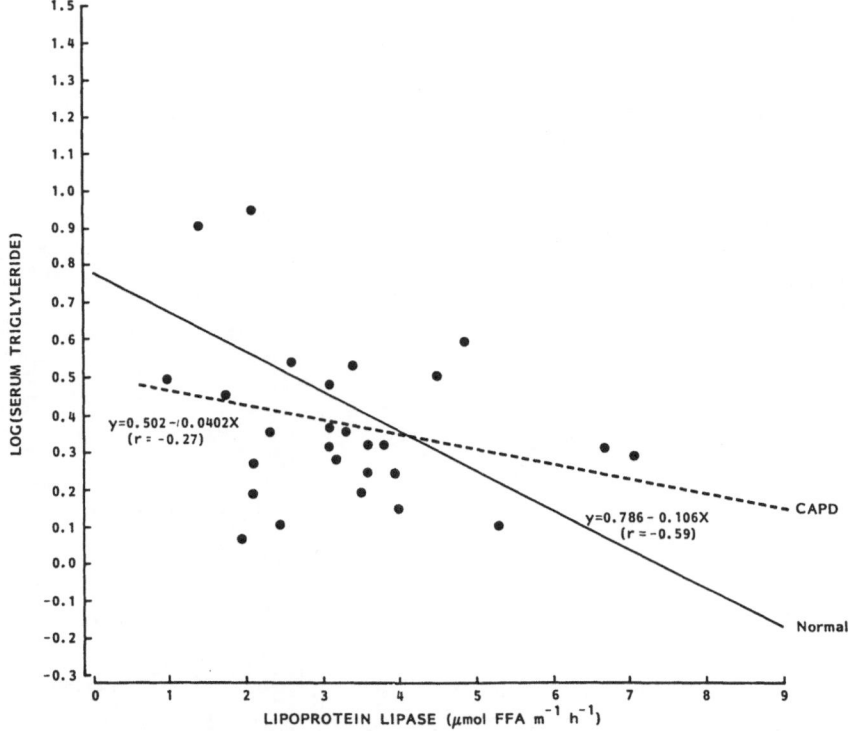

Fig. 1. Correlation between log (TG) and lipoprotein lipase in CAPD patients and normal subjects. The closed circles and interrupted line represent CAPD patients. The solid line is the regression line for normal subjects. Individual data points are not shown for normal subjects.

slightly modified[4] substrate-specific method of Nilsson-Ehle and Ekman.[5] Twenty-two normal subjects served as controls, and the post-heparin lipolytic activities were measured in 21 of them. The results obtained were compared with 46 age- and sex-matched hemodialysis (HD) patients. Details of the latter have been published.[4]

RESULTS

When compared with age- and sex-matched normals or HD patients, female CAPD patients had higher serum TC concentrations than either of the latter (Table 1). However, the mean serum TC concentration of male CAPD patients did not differ significantly from that of normal subjects or HD patients. Female CAPD patients had significantly higher serum TG concentrations than did normal subjects. Their mean serum TG concentration was not significantly different from that of their HD

counterparts. The mean serum TG concentration of male CAPD patients, though higher, was not significantly different from that of normal males. The mean HDL-C of female CAPD patients was not significantly different from that of normal females, but was significantly greater than that of female HD patients. On the contrary, male CAPD patients, like their HD counterparts, had markedly reduced HDL-C concentrations when compared to normal subjects. Both male and female CAPD patients had reduced hepatic lipase and lipoprotein lipase activities. However, the mean lipoprotein lipase activity of female CAPD patients was significantly higher than that of female HD patients (3.70μM FFA/ml/h vs 2.54μM FFA/ml/h).

Figure 1 shows the relation between lipoprotein lipase activities and the log-transformed values of serum TG in CAPD patients and in normal subjects. While a significant inverse correlation ($r = -0.59$) existed between the two parameters of lipid metabo-

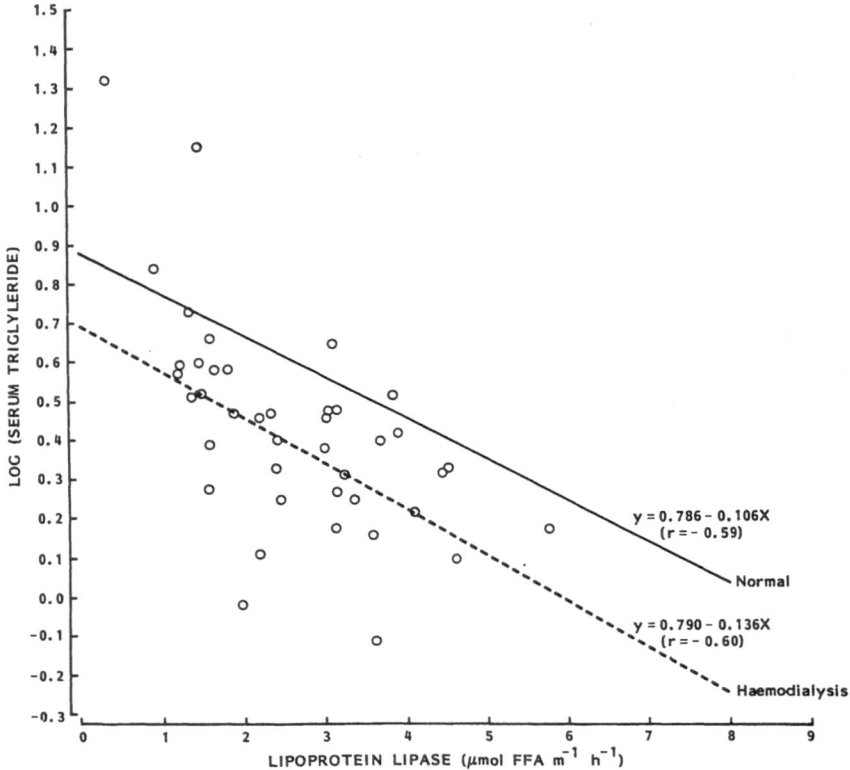

Fig. 2. Correlation between log (TG) and lipoprotein lipase in HD patients and normal subjects. Open circles and the interrupted line represent HD patients. The solid line is the regression line for normal subjects. Individual data points for normal subjects are not shown.

lism in normal subjects, no correlation ($r = -0.27$) could be demonstrated between the same two parameters in CAPD patients. This is in sharp contrast to HD patients who also exhibited a similar inverse correlation between lipoprotein lipase activities and log TG (Fig. 2).

Figure 3 shows the relation between HDL-C and lipoprotein lipase activities in CAPD patients and normal subjects. Although a significant positive correlation ($r = 0.58$) existed between the two parameters in normal subjects, the correlation in CAPD patients was insignificant ($r = 0.22$). Hepatic lipase activities did not correlate with any of the other parameters of lipid metabolism.

DISCUSSION

Defective catabolism of triglyceride-rich lipoproteins in patients with chronic renal failure is a documented phenomenon,[6] and such a defect in lipid

metabolism persists in HD patients[4,6-8] and can be related to the low lipoprotein lipase[4] activities in these patients. Our study revealed that as in HD patients,[4] both hepatic lipase and lipoprotein lipase activities are reduced in patients on CAPD. However, as far as the activities of these two enzymes are concerned, it appears that patients on CAPD carrying out four 2 L exchanges daily fare no worse than those receiving 18–21 hours of intermittent HD per week. Lipoprotein lipase hydrolyzes the triglyceride in the core of triglyceride-rich lipoproteins to free fatty acids and glycerol. It is expected that low lipoprotein lipase activities lead to the accumulation of these lipoproteins and result in hypertriglyceridemia. A poorly dialyzable inhibitor of lipoprotein lipase in uremic plasma has been reported.[9] The molecular characteristic of the inhibitor (or inhibitors) is not known. Since the clearance of "middle molecules" by CAPD far exceeds that achieved by conventional hemodialysis,[10] it is tempting to postu-

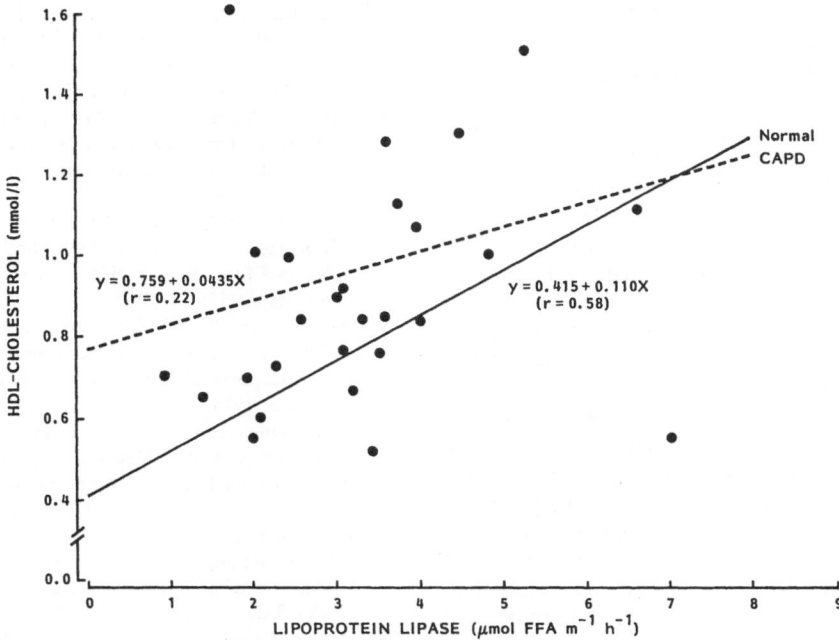

Fig. 3. Correlation between HDL-C concentrations and lipoprotein lipase in CAPD patients and normal subjects. Closed circles and the interrupted line represent CAPD patients. The solid line is the regression line for normal subjects. Individual data points for normal subjects are not shown.

late that CAPD patients will have higher lipoprotein lipase activities than HD patients. The mean lipoprotein lipase activity of female CAPD patients in our study was indeed greater than that of HD patients. However, such an assumption is premature without knowledge of the lipoprotein-lipase-inhibiting activity in the plasma of CAPD patients. Furthermore, it is difficult to explain why the mean lipoprotein lipase activity in male CAPD patients was not significantly different from that of their HD counterparts. It must be remembered that carbohydrate feeding[11] can increase lipoprotein lipase activity, probably by releasing insulin, which has a stimulating effect on lipoprotein lipase.[12, 13] Whether repeated exposure to the glucose load in dialysis solutions is responsible for the significantly higher lipoprotein lipase activity in female CAPD patients cannot be determined from the present data.

In normal subjects as well as in HD patients, a significant inverse correlation exists between lipoprotein lipase and log TG. Since lipoprotein lipase activity was measured *in vitro* under optimal conditions, the inverse correlation cannot be an artefact produced by expansion of the serum TG pool. We have interpreted the inverse correlation between

lipoprotein lipase activities and log TG concentrations in HD patients as evidence that reduced lipoprotein lipase activities cause hypertriglyceridemia.[4] By the same token, the lack of such a relation in CAPD patients implies that the cause of their hypertriglyceridemia lies elsewhere. Perhaps, hepatic synthesis of triglyceride-rich lipoproteins is increased in CAPD patients in response to the hypoalbuminemia resulting from heavy protein loss in the dialysate, a situation analogous to the nephrotic syndrome.[14] The glucose in the dialysis solution is an important source of calories and can be used in hepatic TG synthesis. That the hypertriglyceridemia in our patients is not as severe as reported by other investigators[2] is likely due to our insistence that hypertonic solutions should not be regularly used.

A positive correlation exists between lipoprotein lipase activities and HDL-C concentrations. During the catabolism of triglyceride-rich lipoproteins, some of the surface apoproteins of very low-density lipoproteins are transferred to HDL.[15] Therefore the low HDL concentrations in HD patients is likely the consequence of defective TG catabolism due to low lipoprotein lipase activities.[4] The lack of a positive correlation between

HDL-C and lipoprotein lipase in CAPD patients suggests that other factors, such as increased hepatic synthesis of HDL, may compensate for the low HDL resulting from reduced lipoprotein lipase activities. It is interesting that female CAPD patients had significantly higher HDL-C than did their HD counterparts. This may be related to the higher lipoprotein lipase activities in female CAPD patients. The mean lipoprotein lipase of male CAPD patients is comparable to that of male HD patients, hence also their HDL-C concentrations.

Hepatic lipase is a lipolytic enzyme released in post-heparin plasma.[16] It constitutes the major fraction of total post-heparin lipolytic activity.[17] The role of hepatic lipase remains conjectural, but is widely postulated that it catabolizes intermediate density lipoproteins. Although hepatic lipase has phospholipase A_1 activities *in vitro* and probably plays a role in phospholipid metabolism,[18] whether or not the reduced hepatic lipase activities in CAPD patients cause any abnormalities in lipid metabolism cannot be ascertained from the present study.

REFERENCES

1. Chan MK, Baillod RA, Chuah P, Sweny P, Raftery MJ, Varghese A, and Moorhead JF: Three years' experience of continuous ambulatory peritoneal dialysis. Lancet 1: 1409, 1981
2. Khanna R, Oreopoulos DG, Dombros N, et al.: Continuous ambulatory peritoneal dialysis (CAPD) after three years: Still a promising treatment. Peritoneal Dial Bull 1: 24, 1981
3. Chan MK, Varghese Z, Persaud JW, Baillod RA, and Moorhead JF: Hyperlipidaemia in patients on maintenance haemo- and peritoneal dialysis: The relative roles of triglyceride production and triglyceride removal. Clin Nephrol 17: 183, 1982
4. Chan MK, Persaud JW, Varghese Z, and Moorhead JF: Pathogenic roles of post-heparin lipases in lipid abnormalities in hemodialysis patients. Kidney Int (in press)
5. Nilsson-Ehle P, and Ekman R: Rapid, simple and specific assays for lipoprotein lipase and hepatic lipase. Artery 3: 194, 1977
6. Ibels LS, Reardon MF, and Nestel PJ: Plasma post-heparin lipolytic activity and triglyceride clearance in uremia and hemodialysis patients and renal allograft recipients. J Lab Clin Med 87: 648, 1976
7. Cattran DC, Fenton SSA, Wilson DR, and Steiner G: Defective triglyceride removal in lipemia associated with peritoneal dialysis and hemodialysis. Ann Intern Med 85: 29, 1976
8. Chan MK, Varghese A, Persaud W, Baillod RA, and Moorhead JF: HDL-cholesterol and intravenous fat tolerance in dialysis patients. Proc Eur Dial Transplant Assoc 17: 247, 1980
9. Murase T, Cattran DC, Rubenstein B, and Steiner G: Inhibition of lipoprotein lipase by uremic plasma. A possible cause of hypertriglyceridemia. Metabolism 24: 1278, 1975
10. Oreopoulos DG, Robson M, Faller B, Ogilvie R, Rapoport A, and DeVeber GA: Continuous ambulatory peritoneal dialysis: A new era in the treatment of chronic renal failure. Clin Nephrol 11: 125, 1979
11. Nilsson-Ehle P, Carlstrom S, and Belfrage P: Rapid effects on lipoprotein lipase activity in adipose tissue of humans after carbohydrate and lipid intake. Scand J Clin Lab Invest 35: 373, 1975
12. Borensztain J, Samols DR, and Rubenstein AH: Effects of insulin on lipoprotein lipase activity in the rat heart and adipose tissue. Am J Physiol 223: 1271, 1972
13. Garfinkel AS, Nilsson-Ehle P, and Schotz MC: Regulation of lipoprotein lipase induction by insulin. Biochim Biophys Acta 424: 264, 1976
14. Kaysen GA, and Schoenfield PY: Albumin homeostasis in patients undergoing continuous ambulatory peritoneal dialysis. Kidney Int 25: 107, 1984
15. Tall AR, Greem PHR, Glickman RM, and Riley JW: Metabolic fate of chylomicron phospholipids and apoproteins in the rat. J Clin Invest 64: 977, 1979
16. La Rosa JC, Levy RI, Windmueller HG, and Frederickson DS: Comparison of the triglyceride lipase of liver, adipose tissue and post-heparin plasma. J Lipid Res 13: 356, 1972
17. Huttunen JK, Ehnholm C, Kekki M, and Nikkila EA. Post-heparin plasma lipoprotein: Correlations to sex, age and various parameters of triglyceride metabolism. Clin Sci 50: 249, 1976
18. Jansen H, Van Tol A, and Hulsmann WC: On the metabolic function of heparin-releasable liver lipase. Biochem Biophys Res Comm 92: 53, 1980

N.G. DeSanto, G. Capodicasa, G. Capasso, F. Nuzzi,
V. DeSimone, F. Scoppa, and C. Giordano

84

Body Composition in Uremic Children on CAPD and Hemodialysis

SUMMARY

Twelve prepubertal children with renal failure, half of them treated by CAPD and half by hemodialysis, were studied at the start and after 6 months of dialysis. Weight gain was more substantial with CAPD than with hemodialysis. CADP was associated with a significant increase in intracellular water, while extracellular fluid decreased somewhat, unlike the minimal changes with hemodialysis.

INTRODUCTION

Decreased intracellular water and increased extracellular water have been demonstrated in uremic adults and children undergoing hemodialysis (HD).[1-4] Such changes are more dramatic in prepubertal uremic children.[5] In addition, it has been shown that decreased intracellular water is associated with reduced fat free solids such that the hemodialysis regimen is thought to be responsible for loss of cell mass.

Studies on body composition in uremic patients undergoing CAPD have provided conflicting data in adults,[6] and are still lacking in uremic children. This information might be relevant, since in our experience CAPD was able to correct many of the uremic features associated with stunted growth in uremia.[7-10] The aims of this work were: (1) to collect data on body composition in uremic children undergoing CAPD therapy and (2) to compare the information with that obtained during HD treatment. Data are presented indicating that uremic prepubertal children on CAPD have a nearly normal body composition, while this goal is not achieved with HD treatment.

METHODS

We have studied 12 prepubertal children aged 8–11 years equally divided by sex. The patients all had ESRD and needed dialysis at the time of the study. The patients were divided at random into two groups (Table 1), a CAPD group and a HD group with a comparable glomerular filtration rate (GFR) and nearly identical causes of renal failure. Patients were studied twice: at start of treatment and six months after CAPD or HD treatment. CAPD was performed as usual.[7-10] Hemodialysis was performed with hollow fiber dialyzers with very low priming volume.

GFR was measured according to the method of Guignard et al.[11] GFR = 2 × creatinine clearance + 1 × urea clearance ÷ 3. Total body water was measured by tritium (3 μCi/kg). Extracellular water (ECW) was measured by nonradioactive bromide (0.4 mEq/kg). ICW was measured as the difference (TBW − ECW). Free fat body mass (FFB) was obtained from the nomogram of Moore et al.[12] Fat-

From the Istituto di Medicina Interna e Nefrologia, Cattedra di Nefrologia Pediatrica, I Facoltà di Medicina Università di Napoli and Santobono Hospital, Napoli, Italy.

Table 1. Characterization of Patients
Participating in the Study.

12 prepubertal children
  6 males and 6 females aged 8–11 years with ESRD

Divided in two groups of 6 patients each
  1. CAPD group: GFR 3.0 ± 2.0 ml/min × 1.73 m²
  2. HD group: GFR 2.65 ± 1.98 ml/min × 1.73 m²

Diagnosis Group A: 1 congenital hypoplasia, 2
  glomerulonephritis, 1 Alport's syndrome, 2
  pyelonephritis

Diagnosis Group B: 2 glomerulonephritis, 3 pyelonephritis, 1 hemolytic uremic syndrome

Diets: 100% RDA for protein and energy

free solids (FFS) = FFB − TBW. Predicted data
were calculated as follows: TBW according to Mellits and Cheek[13]; ICW according to Cheek[14]; FFB as
TBW/0.73. Statistical analysis was performed by t
test for paired data.

RESULTS

Data in Table 2 indicate that during CAPD treatment ICW increased significantly, while ECW was
reduced at the same rate ($p < 0.01$). These changes
produced statistically significant changes in the ratios between measured values and predicted values
(O/P). Patients undergoing HD did not show any

significant changes in body composition (Table 3).
During CAPD, body weight gain averaged 1.9 ± 0.5
kg, while during HD the weight gain was 0.6 ±
0.4 kg.

DISCUSSION

The data in Tables 2 and 3 confirm previous data
obtained in uremic children indicating that untreated
children have reduced intracellular water and increased extracellular water,[5] and demonstrate that
CAPD is an anabolic technique that normalizes ICW
and ECW as well as the ratio O/P for FFS. This
effect is important because it was achieved in prepubertal children.[5, 15, 16] The increased body cell
mass is in accord with previous studies from our
laboratory indicating that patients on CAPD may
achieve a positive nitrogen balance.[7, 8] The methodology used in this study may be criticized but,
taken as a whole, it is adequate, as indicated by El-
Bishti et al.[5] The fact that children on CAPD increase their body mass without normalizing stunted
growth is another indicator that renal dwarfism deserves a more rational approach and cannot be explained by the criteria used during the last 15
years.[7–10]

These data are in contrast with those in uremic
adults on CAPD, where water retention occurs without improvement in body cell mass.[17, 18] In fact, as
indicated by Williams et al.,[18] adult patients after 12
months of CAPD showed a mean increase of intracellular water of 7 kg and a loss of 1.69 kg of body

Table 2. Effects of CAPD Treatment on Body Composition. (TBW, ICW,
ECW (L), O/P = Observed/Predicted. Data are Mean ± SE).

Study Period	TBW	ICW	ECW	TBW O/P	ICW O/P	ECW O/P	FFS O/P
Start	13.1 ± 4.28	7.9 ± 3.11	5.2 ± 1.31	1.03 ± 0.02	0.85 ± 0.04	1.26 ± 0.05	0.86 ± 0.04
6 mo CAPD	14.7 ± 4.10	9.8 ± 2.94	4.9 ± 1.62	1.02 ± 0.02	0.96 ± 0.03	1.10 ± 0.04	0.95 ± 0.04
p	0.01	0.01	NS	NS	0.01	0.01	0.05

Table 3. Effects of HD on Body Composition.*

Study Period	TBW	ICW	ECW	TBW O/P	ICW O/P	ECW O/P	FFS O/P
Start	12.9 ± 3.75	7.8 ± 3.27	5.1 ± 1.47	1.04 ± 0.02	0.86 ± 0.03	1.23 ± 0.04	0.85 ± 0.04
6 mo HD	13.4 ± 3.48	8.3 ± 2.75	5.1 ± 1.53	1.02 ± 0.02	0.90 ± 0.03	1.16 ± 0.04	0.89 ± 0.04
p	NS	NS	NS	NS	NS	NS	NS

* Units as in Table 2.

proteins. However, our present data on FFS, as well as previous data from our laboratory,[19] indicate that this is not the case in the younger uremic patients.

ACKNOWLEDGMENTS

Supported by grants of the Ministry of Public Instruction Programs of National and Local Interests.

REFERENCES

1. Coles GA: Body composition in chronic renal failure. Q J Med 41: 25, 1978
2. Comty CM: A longitudinal study of body composition in terminal uremics treated by regular hemodialysis. Canad Med Assoc J 98: 482, 1968
3. Jones RW, El-Bishti M, Bloom SR, Burke J, Carter J, Counahan RC, Dalton N, Morris MC, and Chantler C: The effects of anabolic steroids on growth body composition and metabolism in body with chronic renal failure on regular hemodialysis. J Pediatr 97: 559, 1980
4. Brennan BL, Yasumura S, Letteri JM, and Cohn SH: Total body composition and distribution of body water in uremia. Kidney Int 17: 364, 1980
5. El-Bishti M, Burke J, Gill D, Joner RW, Counahan R, and Chantler C: Body composition in children on regular hemodialysis. Clin Nephrol 15: 53, 1981
6. Panzetta G, Guerra U, D'Angelo A, Sandrini S, Terzi A, Oldrizzi L, and Maiorca R: Body fluid spaces in patients on CAPD. Int J Artif Organs 7: 89, 1984
7. DeSanto NG, Capodicasa G, Pluvio M, and Gilli G: Nitrogen balance and growth in children on CAPD. In Gahl GM, Kessel D, and Nolph K (Eds), Advances in peritoneal dialysis: Proceedings of the 2nd international symposium on peritoneal dialysis. Amsterdam: Excerpta Medica, 1981, p 394
8. DeSanto NG, Capodicasa G, Gilli G, DiLeo VA, Caposso G, and Giordano C: Metabolic aspects of continuous ambulatory peritoneal dialysis with refer-

ence to energy protein input and growth. Int J Pediatr Nephrol 3: 279, 1982
9. DeSanto NG, Capodicasa G, Gilli G, and Giordano C: CAPD in infants and children. In LaGreca G (Ed), Proceedings of the 1st international course on peritoneal dialysis. Milan: Wichtig, 1982, p 344
10. DeSanto NG, Gilli G, Capasso G, DiLeo VA, and Giordano C: Growth during continuous ambulatory peritoneal dialysis (CAPD). Int J Artif Organs 5: 331, 1982
11. Guignard JP, Torrado A, Feldman H, and Gautier F: Assessment of GFR in children. Helv Paediatr Acta 35: 437, 1980
12. Moore FD, Olesen KH, McMurrey JD, Parker HV, Ball MR, and deVeber GA: The body cell mass and its supporting environment. Philadelphia: WB Saunders Co, 1963
13. Mellits DE, and Cheek DB: Growth and body water. In Cheek DB (Ed), Human growth. Philadelphia: Lea and Febiger, 1968
14. Cheek DB: Assessment of protein reserve (cellular mass) in aboriginal children. Am J Clin Nutr 31: 1328, 1978
15. Chantler C, and Holliday MA: Growth in children with renal disease with particular reference in the effects of calorie malnutrition. Clin Nephrol 1: 230, 1973
16. Wass WJ, Barrat M, Howarth RV, Marshal WA, Chantler C, Ogg CS, Cameron JS, Baillod RA, and Moorhead JF: Home dialysis in children. Lancet 1: 242, 1977
17. Rubin J, Flynn MA, and Nolph KD: Total body potassium. A guide to nutritional health in patients undergoing continuous ambulatory peritoneal dialysis. Am J Nutr 34: 94, 1981
18. Williams P, Kay R, Harrison H, McNeil K, Pettit J, Kelman B, Mendez M, Klein M, Olgivie R, Khanna R, Carnichsrl D, and Oreopoulos D: Nutritional and anthropometric assessment of patients on CAPD over one year: Contrasting changes in total body nitrogen and potassium. Peritoneal Dial Bull 1: 82, 1981
19. DeSanto NG, Capasso G, Capodicasa G, Nuzzi F, DeSimone V, and Giordano C: Effects of CAPD on body cell mass in uremic children. Artif Organs (in press)

P. Sandoz, D. Vallance, A.F. Winder, and J. Walls

85

Protein and Amino Acid Losses from the Peritoneum during CAPD and CCPD

SUMMARY

Uremic patients whether dialyzed or not, show some evidence of protein malnutrition. Plasma amino acid profiles in patients treated by CAPD or CCPD significantly differ from normal, but are possibly better than observed hemodialysis patients. Both protein and amino acid losses in CAPD and CCPD are dwell time dependent. Protein losses in CAPD and CCPD average 5 to 6 g/24 h and amino acid losses in CAPD and CCPD are less than 2 g/day.

INTRODUCTION

In the past few years CAPD has become a standard method of treatment for end-stage renal failure (ESRD) and its use is increasing. The metabolic outcome of such patients depends on the underlying uremic state, dietary intake, nutrients supplied in the peritoneal dialysis fluid, and nutrient loss via the peritoneum. At present, in routine CAPD, the only nutrient supplied via the dialysis solution is glucose, and the varying quantities absorbed during dialysis contribute to increased weight gain and lipid abnormalities. In addition to removal of "uremic toxins," the main losses from the peritoneum are protein and amino acids.[1] In continuous cyclic peritoneal dialysis (CCPD), the dwell time varies from 2–40 hours, compared to 4 or

---

From the Area Renal Unit, Leicester General Hospital, and the Department of Biochemistry, Leicester Royal Infirmary, Leicester, England.

8 hours in CAPD, and it is well known that protein and amino acid losses are dwell-time dependent.[2] The aim of the present study was to evaluate the protein and amino acid losses in CAPD and CCPD patients and to compare the nutritional profiles of these patients with nondialyzed and hemodialyzed uremic patients.

PATIENTS AND METHODS

Six patients on CCPD were evaluated and compared with age- and sex-matched CAPD (n = 10) and hemodialysis (n = 10) patients. Ten randomly selected chronic uremic patients and 10 random "normal" controls were also evaluated. The chronic uremic patients were older than the hemodialysis patients and the normal controls were younger. The clinical details of the patients studied are shown in Table 1, together with the dietary protein intake. The daily dietary protein intake was regularly assessed as part of a protocol for another study by the renal unit dietitian, and patients were requested to ingest 1–1.5 g protein/kg body weight/24 h. CAPD and CCPD were performed using previously described techniques.[3] No CAPD or CCPD patient was studied within one month of a peritonitis episode.

All studies were conducted with the patients admitted to the hospital. Fasting blood samples obtained from all subjects were analyzed for urea, creatinine, total proteins, albumin, globulin, and transferrin using standard laboratory techniques. Dialysate was collected after 4 or 8 hour dwell times with either 1.36% or 3.86% (anhydrous) dextrose

Table 1. Clinical Features of Controls and Patients Studied (Mean ± SEM).

	N	Age (yrs)	Sex	Months on Treatment	Body Weight (kg)	Protein Intake/24 h
Controls	10	27.7 ± 1.5	M 6, F 4	—	65.7 ± 2.60	free
Uremics	10	65.8 ± 3.03	M 6, F 4	—	69.1 ± 4.79	40 g
Hemodialysis	10	46.7 ± 3.87	M 5, F 5	18.9 ± 7.05	64.0 ± 4.46	70 g
CAPD	10	50.7 ± 3.25	M 5, F 5	9.5 ± 1.72	67.7 ± 4.32	>100 g
CCPD	6	43.3 ± 4.34	M 3, F 3	21.3 ± 4.42	64.6 ± 2.81	>100 g

concentration in CAPD and after 2, 16, or 40 hours with an (anhydrous) dextrose concentration of 2.16 ± 0.1% in CCPD. The effluent bags were weighed, mixed, and an aliquot removed. Blood and dialysate samples were deproteinized with sulphosalicylic acid (10% w/v) within one hour and stored at −20°C for amino acid analysis. The analysis was performed on an amino acid autoanalyzer (Rank Hilger Chromospek Mk I). In most samples, citrulline could not be differentiated from adjacent amino acids for technical reasons. Statistical analyses were performed by the two tailed Student's t test for paired or unpaired samples.

RESULTS

The nutritional values obtained in this study are shown in Table 2. There was a significant increase in serum creatinine in CCPD compared to CAPD (p < 0.02); serum urea, protein, albumin, and globulin were similar in the two modes of therapy, as was serum transferrin. Although the latter appeared higher in CCPD than in CAPD, this was not significantly different. Serum protein and albumin concentrations were lower in CAPD and CCPD compared

with hemodialysis patients. The plasma amino acid profiles expressed as a percentage of values obtained from the control subjects is given in Table 3. The only significant difference between CAPD and CCPD was a higher serum aspartic acid level in CCPD. The remainder of the amino acids showed similar patterns in both modes of therapy; most were reduced, but some were increased compared to normal values, i.e., glutamic acid, glycine, histidine and arginine. The ratio of tryptophan to phenylalanine was, as expected, low in uremics compared to normal controls (0.54 vs 0.95, p < 0.001). There was an increase with each treatment modality—i.e., hemodialysis 0.62, CAPD 0.65, and CCPD 0.62—but none of these values was significantly different from that of uremia.

The dialysate losses of protein and amino acids in CCPD and CAPD are shown in Table 4. Concentrations were significantly increased by prolonging the dwell time from 2 to 16 to 40 hours in CCPD. Moreover, the dialysate protein significantly increased from 4 to 8 hours in CAPD, but amino acid concentrations did not. Varying dextrose concentrations of the dialysis solution had no effect on protein and amino acid losses. The daily dialysate losses of protein were comparable between CAPD and CCPD

Table 2. Serum Biochemical Parameters of Nutrition in Normal Subjects and Patients (Mean ± SEM).

	Urea (mmol/L)	Creatinine (μmol/L)	Total Protein (g/L)	Albumin (g/L)	Globulins (g/L)	Transferrin (g/L)
Controls	4.85 ± 0.40	91.1 ± 7.37	70.2 ± 1.17	47.8 ± 1.04	22.4 ± 0.82	3.45 ± 0.18
Uremics	46.87 ± 6.22	1115.0 ± 129	58.6 ± 3.34**	31.6 ± 1.87	27.0 ± 2.02	2.11 ± 0.25
Hemodialysis	19.54 ± 1.57	925.6 ± 67.9	66.0 ± 1.1**	39.7 ± 0.90	26.3 ± 0.80	2.7 ± 0.20
CAPD	22.68 ± 2.33	880.9 ± 68.6*	57.8 ± 1.42	33.7 ± 0.97	24.1 ± 1.07	2.81 ± 0.20
CCPD	23.47 ± 3.89	1156.5 ± 67.8*	57.8 ± 3.15	34.3 ± 1.86	23.5 ± 1.43	3.18 ± 0.38

* p < 0.02.
** p < 0.001.

Table 3. Plasma Amino-Acid Values (Expressed as Percentage of Normal Values) in Uremic, Hemodialysis CAPD and CCPD Patients.

	Uremic	Hemodialysis	CAPD	CCPD
Essential Amino-Acids				
Threonine	57.3	46.8	54.5	65.0
Valine	64.7	41.7	54.6	64.0
Iso-leucine	63.1	37.9	81.5	68.9
Leucine	56.9	44.2	73.8	63.9
Histidine	116.3	70.6	111.9	101.1
Tryptophan	40.2	27.6	31.0	29.9
Lysine	71.3	74.5	80.8	66.7
Methionine	94.4	37.0	48.1	40.7
Nonessential Amino-Acids				
Aspartic Acid	142.1	189.4	89.5	155.3
Serine	59.7	49.3	68.2	69.2
Glutamic acid	94.8	58.5	140.0	100.7
Glycine	64.7	80.4	105.2	119.3
Alanine	61.2	52.0	66.5	97.5
Cystine	348	358	88.4	102.3
Tyrosine	48.4	51.5	53.7	55.8
Phenylalanine	89.5	75.2	75.2	80.9
Ornithine	69.7	93.2	100.7	78.8
Arginine	93.8	81.4	100.0	136.5

Table 4. Variation of Protein and Amino-Acid Losses with Time in CAPD and CCPD (Mean ± SEM).

		Protein g/L	Amino-Acid g/L
CCPD	2 h	0.57 ± 0.10	0.138 ± 0.015
	16 h	1.58 ± 0.33*	0.260 ± 0.018***
	40 h	8.4 ± 1.30	0.304 ± 0.017
CAPD	4 h	0.393 ± 0.059	0.181 ± 0.013
	8 h	0.766 ± 0.081***	0.201 ± 0.015

* $p < 0.02$.
*** $p < 0.001$.

Table 5. Daily Protein and Amino-Acid Losses in CAPD and CCPD (Mean ± SEM).

	Protein g/24 h	Amino-Acids g/24 h
CCPD	6.05 ± 0.84*	1.25 ± 0.12**
CAPD	5.92 ± 0.71*	1.962 ± 0.13**

* NS.
** $p < 0.001$.

(Table 5), but the amino acid loss was lower in CCPD (1.26 ± 1.2 g/24 h) compared to CAPD (1.96 ± 1.3 g/24 h).

DISCUSSION

It is generally accepted that uremic patients, whether dialyzed or not, have some degree of protein and calorie malnutrition. In the present study, most biochemical parameters of nutrition measured—i.e., serum protein, albumin, and transferrin—were decreased in uremic patients compared with normal controls; the lower range in the normal control group being unlikely to account for this difference. CAPD and CCPD were as good as if not better than either uremic or hemodialysis patients except in regard to serum proteins in the latter group. CCPD with different dwell times and smaller volumes of dialysate—i.e., 56 L vs 70 L per week—compared favorably with CAPD despite the higher serum creatinine values.

The amino acid profiles for the hemodialysis patients, while comparable with other published data,[4,5] were in general lower than in CAPD, CCPD, or uremic patients. These differences may be accounted for by the increased losses, estimated to be up to 20 g/dialysis in hemodialysis patients, or to different dietary intakes. The amino acid profiles in the CAPD and CCPD patients were similar to those previously described,[6,7] and apart from aspartic acid, no significant difference could be detected between either mode of therapy. Most amino acid concentrations were reduced, but glutamic acid, glycine, histidine, and arginine were increased.

The losses of protein from the peritoneum in this study are lower than most reported data,[8,9] but in keeping with those reported by Katirzoglou et al.[10] The reasons for this decrease are not apparent.[11] The amino acid losses from the peritoneum were less than 2 g/day, confirming previously reported data.[6,7] Both protein and amino acid losses are dwell-time dependent, but no differences were detected between CAPD or CCPD in respect to daily protein losses, although the losses of amino acids in CCPD were less than CAPD despite differing dwell time regimens. Although there was significant nitrogen loss both as protein and amino acids in CAPD and CCPD, the nutritional parameters in these two modes of therapy were comparable with other uremic and dialysis patients, and it is probable that the protein and amino acid losses are compensated by the increased oral protein intake.

REFERENCES

1. Blumenkrantz MJ: Studies of protein and nitrogen metabolism during continuous ambulatory peritoneal dialysis. In Gahl GM, Kessel M, and Nolph KD (Eds), Advances in peritoneal dialysis: Proceedings of the 2nd international symposium on peritoneal dialysis. Amsterdam: Excerpta Medica, 1981, p 391

2. DeSanto NG, Capodicasa G, and DiLeo VA: Kinetics of amino acids equilibrium in dialysate during CAPD. Int J Artif Organs 4: 23, 1981

3. Walls J, Smith BA, Feehally J, Taverner D, and Turgan C: CCPD—An improvement on CAPD? In Gahl GM, Kessel M, and Nolph KD (Eds), Advances in peritoneal dialysis: Proceedings of the 2nd international symposium on peritoneal dialysis. Amsterdam: Excerpta Medica, 1981, p 141

4. Young GA, Swanepoel CR, Croft MR, Hobson SM, and Parsons FM: Anthropometry and plasma valine, amino acids and proteins in the nutritional assessment of haemodialysis patients. Kidney Int 21: 492, 1982

5. Wolfson M, Jones MR, and Kopple JD: Amino acid losses during haemodialysis with infusion of amino acids and glucose. Kidney Int 21: 500, 1982

6. Dombros N, Oren A, and Marliss EB: Plasma amino acid profiles and amino acid losses in patients undergoing CAPD. Peritoneal Dial Bull 2: 27, 1982

7. Giordano C, DeSanto NG, Capodicasa G, DiLeo VA, DiSerafino A, Cirillo D, Esposito R, Fiore R, Damiano M, Buonadonna L, Cocco F, and DiIorio B: Amino acid losses during CAPD. Clin Nephrol 14: 230, 1980

8. Popovich RP, Moncrief JW, Nolph KD, Ghods AJ, Twardowski ZJ, and Pyle WK: Continuous ambulatory peritoneal dialysis. Ann Intern Med 88: 449, 1978

9. Blumenkrantz MJ, Gahl GM, Kopple JD, Kamdar AV, Jones MR, Kessel M, and Coburn JW: Protein losses during peritoneal dialysis. Kidney Int 19: 593, 1981

10. Katirtzoglou A, Oreopoulos DG, Hudsan H, Leung M, Ogilvie R, and Dombros N: Reappraisal of protein losses in patients undergoing CAPD. Nephron 26: 230, 1980

11. Sandoz P, and Walls J: Protein losses in continuous ambulatory peritoneal dialysis (CAPD). Peritoneal Dial Bull (in press)

J. Youmbissi, L. Sellars, A.C. Shore, T. Poon,
and R. Wilkinson

86

Blood Pressure on CAPD: Relationship to Sodium Status, Renin, and Aldosterone, Compared with Hemodialysis

SUMMARY

The control of blood pressure in 44 patients on continuous ambulatory peritoneal dialysis (CAPD) for 7 ± 4 months was studied in relation to measurements of exchangeable sodium (NaE), plasma renin activity (PRA) and plasma aldosterone concentration (PA). Comparisons were made with 21 patients on hemodialysis (HD) for 50 ± 13 months and with 32 normal subjects.

Mean arterial pressure was elevated before dialysis in both groups and fell significantly on dialysis. Blood pressure on dialysis was still significantly elevated in CAPD patients, but not in the HD group. In both dialysis groups mean NaE was normal and PRA and PA were elevated, but there was no difference between dialysis groups. The apparent superiority of HD over CAPD in controlling blood pressure may be related to the greater duration of treatment in the HD patients.

Blood pressure was unrelated to NaE, PRA or PA in either controls or patient groups and there was no relationship between NaE and PRA. There was a direct relationship between PRA and PA in controls and CAPD patients, but not in the HD patients, where PA was directly related to plasma potassium.

From the Department of Medicine and Nephrology, Freeman Hospital, Newcastle upon Tyne, England.

INTRODUCTION

There is evidence that sodium retention, assessed by measurement of exchangeable sodium is important in the hypertension of patients with advanced renal failure.[1,2] In addition, in patients on hemodialysis, a direct relationship between plasma renin and blood pressure has been demonstrated by some groups,[3,4] suggesting a hypertensive role for angiotensin II.

Correction of sodium overload by hemodialysis allows control of hypertension in up to 90% of patients,[5,6] but bilateral nephrectomy may be necessary in the remainder, who usually have very high renin levels.[4] However, blood pressure may fall after bilateral nephrectomy in 80% of hypertensive hemodialysis patients, even in those with normal renin levels,[7] and it has been suggested that the hypertension of uremic patients may be explained by an abnormal relationship between sodium and renin, in that plasma renin levels of whatever value are inappropriately high for the degree of sodium loading.[8]

Hypertensive uremic patients have a similar cardiac output, but they also have increased peripheral resistance compared with normotensive uremic patients.[9] Possible causes of this include whole-body autoregulation,[10] angiotensin II, natriuretic factor,[11] and increased sodium content of the arteriolar wall,[12] which may be influenced by aldosterone.[13]

CAPD is now well established in the management of chronic renal failure.[14] Although blood pressure control has usually been satisfactory,[15-18] there have been few detailed studies. We have therefore examined the control of blood pressure in patients on CAPD and have related this to the renin-aldosterone system and to sodium status, assessed by measurement of exchangeable sodium (NaE). Comparisons have been made with hemodialysis (HD) patients and normotensive controls.

METHODS

Thirty-two normal control subjects, 44 CAPD patients, and 21 HD patients were studied. The CAPD patients were randomly selected after those on dialysis for less than four months and those with peritonitis in the preceding month had been excluded. None of the patients had undergone other forms of dialysis. The HD group was also randomly selected after the exclusion of eight patients previously subjected to bilateral nephrectomy, since none of the CAPD population had undergone this operation. Clinical features and details of dialysis are given in Table 1. Diastolic blood pressure was taken as the disappearance of sounds (phase 5), and mean arterial pressure (MAP) was calculated as diastolic pressure plus one-third pulse pressure. Predialysis MAP was the mean of four readings taken before the start of dialysis. In addition to the above exclusions, some patients from both groups refused to be studied, usually for geographical reasons. In all there were 15 unstudied CAPD patients (7 males, 8 females), mean age 52 ± 11 years (mean ± SD), MAP on dialysis 105 ± 13 mm Hg, four of whom were taking antihypertensives, mean duration of dialysis 3.5 ± 2.0 months. Twenty-three HD patients who had not undergone bilateral nephrectomy were not studied (12 males, 11 females), mean age 49 ± 12 years, MAP on dialysis 96 ± 18 mm Hg, two of whom were on antihypertensives, mean duration of dialysis 42 ± 23 months for 13.2 ± 2 h/week. Within each dialysis group there were no significant differences between the studied and unstudied patients in age, sex, or MAP and within the HD group, there was no significant difference in the duration of dialysis or weekly hours. The normal controls were recruited from healthy clinical and laboratory staff, 14 males and 18 females, mean age 44 ± 16 years.

Antihypertensive medication was withdrawn two weeks before study; patients were seen regu-

Table 1. Clinical Features and Details of Dialysis.

	n	Age (yrs)	Predialysis MAP (mm Hg)	Patients on AHT Predialysis	Duration of Dialysis (months)	Weekly Dialysis Schedule	Dialysate Sodium (mmol/L)	Patients on AHT on Dialysis	Bilateral Nephrectomy
CAPD	44 M = 20 F = 24	46* ± 15	117 ± 23	23	7 ± 4	4 cycles/24 h 1.36% glucose alone in 37 patients	132	9	0
HD	21 M = 11 F = 10	48 ± 13	128 ± 23	14	50 ± 13	13.5 ± 2.5 h in 3 sessions	136	4	0

MAP = Mean arterial pressure.
AHT = Antihypertensive drugs.
* Mean ± SD.

Table 2. Mean Values (±SD) of Measurements in Normal Controls, CAPD and HD Patients (for Plasma-Renin Activity and Plasma-Aldosterone, the Geometric Mean is Given).

	MAP (mm Hg)	Exchangeable Sodium (mmol/kg LBM)	Plasma Renin Activity (pmol/L/min)	Plasma Aldosterone (pmol/L)	Plasma Sodium (mmol/L)	Plasma Potassium (mmol/L)	Plasma Creatinine (µmol/L)
Controls	89 ± 10	53 ± 5	3.5	85	140 ± 3	4.2 ± 0.3	81 ± 14
CAPD	103 ± 18	53 ± 8	8.7	161	139 ± 3	4.2 ± 0.7	976 ± 257
HD	93 ± 19	56 ± 12	14.0	196	138 ± 2	4.4 ± 0.7	820 ± 184

LBM = Lean body mass.

larly and treatment restarted if diastolic pressure reached 130 mm Hg, which occurred in two CAPD patients who were withdrawn from the study. At midday on the first day of study, peritoneal dialysate was drained out, and height, weight, and skinfold thickness measured. Two liters of dialysate were run in and a 24-hour urine collection was started. No further dialysis exchanges were performed for 24 hours. Blood was taken for creatinine and electrolytes and 15 µ Ci (microCuries) [24]Na was given intravenously. At 9:00 AM, after an overnight fast and while supine, blood pressure was measured and venous blood samples were taken for measurement of plasma renin activity (PRA) and plasma aldosterone concentration (PA). At midday the dialysate was drained and the 24-hour urine collection completed: the volume of each was measured and aliquots taken for measurement of sodium concentration and radioactive counting of [24]Na. A second blood sample was taken for measurement of creatinine, electrolytes, and [24]Na. Exchangeable sodium was calculated using the isotope dilution principle[19] after combining the radioactive counts and volumes of urine and dialysate. Lean body mass (LBM) was calculated using the formula of Edwards and Whyte.[20]

Exchangeable sodium in the HD patients was measured during the 24 hours before dialysis. Blood pressure and blood samples for creatinine, electrolytes, [24]Na, PRA, and PA were taken at the start of dialysis, after one hour in the supine position and an overnight fast. Ambulant levels of PRA and PA return to baseline after 30 minutes in the supine position.[21]

Plasma renin activity was measured by radioimmunoassay (New England Nuclear Co.). The coefficient of variation (CV) was 16% intra-assay and 23% interassay, detection limit 0.8 pmol/L/min. Plasma aldosterone was also measured by radioimmunoassay using a modification[22] of the technique of Fraser et al.[23] CV was 15% intra-assay and 21% interassay, detection limit 6 pmol/L.

RESULTS

The results are given in Table 2 and Figures 1–4. Measurements of PRA and PA were positively skewed; the geometric mean is given and statistical tests were done after logarithmic conversion. For other measurements, the arithmetic mean and standard deviation are given. Student's t test was used to compare means.

Predialysis MAP (Table 1) was significantly greater in CAPD and HD groups than MAP in con-

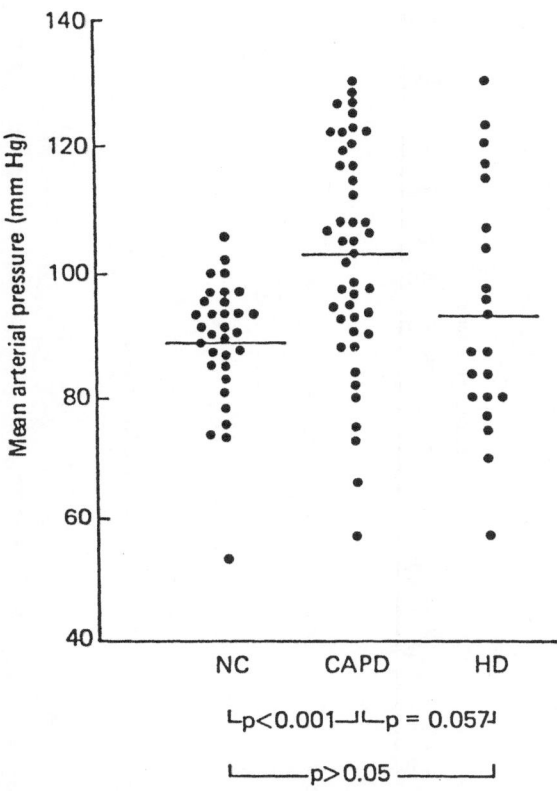

Fig. 1. Mean arterial pressure in normal controls (NC), patients on CAPD, and on hemodialysis (HD). (▬ = mean).

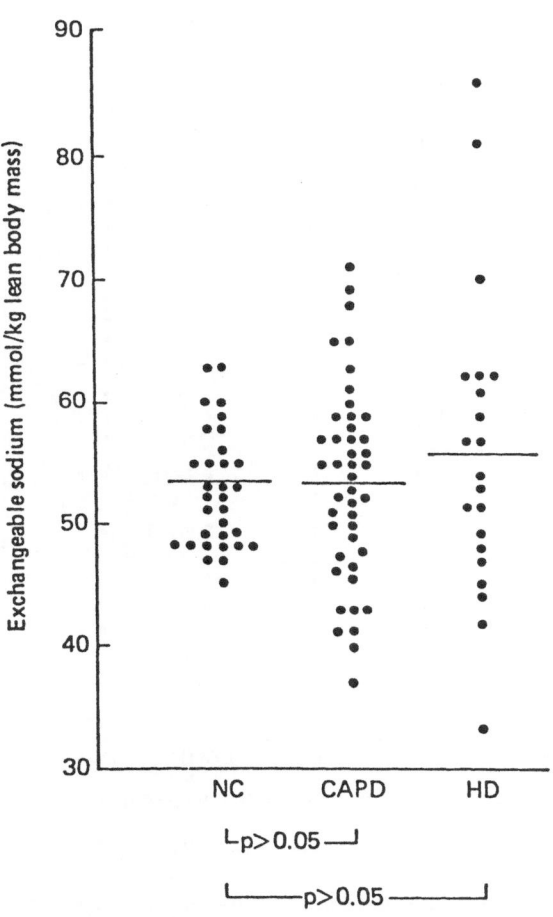

Fig. 2. Exchangeable sodium levels in normal controls (NC), patients on CAPD, and hemodialysis (HD). (▬ = mean).

trols ($p < 0.001$), but there was no significant difference between dialysis groups ($p = 0.08$). MAP on dialysis was significantly lower than the predialysis level in both CAPD (103 ± 18 mm Hg versus 117 ± 23 mm Hg, $p < 0.001$) and HD groups (93 ± 19 mm Hg versus 128 ± 23 mm Hg, $p < 0.001$). On dialysis, there was no significant difference in MAP between the HD group and controls (Fig. 1). MAP was highest in the CAPD group, being significantly different from controls ($p < 0.001$), but not from the HD patients ($p = 0.057$).

There were no significant differences among the mean values of NaE (Fig. 2). The three most extreme values of NaE in the HD group occurred in one obese (NaE = 33 mmol/kg LBM) and two emaciated patients (NaE = 81 and 86 mmol/kg LBM), probably reflecting the limitations of the formula for

calculation of lean body mass at the extremes of body build.

The scatter of PRA and PA levels were much greater in patients than controls. Mean PRA was significantly greater in the CAPD and HD groups than in controls ($p < 0.001$), but there was no significant difference between patient groups ($p > 0.05$), as may be seen in Figure 3. The pattern was the same for PA (Fig. 4). There were no significant differences among the mean values of plasma sodium, or potassium, but plasma creatinine was significantly higher in the CAPD than HD patients ($p < 0.05$).

MAP was unrelated to NaE, PRA, or PA in either controls or dialysis groups (Pearson r, $p > 0.05$). There was no relationship between NaE and PRA or PA in any group. There was a significant direct relationship between PRA and PA in controls

Youmbissi, et al.

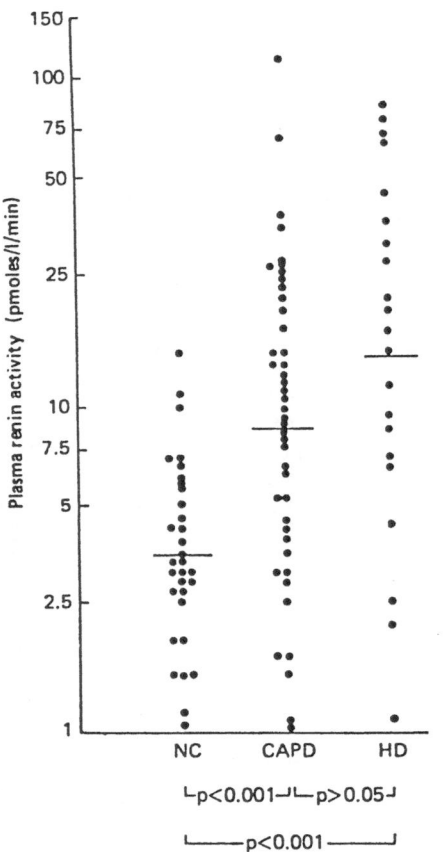

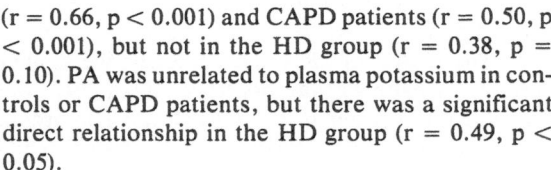

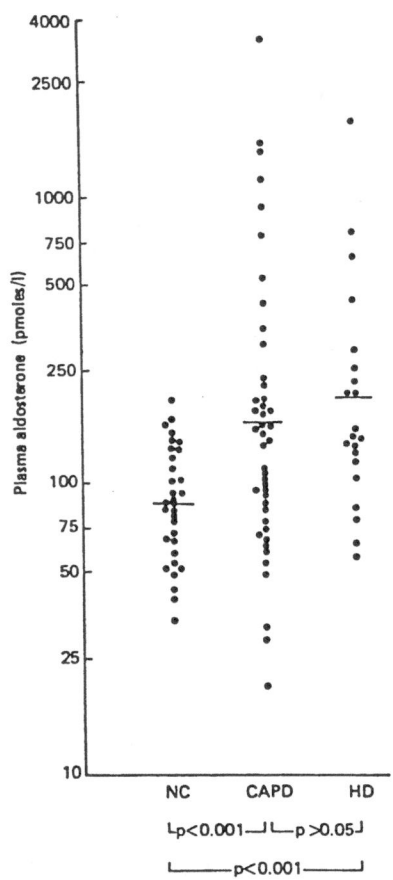

Fig. 3. Plasma-renin activity in normal controls (NC), patients on CAPD, and hemodialysis (HD). (Logarithmic scale, ▬ = geometric mean).

Fig. 4. Plasma-aldosterone concentration in normal controls (NC), patients on CAPD, and hemodialysis (HD). (Logarithmic scale, ▬ = geometric mean).

($r = 0.66$, $p < 0.001$) and CAPD patients ($r = 0.50$, $p < 0.001$), but not in the HD group ($r = 0.38$, $p = 0.10$). PA was unrelated to plasma potassium in controls or CAPD patients, but there was a significant direct relationship in the HD group ($r = 0.49$, $p < 0.05$).

Before starting dialysis, a similar proportion of CAPD (52%) and HD patients (67%) were taking antihypertensive drugs ($p > 0.05$, Fisher's exact test). After establishment on dialysis, the proportion had fallen significantly, to 20% in the CAPD and 19% in the HD patients ($p < 0.01$, Fisher's exact test).

Mean body weight in the CAPD patients at the time of study was 66.6 ± 13.1 kg, significantly greater than the predialysis value of 63.5 ± 12.9 kg ($p < 0.001$, paired t test).

DISCUSSION

Our results show that CAPD lowers blood pressure in patients with end-stage renal failure: MAP fell after starting treatment and fewer patients required antihypertensive drugs. This is probably at least in part due to the maintenance of normal exchangeable sodium levels on dialysis. On the other hand, in a study of seven hypertensive uremic patients,[24] it was possible, after six months on CAPD, to withdraw all antihypertensive drugs with maintenance of normotension: mean body weight remained statistically unchanged, there was an increase in PRA and PA from normal levels predialysis, and there was a reduction in the pressor response to infused angiotenson II. From these findings it was suggested that for some reason there may be reduced vascular sensitivity on CAPD or that CAPD may remove an unidentified middle molecular weight vasopressor substance with a resultant fall in blood pressure and increase in renin secretion. However, it is possible that sodium and water excess were corrected by CAPD and that body weight did not change because of a gain in tissue mass associated with the increase in appetite and the peritoneal glucose load that accompany CAPD. Sodium and water removal would explain the increase in PRA and PA, and also the reduced pressor response to exogenous angiotensin II.[25] In addition, if beta blockers were among the antihypertensive agents withdrawn, then this may have contributed to the elevation of renin levels on CAPD. Our CAPD patients had normal NaE levels on dialysis, presumably having been lowered from elevated levels predialysis. In spite of this, body weight rose significantly, suggesting that long-term changes in weight are an unreliable guide to changes in sodium status on CAPD, although a longitudinal study would be needed to confirm this.

Despite normal NaE levels, blood pressure was higher in our CAPD patients than in controls. Cannaud et al.[26] have also found that hypertension may persist on CAPD. In their study, blood pressure fell in hypertensive patients after one month on CAPD, but after six months, hypertension had returned in association with weight gain, suggesting that control of blood pressure may deteriorate if dietary restrictions are relaxed. As in the study of Glasson et al.,[24] our patients had elevated renin and aldosterone levels, and this may have contributed to the elevation of blood pressure, although the lack of a relationship between MAP and either PRA or PA suggests that these factors are not primary determinants of blood pressure on CAPD. Other groups have failed to demonstrate a relationship between blood pressure and renin in patients on hemodialysis.[6,27–29] It has been shown that the presence of dialysate in the peritoneal cavity increases the MAP of CAPD patients by an average of 4 mm Hg,[30] but this effect would be insufficient to account for our findings.

In this study we confirmed that HD is effective in lowering blood pressure. Hemodialysis appears to be more effective than CAPD, since MAP on HD was not significantly greater than in controls. This could not be explained by lower mean values of NaE, PRA, or PA on HD compared with CAPD, emphasizing that factors other than sodium and the renin-aldosterone system are important in determining blood pressure on dialysis.[31] It has been shown that cardiac output is similar in hypertensive and normotensive patients on HD, but peripheral resistance is higher in the hypertensives.[32] It therefore seems likely that increased peripheral resistance is responsible for the higher blood pressure in our CAPD group compared with the HD group. The HD patients had been on dialysis approximately seven times longer than the CAPD patients, and it is likely that a continuing reduction in peripheral resistance occurs with prolonged dialysis after correction of sodium overload has been achieved and despite elevated renin levels. This may be due to reversal of hypertensive arteriolar changes as blood pressure is lowered.

The direct relationship between PRA and PA on CAPD has been demonstrated by others[24] and indicates that angiotensin II is a major determinant of aldosterone levels in these patients. In the HD group, PA was unrelated to PRA but was directly related to plasma potassium concentration. Others[33,34] have demonstrated that potassium is more important than renin in the regulation of plasma aldosterone in patients on hemodialysis, but a dominant role for renin was found in a longitudinal study.[35]

In conclusion, treatment with CAPD for an average of seven months lowered blood pressure, but not to normal levels. This was associated with a normal mean exchangeable sodium level, but increased levels of renin and aldosterone. Hemodialysis appeared to be more effective than CAPD in controlling blood pressure, despite similar levels of exchangeable sodium, renin, and aldosterone. This may relate to the much greater duration of hemodialysis treatment.

REFERENCES

1. Dathan JRE, Johnson DB, and Goodwin FJ: The relationship between body fluid compartment volumes, renin activity and blood pressure in chronic renal failure. Clin Sci 45: 77, 1973
2. Weidman P, Beretta-Piccoli C, Steffen F, Blumberg A, and Reubi FC: Hypertension in terminal renal failure. Kidney Int 9: 294, 1976
3. Brown JJ, Curtis JR, Lever AF, Robertson JIS, DeWardener HE, and Wing AJ: Plasma renin concentration and the control of blood pressure in patients on maintenance hemodialysis. Nephron 6: 329, 1969
4. Wilkinson R, Scott DR, Uldall PR, Kerr DNS, and Swinney J: Plasma renin and exchangeable sodium in the hypertension of chronic renal failure. QJ Med 39: 377, 1970
5. Vertes V, Cangiano JL, Berman LB, and Gould A: Hypertension in end-stage renal disease. N Engl J Med 280: 978, 1969

6. Craswell PW, Hiro VM, Judd PA, Baillod RA, Varghese Z, and Moorhead JF: Plasma renin activity and blood pressure in 89 patients receiving maintenance haemodialysis therapy. Br Med J 4: 749, 1972

7. Del-Greco F, and Burgess JL: Hypertension in terminal renal failure: Observations pre and post bilateral nephrectomy. J Chron Dis 26: 471, 1973

8. Schalekamp MA, Beevers DG, Briggs JD, et al.: Hypertension in chronic renal failure. An abnormal relationship between sodium and the renin-angiotension system. Am J Med 55: 379, 1973

9. Kim KE, Onesti G, Schwartz AB, Chinitz JL, and Schwartz CD: Hemodynamics of hypertension in chronic end-stage renal disease. Circulation 46: 456, 1972

10. Guyton AC, Coleman TG, Young DB, Lehmeier TE, and Declue JW: Salt balance and long-term blood pressure control. Ann Rev Med 31: 15, 1980

11. Blaustein MP: Sodium ions, calcium ions, blood pressure regulation, and hypertension: A reassessment and a hypothesis. Am J Physiol 232: C165, 1977

12. Tobian L, and Binion JT: Tissue cations and water in arterial hypertension. Circulation 5: 754, 1952

13. Kornel L, Ramsay C, Kanamarlarpudi N, Travers T, and Packer W: Evidence for the presence in arterial walls of intra-cellular molecular mechanism for action of mineralocorticoids. Clin Exp Hyper Theory and Practice A4(9 and 10): 1561, 1982

14. Ramos JM, Gokal R, Siamopoulos K, Ward MK, Wilkinson R, and Kerr DNS: Continuous ambulatory peritoneal dialysis: Three years experience. QJ Med 206: 165, 1983

15. Popovich RP, Moncrief JW, Nolph KD, Ghods AJ, Twardowski ZJ, and Pyle WK: Continuous ambulatory peritoneal dialysis. Ann Intern Med 88: 449, 1978

16. Gokal R, McHugh M, Fryer R, Ward MK, and Kerr DNS: Continuous ambulatory peritoneal dialysis: One year's experience in a UK dialysis unit. Br Med J 281: 474, 1980

17. Rubin J, Barnes T, Burns E, Ray R, Teal N, Hellems E, and Bower J: Comparison of home hemodialysis to continuous ambulatory peritoneal dialysis. Kidney Int 23: 51, 1983

18. Wu G: Cardiovascular deaths among CAPD patients. Peritoneal Dial Bull 3(3 Suppl): S23, 1983

19. Miller H, and Wilson GM: The measurement of exchangeable sodium in man using the isotope ^{24}Na. Clin Sci 12: 97, 1953

20. Edwards KDG, and Whyte HM: Creatinine excretion and body composition. Clin Sci 18: 361, 1959

21. Agabiti-Rosei E, Brown JJ, Cumming AMM, Fraser R, Semple PF, Lever AF, Morton JJ, Robertson AS, Robertson JIS, and Tree M: Is the "sodium-index" a useful way of expressing clinical plasma renin, angiotensin and aldosterone values? Clin Endocrinol 8: 141, 1978

22. Piercy DA: A study of sodium balance and hypertension in acromegaly. PhD Thesis, University of Newcastle upon Tyne, 1977

23. Fraser R, Guest S, and Young J: A comparison of double isotope derivative and radio-immunological estimation of plasma aldosterone concentration in man. Clin Sci 45: 411, 1973

24. Glasson P, Favré A, and Vallotton MB: Response of blood pressure and the renin-angiotension-aldosterone system to chronic ambulatory peritoneal dialysis in hypertensive end-stage renal failure. Clin Sci 63: 207s, 1982

25. Oelkers W, Brown JJ, Fraser R, Lever AF, Morton JJ, and Robertson JIS: Sensitization of the adrenal cortex to angiotensin II in sodium-deplete man. Circulation Res 34: 69, 1974

26. Cannaud B, Mimran A, Liendo-Liendo C, Slingeneyer A, and Mion C: Blood pressure control in patients treated by chronic ambulatory peritoneal dialysis. In Legrain M (Ed), Continuous ambulatory peritoneal dialysis. Amsterdam: Excerpta Medica, 1980, p 212

27. Muenthongchin R, Purnell FM, Jacon GB, and Deane N: Renal vein and peripheral vein renin assay in patients with chronic renal failure on medical and hemodialysis treatment. Proc Eur Dial Transplant Assoc 5: 193, 1968

28. Kotchen TA, Knight EL, Kashgarian M, and Mulrow PJ: A study of the renin-angiotension system in patients with severe chronic renal insufficiency. Nephron 7: 317, 1970

29. Onesti G, Kim KE, Greco JA, DelGuercio ET, Fernandes M, and Swartz C: Blood pressure regulation in end-stage renal disease and anephric man. Circulation Res 36(Suppl 1): 145, 1975

30. Fleming SJ, Powell J, Baker LRI, Cattell WR, and Greenwood R: Influence of intraperitoneal dialysate on blood pressure during continuous ambulatory peritoneal dialysis. Clin Nephrol 19: 132, 1983

31. Cannella G, Castellani A, Mioni G, Usberti M, Guerra U, Albertini A, and Maiorca R: Blood pressure control in end-stage renal disease in man: Indirect evidence of a complex pathogenic mechanism besides renin or blood volume. Clin Sci Mol Med 52: 19, 1977

32. Kim KE, Onesti G, and Schwartz CD: Hemodynamics of hypertension in uremia. Kidney Int 7: S155, 1975

33. Schnurr E, Küppers H, Wiesen K, and Grabensee B: Verhalten des Plasma-Aldosterons Während der Hämodialyse bei terminal niereninsuffizienten Patienten. Deutsche Med Wschr 10I: 1120, 1976

34. Louis F, Zwahlen A, Favré H, and Vallotton M: Contrôle de l'aldostérone plasmatique chez les patients en haemodialyse. Schweiz Med Wschr 110: 1882, 1980

35. Studer A, Zaruba K, Grimm J, Kuhlmann, Siegenthaler W, and Vetter W: Control of plasma aldosterone during chronic haemodialysis. Clin Nephrol 13: 172, 1980

J.A. Diaz-Buxo, W.P. Burgess, M. Greenman,
J.T. Chandler, C.D. Farmer, and P.J. Walker

87

Influence of Hypertension on Vision in Diabetics Undergoing Dialysis: Comparison of Peritoneal and Hemodialysis

SUMMARY

The maintenance of visual function in 41 diabetic patients treated by peritoneal dialysis and 71 treated by hemodialysis was evaluated periodically. Vision was maintained slightly better in the peritoneal dialysis group of adult onset but not that of juvenile onset diabetes when compared to hemodialysis groups. Blood glucose control was not a major determinant of visual outcome; maintenance of vision correlated with control of blood pressure. The major determinant of the visual outcome, however, was the severity of retinopathy at the onset of dialysis.

INTRODUCTION

Blindness is a common and crippling complication observed in diabetic patients undergoing dialysis. The influence of peritoneal dialysis or hemodialysis on deterioration of visual function has not been established. However, observations based on large series of diabetic patients undergoing hemodialysis strongly suggest that control of arterial hypertension may be an important determinant of the rate of progression of diabetic retinopathy.[1]

A prospective, uncontrolled study was designed to evaluate the changes in visual efficiency among insulin-requiring diabetic patients undergoing peritoneal and hemodialysis in our center. The factors potentially responsible for deterioration of vision among these patients were analyzed.

METHODS

All insulin-requiring diabetic patients undergoing peritoneal and hemodialysis in our center between May, 1974, and May, 1981, were included in the study. Juvenile-onset diabetic patients (Type I) were diagnosed prior to age 16 years. Adult-onset patients (Type II) had insulin-requiring diabetes for at least four years prior to initiation of dialysis. Steroid-induced diabetes was excluded from the study. All patients either had a renal biopsy characteristic of diabetic glomerulosclerosis or a clinical picture suggestive of diabetic nephropathy (nephrotic syndrome, neuropathy, and diabetic retinopathy) rather than nephrosclerosis.

One hundred and twelve patients entered the study. The peritoneal dialysis group consisted of 41 patients (20 males, 21 females) of which 18 suffered from juvenile-onset and 23 adult-onset diabetes mellitus. The mean age was 43.5 years and the mean observation period was 20 months. The hemodialysis group included 71 patients (36 males and 35 females) with 24 juvenile-onset and 47 adult-onset diabetics. The mean age was 46.5 years and the mean observation period was 20.2 months. No statistically significant differences were noted between mean age of juvenile and adult-onset diabetics, be-

From the Metrolina Kidney Center and Charlotte Memorial Hospital and Medical Center, Charlotte, North Carolina.

Table 1. Distribution of Diabetic Retinopathy (% of Eyes) at the Initiation of Therapy.

	Peritoneal Dialysis (n = 82)	Hemodialysis (n = 142)
Normal	6	7
Background retinopathy, mild	29	31
Background retinopathy, severe	28	17
Neovascular proliferation	26	29
Involutional, enucleated	11	16

tween the therapeutic groups, and mean observation periods for the different subgroups. There was a predominance of males in the juvenile-onset population and a predominance of females among the adult-onset population for both therapeutic groups. Residual renal function was evaluated by endogenous creatinine clearance, which ranged from 0 to 4.5 ml/min for all patients.

Peritoneal dialysis and hemodialysis were offered to all patients entering the program. Selection between the two modalities of therapy was based primarily on patient preference and family support. Nevertheless, four patients were treated with peritoneal dialysis due to our inability to create adequate vascular access for hemodialysis, and two patients changed to peritoneal dialysis following repeated episodes of arterial hypotension during hemodialysis.

Hemodialysis was performed three times weekly for a total of 12–15 hours per week. Hollow fiber artificial kidneys with surface areas ranging from 1.2–1.5 m² were used.

Peritoneal access was obtained by a permanent Tenckhoff catheter. Thirty-one patients received intermittent peritoneal dialysis (IPD) using a reverse osmosis automated peritoneal dialysis delivery system. All patients started a program consisting of 10 hours every other night using dwell times of 20 min-

utes. Their dialysis prescription was adjusted to provide urea clearances of approximately 60 L/week. Five of the patients dialyzed nightly and left 1–2 L dialysate intraperitoneally during the daytime hours. An additional 10 patients were treated with continuous cyclic peritoneal dialysis (CCPD) since 1980.[2] They received three to four 2 L exchanges at night, with dwell times of 2.0–2.5 hours and a 1–2 L diurnal cycle.

CLINICAL EVALUATION

Ophthalmologic evaluations were performed initially and annually by a retinal specialist. Forty-eight percent of the patients also underwent evaluations at more frequent intervals. The basic ophthalmologic evaluation included funduscopic examination and visual function testing (Snellen rating). Sixty-seven percent of the patients on hemodialysis, 77% of those on IPD, and 90% of patients on CCPD also underwent periodic fluorescent funduscopic angiograms and fundal photographs to evaluate and classify the severity of diabetic retinopathy. The classification and distribution of diabetic retinopathy among the therapeutic groups at the time of the initial evaluation is given in Table 1.

Table 2. Classification According to Arterial Blood Pressure.

Group	Mean BP, mm Hg	Peritoneal Dialysis*	Hemodialysis*
I	≤107	53	38
II	108–120	20	37
III	121–134	17	18
IV	≥135	10	7

* % of patients.

Table 3. Classification According to Glycemic Control.

Group	Glucose, mg/dl	Peritoneal Dialysis*	Hemodialysis*
I	Normal to 180	41	42
II	Normal to 250	35	25
III	Normal to 350	12	19
IV	Often above 350	12	14

* % of patient.

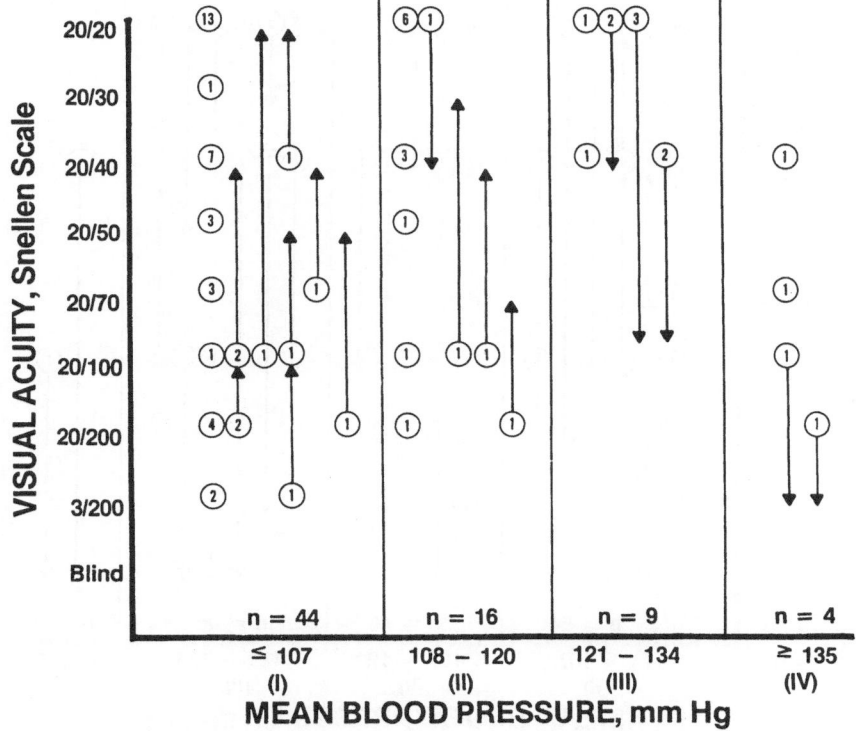

Fig. 1. Visual acuity according to blood pressure control among diabetic patients undergoing peritoneal dialysis. Digits denote number of eyes, isolated circles refer to stable vision, arrows denote change in vision during the observation period.

Vision for all functional eyes was rated with the Snellen scale. The visual acuity was then converted to the percent of visual efficiency using the Snell-Sterling formula.[3]

Blood pressure determinations were obtained before and after each dialytic session. The mean predialysis pressure was used to group patients according to blood pressure control (Table 2).

Blood glucose determinations were performed at least weekly at the time of dialysis in all patients. Furthermore, 40% of the patients used glucometers and evaluated their blood sugar concentrations two to four times daily and as necessary to effect good glucose control. Glycemic control was grouped according to the mode of the blood sugar values (Table 3).

STATISTICAL ANALYSIS

The data were analyzed by paired and unpaired Student's t test where appropriate.[4] The change in visual efficiency over the observation period was correlated with blood pressure by a modified linear regression analysis. The regression analysis of the data assumed that the abscissa (blood pressure group) was a linear function of blood pressure. The formula for the regression is

$$\Delta \text{ visual efficiency} = A + B \text{ (BP group} - 1)$$

From the regression analysis, the slope for visual efficiency change as a function of blood pressure control could be calculated. A comparison of glycemic control and vision change was made in tabular format.

RESULTS

Change in visual acuity during the total observation period according to blood pressure control is given in Figures 1 and 2 for patients undergoing peritoneal and hemodialysis, respectively. It is apparent from these schematic representations that

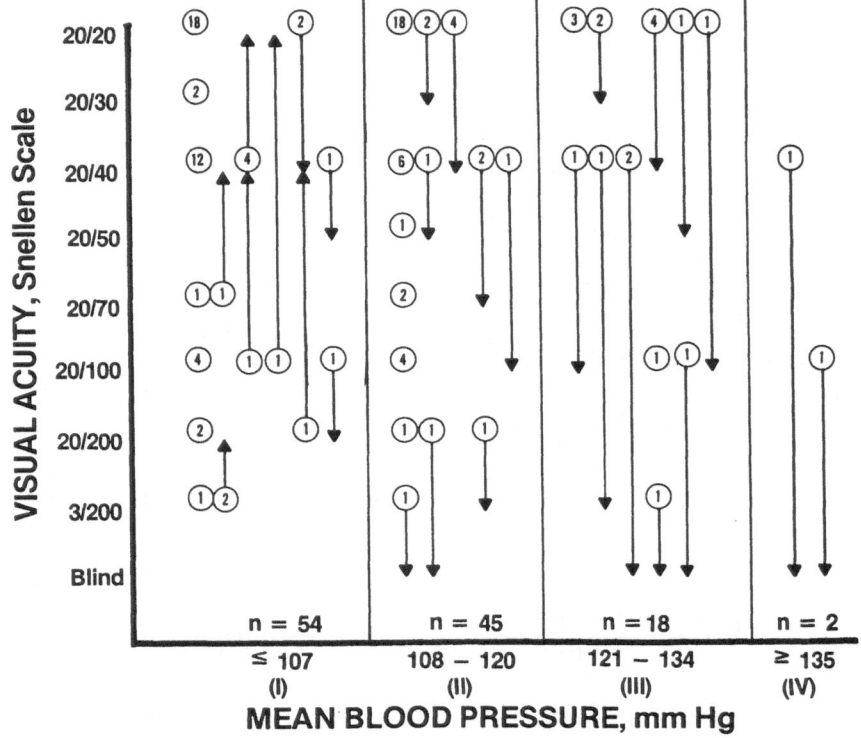

Fig. 2. Visual acuity according to blood pressure control among diabetic patients undergoing hemodialysis. Digits denote number of eyes, isolated circles refer to stable vision, arrows denote change in vision during the observation period.

more patients remained stable or showed improvement in vision among blood pressure groups 1 and 2, and that most patients in groups 3 and 4 showed visual function deterioration, regardless of the dialysis modality.

The average visual efficiency at the time of initi-

Table 4. Mean ± SD Visual Efficiency (% of Normal) at the Time of Initiation of Dialytic Therapy.

Blood Pressure Group	Peritoneal Dialysis	Hemodialysis
I	67 ± 33	76 ± 28
II	76 ± 29	82 ± 26
III	94 ± 8	85 ± 26
IV	54 ± 27	66 ± 24

ation of dialysis failed to show statistical difference between the peritoneal and hemodialysis patients. The initial visual efficiency of the viable eyes of the different blood pressure groups was also similar among patients treated with peritoneal or hemodialysis (Table 4).

The change in visual efficiency over the observation period for juvenile-onset diabetic patients undergoing peritoneal and hemodialysis as a function of blood pressure control is shown in Figure 3. Figure 4 provides similar data for adult-onset diabetic patients. The mean change in visual efficiency according to blood pressure grouping for juvenile-onset patients undergoing peritoneal and hemodialysis was the same and showed a strong correlation with blood pressure (Fig. 3). The average visual efficiency loss was 17% per blood pressure group for juvenile diabetics, regardless of the dialysis modality. A similar correlation between change in visual efficiency and blood pressure was noted for adult-

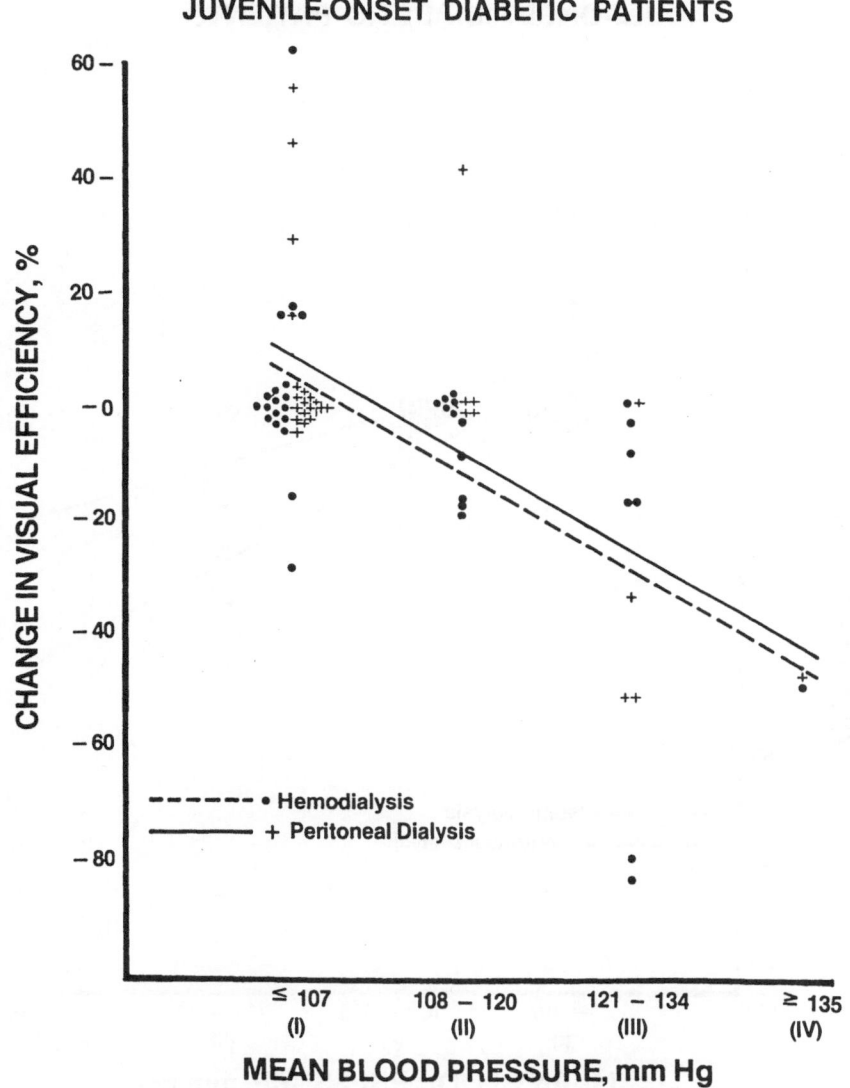

Fig. 3. Changes in visual efficiency according to blood pressure control among juvenile-onset diabetic patients.

onset patients undergoing hemodialysis, with a 16% vision loss per blood pressure group. The adult patients undergoing peritoneal dialysis showed an 8% loss per blood pressure group (Fig. 4).

Table 5 correlates visual function with glycemic control among patients undergoing peritoneal and hemodialysis. No definite relationship between these parameters was noted for either therapeutic group.

DISCUSSION

Peritoneal dialysis has been recommended for the treatment of uremic diabetic patients based on the ability to dialyze without systemic heparinization, the ease of insulin administration through the peritoneal route, and the avoidance of drastic changes in intravascular volume. However, there is no evidence that heparin *per se* is responsible for the

ADULT-ONSET DIABETIC PATIENTS

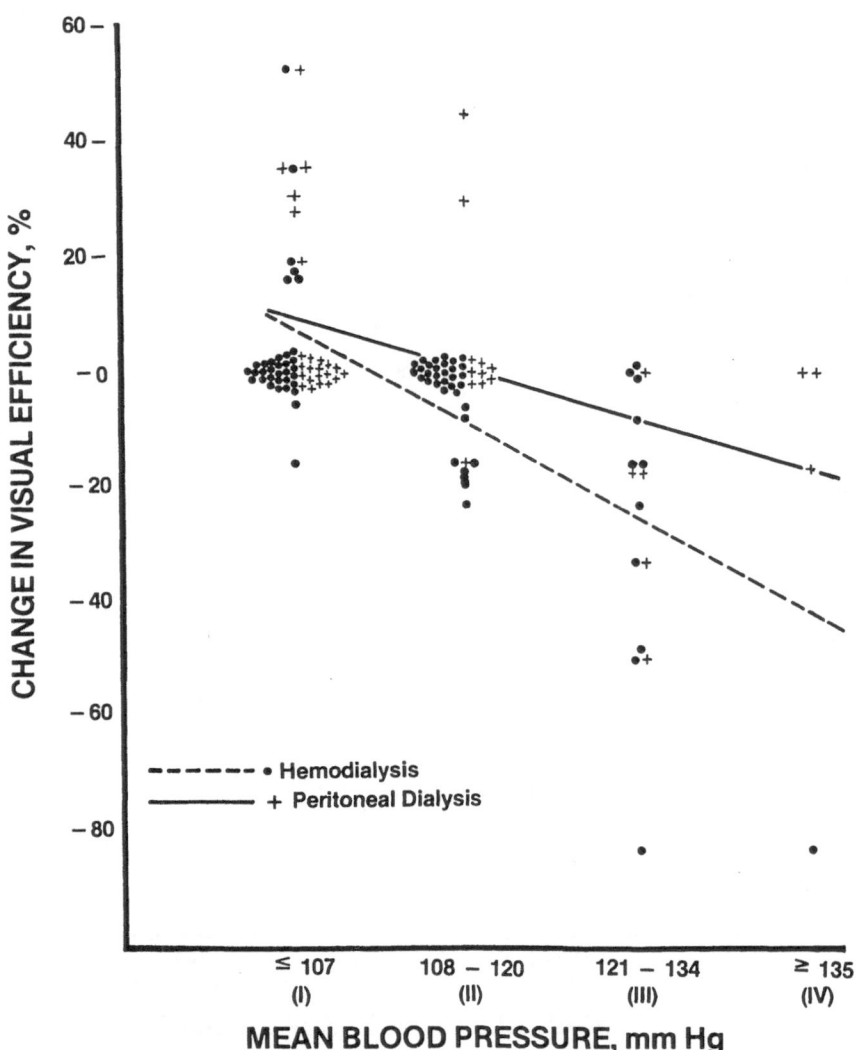

Fig. 4. Changes in visual efficiency according to blood pressure control among adult-onset diabetic patients.

progression of retinopathy in uremic diabetics in the absence of hypertension, nor that peritoneal dialysis is different from hemodialysis in affecting diabetic retinopathy. The studies performed by Shapiro and Comty[1] in diabetic patients undergoing hemodialysis suggest that control of arterial hypertension is the primary determinant of the rate of progression of diabetic retinopathy.

Our data suggest a strong correlation between control of blood pressure and preservation of vision

for patients undergoing both peritoneal and hemodialysis. Furthermore, the correlation was noted for both juvenile and adult-onset diabetic patients. A direct effect of heparin on visual function deterioration in the setting of normal blood pressure is not supported by these observations.

Our studies are limited by their uncontrolled nature and the variation in dialysis prescription among the patients. Nevertheless, the two populations of patients were studied simultaneously, the

Table 5. Changes in Visual Function According to Glycemic Control.

Visual Function	Glycemic Control			
	I	II	III	IV
Peritoneal Dialysis				
Improved	11*	3	3	3
Stable	35	18	5	8
Deteriorated	5	5	3	1
Hemodialysis				
Improved	2**	3	1	2
Stable	31	11	14	8
Deteriorated	9	11	4	4

* Percent of 73 viable eyes.
** Percent of 119 viable eyes.

residual visual function at initiation of the study was similar between the groups, and the distribution of sex, age, and mean length of observation among the two populations were very similar.

The lack of correlation between control of hyperglycemia and preservation of vision is possibly explained by the advanced stage of retinopathy observed in many of the patients and the variable severity of hypertension among the subgroups. Large longitudinal studies will hopefully allow application of multivariant analysis to define the role of glycemic control on preservation of vision among diabetic patients undergoing dialysis.

If ideal control of hypertension is accepted as instrumental for the preservation of vision among diabetics with advanced retinopathy, the rationale may be offered for prescribing continuous peritoneal dialysis to provide constant sodium and fluid removal and maintain steady control of blood pressure. The fact that we are able to prolong by dialysis the life of diabetic patients significantly longer than previously possible, combined with advances in glucose monitoring and therapeutic regimens that allow tighter control of glycemia, will certainly provide the data necessary to define the role of hypertension, hyperglycemia, and other variables in affecting the progression of diabetic retinopathy.

REFERENCES

1. Shapiro FL, and Comty CM: Hemodialysis in diabetics—1979 update. In Friedman EA, and L'Esperance FA, Jr. (Eds), Diabetic renal-retinal syndrome. New York: Grune and Stratton, 1982, p 333

2. Diaz-Buxo JA, Farmer CD, Walker PJ, Chandler JT, and Holt KL: Continuous cyclic peritoneal dialysis: A preliminary report. Artif Organs 5: 157, 1981

3. Newman M: Visual acuity. In Moses RA (Ed), Adler's physiology of the eye, 5th ed. St Louis: CV Mosby Co, 1970, p 561

4. Colton T: Statistics in medicine. Boston: Little, Brown and Co, 1974

P. Nilsson, F. Melsen, N. Grefberg, B.G. Danielson, and B. Lund

88

Bone Histomorphometry during Long-Term CAPD

SUMMARY

Fifteen patients (6 diabetic, 9 nondiabetic) without symptoms of skeletal disease, treated with CAPD without calcium or vitamin D supplements for a mean time of 18 months, were evaluated with serum biochemical variables and trabecular bone histomorphometry after double-labeling with tetracycline and staining for aluminum (Al). Fifteen patients on hemodialysis (HD), matched for age and time on dialysis with the patients on CAPD, and 15 age matched volunteers served as controls.

Histomorphometric data in the CAPD patients were similar to those found in patients on HD. Mean bone formation rates at tissue and basic multicellular unit levels were normal due to the combined effects of a high frequency of activation of remodeling units and a moderately defective mineralization process. Certain differences were noted between diabetic and non-diabetic patients suggesting less resistance to the skeletal actions of parathyroid hormone (PTH) in the diabetic patients.

Serum levels of 25-hydroxycholecalciferal (25-OHD) were reduced in CAPD when compared to HD, but did not relate to histomorphometry. Trabecular bone Al was demonstrable in seven of the 15 patients, five of whom had not been on other forms of dialysis. Positive staining for Al was associated with reduced tetracycline uptake and low bone formation rates.

INTRODUCTION

Since its introduction,[1] CAPD has been established as an attractive method for long-term dialysis treatment, both in diabetic[2,3] and nondiabetic[4,5] patients with end-stage renal disease (ESRD). The literature is less conclusive regarding the effects of CAPD on renal bone disease. Improvement of secondary hyperparathyroidism (HPT), with healing of histological osteitis fibrosa in a majority of patients has been reported,[6] but also persistence or worsening of renal osteodystrophy, including the appearance of Al-associated osteomalacia.[7-9] We have previously reported longitudinal data on calcium-phosphorus homeostasis, PTH levels, and skeletal radiography in patients treated with CAPD without calcium or vitamin D supplements.[10] The present report concerns bone dynamics in a subset of these patients.

METHODS

The study included 15 patients (7 males and 8 females, mean age 43 years, range 23–69 years), treated with CAPD for a mean time of 18 months (range 10–33 months). In six (4 males and 2 females, mean age 40 years), ESRD was caused by diabetic nephropathy secondary to juvenile-onset diabetes mellitus. The remaining patients suffered from

From the Department of Internal Medicine, University Hospital, Uppsala, Sweden, the University Institute of Pathology, Aarhus Amtssygehus, Aarhus, Denmark, and the Department of Rheumatic Diseases, Hvidovre Hospital, Copenhagen, Denmark.

ESRD secondary to chronic glomerulonephritis (n = 5) or chronic interstitial nephritis (n = 4). The time on CAPD was identical in diabetic and nondiabetic patients. Three patients, all nondiabetic had been on HD for 12–36 months before starting CAPD. One patient underwent parathyroidectomy 15 months before starting CAPD. No patient had bilateral nephrectomy and none had symptoms of musculoskeletal disease.

The general management of the patients has been described.[4] Commercially prepared dialysate was used, with four 2 L exchanges per day being the rule. The dialysate calcium concentration was 1.75 mM/L, the magnesium and lactate concentrations 0.75 and 35 mM/L. Calcium or vitamin D supplements were not given. Aluminum-containing phosphate binders were administered to seven patients. The average daily uptake of calcium and phosphate approximated 700 and 1200 mg, respectively.

Histomorphometric and biochemical data were compared to those found in 15 nondiabetic HD patients with a mean age of 49 years (range 20–75 years) and a mean time on HD of 19 months (range 6–66 months). These patients were treated according to the same general principles as those on CAPD. Fifteen healthy volunteers, matched for age with the patients, served as a control group in the evaluation of histomorphometry.[11]

Laboratory Methods

Serum levels of calcium (reference range 2.20–2.60 mM/L), phosphate (0.76–1.44 mM/L), and alkaline phosphatases (0.8–4.8 μkat/L) were determined every four weeks by standard laboratory methods. Serum calcium was adjusted for serum albumin by 0.019 mM/L for each g/L that the individual serum albumin concentration deviated from the normal mean of 46 g/L. Serum Al (normal<10 μg/L) was determined within three months of the bone biopsy using atomic absorption photometry. Serum PTH (reference range 0.40–1.20 arbitrary units/L (U/L)) was determined every three months by an assay measuring intact PTH and the C-terminal 2/3 of the molecule.[12] Serum 25-OHD was measured by a competitive protein-binding assay.[13] All samples were taken during the winter and within three months of the bone biopsy. All biochemical data collected during the 6 mo period preceding, and at the time of the bone biopsy, were pooled, and the average values of the individual biochemical variables were used in the statistical analysis.

Histomorphometric Methods

Demethylchlortetracycline 600 mg/d was given in a 2-10-2-day regime. A transcortical iliac crest biopsy[14] was obtained from 2–6 days after the last does. Undecalcified specimens were embedded in methylmethacrylate, cut and stained as previously described.[11,15] Aurine tricarboxylic acid was used for staining for Al.[16] All measurements were performed on trabecular bone and the following parameters were evaluated:

Fractional trabecular bone volume. ($^tV_{fract(b)}$) μm^3/μm^3—the volume of mineralized and unmineralized trabecular bone as a fraction of a given volume of total trabecular bone tissue.

Fractional formation surfaces. ($S_{fract(f)}$)μm^2/ μm^2—osteoid surfaces as a fraction of total trabecular bone surfaces.

Fractional resorption surfaces. ($S_{fract(r)}$) μm^2/ μm^2—resorption surfaces as a fraction of total trabecular bone surfaces.

Mean width of osteoid seams. (^uW_f)μm—the mean of four extreme measurements in all surfaces covered by osteoid.

Fractional labeled surfaces. ($S_{fract(lab)}$)μm^2/ μm^2—single- and double-labeled surfaces as a fraction of total trabecular bone surfaces.

Fractional labeled formation surfaces. ($S_{fract(lab/f)}$)μm^2/μm^2—single- and double-labeled surfaces as a fraction of the formation surfaces.

Appositional rate. ($^uM/t$)μm/day—the mean distance between tetracycline lines in all double-labeled surfaces, divided by the interval in days (t) between the two labelings.

Fractional aluminum-stained surfaces. ($S_{fract(Al)}$) μm^2/μm^2—trabecular bone surfaces revealing a positive reaction for Al, expressed as a fraction of total trabecular bone surfaces.

Bone formation rate, tissue level, ("turnover"). (^sV_f)μm^3/μm^2/day—

$$^sV_f = S_{fract(lab)} \times {}^uM/t \qquad (1)$$

This represents the amount of new bone mineralized per unit time per unit of trabecular bone surface.

Table 1. Serum Biochemistry
(Mean ± SEM).

	CAPD (n = 15)	HD (n = 15)
Calcium (mM/L)	2.54 ± 0.03	2.46 ± 0.02
Phosphate (mM/L)	1.70 ± 0.10	1.76 ± 0.1
Alk phosphatases (μkat/l)	5.2 ± 1.0	5.6 ± 2.0
PTH (U/l)	5.2 ± 1.0	5.0 ± 1.0
Aluminum (μg/l)	84 ± 8	48 ± 1.0
25-OHD (ng/ml)	10.5 ± 1.0*	19.4 ± 5.0

* p < 0.01 for difference between CAPD and HD.

Trabecular bone volume

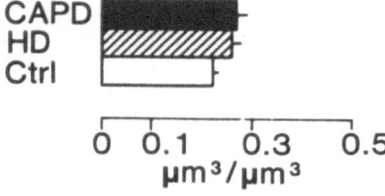

Fract formation surfaces

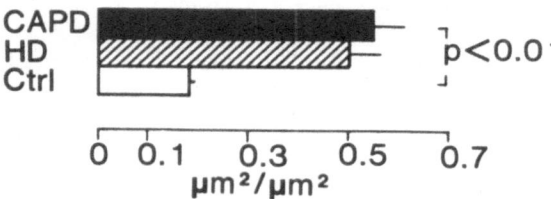

Fract resorption surfaces

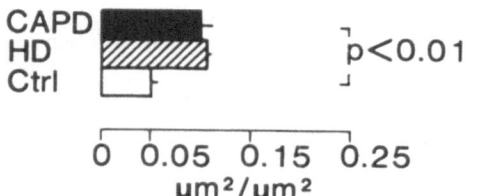

Fig. 1. Fractional trabecular bone volume, fractional formation and resorption surfaces in 15 CAPD patients in comparison to HD patients and controls. Mean, SEM.

Bone formation rate, BMU level. ($^sV_{f(BMU)}$) $\mu m^3/\mu m^2/day$—

$$^sV_{f(BMU)} = \frac{S_{fract(lab)} \times {^u}M/t}{S_{fract(f)}} \qquad (2)$$

The term BMU refers to the basic multicellular unit, the functional group of cells responsible for the turnover of a structural bone unit.[17] The variable represents the amount of new bone mineralized per unit time per unit of osteoid surface.

Mineralization lag time. (t_m) days—

$$t_m = \frac{^uW_f}{^sV_{f(BMU)}} \qquad (3)$$

This defines the average time lag between osteoid formation and subsequent mineralization.[15]

Statistical methods. Conventional nonparametric methods were employed.

RESULTS

Serum Biochemistry

Serum biochemical variables are illustrated in Table 1. All patients were normocalcemic or marginally hypercalcemic. Serum PTH was elevated in all patients. All had elevated serum Al, and mean serum Al in CAPD patients was not different from that in HD patients despite less use of ACPB in the CAPD patients (daily intake of Al(OH)$_3$ (mean ± SEM): CAPD 2.0 ± 0.6 g/day, HD 5.0 ± 0.4 g/day p < 0.01). Serum 25-OHD was decreased in CAPD patients in comparison with a normal material[13] and in comparison with HD patients. In seven patients, serum 25-OHD was analyzed before the start of CAPD and after at least one year of this therapy. In six, serum 25-OHD was lower on CAPD than before the start of dialysis (p < 0.05).

Histomorphometric Analysis

Figures 1–3 illustrate the results of the histomorphometric analysis for the whole group of CAPD patients, with values found in HD patients and controls for comparison. The CAPD patients showed the same deviations from the controls as the HD patients. Thus, mean fractional trabecular bone volume was normal, but fractional formation and

Fract labeled surfaces

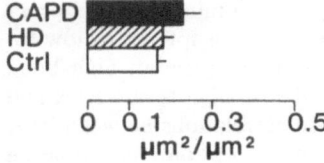

Fract labeled formation surfaces

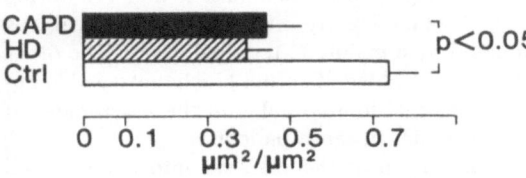

Appositional rate

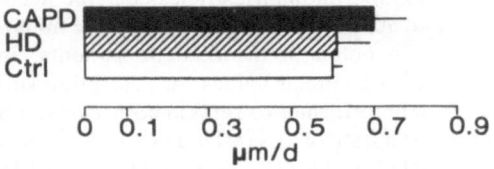

Fig. 2. Fractional labeled trabecular and formation surfaces and appositional rate in 15 CAPD patients in comparison to HD patients and controls. Mean, SEM.

Bone Turnover

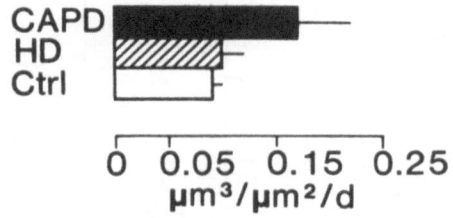

Bone Formation BMU

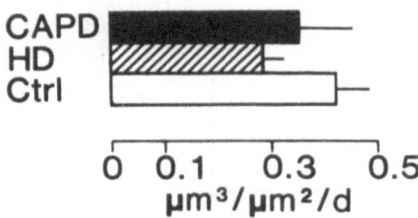

Mineralization lag time

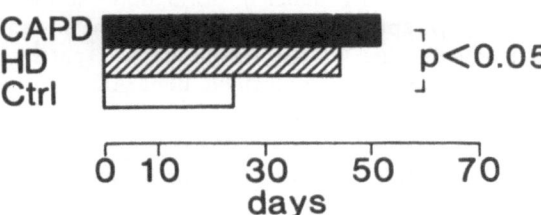

Fig. 3. Bone formation rates at tissue (turnover) and BMU levels and mineralization lag time in 15 CAPD patients in comparison to HD patients and controls. Mean, SEM.

resorption surfaces were increased ($p < 0.01$). Fractional labeled formation surfaces were reduced ($p < 0.05$), but the mean values of appositional rate and of bone formation rates at tissue and BMU levels did not differ from those found in the controls. The mineralization lag-time was moderately prolonged ($p < 0.05$).

Positive bone stain for Al was found in 7 of 15 CAPD patients and in 12 of 15 HD patients. Mean fractional Al-stained bone surfaces were CAPD: $0.08 \pm 0.03 \ \mu m^2/\mu m^2$ (mean $\pm$ SEM), HD: $0.11 \pm 0.03 \ \mu m^2/\mu m^2$. Five of the CAPD patients with demonstrable bone Al had not been exposed to other forms of dialysis. Patients with positive Al staining had a lower tetracycline uptake (fractional labeled formation surfaces) and lower bone formation rates than patients without detectable bone Al (Fig. 4). Positive staining for Al did not correlate with serum Al and could not be related to the duration of treatment with, or to the total ingested dose of ACPB. No

statistically significant correlations could be found between the other variables of serum biochemistry, patient age, or time on CAPD and histomorphometry.

When diabetic (diab) and nondiabetic (non-d) patients were analyzed separately, the diabetic patients were found to have higher serum calcium (diab 2.63 ± 0.02 mM/L, non-d 2.47 ± 0.02 mM/L, mean $\pm$ SEM, $p < 0.01$) and lower serum PTH (diab 2.6 ± 0.4 arbU/L, non-d 7.2 ± 1.6 arbU/L, mean $\pm$ SEM, $p < 0.02$) than the nondiabetic patients. The remaining biochemical variables showed similar similar values in the two groups. Histomorphometrically, the diabetic patients, on the average, had lower frac-

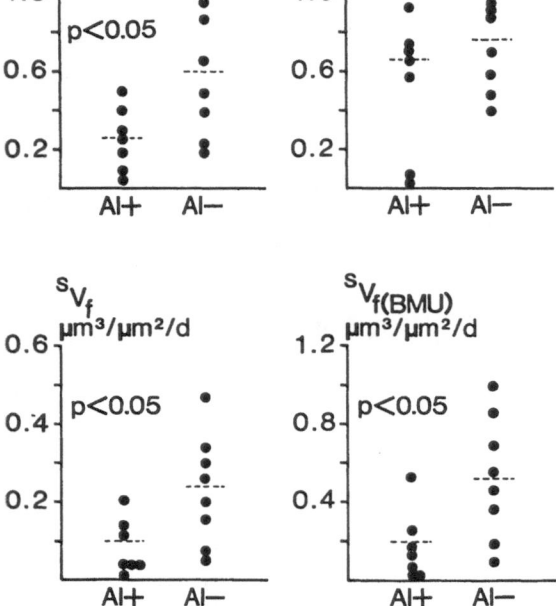

Fig. 4. Fractional labeled formation surfaces ($S_{fract(lab/f)}$), appositional rate ($^{u}M/t$), bone formation rates at tissue ($^{s}V_{f(BMU)}$) levels in CAPD patients with (Al+) and (Al−) detectable bone Al.

tional formation surfaces (diab 0.40 ± 0.07, non-d 0.65 ± 0.06, mean $\pm$ SEM, $p < 0.05$) and mean width of osteoid seams (diab 8.1 ± 1.2 μm, non-d 13.0 ± 0.8 μm, mean $\pm$ SEM, $p < 0.01$), resulting in a lower mean fractional trabecular bone volume ($p < 0.01$). No differences were noted regarding fractional resorption surfaces or any of the variables related to tetracycline labeling. In comparison with the controls, the diabetic patients showed increased mean fractional formation surfaces ($p < 0.05$), but did not otherwise differ from the controls.

DISCUSSION

Trabecular bone histomorphometry in the CAPD patients, the majority of whom had not been exposed to other forms of dialysis, was similar to that found in HD patients treated according to the same general principles. The data agree well with what others have found in HD patients without symptoms of musculoskeletal disease using identi-

cal histomorphometric methods.[18] Individual patients ranged from those with a high bone turnover rate and an essentially normal mineralization process to those with low tetracycline uptake and low-to-absent mineral apposition. In general, high bone turnover was associated with high serum PTH and *vice versa,* but the close correlations between PTH levels and parameters of resorption and formation observed in HD patients, using the same radioimmunoassay for PTH,[19] were not obtained. This might be due to transperitoneal elimination of PTH during CAPD,[20] which clearly must affect PTH levels, as estimated by a mainly C-terminal assay. The other measured variables of serum biochemistry also appeared to be of limited value in the assessment of bone dynamics in these patients.

Subdivision of the material into diabetic and nondiabetic patients provided some additional information. The diabetic patients had higher serum calcium and lower PTH values than the nondiabetic patients. Histomorphometrically less osteoid accumulation and absence of markedly defective mineralization were noted in the diabetic patients. In combination with similar values for resorption surfaces and for bone formation rates at both levels, this could suggest a state of less resistance to the skeletal actions of PTH in the diabetic patients on CAPD. The reason for such a difference remains unknown. A better preserved renal production of 1.25-dihydroxycholecalciferol in end-stage diabetic nephropathy could be one explanation. No data in support of such an assumption have been presented, however. It must also be cautioned that the diabetic patients had suffered a much shorter period of azotemia before starting dialysis treatment than the nondiabetic patients. This may be of importance, even if no relationship between this factor and any of the biochemical or histomorphometric variables could be discerned. It is also noteworthy that we have so far never observed clinical or radiographic signs of progressive hyperparathyroidism in a larger number of diabetic patients on long-term CAPD.[10] Similar observations have been reported for diabetic patients on HD.[21]

Several reports associate bone Al accumulation with low bone turnover and defective mineralization in HD patients.[19, 22] This may continue to be a problem during CAPD. In this study, seven patients (46%) had histochemically demonstrable bone Al. Five of them were on CAPD as their first form of dialysis. As a group, they showed lower tetracycline uptake and lower bone formation rates than patients without detectable bone Al. The close association between fractional Al-stained surfaces and parameters of bone formation found in HD patients[19] was not observed in the CAPD patients, however. Osteomalacia with positive Al staining has also been reported by others[9] in isolated patients on long-term CAPD.

In our experience, the dialysate used for CAPD regularly has contained less than 5–7 μg/L of Al. Moreover, only 7 of 15 patients were currently treated with aluminum containing phosphate binders. Despite this, serum Al in the CAPD patients was at least as high as in the HD patients who were dialyzed against softened water with an Al content of 10–20 μg/L.

Peritoneal Al kinetics have been examined in a few reports suggesting an appreciable Al elimination with CAPD.[23,24] Others,[25] however, have suggested that the low pH of the dialysate may promote transperitoneal Al uptake even with very low dialysate Al. The importance of dialysate pH for Al dialyzability has also been demonstrated in HD.[26] Further investigations are definitely needed concerning the overall Al situation during CAPD treatment.

Several workers[6,9] have reported subnormal and decreasing serum 25-OHD levels in patients on long-term CAPD, and transperitoneal losses of the vitamin have been demonstrated.[27] Similar findings were made in the present study, serum 25-OHD being lower in CAPD patients than in patients treated with HD, and the introduction of CAPD being followed by a significant fall in serum 25-OHD levels. A direct effect of 25-OHD on bone mineralization in the uremic patient has been suggested,[28] while others[29] have failed to find any correlation between serum 25-OHD and bone histomorphometry. The quite similar bone dynamics in CAPD patients and HD patients in this report, and the absence of any correlations between histomorphometric variables and serum levels of 25-OHD seem to argue against a specific role for losses of this vitamin in the pathogenesis of bone disease in CAPD patients.

In conclusion, this study indicates that CAPD, when compared to HD, has no specific effects on bone dynamics in uremic subjects. Despite well regulated serum calcium levels, biochemical and histomorphometric data give evidence of continued parathyroid stimulation, and some patients show a markedly defective mineralization process, which may, at least in part, be due to trabecular bone aluminum accumulation. The possible differences between diabetic and nondiabetic patients are at present the subject of further study.

REFERENCES

1. Popovich RP, Moncrief JW, Decherd JF, Bomar JB, and Pyle WK: The definition of a novel portable/wearable equilibrium peritoneal dialysis technique. Abstracts Am Soc Artif Intern Organs 5: 64, 1976
2. Amair P, Khanna R, Leibel B, Pierratos A, Vas S, Meema E, Blair G, Chisholm L, Vas M, Zingg W, Digenis G, and Oreopoulos D: Continuous ambulatory peritoneal dialysis in diabetics with end-stage renal disease. N Engl J Med 306: 625, 1982
3. Grefberg N, Danielson BG, and Nilsson P: Continuous ambulatory peritoneal dialysis in the treatment of end-stage diabetic nephropathy. Acta Med Scand (in press)
4. Grefberg N, Danielson BG, and Nilsson P: Clinical outcome of 50 patients started on continuous ambulatory peritoneal dialysis in a Swedish centre. Scand J Urol Nephrol 17: 337, 1983
5. Ramos JM, Gokal R, Siampoulos K, Ward MK, Wilkinson R, and Kerr DNS: Continuous ambulatory peritoneal dialysis: Three year's experience. Q J Med 52: 165, 1983
6. Gokal R, Ramos JM, Ellis HA, Parkinson I, Sweetman V, Dewar J, Ward MK, and Kerr DNS: Histological renal osteodystrophy, and 25 hydroxycholecalciferol, and aluminum levels in patients on continuous ambulatory peritoneal dialysis. Kidney Int 23: 15, 1983
7. Calderaro V, Oreopoulos DG, Meema HE, Ogilvie R, Husdan H, Khanna R, Quinton C, Murray T, and Carmichael D: The evolution of renal osteodystrophy in patients undergoing continuous ambulatory peritoneal dialysis (CAPD). Proc Eur Dial Transplant Assoc 17: 533, 1980
8. Tielemans C, Aubry C, and Dratwa M: The effects of continuous ambulatory peritoneal dialysis (CAPD) on renal osteodystrophy. In Gahl GM, Kessel M, and Nolph KD (Eds), Advances in peritoneal dialysis: Proceedings of the 2nd international symposium on peritoneal dialysis. Amsterdam: Excerpta Medica, 1981, p 455
9. Digenis G, Khanna R, Pierratos A, Meema HE, Rabinovich S, Petit J, and Oreopoulos DG: Renal osteodystrophy in patients maintained on CAPD for more than three years. Peritoneal Dial Bull 3: 81, 1983
10. Nilsson P, Danielson BG, Grefberg N, and Wide L: Secondary hyperparathyroidism in diabetic and nondiabetic patients on long-term CAPD. Scand J Urol Nephrol (in press)
11. Melsen F, and Mosekilde L: Tetracycline double-labelling of iliac trabecular bone in 41 normal adults. Calcif Tissue Res 26: 99, 1978
12. Hehrmann R, Nodmayer H, Mohr M, and Hesch R-D: Human parathyroid hormone: Antibody characterization. J Immunoassay 1: 151, 1980
13. Lund B, and Sørensen OH: Measurement of 25-hydroxyvitamin D in serum and its relation to sun-

shine, age and vitamin D intake in the Danish population. Scand J Clin Lab Invest 39: 23, 1979

14. Bordier P, Matrajt H, Miravet L, and Hioco D: Mesure histologique de la masse et de la résorption des travées osseuses. Pathol Biol 12: 1238, 1964

15. Melsen F, and Mosekilde L: Dynamic studies of trabecular bone formation and osteoid maturation in normal and certain pathological states. Metab Bone Dis Rel Res 1: 45, 1978

16. Lillie RD, and Fullmer HM: Histopathologic technic and practical histochemistry. New York: McGraw-Hill, 1976, p 534

17. Frost HM: Tetracycline based histological analysis of bone remodelling. Calcif Tissue Res 3: 211, 1969

18. Nielsen HE, Melsen F, and Christensen MS: Interrelationships between calcium-phosphorus metabolism, serum parathyroid hormone and bone histomorphometry in non-dialyzed and dialyzed patients with chronic renal fialure. Mineral Electrolyte Metab 4: 113, 1980

19. Nilsson P, Melsen F, Malmaeus J, Danielson BG, and Mosekilde L: Relationships between calcium and phosphorus homeostasis, parathyroid hormone levels, bone aluminum and bone histomorphometry in patients on maintenance hemodialysis. Metab Bone Dis Rel Res (in press)

20. Delmez JA, Slatopolsky E, Martin KJ, Gearing BN, and Harter HR: Minerals, vitamin D, and parathyroid hormone in continuous ambulatory peritoneal dialysis. Kidney Int 21: 862, 1982

21. Vincenti F, Hattner R, Amend WJ, Feduska NJ, Duca RM, and Salvatierra O Jr: Decreased secondary hyperparathyroidism in diabetic patients receiving hemodialysis. JAMA 245: 930, 1981

22. Hodsman AB, Sherrard DJ, Alfrey AC, Ott S, Brickman AS, Miller NL, Maloney NA, and Coburn JW: Bone aluminum and histomorphometric features of renal osteodystrophy. J Clin Endocrinol Metab 54: 539, 1982

23. Wolf A, Graf H, Pinggera WF, Stummvoll HK, and Meisinger V: Serum aluminum and continuous ambulatory peritoneal dialysis. Ann Intern Med 92: 130, 1980

24. Sorkin MI, Nolph KD, Anderson HD, Morris JS, Kennedy J, Prowant B, and Moore H: Aluminum mass transfer during continuous ambulatory peritoneal dialysis. Peritoneal Dial Bull 1: 91, 1981

25. Gilli P, Farinelli A, Fagioli F, DeBastiani P, and Buoncristiani U: Serum aluminium levels in patients on peritoneal dialysis. Lancet 2: 742, 1980

26. Gacek EM, Babb AL, Uvelli DA, Fry DL, and Scribner BH: Dialysis dementia: The role of dialysate pH in altering the dialyzability of aluminum. Trans Am Soc Artif Intern Organs 25: 409, 1979

27. Aloni Y, Shany S, and Chaimovitz C: Losses of 25-hydroxyvitamin D in peritoneal fluid: Possible mechanism of bone disease in uremic patients treated with chronic ambulatory peritoneal dialysis. Mineral Electrolyte Metab 9: 82, 1983

28. Fournier A, Bordier P, Gueris J, Sebert JL, Marie P, Ferriére C, Bedrossian J, and DeLuca HF: Comparison of 1-hydroxycholecalciferol and 25-hydroxycholecalciferol in the treatment of renal osteodystrophy: Greater effect of 25-hydroxycholecalciferol on bone mineralization. Kidney Int 15:196, 1979

29. Nielsen HF, Melsen F, Lund B, Sørensen HO, and Christensen MS: Serum-25-hydroxycholecalciferol and renal osteodystrophy. Lancet 1: 754, 1977

J.A. Pederson, A.J. Felsenfeld, A.L. Voigts, and F. Llach

89

Effect of CAPD on Renal Osteodystrophy in Unmodified Patients Moving from Hemodialysis to CAPD

SUMMARY

The effect of one year of CAPD on bone histology was studied in seven hemodialysis patients changing to CAPD. The course of these patients was not modified by oral calcium supplements, vitamin D or parathyroid ablation. An existing pattern of dialysis osteomalacia in three patients changed in two to osteitis fibrosa. This change was associated with decreased stainable aluminum in the bone biopsies obtained during CAPD. The specific role played by CAPD in effecting this change is uncertain. Progression and development of osteitis fibrosa in these patients was not prevented by a 7.0 mg/dl calcium containing dialysis solution. The observed persistence of abnormally high parathyroid hormone levels and increasing alkaline phosphatase concentrations supports the concept that a negative calcium balance may be a critical factor in progression of osteitis fibrosa among CAPD patients.

INTRODUCTION

Renal osteodystrophy, potentially disabling patients with end stage renal disease, is multifactorial in origin. At least four subtypes have been described with variable frequency among dialysis patients.[1-5] The most frequent lesion is osteitis fibrosa, a result of secondary hyperparathyroidism. Another type, a mixed disorder, has features of osteitis fibrosa and osteomalacia. Both osteitis fibrosa and the mixed type lesions may respond favorably to vitamin D. Osteomalacia alone is also seen, usually associated with heavy deposits of aluminum. This type, referred to as dialysis osteomalacia does not respond to vitamin D therapy and is generally attributed to bone lesions induced by elevated aluminum concentrations in the water used to prepare hemodialysis solutions.[6-8] Less widely recognized, enteric aluminum exposure especially aluminum containing antacids, may also contribute to aluminum deposition.[9-12] Finally, aplastic bone disease that shows little evidence of either cellular proliferation or mineralization activity has been described.

Osteitis fibrosa, mixed osteitis fibrosa-osteomalacia, and osteomalacia have all been reported in patients treated with CAPD.[13-15] Changes in the bone histology are reported following CAPD, but the specific influence on renal osteodystrophy by CAPD in these reports is not clear. Other factors such as the duration of prior dialysis treatment, antecedent or concurrent treatment with vitamin D and calcium supplements, parathyroidectomy, and the calcium concentration of dialysis solutions may also influence the histologic pattern.

The present study attempts to define the effects on renal osteodystrophy of CAPD among patients transferring from maintenance hemodialysis treatment. None of the patients included in this study were treated with agents that affect bone metabolism except dialysis and aluminum containing antacids.

From the Department of Medicine, University of Oklahoma Health Sciences Center and VA Medical Center, Oklahoma City, Oklahoma.

METHODS

Seven men, 52 ± 12 years, (mean ± SD), electing CAPD after 32 ± 26 months of hemodialysis were studied. Eighteen, double tetracycline labeled, transcortical anterior iliac crest bone biopsies were obtained in these patients using a biopsy needle with a 7.5 mm I D. A tetracycline label was administered orally twice, 250 mg qid for two consecutive days at 10-day intervals prior to each biopsy to assess mineralization.

Baseline bone biopsies were obtained 10 ± 8.7 months prior to beginning CAPD, but this figure includes a specimen from one patient within the month treatment started. Comparative biopsies were performed after 12 ± 1.5 months of CAPD. Four additional biopsies not considered in the statistical analysis of the data were obtained in four of the patients at 1–30 months after starting CAPD. Concurrent data included routine skeletal X-rays plus determinations of the serum calcium, phosphorus, alkaline phosphatase, parathyroid hormone, and aluminum concentrations.

Parathyroid hormone (PTH), carboxy- and amino-terminal, was assayed with a radioimmunologic technique previously detailed.[16] Serum aluminum, measured by atomic absorption and graphite furnace,[17] was determined after 12 ± 1.5 months of CAPD and compared to levels in a contemporary group of hemodialysis patients and normal controls.

None of the patients had undergone parathyroidectomy nor received treatment with either calcium or vitamin D preparations prior to or during treatment with CAPD. Aluminum antacids were prescribed throughout in doses sufficient to control serum phosphorus concentrations. Approximately one-fourth to one-third less antacid was required after converting from hemodialysis to CAPD. Hemodialysis for each patient was conducted using a 7.0 ± 0.5 mg/dl calcium bath prepared with treated water containing less than 5 g/L aluminum. During each day of CAPD, 2 L exchanges (1.5% dextrose times 3 and 4.25% dextrose once) also contained 7.0 mg/dl calcium (Travenol Dianeal 137 or PD2).

The undecalcified bone samples were dehydrated, defatted, and embedded in methyl methacrylate before sectioning with a Jung model K sledge microtome. Goldner stained 5 μm sections were examined with a Leitz Ortholux II microscope and quantified with a Merz Schenk reticle. Additional 5 μm sections were stained for aluminum by the method of Maloney et al.[18] Unstained 15 μm sections were examined in fluorescent light to evaluate the extent of mineralization as demarcated by the tetracycline labels.

Morphometric analysis of the biopsies included the following parameters with reference to normal values (M ± SD)[19]: osteoblastic osteoid, the fraction of trabecular bone surface covered by osteoblasts (0.76 ± 0.76%); total osteoid surface, the fraction of trabecular bone surface covered by osteoid (15.5 ± 5.5%); osteoclastic resorption, the fraction of trabecular bone surface covered by osteoclasts (0.15 ± 0.12%); osteoclast count, the number of osteoclasts per square millimeter of cancellous bone (2.5 ± 1.2 cells); relative osteoid volume, the fraction of trabecular bone volume occupied by osteoid (2.5 ± 1.2%); bone volume, the fraction of cancellous bone volume occupied by bone matrix (23 ± 5%); and endosteal fibrosis volume, the fraction of cancellous bone volume occupied by fibrosis (0%).

Each biopsy was classified in one of two diagnostic categories as follows: (1) osteitis fibrosa displaying endosteal fibrosis, increased osteoclastic bone resorption and osteoblastic activity with active mineralization as demonstrated by broad or distinct double tetracycline bands; (2) osteomalacia showing large, acellular deposits of osteoid, less than 0.5% endosteal fibrosis, minimal osteoclastic activity, and the cessation of bone formation as judged by the absence of other than trace tetracycline fluorescence. For purposes of this study, biopsies containing mixed features of osteitis fibrosa and osteomalacia were classified as osteitis fibrosa. Aplastic bone disease, which contains a normal ratio of osteoid to mineralized bone but no active mineralization, cellular activity, or endosteal fibrosis was not observed. Aluminum staining, more prominent in the sections showing osteomalacia, was not considered as a criterion for diagnostic classification.

The data were evaluated for significant change by signed rank analysis[20] of the differences between values concurrent with the baseline biopsy and those 12 ± 1.5 months after beginning CAPD. Change was accepted as significant at the 95% probability level. All values are presented as the mean ± SD unless otherwise specified.

RESULTS

The histologic data are detailed in Table 1. Patients 1, 4, and 6 have dialysis osteomalacia in biopsies obtained prior to beginning CAPD. No change occurred in subsequent samples obtained during CAPD from patient 4, but patient 1 demonstrated a

Table 1. Bone Histology in CAPD Patients.

Patient	Months CAPD at Time of Biopsy*	Diagnosis	Osteoblastic Osteoid %	Total Osteoid Surface %	Osteoclastic Resorption %	Number Osteoclasts per mm^2	Relative Osteoid Volume %	Bone Volume %	Endosteal Fibrosis Volume %	Tetracycline Bands	Intensity Aluminum Staining (0–4)
1	− 6	Osteomalacia	0.0	72.7	0.7	0.1	17	15.6	0.0	Trace	1.0
	+ 12	Osteitis fibrosa	13.3	48.7	10.1	3.9	12	23.5	3.8	Double	0.5
2	− 5	Osteitis fibrosa	5.2	40.7	7.0	2.0	10	19.1	2.1	Broad	0.5
	+ 14	Osteitis fibrosa	16.6	64.0	11.6	4.2	12	21.1	6.9	Double	0.0
	+ 30	Osteitis fibrosa	41.0	70.1	11.2	4.8	21	18.5	8.6	Double	0.0
3	− 11	Osteitis fibrosa	2.3	82.5	4.6	1.3	35	7.9	0.7	Broad	2.0
	+ 10	Osteitis fibrosa	4.6	77.3	5.3	2.0	20	16.2	1.3	Double	0.5
4	− 6	Osteomalacia	0.0	81.0	0.6	0.1	29	13.6	0.0	Trace	4.0
	+ 14	Osteomalacia	0.1	85.5	1.7	0.5	33	16.3	0.0	Trace	3.0
	+ 28	Osteomalacia	0.1	73.8	0.1	0.2	35	17.4	0.0	Trace	3.0
5	− 19	Osteitis fibrosa	27.1	58.1	14.3	2.9	11	9.4	4.9	Broad	1.0
	+ 1	Osteitis fibrosa	35.5	66.7	11.8	4.6	16	16.8	15.8	Broad	0.0
	+ 11	Osteitis fibrosa	35.5	67.4	10.0	5.7	17	16.8	15.2	Double	0.0
6	− 24	Osteomalacia	0.0	59.7	0.3	0.1	17	8.3	0.0	Trace	1.0
	+ 1	Osteitis fibrosa	7.8	76.7	8.5	2.5	26	12.5	1.3	Broad	0.0
	+ 11	Osteitis fibrosa	3.7	58.3	6.1	4.0	14	21.0	2.6	Double	0.0
7	+ 1	Osteitis fibrosa	4.2	49.0	1.1	0.4	9	19.3	0.4	Double	0.0
	+ 11	Osteitis fibrosa	2.1	36.7	2.0	1.0	3	20.9	1.1	Double	0.0
Mean‡			+5.3	−0.8	+2.6	+2.1	−2.4	+6.1	+3.3		−0.8
±SD			5.8	15.3	4.4	1.1	7.2	4.1	3.5		0.8
p <			0.05	ns	0.05	0.05	ns	0.05	0.05		0.05

* (−) Months prior to; (+) Months after starting CAPD treatment.
‡ Mean ± SD of the difference between baseline data at 10 ± 8.7 months prior to the start of CAPD and comparison data, 12 ± 1.5 months after starting treatment.

pattern of osteitis fibrosa upon repeating the biopsy after 12 months of CAPD. Patient 6, however, on whom the baseline biopsy was performed 24 months before CAPD, already had prominent osteitis fibrosa only one month after leaving hemodialysis. In patients 2, 3, 5, and 7, baseline specimens all showed osteitis fibrosa, the severity increasing after variable periods of treatment with CAPD.

Comparison of the data for all patients at 10 ± 8.7 months prior to beginning CAPD with that after 12.0 ± 1.5 months of treatment, reveals significant increases in osteoblastic osteoid, osteoclastic resorbtion, osteoclasts/mm², bone volume, the volume of endosteal fibrosis, and a decrease in the intensity of aluminum staining.

Osteitis fibrosa is present in all specimens from patients 2, 3, and 5. Broad tetracycline bands, indicative of disorganized mineralization, were seen in the initial biopsies from these patients. Subsequently, with progression of this pathology and its *de novo* appearance in patients 1 and 6, mineralization and bone formation becomes more organized. This is documented by the presence of two distinct bands of tetracycline fluorescence. The improved mineralization is also associated with decreased aluminum staining. Thus, except for patient 4, with severe dialysis osteomalacia and dense aluminum deposits, all patients either lose or demonstrate appreciably less intense aluminum staining as mineralization improves and osteitis fibrosa becomes progressively severe.

Table 2 lists the biochemical and radiographic data at the time of each biopsy. In patients with osteitis fibrosa, only 6 of 13 skeletal X-rays were reported to have features such as subperiosteal bone resorption consistent with the diagnosis of osteitis fibrosa. Among these, patient 5 also demonstrated old fractures on two films, while apparent pseudo fractures were seen after one month of CAPD in patient 6. In the three patients with osteomalacia, X-rays at the time of the biopsies were normal in two cases and showed old fractures in all three films from patient 4.

The serum calcium concentration increased in five patients and decreased in two during the initial 12 ± 1.5 months of CAPD. The mean increase for all patients, 0.3 ± 0.7 mg/dl is not significant and no differences are apparent between the concentrations associated with osteomalacia, 9.3 ± 0.5 mg/dl, and those with osteitis fibrosa, 9.4 ± 0.7 mg/dl. The average serum phosphorus concentration, lower after one year of CAPD, 1.3 ± 1.8 mg/dl, and lower in patients with osteitis fibrosa, 5.4 ± 1.9 mg/dl

versus 6.3 ± 1.7 mg/dl in those with osteomalacia, does not significantly change with CAPD

The concentration of both the carboxy and amino PTH terminals were lower in the samples during CAPD. The carboxy terminal levels are however abnormally high in all samples (normal = 0.1–0.3 ng/ml) except in patient 4, with severe osteomalacia and intense aluminum staining after 28 months of CAPD. The concentration of the carboxy terminal increases in relationship to the alkaline phosphatase concentration, i.e., $Y = 0.09$ alkaline phosphatase$^{0.6}$, ($r = 0.86$). Amino terminal concentrations are variably elevated in patients 1, 5, and 6 (normal = 0.05–0.3 ng/ml). The serum alkaline phosphatase activity increased, 71.6 ± 96.5 IU/L, in a linear relationship to the endosteal fibrosis volume, i.e., $Y = 79$ fibrosis volume + 15, ($r = 0.84$).

Serum aluminum was measured after 12 ± 1.5 months of CAPD treatment, and like the other data varied individually. The mean aluminum concentration, 99 ± 81 μg/L is not different from that for contemporary patients treated by hemodialysis, 120 ± 80 μg/L, but greatly exceeds the level from 29 normal individuals, 3.9 ± 1.0 μg/L. Although no statistical correlation exists between the serum aluminum concentrations and the intensity of the histologic staining for aluminum, the highest serum levels are noted in patients 1, 3, and 4, all with residual aluminum staining in the bone after one year of CAPD.

DISCUSSION

In the present study, two of the three patients with osteomalacia in biopsies taken during hemodialysis demonstrated a change to osteitis fibrosa when the biopsy was repeated during CAPD. The other four displayed progressive osteitis fibrosa. The specific role CAPD played in effecting these changes remains uncertain, however, due to the time lag between the initial biopsy and the start of CAPD. This is especially prominent in patient 6, where osteitis fibrosa is already present after only one month of CAPD.

No patient in this study received either oral calcium or vitamin D preparations, and all had intact parathyroid glands for thē duration of the study. This contrasts with other reports of bone histology in CAPD patients in which calcium was supplemented, vitamin D prescribed, or parathyroidectomies performed.[13–15]

The apparent tendency toward resolution of osteomalacia in our patients resembles that ob-

Table 2. Biochemical and Radiographic Data in CAPD Patients.

Patient	Months CAPD at Time of Biopsy*	Serum				Parathyroid Hormone		Clinical Reports of Skeletal‡ X-rays
		Calcium mg/dl	Phosphorus mg/dl	Alkaline Phosphatase IU/L	Aluminum µg/L	Carboxy ng/ml	Amino ng/ml	
1	− 6	9.4	7.5	60	—	2.66	1.75	Normal
	+12	9.9	4.2	129	255	1.46	0.26	SPR
2	− 5	9.9	5.3	115	—	2.00	0.06	SPR
	+14	10.1	4.5	119	65	1.56	0.05	Normal
	+30	10.1	4.5	205	—	0.99	0.05	Normal
3	−11	9.7	9.0	70	—	1.56	0.05	SPR
	+10	9.1	4.7	64	86	1.00	0.05	SPR
4	− 6	9.2	7.6	78	—	0.89	0.05	FRAC
	+14	9.9	6.5	130	155	0.90	0.08	FRAC
	+28	8.5	6.4	94	—	0.05	0.05	FRAC
5	−19	8.9	7.2	157	—	2.52	0.26	Normal
	+ 1	9.8	8.6	220	—	1.62	1.09	FRAC + SPR
	+11	10.2	7.1	429	77	2.09	0.65	FRAC + SPR
6	−24	9.4	3.4	56	—	2.04	0.69	Normal
	+ 1	8.5	4.1	160	—	2.18	1.02	PF
	+11	9.5	3.7	157	44	1.71	0.66	FRAC
7	+ 1	8.5	3.5	70	—	1.23	0.05	Normal
	+12	8.4	3.5	81	12	—	—	Normal
Mean§		+0.3	−1.3	+71.6	—	−0.5	−0.2	
±SD		0.6	1.8	96.5	—	0.4	0.7	
p <		ns	ns	0.05	—	ns	ns	

* (−) Months prior to, (+) months after start of CAPD treatment.
‡ SPR = subperiosteal resorption; FRAC = healed fracture; PF = pseudo fracture.
§ Mean ± SD of the difference between baseline data at 10 ± 8.7 mos prior to start of CAPD and comparison data, 12 ± 1.5 mos after starting treatment.

served among five of six patients after one year of CAPD reported by Teitelbaum et al.[13] These patients, however, were given oral calcium supplements and additionally showed improvement in concommitant osteitis fibrosa, which the authors attributed to decreased parathyroid hormone concentrations.

In contrast to the progression of osteitis fibrosa observed in the present study, Gokal et al.[14] reported decreased osteitis fibrosa in 15 patients followed on CAPD for at least 12 months. However, only 26% of these patients received prior hemodialysis, many took oral calcium supplements, four were treated with vitamin D preparations, and several required parathyroidectomy. Additionally, in a number of the patients, osteitis fibrosis was absent or minimal in both the initial and one-year biopsies.

The concentration of serum calcium for our patients, 9.4 ± 0.6 mg/dl, was normal, while that for phosphorus was elevated, 5.6 ± 1.9 mg/dl. Like the report by Gokal et al.,[14] neither value changed remarkably after a period of CAPD. The progressive osteitis fibrosa and unchanging serum calcium levels in the present study suggest that serum calcium may be sustained by bone resorption. Further, this implies that augmented calcium intake may be essential for patients treated with CAPD. This concept is supported by reports where impaired calcium balance was altered with oral calcium or vitamin D supplements, with resultant increases in serum calcium concentrations.[13,15,21,22]

In the present study, the concentration of PTH tends to decrease after starting CAPD. Increased peritoneal clearance of PTH, as reported by others,[23-25] may play a role. Parathyroid hormone concentrations are abnormally elevated, however, consistent with secondary hyperparathyroidism in renal failure. Enhanced biologic activity of PTH is suggested by the relationships between PTH, alkaline phosphatase, and endosteal fibrosis. While similar biochemical results correlated with X-ray abnormalities in the report by Digenis et al.,[15] skeletal films in the present study failed to accurately reflect PTH, alkaline phosphatase activity, or bone histopathology.

Serum aluminum measured after one year of CAPD was elevated and similar to levels previously reported.[22,26] Concentrations were greatest in the three patients showing residual aluminum staining of the bone after a year of CAPD. These data are consistent with reports linking tissue aluminum to osteomalacia and impaired parathyroid hormone secretion.[27-29]

A decrease in stainable bone aluminum was observed in the present study. This may result from the combined influence of peritoneal aluminum clearance[30] and reduced aluminum antacid intake by CAPD patients.[26]

REFERENCES

1. Ellis HA, Pierides AM, Feest TG, Ward MK, and Kerr DNS: Histopathology of renal osteodystrophy with particular reference to the effects of 1-hydroxyvitamin D_3 in patients treated with long term haemodialysis. Clin Endocrinol 7(Suppl): 315, 1977
2. Coburn JW, Brickman AS, Sherrard DJ, Singer FR, Wang EGC, Baylink DJ, and Norman AW: Use of 1-25(OH)2 vitamin D_3 to separate types of renal osteodystrophy. Proc Eur Dial Transplant Assoc 14: 442, 1977
3. Hodsman AB, Sherrard DJ, Wang EC, Brickman AD, Lee DBN, Alfrey AC, Singer FR, Norman AW, and Coburn JW: Vitamin D resistant osteomalacia in hemodialysis patients lacking secondary hyperparathyroidism. Ann Intern Med 94: 629, 1981
4. Cournot-Witmer G, Zingraff J, Plachot JJ, Escaig F, Lefevre R, Boumati P, Bourdeau A, Garabédian M, Galle P, Bourdon R, Drüeke T, and Balson S: Aluminum localization in bone from hemodialysis patients: Relationship to matrix mineralization. Kidney Int 20: 375, 1981
5. Ott SM, Maloney NA, Coburn JW, Alfrey AC, and Sherrard DJ: The prevalence of bone aluminum deposition in renal osteodystrophy and its relation to the response to calcitrol therapy. N Engl J Med 307: 709, 1982
6. Ward MK, Feest TG, Ellis HA, Parkinson IS, Kerr DNS, Herrington J, and Goode GL: Osteomalacia dialysis osteodystrophy: Evidence for a water-borne aetiological agent, probably aluminium. Lancet 1: 841, 1978
7. Parkinson IS, Ward MK, and Kerr DNS: Dialysis encephalopathy, bone disease and anaemia: The aluminium intoxication syndrome during regular haemodialysis. J Clin Pathol 34: 1285, 1981
8. Hodsman AB, Sherrard DH, Alfrey AC, Ott S, Brickman AD, Miller NL, Maloney HA, and Coburn JW: Bone aluminum and histomorphometric features of renal osteodystrophy. J Clin Endocrinol Metab 54: 539, 1982
9. Andreol SP, Bergstein JM, and Sherrard DJ: Aluminum intoxication from aluminum-containing phosphate binders in children with azotemia not undergoing dialysis. N Engl J Med 310: 1079, 1984
10. Griswold WR, Reznik V, Mendoza A, Trauner D, and Alfrey AC: Accumulation of aluminum in a nondialyzed uremic child receiving aluminum hydroxide. Pediatrics 71: 56, 1983

11. Kaye M: Oral aluminum toxicity in a non-dialyzed patient with renal failure. Clin Nephrol 20: 208, 1983

12. Felsenfeld A, Gutman RA, Llach F, and Harrelson JM: Osteomalacia in chronic renal failure: A syndrome previously reported only with maintenance dialysis. Am J Nephrol 2: 147, 1982

13. Teitelbaum SL, Fallon MD, Gearing BK, Dougan CS, and Delmez JA: The effects of continuous ambulatory peritoneal dialysis (CAPD) on bone histomorphology. Kidney Int (Abstract) 21: 180, 1982

14. Gokal R, Ramos JM, Ellis H, Parkinson I, Sweetman V, Dewar J, Ward MK, and Kerr DNS: Histological renal osteodystrophy and 25 hydroxy cholecalciferol and aluminum levels in patients on continuous ambulatory peritoneal dialysis. Kidney Int 23: 15, 1983

15. Digenis G, Khanna R, Pierratos A, Meema HE, Rabinovich S, Pettit J, and Oreopoulos DG: Renal osteodystrophy in patients maintained on CAPD for more than three years. Peritoneal Dial Bull 3: 81, 1983

16. Llach F, Felsenfeld A, and Haussler MR: The pathophysiology of altered calcium metabolism in rhabdomyolysis-induced acute renal failure: Interactions of parathyroid hormone, 25-hydroxycholecalciferol and 1-25 dihydroxycholecalciferol. N Engl J Med 305: 117, 1981

17. LeGendre GR, and Alfrey AC: Measuring picogram amounts of aluminum in biological tissues by flameless atomic absorption analysis of a chelate. Clin Chem 22: 53, 1976

18. Maloney NA, Ott SM, Alfrey AC, Miller NL, Coburn JW, and Sherrard DJ: Histological quantitation of aluminum in iliac bone from patients with renal failure. J Lab Clin Med 99: 206, 1982

19. Felsenfeld AJ, Harrelson JM, and Gutman RA: A quantitative histomorphometric comparison of 40 micron thick paragon sections with 5 micron thick goldner sections in the study of undecalcified bone. Calcif Tissue Int 34: 232, 1982

20. Sokal RR, and Rahlf FJ: Biometry, 2nd Ed. New York: WH Freeman, 1981, p 448

21. deFremont JF, Morinière P, Kechzmareck P, Fievet P, Bataille P, and Fournier A: Hypercalcemia in continuous peritoneal dialysis patients (Abstract). Int Congr Nephrol 8: 399, 1981

22. Kurtz SB, Wong VH, Anderson CF, Vogel JP, McCarthy JT, Mitchell JC, Kumar R, and Johnson WJ: Continuous ambulatory peritoneal dialysis: Three years experience at the Mayo clinic. Mayo Clin Proc 58: 633, 1983

23. Alonso JLM, Martinez ME, Selgas R, Casares I, and Gomez P: Peritoneal clearance of parathyroid hormone (Abstract). Int Congr Nephrol 8: 420, 1981

24. Delmez JA, Slatopolsky E, Martin KJ, Gearing BN, and Harter HR: Minerals, vitamin D, and parathyroid hormone in continuous ambulatory peritoneal dialysis. Kidney Int 21: 862, 1982

25. Delmez JA, Martin KJ, Harter HR, Gearing B, and Slatopolsky E: Effects of continuous ambulatory peritoneal dialysis on the removal of PTH in renal failure (Abstract). Am Soc Artif Intern Organs 9: 44, 1980

26. Thomson NM, Stevens BJ, Humphrey TJ, and Atkins RC: Comparison of trace elements in peritoneal dialysis, hemodialysis, and uremia. Kidney Int 23: 9, 1983

27. Ihle BU, Buchanan MCR, Stevens B, Becker GJ, and Kincaid-Smith P: The efficacy of various treatment modalities on aluminum associated bone disease. Proc Eur Dial Transplant Assoc 19: 195, 1982

28. Morrisey J, Rothstein M, Mayor G, and Slatopolsky E: Suppression of parathyroid hormone secretion by aluminum. Kidney Int 23: 699, 1983

29. Hercz G, Milliner DS, Shinaberger JH, Nissenson AR, Cutler RE, Goodman WG, Gentile DE, Kraus AP, and Coburn JW: Aluminum metabolism and record during CAPD (Abstract). Am Soc Nephrol 16: 120A, 1983

30. Sorkin MI, Nolph KD, Anderson HO, Morris JS, Kennedy J, Prowant B, and Moore H: Aluminum mass transfer during continuous ambulatory peritoneal dialysis. Peritoneal Dial Bull 1: 91, 1981

B. Wallaeys, R. Cornelis, and N. Lameire

90

The Trace Elements Br, Co, Cr, Cs, Cu, Fe, Mn, Rb, Se and Zn in Serum, Packed Cells, and Dialysate of CAPD Patients

SUMMARY

Trace element homeostasis has been studied in five patients undergoing CAPD. Neutron activation analysis was used to quantify trace elements in carefully handled specimens of blood, dialysis fluid and urine. Serum and erythrocyte bromide concentrations were significantly below normal and bromide was removed in peritoneal dialysate. Rubidium also was removed by peritoneal dialysis and erythrocyte concentrations were low. A modest decrease in serum selenium accompanied by a slight increase in the dialysate concentration was observed. The decrease in serum cobalt concentrations could not be explained by the data, whereas changes in zinc concentrations could be ascribed to altered distribution. An accumulation of chromium in plasma was associated with a decrease in the dialysate concentration. No abnormalities were detected in the concentrations of cesium, copper, iron or manganese.

INTRODUCTION

Over the last few years, much interest has been focused on alterations of trace element concentrations in serum and packed cells of the uremic patient. In this study, the effect of CAPD on trace element profiles in serum and packed cells was investigated. The peritoneum represents the site for transit of waste products and electrolytes from the blood to the dialysate. Trace element exchanges occur both ways, which might cause an extreme and uncontrolled accumulation or depletion of some elements.

METHODS

Trace elements in serum and packed blood cells of five CAPD patients were studied. Alterations in trace elements in one patient before initial dialysis and after two months of treatment were also studied. The data on the patients are summarized in Table 1.

Two blood samples were considered: one before the dialysis fluid was introduced into the peritoneum and one after the sixth dwell period. Fresh dialysis fluid and the sixth dwell dialysate were also sampled. The analytical technique used for the determination of the trace elements was neutron activation analysis (NAA).

Experimental

The blood samples were collected with the aid of a plastic cannula trocar (intranule 110 16, Vygon), flushed with 20 ml blood before actual sampling in ultra-clean Suprasil Heraeus quartz vials. The dialysis fluid was sampled directly from the storage bag before treatment, and six hours later a sample was taken from the effluent dialysate. All further sample handling was performed in a dust-poor room.

From the Laboratory for Analytical Chemistry, Rijksuniversiteit Gent, Proeftuinstraat 86, and the Division of Nephrology, Department of Medicine, University Hospital, De Pintelaan 185, B-9000 Gent, Belgium.

Table 1. CAPD Patient Characteristics.

Patient No.	Age (yrs)	Sex	Start of Dialysis	Sampling Date	Diagnosis
1	65	M	03/01/79	14/07/80	Chronic pyelonephritis (phenacetin)
2	60	M	20/02/80	23/01/81	Chronic interstitial nephritis (phenacetin)
3	67	F	13/09/79	09/03/81	Chronic interstitial nephritis (phenacetin)
4	64	M	05/01/82	12/03/82	Urate nephropathy
5	37	F	12/10/82	15/12/82	Alport's syndrome

The blood was allowed to clot spontaneously for one hour, and afterward was centrifuged and the serum was separated from the packed cells. All samples were deep-frozen and lyophilized.

For the determination of Cu and Mn, short irradiations (3 hours) at a thermal neutron flux of $10^{12} \cdot cm^{-2} \cdot sec^{-1}$ (Thetis reactor Gent, Belgium) were performed, followed by radiochemical separation. Determination of Br was performed in a purely instrumental way, after irradiation (3 hours) at a flux of $10^{12} n \cdot cm^{-2} \cdot sec^{-1}$ (Thetis reactor Gent, Belgium). The simultaneous determination of Co, Cs, Fe, Rb, Se, and Zn requires irradiation for 12 days at a thermal neutron flux of $10^{13} n \cdot cm^{-2} \cdot sec^{-1}$ (BR-II reactor Mol, Belgium). The irradiated samples were wet-ashed and measured for γ-activity. Analysis for Cr was performed after radiochemical separation on dry-ashed serum samples and dialysates, which were irradiated for 12 days at a thermal neutron flux of $10^{14} n \cdot cm^{-2} \cdot sec^{-1}$ (BR-II reactor Mol, Belgium). Cr in packed cells was not possible by NAA.

DISCUSSION

For the elements Br, Co, Cs, Cu, Fe, Mn, Rb, Se, and Zn in serum and packed cells, and for Cr in serum, there was no significant difference between the concentrations at the start and end of a single dialysis session. Therefore the results, given in Table 2, are the means of those data. The normal levels in healthy individuals for Br,[1] Co,[2,3] Cr,[3] Cs, Fe, Rb, Se, Zn,[4] and Cu and Mn[5] are also listed.

Analysis of variance (using a t-distribution with 95% confidence intervals) was applied as a criterion for testing the null hypothesis that the population means were the same in both classes, i.e., CAPD patients versus healthy individuals.

The element Br, both in serum and in packed cells, fell far below the normal range. The increase in Br content of the dialysate indicates that some Br leaves the body through the peritoneum. It is possible that the Br store of these patients becomes depleted by this continuous dialysis treatment. A similar low blood Br status has previously been studied in hemodialysis patients.[6]

Serum Co concentrations in the CAPD patients appeared to be significantly higher than in normals, whereas Co in the packed cells was normal. Co was low in the dialysate and remained unchanged over the dwell period.

The mean Cr values in the sera of these CAPD patients was about 26 times higher than the normal mean. The mean concentration of Cr in dialysis fluid was exceptionally high, up to eight times the normal serum concentration. It was the only trace element in dialysis fluid to exceed the normal mean serum value. Cr in dialysis fluid seems to be absorbed into the body.

The Cs, Cu, Fe, and Mn concentrations, both in serum and in packed cells, were around values seen in normals. Cs in fresh dialysis fluid was extremely low, but increased nearly 11 times by the end of the dwell. The original Cu concentrations in dialysis fluid were about 100 times lower than the normal mean serum Cu value, and doubled after the dwell time. Fe was not detected in the dialysis fluid. The original Mn content of the dialysis fluid was comparable to that of serum, but decreased to half its original value by the end of the dwell period.

Serum Rb was normal, but in packed cells was distinctively below normal. Rb was hardly detectable in fresh dialysis fluid, but increased after exposure to the peritoneum.

Serum Se was low and in packed cells was normal. This element was very low in the dialysis fluid and the concentration tripled after the dwell period.

Zn in serum of CAPD patients was significantly lower than in healthy individuals, whereas Zn in packed cells was significantly higher than in normals. The Zn content of the dialysis fluid was very low and fell by more than half by the end of the dwell time. Similar deviations from normality have been

Table 2. Mean ± SD Trace Element Concentrations in Serum Packed Cells and Dialysis Fluid of CAPD Patients versus Normal Values.

Element	Serum (ml)		Packed Cells (g)		Dialysis Fluid (ml)	
	Patient	Normal	Patient	Normal	Fresh	Spent
Br (µg)	1.23 ± 0.63* (n = 9)	4.87 ± 2.02 (n = 10)	0.47 ± 0.09* (n = 8)	4.14 ± 1.44 (n = 10)	0.44 ± 0.14 (n = 3)	1.09 ± 0.46 (n = 3)
Co (ng)	0.31 ± 0.10* (n = 10)	0.108 ± 0.060 (n = 17)	0.55 ± 0.22 (n = 8)	0.59 ± 0.23 (n = 6)	0.08 ± 0.07 (n = 5)	0.09 ± 0.06 (n = 5)
Cr (ng)	4.25 ± 1.72* (n = 10)	0.160 ± 0.083 (n = 20)			1.22 ± 0.47 (n = 5)	0.74 ± 0.15 (n = 5)
Cs (ng)	1.01 ± 0.28 (n = 10)	0.74 ± 0.25 (n = 36)	5.64 ± 1.65 (n = 10)	4.82 ± 2.10 (n = 36)	<0.07 (n = 5)	0.74 ± 0.28 (n = 5)
Cu (µg)	1.31 ± 0.39 (n = 6)	1.07 ± 0.24 (n = 46)	0.68 ± 0.17 (n = 6)	0.66 ± 0.08 (n = 46)	0.011 ± 0.001 (n = 3)	0.023 ± 0.002 (n = 3)
Fe (µg)	1.21 ± 0.37 (n = 10)	1.63 ± 0.43 (n = 36)	1025 ± 136 (n = 10)	(n = 36)	N.D.	N.D.
Mn (ng)	0.58 ± 0.10 (n = 6)	0.57 ± 0.13 (n = 46)	10.3 ± 3.8 (n = 6)	15.0 ± 4.9 (n = 46)	0.44 ± 0.09 (n = 3)	0.21 ± 0.04 (n = 3)
Rb (µg)	0.164 ± 0.021 (n = 10)	0.173 ± 0.036 (n = 36)	3.49 ± 0.17* (n = 10)	4.28 ± 0.98 (n = 36)	N.D.	0.40 ± 0.17 (n = 5)
Se (µg)	0.095 ± 0.018* (n = 10)	0.130 ± 0.021 (n = 36)	0.142 ± 0.014 (n = 10)	0.163 ± 0.030 (n = 36)	$(0.9 ± 0.8)10^{-3}$ (n = 5)	$(2.6 ± 1.5)10^{-3}$ (n = 5)
Zn (µg)	0.74 ± 0.14* (n = 10)	1.13 ± 0.20 (n = 36)	14.0 ± 1.0* (n = 10)	11.1 ± 1.8 (n = 36)	0.056 ± 0.013 (n = 5)	0.019 ± 0.009 (n = 5)

n = number of samples: start + end of CAPD treatment.
* significant versus normals: p 0.05; ND = not detected.

reported for Zn in serum and packed cells of hemodialysis patients.[7]

There is some question whether the observed trace element abnormalities for Br, Co, Cr, Rb, Se, and Zn already existed in the uremic patients prior to the start of the CAPD treatment, or whether they were induced by it.

One patient was sampled one day before the onset of continuous dialysis (the analyses are still in progress). The serum Br value was 6.09 μg/ml, whereas after two months CAPD it was reduced to 2.88 μg/ml. The serum Cr value appeared to be normal (0.28 ng/ml) prior to CAPD treatment; two months later, however, the value had risen to 4.0 ng/ml. As Cr is an essential element, a more profound investigation seems warranted.

CONCLUSION

The investigation of Cs, Cu, Fe, and Mn in the sera and packed cells of five CAPD patients showed that they were maintained within the normal range. The elements Co and Se in packed cells were also normal. On the contrary, Co in serum was significantly higher than normal, whereas Se in serum was significantly lower than in healthy individuals. Rb was normal in serum, but slightly lower than normal in packed cells. Zn was significantly lower in serum, but somewhat higher than normal in packed cells. An important alteration, however, was the depletion of Br in serum and packed cells. Subnormal blood Br levels, resulting in insomnia, have already been reported for patients on hemodialysis.[6,8] The dramatic increase of serum Cr in these CAPD patients is a most intriguing finding. As the main excretory pathway for this element is the urinary tract, which is impaired in these patients, it is likely that accumulation of Cr in different organs might occur.

Study of trace elements in human serum has until now been restricted to determination of their total content. Although this knowledge is very important, it is necessary to establish a link between trace elements and serum proteins. This research requires biochemical separation techniques, coupled to an elemental detection method possessing high sensitivity and accuracy (e.g., NAA). The element Cr will be the first one to be studied in this way, and may give valuable clinical information for the CAPD patient.

REFERENCES

1. Cornelis R, Mees L, Lemey G, and Versieck J: Unpublished results
2. Krivan V, Geiger H, and Franz HE: Determination of Fe, Co, Cu, Zn, Se, Rb and Cs in NBS bovine liver, blood plasma and erythrocytes by INAA and AAS. Fres Z Anal Chem 305: 399, 1981
3. Versieck J, Hoste J, Barbier F, Steyaert H, DeRudder J, and Michels H: Determination of Cr and Co in human serum by neutron activation analysis. Clin Chem 24: 303, 1978
4. Versieck J, Hoste J, Barbier F, Michels H, and DeRudder J: Simultaneous determination of iron, zinc, selenium, rubidium and cesium in serum and packed blood cells by neutron activation analysis. Clin Chem 23: 1301, 1977
5. Versieck J, Speecke A, Hoste J, and Barbier F: Determination of manganese, copper and zinc in serum and packed blood cells by neutron activation analysis. Z Klin Chem Klin Biochem 11: 193, 1973
6. Cornelis R, Ringoir S, Lameire N, Mees L, and Hoste J: Blood bromine in uremic patients. Mineral Electrolyte Metab 2: 186, 1979
7. Cornelis R, Mees L, Ringoir S, and Hoste J: Serum and red blood cell Zn, Se, Cs and Rb in dialysis patients. Mineral Electrolyte Metab 2: 88, 1979
8. Oe PL, Vis RD, Meijeer JM, van Langevelde F, Allon W, van deMeer C, and Verheul H: Bromine deficiency and insomnia in patients on dialysis. In Howell JMcC, Gawthorne JM, and White CL (Eds), Trace element metabolism in man and animals (TEMA-4). Australian Academy of Sciences, 1981, p 526

A. Cantaluppi, S. Casati, G. Graziani, A. Citterio,
I. Simoni, L. Borghi, A. Montanari, and A. Novarini

91

High Muscle Magnesium and Potassium in Long-Term Regular Dialysis Treatment

SUMMARY

Muscle potassium and magnesium concentrations were studied in 35 healthy subjects, 24 patients with chronic renal failure not treated by dialysis, and 35 patients on RDT subdivided according to the type of dialysis. The low muscle potassium in chronic renal failure is corrected by either hemodialysis or CAPD. In dialysis patients there is a progressive increase in muscle K and Mg that depends on the duration of RDT.

INTRODUCTION

Abnormalities of water and electrolyte equilibrium are common in chronic renal failure (CRF); however, extracellular electrolyte concentrations have little value in predicting water and electrolyte status of the intracellular compartment. This has special importance for potassium (K) and magnesium (Mg), which are high in concentration in intracellular fluid and low in concentration in extracellular fluid. Since skeletal muscle is the most abundant cellular tissue, analysis of muscle tissue in uremic patients is thought to give direct information of cell composition of the body in CRF. In terminal renal failure, body water and plasma electrolyte composition are controlled by dialysis; however, information on the effects of dialysis on muscle water and electrolyte is available only for short periods of regular dialysis treatment (RDT).[1] Since RDT is able to prolong the survival of uremic patients, it is conceivable that, under such long-term unphysiological conditions, other factors such as the dialysis procedure *per se* (e.g., dialysis solution composition) or pharmacological treatment (e.g., Mg-containing phosphate-binding antacids or vitamin D preparations) may affect the water and electrolyte content of skeletal muscle.

In this study, muscle K and Mg were measured in control subjects, in patients with advanced CRF not on RDT, and in patients on hemodialysis (HD) or CAPD.

METHODS

We studied 35 healthy control subjects, 24 patients with advanced chronic renal failure (plasma creatinine > 7 mg/dl) not treated by dialysis (CRF), and 35 uremic patients begun on RDT (Table 1). Dialysis patients were divided into four groups according to the type of RDT (HD; CAPD; CAPD after a period of HD, HD + CAPD) and the duration of RDT (<48 months HD_I and >98 months HD_{II}).

Prior to muscle biopsy, none of the patients of CRF group had dietary bicarbonate or steroid treatment. In this group, diuretic therapy in seven hypertensive patients had been stopped at least eight

From the Divisione di Nefrologia, Ospedale Maggiore Policlinico, Milano and Istituto di Semeiotica Medica, Università di Parma, Italy.

Table 1. Patient Characteristics.

	Controls	CRF	HD$_I$	CAPD	HD$_{II}$	HD $\pm$ CAPD
No. of pts	35	24	7	9	15	4
M/F	19/16	14/10	5/2	5/4	13/2	3/1
Age (years)	58 $\pm$ 6	59 $\pm$ 14	52 $\pm$ 5	64 $\pm$ 6	55 $\pm$ 11	62 $\pm$ 9
Body weight (Kg)	66 $\pm$ 5	58 $\pm$ 8	63 $\pm$ 9	62 $\pm$ 10	58 $\pm$ 8	58 $\pm$ 14
Months of RDT	—	—	12–48	12–24	98–186	78–178

Data as mean $\pm$ SD.

months prior to observation. These latter patients were receiving hypotensive therapy, with beta-blockers or methyldopa at the time of observation. In the RDT group, 30 of 35 patients chronically received vitamin D preparations and an antacid mixture of Mg $(OH)_2$ and Al $(OH)_3$ as an intestinal phosphate-binder. Hemodialysis treatment, in the last 10 years, was carried out three times a week for 4–5 hours with single-pass technique using either disposable hollow fiber or parallel plate dialyzers with surface area of 1 m^2. Dialysis solution composition (mM/L) was Na 136–142, K 0–2, Mg 0.75, Ca 2, Cl 106–110.5, Acetate 38, Glucose 5.55. Dialysate flow was 500 ml/min and blood flow 250–300 ml/min. CAPD was performed with three to four daily exchanges of 2 L solutions with the following composition (mM/L): Na 132, Mg 0.75, Ca 1.75, Cl 102, Lactate 35. Different dextrose monohydrate concentrations (1.5, 2.5, and 4.25 g/dl) were used according to clinical requirements. In all the subjects, plasma and muscle tissue were obtained after an overnight fast: the HD patients were studied before dialysis and those on CAPD, three hours after the first morning peritoneal exchange.

Skeletal muscle tissue was obtained, after local anesthesia of the skin, by needle biopsy of quadriceps, using the needle described by Bergström,[2] or during surgery for arteriovenous fistula at the fore-arm. Techniques of analysis of plasma and muscle K and Mg have been already described.[3]

RESULTS

In Table 2 the results of muscle K and Mg (Km and Mgm) and of serum Mg are reported for control subjects, patients with advanced renal failure not on RDT (CRF), and patients treated by dialysis according to the type and the duration of RDT. Results are expressed as mM/kg of muscle fat free solids for Km and Mgm and as mM/L for serum Mg.

Plasma K was normal in all the groups. As reported in Table 2, serum Mg was significantly higher than normal in CRF and markedly elevated in all RDT groups. It is also apparent that both K and Mg in the muscle were increased only in the groups with long duration of RDT (HD$_{II}$ and HD + CAPD), while HD$_I$ and CAPD groups showed normal muscle K and Mg.

DISCUSSION

Our findings show that low Km in CRF is normalized in early RDT, either with HD or CAPD; Mgm is normal in CRF and early RDT; however,

Table 2. Results.

	Months of RDT	Km	Mgm	Mg Serum
Controls (35)	—	458 $\pm$ 36	40 $\pm$ 5	0.6 – 0.9
CRF (24)	—	409 $\pm$ 62*	43 $\pm$ 6	1.0 $\pm$ 0.2*
HD$_I$ (7)	12–48	439 $\pm$ 49	38 $\pm$ 6	1.4 $\pm$ 0.6*
CAPD (9)	12–24	467 $\pm$ 60	38 $\pm$ 5	1.4 $\pm$ 0.2*
HD$_{II}$ (15)	98–186	504 $\pm$ 47*	54 $\pm$ 6*	1.6 $\pm$ 0.4*
HD + CAPD (4)	78–178	498 $\pm$ 38*	60 $\pm$ 6*	1.3 $\pm$ 0.1*

Number in parentheses indicate the number of patients studied. Data as a mean $\pm$ SD.
* $p < 0.001$ versus Controls, Student t test.

484

Cantaluppi, et al.

Km and even more apparently Mgm are higher than normal in long-term RDT, irrespective of the type of RDT. This suggests that in dialysis patients there is a progressive increase in muscle K and Mg that depends on the duration of RDT.

Potassium status has been extensively studied in CRF; in undialyzed uremia it is generally accepted that muscle K is low.[4,5] Several factors, such as chronic acidosis and malnutrition, may contribute to K depletion in CRF.[5] However, it is thought that low cell K with normal plasma K is mainly related to the specific disturbances of cell function of CRF, including impaired Na/K pump activity,[6] increased passive permeability to Na,[7] and reduced membrane potential.[4] These dysfunctions have been shown to undergo early reversal by HD,[6] with normalization of K in both muscle and leucocytes,[4,6] as confirmed by the present data. However, in long-term RDT, muscle K was not only normalized, but was also higher than normal. This finding is unexplained; a normal intake of nutrients, including K, and good control of acidosis may actually contribute to a chronic positive K balance, perhaps through an increase of cell K capacity.[5,8] However, other mechanisms acting on membrane function would be expected to be involved. Indeed, a membrane potential higher than normal has been found in RDT patients on thrice weekly dialysis.[9] It may be inferred that, in RDT, muscle plasma membrane becomes hyperpolarized due to an increased Na/K pump activity in response to the high passive influx of Na. This would result in an increase in both muscle K and membrane potential. Simultaneous measurements of muscle K and membrane potential are required to further clarify this point.

Normal muscle Mg has been previously found in undialyzed CRF[10]; we confirm this issue despite significantly high plasma Mg. Hypermagnesemia was even more marked in RDT; however, it seemed to be associated with high muscle Mg only in patients on long duration RDT. Previous studies have shown that muscle Mg may be relatively independent of both the size of the other body Mg pools (such as bone and erythrocytes) and plasma Mg.[11-12] In addition, significant changes in muscle Mg have been observed at zero external balance.[12] This has suggested that factors other than total body Mg are the major determinant of muscle Mg levels. On the other hand, not only hypermagnesemia but also a sustained positive external Mg balance would occur in RDT through a number of mechanisms, including abolished urine Mg excretion, high oral intake of Mg (Mg-rich antacids), and vitamin D-induced high in-

testinal absorption of Mg. In addition, the usual dialysate Mg of 0.75 mM/L does not seem to have a significant effect on plasma Mg in RDT.[13] Finally, a measured positive daily Mg balance has been shown recently in CAPD patients.[14] Thus, the long-term Mg excess in RDT seems to be reflected not only by hypermagnesemia and high bone Mg,[15] but also by an accumulation of Mg in skeletal muscle cells. RDT, therefore, seems to be a unique experimental model in which the changes in total body Mg result in variations in muscle Mg.

The physicochemical status of Mg in the cells must be considered to explain the high muscle Mg in RDT; indeed, only a minor fraction of cell Mg is ionized, while the rest is mostly in "bound" form to creatine, proteins, and ATP.[16] It is worth noting that cell ATP has been found to be elevated in CRF.[17] High cell ATP or changed affinity to cell proteins for Mg might contribute, at least hypothetically, to the increase in muscle Mg. However, the mechanism by which muscle cells in uremia become able to store more Mg than under physiological conditions is unknown. This finding deserves further investigation. Finally, from the studies on the interactions between K and Mg in the cells,[12,18] it has been well demonstrated that each of the cations plays a permissive role in the ability of muscle cells to store the other. This issue could also explain the changed pattern of muscle composition in RDT.

REFERENCES

1. Bergström J, and Hultman E: Water, electrolyte and glycogen content of muscle tissue in patients undergoing regular dialysis treatment. Clin Nephrol 2: 24, 1974
2. Bergström J: Muscle electrolytes in man. Scand J Clin Lab Invest 14(Suppl 68): 7, 1962
3. Montanari A, Borghi L, Curti A, Mergoni M, Sani E, Elia G, Canali M, Novarini A, and Borghetti A: Skeletal muscle cell abnormalities in acute hypophosphatemia during total parenteral nutrition. Mineral Electrolyte Metab 10: 52, 1984
4. Bilbrey GL, Carter NW, White MG, Schilling JF, and Knochel JP: Potassium deficiency in chronic renal failure. Kidney Int 4: 423, 1973
5. Montanari A, Borghi L, Canali M, Novarini A, and Borghetti A: Studies on cell water and electrolytes in CRF. Clin Nephrol 9: 200, 1978
6. Patrick J, Jones NF, Bradford B, and Gaunt J: Leucocyte potassium in uraemia: Comparisons with erythrocyte potassium and total exchangeable potassium. Clin Sci 43: 669, 1972

7. Swaminathan R, Clegg G, Cumberbatch M, Zareian Z, and McKenna F: Erythrocyte sodium transport in chronic renal failure. Clin Sci 62: 489, 1981

8. Scribner BH, and Burnell JM: Interpretation of the serum potassium concentrations. Metabolism 5: 468, 1956

9. Cotton JR, Woodard TA, Carter NW, and Knochel JP: Resting skeletal muscle membrane potential as an index of uremic toxicity. J Clin Invest 63: 501, 1979

10. Maschio G, Campanacci L, Mioni G, Bazzato G, Bruschi E, Riz G, and Gianfranceschi G: Acqua ed elettroliti tissutali nell'uremia cronica. Minerva Nefrol 16: 41, 1969

11. Alfrey AC, Miller NL, and Butkus D: Evaluation of body magnesium stores. J Lab Clin Med 84: 153, 1974

12. Montanari A, Borghi L, Canali M, Curti A, Bucciero G, Perinotto P, Novarini A, and Borghetti A: Effets du potassium et des proteines cellulaires sur le magnesium musculaire chez des patients atteints de troubles hydroelectrolytiques. Rev Franc Endo Clin Metab Nutr 20: 531, 1979

13. Burnell JM, and Teubner E: Effects of decreasing magnesium in patients with chronic renal failure. Proc Clin Dial Transplant Forum 5: 191, 1976

14. Delmez JA, Slatopolsky E, Martin KJ, Gearing BN, and Harter HR: Minerals, vitamin D, and parathyroid hormone in continuous ambulatory peritoneal dialysis. Kidney Int 21: 862, 1982

15. Coburn JW, Kurokawa K, and Llach F: Altered divalent ion metabolism in renal disease and renal osteodystrophy. In Maxwell MH, and Kleeman CR (Eds), Clinical disorders of fluid and electrolyte metabolism. New York: McGraw-Hill, 1980, p 1153

16. Veloso D, Guynn RW, Oskarsson M, and Veech RL: The concentrations of free and bound magnesium in rat tissues. J Biol Chem 248: 4811, 1973

17. Kramer HJ, Gospodinov D, and Kruck F: Functional and metabolic studies on red blood cell sodium transport in chronic uremia. Nephron 16: 344, 1976

18. Whang R, and Aikawa JK: Magnesium deficiency and refractoriness to potassium repletion. J Chron Dis 10: 65, 1977

N. DiPaolo, G. Pula, U. Buoncristiani, P.P. Giomarelli,
M. DeMia, B. Biagioli, E. Zei, F. Manescalchi, and P. Rossi

92

Respiratory Function in CAPD

SUMMARY

Respiratory function was studied in 15 CAPD patients with indwelling dialysate and in 10 patients before and after hemodialysis. Respiratory volumes and flow rates were normal in CAPD patients but oscillated with hemodialysis. CAPD was characterized by hyperventilation and increased O_2 consumption while hemodialysis induced a restrictive defect attributed to pulmonary leukocyte sequestration. A modest restrictive defect in CAPD patients may relate to the intraabdominal fluid volume.

INTRODUCTION

Respiratory pathophysiology (RP) has been studied in uremic patients under both conservative and substitution therapy.[1-3] There are several studies concerning patients in hemodialysis (HD) and in peritoneal dialysis. Even though the published data do not agree totally, on review it emerges that peritoneal dialysis and, in particular, CAPD, does not cause important variations in spite of the constant presence of 2 L of fluid in the peritoneal cavity.[4] Several studies of CAPD and RP have revealed differences in RP between an empty abdomen and a full one.[5] It has not been possible to find any controlled study of respiratory function (RF) in CAPD and HD, and therefore it is impossible to compare the effect of the two treatments. The purpose of these studies

was to elucidate differences, and if so, of what type, between a population of patients on CAPD and one on HD.

METHODS

For at least two years, 25 uremic patients in substitution therapy have been studied. Fifteen of these were on CAPD and 10 on HD. All were chosen randomly, taking care to exclude those with diseases of the respiratory tract and malformations of the thoracic cage. Patients were from 16–67 years old (average 45.24 ± 14.22 years). HD was performed four hours thrice weekly with a dialysis solution containing 140 mEq/L Na, and 38 mEq/L of acetate. CAPD was done seven days a week with four exchanges a day. Before and after HD there was an average body weight variation of 2.2 ± 1.4 kg. The RP studies were done on days chosen at random with a full abdomen in CAPD, before and after dialysis in HD.

The RP was analyzed with the following equipment: Beckman MMC metabolic measurement cart, ABL 2 acid base laboratory radiometer (Copenhagen), and an OSM 2 hemoximeter radiometer (Copenhagen and Siregnost FD Siemens). The following data were evaluated.

Pulmonary Volumes and Flows

Pulmonary volumes and flows were obtained by spirometry, with the patient at rest, before and after giving terbutaline, three tests of forced vital capacity (FVC), maximal ventilation (MMV), nitrogen wash

From the Nephrology and Dialysis Department, USL 30 Siena, and Perugia, Institute of Thoracic and Cardiovascular Surgery, University of Siena, Italy.

out, and the single breath nitrogen test to establish the closing volume (CV).

Analysis of Expired Gases

The following data were evaluated: inspired fraction of O_2 (FIO_2), partial pressure of alveolar gases (PA_{O_2}, PA_{CO_2}) measured at the end of expiration, minute volume (VM) corrected in BTPS, tidal volume (VT) also corrected in BTPS, respiratory rate (RR), metabolic production of CO_2/min (VCO_2), Uptake of O_2/min (VO_2), respiratory quotient, dead space (Vd/Vt) in BTPS, and respiratory equivalents for O_2 (Veq_{O_2}), and for CO_2 (Veq_{CO_2}).

Blood Gas Analysis

The data evaluated were pH, P_{O_2}, P_{CO_2} and bicarbonate, the base excess, the CO_2 content, the standard bicarbonate, and the standard bicarbonate excess.

Oximetry

Data on the saturation and concentration of the hemoglobin and CO were obtained.

Bronchial Resistance

Data have been calculated evaluating the oscillating resistances, expressed in mbar/sec (Ros). Using a calculator, the data have been established in real time, and the statistical significance of paired data was studied.

RESULTS

Static and Dynamic Volumes

In CAPD a slight ventilatory deficit of the restrictive type exists with a vital capacity (VC) of 71.4% (Fig. 1) and a Tiffeneau Index of 78.1% (FEV_1/FVC), Miller's Quadrant (Fig. 2). During CAPD the residual volume (RV), the functional residual capacity (FRC), and the total lung capacity (TLC) are in the normal range (Fig. 3). The bronchial resistances were 35% above average values. During HD a mixed ventilatory deficit was observed; before HD VC was 60.3% and Tiffeneau index was 61.1%, and after HD VC was 70.2% and Tiffeneau index was 69.7%. The expiratory flows (FEV 25–75) were normal in CAPD, were lower before HD (p < 0.01),

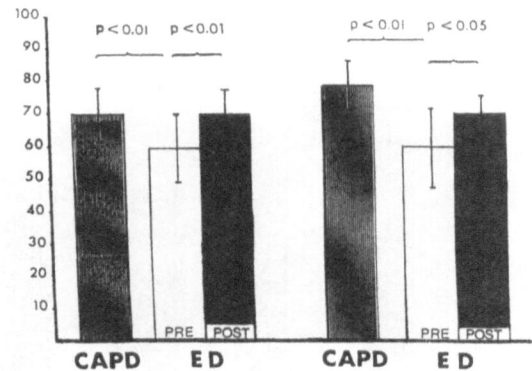

Fig. 1. Mean values, SD, and significance for Vital Capacity (VC) and for FEV_1/VC (Tiffeneau index) in CAPD and hemodialysis (ED) patients.

and became significantly higher after HD. FRC and TLC were normal before HD and became significantly lower after HD.

The CV (Fig. 4) during the phase before HD increased as compared to CAPD (p < 0.01) and decreased partially after HD. Before HD (+60%) with respect to CAPD (p < 0.01), the bronchial

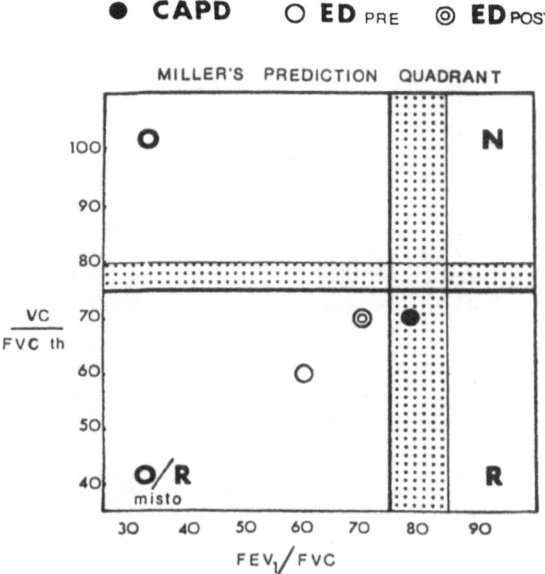

Fig. 2. In CAPD there is a slight respiratory deficit of the restrictive type, but before hemodialysis (ED pre), the deficit is marked, and regresses only in part after hemodialysis.

488   DiPaolo, et al.

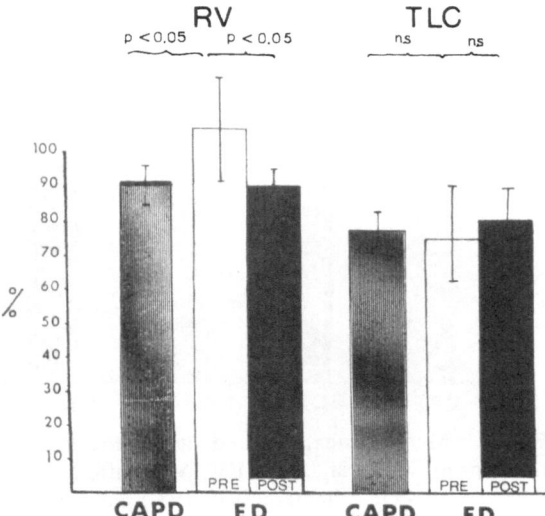

Fig. 3. Mean values, SD, and significance for residual volume (RV), and total lung capacity (TLC) in CAPD and hemodialysis (ED) patients.

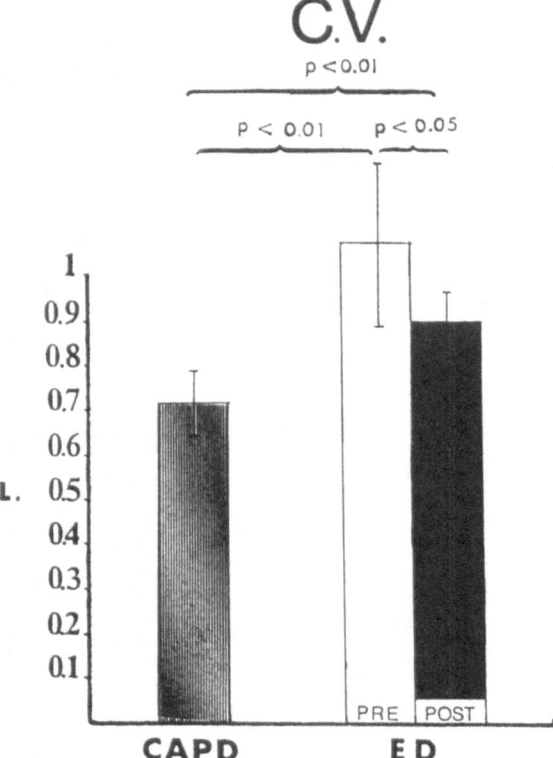

Fig. 4. Mean values, SD, and significance for the closing volume (CV) during CAPD with respect to hemodialysis (ED).

resistances were considerably increased and showed a recovery of 12% after HD, still remaining inferior to the values for CAPD (p < 0.01).

Ventilation-Metabolic and Blood Gas Data

A minute volume (VM) of 9.3 L/min with a respiratory rate (RR) of 14/min indicated a state of hyperventilation in CAPD. The consequence was that the alveolar ventilation was at the highest value within normality, with an alveolar PA_{O_2} of 98 mm Hg, a Pa_{CO_2} of 77 mm Hg, and an alveolar-arterial O_2 difference of 21 mm Hg. The PA_{CO_2} was 33 mm Hg, with a low Pa_{CO_2} (31 mm Hg) (Figs. 5 & 6). The O_2 consumption (VO_2) (Fig. 7) with a respiratory quotient ($R = VCO_2/VO_2$) of 0.73 and a normal production of CO_2 (VCO_2) was also at the highest limit of normal. The arterial pH (7.41), oxygen saturation (98.3%), dead space (0.27 L), and the shunt fraction were all within the normal range, but the respiratory equivalents for O_2 ($VeqO_2$) and for CO_2 ($VeqCO_2$) were increased. Terbutaline-induced bronchodilatation did not cause significant variations in these values.

Unlike CAPD, HD did not induce hyperventilation. The VE was clearly decreased before HD compared to CAPD (p < 0.01), and improved only slightly after HD. At the alveolar level, before HD, the PA_{O_2} increased from 91 ± 5 mm Hg to 99 ± 4 mm Hg after HD (p < 0.05), whilst the Pa_{O_2} remained modestly hypoxic (68.6 ± 6 mm Hg before HD and 69 ± 7 mm Hg after HD) with an alveolar-arterial O_2 difference that increased significantly from 23 to 29 mm Hg, compared to 21 mm Hg in CAPD (p < 0.05). At the alveolar level, CO_2 remained almost unchanged, whilst it became significantly lower at the arterial level. The uptake of O_2 before HD was less than the volume taken up during CAPD, and although it improved after HD, it still remained lower with respect to the values in CAPD (p < 0.01) production of CO_2. As in the population on CAPD, there was an elevation in the QR to 0.85. The dead space was higher before HD than it was in CAPD, and this was reduced after HD.

The pH rose from 7.35 before HD, to 7.39 after. Such values always exceeded those of CAPD patients. The shunt fraction in HD was always slightly higher than in CAPD, both before and after HD. Before and after HD, Veq_{CO_2} and Veq_{O_2} were slightly lower than the values obtained in CAPD. The correlation between the Pa_{O_2} and CV (Fig. 8) demonstrates an inverse relationship between the two,

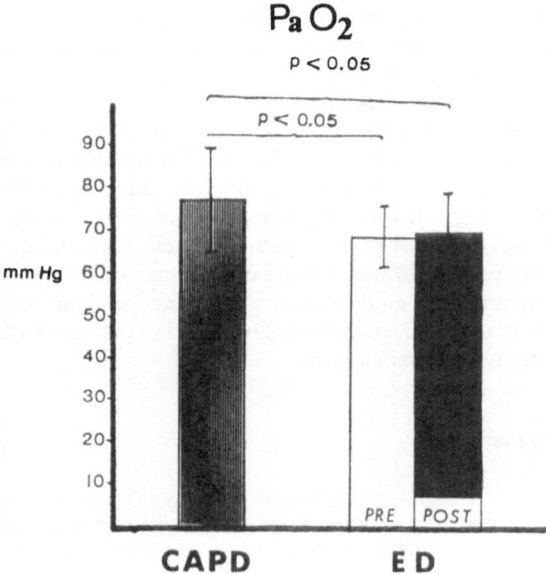

Fig. 5. Mean values, SD, and significance for Pa_{O_2} in CAPD and hemodialysis (ED) patients.

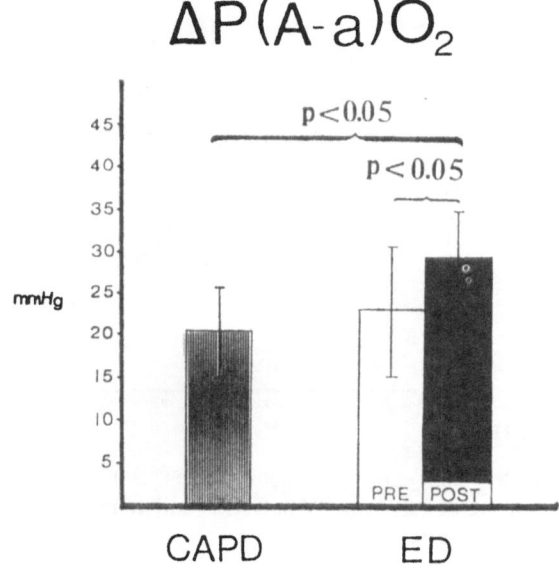

Fig. 6. Mean values, SD, and significance for $P(A-a)O_2$ in CAPD and hemodialysis (ED) patients.

each assuming a different slope in the three groups studied.

DISCUSSION

Our results clearly show that RF in patients on CAPD is much more efficient than RF in patients on HD, either in terms of static or dynamic volumes or in terms of ventilation and blood gases. Another consideration is that we chose patients that had at least two years of treatment, and did not show alterations of respiratory function, which are easily found in uremic patients in the first days and months of substitution therapy (the alterations are due to pleural, pericardial, and bronchopulmonary diseases). Regarding CAPD, those who have studied RP have observed a modest restrictive defect. This is possibly due to reduction of closure volume,[5] subclinical pulmonary edema, and fibrotic modifications of the parenchyma.[6] In addition, compensatory hyperventilation to eliminate CO_2 is offset by an increased consumption of O_2, maintaining a normal Pa_{O_2}.[7,8]

Prefaut et al.[9] realized that in CAPD a decrease in CV in relation to loss of pulmonary interstitial water was related to the absence of the characteristic peribronchial edema of the uremic patient, which is responsible for trapping alveolar gases. Ahluwalia

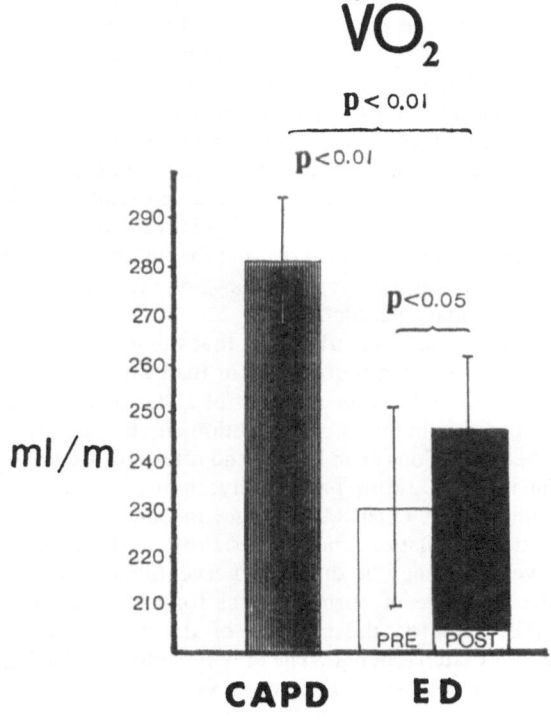

Fig. 7. Mean values, SD, and significance for O_2 consumption in CAPD and hemodialysis (ED) patients.

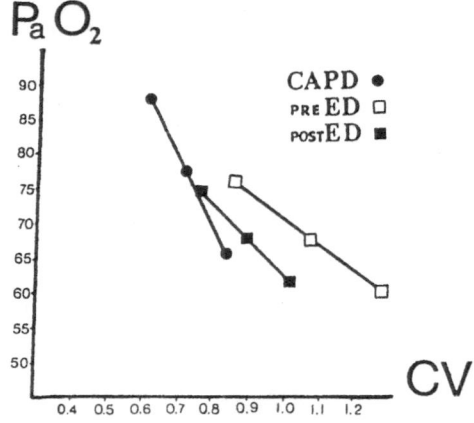

Fig. 8. Correlation of mean values, SD, and significance of Pa_{O_2} and CV in CAPD and hemodialysis (ED) patients.

et al.[10] have compared CAPD to a state of advanced pregnancy because the elevation of the diaphragm (due to the presence of the peritoneal dialysate) contributes to the decreases in PV, FRC, ERV, and TLC. HD patients have a restrictive defect associated with hypoxia, probably due to hyperventilation due to the fall in Pa_{CO_2}, or due to an increased alveolar-arterial O_2 difference due to ventilation perfusion mismatching. This seems to be due to intravascular leucocyte microembolization and correlates with the significant decrease in circulating leucocytes. Romaldini et al. also agree that the fall in CO_2 after HD provokes a decrease in Pa_{CO_2} due to a decrease in pulmonary ventilation.

Our results clearly show that the RF in CAPD patients is much more efficient than the RF in patients on HD, either in terms of static or dynamic volumes or in terms of ventilation and blood gases. The oscillations seen before and after HD are missing in CAPD. More particularly, there is better consumption of O_2 in CAPD due, in our opinion, to better ventilation and oxygenation at the arterial level. This may be due to hyperventilation that, in the presence of normal values for CV (altered in HD), supports the absence of the parabronchial compression (edema). The only pathological finding we have observed is the modest ventilatory deficit of the restrictive type. This is significantly lower than that observed both before and after HD, where there was also an obstructive component.

We can hypothesize that in CAPD, since all other functional parameters were normal (clearly different from the situation in HD patients), this modest ventilatory deficit may be due to uremic pathology (fibrin deposits, microemboli, myopathy), and not to the treatment itself. Our findings exclude that a liter or more of fluid may in some way significantly modify respiratory function from normal, since all studies were obtained in patients with full abdominal cavities.

REFERENCES

1. Romaldini H, Stabile C, Faro S, DosSantos M, Ramos O, and Tiberio O: Pulmonary ventilation during hemodialysis. Nephron 32: 131, 1982
2. DeBaker W, Verpootten G, Borgongon D, Vermiere P, Lins I, and DeBore M: Hypoxemia during hemodialysis. Kidney Int 23: 738, 1983
3. Goggin MJ, and Joekes AM: Gas exchange in renal failure II. Br Med J 2: 247, 1971
4. Singh S, Dale SH, and Morgan AB: Pulmonary function tests (PFT) in patients on CAPD. Abstr Am Soc Artif Organs 10: 59, 1981
5. Winchester JF, DaSilva AMT, Davis W, Clarence W, Barnard W, Rakowski TA, and Schreiner GE: Altered pulmonary function with CAPD. In Gahl GM, Kessel M, and Nolph KD (Eds), Advances in peritoneal dialysis: Proceedings of the 2nd international symposium on peritoneal dialysis. Amsterdam: Excerpta Medica, 1981, p 329
6. Berlyne GM, Lee HA, Ralston AJ, and Woodcock JA: Pulmonary complications of peritoneal dialysis. Lancet 2: 75, 1966
7. LaGreca G, Biasioli S, Chiaromonte S, Dari M, Fabris A, Feriani M, Pisani E, Ronco C, and Zen F: Acid-base balance on peritoneal dialysis. Clin Nephrol 16: 1, 1981
8. Biasioli S, Chiaramonte S, Cantarella G, Fabris A, Feriani M, Pisani E, Ronco C, and LaGreca G: Compensatory hyperventilation in CAPD patients. Peritoneal Dial Bull 2: 189, 1982
9. Prefaut CH, Monteil A, Ramonatxo M, and Slingeneyer A: Closing volume and pulmonary gas exchange during peritoneal dialysis. Bull Eur Phys Resp 14: 755, 1978
10. Ahluwalia M, Ishirawa S, Gellman M, Shah T, Sekar T, and MacDonnell KF: Pulmonary functions during peritoneal dialysis. Clin Nephrol 18: 251, 1982

S. Lamperi, S. Carozzi, A. Icardi, and G. Reali

93

Effect on Erythropoiesis of Normal Monocytes and Peritoneal Macrophages from CAPD Patients

SUMMARY

The morphology and function of macrophages isolated from peritoneal fluid at the start of CAPD (M_0) and at the 9th month (M_9) have been compared with normal macrophages (NM).

M_0 had a greater morphologic heterogeneity by scanning electron microscopy (SEM), but M_9 were similar to normal. The reduced number of primitive erythroid progenitors (BFU-E) developed per plate in *in vitro* cultures with bone marrow cells drawn from CAPD patients at the start of therapy, showed a significant increase with the addition of NM or M_9. No modification was observed with the coincubation of monocytes drawn from the predialysis phase or from HD patients.

Normal monocyte infusions *in vivo* in four elderly CAPD patients with resistant anemia were followed by an improvement in the hematocrit (31%), hemoglobin (61%), reticulocytes (816%) and by an increase in the number of BFU-E in *in vitro* cultures (174%).

These results suggest that the interactions between early erythroid progenitors and the stromal cells, such as monocytes or macrophages which are responsible for BFU-E growth, are abnormal in uremic patients.

CAPD, induced an improvement in the structure and function of these cells, and may be responsible for the hematopoietic recovery observed with this therapy.

INTRODUCTION

Some studies have shown that the growth of human erythroid colonies (BFU-E) in the early maturation of the old cell depends not only on erythropoietin, but also on the presence of cells such as T-lymphocytes or monocytes in the cell culture.[1,2] These cells belonging to the immunological system are notoriously impaired in chronic renal failure and improve only with CAPD.[3,4] Since hypoproliferative anemia of uremic patients can be corrected by CAPD,[5,6] it may be that this improvement is connected with the cellular modifications that may occur with this therapy. In view of these possibilities, we studied the morphology of macrophages isolated from peritoneal fluid at the start of CAPD and in the ninth month, as well as the behavior *in vitro* and *in vivo* of these cells of uremic subjects in the predialysis phase (PDP) and under several therapies.

METHODS

Studies were performed in two groups of patients: Group 1 consisted of 38 subjects, of whom six were hematologically normal nonuremic, and 32 with chronic renal disease, of whom ten were in the predialysis phase (PDP), ten were on hemodialysis (HD), and 12 on continuous ambulatory peritoneal

From the Division of Nephrology, St. Martin Hospital, and the Service of Immunohematology, Galliera Hospital, Genoa, Italy.

dialysis (CAPD). Blood, peritoneal fluid, and bone marrow cell samples were collected from these subjects in order to separate the T-lymphocytes, monocytes, macrophages, and T-cell subsets, to determine the T-cell growth factor activity (TCGF), to perform scanning electron microscopy (SEM) study and bone marrow cell cultures capable of identifying the number of BFU-E per plate. Informed consent was obtained.

SEM Study

Macrophages isolated from peritoneal fluid with the method described below, at the start of therapy (M_0) and after nine months (M_9) were studied by SEM. The cells were fixed in 0.5% glutaraldehyde in phosphate buffer (pH 7.4), dehydrated in increasing concentrations of buffered acetone, and dried in a stream of warm air. Slides were coated under vacuum with a thin film of gold. All specimens were examined in an ISM-35 scanning electron microscope.[7]

Model for Separation of Cellular Lines

Mononuclear cells were obtained from heparinized blood samples by separation on Ficoll-Hypaque gradient. T-lymphocytes were enriched from suspensions of nonadherent mononuclear cells by the E-rosette method.[8] Monocytes were obtained by the technique described by Shaw et al.[9] Pure populations of macrophages from peritoneal fluid samples were obtained by glass adhesiveness.[10]

The unseparated T-lymphocyte sets were depleted of the OKT4 positive component by OKT4 antibody C'-mediated T-cell lysis.[11]

T-cell Subset Identification

T-cell subsets, identified by the reactivity with OKT3, OKT4, and OKT8 monoclonal antibodies (Ortho Pharmaceutical Corp., Raritan, NJ) were determined by indirect immunofluorescence staining using fluorescein isothiocyanate-conjugated goat anti-mouse IgG (G/M FITC; Meloy Laboratories).[12]

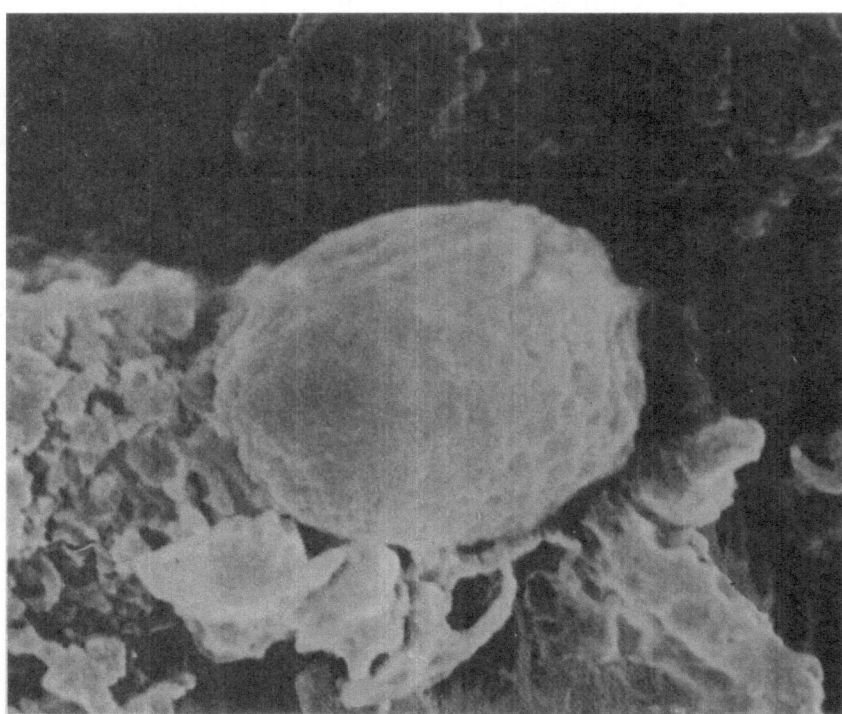

Fig. 1. SEM surface characteristics of peritoneal macrophages isolated from peritoneal fluid from a CAPD patient (B.G.) at the start of therapy (original magnification × 10,000).

TCGF Assay

The TCGF activity in culture supernatants from peripheral blood lymphocytes was measured by the quantitative microassay introduced by Gillis et al.[13]

Erythroid Colony Assay (BFU-E)

Bone marrow cell cultures were performed using the Iscove et al. method,[14] incubating only 2×10^5 mononuclear bone marrow cells, separated on Ficoll-Hypaque gradient, drawn from normal subjects, uremic in PDP, on HD or on CAPD, or with the addition of unseparated T-lymphocytes or monocytes belonging to the same subjects, or by adding peritoneal macrophages from CAPD patients having had 9 ± 2 months of therapy. The number of T-lymphocytes, monocytes, or macrophages incubated in the various cultures was 2×10^5 cells per plate, and the results were expressed as number of BFU-E developed per 2×10^5 cells cultured.

In Vivo Studies

Group 2, which was picked out from 90 hemodialyzed or CAPD patients, included eight very elderly patients with mean age 79 ± 3 years, four undergoing HD, and four CAPD. Over several months of observation, these subjects had repeated

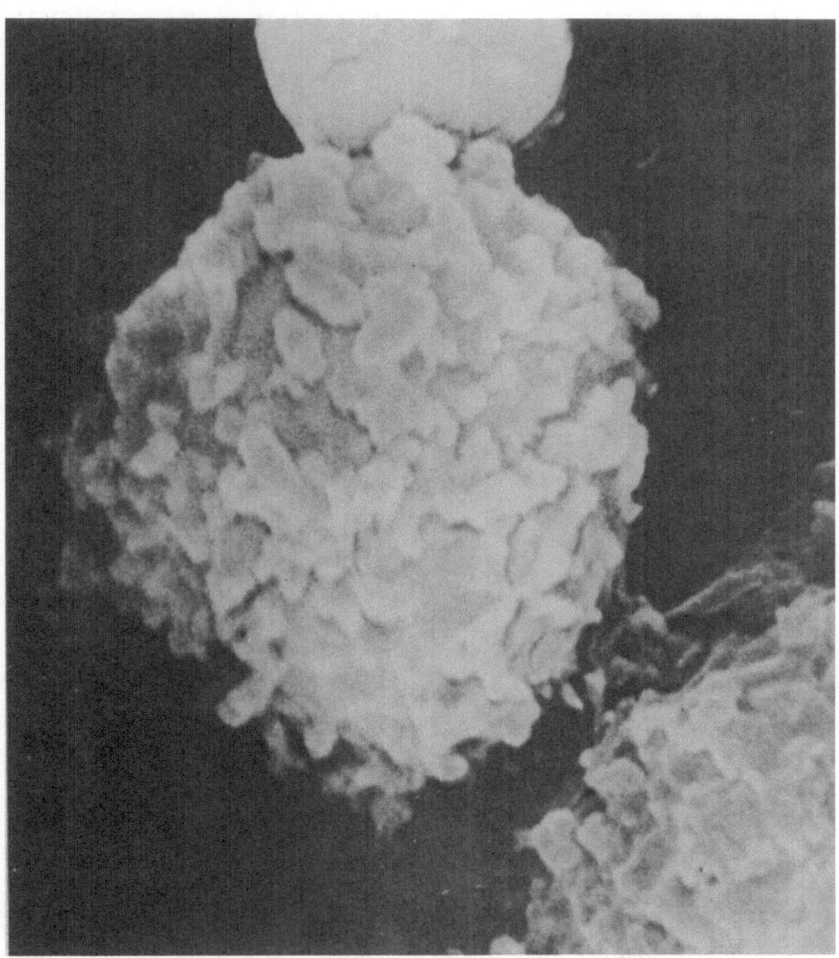

Fig. 2. SEM surface characteristics of peritoneal macrophages isolated from peritoneal fluid from a CAPD patient (B.G.) at the ninth month of therapy (original magnification × 10,000).

infectious diseases in the presence of some immuno-hematological abnormalities such as a noticeable and resistent anemia with granulocytopenia, very high depression of immunological defense. Since these patients needed granulocyte transfusions before beginning this therapy, infusions of irradiated monocyte-macrophage cells, such as buffy coat isolated by leukopheresis, were administered for a total of four units for each patient, performed every 10 days.[15] Informed consent was obtained.

Before the infusions, for a period of 180 days during and after therapy, the hematocrit (Ht%), hemoglobin (Hb g/dl), reticulocytes (Retic/μl) by using usual methods, serum erythropoietin (ESF mU/ml) values, and BFU-E development in *in vitro* cultures, respectively determined by Wardle modified by Dunn et al.[16] and Iscove et al.[14] methods, were evaluated each month.

Statistics

The data were expressed as mean ± SD, and the comparison between cohorts was made using Student's test. Statistical significance was accepted at 0.05 level.

RESULTS

SEM Surface Characteristics of Peritoneal Macrophages

Compared to normal cells of the same type, the macrophages, isolated from peritoneal fluid at the start of therapy, showed some abnormalities, such as decrease or disappearance of microvilli on the exterior surface and a tendency to adhere to each other and to form clumps (Fig. 1). The macrophages,

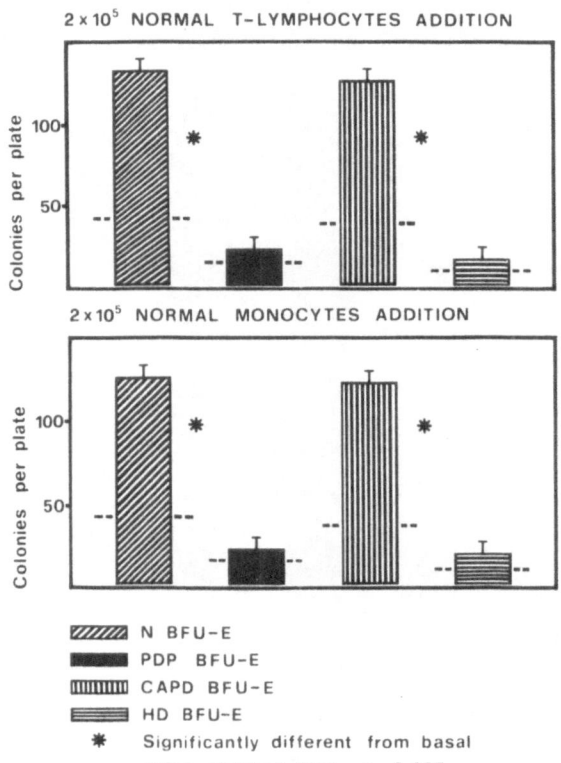

Fig. 3. Effects of normal T-lymphocyte or monocyte addition on normal (N), predialysis phase (PDP), CAPD, and hemodialysis (HD) BFU-E growth.

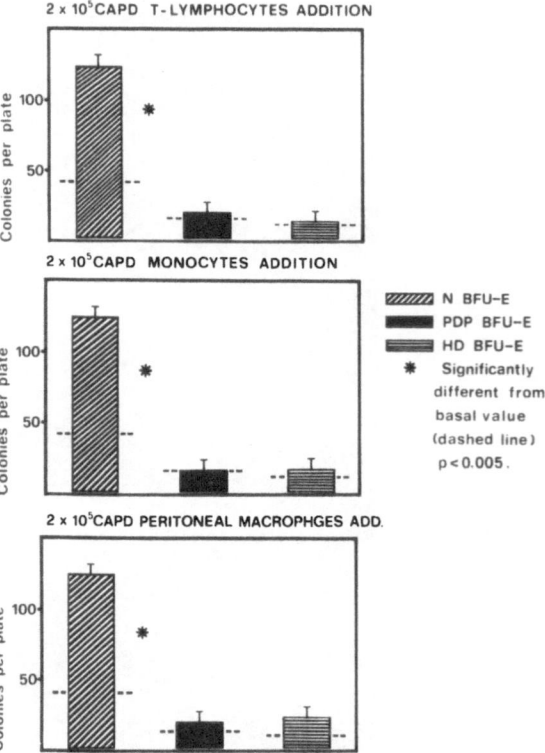

Fig. 4. Effects of CAPD T-lymphocyte, monocyte, or peritoneal macrophage addition on normal (N), predialysis phase (PDP), or hemodialysis (HD) BFU-E growth.

isolated from peritoneal fluid in the ninth month of therapy, demonstrated recovery of the above alterations characterized by the reappearance of slender microvilli on the cell surface, which appears relatively smooth (Fig. 2).

Normal or Uremic Patients in PDP, on HD or CAPD: BFU-E Cell Development in *in Vitro* Cultures

Under these experimental conditions, the development of BFU-E colonies per plate in the uremic patients on CAPD (mean value 44.3 ± 5) was similar to that observed in normal subjects in whom the mean level was 45 ± 3.5. The number of BFU-E colonies developed in culture of bone marrow cells drawn from uremic patients in PDP (mean value 16 ± 3.8 colonies per plate) and HD (mean value 12 ± 2.8 colonies per plate) was below normal, respectively 64.44% and 73.33% (p < 0.005).

Studies on the Various Coincubations

When T-lymphocytes isolated from normal subjects were added to normal or CAPD bone marrow cell cultures, we observed an increased development in the number of BFU-E colonies per plate, respectively 211.36 ± 21% and 184.09 ± 23% as compared to basal levels. Results similar to those of T-lymphocytes were obtained using normal monocytes. On the contrary, when normal lympho-monocytes were added to PDP or HD bone marrow cell cultures, there were no significant variations in the

number of BFU-E colonies per plate in comparison to basal values (Fig. 3).

The addition of CAPD lymphocytes, monocytes, or peritoneal macrophages to bone marrow cell cultures caused an increased BFU-E development of 186.4 ± 23%, 189.5 ± 12%, 191.5 ± 18% (p < 0.005), respectively, in comparison to basal conditions. When the same cells were added to PDP bone marrow cell cultures, we did not observe any significant variation in the number of BFU-E compared to basal levels (Fig. 4). The addition of PDP or HD lympho-monocytes to normal, PDP, HD, CAPD bone marrow cell cultures did not produce any significant variation in BFU-E development.

The addition of normal or CAPD OKT4-depleted T-lymphocytes to BFU-E cultures of the same subjects, produced a significant reduction in the number of colonies in comparison to the values observed when the incubation was performed with unseparated T-lymphocytes. This reduction with normal BFU-E was 50.33%, 52%, and 49.6%, respectively, with BFU-E from CAPD patients (p < 0.005) (Fig. 5).

Study on the T-cell Subsets Identified by Monoclonal Antibodies on Normal Subjects and in Uremic Patients in PDP, on HD and CAPD

The evaluation of T-cell subsets OKT3, OKT4, OKT8, expressed as the percentage of positive T-lymphocytes did not show any significant difference between the results obtained in the patients on PDP,

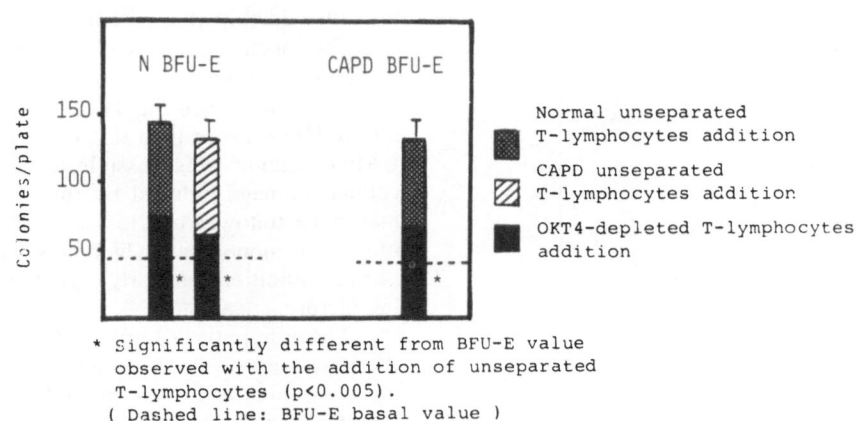

* Significantly different from BFU-E value
  observed with the addition of unseparated
  T-lymphocytes (p<0.005).
  (Dashed line: BFU-E basal value)

Fig. 5. Effects of normal (N) or CAPD OKT4-depleted T-lymphocyte addition on N or CAPD BFU-E growth.

or on HD and CAPD, and those observed in normal subjects.

Study on TCGF Activity

In uremic patients on PDP or on HD, the TCGF activity showed reduced values of 70% and 60% in comparison to those observed in normal controls (p < 0.005). The TCGF activity in the uremic patients on CAPD demostrated a nonsignificant reduction (0.5%) (Fig. 6).

Study on Buffy-coat Cell Infusions
"in Vivo"

The buffy-coat cell infusions in the four CAPD elderly patients were followed, in the course of observation, by an increase in Ht, Hb, and Retic values 31%, 61%, 81.6%, respectively, as compared to basal levels and by no significant ESF modifications.

Simultaneously, the number of BFU-E developed per plate increased in comparison to initial values. Such improvements remained steady until 150 days after the interruption of therapy. At this point, in fact, the reduction in the Ht, Hb, Retic values, in comparison to those observed in the period of maximum increase, was 10.3%, 10.5%, 27%, respectively.

In hemodialyzed elderly patients, the buffy-coat cell infusions were not followed by any significant modifications in the various parameters during the same period of study (Fig. 7).

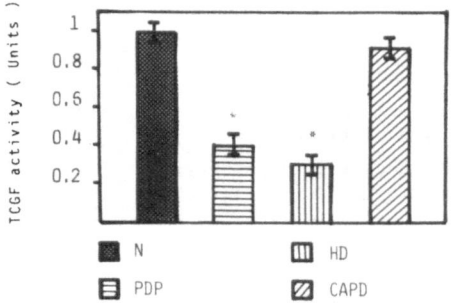

* Significantly different from N value (p<0.005)

Fig. 6. TCGF activity in normal subjects (N) and in uremic patients in predialysis phase (PDP), on hemodialysis (HD), and CAPD.

DISCUSSION

In uremic patients, erythropoiesis is depressed in PDP on HD, and this abnormality is associated with an incapacity of lympho-monocytes of the same subjects to stimulate BFU-E growth, as the BFU-E are incapable of responding to the stimulating activity of normal lympho-monocytes. The lympho-monocytes or macrophages of patients on CAPD show a stimulating activity on normal BFU-E development, as the BFU-E of the same patients appear capable of responding to the stimulating action of normal lymph-monocytes. It is unlikely that this is due to the enrichment of peripheral BFU-E introduced into the "in vitro" cultures with lympho-monocyte population. In fact, in other work, it was seen that the cell preparations themselves exhibited virtually no BFU-E colony expression, showing that the T-lymphocytes were minimally contaminated with BFU-E.[17] On the other hand, the cultures prepared with macrophages drawn from peritoneal fluid, and therefore surely not contaminated with peripheral BFU-E, gave the same results as the lympho-monocytes isolated from peripheral blood.

These results suggest the presence, in uremic patients in PDP or on HD, of an inhibition of normal stimulating activity exercised by lympho-monocytes on bone marrow erythroid progenitors, which causes a hypoproliferative state. Both the loss of this activity of lympho-monocytes and T-cell subsets and the BFU-E response appears to regenerate with CAPD and not with other dialytic techniques. Therefore it is possible to assume the presence, in renal insufficiency, of a material that is preferentially removed by CAPD, capable of inducing a deterioration in both BFU-E cells and lympho-monocytes, the latter documented by our SEM study.

The mechanism by which such a material impairs the activity of the immunocompetent cells appears unclear. Since the TCGF activity in PDP or during HD is lower than that in normal subjects or CAPD patients, it is possible to suppose that the cellular damage induced by the above-mentioned material is followed by a loss of production capacity of lympho-monokines, which may represent, under normal conditions, an early erythropoietic stimulating factor.

These hypotheses appear to be confirmed by the improvement of the hematological parameters (in vivo) obtained with the infusions of normal lympho-monocytes from the patients treated by peritoneal dialysis who showed, before therapy, a hypoproliferative anemia.[18]

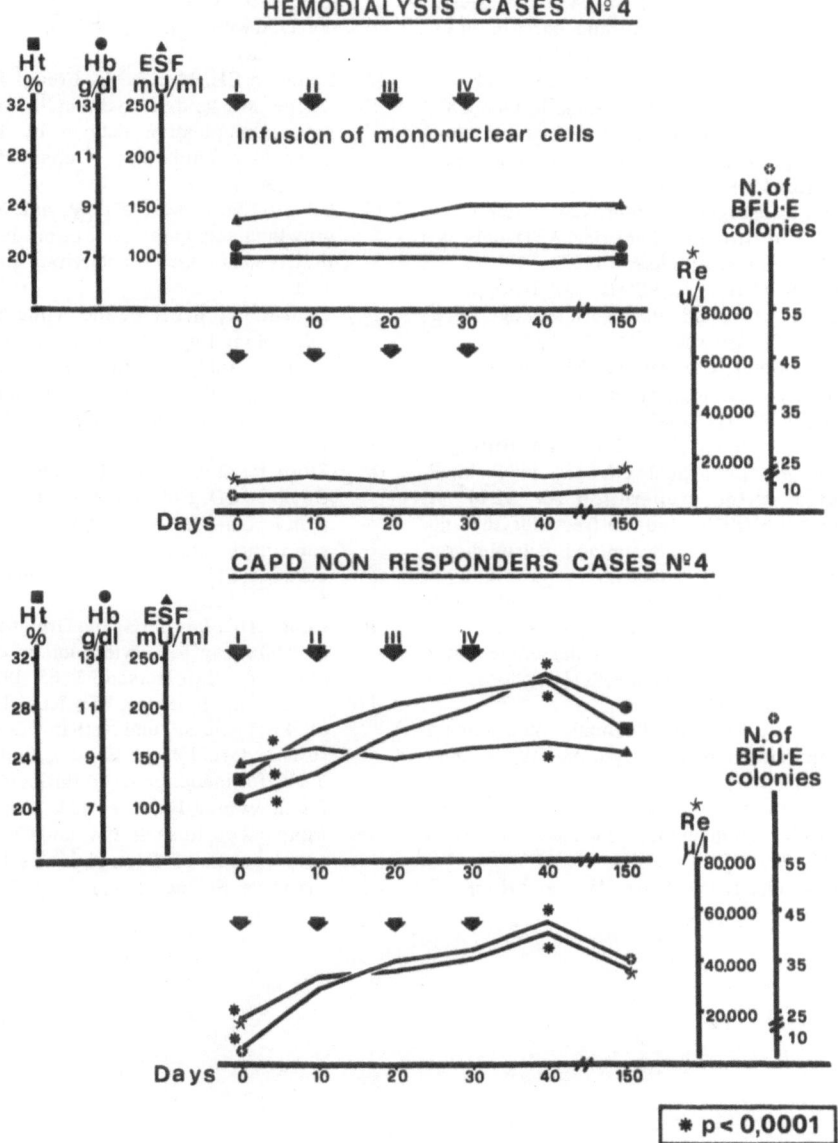

Fig. 7. Hematocrit (Ht%), hemoglobin (Hb, g/dl), erythropoietin (ESF mU/ml), reticulocyte (Ret/μL), and BFU-E growth behavior in hemodialysis (HD) or CAPD patients who underwent buffy-coat infusions.

There are no convincing data that the recovery of BFU-E growth under these conditions may be attributed to a direct effect of the immunocompetent cells or to the presence in the infusions of the peripheral BFU-E contaminating the lympho-monocyte preparation, since the buffy-coat cells were irradiated before administration, and therefore any cellular activity was interrupted. The most convincing hypothesis is that the restored proliferative development of bone marrow cells is attributable to the products of their secretion.

REFERENCES

1. Linch DC, Boyle D, and Beverley PCL: T-cell and monocyte requirements for erythropoiesis. Acta Haematol 67: 34, 1982

2. Kurland JI, Meyers PA, and Moore MAS: Synthesis and release of erythroid colony and burst-potentiating activities by purified populations of murine peritoneal macrophages. J Exp Med 151: 835, 1980

3. Osaki K, Otsuka H, Uomizu K, Harada R, Otsuji Y, and Hashimoto S: Monocyte-mediated suppression of mitogen responses of lymphocytes in uremic patients. Nephron 34: 87, 1983

4. Langhoff E, Ladefoged J: Improved lymphocyte transformation in vitro of patients on CAPD dialysis. Abstr Eur Dial Transplant Assoc 1983, p 19

5. Zappacosta AR, Caro J, and Erslev AJ: Normalization of hematocrit in patients with end stage renal disease or CAPD. Am J Med 72: 53, 1982

6. Lamperi S, Icardi A, Carozzi, S, and Trasforini D: Erythropoietin behaviour and renal anemia in CAPD. Excerpta Med 567: 311, 1981

7. Schneider GB, Poewwinse SM, and Billings-Gagliardi S: Morphological changes in isolated lymphocytes during preparation for SEM: A comparative TEM/SEM study in freeze drying and critical drying point drying. Scanning Electronmicroscopy 2: 77, 1978

8. Mendes NF, Tolnai MEA, Silveira SB, Gilbertsen SB, and Metizgar RS: Technical aspects of the rosette tests used to direct human complement receptor (B) and sheep erythrocyte binding (T) lymphocytes. J Immunol 11: 860, 1973

9. Shaw GM, Levy PC, and LoBuglio AF: Human monocyte antibody-dependent cytotoxicity to human cell. J Clin Invest 62: 1172, 1978

10. Boyum A: Isolation of mononuclear cell and granulocytes from human blood. Scand J Lab Invest 21(Suppl 97): 77, 1968

11. Zarling JM, Clouse KA, Biddison WE, and Kung PC: Phenotypes of human natural killer cell populations detected with monoclonal antibodies. J Immunol 127: 2575, 1981

12. Reinherz EL, Moretta L, Breard JM, Mingari MC, Cooper MD, and Schlossman SF: Human T-lymphocyte subpopulation defined by Fc receptor and monoclonal antibodies. A comparison. J Exp Med 151: 696, 1980

13. Gillis S, Ferm MM, Ou W, and Smith KA: T-cell growth factor: Parameters of production and a quantitative microassay for activity. J Immunol 120: 2027, 1978

14. Iscove NN, Sieber F, and Winterhalter KH: Erythroid colony formation in culture of mouse and bone marrow: Analysis of the requirement for erythropoietin by gel-filtration and affinity chromatography on agarose Concanavalin-A[1]. J Cell Physiol 83: 309, 1974

15. Storb R, Doney CK, Thomas ED, Appelbaum F, Buckner CD, Clift RA, Deeg J, Goodell BW, Hackman R, Hansen JA, Sanders J, and Sullivan K: Marrow transplantation with or without donor buffy-coat cells for 65 transfused aplastic anemia patients. Blood 59: 236, 1982

16. Dunn CDR, Jarvis JH, and Grenman JM: A quantitative bioassay for erythropoietin using mouse fetal liver cells. Exp Hematol 3: 65, 1975

17. Lipton JM, Reinherz EL, Kudish M, Jackson PL, Schlossmann SF, and Nathan DG: Mature bone marrow erythroid burst-forming units do not require T-cell for induction of erythropoietin-dependent differentiation. J Exp Med 152: 350, 1980

18. Morgan DA, Ruscetti FW, and Gallo RC: Selective in vitro growth of T-lymphocytes from normal bone marrows. Science 193: 1007, 1976

J. Rahmat, J.F. McAnally, J.F. Winchester, T.A. Rakowski,
N. Perri, W.P. Argy, and G.E. Schreiner.

94

Creatine Kinase, Amylase, and Parathyroid Hormone in Stable CAPD and Hemodialysis Patients

SUMMARY

Since there are conflicting reports on elevation of plasma creatine kinase and amylase above normal in dialysis patients we studied total and isoenzyme fractions of creatine kinase and amylase. In addition since hyperparathyroidism and pancreatitis are associated we also studied plasma-n-terminal parathyroid hormone levels. Studies were performed in 35 stable CAPD patients, and creatine kinase alone was studied in 11 stable hemodialysis patients. Total creatine kinase was elevated in nine of 35 CAPD patients (25.7%); elevated isoenzyme fractions of CK were as follows: nine of nine patients had elevated MM band, one of nine had elevated MB and one of nine had elevated BB band. In the hemodialysis patients two of 11 had elevated CK (MM bands). Total amylase was elevated in 17 of 26 CAPD patients with ten of these patients having an elevated pancreatic isoenzyme fraction; in six of 17, the salivary isoenzyme fraction equalled the pancreatic enzyme fraction in one patient. Parathyroid hormone was elevated in 24 of 35 CAPD patients, but no correlation existed between parathyroid hormone levels, creatine kinase and amylase, although there was a significant correlation between creatine kinase and amylase levels in CAPD patients ($r = 0.4$, $n = 23$, $p < 0.05$). These findings suggest a common etiology for elevated creatine and amylase in otherwise stable CAPD patients such as inadequate dialysis, subclinical skeletal myopathy, or metabolic complications. These findings warrant further study.

INTRODUCTION

A number of human enzymes occur in different body tissues as distinct isomeric species. Creatine kinase (CK) is a dimer molecule with three isoenzymes.[1] Each isoenzyme is composed of a combination of monomers referred to as B or M. The resulting polypeptides are CK-MM, CK-MB, and CK-BB. They are respectively referred to clinically as muscle band, cardiac band, and brain band enzymes, the names denoting the tissue where the enzyme is found in the highest concentration. Tsung[2] assayed human tissue obtained at surgery for CK isoenzymes and found small quantities of CK-BB in urinary bladder, lung, prostate, uterus, thyroid, stomach, and intestine (in decreasing order). The CK-MM isoenzyme is detectable in serum and reflects normal skeletal muscle metabolism in which creatine is converted to creatinine. In contrast, CK-MB and CK-BB are not normally present in serum. Levels of CK are higher in blacks than in whites and in men than in women.[3]

Elevated levels of CK are well demonstrated in neuromuscular disorders,[4] hypoparathyroidism,[5] and in the CSF of some psychotic patients.[6] Elevation of CK-MB activity is believed to be highly specific for the diagnosis of myocardial infarction.[7,8]

From Georgetown University Hospital, Washington, D.C., and St. Elizabeth's Hospital, Elizabeth, New Jersey.

There are, however, reports of increased CK-MB activity noted with muscular dystrophy,[9] myositis,[10] hypothyroidism,[11] hypothermia,[12] cardiac arrythmia,[13] following minor iatrogenic cardiac trauma,[14] after subarachnoid hemorrhage,[15] and with pericarditis.[8]

The presence of elevated levels of CK in uremic patients was first reported by Eschar and Zimmerman.[16] Since then several reports have appeared in the literature with conflicting results. Galen[17] found high CK levels in 20 of 43 dialysis patients, 19 of whom had elevated CK-BB fractions. Weseley et al.[18] and Pascual et al.[19] reported the presence of CK-BB isoenzymes in the serum of patients with chronic renal failure and implicated the neurologic damage of uremia as the cause. However, the occurrence of CK-BB in uremia has not been confirmed by other investigators, who have shown that methodologic problems exist that may lead to artifactual measurement of the isoenzymes.[20,21] On the other hand, Ma et al.[22] and Martinez-Vea et al.[23] have demonstrated elevated CK-MB isoenzyme activity in 28.3% and 26% respectively of their long-term maintenance hemodialysis patients who did not have evidence of myocardial infarction. Cohen et al.[24] and Soffer et al.[25] reported elevation of CK-MM isoenzyme fractions in their hemodialysis population and attributed that to skeletal muscle abnormalities in uremia.

To our knowledge, the CK activity in CAPD patients has not been studied. Weseley et al.,[18] however, in their group of ESRD patients had 14 who were treated by intermittent peritoneal dialysis for one week to three months, 13 of 14 patients had positive CK-BB bands in plasma.

Morton et al.[26] had shown that in renal failure, even in the absence of acute pancreatitis, the clearance of amylase rises in relation to the clearance of creatinine. Pasternack and Klockars[27] observed that only in severe renal failure was the enzyme consistently elevated and that salivary and pancreatic isoenzymes contributed almost equally to the increase, indicating that the diseased kidney was unable to handle the isoenzymes. Since hyperparathyroidism and pancreatitis are associated and since thyroid and parathyroid status have been linked to the etiology for elevation in total CK levels,[25] we studied parathyroid hormone levels, amylase isoenzymes, and CK levels in CAPD patients, and for comparison we chose to examine CK levels in hemodialysis patients.

METHODS

Thirty-five unselected stable CAPD patients and 11 hemodialysis patients undergoing regular incenter hemodialysis were studied. None had recent myocardial infarction, angina, cardiac arrhythmia, or evidence of hypothyroidism, hypothermia, myositis, or muscular dystrophy. No patient had a recent history of accelerated hypertension, hypotension, or pulmonary edema, or had received intramuscular injections one week prior to the study. No patients had intercurrent viral infection, peritonitis or received drugs known to have caused myopathy. The mean age of the CAPD patients was 45.8 ± 13.6 yrs

Table 1. Mean $\pm$ SD Enzyme and Isoenzyme Fractions and Parathyroid Hormone Concentrations in CAPD and HD Patients.

	CAPD	HD
CK (Total)	127 ± 89 IU/L	172 ± 196 IU/L
(Raised Concentrations)	(↑ 9/35)	(↑ 2/11)
CK MM	9/9	2/2
CK MB	1/9	0
CK BB	1/9	0
Amylase	176 ± 108 IU/L	
(Raised Concentrations)	(↑ 17/26)	
P	10/17	
S	6/17	
P = S	1/17	
PTH (N-terminal)	1673 ± 1198 pg/ml	
	(↑ IN 24/35)	

($\bar{x} \pm$ SD, 16 males, 19 females; 14 blacks, 21 whites). The etiology of the ESRD was diabetic nephropathy (2), polycystic kidney disease (6), nephrosclerosis (11), chronic glomerulonephritis (9), glomerulonephritis (4), and unknown (3). Duration of CAPD was 4–60 months. Seven of the hemodialysis patients were male and four were female, and the 11 patients had a mean age of 50.6 ± 13.9 years.

Venous blood was obtained for the determination of serum activity of all three CK isoenzymes (total and isoenzyme fractions), amylase (total and isoenzyme fractions), and n-terminal PTH. Total CK and total amylase were measured by enzymatic methods, CK isoenzyme fractions, and amylase isoenzyme fractions (Pancreatic-P, Salivary-S) were measured by gel electrophoresis, and parathyroid hormone was estimated by radioimmunoassay. The values in normal controls in our laboratory were CK total 22–180 IU/L, CK-MM 95–100%, CK-MB 0–3%, CK-BB 0–1%; total amylase 20–128 IU/L, A-P 50%, A-S 50%, PTH (n-terminal) 230–630 pg/ml as bovine PTH.

RESULTS

In nine of 35 CAPD patients, elevations of total CK activity above 180 IU/L (25.7% of patients) was found. The range was 51–410 IU/L with a mean of 127 ± 89 IU/L (Table 1). All nine patients had 100% CK-MM isoenzyme activity, and in addition, one patient had 4% MB band. Another CAPD patient whose total CK activity was in the normal range had a 32% BB band. The serum amylase in CAPD patients was elevated above 128 IU/L in 17 of 26 patients (65.3%); the range was 150–508 IU/L with a mean of 176 ± 108 IU/L. Ten of 17 amylase enzymes were predominantly pancreatic isoenzymes, and six were predominantly salivary isoenzymes. One patient had an equal amount of pancreatic and salivary fractions. Among the 11 hemodialysis patients, CK was elevated in two (18.1%), with a range of 27–630 IU/L and a mean of 171.7 ± 196.3 IU/L. Both patients had 100% MM isoenzyme activity. PTH (n-terminal) was elevated in 24 of 35 CAPD patients (68.6%) with a range of 100–4700 pg/ml and a mean of 1673 ± 1198 pg/ml.

In two patients CK and amylase clearance by the peritoneum were calculated (Table 2). In patient 1, total CK clearance was 0.33 ml/min and total amylase clearance was 4.3 ml/min; in patient 2, total CK clearance was 0.39 ml/min and total amylase clearance was 6.8 ml/min. There was no correlation

between the concentration of parathyroid hormone, creatine kinase, and amylase. However, there was a significant correlation between creatine kinase and amylase concentrations (r = 0.4, N = 23, p < 0.05) in CAPD patients.

DISCUSSION

Our study demonstrates that elevation of total serum CK activity can occur in stable CAPD patients without known causes for its rise. Since the enzymes are cleared by the reticuloendothelial system,[28] it is possible that in uremia the catabolic function of the reticuloendothelial system is affected. To our knowledge this has not been systematically studied, and since the predominant CK isoenzyme abnormality is an elevation of CK-MM band, we conclude that the elevation is related to some abnormality of skeletal muscle associated with ESRD. Uremic myopathy is an ill defined entity encompassing a variety of muscle disorders seen in renal failure. Muscle weakness is not uncommonly found in uremic patients and is similar to the myopathy associated with nonuremic osteomalacia. There is predominant involvement of proximal muscles, and occasionally this is selective and/or asymmetric. The lower extremities and lower limb girdle are more commonly affected than the upper extremity muscle, and muscles of the neck are rarely involved, while bulbar, facial, and ocular muscles are usually spared.[29] The myopathic nature of the muscle weakness can be demonstrated on electromyography. We have previously demonstrated a relationship between hyperferritinemia and myopathy in association with HLA subtypes,[30] but we did not study the relationship between the CK-MM band elevation, HLA subtypes, and ferritin levels in this group of CAPD patients.

Muscle weakness and elevated CK levels have been reported in primary and secondary hyperparathyroidism[31] and hypoparathyroidism.[5] We were unable to demonstrate any relationship between PTH levels and CK, and no correlation was found between calcium x phosphorus products greater than

Table 2. CK and A Clearances in Two CAPD Patients.

Patient 1	Patient 2
C_{CK} (Tot) 0.33 ml/min	C_{CK} (Tot) 0.934 ml/min
C_A (Tot) 4.3 ml/min	C_A (Tot) 6.8 ml/min

70 and CPK in our patients. Vitamin D_3 deficiency independent of its effect on calcium and PTH may be involved in the development of myopathy. None of our patients had clinical signs of muscle weakness, although formal electromyographs were not performed as part of this study. In contrast to some reports, but in agreement with others, we did not find elevation of CK-MB band isoenzyme, possibly because the methodology used is able to differentiate CPK variant bands from normal CK-MB, which might otherwise factitiously elevate these levels. In hemodialysis patients we were only able to find elevation in CK-BB band in our otherwise stable CAPD patients, which agrees with the findings of Ma et al.[22]

Acute pancreatitis and hyperparathyroidism have long been clinically associated.[32] To our surprise, 65.3% of the CAPD patients in this study had elevation of serum amylase, with approximately two-thirds of the enzymes being pancreatic in origin and the other third salivary in origin. This finding is difficult to explain. Additionally, in the two patients studied here, the amylase clearance was slightly lower than that reported by Glenn and Nolph,[33] who found amylase clearance values between 5.0 and 13.52 ml/min. It is, however, known that endocrine functions of the pancreas respond to stimulation by the high glucose load from CAPD solutions,[34] but to date no studies of exocrine function have been reported.

Since there was significant correlation between the total CK and total amylase concentrations in CAPD patients, it might be considered that a common etiology for elevation of CK and amylase in otherwise stable CAPD patients exists. In conclusion, elevated CK-MM may occur in otherwise stable CAPD patients and may represent a subclinical skeletal myopathy, or deranged protein-muscle wasting noted in some uremic patients. Additionally, elevation of serum amylase was an unexpected finding, the isoenzyme being predominantly from the pancreas. There was a significant correlation between total CK and total amylase concentrations in these stable CAPD patients, suggesting a common etiology such as inadequate dialysis. These findings warrant further investigation.

REFERENCES

1. Van-der-Veen KJ, and Willibrands AF: Isoenzymes of creatinine phoskinase in tissue extracts and in normal and pathological sera. Clin Chim Acta 12: 312, 1966
2. Tsung SH: Creatine kinase isoenzyme patterns in human tissue obtained at surgery. Clin Chem 22: 173, 1976
3. Meltzer HY: Factors affecting serum creatinine phosphokinase levels in the general population: The role of race activity and age. Clin Chim Acta 33: 165, 1971
5. Wolf MA: Creatinine phosphokinase activity in hypoparathyroidism. N Engl J Med 288: 215, 1973
6. Vale S, Espejel MA, Calcaneo F, Ocampo J, and Diaz-de-Leon J: Creatinine phosphokinase. Increased activity of the spinal fluid in psychotic patient. Arch Neurol 30: 103, 1974
7. Roberts R, and Sobel BE: Creatine kinase isoenzymes in the assessment of heart disease. Am Heart J 95: 521, 1978
8. Smith AF, Radford D, Wong CP, and Oliver MF: Creatine kinase MB isoenzyme studies in the diagnosis of myocardial infarction. Br Heart J 38: 225, 1976
9. Silverman LM, Mendell JR, Sahenk Z, and Fontana MB: Significance of creatine kinase isoenzyme in Duchenne dystrophy. Neurology 26: 561, 1976
10. Brownlow K, and Elevitch FR: Serum creatinine phosphokinase isoenzyme in myositis. JAMA 230: 1141, 1976
11. Goldman J, Matz R, Mortimer R, and Freeman R: High elevations of creatine phosphokinase in hypothyroidism. JAMA 238: 325, 1977
12. Carlson CJ, Emilson B, and Rapaport E: Creatine phosphokinase MB isoenzyme in hypothermia; case reports and experimental studies. Am Heart J 95: 352, 1978
13. Mercer DW, and Varat MA: Detection of cardiac-specific creatine kinase isoenzyme in sera with normal or slightly increased total creatine kinase activity. Clin Chem 21: 1088, 1975
14. Tonkin AM, Lester RM, Guthrow CE, Roe CR, Hackel DB, and Wagner GS: Persistence of MB isoenzyme in serum after minor iatrogenic cardiac trauma. Circulation 51: 627, 1975
15. Fabinyi G, Hunt D, and McKinley L: Myocardial creatine kinase isoenzyme in serum after subarachnoid hemorrhage. J Neurol Neurosurg Psychiatry 40: 818, 1977
16. Eschar J, and Zimmerman HJ: Creatine phosphokinase in disease. Am J Med Sci 253: 272, 1967
17. Galen RS: Creatine kinase isoenzyme BB in serum of renal disease patients. Clin Chem 22: 120 1976
18. Weseley SA, Byrnes A, Alter S, Solangi KB, and Goodman AI: Presence of creatine phosphokinase brain band in the serum of chronic renal disease patients. Clin Nephrol 8: 345, 1977
19. Pascual C, Segura RM, and Schwartz S: Situations that can lead to increased creatine kinase isoenzyme BB activity in serum. Clin Chem 24: 729, 1978
20. Coolen RB, Herbstman R, and Hermann P: Spurious brain creatine kinase in serum from patients with renal disease. Clin Chem 24: 1636, 1978
21. McKenzie D, and Henderson AR: An artifact in lactate dehydrogenase isoenzyme patterns assayed by

fluorescence occurring in the serum of patients with end-stage renal disease requiring maintenance hemodialysis. Clin Chem Acta 70: 33, 1976

22. Ma KW, Brown DC, Steele BW, and From AH: Serum creatine kinase MB isoenzyme activity in long-term hemodialysis patients. Arch Intern Med 141: 164, 1981

23. Martinez-Vea A, Montoliu J, Company X, Vives A, Lopez-Pedret J, and Revert L: Elevated CK-MB with normal total creatine kinase levels in patients undergoing maintenance hemodialysis. Arch Intern Med 142: 2346, 1982

24. Cohen IM, Griffiths J, Stone RA, and Leech T: The creatine kinase profile of a maintenance hemodialysis population. A possible marker of uremic myopathy. Clin Nephrol 13: 235, 1980

25. Soffer O, Fellner SK, and Rush RL: Creatine phosphokinase in long-term dialysis patients. Arch Intern Med 141: 181, 1981

26. Morton WJ, Tedesco FJ, Harter HR, and Alpers DH: Serum amylase determinations and amylase to creatinine clearance ratio in patients with chronic renal insufficiency. Gastroenterology 71: 594, 1976

27. Pasternack A, and Klockars M: Clearance ratios of amylase and isoenzyme to creatinine in renal disease. Clin Nephrol 9: 25, 1978

28. Roberts R, Henry PD, and Sobel BE: An improved basis for enzymatic estimation of infarct size. Circulation 52: 743, 1975

29. Floyd M, Ayyas DR, Baswick DD, Hudgson P, and Weightman D: Myopathy in chronic renal failure. Q J Med 43: 508, 1974

30. Bregman H, Gelfand MC, Winchester JF, Manz HJ, Knepshield JH, and Schreiner GE. Iron overload associated myopathy in patients on maintenance hemodialysis. A histocompatibility linked disorder. Lancet 2: 882, 1980

31. Mallette LE, Patten BM, and Engle WK: Neuromuscular disease in secondary hyperparathyroidism. Ann Intern Med 82: 474, 1975

32. Shoji T, Sasaoka T, Kanayama M, Nakagawa W, and Hayashi Y: Possibility of peritoneal dialysis as inducing factor of acute pancreatitis. Abstracts, 1st International Symposium on Peritoneal Dialysis, Chapala, 1978, p 2

33. Glenn LD, and Nolph KD: Treatment of pancreatitis with peritoneal dialysis. Peritoneal Dial Bull 2: 63, 1982

34. von Baeyer H, Gahl GM, Riedinger H, Borowzak R, Averdunk R, Schurig R, and Kessel M: Adaptation of CAPD patients to the continuous peritoneal energy uptake. Kidney Int 23: 29, 1983

E.A. Ross, D.O. Rodgerson, and A.R. Nissenson

95

CK Isoenzymes in CAPD and Hemodialysis Patients

SUMMARY

The high incidence of elevated CK-MM isoenzyme in CAPD patients suggests that subclinical myopathy may be more common in such patients than in those on hemodialysis. A high absolute quantity of CK-MB may be of noncardiac origin, when it represents a normal percent of an elevated total CK value. Knowledge of assay methodology is important in avoiding misinterpretation of elevations in CK-MB levels that are in reality factitious.

INTRODUCTION

Serum creatine phosphokinase (CK) abnormalities have frequently been reported in patients with chronic renal failure.[1-3] Studies of healthy hemodialysis (HD) patients have found elevations in the total CK, as well as the MM, MB, and BB isoenzyme fractions, suggesting occult myopathy, myocardial ischemia, or neuropathy, respectively. Recent advances in the laboratory assays, however, indicate that some of the older methods can factitiously elevate the isoenzyme determinations. Thus, increases in ''MB'' that are in reality of noncardiac origin could confound clinical efforts to diagnose myocardial infarction, especially in the HD popula-

tion, which is prone to ischemic heart disease. It is not clear whether similar phenomena occur in CAPD patients. The purpose of this study was to further examine CK levels in clinically healthy CAPD and HD patients. Up to three different isoenzyme assay techniques were used to assess their validity.

METHODS

Patients

All stable chronic outpatients on dialysis in the UCLA Dialysis Program were candidates for inclusion in the study. Subjects were excluded if they had any intramuscular injection, surgical procedure, known muscle trauma, unusually strenuous physical exertion, known (nonuremic) myopathy, or severe angina within one week of study.

Blood Sampling

Random morning specimens were drawn on the CAPD patients. Sampling was done 48 hours after the last dialysis for the HD patients. The blood was tested for total CK, CK-MM, CK-BB, CK-MB, and aldolase.

Blood Assays

Total CK was measured using a modified Rosalki method by an SMAC autoanalyzer. CK-MM was assayed by DEAE-Sephadex column chroma-

From the Department of Medicine, Division of Nephrology, UCLA School of Medicine, and the Department of Pathology, UCLA Medical Center, Los Angeles, California.

505

tography using a modified Mercer method. CK-BB
was also measured by column separation. CK-MB
was assessed by (1) column separation, as above; (2)
RIA, radioimmunometric technique using the Em-
bria method; and (3) electrophoresis (agarose).
Aldolase was measured using routine kinetic
techniques.

RESULTS

Patient Characteristics

A total of 35 patients were studied between
August 1983 and May 1984: Fourteen CAPD patients, six males and eight females, with a mean time
on CAPD of 17 months, and 22 HD patients, 12
males and 10 females, with a mean time on HD of 4
years. The etiology of ESRD is listed in Table 1.

CK Assay Results

CAPD PATIENTS

Total CK was elevated (up to 5 times normal) in
nine of 13 (69.2%) patients tested (Table 2). The
range was <10 to 627 U/L, with a mean of 217 U/L
(normal <120). In eight of these, the MM fraction
was also elevated, and in the other patient it was high
normal. Only one patient had an elevated MB fraction (4 times normal by column separation, 8% of the
total level) when initially assayed. When repeated 6
months later, the MB level by RIA was normal. No
CAPD patient had an elevated BB fraction.

HD PATIENTS

Total CK was elevated (5 times normal) in one
of 22 (4.5%) patients tested (the range was <10 to
539 U/L, with a mean of 67 U/L) (Table 2). This
subject was also the only one to have an elevated
MM, as well as a twice normal MB by column separation (confirmed by mildly elevated MB values by
RIA). Although the absolute level was high, the MB
fraction was only 2% of the total CK value, within
the normal range.

One additional HD patient demonstrated an elevated "MB" by column separation; however, total
CK was normal. Electrophoresis revealed an atypical (variant) CK band, with an MB level that was
normal. Repeat assays on fresh blood two and four
months later failed to show the electrophoretic variant, and the MB fraction was normal by RIA. The
CK-BB fraction was normal in all HD patients.

Table 1. Study Patient Characteristics.

	CAPD	HD
Number	14	22
Male/Female	6/8	12/10
Mean time on dialysis modality	17 mo	4 yrs
Etiology of ESRD		
Diabetes	6	6
Hypertension	4	3
Glomerulonephritis	0	6
Obstructive uropathy	0	3
Other	3	3
Unknown	1	1

Aldolase Assay Results

Only one CAPD patient had an abnormal
aldolase, which occurred concurrent with twice normal total CK as well as CK-MM levels (Table 2). No
HD patient had an elevated aldolase.

DISCUSSION

Elevated total CK has been previously reported
in HD patients. Galen[1] reported that 20 of 43 patients
had an abnormally high total CK level. Cohen et al.[2]
showed and elevated value in 26 of 100 subjects, and
suggested that CK was a possible marker for uremic
myopathy, since there was a correlation with the
level of BUN. Similarly, Ma et al.[3] showed that in 11
of 46 (23.9%) HD patients the MM fraction was

Table 2. Blood Assay Results.

	CAPD	HD
↑ Total CK	9/13	1/22
↑ MM	4/8	1/22
↑ MB with Total CK	1/12*	1/22
↑ MB with normal CK	0/11	1/22**
↑ Aldolase	1/9	0/22
↑ BB	0/9	0/22

* Four-fold by column, upper normal limit by RIA when repeated.
** One patient with normal total, three-fold MB (col-umn), normal MB (RIA), atypical band present.

elevated, suggesting a skeletal muscle source. Such abnormalities in the total and isoenzyme fractions of CK in seemingly healthy ESRD patients on chronic dialysis are of clinical concern. These findings have led previous investigators to suggest the existence of an occult myopathy or neuropathy in such patients. However, those disturbing reports are now difficult to interpret; recent advances in laboratory methodology reveal the possibility of factitious results from some of the older methods. The present study compares the results from different assay techniques and extends the analysis to CAPD patients.

This study shows that while only one of 22 (4.5%) HD patients had a high total CK level, 9 of 13 (69.2%) CAPD patients had this abnormality. Ion-exchange chromatography revealed that the source of that elevation was predominantly in the MM fraction. Although there are other potential sources of CK-MM (e.g., gastrointestinal tumor), this finding is most suggestive of a muscle abnormality. Indeed, one such CAPD patient did have an elevated aldolase level. No patient, however, had any clinical evidence or history of myopathy. Electrophysiological studies are presently underway in these patients in an attempt to clarify this issue.

With refinements in assay methodology and with greater knowledge of CK structure, it is now clear that many of the older assay techniques can yield misleading results for the isoenzyme levels.[4] Certain CK variants can be factitiously measured as "CK-MB" using some of the older immunoinhibition assays. In particular, two CK "Macro" variants have been well-described. Type I (accounting for two-thirds of these cases) is usually CK-BB linked to immunoglobulins. It has been found in 3% to 6% of hospitalized patients without correlation to specific diseases and may persist for long periods of time. Type II is thought to be an oligomer of the distinct mitochondrial form of CK, in a variable state of aggregation. It can be seen in seriously ill patients, often with malignancies. Ion exchange chromatography (one of the currently available clinical methods) can misinterpret the Type I variant, reporting it as "MB." Electrophoresis will, however, reveal it as an atypical band migrating between MM and the actual MB. The variants do not crossreact in the new commercially available RIA techniques. In addition, some fluorescence methods can factitiously elevate the BB level.

Using cellulose acetate electrophoresis for CK separation, Galen[1] showed that 19 of 100 HD patients had high MB fractions. However, he used "3% of total CK" as the upper limit of normal MB

(6% was the limit in the present study), and it is not clear to what degree his patients exceeded that level. No mention was made of possible atypical bands. Ma et al.[3] used ion-exchange chromatography to demonstrate an elevated MB in 13 of 46 (28.3%) HD subjects. A skeletal muscle source was suggested because the abnormality correlated with a high MM fraction, but CK variants were not specifically sought. Therefore, the possibility of factitious CK-MB elevations was not explored.

In the present study of the 22 HD patients, only two (9.1%) had elevated "MB" levels by ion-exchange chromatography. One of 22 (4.5%) subjects had an elevated absolute MB level at five times normal, but the total CK was increased proportionately, yielding a normal MB of 2%. Thus, in patients without myocardial ischemia, but with marked elevations in the total CPK level, a normal percent of CPK-MB may occur concomitantly with an abnormally high absolute quantity. Therefore, both total CK and CK-MB need to be measured to avoid misdiagnosis of myocardial infarction.

The other HD subject with a high "MB" by column separation had a normal total value. Indeed, electrophoresis revealed an atypical CK variant band that had factitiously elevated the other assay's "MB" result; there was no actual MB abnormality. Knowledge of the methodology is therefore crucial in avoiding misinterpretation of the "CK-MB" result.

Of our CAPD patients, only one of 12 had a high (four times normal) MB level by column chromatography (8% of a two-fold elevated total CK); unfortunately, electrophoresis was not performed at that time. Later, however, no atypical band was present, concurrent with a high normal MB by RIA.

Using fluorometric techniques, Galen[1] and Weseley et al.[5] showed increased levels of CK-BB in HD and PD patients. However, Homberger et al.,[6] using a more specific RIA, reported that 15 of 60 azotemic subjects had a high BB fraction. Although some of these individuals had chronic renal failure, most had either acute renal failure (with the possibility of renal tubular release of BB) or had associated malignancies (which could produce BB). Using ion-exchange chromatography separation, none of our CAPD or HD patients had high BB fractions. The disparity between our study and previous studies, could at least be due in part to differences in the study populations, all of our subjects had chronic renal failure and none had malignancy. Indeed Ma et al.[3] found normal CK-BB levels by column separation in 46 "healthy" chronic HD patients.

REFERENCES

1. Galen RS: Creatine kinase isoenzyme BB in serum of renal-disease patients. Clin Chem 22: 120, 1976
2. Cohen IM, Griffiths J, Stone RA, and Leech T: The creatine kinase profile of a maintenance hemodialysis population: A possible marker of uremic myopathy. Clin Nephrol 13: 235, 1980
3. Ma KW, Brown DC, Steele BW, and From AHL: Serum creatine kinase MB isoenzyme activity in long-term hemodialysis patients. Arch Intern Med 141: 164, 1981
4. Lang H, and Wurzburg U: Creatine kinase, an enzyme of many forms. Clin Chem 28: 1439, 1982
5. Weseley SA, Byrnes A, Alter S, Solangi KB, and Goodman AI: Presence of creatine phosphokinase brain band in the serum of chronic renal disease patients. Clin Nephrol 8: 345, 1977
6. Homburger HA, Miller SA, and Jacob GL: Radioimmunoassay of creatine kinase B-isoenzymes in serum of patients with azotemia, obstructive uropathy, or carcinoma of the prostate or bladder. Clin Chem 26: 1821, 1980

Z. Sasson, H.D. Strauss, M.N. Druck, G. Wu,
M. Jutkovich, and D.G. Oreopoulos

96

Total CK and CK-MB Elevation in Dialysis Patients without Acute Myocardial Infarction

SUMMARY

The prevalence of total creatine kinase (CK) and CK-MB isoenzyme elevation in chronic dialysis patients remains controversial.

We studied 135 patients undergoing chronic hemodialysis (HD) or peritoneal (PD) dialysis. Mean age was 55.4 years (range 20 to 85 years). All had an ECG and blood drawn concurrently. No patient had chest pain in the preceding 24 hours or ECG changes of acute myocardial infarction. Total CK was measured by the Rosalki method, and CK-MB qualitatively by electrophoresis (Method I) and quantitatively by glass bead adsorption (Method II).

Twenty of 135 patients (14.8%) had elevated total CK; 5/135 (3.7%) had elevated CK-MB of which only one had normal total CK. Results were similar for HD and PD patients. We conclude that in chronic dialysis patients CK-MB is elevated in a small proportion without other clinical evidence of acute myocardial infarction and that total CK is commonly elevated. In light of these findings, CK and CK-MB elevations should be interpreted with caution in dialysis patients in whom a diagnosis of myocardial infarction is suspected.

INTRODUCTION

Creatine kinase is a large molecular weight enzyme of approximately 80,000 daltons catalyzing the transfer of phosphate from creatine phosphate (CP) to ADP, thus forming free creatine (C) and the high energy ATP required for efficient muscle contraction:

$$ADP + CP \xrightleftharpoons{\quad CK \quad} ATP + C$$

Three isoenzymes of CK have been identified by electrophoresis and designated MM, MB, and BB.[1] MM has a wide tissue distribution and is detectable in normal serum. MB and BB have more limited tissue distribution, and normally contribute less than 5% to the total CK activity (TCK).

MB is found in greatest concentrations in myocardial cells and in very small concentrations in skeletal muscle and the GI tract. Thus, because the heart is the only organ with sufficient concentrations of MB, serum MB elevation has generally been accepted as a specific and sensitive marker of myocardial necrosis.[2,3] MB elevations have also been reported in a number of noncardiac conditions, generally in association with extensive MM release or diminished clearance.[4-8]

The presence of elevated TCK in uremic patients was first reported in 1967 by Eschar and Zimmerman,[9] and repeatedly confirmed in dialysis patients with varying prevalence rates of 19–42%. More recently, MB elevations in dialysis patients have been reported with varying prevalence rates of 1–28% without evidence of uremic pericarditis.[10-13] An important reason for the variability may relate to methodology in that some methods do not distinguish between BB and MB, others may have false elevations of MB in the presence of high MM levels, and yet others may falsely detect complexing of

From the Toronto Western Hospital, Toronto, Ontario, Canada.

immunoglobulins to BB (macro CK) as MB.[14–17] Agarose gel electrophoresis[18] and glycophase glass bead adsorption[19] have been widely accepted as highly sensitive and specific techniques for the qualitative and quantitative detection of MB isoenzyme elevations, respectively.

The present study assessed the true prevalence of MB and TCK elevations in a stable patient population on chronic peritoneal dialysis (PD) and hemodialysis (HD) in the absence of suspected acute myocardial infarction by applying these two methods of isoenzyme detection.

METHODS

The study population consisted of 135 patients undergoing regular chronic dialysis, 94 on PD and 41 on HD. Mean age was 55.4 years, with a range of 20–85 years, and mean dialysis duration was 21.3 months with a range of 1–100 months. No patient had chest pain in the preceding 24 hours. All patients had a standard 12 lead ECG, and blood samples were drawn during the same visit.

Total CK was assayed spectrophotometrically by the Rosalki method.[20] MB was qualitatively assessed by agarose gel electrophoresis using the Corning medical CK isoenzyme substrate set (CK-MB I), and quantitatively measured by glycophase glass bead adsorption using the Lancer MB/CK isoenzyme separation kit (CK-MB II). This method has a reproduceability in our laboratory of ±4%. The upper limit of normal for MB in our laboratory is 7 IU/L, which is the mean +2 standard deviations on determination in 51 normal individuals.[23] As all normal values were <8 IU/L, we counted only values ≥8 IU/L as elevated.

RESULTS

The results are depicted in Figure 1. In all, 20/135 (14.8%) of patients had elevated TCK; 5/135 (3.7%) had MB elevations by both methods I and II (mean 10.4 IU/L, range 8.8–11.7 IU/L). Only one patient with elevated MB had normal TCK. No patient had ECG changes of acute myocardial infarction, although there were a variety of other

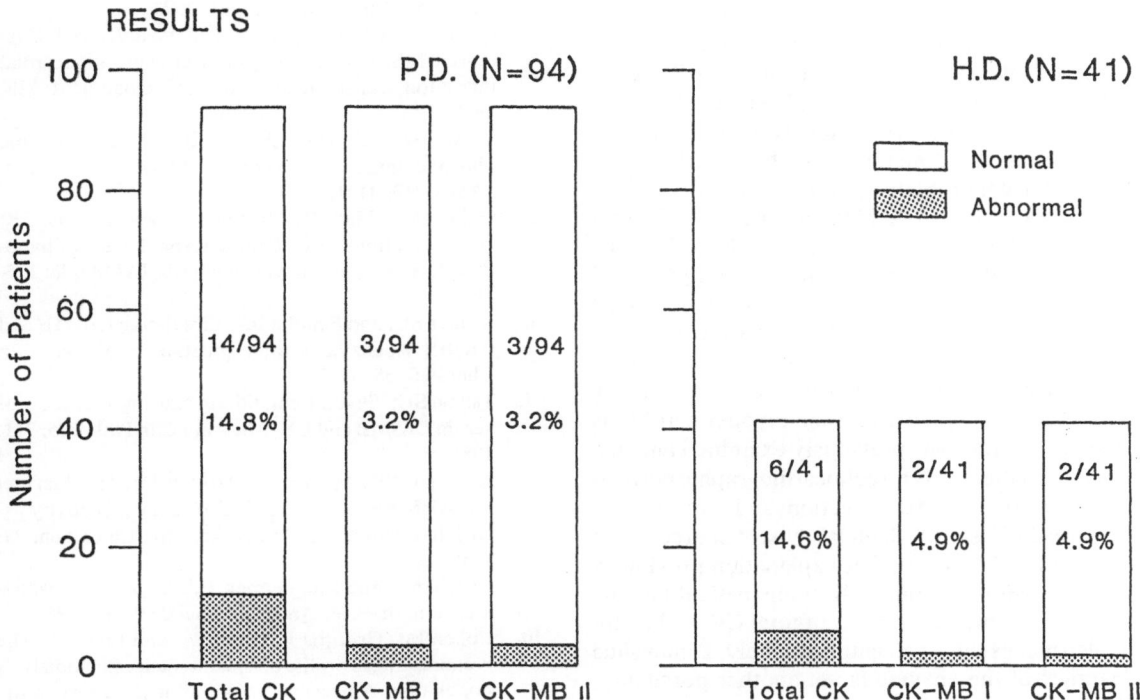

Fig. 1. Result of present study. No difference between the PD and HD populations. Only 1 patient with elevated CK-MB had normal total CK. No patient had ECG changes of acute myocardial infarction.

abnormalities including hypertrophy patterns, conduction disturbances, and other nonspecific repolarization changes. Results were similar for HD and PD patients. Only two of the five patients with MB elevations had a clinically significant history of coronary disease. The etiology, duration of renal failure, thyroid status, parathyroid status, or other enzymatic levels did not correlate with either TCK or MB elevations.

DISCUSSION

Our study demonstrates the true prevalence of total CK and the CK-MB isoenzyme elevation in a large, stable, outpatient population of peritoneal and hemodialysis patients at one point in time. The finding of total CK elevation in approximately 15% of this population was slightly lower but still in keeping with previously published reports.[10,12,21] This abnormality did not correlate with the underlying etiology of renal failure, with the BUN level, nor with thyroid and parathyroid status of our patients, as has been previously suggested.[12] The underlying mechanism for this elevation remains unexplained, although it has variously been attributed to uremic myopathy, diminished clearance, coexistent hypothyroidism, and several other metabolic derangements, none of which have been well-substantiated.

The finding of CK-MB elevation in 3.7% by both electrophoresis and glycophase adsorption is similarly unexplained. It is unlikely to be a factitious elevation, as these methods are free of the other methodological problems referred to above, including the carryover of CK-MM into the CK-MB fraction and the false detection of macro-CK as CK-MB. It is equally unlikely to be secondary to a myocardial ischemic event, as these were stable, ambulatory outpatients free of recent ischemic pain with otherwise unremarkable electrocardiograms, and most did not have a clinical history of coronary artery disease. Uremic pericarditis or myopericarditis is possible, but this was previously examined and discounted, as there was no echocardiographic correlation between CK-MB elevation and presence of pericardial effusion.[13] Skeletal muscle source of the elevated CK-MB is another explanation previously put forth, but the normal CK in one patient and the lack of substantial elevations of total CK in the others also makes this explanation unlikely. Diminished clearance of the enzyme is yet another possibility. Although creatine kinase is cleared by the reticuloendothelial system,[22] it is known that various parts of this system are adversely affected by chronic renal failure by an as yet unclear mechanism. Whether the normal turnover of CK and CK-MB can result in mild serum elevations of these enzymes in the presence of a deranged clearance system is an attractive hypothesis that remains to be tested.

In conclusion, we have demonstrated that in chronic dilaysis, patients total CK is commonly elevated, and CK-MB is mildly elevated in a small proportion of patients without other clinical evidence of acute myocardial infarction. In light of these findings, CK and CK-MB elevations should be interpreted with caution in dialysis patients in whom a diagnosis of acute myocardial infarction is suspected, and the typical pattern of rise and disappearance of this enzyme over a period of days rather than its isolated evaluation should be observed.

REFERENCES

1. Van der Veen KJ, and Willebrands AF: Isoenzymes of creatine phosphokinase in tissue extracts and in normal and pathological sera. Clin Chim Acta 13: 312, 1966
2. Wagner GS, Roe CR, Limbird LE, Rosati RA, and Wallace AG: The importance of identification of the myocardial specific isoenzyme of creatine phosphokinase (MB ferm) in the diagnosis of acute myocardial infarction. Circulation 47: 263, 1973
3. Grande P, Christiansen C, Pedersen A, and Cristensen MS: Optimal diagnosis in acute myocardial infarction, a cost effective study. Circulation 61: 723, 1980
4. Brownlow RB, and Eleriten FR: Serum creatine phosphokinase isoenzyme (CPK_2) in myositis. JAMA 230: 1141, 1974
5. Goldman J, Matz R, Mortimer R, and Freeman R: High elevations of creatine phosphokinase in hypothyroidism: An isoenzyme analysis. JAMA 238: 325, 1977
6. Kimler SC, and Sandhu RS: Circulating CK-MB and CK-BB isoenzymes after prostate resection. Clin Chem 26: 55, 1980
7. Tsung SH: Several conditions causing elevation of serum CK-MB and CK-BB. Am J Clin Pathol 75: 711, 1981
8. Hickman PE, Massina S, Trotter JM, and Masarei JR: High creatine kinase MB isoenzyme activity associated with a rhabdomyosarcoma. Clin Chem 29: 1549, 1983
9. Eshchar J, and Zimmerman HJ: Creatine phosphokinase in disease. Am J Med Sci 253: 272, 1967
10. Cohen IM, Griffiths J, Stone RA, and Leech T: The creatine kinase profile of a maintenance hemodialysis population: A possible marker of uremic myopathy. Clin Nephrol 13: 235, 1980
11. Homburger HA, Miller SA, and Jacob GL: Radioimmunoassay of creatine kinase B isoenzyme in serum

of patients with azotemia, obstructive uropathy, or carcinoma of the prostate or bladder. Clin Chem 26: 1821, 1980

12. Sofer O, Fellner SK, and Rush RL: Creatine phosphokinase in long-term dialysis patients. Arch Intern Med 141: 181, 1981

13. Ma KW, Brown DC, Steele BW, and From AH: Serum creatine kinase MB isoenzyme activity in long-term hemodialysis patients. Arch Intern Med 141: 164, 1981

14. Lott JA, and Stang JM: Serum enzymes and isoenzymes in the diagnosis and differential diagnosis of myocardial ischemia and necrosis. Clin Chem 26: 1241, 1980

15. Wicks R, Usategui-Gomez M, Miller M, and Warshaw M: Immunochemical determinations of CK-MB isoenzyme in human serum. II. An enzymatic approach. Clin Chem 28: 54, 1982

16. Seckinger DL, Vazquez AD, Rosenthal PK, and Mendizabal RC: Cardiac isoenzyme methodology and the diagnosis of acute myocardial infarction. Am J Clin Pathol 80: 164, 1983

17. Devine JE: Macro-creatine kinase as an interference in CK isoenzyme determinations. Enzyme 30: 139, 1983

18. Corning Medical: Corning CK isoenzyme substrate set. For use in quantitative and qualitative fluorometric determination of creatine kinase isoenzymes by electrophoresis. Corning Medical, Palo Alto, CA

19. Henry PD, Roberts R, and Sobel BE: Rapid separation of plasma creatine kinase isoenzymes by batch adsorption on glass beads. Clin Chem 21: 844, 1975

20. Rosalki SB: An improved procedure for serum creatine phosphokinase determination. J Lab Clin Med 69: 696, 1967

21. Galen RS: Creatine kinase isoenzyme BB in serum of renal disease patients. Clin Chem 22: 120, 1976

22. Roberts R, Henry PD, and Sobel BE: An improved basis for enzymatic estimation of infarct size. Circulation 52: 743, 1975

23. Buda AJ, Macdonald IL, Dubbin JD, Orr SA, and Strauss HD: Myocardial infarct extension: Prevalence, clinical significance and problems in diagnosis. Am Heart J 105: 744, 1983

R.S.C. Rodger, K. Fletcher, D. Genner, J. Dewar,
M.K. Ward, and D.N.S. Kerr

97

Sexual Dysfunction in Patients Treated by CAPD

SUMMARY

A comparison of sexual function in 27 male CAPD patients with that of 73 male hemodialysis patients revealed impotence in more than half of each group and testicular atrophy in the vast majority. Gynecomastia was infrequent. Plasma testosterone levels were higher in the CAPD population but differences in prolactin, FSH, TH and PTH were minor. The similarities in sexual function of hemodialysis and CAPD patients do not support middle molecule toxicity as a major pathogenetic factor in uremic sexual dysfunction.

INTRODUCTION

Pituitary testicular axis disturbance in chronic renal failure may be a feature of middle molecule toxicity.[1] Although hyperprolactinemia is often also present,[2] the pattern of disturbance predominantly reflects primary gonadal failure and may be one of the factors causing sexual dysfunction in male dialysis patients. As CAPD has been shown to improve middle molecule clearance compared with other forms of dialysis therapy,[3] patients undergoing this treatment might have less marked hormonal imbalance and sexual dysfunction.

From the Departments of Medicine and Clinical Biochemistry, Royal Victoria Infirmary, Newcastle upon Tyne, United Kingdom, and Royal Postgraduate Medical School, London, United Kingdom.

METHODS

Twenty-seven CAPD patients selected at random from the male dialysis population were assessed and compared with 73 male patients undergoing hemodialysis (HD). The distribution of age and of primary renal disease, and the incidence of previous renal transplantation and of the ingestion of drugs associated with sexual dysfunction, were similar in both groups. The mean duration of dialysis, however, was significantly greater in the HD group ($p < 0.001$). Patients were interviewed using a standard questionnaire and examined to identify testicular atrophy and gynecomastia. Serum zinc was measured by flameless absorption spectrophotometry, and plasma testosterone (T), serum prolactin, follicle stimulating hormone (FSH), luteinizing hormone (LH), and parathormone (PTH) levels were measured by radioimmunoassay. Statistical analysis was performed by the regression equation and the Students t test. FSH, LH, and PTH levels were log transformed prior to comparative analysis to normalize their skewed distribution. Prolactin levels were compared using the Mann-Whitney U test.

RESULTS

Sixty-six percent of CAPD patients complained of erectile impotence following the onset of uremia and regular dialysis therapy. Gynecomastia and testicular atrophy were noted in 12% and 92% of

Table 1. Sexual Function in 100 Male Dialysis Patients.

	Impotent		Partial		Complete		Testicular Atrophy		Mild		Severe
HD	44/73	(60%)	18/73	(25%)	26/73	(35%)	51/62 (82%)		43/62	(69%)	8/62 (13%)
CAPD	18/27	(66%)	6/27	(22%)	12/27	(44%)	23/25 (92%)		18/25	(72%)	5/25 (20%)
Total	62/100 (62%)		24/100 (24%)		38/100 (38%)		74/87 (85%)		61/87 (70%)		13/87 (15%)

Erectile impotence: partial   =   erections $\leq$1/week
                           complete =   erections <1/month.
Testicular atrophy: mild   =   testicular volume <15 mls
                           severe   =   testicular volume $\leq$6 mls.

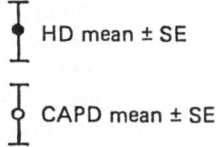

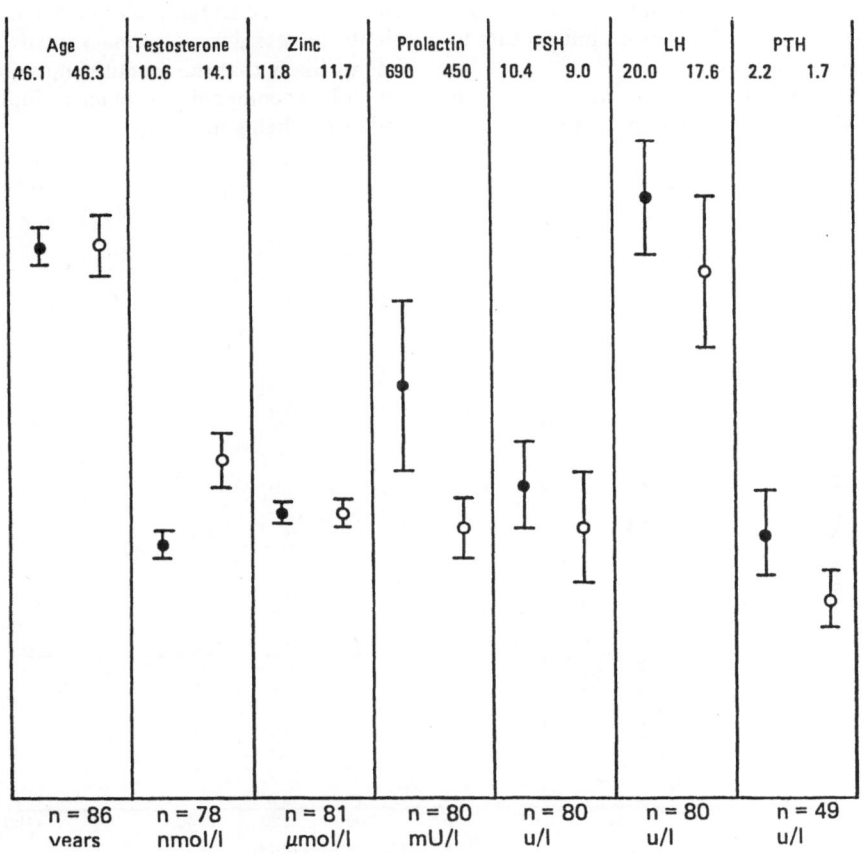

Fig. 1. Age, time, and hormone levels in dialysis patients.

CAPD patients, respectively. The findings were not significantly different in HD patients (Table 1).

Plasma T levels were higher in CAPD patients compared with patients treated by HD (Fig. 1, p = 0.006) and did not correlate with serum zinc, prolactin, or PTH levels, or with the duration of ESRD (Fig. 2). Serum prolactin, FSH, LH, and PTH levels were lower in patients treated by CAPD, but these differences did not reach statistical significance (Fig. 1).

DISCUSSION

Despite the advances in the management of ESRD in recent years, male dialysis patients continue to complain of reduced libido and erectile impotence and there was no evidence from this study that these symptoms were ameliorated by CAPD. Sexual activity and fertility may be restored following successful renal transplantation, but maintenance HD does not have this effect.[4] The similarities that we have observed between HD patients and those treated by CAPD does not support middle molecule toxicity as a major factor contributing to sexual dysfunction in uremia.

The male hormone profile is apparently improved by CAPD, although most patients also have testicular atrophy consistent with chronic or continuing gonadal damage. Sex hormone binding globulin (SHBG) levels are elevated in patients undergoing maintenance dialysis,[5] demonstrating that "free testosterone" levels are lower than indicated by plasma testosterone levels in ESRD. However, no significant difference between patients treated by CAPD and HD was found, and so the differences in the plasma testosterone levels that we have observed probably reflect differences in "free testosterone" levels. The duration of dialysis was greater in HD patients, but this has been shown not to influence their male hormone status.[4]

Although a sufficient amount of circulating androgen is required to maintain male sexual function, there is no evidence for a relation between circulating androgen levels and differences in sexual behavior.[6] Erectile function may remain intact even several years following castration.[7] It is thought that testosterone facilitates the erectile mechanism, indirectly acting as a libido factor.[8] There is no correlation between plasma testosterone levels and sexual function in ESRD and although many dialysis patients have signs of primary testicular failure, it seems likely that the erectile impotence that so frequently accompanies uremia is induced by some other mechanism.

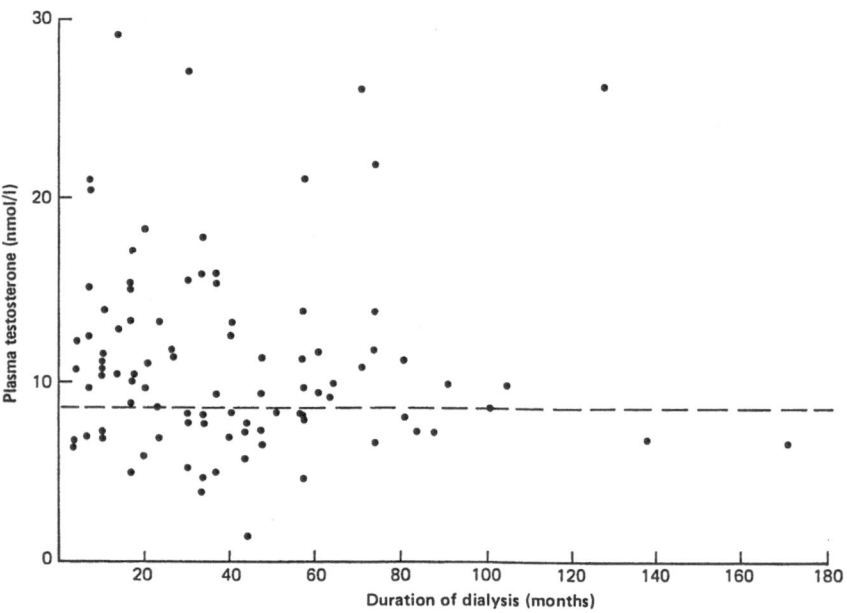

Fig. 2. Relation of plasma testosterone levels with duration of dialysis.

ACKNOWLEDGMENTS

Dr. Fletcher's research was supported by grants from the Northern Regional Health Authority and the Northern Regional Research Fund.

REFERENCES

1. Holdsworth S, Atkins RC, and DeKretser DM: The pituitary testicular axis in men with chronic renal failure. N Engl J Med 296: 1245, 1977
2. Gomez F, DeLaCueva R, Wauters J, and Lemarchand-Beraud T: Endocrine abnormalities in patients undergoing long-term hemodialysis. Am J Med 68: 522, 1980
3. Bergström J, Asaba H, Fürst P, and Lindholm B: Middle molecules in chronic uremic patients treated with peritoneal dialysis. In Gahl GM, Kessel M, Nolph KD (Eds), Advances in peritoneal dialysis: Proceedings of the 2nd international symposium on peritoneal dialysis. Amsterdam: Excerpta Medica, 1981, p 47
4. Holdsworth SR, DeKretser DM, and Atkins RC: A comparison of hemodialysis and transplantation in reversing the uremic disturbance of male reproduction function. Clin Nephrol 10: 146, 1978
5. Semple CG, Beastall GH, Henderson IS, Thomson JA, and Kennedy AC: The pituitary testicular axis of uraemic subjects on haemodialysis and CAPD. Acta Endocrinol 101: 464, 1982
6. Schiavi RC, and White D: Androgens and male sexual function: A review of human studies. J Sex Marital Ther 2: 214, 1976
7. Eibl E: Treatment and after care of 300 sex offenders. Proceedings on the German conference on treatment possibilities for sex offenders in Eppengen. Justizministerium Baden Wurtemberg, 1978
8. Davidson JM, Kwan M, and Greenleaf WJ: Hormone replacement and sexuality in men. Clin Endocrinol Metab 11: 599, 1982

Complications, Peritonitis, and Response to Infection

B. Spinowitz, A. Leggio, M. Galler, R. Golden,
J. Rascoff, and C. Charytan

98

Prognostic Indicators of Hernia Development in Patients Undergoing CAPD

SUMMARY

Among 157 patients trained for CAPD, 81 hernias developed in 44 of them. The hernias were 30% incisional, 38% umbilical, 17% inguinal and 15% ventral. Most hernias developed within the first year. Parous females, patients with polycystic kidney disease, and those with prior hernia surgery were at highest risk of this complication and deserve special vigilance. Hernias should be treated promptly to avoid incarceration which occurred in 19% of this series.

INTRODUCTION

The development of abdominal hernias is a recognized, though underrated, cause of morbidity and dropout in patients on continuous ambulatory peritoneal dialysis (CAPD).[1-8] We report a retrospective study performed to determine the incidence of abdominal hernia formation and to delineate any factors that may place CAPD patients at an increased risk of this complication.

METHODS

A chart review was done on all end stage renal disease (ESRD) patients trained for CAPD at the Booth Memorial Medical Center between January

_____
From the Booth Memorial Medical Center Flushing, New York.

1980, and December 1983. Localization of the abdominal hernias and the type of peritoneal dialysis catheter used was gleaned from the operative reports when available. The potential risk factors studied included sex, age, parity, underlying diseases, steroid therapy, previous surgery, a serum albumin level greater than or less than 3.5 g/dl and the CAPD break-in technique used.

RESULTS

Among 157 patients trained for CAPD, 81 hernias developed in 44 patients during a follow-up of 2513 patient months. One third of all hernias occurred during the first 6 months on CAPD and two-thirds were noted within the first year of CAPD. Thirty percent of the hernias were incisional, 38% umbilical, 17% inguinal, and 15% ventral. Fifteen hernias became incarcerated and required emergency surgery.

Twenty two of 77 males had 29 hernias (36% of all hernias) and 22 of 80 females had 52 hernias (64% of all hernias) $p < 0.01$. There was no correlation between parity and hernia formation although nulliparous patients had a significantly lower incidence of hernia formation (11.1%) as compared to patients who had any pregnancies (29.5%).

There was no correlation between hernia formation and the age of the patient, their activity prior to or during dialysis, prior surgery, steroid therapy, serum albumin levels, type of catheter used for CAPD, or the CAPD break-in technique utilized. Six of 13 patients with polycystic kidney disease (46.2%)

developed abdominal hernias, in contrast to 38 of 144 patients (26.4%) of patients with all other ESRD etiologies. Twelve of 26 patients who had undergone a prior hernia repair developed abdominal hernias while on CAPD. Five patients (3% of the total CAPD population) required a change of dialysis modality because of recurrent hernia formation. Two patients required a decrease in volume and an increase in frequency of their CAPD exchange regimen.

DISCUSSION

Although abdominal hernia formation is a recognized complication of CAPD,[1-8] we believe that its frequency and significance has been underrated. Other authors have reported a frequency of hernia formation varying from 9 to 28%. Despite the potentially high incidence of this complication, it is generally not reported nor recognized as a significant cause of CAPD dropout or major morbidity.[1,5,8]

The development of hernias in 28% of our CAPD population with 15 patients requiring emergency surgery for incarceration and 18 patients having recurrent hernias requiring repeated surgery is adequate proof of the significance and importance of this CAPD complication. Furthermore, the frequent interruption of CAPD therapy necessitated by this complication and the subsequent 3% dropout rate further underscores the significance of this complication.

From our retrospective review, it would appear that parous females, patients with polycystic kidney disease and those with prior hernia surgery are at greatest risk of this complication. This finding is further supported by a recent study suggesting a collagen defect in patients with polycystic kidney disease.[9] Although these patients should not be denied access to this treatment modality, they should be carefully observed for this complication and its recurrence post surgical correction. Once hernias develop, they should be quickly corrected in view of the demonstrated risk of incarceration.

Alternative surgical implantation techniques may decrease the incidence of hernia development in CAPD. Further, patients at high risk of hernia development might benefit from a decrease in intra-abdominal pressure through the use of more frequent smaller volume exchanges.[10] These approaches are being presently investigated to determine their effect on the incidence of abdominal hernia formation in CAPD patients.

REFERENCES

1. Khanna R, Oreopoulos DG, Dombros N, Vas S, Williams P, Meema HE, Hudsan H, Ogilvie R, Zellerman G, Roncari DAK, Clayton S, and Izatt S: Continuous ambulatory peritoneal dialysis after three years: Still a promising treatment. Peritoneal Dial Bull 1: 24, 1981
2. Chan MK, Baillod RA, Tanner A, Raftery M, Sweny P, Fernando ON, and Moorhead JF: Abdominal hernias in patients receiving continuous ambulatory peritoneal dialysis. Br Med J 283: 826, 1981
3. Griffin PJA, and Coles GA: Strangulated hernias through Tenckhoff catheter sites. Br Med J 284: 1837, 1982
4. Rubin J, Raju S, Teal N, Hellems E, and Bower JD: Abdominal hernias in patients undergoing continuous ambulatory peritoneal dialysis. Arch Intern Med 142: 1453, 1982
5. Gloor HJ, Nichols WK, Sorkin MI, Prowant B, Kennedy JM, Baker B, and Nolph KD: Peritoneal access and related complications in continuous ambulatory peritoneal dialysis. Am J Med 74: 593, 1983
6. Orkin BA, Foukalsrud EW, Salusky IB, Ettinger RB, Hall T, Jordan SC, and Fine RN: Continuous ambulatory peritoneal dialysis catheters in children. Arch Surg 118: 1398, 1983
7. Digenis GD, Khanna R, Mathews R, Oreopoulos DG: Abdominal hernias in patients undergoing continuous ambulatory peritoneal dialysis. Peritoneal Dial Bull 2: 115, 1982
8. Oreopoulos DG, Khanna R, Williams P, Vas SI: Continuous ambulatory peritoneal dialysis, 1981. Nephron 30: 293, 1982
9. Leier CV, Baker PB, Kilman JW, Wooley CF: Cardiovascular abnormalities with adult polycystic kidney disease. Ann Intern Med 100: 683, 1984
10. Gotloib L, Mines M, Garmizo L, and Varka I: Hemodynamic effects of increasing intraabdominal pressure in peritoneal dialysis. Peritoneal Dial Bull 1: 41, 1981

G. Fang

99

Peritoneal Catheter Perforating into the Colon—A Serious Complication of Peritoneal Dialysis

SUMMARY

This paper presents a young man who developed a serious complication of peritoneal dialysis, peritoneal catheter perforation of the colon in the 10th month of continuous ambulatory peritoneal dialysis. The diagnosis in this patient with end-stage renal failure secondary to chronic glomerulonephritis, was made after the patient experienced recurrent episodes of bacterial peritonitis for two months prior to the manifestation of the colonic perforation. Our data indicated that peritonitis played a role in the development of colonic perforation by the indwelling peritoneal catheter, and our observations support the opinion of Diaz-Buxo who emphasized the need for modification of the traditional dialysis catheter design.

INTRODUCTION

Continuous ambulatory peritoneal dialysis (CAPD) can result in many unusual complications. Ramos et al.[1] reported a patient who developed a Morgagni hernia during CAPD. Spadaro et al.[2] used Technetium-99m-labeled macroaggregated albumin and demonstrated the transdiaphragmatic leakage of dialysate in patients on peritoneal dialysis. A peritoneovaginal fistula had also been previously reported.[3] Although erosion of the colon had been reported, most instances of colonic perforation occurred shortly after peritoneal catheterization, and delayed perforation due to a Tenckhoff catheter is rare.

This paper reports a patient who had undergone CAPD for 10 months. At the 10th month of CAPD he developed colonic perforation, the peritoneal catheter perforating into the colonic lumen for about 5 cm in length. The patient experienced recurrent episodes of bacterial peritonitis 2 months prior to discovery of the perforation. We therefore consider that the peritonitis might be the main cause of the colonic perforation. The purpose of this paper is to emphasize that CAPD could produce the serious complication of intestinal perforation. One should be aware that perforation could occur during CAPD, particularly in those patients who suffered from peritonitis. In order to prevent this complication we suggest that the tip of the peritoneal catheter should be modified and the catheter should be selected according to the size of the patient.

CASE REPORT

A 24-year-old Chinese male with a diagnosis of end stage renal failure secondary to chronic glomerulonephritis was admitted to the hospital for CAPD. On physical examination, his blood pressure was 140/90 mm Hg. He was chronically ill, pale, undernourished, and edematous. No rash or lymphadenopathy were found on general examination. The eyelids were puffy. The lungs were normal, and

From the Department of Internal Medicine, Guiyang Medical College Hospital, Guizhou, People's Republic of China.

522

Fang

the heart was dilated. The abdomen was normal. There was ++ peripheral edema extending to the thighs and sacral area. Neurologic examination was negative.

The urine gave a +++ test for protein and had a specific gravity of 1.014; the sediment contained 5 white cells, 10 red cells, and few casts occasionally were seen under high-power field. Blood analysis: the hemoglobin was 6.0 g/dl; the white cell count was 7100/mm³, with 70% neutrophils, 28% lymphocytes and 2% eosinophils. The platelet count was 74,000/mm³. The levels of serum urea nitrogen and creatinine were 91 mg/dl and 22 mg/dl, respectively. The concentration of calcium was 8 mg/dl, and that of protein was 4.9 g/dl (albumin, 2.0 g/dl and globulin, 2.9 g/dl). The sodium was 140 mEq/L, the potassium was 5.6 mEq/L, the chloride was 118 mEq/L, and the carbon dioxide was 16 mEq/L. An electrocardiogram demonstrated a normal rhythm at a rate of 97 beats/min, and possible left ventricular hypertrophy. X-ray films of the chest showed slight cardiac enlargement, with left ventricular predominance. The creatinine clearance was 1.8 ml/min. Otherwise, the examination was unremarkable.

On January 4, 1982, under local anesthesia we inserted a single-cuffed adult Tenckhoff peritoneal catheter into the patient's peritoneal cavity and then the catheter was aimed down into the pelvis. The catheter was passed as far as it would comfortably go. The point of insertion of the catheter was one-third superior to the midline from the umbilicus to the symphysis pubis. The operation was uncomplicated. After insertion the drainage from the catheter was good and the dialysate outflow was clear and complete. Early in CAPD, there were no apparent complications. The patient's general condition and the blood chemistries improved gradually. The patient remained active and free of symptoms for 7 months and his general nutritional status remained stable. At the 8th month of CAPD, he had a typical picture of bacterial peritonitis. Peritoneal fluid culture grew E. Coli The leucocyte count of the fluid was 15,000 mm³ with 85% polymorphonuclears. Intraperitoneal gentamicin 160,000 units per day was administered for 10 days. After 3 days the fluid became clear and the cell count dropped to 150/mm³. No organism grew by culture. Several days later peritonitis recurred. After that, the peritonitis recurred for several times within 2 months, but the patient was still maintained on peritoneal dialysis. At the 10th month of CAPD, the patient complained of lower abdominal discomfort. The CAPD was discontinued and hemodialysis was instituted. A few days later the patient complained of anal discomfort.

The peritoneal catheter was touched by digital examination, and a partial catheter about 5 cm in length in the colon lumen was seen by rectoscopy. We found that the site of the perforation was about 10 cm proximal to the anus. The peritoneal catheter was removed and the patient was kept on hemodialysis. Five months later the patient died of recurrent peritonitis and exhaustion resulting from malnutrition.

DISCUSSION

Although the complications of intestinal perforation has been reported,[3,4] most instances of intestinal perforation occurred shortly after peritoneal catheter insertion. Delayed perforation is extremely unusual. Intestinal perforation shortly after peritoneal catheter insertion, and, therefore, injury to the intestinal wall during the operative procedure might be considered. In our case, the colonic perforation occurred after 9 months of CAPD. Before colonic perforation the peritoneal catheter functioned normally. We therefore consider that the perforation induced by the injury of the peritoneal catheter insertion was less possible. Our patient had recurrent episodes of bacterial peritonitis 2 months before the colonic perforation, thus we believe that peritonitis might be the leading cause of the colonic perforation. We agree with the mechanisms for peritonitis leading to visceral perforation, suggested by Diaz-Buxo.[3] They are that peritonitis can weaken the visceral wall by the direct inflammatory process which facilitates pressure necrosis; peritonitis may also affect the patient's nutritional status by provoking increased losses of protein via the effluent, by accelerating catabolic processes; and by interfering with adequate nutrition due to anorexia, nausea and emesis. We consider another mechanism, that is, that perforation may be due to the peritoneal adhesion and limitation of the intestinal movement caused by peritonitis, thus facilitating the tip of the catheter perforating into the intestine.

Although peritoneal catheter perforation into the colon is an unusual event reported in the literature, it was a serious complication of continuous ambulatory peritoneal dialysis. Although the peritonitis was the leading cause of the colonic perforation, the bacteria and waste materials in the colonic lumen entered the peritoneal cavity through the site of perforation following the perforation. This condition led to recurrent episodes of peritonitis and caused the pernicious cycle and also resulted in difficulty of treatment. Our patient finally died from recurrent episodes of peritonitis and exhaustion. We suggest, therefore, one should be alert that intestinal perforation could occur during CAPD, since intestinal perforation may occur in the earlier stage or after several months of the CAPD, particularly in those patients who suffer from peritonitis.

In order to prevent this complication we suggest that during the period of CAPD one should conscientiously prevent and treat peritonitis, and should provide enough nutrients including appropriate proteins, vitamins, and sufficient calories to increase host resistance to bacterial infection. In addition, the tip of the peritoneal catheter should be modified and the catheter should be selected according to the size of the patient.

REFERENCES

1. Ramos TM, Burke DA, and Veitch PS: Hernia Morgagni in patients on continuous ambulatory peritoneal dialysis. Lancet 1: 161, 1982
2. Spadaro JJ, Thakur V, and Nolph KD: Technetium-99m-labeled macroaggregated albumin in demonstration of trans-diaphragmatic leakage of dialysate in peritoneal dialysis. Am J Nephrol 2: 36, 1982
3. Diaz-Buxo JA, Burgess PB, and Walker PJ: Peritoneovaginal fistula. Unusual complication of peritoneal dialysis. Peritoneal Dial Bull 3: 142, 1983
4. Valles M, Cantarell C, Vila J, and Tovar JL: Delayed perforation of the colon by a Tenckhoff catheter. Peritoneal Dial Bull 2: 190, 1982

R.H.J. Beelen, J. van der Meulen, H. Verbrugh,
E.C.M. Hoefsmit, P.L. Oe, and J. Verhoef

100

CAPD, a Permanent State of Peritonitis:
A Study on Peroxidase Activity

SUMMARY

In vivo in the animal model peritoneal
macrophages can be divided by their peroxidase
activity (PA) pattern in exudate-, exudate-resident-,
resident- and PA-negative macrophages. In the normal steady state 90% of the macrophages are resident cells. After acute inflammation, exudate and
exudate-resident macrophages appear, whereas
after chronic inflammation exudate and PA-negative
macrophages appear. CAPD patients with clear
peritoneal effluent were studied because they are
considered to be in a normal steady state. However,
in only one of six patients resident macrophages
were found. Exudate and PA-negative macrophages
were always found, suggesting that in otherwise
asymptomatic CAPD chronic inflammation exists.
The clinical significance of the presence of resident
macrophages is discussed.

INTRODUCTION

The diaminobenzidine (DAB) technique developed by Graham and Karnovsky[1] to localize (extracellular) horseradish peroxidase has also been used

From the Departments of Electron Microscopy and
Internal Medicine, Medical Faculty and University Hospi-
tal, Free University, Amsterdam, The Netherlands, and
Department of Infectious Diseases, University Hospital,
Utrecht, The Netherlands.

to study the localization of endogenous peroxidase
activity (PA) in various types of cells, including
blood monocytes and tissue macrophages.

Extensive morphologic and cytochemical studies in the animal model have shown, that peritoneal
fluid contains macrophages with divergent PA, the
relative proportions of the different types of
macrophages varying with the state of inflammation
in the peritoneum. Macrophages derived from a
normal unstimulated peritoneal cavity show PA
exclusively in the nuclear envelope and rough
endoplasmic reticulum (RER).[2-5] They are called
resident macrophages and have never been discovered *in vivo* in man,[6-8] however, they have been seen
in vitro after culturing human blood monocytes.[6,9]

In peritoneal exudates of animals, macrophages
show PA only in some of the lysosomal granules,[2-4]
as in blood monocytes[2,3,10] and are called exudate
macrophages. In human blood, monocytes and
macrophages from pleural exudates this PA localization is also seen.[6] This difference in PA pattern between monocytes and resident macrophages has
been used to challenge the monocytic origin of resident macrophages.[11] However, recently we identified transitional exudate-resident and PA-negative
cells during acute inflammation in rats and
mice,[2,12,13] which is in agreement with derivation of
all macrophages from one lineage according to the
concept of the mononuclear phagocyte system
(MPS).[14]

The present study further investigates the
dynamics of the four types of PA pattern in perito-

neal macrophages seen in the animal model. The dynamics are related to the type of inflammation induced.

Moreover, in this study we have investigated the PA pattern of the peritoneal macrophages isolated from CAPD patients without peritonitis. We compare these human results with the animal experiments. This comparison suggests that inspite of the clinical impression of absence of peritonitis a peritoneal inflammatory state exists.

MATERIAL AND METHODS

Peritoneal Cells

Male Wistar rats weighing 180 to 200 g were used. Cell suspensions from the unstimulated peritoneal cavity were obtained after gentle kneading of the abdomen. Peritoneal exudates were induced by intraperitoneal administration of sterile newborn calf serum (NBCS), according to Beelen et al.[2] and van Furth and Cohn,[15] which caused acute inflammation. Chronic inflammation was induced by intraperitoneal administration of paraffin oil. The cells from the peritoneal cavity were isolated up to 8 days as described in detail elsewhere.[2]

CAPD patients. Six patients, treated with CAPD for 1 to 6 months, were investigated. At time of investigation the leukocyte count of the effluent peritoneal fluid was below $100 \times 10^6/L$. In the previous two weeks the effluent had always been clear. The peritoneal fluid was collected after a dwell time varying from 6 to 10 hours.

The cells were counted and differential counts were done from slides made with a cytospin. The number of different types of peritoneal macrophages was determined by counting the cells observed in electron microscopic sections; a minimum of 200 macrophages were counted that represented 3 to 6 experiments.

Cytochemical Procedures

Cells were fixed immediately after collection for 10 minutes in 1.5% glutaraldehyde at 4°C, washed three times and reacted for PA in DAB,[2] i.e., pH 6.5, preincubation and incubation (0.01%) one hour at 20°C. The cells were postfixed with OsO_4 for 30 minutes at 4°C, processed for electron microscopy and embedded in Araldite, since the oxidized DAB-polymer becomes electron opaque with OsO_4,[16] staining with lead citrate was omitted.

Staining with uranyl acetate was omitted because it could have extracted or masked the reaction product.[5] Control preparations consisted of preparations in which H_2O_2 was omitted.

RESULTS

Localization of Peroxidase Activity in Rat Peritoneal Macrophages *in Vivo*

Cell suspensions from the unstimulated peritoneum mainly contain macrophages (~70%) and granulocytes. The macrophages from the normal steady-state rats predominantly (>90%) show PA in the nuclear envelope and RER (Fig. 1A). These are resident macrophages.

After induction of an acute inflammatory reaction with NBCS or a chronic inflammatory reaction with paraffin oil, four populations of macrophages can be distinguished on the basis of their different patterns of PA. First, some macrophages of the peritoneal exudates show the PA pattern of normal resident macrophages. Second, macrophages of the peritoneal exudates show reaction product in a varying number of lysosomal granules (Fig. 1B) and so show the PA pattern of blood monocytes and exudate macrophages. Third, some macrophages of the peritoneal exudate, however, show reaction products both in the nuclear envelope and the RER and in a varying number of lysosomal granules (Fig. 1C). The granules of these cells show exactly the same localization (preferentially Golgi area), dimensions (100 to 450 nm), morphologic characteristics (i.e., oval or spherical and occasionally elongated), and cytochemical characteristics as those of the exudate macrophages. The reactivity of the nuclear envelope and RER in these cells behave just like those in resident macrophages. Since these cells have the combined morphologic and cytochemical features of both the exudate and the resident macrophages, we have called them exudate-resident macrophages.[2] In addition, there is a fourth population of macrophages in the peritoneal exudates; these cells show no reaction product at all and are called PA-negative macrophages.

Quantitative Aspects of These Four Types of Macrophages

After induction of an acute inflammation (Fig. 2A) the total number of resident macrophages decreases to 2×10^6 cells at 24 hours and then in-

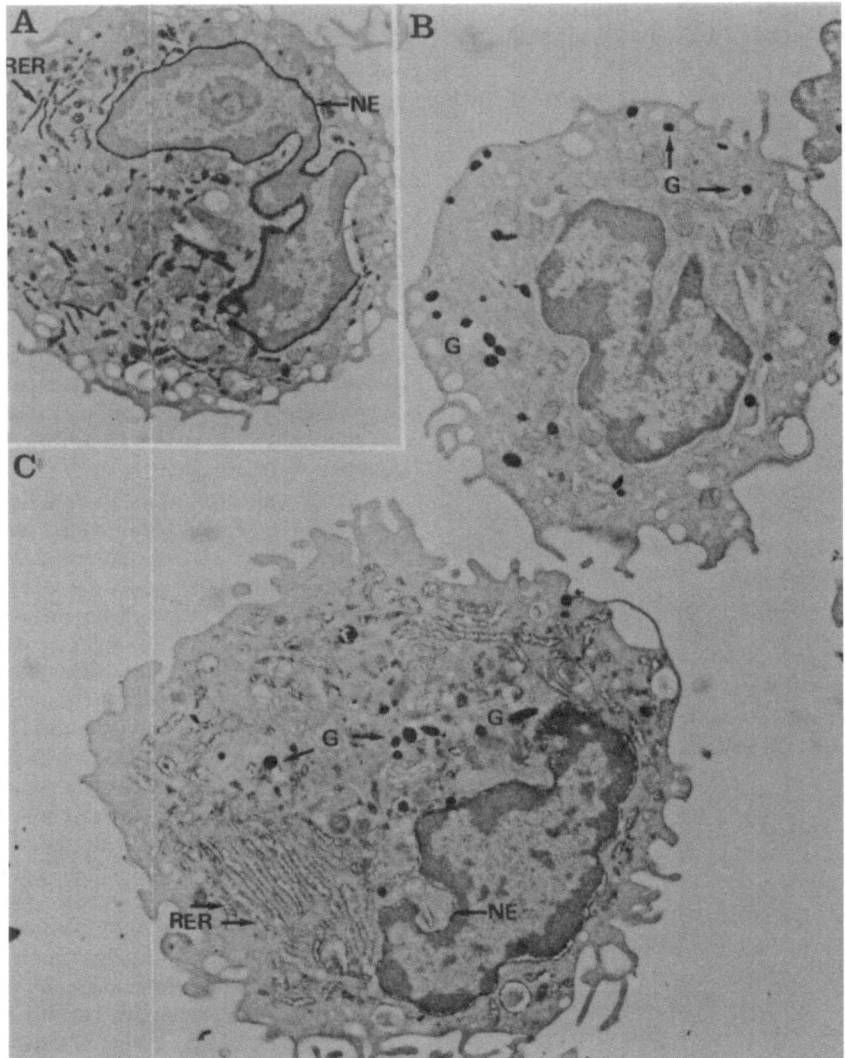

Fig. 1. Three patterns of peroxidase activity representing three types of macrophage. (**A**) Resident macrophages with reaction product in the nuclear envelope (NE) and RER (RER). (**B**) Exudate macrophages with reaction product in cytoplasmic granules (G) (lysosomal vesicles). (**C**) Exudate-resident macrophages with reaction product in the lysosomal vesicles as well as in the nuclear envelope and RER (x 9000).

creased until the normal level is regained 8 days after induction. The number of exudate macrophages rises sharply, with a peak at 24 hours and then decreases, returning to the normal level after 8 days. The exudate-resident macrophages, which first appear 24 hours after induction of inflammation, reach a maximum of about 2×10^6 cells at 48 to 96 hours and then decrease (Fig. 2A). The kinetics of these three types of macrophages during acute inflammation clearly show that the maxima of exudate-resident cells coincide with the sharp decrease in the number of exudate macrophages and the rapid increase in the number of resident macrophages, which indicates that exudate-resident macrophages are indeed a transitional form between exudate and resident macrophages. PA-negative macrophages are present only in low and fairly constant numbers during an acute inflammation.

After the induction of a chronic inflammation (Fig. 2B), the number of exudate macrophages and PA-negative macrophages rises sharply to about 12 × 10⁶ cells at 2 days and remains at that level up to 8 days. The number of resident macrophages, which decreases after induction of the inflammation, remains at a constant level of about 2×10^6 cells. Exudate-resident macrophages, which first appear after induction of the inflammation, also remain at a fairly constant level of 2×10^6 cells for at least 8 days. The kinetics of these four types of macrophage during chronic inflammation suggest a constant influx of monocyte-derived exudate macrophages due to the chronic inflammatory conditions. These exudate macrophages may subsequently lose the PA in their lysosomal granules and become PA-negative.

Localization of PA in and Quantitative Aspects of Peritoneal Macrophages from CAPD Patients

The peritoneal effluents from the 6 CAPD patients contained 3.5 to 27×10^6 cells/L. In the differential count all patients had at least 50% macrophages and varying percentages of other cells

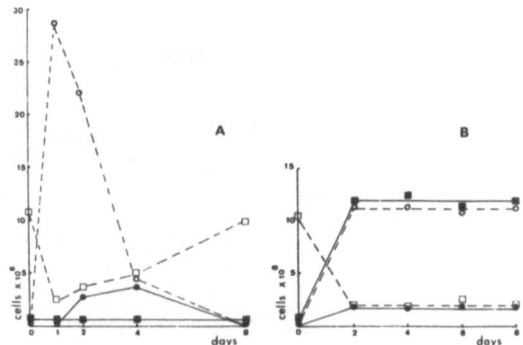

Fig. 2. Absolute numbers of exudate (—○—), exudate-resident (—●—), resident (—□—), and peroxidase activity-negative macrophages (—■—) in the inflammatory peritoneal exudates elicited with (**A**) newborn calf serum (acute inflammation) or (**B**) paraffin oil (chronic inflammation) in rat.

(mainly lymphocytes, granulocytes, and mesothelial cells).

With respect to the cytochemistry the macrophages are exudate macrophages (PA in the lysosomal granules) or PA-negative macrophages (Fig. 3). The distribution of PA may suggest that a chronic inflammatory state in all six patients is present as compared with the inflammation induced with paraf-

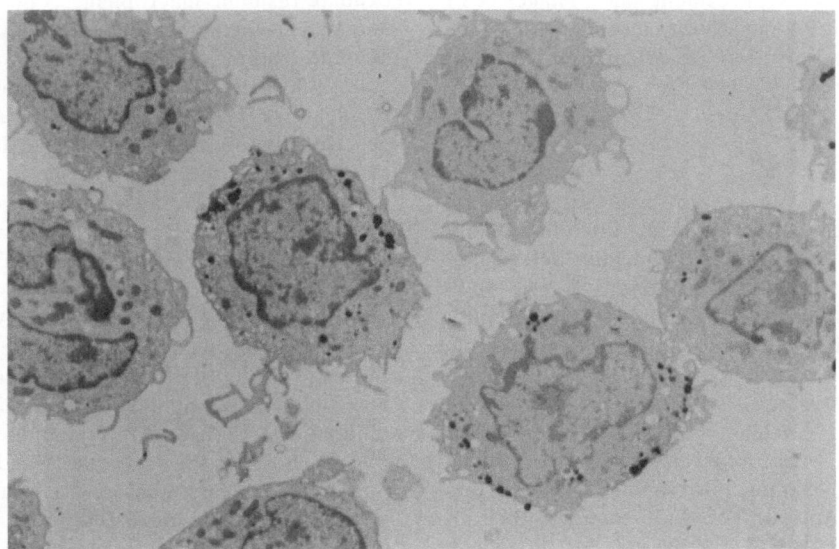

Fig. 3. Three patterns of PA as observed in peritoneal macrophages from CAPD patients. Exudate macrophages and PA-negative macrophages (x 4500). See Figure 4.

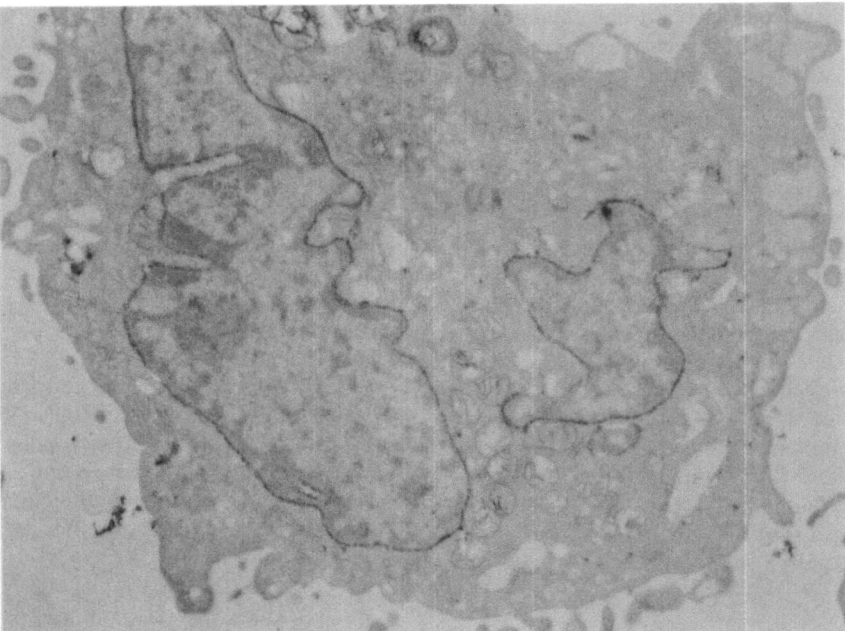

Fig. 4.   Human resident macrophage *in vivo* (x 14,500).

fin oil in the rat. In one patient, however, we clearly demonstrate the existence of resident macrophages *in vivo* (PA in the nuclear envelope and RER; Fig. 4). The relative percentages of the exudate, PA-negative and resident macrophages are shown in Fig. 5. In the one patient with resident macrophages (4%), the number of PA-negative macrophages is 22%, which is relatively low as compared to other patients.

DISCUSSION

Populations of macrophages are functionally, morphologically and cytochemically heterogeneous,[17] but the basis for this diversity has yet to be resolved,[18] but are best explained by stage of maturation-differentiation of cells belonging to one lineage.[14,19]

Our ultrastructural studies in the rat revealed the presence of at least 4 types of macrophages differing in PA staining characteristics,[2] which prompted us to examine the dynamics of the subpopulations with the aim of understanding their interrelationship also in comparison to the type of inflammation induced.

Under normal steady state conditions we found predominance of resident macrophages that agrees with findings of others in the animal model.[2,4,5,20] After inducing acute inflammation there was a rapid influx of blood monocytes that are classified as exudate macrophages, and these cells transform into resident macrophages via the transitional stage of exudate-resident macrophage (Fig. 2A). After inducing chronic inflammation a constant influx of exudate macrophages was seen. These cells subsequently lost the PA in their lysosomes and became PA-negative (Fig. 2B). This loss of PA has also been described by others.[7,14,20,21] These data correspond exactly with earlier experiments in which we[3,6,13] and others[5,9] have shown that *in vitro* blood monocytes and exudate macrophages transform into exudate-resident macrophages and PA-negative cells and subsequently into resident macrophages. We therefore strongly suggest that the divergent PA patterns as seen *in vivo* and *in vitro* represent changes in the stage of activation or stage of development of the macrophage subpopulations that all belong to the mononuclear phagocyte population.[2,14,19,22] As clearly shown in the rat model, the dynamics of the macrophage subpopulations are related to the state of inflammation induced (Fig. 2).

In humans until now no resident macrophages have been described.[6-8] The absence of these cells in the human system could be due to the fact that the cells are mostly withdrawn from patients suffering

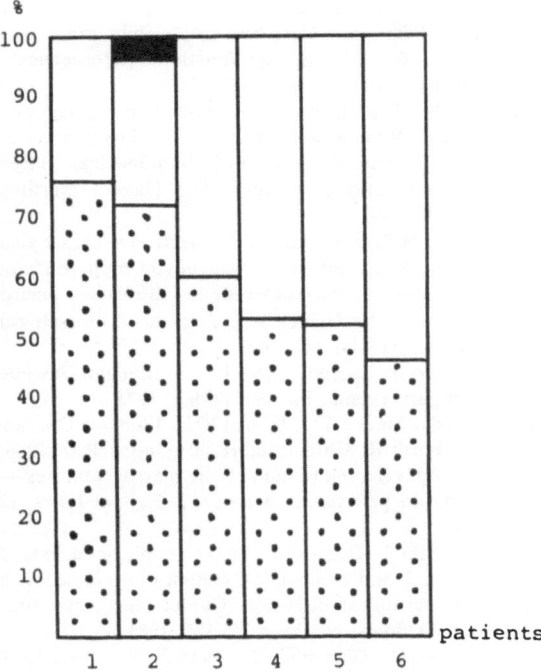

Fig. 5. The distribution (%) of *in vivo* exudate (▣), PA-negative (□) and resident macrophages (■) in six CAPD patients.

from chronic inflammation.[6] Alternatively resident macrophages may remain adherent to the wall of the peritoneal serous cavity, when they are recovered (in animals the abdomen is kneaded, which may result in detachment of the resident macrophages when the cells are withdrawn). Finally, their absence could be due to the fact that in human *in vivo* resident macrophages do not exist.

In this study we have looked at the content of the peritoneal effluent of CAPD patients without peritonitis in the previous 2 weeks, since we expected them firstly to be a rich source of macrophages and second, because their cellularity might be of diagnostic value indicating early bacterial peritonitis.[23,24] As shown in this paper (Fig. 4), resident macrophages were found *in vivo* in this study, which at least shows that it is possible to find this type of cell in men.

Only in one of six patients studied were resident macrophages found (Fig. 5), and we conclude that in CAPD patients a chronic inflammatory state exists.

The clinical significance of the presence of resident macrophages in CAPD patients is purely specu-

lative. One may claim that the aim should be to have a high percentage of resident macrophages during CAPD treatment because this presence reflects an unstimulated peritoneum. On the other hand resident macrophages represent an end-stage of a phagocytic cell line, most probably less able to attack invading microorganisms. A high percentage of these aged cells could mean a lack in mobilizing exudate macrophages, necessary to attack invading microorganisms. The functional differences in immune effector functions as killing of *Staphylococcus epidermis in vitro*[25] between these macrophage subpopulations are presently under study.

ACKNOWLEDGMENTS

The authors would like to thank Inge Eestermans for technical assistance, Shimon Paniry for preparing the micrographs and Anjo Steenvoorden-Bosma for typing the manuscript. Supported in part by the Kidney Foundation, Amsterdam, The Netherlands.

REFERENCES

1. Graham RC, and Karnovsky MJ: The early stages of absorption of injected horseradish peroxidase in the proximal tubules of mouse kidney: Ultrastructural cytochemistry by a new technique. J Histochem Cytochem 14: 291, 1966
2. Beelen RHJ, Broekhuis-Fluitsma DM, Korn C, and Hoefsmit ECM: Identification of exudate-resident macrophages on the basis of peroxidatic activity. J Reticuloendothel Soc 23: 103, 1978
3. Beelen RHJ, Fluitsma DM, van der Meer JWM, and Hoefsmit ECM: Development of the different peroxidatic activity patterns in peritoneal macrophages in vivo and in vitro. J Reticuloendothel Soc 25: 513, 1979
4. Lepper AWD, and D'Arcy Hart P: Peroxidase staining in elicited and non-elicited mononuclear cells from BCG-sensitized and non-sensitized mice. Infect Immunol 14: 522, 1976
5. Bodel PT, Nichols BA, and Bainton DF: Differences in peroxidase localization of rabbit peritoneal macrophages after surface adherence. Am J Pathol 91: 107, 1978
6. Beelen RHJ, van 't Veer M, Fluitsma DM, and Hoefsmit ECM: Identification of different peroxidatic activity patterns in human macrophages in vivo and in vitro. J Reticuloendothel Soc 24: 355, 1978
7. Watanabe N, Masubuchi S, and Kageyama K: Ultrastructural localization of peroxidase in mononuclear phagocytes from the peritoneal cavity, blood, bone

marrow and omentum, with a special reference to the origin of peritoneal macrophages. Rec Adv RES Res 11: 120, 1973

8. Bainton DF, and Golde DW: Differentiation of macrophages from normal human bone marrow in liquid culture—electron microscopy and cytochemistry. J Clin Invest 61: 1555, 1978

9. Bodel PT, Nichols BA, and Bainton DF: Appearance of peroxidatic reactivity within the rough endoplasmic reticulum of blood monocytes after surface adherence. J Exp Med 145: 264, 1977

10. Van der Rhee HJ, de Winter CPM, and Daems WT: Fine structure and peroxidatic activity of rat blood monocytes. Cell Tissue Res 185: 1, 1977

11. Daems WT, and Koerten HK: The effects of various stimuli on the cellular composition of peritoneal exudates in the mouse. Cell Tissue Res 190: 47, 1978

12. Beelen RHJ, and Fluitsma DM: What is the relevance of exudate-resident macrophages? Immunobiology 161: 266, 1982

13. Hoefsmit ECM, and Beelen RHJ: The expression of F4/80 and Ia on peritoneal macrophages in normal and BCG immunized mice. In van Furth R (Ed), Mononuclear phagocytes in inflammation. The Hague: Martinus Nijhoff, 1984

14. Van Furth R, Cohn ZA, Hirsch JG, Humphrey JH, Spector WG, and Langevoort HL: The mononuclear phagocyte system: A new classification of macrophages, monocytes and their precursor cells. Bull WHO 46: 845, 1972

15. Van Furth R, and Cohn ZA: The origin and kinetics of mononuclear cells. J Exp Med 128: 415, 1968

16. Tice LW: Effect of hypophysectomy and TSH replacement on the ultrastructural localization of thyroidperoxidase. Endocrinology 95: 421, 1974

17. Förster O, and Landy M: Heterogeneity of mononuclear phagocytes. New York: Academic Press, 1981

18. Walker WS: Macrophage functional heterogeneity. Adv Exp Med Biol 155: 435, 1982

19. Van Furth R: Cells of the mononuclear phagocyte system. Nomenclature in terms of sites and conditions. In van Furth R (Ed), Mononuclear phagocytes—functional aspects. The Hague: Martinus Nijhoff, 1980, p 1

20. Daems WT, and Brederoo P: Electron microscopical studies on the structure, phagocytic properties and peroxidatic activity of resident and exudate macrophages in the Guinea pig. Zeitschr Zellforsch Mikrosk Anat 144: 247, 1973

21. Büchner T: Entzündungszellen im Blut und Gewebe. Stuttgart, Gustav Fischer Verlag, 1971

22. Van der Meer JWM, Beelen RHJ, Fluitsma DM, and van Furth R: Ultrastructure of mononuclear phagocytes developing in liquid bone marrow cultures—a study on peroxidatic activity. J Exp Med 149: 17, 1979

23. Cichocki T, Hanicki Z, Sulowicz W, Smoleński O, Kopeć J, and Zembala M: Output of peritoneal cells into peritoneal dialysate. Cytochemical and functional studies. Nephron 35: 175, 1983

24. Piccoli G, Giacchino F, Belardi P, Quarello F, Alloatti S, Giacchino M, and Musso A: Immune response in peritoneal dialysis (CAPD). In LaGreca G, Biasioli S, and Ronco C (Eds), Peritoneal dialysis. Milan: Wichtig Editore, 1982, p 479

25. Verbrugh HA, Hoidal JR, Nguyen BYT, Verhoef J, Quie PG, and Peterson PK: Human alveolar macrophage cytophilic immunoglobulin G-mediated phagocytosis of protein A-positive Staphylococci. J Clin Invest 69: 63, 1982

H.E. Leichter, I.B. Salusky, M. Wilson, T. Hall, S.C. Jordan,
R.B. Ettenger, and R.N. Fine

101

A 3 1/2 Year Experience with Peritonitis in Children Undergoing CAPD and CCPD

SUMMARY

In 3 1/2 years 68 children, mean age 11.1 years, were trained for CAPD or CCPD. Sixty-three episodes of peritonitis occurred during 654 patient months of CAPD (one every 10.4 months) and 31 during 256 patient months of CCPD (one every 8.3 months). At 12 months, 46% were free of peritonitis. Sterile cultures were frequent. When identified, organisms were usually gram positive. Infections responded to antibiotic therapy alone in most cases. Cefazolin was used as initial therapy but tobramycin was added for gram negative organisms. Persistent or recurrent infections were managed by transient catheter removal. The overall catheter survival rate was 69% at one year.

INTRODUCTION

Since the initial use in children in 1979,[1-2] continuous ambulatory peritoneal dialysis (CAPD) has been shown to be an effective dialytic modality for treatment of children with end-stage renal disease (ESRD).[3-8] Although renal transplantation is the ultimate treatment goal in such patients, CAPD remains an acceptable alternative while awaiting a renal transplant.

The major advantage of CAPD is the adequate control of the clinical manifestations of uremia,

blood pressure, and decreased blood transfusion requirements. Increased freedom and mobility are significant benefits associated with CAPD. Unfortunately, there are both psychosocial and medical disadvantages. Repetitive performance of the exchange procedures can lead to patient and parent "burnout." Peritonitis and catheter related problems are the major medical disadvantages. In an attempt to decrease the risk of peritonitis secondary to multiple connections and disconnections, and to avoid potential patient or family burnout, continuous cycling peritoneal dialysis (CCPD) was introduced.[9]

This present study reports our experience with peritonitis in children undergoing CAPD, and CCPD during the past 3 1/2 years.

MATERIALS AND METHODS

Patient Population

In the 3 1/2 years since the initiation of our program in August 1980, 68 patients (35 males, 33 females), aged 3 months to 21 years (mean 11.1 ± 7 (SEM) years) have been trained for CAPD and/or CCPD. We evaluated the incidence of peritonitis in these 68 patients who had undergone CAPD and CCPD for 11.1 ± 1.0 and 8.4 ± 1.2 months, respectively (range 1 to 38 months). Sixty-two patients (91%) were initially trained for CAPD and 21 (34%) were subsequently switched to CCPD after 12.7 ± 2.0 months of CAPD; only one patient returned to

From the UCLA School of Medicine, Division of Pediatric Nephrology, Los Angeles, California.

CAPD. In six patients (9%), CCPD was the initial dialysis modality.

Dialysis Technique and Peritoneal Access

CAPD was accomplished with four to five daily exchanges, with a volume ranging from 30 to 50 ml/Kg body weight per exchange, depending upon commercially available dialysate volumes (Dianeal®, Travenol Laboratories, Deerfield, IL). CCPD was performed with five, 2 hour nighttime exchanges (AMP 80/2 cycler, American Medical Products Corporation, Freehold, NJ) followed by a single diurnal dwell at one-half the nocturnal volume, or with no daytime dwell. The dialysis fluid dextrose concentration was adjusted to the desired degree of ultrafiltration, which depended upon the patient's blood pressure and body weight. According to the degree of acidosis, either PD 1 or PD 2 (Travenol Laboratories) was used to maintain the serum bicarbonate level within normal limits.

All patients were dialyzed through a permanent indwelling catheter. Partial omentectomy was performed at the time of catheter placement. Single-cuff, double-cuff Tenckhoff and column disc (Life cath) catheters were used.

For the first 48 to 72 hours following catheter insertion, automated peritoneal dialysis with low volumes and frequent exchanges was initiated. Antibiotics (cefazolin 250 mg/L) and heparin (250 U/L) were added to the dialysate for the first 48 hours following surgery. If uremic symptoms did not necessitate the immediate initiation of CAPD, the patients or their parents were trained in ten sessions to perform CAPD or CCPD. Patients who required immediate dialysis to relieve symptoms had intermittent peritoneal dialysis (IPD) for 8 hours three times a week until appropriate training was accomplished.

Diagnosis and Initial Management of Peritonitis

During the training period, each patient and/or parent was instructed to recognize the signs and symptoms of peritonitis. These are cloudy dialysate fluid, abdominal pain, fever, and vomiting. If any of the latter occurred, the patient and/or parent was instructed to call the CAPD nurse, who was available 24 hours a day, 7 days a week. The nurse instructed patients to drain the dialysate solution from the abdominal cavity, save the bag in the refrigera-

tor, and proceed with three rapid exchanges with the usual volumes, followed by 4–6 hour exchanges with dialysate containing heparin (250 U/L) and cefazolin (250 mg/L). The first and fourth bag were saved and brought to the hospital. The decision to hospitalize the patient and to initiate parenteral treatment depended on the severity of the clinical symptoms.

Peritoneal dialysate (10 ml) was obtained from each bag for cell count, Gram stain and culture. The diagnosis of peritonitis was based on clinical findings and an increased cell count (>100 cells/mm^3) in the dialysate. CAPD patients continued with their regular exchanges. CCPD patients were switched to CAPD for at least 4 to 6 days. Recurrent peritonitis was defined as the presence of the same organism within 2 weeks after stopping antibiotic therapy. Persistent infection was defined as persistence of positive dialysate cultures with the same organism, despite appropriate antibiotic treatment.

Treatment of Peritonitis

Initially, all patients were placed on cefazolin (250 mg/L) and heparin (250 U/L) intraperitoneally (IP). If the smear indicated Gram-negative bacteria, or the cloudy bags did not clear up within 48 hours treatment, intraperitoneal therapy with tobramycin (8 mg/L) was initiated. Repeated cultures were taken at days 5 and 10, and if the last culture (day 10) was negative, 48 hours after therapy was discontinued.

Uncomplicated "no growth" and Gram-positive infections were treated with cefazolin intraperitoneally for 12 to 14 days. If tunnel infections coincided with the peritonitis, additional parenteral oxacillin was given for 3 to 5 days, followed by oral therapy according to the clinical situation.

Peritonitis with Gram-negative organisms was treated for 21 days intraperitoneally. Antibiotics were used according to the different sensitivities. Tobramycin was used in all patients with Gram-negative episodes. In three instances, additional 10 days of parenteral therapy with ticarcillin, which is synergistic with aminoglycosides, was used in recurrent peritonitis. In fungal infections, catheter removal and switching to hemodialysis was carried out for at least three weeks. Indications for removal of the peritoneal catheter were recurrent or persistent peritonitis and tunnel infections resistant to therapy.

Data are expressed as mean ± SEM. Life table analysis was used to describe the catheter survival and the interval to the first episode of peritonitis.

Table 1. Etiology of Peritonitis Episodes (n = 94).

Organism	CAPD	CCPD	Total		%
No growth	30	12	42		44
Staph. aureus	9	5	14		
Coag neg Staph.	8	2	10		
				29	31
Strep. viridans	3	—	3		
Beta streptococcus	1	1	2		
Pseudomonas aeruginosa	2	3	5		
Enterobacteria	1	3	4		
Klebsiella pneumoniae	1	2	3		
				20	22
Serratia marcescens	2	1	3		
E. coli	2	2	4		
Hemophilus influenzae	1	0	1		
Candida albicans	2	0	2		2
Anaerobic bacteria	1	0	1		1
Number of Episodes	63	31	94		100

RESULTS

There were 94 peritonitis episodes during 910 patient months in the 68 patients. Sixty-three occurred during 654 patient months of CAPD (1 every 10.4 patient months) and 31 during 256 patient months of CCPD (1 every 8.3 patient months) with an overall CAPD and/or CCPD incidence of 1 every 9.7 patient months. Thirty-one children had the first peritonitis episode after 6 ± 1.0 months of CAPD and 15 children after 6.3 ± 1.4 months of CCPD. Forty-six percent of the patients were peritonitis free at 12 months of CAPD/CCPD and 33% at 24 months, by life table analysis. Cloudy bags, abdominal pain, vomiting, and fever were the primary symptoms, although in nine episodes (9.6%), only one of these symptoms was present.

In 42 episodes (44%), the cultures revealed no growth, while 29 (31%) yielded Gram-positive organisms. Gram-negative bacteria accounted for 20 (22%) episodes. Candida albicans was present in two patients (2%) while anaerobic bacteria were seen in one patient. The etiology of peritonitis is shown in Table 1.

Sixteen episodes (16/94, 17%) were associated with recurrent or persistent infections in 15 patients (15/68, 22%). The etiology is shown in Table 2.

Despite appropriate antibiotic treatment, these infections were not eradicated and, in all but one instance, replacement of the catheter was necessary.

Two patients with Pseudomonas aeruginosa peritonitis were switched temporarily to hemodialysis for 4 weeks. One Pseudomonas infection responded to intraperitoneal antibiotic therapy and two children with residual renal function had a catheter removal and were off dialysis for 10 days before reinsertion of a new catheter. Fungal infections (Candida albicans) occurred in two patients without any previously treated bacterial peritonitis. In both cases, the catheter was removed.

Membrane loss occurred in three children. Two of them experienced significant damage to the peritoneum after Candida albicans peritonitis. The remaining patient had a second Staphylococcus aureus peritonitis episode within 1 year, precluding

Table 2. Etiology of Recurrent or Persistent Peritonitis.

Organism	CAPD	CCPD	Total
Staph. aureus	2	3	5
Pseudomonas	1	3	4
Candida albicans	2	—	2
Enterobacter	1	—	1
E. coli	—	1	1
Serratia marcescens	—	1	1
Coag neg Staph.	1	—	1
Strep. viridans	1	—	1

continuation of peritoneal dialysis. Each lost ultra-filtration capacity and were switched to hemodialy-sis. Death occurred in two patients (3%), unrelated to peritonitis.

A total of 97 dialysis catheters were inserted. Double-cuff Tenckhoff catheters were used initially and a total or 51 were inserted. Twenty single cuff Tenckhoff catheters were used. Recently, we have used 26 column discs (Lifecath). The catheter sur-vival for two cuff catheters was 87% at 1 year, com-pared to 52% with one-cuff Tenckhoff and Lifecath catheters. The difference was significant (p < 0.006). The overall survival rate for 1 year was 69%.

DISCUSSION

Since the first description of CAPD in 1976 by Popovich et al.,[10] peritonitis has been a major prob-lem. The initial use of dialysate containing bottles which necessitated "breaking" of the system twice during each exchange led to high rates of peritonitis. In 1978, Oreopoulos et al.,[11] introduced the use of dialysate in plastic bags. Following the instillation of the dialysate solution into the peritoneal cavity, the bag could be attached to the body and utilized for efflux of the spent dialysate several hours later. By this modification, the number of disconnections was reduced by 50%, thereby decreasing the incidence of peritonitis. There are only a few reports detailing the incidence of peritonitis in children.[12–15] Potter et al.[12] and Alexander,[13] reported one episode every 3.3 and 4.1 patient months, respectively. However, this was prior to the availability of smaller volumes of dialysate in bags in the United States. Subsequent studies demonstrated major improvements. The peritonitis rate reported by Balfe et al.[14] and that from our center[15] were one episode every 13.1 pa-tient months and one every 12.5 patient months, respectively. The present report indicates an overall peritonitis rate of one episode every 9.7 patient months. Despite the use of CCPD, the infection rate was not improved (1/8.3 CCPD, 1/10.4 CAPD), indi-cating that fewer connections do not necessarily decrease the risk of peritonitis. More recent studies by Keane et al.,[16] have indicated that other factors, such as the host defense system or other immuno-logic parameters, play a significant role in the perito-nitis rate. It has been shown that the degree of bacterial opsonization, which is critical to the effec-tive defense of the peritoneal cavity by phagocytic cells, may predispose patients to develop peritoni-tis. The peritonitis rate with Staphylococcus epider-midis in patients with "high" peritoneal dialysate

opsonic activity against this bacterial species was lower than in patients with "low" peritoneal dialysis opsonic activity.

Our study shows a relatively high percentage of cultures (44%) with no growth. This may be related to the culture method. No attempt was made to concentrate the dialysate in order to increase the yield as previously described.[17–18] Another factor contributing to the low yield may be the lag-time between the initiation of the symptoms and the time of culturing. Because of long distances from the hospital, the "infected" dialysate was frequently refrigerated overnight prior to culturing.

Gram-positive infections responded to cefa-zolin treatment, yet 7 of the 16 recurrent or persistent peritonitis episodes were caused by Staphylococci and Streptococci, requiring catheter removal. Gram-negative infections were present in seven recurrent peritonitis episodes. It is interesting to note that no patient with a Gram-negative infec-tion had to be transferred to hemodialysis.

Fungal infections are the most serious cause of peritonitis. They do not respond to antifungal ther-apy, and catheter removal with subsequent switch-ing to hemodialysis is necessary for at least 2 to 3 weeks. There is no doubt that fungal infections strongly indicate prompt catheter removal. This can be emphasized by our finding that peritoneal damage consequent to fungal peritonitis led to discontinua-tion of peritoneal dialysis in two patients.

Therapy for peritonitis in patients on CAPD has not been standardized. Our regimen for uncomplica-ted peritonitis episodes seems to be effective. In complicated peritoneal infections (i.e., Gram-nega-tive peritonitis) even a prolonged course of intraperi-toneal and parenteral treatment could not prevent early catheter removal. As indicated in another study,[19] catheter removal is the treatment of choice in some patients.

Initially, we used double-cuff Tenckhoff cath-eters, but the prevalence of exit site infections, as well as extrusion of the proximal cuff through the skin exit site precipitated switching to the single-cuff catheter. With the column disc catheter, problems developed in small children, because of the large size of the elbow where the catheter inserts into the peritoneal cavity. In this area, there was a high inci-dence of traumatic hematoma; because of the lack of subcutaneous tissue, leading to an increased risk of infection.

Peritonitis still remains a major medical disad-vantage in addition to catheter related problems. The long-term efficiency of the peritoneum as a dialyzing membrane, especially after several peritonitis episodes, can ultimately limit the prolonged use of peritoneal dialysis. Further studies are necessary to detect patients at risk to develop peritonitis and to determine the immunologic factors which may predispose to peritonitis. Efforts to further decrease the incidence of peritonitis by using inline filters or ultraviolet radiation have not as yet proven to be effective.[20] At present, despite these problems, the use of CAPD/CCPD is an adequate dialysis modality for children until a transplant becomes available.

ACKNOWLEDGMENTS

We thank Amy Landsberg for her excellent secretarial assistance. Heinz E. Leichter is supported by a grant from the "Deutsche Forschungsgemeinschaft." Supported in part by the Peter Y. Boxembaum Research Fund.

REFERENCES

1. Oreopoulos DG, Katirtzoglou A, Arbus G, and Cordy P: Dialysis and transplantation in young children. Br Med J 1: 1628, 1979
2. Balfe JW, and Irwin MA: Continuous ambulatory peritoneal dialysis in pediatrics. In Legrain M (Ed), Continuous ambulatory peritoneal dialysis. Amsterdam: Excerpta Medica, 1980, p 131
3. Alexander SR, Tseng CH, Maksym KA, Campbell RA, Talwalkar YB, and Kohaut EC: Clinical parameters in CAPD for infants and children. In Moncrief JW, and Popovich RP (Eds), CAPD update. New York: Masson Publishing, 1981, p 195
4. Potter DE, McDaid TK, McHenry K, and Mar H: Continuous ambulatory peritoneal dialysis in children. Trans Am Soc Artif Intern Organs 27: 64, 1981
5. Salusky IB, Lucullo L, Nelson P, and Fine RN: Continuous ambulatory peritoneal dialysis in children. Pediatr Clin North Am 29: 1005, 1982
6. Baum M, Powell D, Calvin S, McDaid T, McHenry K, Mar H, and Potter D: Continuous ambulatory peritoneal dialysis in children. N Engl J Med 307: 1537, 1982
7. Salusky IB, Kopple JD, and Fine RN: Continuous ambulatory peritoneal dialysis in pediatric patients. A 20 month experience. Kidney Int 24(Suppl 15): 101, 1983
8. Leichter HE, Salusky IB, Alliapoulos JC, Hall T, Jordan SC, Ettenger RB, and Fine RN: CAPD and CCPD in children: An experience of 3 1/2 years. Dial Transpl 13: 382, 1984
9. Diaz-Buxo JA, Walker PJ, Farmer CD, Chandler J, and Holt K: Continuous cyclic peritoneal dialysis. Kidney Int 19: 145, 1981
10. Popovich RP, Moncrief JW, Decherd JB, Bomar JB, and Pyle WK: The definition of a novel portable/wearable equilibrium peritoneal dialysis technique. Abstr Am Soc Artif Intern Organs 5: 64, 1976
11. Oreopoulos DG, Robson M, Izatt S, Clayton S, and deVeber GA: A simple and safe technique for continuous ambulatory peritoneal dialysis (CAPD). Trans Am Soc Artif Intern Organs 24: 484, 1978
12. Potter DE, McDaid TK, and Ramirez JA: Peritoneal dialysis in children. In Atkins RC, Thomson NM, and Farrell PC (Eds), Peritoneal dialysis. Edinburgh, Churchill Livingstone, 1981, p 356
13. Alexander S: CAPD in children. 2nd national conference on CAPD. Kansas City, MO, Feb 15–17, 1982 (unpublished)
14. Balfe JW, Vigneux A, and Williamsen J: The use of CAPD in the treatment of children with end-stage renal disease. Peritoneal Dial Bull 1: 35, 1981
15. Fine RN, Salusky IB, Hall T, Lucullo L, Jordan SC, and Ettenger RB: Peritonitis in children undergoing continuous ambulatory peritoneal dialysis. Pediatrics 71: 806, 1983
16. Keane WF, Comty CM, Verbrugh HA, and Peterson PK: Opsonic deficiency of peritoneal dialysis effluent in continuous ambulatory peritoneal dialysis. Kidney Int 25: 539, 1984
17. Rubin J, Rogers WA, Taylor HM, Everett ED, Prowant BF, Fruto LV, and Nolph KD: Peritonitis during continuous ambulatory peritoneal dialysis. Ann Intern Med 92: 7, 1980
18. Vas S: Microbiological aspects of peritonitis. Peritoneal Dial Bull 1(Suppl): S11, 1981
19. Krothapalli R, Duffy WB, Lacke C, Payne W, Patel H, Perez V, and Senekjian HO: Pseudomonas peritonitis and continuous ambulatory peritoneal dialysis. Arch Intern Med 142: 1862, 1982
20. Ash SR, Horswell R Jr, Heeter EM, and Bloch R: Effect of the Peridex filter on peritonitis rates in a CAPD population. Peritoneal Dial Bull 3: 89, 1983

D.J. Tsakiris, T.C. Aitchison, J.D. Briggs, B.J.R. Junor, W.G.J. Smith, and M.A. Watson

102

Incidence of Peritonitis and Delayed-Type Hypersensitivity in Patients on CAPD

SUMMARY

Analysis of the incidence of peritonitis over a 3 year period was carried out, using techniques of survival data, in two groups of continuous ambulatory peritoneal dialysis (CAPD) patients who were separated on the basis of their cell-mediated immune response assessed by the skin reaction to dinitrochlorobenzene (DNCB). There were 28 weak and 23 strong DNCB reactors. Thirty-five percent of the first group remained free of peritonitis during the first 12 weeks of CAPD, compared to 75% of the latter group. Strong DNCB reactors also had a consistently higher probability of remaining free of peritonitis for longer before developing second and third episodes of peritonitis in comparison to the weak DNCB reactor group. Estimates of the mean times to the first, second and third episodes of peritonitis were 22, 43, and 70 weeks respectively for the weak DNCB group and 25, 84, and 109 weeks respectively for the strong reactor group. Although these differences between the groups failed to achieve statistical significance, there was a significant difference between the two groups in the number of patients requiring catheter removal following failure of antimicrobial therapy for bacterial peritonitis (67% vs 38%, $p < 0.05$). These results suggest that differences in the host immune response may influence susceptibility to peritonitis in CAPD patients.

From the Renal Unit, Western Infirmary and the Department of Statistics, University of Glasgow.

INTRODUCTION

CAPD has expanded rapidly in the UK over the last 5 years, but despite improvements in technique and equipment, peritonitis still remains the major complication. Although Corey[1] reported that peritonitis is distributed randomly, some patients develop this complication more often than others. Recently there has been an increasing interest in peritoneal defense mechanisms,[2-5] aiming to clarify the pathogenesis of peritonitis and identify characteristics of patients with high infection rates. Delayed-type hypersensitivity (DTH) responses to recall antigens have been used before to detect high risk patients in the general surgical population,[6] in critically ill patients,[7] and following renal transplantation.[8,9] The DNCB skin test has the advantage over those using recall antigens of not testing immunologic memory, since it is a new antigen to which patients will not previously have been exposed.[10] The object of this study was to determine whether there was any correlation between the incidence of peritonitis in CAPD patients and the host immune response measured by the DNCB skin test.

PATIENTS AND METHODS

Between November 1979 and October 1982, 66 patients were treated by CAPD in our unit. In 51 of these, (23 males, 28 females) whose ages ranged from 19 to 69 years, the DNCB test was performed within 2 months of the start of treatment. The technique of the test has been described previously.[10] The result is expressed as a score of 0 to 15 with scores of >3 being classed as indicating strong DTH reactors and 0 to 3 as weak reactors.

CAPD Technique

Access to the peritoneal cavity was gained with a single or double-cuffed Tenckhoff catheter inserted under general anesthesia. Patients used three or four 2 L exchanges/day (Travenol® or Fresenius®) according to individual needs, and the administration sets (Travenol® or Fresenius®) were changed every 4 weeks in hospital. The period of the survey extended until March 1983.

Peritonitis

Peritonitis was diagnosed on the basis of abdominal pain and a cloudy effluent. Dialysate white cell counts were only available from September 1982 and their results were not analyzed in this study. Gram stain and culture of dialysate were performed in all cases. We defined recurrence of peritonitis as an episode due to the same organism occurring within 2 weeks of discontinuing antibiotic therapy. These were considered as a single entry in the statistical analysis. Initial treatment of peritonitis consisted of intraperitoneal cefuroxime with the

addition of gentamicin and/or flucloxacillin later if indicated by the microbiological findings. When peritonitis failed to respond to antibiotics the catheter was removed and usually reinserted after 2 weeks.

Statistical Analysis

The incidence of the first, second, and third episodes of peritonitis in the two DNCB groups was analyzed separately, using techniques of survival data[11]: (1) the Kaplan-Meier method, which gives the estimated probability of surviving at least 't' weeks before each episode of peritonitis, against the exposed time 't' of treatment. (2) The log-rank test, with which we carried out a hypothesis test of whether the distribution of the time to each episode of peritonitis is the same in the two DNCB groups, and (3) we calculated the estimates of the mean times (with standard errors) to each episode based on the survival curves. All survival data computations were carried out using the statistical computing package BMDP, and in particular programs P1L and P2L.[12] The effects of age and sex on the probability of suffering an episode of peritonitis at any time were considered through a proportional hazards model.[11] The comparability of the two groups and the response of peritonitis to chemotherapy were assessed using the chi-square and Student's t tests.

Table 1. Characteristics of Patients of the Two DNCB Groups.

DNCB Score	Weak Reactors 0–3	Strong Reactors >3
Number of patients	28	23
Age: (yrs) mean ± SD	46.5 ± 12.9	51 ± 9.6
Sex: females	19 (68%)*	9 (39%)*
Primary renal disease		
Glomerulonephritis	8	7
Chronic pyelonephritis	7	1
Hypertensive nephrosclerosis	3	3
Diabetes	2	4
Polycystic kidneys	2	3
Miscellaneous	4	4
Unknown	2	2
Duration of CAPD (patient weeks)		
Total	1816	1820
Range	4–148	38–168
Mean ± SD	64.9 ± 45.5	79.1 ± 33.8

* $p < 0.05$.

Table 2. Peritonitis Episodes in the Two DNCB Groups.

DNCB Score	Weak Reactors 0–3	Strong Reactors >3
Number of patients	28	23
Total number of episodes	72	51
Fungal	4	3
Recurrences	20	9
Antimicrobial failure		
Number of patients needing catheter removal (for bacterial peritonitis only	18/27 (67%)*	8/21 (38%)*

* p < 0.05.

RESULTS

Twenty-eight patients had DNCB scores of 0 to 3, while 23 had scores of >3 (Table 1). The mean ages, duration of CAPD, and primary renal disease in the two groups were comparable. Females accounted for 68% of weak reactors and only 39% of strong reactors. This difference is significant (p < 0.05) and in keeping with previous studies.[10]

Seventy-two and 51 episodes of peritonitis occurred in the weak and strong reactors respectively (Table 2). There were more episodes of recurrent peritonitis among the weak reactors. Also there was a significant difference in the number of patients needing catheter removal following failure of antimicrobial therapy between the weak and strong reactors (67% versus 38% = p < 0.05). Other factors that might have influenced the development of peritonitis were comparable between the two groups (Table

3). The incidence of first, second, and third episodes of peritonitis in the two groups are shown in Figures 1, 2, and 3 respectively. At 12 weeks, approximately 35% of the weak reactors were free of peritonitis compared to 75% of the strong reactors at that stage. Strong reactors tended to have their first episode within 16 to 28 weeks and beyond 28 weeks the pattern appeared to be similar with approximately 25% of patients free of peritonitis in both groups. The strong reactors also had a higher probability of remaining free of second and third episodes for longer. Approximately 30% of the weak reactors were free of the second episode of peritonitis after 40 weeks of treatment compared to 60% of the strong reactors. After 60 weeks of treatment, 40% of the weak reactors were free of the third episode compared to 65% of the strong reactors. The differences between the two groups are not significant for any episode of peritonitis, although the suggestion from

Table 3. Other Factors Predisposing to Development of Peritonitis in the Two DNCB Groups.

DNCB Score	Weak Reactors 0–3	Strong Reactors >3
Number of patients	28	23
With poor compliance*	11	5
On hemodialysis prior to CAPD	10	7
With exit site infection associated with peritonitis	4	4
With fecal peritonitis	2	2
Serum albumin, mean ± SD (g/dl)	33.8 ± 4.4	31.9 ± 5.4

* Poor compliance was defined according to criteria cited in reference 14.

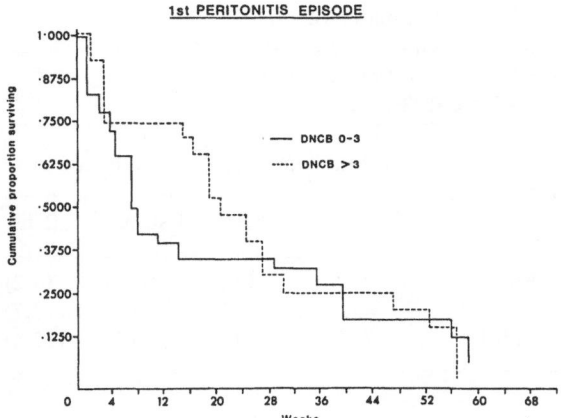

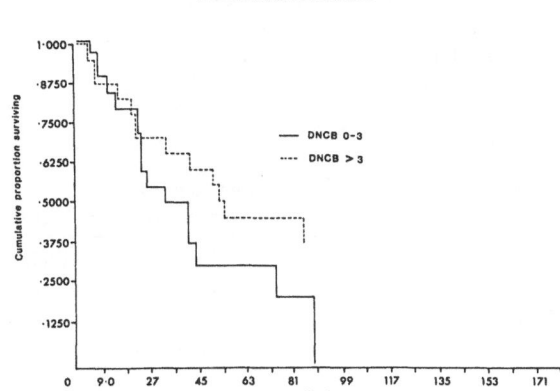

Fig. 1. Probability of remaining free of the first episode of peritonitis against the exposed time of treatment of the two DNCB groups of CAPD patients.

Fig. 2. Probability of remaining free of the second episode of peritonitis against the exposed time of treatment of the two DNCB groups of CAPD patients.

the p values (Table 4) and the estimated mean survival times (Table 5), is clear. Although sex clearly showed no effect at all on the probability of suffering any episode of peritonitis, there was an almost significant effect of age on the probability of suffering the third episode, but surprisingly as age increased the instantaneous probability of an episode of peritonitis decreased. This may be just an artefact of the data, since the strong reactors tended to be older than the weak reactors. Twenty-nine percent (8 of 28) of the weak reactors and 17% (4 of 23) of the strong reactors had more than three episodes of peritonitis but these numbers were too small for such episodes to be analyzed.

DISCUSSION

Corey[1] reported that the distribution of peritonitis in CAPD patients is random, and Pierratos et al.[13] supported this view by finding that the probability curve of the first episode of peritonitis is almost identical to that constructed from all episodes of peritonitis. However, both authors implied that their data did not exclude the fact that identifiable characteristics which predispose some patients to high infection rates may exist. Coward et al.[14] reported that poor compliers have a higher incidence, and persistent exit site infection due to *Staphylococcus aureus* may also predispose to peritonitis.[15] Secondary peritonitis may develop subsequent to chronic intra-abdominal infection or surgery.[16] Apart from these

factors it is reasonable to speculate that differences in the host immune response and particularly differences in the bactericidal activity of the mononuclear phagocytes may exist. Plant and Glynn[17] found that inbred mice strains, like BALB/c, which are susceptible to *Salmonella* infections had negative DTH responses, while more resistant strains, like CBA, gave positive ones. In humans Magliulo et al.[18] reported that macrophages from subjects hypersensitive to PPD had better phagocytic and bactericidal activity for *Paracolonbacter aeroginoides* com-

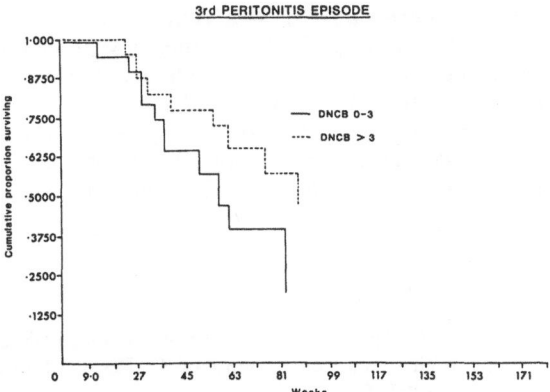

Fig. 3. Probability of remaining free of the third episode of peritonitis against the exposed time of treatment of the two DNCB groups of CAPD patients.

Table 4. Log-Rank Test of Equality of Distributions of Time to n^{th} Episode of Peritonitis in the Two DNCB Groups.

Episode of Peritonitis	Observed Value of Test Statistic	Degrees of Freedom	P-Value
First	0.04	1	0.84
Second	1.99	1	0.16
Third	23.4	1	0.13

Table 5. Estimates of Mean "Survival Times" (Weeks) until the nth Episode of Peritonitis in the Two DNCB Groups.

Episode of Peritonitis	Weak Reactors		Strong Rectors	
	Estimate	(SE)	Estimate	(SE)
First	21.5	(4.6)	108.9	(4.2)
Second	43.4	(6.5)	83.9	(15.7)
Third	70.1	(13.8)	108.9	(15.4)

pared to macrophages from subjects unreactive to PPD, while Lenzini et al.[19] found that patients with tuberculosis reactive to PPD had a marked early response to antituberculous drugs, whereas unreactive ones presented a poor response to treatment. Furthermore, in other reports[6-9] there is evidence of a correlation between DTH responses and resistance to infection in various types of high risk patients.

Our results, although not conclusive, suggest that differences may exist in the host immune response among CAPD patients in that strong DNCB reactors have a better chance of remaining free of peritonitis for longer, and also may have a better response to antibiotic therapy. Therefore, one can suggest that the response to DNCB may indicate differences in the peritoneal defense mechanisms. Diskin et al.[5] reported that bactericidal activity for *Staphylococcus aureus* was retained selectively only in four of the 12 CAPD patients they studied. It would be interesting to know whether this might correlate with DTH responses and in order to look at this question we are now studying phagocytic and bactericidal activity of peritoneal macrophages in relation to these patients' DTH responses.

REFERENCES

1. Corey P: An approach to the statistical analysis of peritonitis data from patients on CAPD. Peritoneal Dial Bull 1: 529, 1981
2. MacGowen QP, Peterson PK, Keane W, and Quie PG: Human peritoneal macrophage phagocytic, killing and chemiluminescent responses to opsonised Listeria monocytogenes. Infect Immunol 40: 440, 1983
3. Verbugh HA, Keane WF, Hoidal JR, Freiberg MR, Elliot GR, and Peterson PK: Peritoneal macrophages and opsonins: Antibacterial defense in patients undergoing chronic peritoneal dialysis. J Infect Dis 147: 1018, 1983
4. Rubin J, Lin LM, Lewis R, Cruse J, and Bower JD: Host defense mechanisms in CAPD. Clin Nephrol 20: 140, 1983
5. Diskin CJ, Coplon N, Feldman C, and Vosti K: Antimicrobial activity in CAPD. Peritoneal Dial Bull 3: 150, 1983
6. Christou NV, Meakins JL, and MacLean LD: The predictive role of delayed hypersensitiviy in preoperative patients. Surg Gynecol Obstet 152: 297, 1981
7. Bradley JA, Ledingham IMcA, and Hamilton DNH: Assessment of host resistance in critically ill surgical patients by the reponse to recall skin antigens. Intensive Care Med 7: 105, 1981
8. Guttman RD, Meakins JL, Morehouse DD, and Milne C: Development of anergy to delayed-type hypersensitivity antigens following renal allotransplantation. Kidney Int 20: 275, 1981
9. Milne CA, Guttman RD, and Meakins JL: Short-term implications of delayed-type hypersensitivity responses in renal transplant recipients. Transplant Proc 14: 673, 1982
10. Watson MA, Briggs JD, Diamandopoulos AA, Hamilton DNH, and Dick HM: Endogenous cell-mediated immunity, blood transfusion, and outcome of renal transplantation. Lancet 2: 1323, 1979
11. Brown BW, Lagakos SW, and Byar DP: Statistical methodology. In Mike V, arid Stanley K (Eds), Statistics in medical research. New York: John Wiley and Sons, 1982, p 317
12. Bendetti J, and Yuen K: Life tables and survival functions. In Dixon WJ, and Brown MB (Eds), BMDP-81, Bio-Medical computer programs, P-series, user's manual. Los Angeles: University of California Press, 1981, p 557

13. Pierratos A, Amair P, Corey P, Vas SI, Khanna R, and Oreopoulos DG: Statistical analysis of the incidence of peritonitis on CAPD. Peritoneal Dial Bull 2: 32, 1982

14. Coward RA, Uttley L, Murray Y, Greenwood E, and Mallick NP: The importance of patient selection for CAPD. Peritoneal Dial Bull 2: 8, 1982

15. Vas S: Microbiological aspects of peritonitis. Peritoneal Dial Bull 1: S11, 1981

16. Slingeneyer A, Mion C, Beraud JJ, Oules R, Brauyer B, and Balmes M: Peritonitis, a frequently lethal complication of intermittent and continuous ambulatory peritoneal dialysis. Proc Eur Dial Transplant Assoc 18: 212, 1981

17. Plant J, and Glynn AA: Natural resistance to salmonella infection, delayed hypersensitivity and Ir genes in different inbred strains of mice. Nature 248: 345, 1974

18. Magliulo E, DeFeo V, Stirpe A, Riva C, and Scevola D: Enhanced in vitro phagocytic power of macrophages from PPD-stimulated skin sites in human subjects hypersensitive to PPD. Clin Exp Immunol 14: 371, 1973

19. Lenzini L, Rottoli P, and Rottoli L: The spectrum of human tuberculosis. Clin Exp Immunol 27: 230, 1977

L.L. Bloodworth and M.J. Harber

103

The Importance of Iron for Bacterial Growth in Peritoneal Dialysis Fluid

SUMMARY

Iron is an essential nutrient for microbial growth and is the usual growth limiting factor *in vivo*. We have examined the influence of iron and the iron binding drug deferrioxamine on the growth of common peritoneal pathogens in peritoneal dialysis effluent, sterilized by filtration, obtained from patients on CAPD. The bacteria selected for study were *Staphylococcus epidermidis*, *Escherichia coli*, *Pseudomonas aeruginosa*, and *Proteus mirabilis*. Growth was assessed turbidimetrically and by measurement of bacterial ATP using firefly bioluminescence. Addition of 10 μM ferric chloride, or hemoglobin to give an equivalent increment in iron concentration, produced a considerable increase in both bacterial growth rate and growth yield for all four strains. Deferrioxamine stimulated a concentration dependent enhancement of growth indicating that the bacteria were able to use this substance (which is of microbial origin) for iron uptake. These observations suggest that the treatment of iron overload in patients on CAPD with deferrioxamine might enhance susceptibility to peritonitis but that incorporation of a more powerful or irreversible iron chelator into peritoneal dialysis fluid could be of value in preventing peritonitis.

From the Department of Renal Medicine, Welsh National School of Medicine, KRUF Institute, Royal Infirmary, Cardiff, Wales.

INTRODUCTION

Despite major advances in the development of aseptic techniques designed to prevent the entry of microorganisms into the peritoneal cavity, bacterial peritonitis continues to be one of the most troublesome complications of CAPD.[1] This study was initiated in an attempt to determine if the pattern of bacterial growth in peritoneal dialysis effluent could be modified by deprivation of iron, which is an essential nutrient for microbial growth.[2,3] We have examined the effects of iron, as ferric chloride or hemoglobin, and the iron chelating agent deferrioxamine (DFO) on bacterial growth *in vivo*. DFO has been widely used in the management of iron overload states in man, and has recently been incorporated into peritoneal dialysis fluid for this purpose.[4]

Preliminary experiments by ourselves and others have revealed that peritoneal dialysis fluid containing either lactate or acetate as a buffering agent possesses an inherent antibacterial activity.[5] This fluid has no measurable iron content, nor does it contain a nitrogen source. Moreover it has a low pH and high osmolality. During dialysis, amino acids and plasma proteins cross the peritoneal membrane into the fluid within the peritoneal cavity. In inflammatory states, such as with bacterial peritonitis, the exudation of plasma constituents is increased and allows for the development of a nutrient medium that will support microbial growth. Chelation of available iron might reasonably be expected to deprive growing bacteria of an essential nutrient, thereby delaying, or even preventing, further growth.

In this preliminary communication we have demonstrated the importance of iron for bacterial growth in peritoneal dialysis effluent, and also show that DFO can enhance bacterial growth in the presence of iron.

MATERIALS AND METHODS

Four common peritoneal pathogens isolated in our laboratory were selected for study: *Staphylococcus epidermidis*, *Escherichia coli*, *Proteus mirabilis*, and *Pseudomonas aeruginosa*. The bacteria were subcultured in Oxoid nutrient broth no. 2 for 18 hours, washed in sterile unused peritoneal dialysis fluid (Dianeal 137®, Travenol Laboratories, UK), resuspended in this fluid to an E560 of 0.1, and then further diluted 1 in 100 to prepare the inoculum for experimental use.

Effluents for use as culture media were collected from eight patients both with and without bacterial peritonitis while undergoing routine CAPD with 1.36% (anhydrous) dextrose dialysis solutions. Equal volumes from each of the ''infected'' and ''uninfected'' effluents were pooled to give two collections, both of which were prefiltered using a Millipore AP20 filter to remove cellular elements and fibrin, and sterilized by filtration through a Millipore 0.45 μM filter.

In one series of experiments, 5 ml quantities of each of the ''infected'' and ''uninfected'' effluent pools, both with and without added ferric chloride at

Table 1. Bacterial Growth in ''Uninfected'' and ''Infected'' Peritoneal Dialysis Effluent with and without Added Iron (10 μm FeCl$_3$).

Sample	ATP(RLU)						OD
	1 hr	2 hr	4 hr	6 hr	8 hr	24 hr	24 hr
Control cultures							
uninfected dialysate	19	24	22	31	58	88	0.064
uninfected dialysate +FeCl$_3$	19	34	23	32	72	97	0.017
infected dialysate	23	28	24	33	68	95	0.077
infected dialysate +FeCl$_3$	22	31	25	32	96	179	0.00
E. coli							
uninfected dialysate	27	26	46	43	91	141	0.00
uninfected dialysate +FeCl$_3$	18	37	113	169	572	5736	0.144
infected dialysate	18	34	38	106	136	5684	0.135
infected dialysate +FeCl$_3$	30	71	2536	17,337	16,906	5770	0.479
Staph. epidermis							
uninfected dialysate	16	18	20	28	36	127	0.035
uninfected dialysate +FeCl$_3$	32	28	25	34	41	180	0.020
infected dialysate	24	26	28	46	75	99	0.036
infected dialysate +FeCl$_3$	23	28	37	83	162	19,326	0.164
Proteus mirabilis							
uninfected dialysate	20	23	53	42	83	10	0.00
uninfected dialysate +FeCl$_3$	21	27	83	113	232	5745	0.185
infected dialysate	22	31	51	98	244	1921	0.003
infected dialysate +FeCl$_3$	24	41	209	3563	1444	22,613	0.448
Pseudo aeruginosa							
uninfected dialysate	17	39	36	31	54	849	0.079
uninfected dialysate +FeCl$_3$	17	44	83	40	1473	9399	0.357
infected dialysate	26	46	70	61	397	4373	0.073
infected dialysate +FeCl$_3$	47	37	100	668	2075	11,920	0.339

OD = optical density at 560 nM.

a final concentration of 10 μM, were inoculated with 100 ml of diluted bacterial suspension to give an initial viable count of about 10^4 colony forming units (cfu)/ml. The cultures were incubated in a water bath at 37° C, and 100 ml samples were withdrawn at timed intervals up to 24 hours for the assay of intracellular ATP, which was used as an index of viable cell numbers.[6] ATP was extracted by vortex mixing 100 μl culture with 100 μl Lumac NRB reagent for 10 seconds, followed by the addition of 800 μl 25 mM Hepes buffer pH 7.75 containing 3 mM EDTA. For assay, 100 μl of extract was treated with 50 μl ATP bioluminescence reagent (Boehringer Mannheim), and light emission was measured in relative light units (RLU) using a Lumac Biocounter M2010. Bacterial growth after 24 hours incubation was also assessed turbidimetrically at 560 nm.

In a second experiment deferrioxamine was added at a range of concentrations (1 to 1000 μM) to 4 ml quantities of "infected" effluent supplemented with either 10 μM ferric chloride or hemoglobin at a final concentration of 0.016% (w/v), which gave an equivalent increment in iron content. These solutions were inoculated with *S. epidermidis* and treated as above.

RESULTS AND CONCLUSIONS

Bacterial growth rate and overall growth yield were both markedly enhanced for all test organisms except *S. epidermidis* when "uninfected" peritoneal dialysis effluent was supplemented with ferric chloride, and these stimulatory effects were observed with all four test strains using "infected" effluent as the culture medium (Table 1). Addition of hemoglobin instead of ferric chloride produced a similar pattern of growth enhancement (data for *S. epidermidis* in Table 2).

The addition of deferrioxamine to iron-stimulated cultures in "infected" effluent produced a further increase in bacterial growth rate for *S. epidermidis* (Table 2). Hence this organism would appear to be able to use this substance, which is a microbial siderophore,[7] to enhance iron acquisition.

The implications of these observations are three-fold. First, treatment of CAPD patients with iron-overload by deferrioxamine—particularly when administered intraperitoneally—may increase the incidence of bacterial peritonitis in susceptible patients. Second, patients on CAPD who have minor, possibly even subclinical, hemorrhage into the

Table 2. Growth of *Staph Epidermidis* in "Infected" Peritoneal Dialysis Effluent With Either Ferric Chloride (= 10 μM Fe_3+) or Hemoglobin (= 10 μM Fe_3+), and Deferrioxamine.

Sample		ATP (RLU)						OD
		2 hr	4 hr	6 hr	8 hr	10 hr	24 hr	24 hr
Control Culture		0	0	19	0	8	291	0.036
FeCl$_3$	DFO							
10 μM	—	0	0	2	2	14	5720	0.174
10 μM	1 μM	2	0	0	23	67	25,990	0.440
10 μM	10 μM	0	0	2	26	82	24,199	0.423
10 μM	100 μM	0	1	5	40	154	25,882	0.462
10 μM	1000 μM	0	2	24	303	1657	33,943	0.420
Hemoglobin	DFO							
10 μM Fe	—	0	0	7	36	139	33,086	0.788
10 μM Fe	1 μM	0	4	12	42	149	28,377	0.782
10 μM Fe	10 μM	0	3	6	41	175	28,832	0.747
10 μM Fe	100 μM	0	6	7	59	247	33,268	0.762
10 μM Fe	1000 μM	0	7	42	402	2070	36,351	0.790

DFO = deferrioxamine.
OD = optical density at 560 nM.

peritoneal dialysis fluid may also be more suscep-tible to infection and we feel that this point, in par-ticular, requires further evaluation. Last, it may be possible to inhibit bacterial growth in peritoneal dialysis effluent by the incorporation of a more pow-erful, irreversible iron chelating agent, and we are currently evaluating alternative agents for this purpose.

REFERENCES

1. Rubin J, Rogers WA, Taylor HM, Everett ED, Prowant BF, Fruto LV, and Nolph KD: Peritonitis during continuous ambulatory peritoneal dialysis. Ann Intern Med 92: 7, 1980

2. Weinberg ED: Iron and infection. Microbiol Rev 42: 45, 1978

3. Bullen JJ, Rogers HJ, and Griffiths E: Role of iron in bacterial infection. Curr Topics Microbiol Immunol 80: 1, 1978

4. Stanbaugh GN, Holmes AW, Gillit D, Reichel GW, and Stranz M: Iron chelation therapy in CAPD. A new and effective treatment of iron overload disease in ESRD patients. Peritoneal Dial Bull 3: 99, 1983

5. Richardson JA, and Borchardt KA: Adverse effect on bacteria of peritoneal dialysis solutions that contain acetate. Br Med J 3: 749, 1969

6. Harber JM: Applications of luminescence in medical microbiology and hematology. In Kricka LJ, and Carter TJN (Eds), Clinical and biochemical lumines-cence. New York: Marcel Dekker, 1982, p 189

7. Keberle H: The biochemistry of desferrioxamine and its relation to iron metabolism. Ann NY Acad Sci 119: 758, 1964

M.F. Kleiman, R.O. Doehring, K.I. Furman, and G.J. Koornhof

104

The Importance of Intracellular Organisms in CAPD

SUMMARY

Conventional culture frequently yields no or scanty growth of organisms from infected dialysate. In a series of 45 episodes of peritonitis on continuous ambulatory peritoneal dialysis, osmotic lysis of phagocytic cells in a centrifuged pellet of dialysis fluid increased the rate of positive cultures from 76% to 98%. Planting of an unlysed concentrate on media containing surface active agents was of intermediate efficacy in increasing the positive culture rate.

Osmotic lysis not only increases the yield of positive cultures, but also the heaviness of growth on primary plating media, enhancing the degree of confidence with which infection can be ascribed to a given isolate.

INTRODUCTION

The organisms responsible for CAPD peritonitis derive from a wide range of bacterial, mycobacterial, and mycotic species, and are frequently multiply drug-resistant.[1] Identification and susceptibility testing is therefore essential for rational therapy.

This ideal is compromised by the fact that between 4% and 28% of cases no organism is cultured (culture negative or "sterile" peritonitis).[2-5] A more worrisome, nonquantifiable problem is that in many cases the organism ascribed an etiologic role, is grown only in broth culture,[7] or as only one to a few colonies on primary solid media. Such growth must always be suspected of deriving from contamination.

On the basis of our observation of the paradoxically heavier growth on MacConkey than on blood agar from an equal inoculum, and of the finding that in cases positive on Gram staining, the organisms are almost exclusively intracellular[6]; we have looked at the effect on recovery of organisms of lysing phagocytic cells either before plating on agar, using distilled water or Triton X, or by the incorporation of surface active agents into the agar medium.

MATERIALS AND METHODS

Patients

The Microbiology Laboratory of the Johannesburg Hospital serves a continuous ambulatory peritoneal dialysis (CAPD) unit that had between 40 and 48 patients during the study period.

For the period April 1983 to April 1984, the first returns of dialysis fluid from all patients presenting with episodes of clinically diagnosed peritonitis were processed without delay according to our study protocol. Returns from patients who had had antimicrobial therapy prior to presenting to the unit were excluded from the study group. A total of 45 peritonitis episodes were available for study.

Culture Methods

Three 100 ml aliquots were withdrawn asceptically from the dialysis bag and centrifuged at 4000 rpm for 10 minutes. A drop (Pasteur pipette) of de-

From the South African Institute for Medical Research and University of the Witwatersrand, Medical School, Johannesburg, South Africa.

posit from one tube was spread directly onto each agar medium using a sterile glass spreader. The deposits in the other two tubes were lysed by adding 100 ml sterile distilled water and 2% Triton X respectively, immediately recentrifuged at 4000 rpm for 10 minutes and the deposit planted onto agar media as for the unlysed deposit.

The distilled water and Triton solution were controlled for sterility each time they were used.

Media used were 5% horse blood Columbia agar, Chocolatized agar, 10% laked horse blood agar, MaConkey agar, and Sabouraud dextrose agar. In addition, 28 of the specimens were planted on chocolatized agar containing 2% polysorbate 80 (Tween 80). Chocolatized blood media were incubated under 10% CO_2, the laked blood anerobically, and other media aerobically, all at 35°C and read at 24 hours, 48 hours, and one week of incubation. Colony counts were performed and isolates identified by standard methods. A separate aliquot of each dialysate specimen was cultured for mycobacteria. Statistical analysis was by the Wilcoxon test for paired data.

RESULTS

Gram Stain

Of 45 specimens, 21 (47%) were positive on gram staining, though often only after prolonged search. Seventeen showed gram-positive cocci, two gram-positive bacillic, and two gram-negative bacilli. Organisms were typically intracellular, in clumps with only the occasional slide also showing a few organisms outside phagocytic cells.

Culture

One specimen grew *Mycobacterium tuberculosis*. Of the remaining 44, a bacterium or yeast was isolated from 43 (98%). The specimen positive for tuberculosis will be omitted from further discussion and from the denominators of positivity rates.

Unlysed Deposit

The colony counts on blood and MacConkey agar are shown in the first two columns of Table 1. An organism isolated on blood agar in 33 cases (75%) and on MacConkey in 39 cases (89%). This difference is significant (p < 0.001). The colony count was increased eightfold on average on MacConkey for specimens positive on both media. Tween 80 choco-

late agar (results not shown) produced positivity rates and colony counts intermediate between those of blood and MacConkey.

Water Lysed Deposit

Colony counts are shown in the third and fourth columns of Table 1. The rate of positive isolates on blood agar is here raised to 43 out 44 (98%), and colony counts increased on average 37-fold. The difference is significant (<0.001). After water lysis there is no significant difference in positivity rate or colony count between blood agar and MacConkey agar.

Triton Lysed Deposit

Colony counts on blood and MacConkey agar are shown in the fifth and sixth columns of Table 1. While essentially equivalent to water lysis in the recovery of *Staphylococcus epidermidis* Triton lysis inhibited the recovery of other organisms.

Media and Growth Conditions

None of the organisms isolated during the course of this study failed to grow on 5% blood agar incubated aerobically.

DISCUSSION

The culture of large volumes of peritoneal fluid, concentrated by centrifugation[7-9] or filtration,[2,9,10] is widely recommended for improved isolation rates in CAPD peritonitis. We believe that we have shown that a further quantum step in improved rate and quality of isolation can be achieved by lysis of phagocytic cells present in the dialysate.

We were initially interested in the use of surface active agents for cell lysis, but have found osmotic lysis with distilled water superior, as all surface active agents will inhibit the growth of some potential isolates.

Two independent events can be recognized that improve colony counts, firstly the "rescue" of organisms from their intracellular location, which is seen when a surface active agent such as bile is incorporated in the solid media, and a further increase due to dispersion of packets of organisms from the lysed cells, resulting in more colony forming units being available, when lysis is performed prior to plating, this being an added advantage to osmotic lysis.

Table 1. Colony Counts from Unylsed and Lysed Dialysate Deposits.

Organism Isolated	Unlysed		Water Lysis		Triton Lysis	
	Blood Agar	MacConkey Agar	Blood Agar	MacConkey Agar	Blood Agar	MacConkey Agar
Staphylococcus	11	132	800	1168	260	604
epidermidis	3	34	106	110	62	9
	3	60	808	740	508	508
	0	3	1	2	0	0
	316	1104	692	480	556	282
	0	44	172	172	110	124
	21	414	620	540	604	1000
	11	102	388	268	496	144
	185	>2000	>2000	>2000	>2000	>2000
	468	900	1271	2000	1176	2000
	2	15	163	68	95	4
	1080	1560	2000	>2000	>2000	>2000
	0	12	56	39	105	65
	55	351	312	276	356	360
	26	53	680	356	436	226
	104	1840	558	1440	1140	1280
	39	162	1044	560	360	224
	5	124	420	672	210	240
	1	0	2	1	0	1
	7	126	480	420	96	144
	4	23	88	60	88	38
	324	>2000	>2000	>2000	>2000	>2000
	0	5	27	22	5	3
	0	0	1	0	0	0
	44	232	160	112	ND*	ND
Streptococcus	3	30	144	18	0	0
viridans	0	0	20	28	0	0
	0	2	10	28	5	1
Bacillus sp	1	2	42	27	0	0
	140	146	268	250	200	51
Lactobacillis sp	14	86	420	108	8	7
	0	3	10	13	5	2
Acinetobacter sp	0	0	5	3	0	2
	21	208	660	1080	11	86
	210	>2000	>2000	>2000	228	244
	1	5	1	3	0	6
	0	55	196	128	ND	ND
Escherichia coli	82	960	>2000	>2000	132	90
	21	59	229	287	32	123
	61	187	149	190	3	3
Proteus sp	69	246	408	330	46	9
Alkaligenes sp	200	720	>2000	>2000	ND	ND
Candida sp	150	144	1116	1440	492	420

Improved isolation following lysis was most marked for the gram-positive organisms and *Acinetobacter*, with that of other gram-negative bacilli and of yeasts being less enhanced.

It may be speculated that organisms of less inherent pathogenicity are more susceptible to phagocytosis and intracellular killing, and therefore need to be "rescued" as soon as possible by destruction of the phagocyte. An investigation of this hypothesis has been started in our laboratory.

When contrasted with other series,[2,5,7,10,] our series is remarkable for paucity of such organisms as *Staphylococcus aureus* and *Pseudomonas*, which might be expected to be of high virulence.

The finding that colony counts on blood and MacConkey agar were not significantly different when planted with a lysed inoculum indicates that the poor growth on a conventionally planted blood agar plate is not due to an organism characteristic, such as inhibition by a toxic substance in the agar.

CONCLUSION

We would strongly recommend the inclusion of an osmotic lysis step in the processing of peritoneal dialysate. This method allows a recovery rate of organisms at least as good as, if not better than that claimed for broth culture,[7] with the great advantage for interpretation that heavy growths are seen in primary plating media.

The implication of the predominantly intracellular location of the bacteria in CAPD peritonitis deserves further study with regard to treatment and the natural history of the disease.

REFERENCES

1. Gray HH, and Eykyn SJ: CAPD peritonitis (Letter). Lancet 1: 349, 1983
2. Gokal R, Ramos JM, Francis DMA, Ferner RE, Goodship THJ, Proud G, Bint A, Ward MK, and Kerr DNS: Peritonitis in continuous ambulatory peritoneal dialysis: Laboratory and clincial studies. Lancet 2: 1388, 1982
3. Krothapalli R, Duffy B, Lacke C, Payne W, Patel W, and Perez V: Pseudomonas peritonitis and continuous ambulatory peritoneal dialysis. Arch Intern Med 142: 1862, 1982
4. Prowant BF, Nolph KD: Clinical criteria for diagnosis of peritonitis. In Atkins RC, Thomson NM, and Farrell PC (Eds), Peritoneal dialysis. Edinburgh: Churchill Livingston, 1981, p 257
5. Fenton S, Wu G, Cattran D, Wadgymar A, Allen AF: Clinical aspects of peritonitis in patients on CAPD. Peritoneal Dial Bull 1: 54, 1981
6. Doehring RO, Kleiman MF, Koornhof HJ: Intracellular organisms as a cause of culture negative peritonitis in continuous ambulatory peritoneal dialysis. Proc Int Congr Infect Dis 1983, p 72
7. Knight KR, Polak A, Crump J, Maskell R: Laboratory diagnosis and oral treatment of CAPD peritonitis. Lancet 2: 1301, 1982
8. Fenton P: Laboratory diagnosis of peritonitis in patients undergoing continuous ambulatory peritoneal dialysis. J Clin Pathol 35: 1181, 1982
9. Vas SI: Microbiological aspects of peritonitis. Peritoneal Dial Bull 1(Suppl): S11, 1981
10. Vas SI: Microbiological aspects of chronic ambulatory peritoneal dialysis. Kidney Int 23: 83, 1983

S. Lamperi and S. Carozzi

105

Immunologic Pattern in CAPD Patients with Low or High Peritonitis Incidence

SUMMARY

In 38 patients on CAPD, 30 with a low and eight with a high peritonitis incidence, before and after the prophylactic use of intravenous human SRK immunoglobulins, some humoral and cellular immunological parameters were studied. Those studied were B-lymphocyte surface immunoglobulin percentage, IgG, IgA, IgM, C3 levels, E-rosette and active E-rosette percentages. DNCB and PPD skin positivities, OKT4/OKT8 ratio, T-cell growth factor and interleukin 1 activities, lymphocyte transformation index, peripheral neutrophil chemotaxis, direct phagocytosis, bacterial killing, indirect phagocytosis, random migration and peritoneal macrophage spontaneous migration and quantitative indirect phagocytosis.

The results confirm that renal failure impairs humoral and cellular immunological activities. CAPD treatment is followed by a positive effect on the various immunological parameters, particularly on the peritoneal macrophages which show a recovery of their activities as has never been seen with other dialytic techniques.

The prophylactic use of human SRK immunoglobulin appears suitable particularly in the patients in whom the preliminary examination reveals a greater immunological abnormality before starting CAPD.

From the Division of Nephrology, St. Martin Hospital, Genoa, Italy.

INTRODUCTION

Various aspects of humoral and cellular immunity have been studied in uremic patients and animals with experimentally induced uremia, and have shown that the immune responsiveness is significantly impaired in uremia.[1,2]

Such a situation results in impaired host defenses and may facilitate the appearance of peritonitis in CAPD patients.

In the previous studies, different investigators implicated depression of both leukocytes and humoral factors in causing of the high incidence of infections in patients on chronic hemodialysis,[3,4] while less is known about the *in vitro* and *in vivo* activities, in patients on CAPD.

This study examines some aspects of cellular and humoral immune functions in CAPD patients with a different incidence of peritonitis, a few of them were treated with immunoglobulin therapy.

PATIENTS AND METHODS

This study was performed in 38 uremic patients on CAPD, (20 males, 18 females, age range 41 to 65 years [mean 54 ± 10.2]) and in 50 normal subjects.

The primary renal diseases were: chronic glomerulonephritis in 16, malignant nephrosclerosis in 18, polycystic disease in 2, and chronic pyelonephritis in 2 patients.

The dialysis schedule was four daily exchanges of 2 L dialysis fluid (Viaflex®, Travenol Laboratories, Deerfield, IL).

The patients were subdivided into two groups, depending on their peritonitis frequency: Group 1 (n = 30 subjects) with 1.5 ± 0.5 episodes/patient/ year, and Group 2 (n = 8 subjects) with 5.0 ± 0.8 episodes/patient/year.

At the start of treatment the mean serum creatinine levels were respectively, in the two groups, 11.3 ± 1.2 and 11.7 ± 1.7 mg/dl, serum proteins 6.5 ± 0.4 and 6 ± 0.6 g/dl, the hematocrit values 22 ± 1 and 21 ± 1.5%, the hemoglobin 7.1 ± 0.4 and 7 ± 0.2 g/dl, the leukocytes 6850 ± 1200 and 6200 ± 1100/mm^3, the neutrophils 5304 ± 850 and 4860 ± 630/mm^3, the lymphocytes 1166 ± 215 and 1153 ± 177/mm^3.

The two groups did not differ in mean age, and the observation period was from the start of the treatment (PDP) until the 24th month. In the two groups the following parameters were studied every 3 months.

Humoral immunologic pattern. Serum immunoglobulins (IgG, IgA, IgM, mg/dl) and complement (C3 mg/dl) were determined by radial immunodiffusion,[5] peripheral B-lymphocytes were counted by membrane immunofluorescence for surface immunoglobulins (S-Ig%).[6]

Cellular immunologic pattern. E-rosettes and active E-rosettes were assessed by the usual techniques.[7] The OKT4/OKT8 ratio, using OKT4 and OKT8 monoclonal antibodies (ORTHO Pharmaceutical Corp, Raritan, NJ) was determined by indirect immunofluorescence.[8] The lymphocyte transformation reported as stimulation index was assayed by the method described by Lewis.[9]

The T-cell growth factor (TCGF U/ml) and the interleukin 1 activities (IL 1 U/ml) were measured respectively by the methods of Gillis et al.[10] and Conlon.[11]

The peripheral neutrophils collected by the usual method[12] were tested for random migration and chemotaxis by the modified Boyden chamber method of Wilkinson[13] and the results were expressed as the distance (μm) traveled by the leading front of the cells.

Bacterial killing and direct phagocytosis, tested against *Staphylococcus aureus* (A8 strain) were studied using the Solberg method.[14]

For indirect phagocytosis the nitroblue tetrazolium (NBT) test was performed using the technique described by Windhorst et al.[15] Polymorphs containing at least ten colored granules were counted as NBT positive cells (%).

The delayed hypersensitivity skin tests were performed using two antigens: Tuberculin (PPD-Beheringwerke) and dinitrochlorobenzene (DNCB-Merck).[16]

Finally peritoneal macrophages were collected from dialysate bags with the method described by others,[17] isolated by glass adhesiveness, tested for indirect phagocytosis by quantitative NBT test, expressed as μg of formazan formed by 10^6 cells[18] and for spontaneous migration (Migration Index—MI).[18]

Six patients of Group 2 (Group 3) were submitted to a prophylactic treatment of recurrent bacterial peritonitis with intravenous human immunoglobulins (Swiss Red Cross Immunoglobulin, SRK-Ig) administered every 3 weeks for 1 year at the dosage of 0.2 g/Kg body weight. Informed consent was obtained.

All the above mentioned parameters were determined in the patients on treatment, at the start of the study and after each immunoglobulin administration (15 times).

Statistics. The data, expressed as mean ± SD were analyzed by the Student t test. Statistical significance was accepted at 0.05 level or less.

RESULTS

Humoral Immunologic Pattern in Group 1

In the PDP the S-Ig, IgG, IgA, IgM values did not differ and the C3 levels were low 34.44% (p < 0.05) in comparison to normal. This parameter, however, normalized by the 6th month of CAPD (Table 1).

Humoral Immunologic Pattern in Group 2

In Group 2 in the PDP the humoral immunity had the same behavior as Group 1. In the successive months, however, C3 fell below normal 45.55% (p < 0.05). In addition in IgG, at normal levels at the start, decreased 34.38% in the 24th month (p < 0.05) (Table 2).

Cellular Immunologic Pattern in Group 1

In PDP significant respective decreases in E-rosette percentage, DNCB and PPD positivities, TCGF and IL 1 activities, lymphocyte transforma-

Table 1. Humoral Immunologic Pattern in Group 1.*

	Control†	PDP	Months							
			3	6	9	12	15	18	21	24
S-Ig %	12 ±3	9.2 ±1.5	10.3 ±2	10.5 ±2.8	10.6 ±3.5	10.3 ±4.1	10.2 ±2.1	10.4 ±1.5	10.3 ±1.9	10.9 ±2.6
IgG mg/dl	1300 ±150	1198 ±210	1245 ±225	1263 ±195	1190 ±175	1242 ±150	1200 ±18	1275 ±175	1225 ±215	1295 ±240
IgA mg/dl	200 ±100	260 ±143	217 ±130	230 ±135	235 ±140	225 ±130	223 ±115	205 ±95	215 ±75	195 ±80
IgM mg/dl	160 ±65	175 ±55	172 ±48	188 ±53	175 ±59	183 ±45	175 ±65	168 ±55	175 ±49	170 ±59
C₃ mg/dl	90 ±15	59‡ ±19	79§ ±2	83§ ±8	91§ ±5	93§ ±7	89§ ±6	88§ ±8	91§ ±4	94§ ±4

* Values are the Mean ± SD for 30 patients.   ‡ Significantly different from control value (p < 0.05).
† Values are the Mean ± SD for 50 normal subjects.   § Significantly different from PDP value (p < 0.05).

Table 2. Humoral Immunologic Pattern in Group 2.*

	Control†	PDP	Months							
			3	6	9	12	15	18	21	24
S-Ig %	12 ±3	9.2 ±2.5	9 ±3	8.7 ±2.9	8.2 ±4.5	8.5 ±4	8.1 ±3.7	8 ±3.9	8.3 ±2.9	8.5 ±2.6
IgG mg/dl	1300 ±150	1143 ±110	1207 ±125	1168 ±150	1041 ±100	905 ±80	806‡ ±85	800‡ ±65	810‡ ±75	750‡§ ±80
IgA mg/dl	200 ±100	230 ±115	243 ±125	250 ±105	262 ±137	220 ±164	217 ±143	235 ±139	225 ±143	235 ±148
IgM mg/dl	160 ±65	163 ±73	169 ±86	198 ±97	237 ±51	242 ±59	281 ±79	275 ±149	218 ±117	234 ±98
C₃ mg/dl	90 ±15	54 ±7	51 ±4	53 ±5	55 ±8	49 ±5	56 ±7	50 ±9	55 ±10	49 ±12

* Values are the Mean ± SD for 8 patients.   ‡ Significantly different from control value (p < 0.05).
† Values are the Mean ± SD for 50 normal subjects.   § Significantly different from PDP value (p < 0.05).

Table 3. Cellular Immunologic Pattern in Group 1.*

	Control†	PDP	Months							
			3	6	9	12	15	18	21	24
Lymphocytes mm³	1450 ±350	1166 ±215	1210 ±233	1343 ±214	1380 ±297	1410 ±290	1390 ±310	1370 ±300	1383 ±281	1340 ±244
E-rosettes %	59 ±6	22‡ ±5	39‡ ±6	45§ ±4	53§ ±5	49§ ±4	54§ ±3	51§ ±5	50§ ±7	53§ ±5
Active E-rosettes %	31 ±2	26 ±5	27 ±8	31 ±11	30 ±13	30 ±9	31 ±10	30 ±7	32 ±4	30 ±5
OKT4/OKT8 (ratio)	2.1 ±0.3	1.8 ±0.4	1.7 ±0.3	1.9 ±0.4	2.1 ±0.5	2.3 ±0.7	2.2 ±0.5	2.1 ±0.7	2.2 ±0.4	2 ±0.3
DNCB positive %	90	20‡	40‡§	53.3‡§	66.6§	66.6§	73.3§	73.3§	73.3§	73.3§
PPD positive %	92	23‡	43.3‡§	60§	76.6§	80§	80§	80§	80§	80§
TCGF (U/ml)	0.90 ±0.1	0.41‡ ±0.1	0.57‡ ±0.09	0.78§ ±0.2	0.83§ ±0.1	0.85§ ±0.1	0.86§ ±0.07	0.82§ ±0.07	0.85§ ±0.9	0.85§ ±0.05
IL-1 (U/ml)	5 ±0.7	2.3‡ ±1.2	3.8§ ±1.4	3.9§ ±1.3	4§ ±1.5	4.3§ ±1.3	4.1§ ±1.4	4.6§ ±1.7	4.4§ ±1.6	4.7§ ±1.8
Lymphocyte transformation (Index)	112 ±15	29‡ ±6	54‡ ±5§	63‡ ±6§	72§ ±7	78§ ±8	79§ ±5	83§ ±9	80§ ±9	85§ ±7

* Values are the Mean ± SD for 30 patients.
† Values are the Mean ± SD for 50 normal subjects.
‡ Significntly different from control value (p < 0.05).
§ Significantly different from PDP value (p < 0.05).

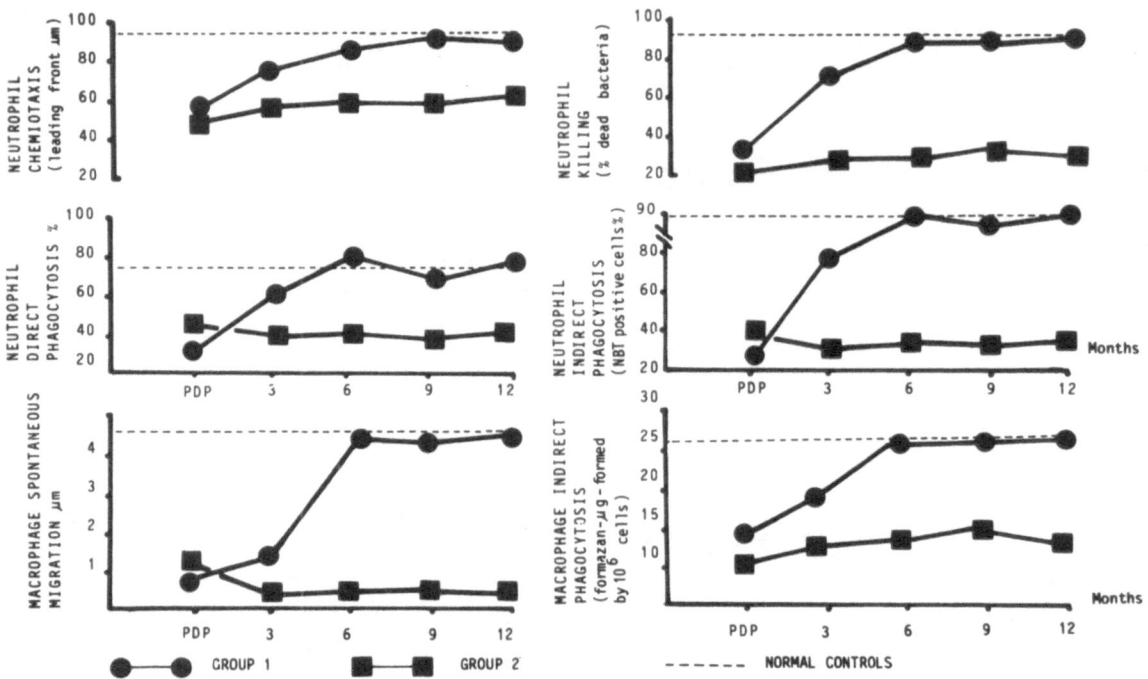

Fig. 1. Neutrophil chemotaxis, direct phagocytosis, bacterial killing, indirect phagocytosis, macrophage spontaneous migration, and indirect phagocytosis behavior in Groups 1 and 2.

tion indices as a percent of normal controls (62.71%, 77.77%, 75%, 54.44%, 54%, and 74.10%; p < 0.05) were observed. Other parameters such as active E-rosette percentage, OKT4/OKT8 ratio and lymphocyte count did not show any significant change. In the months of therapy a progressively significant increase in the above mentioned parameters respectively occurred (145.45%, 266.5%, 247,82%, 109.75% 104.34%, and 193.10%; p < 0.05) starting from the 3rd month (Table 3).

Peripheral neutrophil chemotaxis, direct phagocytosis, bacterial killing NBT test demonstrated a significant decrease respectively (40.81%, 58.66%, 66.66%, and 61.11%; p < 0.05) in comparison to normal levels, and an increase respectively of 68.96%, 168.96%, 200%, and 160% (p < 0.05) in comparison to PDP values. As regards random migration no significant differences were found in Group 1 CAPD patients in comparison to controls. The peritoneal macrophages drawn at the start of treatment demonstrated a significant decrease in spontaneous migration and indirect phagocytosis, respectively, of 78.88% and 48.14% (p < 0.05) in comparison to normal.[18]

These abnormalities were restored in the course of CAPD with an increase respectively of 388.88% and of 85.71% (p < 0.05), which reached maximum at the 6th month (Fig. 1).

Cellular Immunologic Pattern in Group 2

In PDP a significant respective decrease, more evident than in Group 1, of E-rosette percentage, DNCB and PPD positivities, TCGF, and IL 1 activities and lymphocyte transformation index in comparison to normal (66.10%, 86.11%, 86.41%, 63.33%, 62%, and 80.35%; p < 0.05) was observed, without any modification in lymphocyte count, active E-rosette percentage and OKT4/OKT8 ratio.

All above mentioned abnormalities persisted unchanged in the course of the various months of therapy (Table 4).

In PDP the peripheral neutrophil chemotaxis, direct phagocytosis, bacterial killing, and indirect phagocytosis showed a significant decrease in regard to normal respectively of 51.02%, 42.66%, 77.77%, and 58.88% (p < 0.05) without any improvement in the successive months of CAPD. Similar

Table 4. Cellular Immunologic Pattern in Group 2.*

| | Control† | PDP | | | | | Months | | | |
			3	6	9	12	15	18	21	24
Lymphocytes mm³	1450 ±350	1153 ±177	1259 ±134	1034 ±153	954 ±139	1109 ±204	1153 ±208	1074 ±197	977 ±179	950 ±210
E-rosettes %	59 ±6	20‡ ±4	29 ±6	22 ±8	23 ±9	16 ±7	19 ±7	18 ±5	16 ±8	20 ±9
Active E-rosettes %	31 ±2	28 ±3	32 ±4	25 ±8	22 ±7	27 ±5	29 ±9	31 ±9	30 ±5	24 ±3
OKT4/OKT8 (ratio)	2.1 ±0.3	1.7 ±0.2	1.9 ±0.4	1.8 ±0.2	1.8 ±0.6	1.7 ±0.1	1.9 ±0.2	1.7 ±0.1	1.8 ±0.3	1.9 ±0.3
DNCB positive %	90	12.5‡	12.5	12.5	12.5	12.5	12.5	12.5	12.5	12.5
PPD positive %	92	12.5‡	12.5	12.5	12.5	12.5	12.5	12.5	12.5	12.5
TCGF (U/ml)	0.90 ±0.1	0.33‡ ±0.1	0.37 ±0.08	0.29 ±0.09	0.25 ±1.1	0.28 ±1.5	0.38 ±1.2	0.30 ±0.07	0.22 ±0.09	0.39 ±1
IL-1 (U/ml)	5 ±0.7	1.9‡ ±0.3	1.5 ±0.5	1.7 ±0.7	2.1 ±0.1	1.4 ±0.8	1.6 ±0.9	1.6 ±0.4	1.5 ±0.7	1.7 ±0.5
Lymphocyte transformation	112 ±15	22‡ ±5	20 ±3	18 ±8	23 ±6	20 ±7	16 ±5	24 ±4	18 ±4	19 ±6

* Values are the Mean ± SD for 8 patients.

† Values are the Mean ± SD for 50 normal subjects.

‡ Significantly different from control value (p < 0.05).

results were obtained on study of spontaneous migration and quantitative indirect phagocytosis behavior of peritoneal macrophages which demonstrates, in PDP a decrease, in comparison to normal controls, respectively of 66.66% and 62.69% (p < 0.05) (Fig. 1).

Humoral and Cellular Immunologic Patterns in Group 3

In Group 3 a significant increase in serum IgG and C3 levels and in the number of postive DNCB and PPD patients, in comparison to the basal values,

starting from the 3rd month of SRK immunoglobulin treatment, respectively of 91.78%, 104.25%, 150%, and 150% (p < 0.05) was observed. All other evaluations did not show any significant modification (Table 5).

Contemporarily the chemotaxis, direct phagocytosis, bacterial killing, and indirect phagocytosis of the peripheral neutrophils increased respectively to 96%, 150%, 340%, and 350% (p < 0.05). A similar increase, respectively 700% and 130% (p < 0.05) was seen in spontaneous migration and indirect phagocytosis of peritoneal macrophages (Fig.2). In the same period of observation a significant de-

Table 5. Humoral and Cellular Immunologic Patterns in Group 3.*

	Control†	B	Months 3	6	9	12
S-Ig %	12 ±3	8.5 ±1.5	9.3 ±1.5	9.4 ±1.7	9.5 ±1.3	9.8 ±1.5
IgG mg/dl	1300 ±150	730 ±170	1155‡ ±193	1358‡ ±212	1379 ±155	1400‡ ±147
IgA mg/dl	200 ±100	230 ±137	217 ±121	223 ±100	240 ±90	249 ±130
IgM mg/dl	160 ±65	240 ±52	203 ±80	187 ±58	160 ±40	152 ±30
C₃ mg/dl	90 ±15	47 ±5	79 ±8	84‡ ±4	91‡ ±9	96‡ ±11
E-rosettes %	59 ±6	19 ±7	27 ±9	31 ±13	25 ±11	30 ±12
Active E-rosettes %	31 ±2	21 ±4	23 ±3	28 ±5	26 ±3	26 ±4
OKT4/OKT8 (ratio)	2.1 ±0.3	1.7 ±0.4	1.8 ±0.5	1.7 ±0.5	1.9 ±0.7	1.8 ±0.8
DNCB positive (patients)	45	2	3	4	4	5‡
PPD positive (patients)	46	2	2	3	3	5‡
TCGF (U/ml)	0.90 ±0.1	0.30 ±0.09	0.35 ±0.08	0.43 ±1	0.41 ±0.07	0.45 ±0.09
IL-1 (U/ml)	5 ±0.7	1.7 ±0.3	1.9 ±0.5	2.1 ±0.2	2.3 ±0.8	2.3 0.4
Lymphocyte transformation (Index)	112 ±15	18 ±5	23 ±4	25 ±6	23 ±3	25 ±6

* Values are the Mean ± SD for 6 patients.
† Values are the Mean ± SD for 50 normal subjects.
‡ Significantly different from <B> value (p < 0.05).
B: Values are the Mean ± SD observed before SRK-Ig treatment.

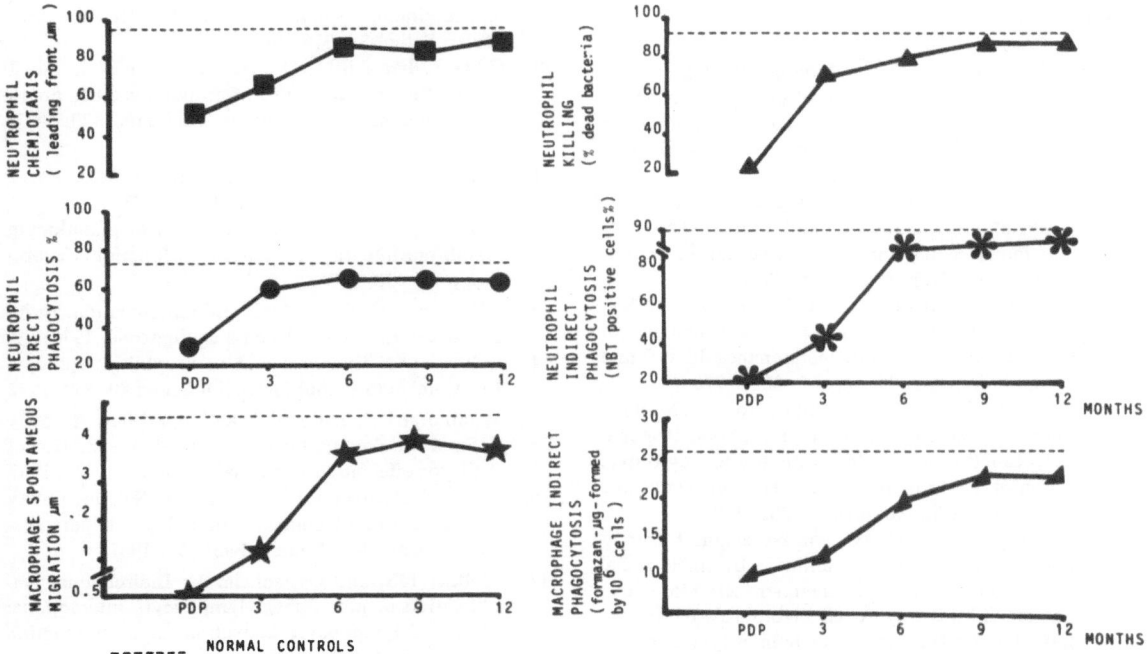

Fig. 2. Neutrophil chemotaxis, direct phagocytosis, bacterial killing, indirect phagocytosis, macrophage spontaneous migration, and indirect phagocytosis behavior in Group 3.

crease ($p < 0.05$) in the peritonitis occurrence was obtained with an average incidence of 2.5 ± 0.8 episodes/patient/year.

DISCUSSION

The results in uremic patients in end stage renal disease demonstrate a significant decrease in immunologic defenses, particularly cellular immunity, including the delayed hypersensitivity and lymphokine production such as interleukin 1 and 2. This situation indicates defective function of immunocompetent cells both directly and via their secretions. These abnormalities are evident not only at the peripheral level but, above all, in peritoneal macrophages, which represent the first stage of host-defense against external insults.

The above mentioned abnormalities improve during CAPD in most patients but are unchanged in CAPD patients suffering from recurrent bacterial peritonitis episodes, independent of age, primary renal disease and degree of dialysis and may be linked, on the contrary to a constitutionally impaired responsiveness to the stimuli.

In some cases the prophylactic use of intravenous SRK immunoglobulin supplement provokes a satisfactory enhancement,[19] not only of humoral immunity, but also of some aspects of cellular response, confirming that some aspects of impaired immunity in uremic patients consists of defective cooperation between the T and B lymphocyte systems.

In conclusion our studies confirm that renal failure alters immunologic, humoral and cellular activities. CAPD treatment has a beneficial effect on the various immunologic parameters but in particular on the macrophages, which show a recovery of their activities as has never been verified with other dialytic techniques.[20]

Notwithstanding these results a few CAPD patients do not show any of the above mentioned positive effects. But it is unclear if such a situation is attributable to a previous predisposition to immunologic abnormalities or to impairment of the immunologic system acquired in the course of peritonitis.

The prophylactic use of SRK immunoglobulin appears indicated particularly in patients in whom early evidence of a greater than usual immunologic alteration exists before starting CAPD.

REFERENCES

1. Ringoir S, Van Looy L, Van deHeyning P, and Leroux-Roels G: Impairment of phagocytosis activity of macrophages as studied by the skin window test in patients on regular hemodialysis. Clin Nephrol 4: 234, 1975

2. Mezzano S, Pesce AJ, Pollak VE, and Michael JG: Analysis of humoral and cellular factors that contribute to impaired immune responsiveness in experimental uremia. Nephron 36: 15, 1984

3. Hosking CS, Atkins RC, Scott DF, Holdsworth SR, Fitzgerald MG, and Shelton MJ: Immune and phagocytic function in patients on maintenance dialysis and transplantation. Clin Nephrol 6: 501, 1976

4. Charpentier B, Lang PH, Martin B, Noury J, Mathieu D, and Fries D: Depressed polymorphonuclear leukocyte function associated with normal cytotoxic function of T and natural killer cells during chronic hemodialysis. Clin Nephrol 19: 288, 1983

5. Mancini G, Carbonara AO, and Heremans J: Immunochemical quantitation of antigens by single radial immunoglobulins. Immunochemistry 21: 235, 1965

6. Papamichail M, Brown JC, and Holborow EJ: Immunoglobulins on the surface of human lymphocytes. Lancet 1: 850, 1971

7. Mendes NF, Tolnai MEA, Silveira SR, Gilbertsen SB, and Metizgar RS: Technical aspects of the rosette tests used to direct human complement receptor (B) and sheep erythrocyte binding (T) lymphocytes. J Immunol 11: 860, 1973

8. Reinherz EL, Moretta L, Breard JM, Mingari MC, Cooper MD, and Schlossman SF: Human T-lymphocyte subpopulation defined by Fc receptor and monoclonal antibodies. A comparison. J Exp Med 151: 696, 1980

9. Lewis R: Histopathology and cell-mediated immune reactivity in halothane-associated lymphomagenesis and autoimmunity in BXSB/ and MRL/MP mice. Exp Molec Pathol 36: 378, 1982

10. Gillis S, Ferm MM, Ou W, and Smith KA: T-cell growth factor: Parameters of production and a quantitative microassay for activity. J Immunol 120: 2027, 1978

11. Conlon PJ: A rapid biologic assay for the detection of Interleukin 1. J Immunol 31: 1280, 1983

12. Dankberg F, Persidsky MD: A test of granulocyte membrane integrity and phagocytic function. Cryobiology 13: 430, 1976

13. Wilkinson PC: Chemotaxis and inflammation. Edinburgh and London: Churchill Livingstone, 1974, p 3

14. Solberg CO: Evaluation of neutrophil granulocyte function. Acta Pathol Microbiol Scand 80: 559, 1972

15. Windhorst DB, Holmes B, and Good RA: A newly defined X-linked trait in a man with demonstration of the Lyon effect in carrier females. Lancet 1: 737, 1967

16. Cohen S, Bernacerraf B, McCluskey RT, and Ovary Z: Effects of anticoagulants on delayed hypersensitivity reactions. J Immunol 98: 351, 1967

17. Meltzer MS, and Oppenheim JJ: Bidirectional amplification of macrophage-lymphocyte interactions: enhanced lymphocyte activation factor production by activated adherent mouse peritoneal cells. J Immunol 118: 77, 1977

18. Alföldy P, and Lemmel EM: Reduction of nitroblue of tetrazolium for functional evaluation of activated macrophages in the cell-mediated immune reaction. Clin Immunol Immunopathol 12: 263, 1979

19. Fisher GW, Hunter KW, Hemming VG, and Wilson SR: Functional antibacterial activity of intravenous immunoglobulin preparation: in vitro and in vivo studies. Vox Sang 44: 296, 1983

20. Rubin J, Lin LM, Lewis R, Cruse J, and Bower JD: Host defense mechanisms in continuous ambulatory peritoneal dialysis. Clin Nephrol 20: 140, 1983

H.A. Verbrugh, R.P. Verkooyen, J. Verhoef, P.L. Oe, and J. van der Meulen

106

Defective Complement-Mediated Opsonization and Lysis of Bacteria in Commercial Peritoneal Dialysis Solutions

SUMMARY

Complement-mediated opsonization and lysis of bacteria were studied in peritoneal dialysis solutions. Opsonization was assessed by the uptake of ^{3}H-labeled *E. coli* (serum-resistant strain ON2) by human blood leukocytes. Bacteriolysis was evaluated by the release of label from ^{3}H-labeled *E. coli* (serum-sensitive strain K12). Uptake of ON2 was 46% after opsonization with 1% serum in control buffer, but only 2 to 15% of the bacteria were taken up after opsonization in peritoneal dialysis solutions. In contrast to complement-mediated opsonization bacterial opsonization with antibody was not reduced in dialysis solutions. Lysis of K12 was 26% and 78% in control buffer with 10% and 20% serum, respectively. In contrast, serum did not lyse K12 in dialysis solutions. Both the classical and alternative complement pathways functioned poorly in peritoneal dialysis solutions. Complement-mediated opsonization and lysis of *E. coli* was not dependent on the glucose concentration of the media but could largely be restored by increasing the pH of dialysis solutions from <5.5 to over 6.5. The amount of titrateable acid in commercial dialysis solutions varied from 0.055 to 0.167 mEq NaOH/dl among different suppliers. We conclude that commercial peritoneal dialysis solutions severely compromise the opsonic and bacteriolytic functions of serum complement which may be important in the peritoneal defense against infection.

From the Laboratory for Microbiology, University of Utrecht Medical School, Utrecht; the Department of Medicine, Free University of Amsterdam Medical School, Amsterdam, the Netherlands.

INTRODUCTION

The complement system plays an important role in host defense against microbial invasion. Bacteria that have reacted with serum complement are much better recognized and ingested by phagocytic cells; this phenomenon is called opsonization of bacteria and is crucially dependent on the binding of complement factor C3 to the bacterial surface.[1,2] In addition, complement is essential in the lytic activity of serum toward Gram-negative bacterial species. In this reaction complement components C5-C9 together with serum lysozyme can pierce the Gram-negative cell wall and thereby trigger bacteriolysis.[3]

The high incidence of bacterial peritonitis in patients treated with chronic ambulatory peritoneal dialysis (CAPD) suggests that accidental bacterial contamination of the peritoneal cavity is not effectively handled by the local defense mechanisms in these patients. We previously reported the relative lack of opsonins and phagocytic cells in the dialysis effluents from CAPD patients, and noted that patients with low opsonic titers were at increased risk of developing peritonitis.[4,5] Results of this study suggest that currently available peritoneal dialysis solutions further hamper the peritoneal defense mechanisms by antagonizing the opsonic and bacteriolytic activity of serum complement.

MATERIALS AND METHODS

Bacteria

Staphylococcus epidermidis L (a clinical isolate), *Escherichia coli* ON2 (serum-resistant), and *E. coli* K12 (serum-sensitive) were used in this study. Radiolabeling of bacteria was achieved by growing them in Mueller-Hinton broth (Difco Laboratories, Detroit, MI) containing (methyl-^{3}H) thymidine (ICN, Irvine, CA), as previously described.[6]

Media

CAPD solutions containing 1.5%, 2.5%, or 4.25% glucose were kindly donated by Travenol GMBH (München, FRG), Fresenius AG (Bad Homburg v.d. H., FRG) and B. Braun Melsungen AG (Melsungen, FRG). Hank's balanced salt solution containing 0.1% gelatin (GHBSS) was used as control medium throughout the study.

Serum Complement

A pool of serum was obtained from 12 healthy donors. Serum was stored at −70°C until use. For each experiment serum was equilibrated with the experimental media by dialysis (18 hours at 4°C) against excess amounts of the respective media. Thereafter dilutions of dialyzed serum were made in the same medium. In some experiments activation of the classical complement pathway was blocked by chelating serum with 10 mM ethylene glycol tetraacetic acid (Sigma Chemical Co., St. Louis, MO) in the presence of 5 mM MgCl$_2$ (MgEGTA serum). To completely inactivate complement, serum was heated (30 minutes at 56°C) prior to use.

Assessment of Bacterial Opsonization

Opsonization of bacteria was studied in a two-step assay. First, radiolabeled bacteria were incubated in dilutions of serum in various experimental media for 15 minutes at 37°C. Bacteria were then washed once and subsequently mixed with human blood polymorphonuclear leukocytes (PMN). The bacteria-PMN mixtures were incubated in a 37°C shaking waterbath. The uptake of bacteria by PMN, after indicated incubation times, was determined by measuring PMN-associated radioactivity. Phagocytosis was expressed as a percentage of total added radioactivity and was taken as a measure of bacterial opsonization, as previously described.[2,6]

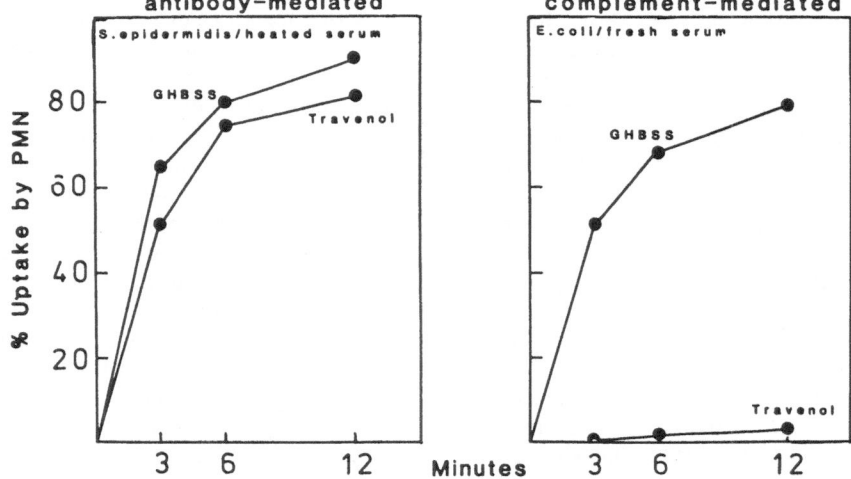

Fig. 1. Defective complement-mediated opsonization of *Escherichia coli* ON2 (right panel) but normal antibody-mediated opsonization of *S. epidermidis* (left panel) in CAPD solution (Travenol). Bacteria were preopsonized with 5% fresh serum or heated serum in either GHBSS or Travenol solution for 15 min at 37°C. After opsonization bacteria were washed and mixed with polymorphonuclear leukocytes (PMN) Phagocytosis was measured after 3, 6 and 12 min incubation. Symbols represent the means of two separate experiments.

Assesment of Bacteriolysis

The bacteriolytic action of serum complement was studied in an assay modified from Friedlander[7] as previously described.[8] Briefly, ^{3}H thymidine-labeled *E. coli* K12 were incubated with serum diluted in the experimental media. After incubation at 37°C for 0 minutes and for indicated times thereafter the bacteria were sedimented by centrifugation. The radioactivity in the pellets was determined by liquid scintillation counting. The loss of radioactivity from bacterial pellets with time was taken to indicate bacteriolysis and is expressed as a percentage of lysis compared to zero minutes.

RESULTS

The ability of serum to opsonize bacteria was greatly influenced by the medium under study. Thus, *E. coli* ON2 opsonized with 5% fresh serum in GHBSS were rapidly taken up by human PMN (Fig. 1, right panel). Greater than 75% of the *E. coli* were PMN-associated after 12 minutes incubation. In sharp contrast, less than 5% uptake was recorded when *E. coli* had been opsonized with fresh serum in Travenol CAPD solution. When phagocytosis was allowed to proceed for 60 minutes, more bacteria became PMN-associated. However, the mean (range) uptake of *E. coli* at 60 minutes was 90% (83%–98%) after opsonization in GHBSS, compared to 50% (14%–74%) after opsonization in Travenol CAPD solutions (not shown in Fig. 1). The uptake of *E. coli* ON2 depends on complement-mediated opsonization as evidenced by the com-

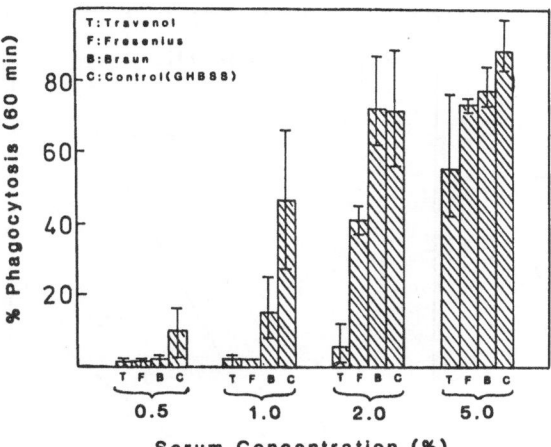

Fig. 2. Effect of CAPD solutions from three different manufacturers on complement-mediated opsonization of *E. coli* ON2. Bacteria were opsonized with indicated concentrations of serum in CAPD solutions from Travenol (T), Fresenius (F) or Braun (B). GHBSS was used as control medium (C). After opsonization bacteria were washed and mixed with PMN. Phagocytosis was determined after 60 min. Bars indicate the means of at least three separate experiments; brackets represent the total ranges.

plete lack of bacterial uptake when heat-inactivated serum was used (not shown in Fig. 1), as previously reported.[4]

Antibody-mediated opsonization, on the other hand, was little affected by CAPD solutions. Thus, the uptake of *S. epidermidis* L by human PMN was

Table 1. Effect of CAPD Solution on Bacterial Opsonization via the Alternative Complement Pathway.

Serum Concentration	*Escherichia coli* ON2 Opsonized* with			
	Normal Serum in		MgEGTA Serum† in	
	GHBSS‡	Braun§	GHBSS	Braun
	% Uptake by PMN (60 minutes)			
1.0%	52	13	3	4
5.0%	85	73	24	7
10.0%	82	79	66	15
20.0%	nt‖	nt	75	70

* Opsonization time was 15 min at 37°C.
† Serum chelated with MgEGTA to block the classical complement pathway.
‡ GHBSS, Hank's balanced salt solutions with 0.1% gelatin.
§ Braun, CAPD solution (1.5% glucose).
‖ nt, not tested.

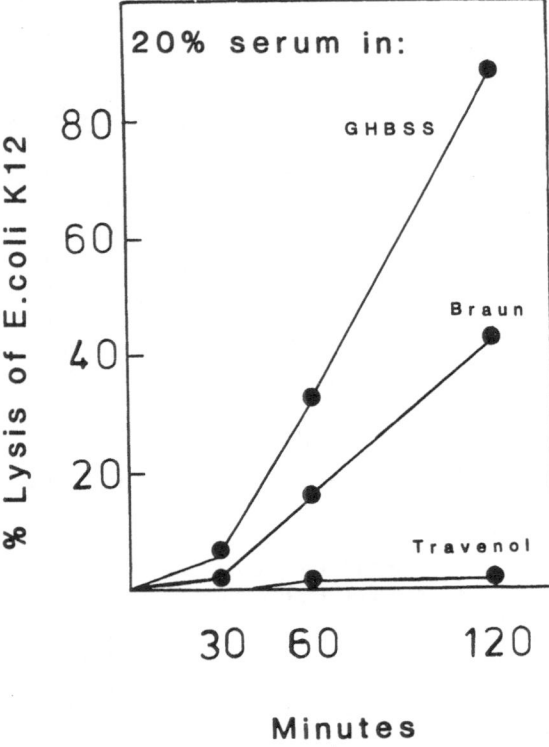

Fig. 3. Defective complement-mediated lysis of *Escherichia coli* K12 in CAPD solutions (Braun, Travenol). Radiolabeled bacteria were incubated with 20% fresh serum in either GHBSS or CAPD solutions at 37°C. At indicated times the release of radiolabel from the bacteria was determined and expressed as percent lysis. Results are from one representative experiment.

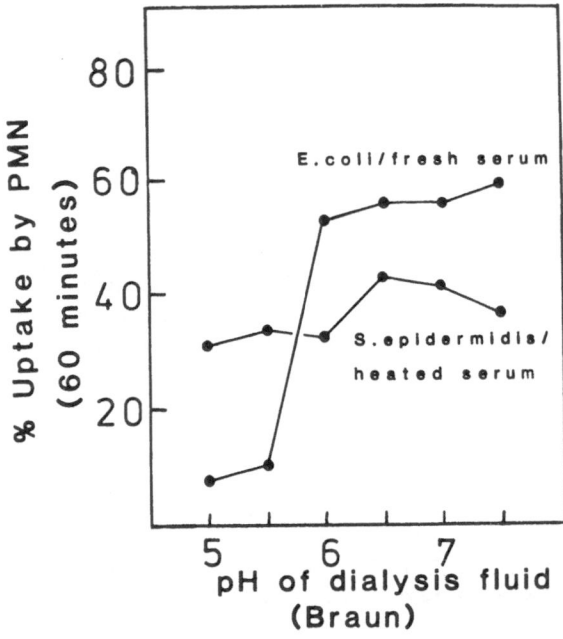

Fig. 4. Effect of pH on bacterial opsonization in CAPD solutions. *Escherichia coli* ON2 was opsonized (15 min at 37°C) with 1% fresh serum and *Staphylococcus epidermidis* was opsonized with 1% heated serum. The CAPD solution (Braun, 1.5% glucose) was adjusted to indicated pH with either 0.1 N HCL or 0.1 N NaOH. After opsonization bacteria were washed and mixed with PMN. Phagocytosis was determined after 60 min. Note the striking effect of pH on *E. coli* opsonization by complement and the lack of pH effect on *S. epidermidis* opsonization by antibody.

greater than 80% after opsonization with 5% heated serum in either GHBSS or Travenol CAPD solution (Fig. 1, left panel). *S. epidermidis* opsonization by heated serum has previously been noted and is presumed to be largely due to serum antibody.[4] Thus, complement-mediated, but not antibody-mediated, opsonization of bacteria is severely compromised by CAPD solutions.

To investigate the effects of CAPD solutions further we examined supplies from different manufacturers and solutions with different dextrose concentrations. Travenol solutions more severely hampered complement-mediated opsonization than similar solutions from the other two suppliers; Braun CAPD solutions were least antagonistic (Fig.

2). The glucose concentration did not influence complement-mediated opsonization (data not shown).

Opsonization of *E. coli* ON2 was also studied in MgEGTA chelated serum. Bacterial opsonization did occur using MgEGTA serum, although higher concentrations of serum were needed (Table 1). However, the opsonic activity of MgEGTA serum was further reduced when CAPD solutions instead of GHBSS were used as the experimental media (Table 1). Thus, both the classical and alternative complement pathways are affected by the conditions present in the CAPD milieu.

The complement-mediated lysis of *E. coli* K12 was likewise severely compromised in CAPD solutions. Lysis of *E. coli* K12 was greater than

85% after incubation (2 hours) with 20% serum in GHBSS. In sharp contrast, only 42% of the bacteria were lysed in the presence of Braun CAPD solutions and virtually no lysis occured in Travenol CAPD solutions (Fig. 3). Even at 40% serum concentration *E. coli* K12 lysis in Travenol CAPD solutions remained less than 10% after 2 hours incubation (data not shown).

In efforts to restore complement-mediated opsonization and lysis of bacteria in CAPD solutions it was found that the acidity of the CAPD solutions was largely responsible for the poor action of complement in these buffers. Thus, increasing the pH of CAPD solutions from their usual range of 5.0 to 5.5 to over 6.5 resulted in media that supported both complement-mediated opsonization of *E. coli* ON2 (Fig. 4) as well as lysis of *E. coli* K12 (Table 2).

Interestingly, the amount of titrateable acid in CAPD solutions varied considerably among commercial suppliers. Thus, Braun CAPD solutions contained 0.055 to 0.078 mEq/ml of titrateable acid compared to 0.154 to 0.167 mEq/dl for Travenol CAPD solutions (Fig. 5). Fresenius CAPD solutions contained intermediate amounts of titrateable acid (Fig. 5). The different acid contents correlated well with the differences between CAPD solutions noted in the opsonization and lysis experiments (*vide supra*).

DISCUSSION

Patients undergoing CAPD are at increased risk of developing bacterial peritonitis.[9] These results suggest that their increased susceptibility may, in part, be due to the use of CAPD solutions that severely hamper the antibacterial activity of serum complement. Generalized complement deficiencies affecting bacterial opsonization (C3-deficiency) and those affecting bacteriolysis (deficiencies in C5, C6, C7, or C8) predispose patients to serious infections.[10–12] In addition, localized deficiencies of complement at certain sites of the body, including the peritoneal cavity, have been suggested to predispose patients to infection at those sites.[13–16] Our previous data showed that in contrast to normal serum, peritoneal dialysate obtained from daily exchanges of CAPD patients contained low titers of opsonic activity for *S. epidermidis*.[4] Many patients did not have any detectable opsonic activity. *S. epidermidis* opsonic activity was predominantly heat-stable (i.e., antibody-mediated) and, when present, seemed to protect CAPD patients from peritonitis with these organisms.[5]

Table 2. Effect of pH on Complement-Mediated Lysis of *Escherichia Coli* K12.

pH of Buffer*	E. coli K12 Lysis by 20% Serum in (% lysis after 2 hours)	
	GHBSS†	Travenol‡
5.0	0	0
5.5	44	5
6.0	87	41
6.5	88	52
7.0	90	80

* Adjusted with 0.1 N HCL or 0.1 N NaOH.
† GHBSS, Hank's balanced salt solution with 0.1% gelatin.
‡ Travenol, CAPD solution (1.5% glucose).

In contrast, heat-labile (i.e., complement-mediated) peritoneal opsonins were much less frequently detected in CAPD patients and *E. coli* could not be opsonized by the CAPD effluents.[4] The present study would indicate that complement, even when present immunochemically, may not be functionally active in this milieu. However, the low levels of complement factor C3 in CAPD effluents would argue that a quantitative lack of complement probably also exists.[4,5]

Inactivation of complement by CAPD solutions was demonstrated in this study. Largely due to the

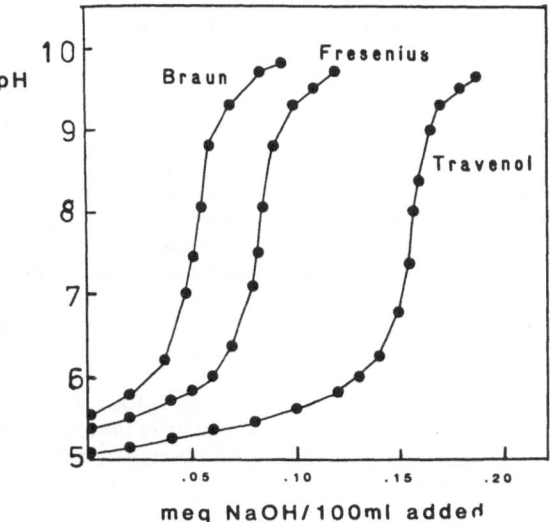

Fig. 5. Titrateable acid in commercial CAPD solutions obtained from three different suppliers.

low pH of these solutions complement-mediated opsonization and lysis of bacteria was severely compromised. Although the pH of the dialysate at the end of the dwell usually exceeds 7.0, complement may not be active in the peritoneal cavity during the initial period of the dialysis. In addition, complement components exposed to a low pH may become irreversibly inactivated resulting in immunochemically detectable but functionally inactive complement factors.[17] The low pH of dialysis solutions has previously been demonstrated to reduce the activity of phagocytic cells such as human PMN and peritoneal macrophages.[4, 18]

Thus, removal of bacteria from the peritoneal cavity, through opsonization, phagocytosis and bacteriolysis may be compromised by highly acidic CAPD solutions. Surprisingly, the amount of acid added to CAPD solutions has not been standardized. We found a 3-fold difference in the amount of titrateable acid among CAPD solutions from three different manufacturers. The differences in the acidity of the dialysis solutions correlated with the extent of their deleterious effects on the complement system. Since the need to acidify these solutions rests solely with the manufacturing process we conclude that dialysis solutions should be modified to support rather than antagonize the peritoneal defense mechanisms of CAPD patients.

ACKNOWLEDGMENT

This study was supported by a grant from the Kidney Foundation of the Netherlands.

REFERENCES

1. Stossel TP, Field RJ, Gitlin JD, Alper CA, and Rosen FS: The opsonic fragment of the third component of human complement (C3). J Exp Med 141: 1329, 1975
2. Verbrugh HA, Van Dijk WC, Van Erne ME, Peters R, Peterson PK, and Verhoef J: Quantitation of the third component of human complement attached to the surface of opsonized bacteria: Opsonin-deficient sera and phagocytosis-resistant strains. Infect Immunol 26: 808, 1979
3. Schreiber RD, Morrison DC, Podack ER, and Müller-Eberhard HJ: Bactericidal activity of the alternative complement pathway generated from eleven isolated plasma proteins. J Exp Med 149: 870, 1979
4. Verbrugh HA, Keane WF, Hoidal JR, Freiberg MR, Elliott GR, and Peterson PK: Peritoneal macrophages and opsonins: Antibacterial defense in patients undergoing chronic peritoneal dialysis. J Infect Dis 147: 1018, 1983
5. Keane WF, Comty CM, Verbrugh HA, and Peterson PK: Opsonic deficiency of peritoneal dialysis effluent in continuous ambulatory peritoneal dialysis. Kidney Int 25: 539, 1984
6. Peterson PK, Verhoef J, Schmeling D, and Quie PG: Kinetics of phagocytosis and bacterial killing by human polymorphonuclear leukoctyes and monocytes. J Infect Dis 136: 502, 1977
7. Friedlander AM: DNA release as a direct measure of microbial killing. I. Serum bactericidal activity. J Immunol 115: 1404, 1975
8. Van Dijk WC, Verbrugh HA, Peters R, Van Erne ME, Peterson PK, and Verhoef J: *Escherichia coli* K antigen in relation to serum-induced lysis and phagocytosis. J Med Microbiol 12: 123, 1979
9. Harrington JT: Chronic ambulatory peritoneal dialysis. N Engl J Med 306: 670, 1982
10. Nicholson A, and Lepow IH: Host defense against *Neisseria meningitidis* requires a complement-dependent bactericidal activity. Science 205: 298, 1979
11. Leddy JP, and Steigbigel RT: Complement, serum bactericidal activity, and disseminated Gram-negative infection (editorial). Ann Intern Med 90: 984, 1979
12. Johnston RB, and Stroud RN: Complement and host defense against infection. J Pediatr 90: 169, 1977
13. Fromkes JJ, Thomas FB, Mekkjian HS, and Evans M: Antimicrobial activity of human ascitic fluid. Gastroenterology 73: 668, 1977
14. Akalin HE, Laleli Y, and Telatar H: Bactericidal and opsonic activity of ascitic fluid from cirrhotic and noncirrhotic patients. J Infect Dis 147: 1011, 1983
15. Lew PD, Zubler R, Vaudaux P, Farquet JJ, Waldvogel FA, and Lambert PH: Decreased heat-labile opsonic activity and complement levels associated with evidence of C3 breakdown products in infected pleural effusions. J Clin Invest 63: 326, 1979
16. Bernstein JM, Schenkein HA, Genco RJ, and Bartholomew WR: Complement activity in middle ear effusions. Clin Exp Immunol 33: 340, 1978
17. Hemmer CH, Hänsch G, Gresham HD, and Shin ML: Activation of the fifth and sixth components of the human complement system: C6-dependent cleavage of C5 in acid and the formation of a bimolecular lytic complex, C5b,6[a]. J Immunol 131: 892, 1983
18. Duwe AK, Vas SI, and Weatherhead JW: Effects of composition of peritoneal dialysis fluid on chemiluminescence, phagocytosis, and bactericidal activity in vitro. Infect Immunol 33: 130, 1981

S. Steen, P. Brenchley, J. Manos, R. Pumphrey,
and R. Gokal

107

Opsonizing Capacity of Peritoneal Fluid and Relationship to Peritonitis in CAPD Patients

SUMMARY

Peritoneal dialysate of 45 patients was examined for opsonic activity. The opsonizing capacity of dialysate from patients with a history of peritonitis was lower than that of patients never experiencing peritonitis, but did not correlate with numbers of episodes of peritonitis. The duration of CAPD did not correlate with dialysate IgG and C_3 levels or with opsonizing capacity. IgG and C_3 concentrations are about 40–50 times lower in dialysate than in serum. The correlation of dialysate opsonic activity with peritonitis allows early identification of patients at high risk.

INTRODUCTION

CAPD is increasingly being used to treat patients with end-stage renal failure. Peritonitis remains a major complication of the treatment, occuring at least once every 6 to 12 patient months.[1]

Immunologic mechanisms are of prime importance in protecting the host against pathogenic bacterial and fungal organisms. A fundamental role for phagocytic cells (polymorphonuclear leukocytes and macrophages) and humoral opsonizing factors (IgG and C_3) in host immunity has been established in a range of diseases.[2,3] These defenses may also protect the peritoneal cavity from infection under normal circumstances but impairment of these mechanisms may predispose an individual to peritonitis.

In order for most pathogens to be phagocytosed efficiently, it is essential that they are opsonized, a process dependent on the concentration of specific IgG and/or alternate pathway complement components. We have measured the capacity of peritoneal dialysate (PD) to opsonize a standard preparation of zymosan particles, and the dialysate concentration of total IgG and C_3. Dialysate from patients with and without previous history of peritonitis were examined in this study to determine the relationship of opsonization capacity and history of peritonitis.

PATIENTS

We have studied 45 patients (mean age 44 years, range 20–71 years) on CAPD for 15.8 months (range 1–37 months). Nine patients had no history of peritonitis, 27 had 1 to 2 episodes and nine had three or more episodes. Studies were done at least 1 month beyond an episode of peritonitis on fluid (1.36% anhydrous dextrose) from an overnight dwell (Table 1).

METHODS

The ability of the PD fluid to opsonize zymosan particles was quantitated by a luminol-amplified, chemiluminescence assay of phagocytosis using

From the Departments of Renal Medicine and Immunology, Manchester Royal Infirmary, Manchester, England.

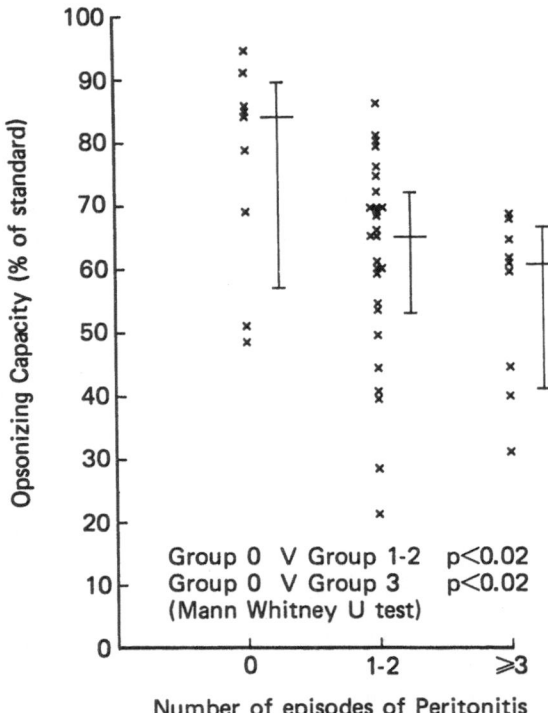

Group 0 V Group 1-2   p<0.02
Group 0 V Group 3   p<0.02
(Mann Whitney U test)

Fig. 1. Relationship of opsonizing capacity to peritonitis.

polymorphonuclear leukocytes isolated from normal peripheral blood.[4] Briefly PD fluid (concentrated 5-fold) was incubated with 4 mg zymosan at 37°C for 30 minutes. The washed, opsonized zymosan was added to 0.5×10 PMN cells and the chemiluminescence generated during phagocytosis was measured in a liquid scintillation counter in out of coincidence mode (LKB Rackbeta). Results are expressed as time (minutes) to peak response relative to a standard preparation of zymosan opsonized with a pool of normal human serum (10% concentration).

C_3 and IgG concentrations in serum and dialysate were quantitated by rate nephelometry (Beckman Instruments).

RESULTS

Unconcentrated dialysate showed detectable opsonic activity. After 5-fold concentration, the opsonization was reproducible and more easily quantifiable and all results relate to the use of concentrated PD fluid.

The opsonizing capacity of PD fluid from patients with a history of peritonitis was significantly lower than that of patients with no incidence of peritonitis ($p < 0.02$, Mann Whitney U test, 2 tailed,

Table 1. Patient Groups.

Episodes of Peritonitis	Number of Patients	Mean Age (years)	Time on CAPD (Median, months)
0	9	48 (25–71)	6 (1–20)
1–2	27	44 (21–65)	15* (7–36)
>3	9	47 (24–62)	21* (8–37)

* $p < 0.02$.

Table 2. Relation between Peritonitis Episodes and Opsonizing Proteins.

Episodes of Peritonitis	Serum IgG (g/L)	Fluid IgG (mg/L)	Serum C_3 (g/L)	Fluid C_3 (mg/L)
0	8.4 (5.9–12.0)	117 (72–208)	1.0 (0.92–1.32)	20.1)10–38)
1–2	8.2 (3.4–17.6)	102 (69–146)	0.99)0.46–2.29)	13.8 (6–27)
>3	8.2 (4.5–16.8)	90 (52–102)	0.99 (0.6–2.21)	15.2 (6–24)

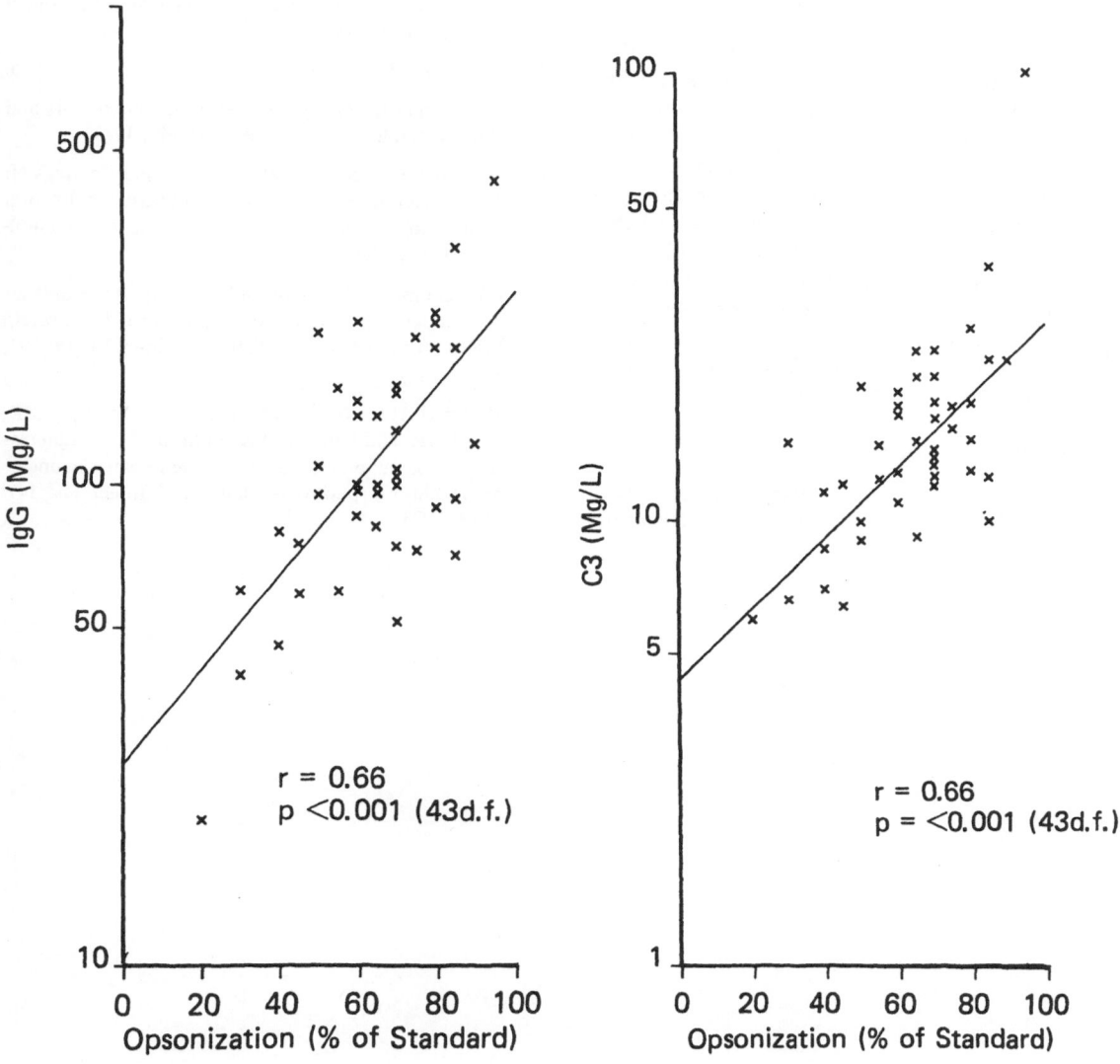

Fig. 2. Correlation of PD fluid IgG and opsonizing capacity.

Fig. 3. Correlation of PD fluid C3 and opsonizing capacity.

Fig. 1). There was no significant difference in PD fluid opsonization between patients with 1–2 episodes of peritonitis compared to patients with three or more episodes.

Patients with peritontis had been on CAPD for a significantly longer time than patients who had no history of peritonitis (Table 1, $p < 0.02$). However, there was no significant difference in PD fluid IgG and C_3 concentrations between the groups (Table 2) and there was no correlation between the length of time on CAPD and IgG and C_3 levels ($r = -0.18$, $p > 0.05$, data not shown). Likewise, there was no correlation between time on CAPD and opsonization capacity.

A correlation was observed between opsonizing capacity and PD fluid IgG concentration (Fig. 2) and between opsonizing capacity and PD fluid C_3 values (Fig. 3). PD fluid concentrations of IgG and C_3 were found to be 40 to 50 times lower than the serum values (Table 2).

DISCUSSION

We have confirmed previous reports[5,6] that peritoneal dialysate contains immunologically important molecules, i.e. IgG and C_3, although the concentrations are approximately 40 to 50 times lower than serum values. These components are detectable by a functional assay of opsonization in CAPD effluent but are more readily quantifiable after 5-fold concentration. We have identified low PD fluid opsonization capacity as a factor related to the incidence of peritonitis in patients on CAPD. We suggest that monitoring PD fluid opsonization capacity early in the course of CAPD may identify patients at risk of repeated peritonitis.

REFERENCES

1. Fenton SS, Wu G, Cattran C, Wadgymar A, and Allen AF: Clinical aspects of peritonitis in patients on chronic ambulatory peritoneal dialysis. Peritoneal Dial Bull 1: 51, 1981

2. Stossel TP: Phagocytosis. Sem Haematol 12: 83, 1975

3. Winkelstein JA: Opsonins, their function, identity and clinical significance. J Pediatr 82: 747, 1973

4. Easmon CSF, Cole PJ, Williams AJ, and Hastings N: The measurement of opsonic and phagocytic function by luminol-dependent chemiluminescence. Immunology 41: 67, 1980

5. Blumenkrantz MJ, Gahl GM, Kopple JD, Kamadar AV, Jones MR, Kessel M, and Coburn JN: Protein losses during peritoneal dialysis. Kidney Int 19: 593, 1981

6. Verbrugh HA, Keane WN, Hoidal JR, Freiberg MR, Elliot GR, and Peterson PK: Peritoneal macrophages and opsonins; antibacterial defense in patients undergoing chronic peritoneal dialysis. J Infect Dis 147: 1018, 1983

F. Giacchino, M. Rotunno, M. Pozzato, M. Formica,
P. Belardi, F. Bonello, and G. Piccoli

108

Opsonization Capacity of Plasma and Peritoneal Dialysate in CAPD Patients

SUMMARY

Plasma fibronectin concentrations in CAPD patients were found not to be different from healthy controls. During peritonitis plasma fibronectin concentration was lowered and the plasma fibronectin/peritoneal fibronectin ratio increased. In two patients with recurrent peritonitis the plasma fibronectin/peritoneal fibronectin ratio remained very low. Since fibronectin is an important opsonic protein for staphylococcal destruction, its low concentration in some patients with frequent peritonitis suggests a causal role in these patients.

INTRODUCTION

Fibronectins are glycoproteins present in plasma, extracellular fluid and connective tissue.[1,2] Fibronectin (molecular weight 400,000 daltons) is synthesized by a variety of different cells, such as fibroblasts, macrophages and endothelial cells.[3-5] Its importance lies in its role as a non-immunologic opsonic protein in the host defense system, promoting particle ingestion by phagocytic cells of the reticuloendothelial system.[6] Recently it has been shown that fibronectin promotes the attachment of some bacteria, especially *Staphylococcus* strains, to neutrophils, whereas ingestion of bacteria requires

From the Medical Nephrology Institute of the University of Turin and Nephrology and Dialysis Departments, San Giovanni Hospital, Turin, Italy.

other opsonins (immunoglobulin G or complement). On the other hand it has been found that fibronectin binds many strains of coagulase-negative *Staphylococci*, which lack IgG receptors. There is often a fall in the level of circulating fibronectin in patients who have had surgery, trauma or sepsis; in these cases the prognosis is poor.[9] In a previous study[10] we found that peritonitis in peritoneal dialysis (CAPD) patients was not correlated with cell-mediated mechanisms of the immune response. To evaluate the influence of opsonic capacity on peritonitis in patients treated by CAPD, we determined the concentration of fibronectin in both plasma and peritoneal dialysate of 25 CAPD patients.

MATERIALS AND METHODS

Patients

Twenty five patients (10 males, 15 females; mean age 55 ± 9 years) undergoing peritoneal dialysis (mean duration of treatment 16 ± 4 months) were studied. Three to five exchanges a day were made with Dianeal® bags (1.5 or 2.5 or 4.25 g/L dextrose). Ten healthy individuals (5 males, 5 females; mean age 30 ± 5 years) served as controls for plasma fibronectin.

Plasma Fibronectin

Fibronectin was determined by using a nephelometric immunoassay (ICS Immunochemistry analyzer).[11] Blood was collected in sodium citrate and

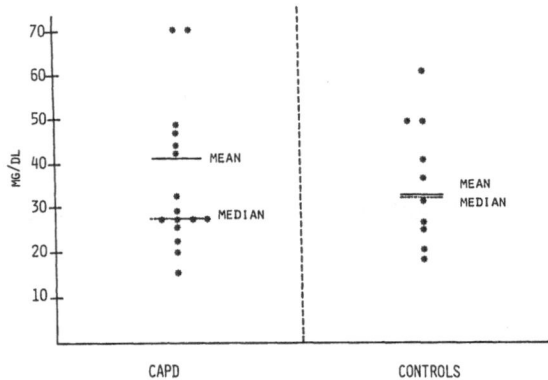

Fig. 1. Plasma fibronectin in CAPD patients and healthy controls.

plasma was separated by centrifugation at room temperature. Plasma from CAPD patients and controls was cleared through a Millipore® filter. A standard plasma (Behringwerke) with known concentration of fibronectin was also used. Anti-human fibronectin rabbit serum (Behringwerke) was also cleared by filtration through a Millipore® filter before use.

The final test consists of 200 μl of plasma, dilution 1:10 in 0.15 Mol NaCl was incubated with 400 μl of antiserum, dilution 1:5 in 0.15 Mol NaCl. Reaction time was 60 minutes.

Peritoneal Fibronectin

Three hundred milliliters of peritoneal dialysate from the first bag of the morning were filtered and concentrated 60 to 100 times using dialyzer tubing

(molecular weight cut-off 12,000 daltons, Spectrapor). Dilution 1:2 of peritoneal dialysate was also used. Fibronectin was determined using the above method.

Statistics

The data obtained were stored in a Packard computer and statistical analyses were stored in a Packard computer and statistical analyses were made by Student's and two tailed Fisher's tests.

RESULTS

The plasma concentration of fibronectin of the CAPD patients did not differ significantly from the control group (Fig. 1). Four patients had several episodes of peritonitis (Fig. 2): in these patients plasma fibronectin was significantly lower than in the others, and the increased plasma fibronectin/ peritoneal fibronectin ratio increased. In 6/10 cases, peritonitis was caused by a coagulase-negative *Staphylococcus*.

During peritonitis, plasma fibronectin increased slightly (55.3 ± 19.9 mg/dl; $p < 0.05$); and plasma fibronectin/peritoneal fibronectin ratio increased ($p < 0.02$) compared to values before infection (Fig. 3).

When patients recovered from peritonitis, plasma fibronectin remained high (65.5 ± 8 mg/dl) in those patients in whom no further peritonitis episodes developed within 3 to 6 months, but in two patients in whom peritonitis recurred, the fibronectin level remained low (9 ± 3 mg/dl).

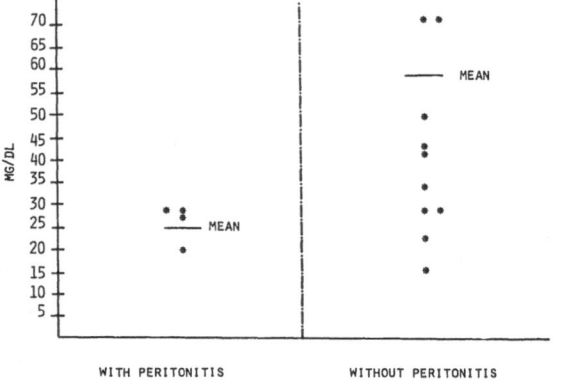

Fig. 2. Plasma fibronectin in CAPD patients with and without peritonitis. Plasma fibronectin concentration was significantly lower ($p < 0.01$) in patients with peritonitis.

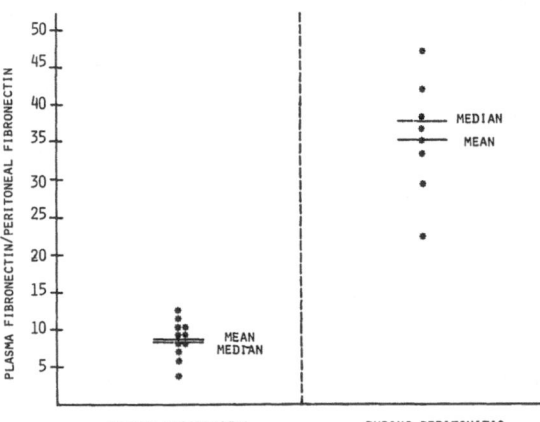

Fig. 3. Plasma fibronectin/peritoneal fibronectin ratio in CAPD patients. This ratio increased significantly during peritonitis ($p < 0.02$).

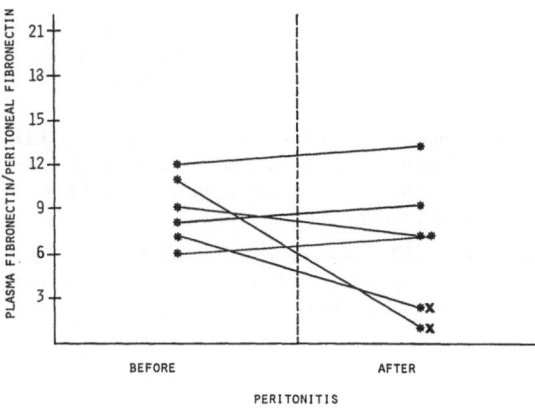

Fig. 4. Plasma fibronectin/peritoneal fibronectin ratio after peritonitis. **X** = patients who developed recurrent peritonitis.

Figure 4 shows the plasma fibronectin/peritoneal fibronectin ratio after the peritonitis episode. Peritoneal fibronectin returned to the values before infection and there was an increase in the plasma fibronectin/peritoneal fibronectin ratio except in the patients who later developed peritonitis.

DISCUSSION

The fact that plasma fibronectin concentration is reduced in severe disseminated intravascular coagulation syndrome[12] is consistent with its important role in mediating clearance of circulating fibrin complexes from the blood via the reticuloendothelial system. A reduced plasma concentration of fibronectin has also been described in patients with severe trauma or sepsis[9-13] and it has also been shown to play a role in host defense mechanisms against *Staphylococcus*.[7]

In our study, plasma fibronectin of CAPD patients did not significantly differ from the control group. The ratio of plasma fibronectin to peritoneal fibronectin averaged 8.87. No differences in fibronectin concentrations were found in our study in regards to sex or age as those described for healthy people.[14]

During peritonitis we observed an increase in the plasma concentrations of fibronectin and in the fibronectin/peritoneal fibronectin ratio; this phenomenon may be due to the increased consumption of peritoneal fibronectin or to its reduced production by peritoneal macrophages, even though plasma concentrations were increased. On the other hand reduced permeability of the peritoneal membrane to fibronectin cannot be excluded.

The opsonic activity of immunoglobulins is directed particularly against Gram positive bacteria; in some strains of coagulase negative *Staphylococci* in which a lack of IgG receptors has been observed,[7] fibronectin has been found to play a major defense role. The fact that a reduction in both plasma and peritoneal fibronectins have been observed in patients who had had several episodes of peritonitis supports these findings.

In our study, plasma and peritoneal fibronectins were very low in patients who had suffered from coagulase-negative *Staphylococcus* peritonitis, suggesting that a lack of opsonic activity in the plasma and in the peritoneal dialysate may constitute one of the principal causes of infection.

ACKNOWLEDGMENT

This work was supported by a grant from Travenol Laboratories.

REFERENCES

1. Mosesson MW, Umfleet RA: The cold insoluble globulin of human plasma. I. Purification, primary characterization, and relationship to fibrinogen and cold insoluble fraction components. J Biol Chem 245: 5728, 1970
2. Yamada KM, and Olden K: Fibronectins—adhesive glycoproteins of cell surface and blood. Nature 275: 179, 1978
3. Johansson S, Rubin K, Hook M, Ahgren T, and Seljelid R: In vitro biosynthesis of cold insoluble globulin (fibronectin) by mouse peritoneal macrophages. FEBS Letter 105: 313, 1979
4. Rouslahti E, and Engvall E: Immunochemical and collagen-binding properties of fibronectin. Ann NY Acad Sci 312: 178, 1978
5. Rouslahti E, and Vaheri A: Novel human serum protein from fibroblast plasma membrane. Nature 248: 790, 1974
6. Fibronectin and infection. Lancet. 1: 106, 1983
7. Mosesson MW, and Amrani DL. The structure and biologic activities of plasma fibronectin. Blood 56: 145, 1980
8. Nord CE, Holta-Oie S, Ljungh A, and Wadstrom T: Characterization of coagulase-negative staphylococcal species from human infection. In Jeliaszewicz J (Ed), Staphylococci and staphylococcal diseases. Stuttgart: Gustav Fischer Verlag, W Germany, 1976 p 105

9. Saba TM, and Jaffe E: Plasma fibronectin (opsonic glycoprotein); its synthesis by vascular endothelial cells and role in cardiopulmonary integrity after trauma as related to reticuloendothelial function. Am J Med 60: 577, 1980

10. Giacchino F, Alloatti A, Quarello F, Coppo R, Pellerey M, and Piccoli G: The influence of peritoneal dialysis on cellular immunity. Peritoneal Dial Bull 2: 165, 1982

11. Pott G, and Meyering M: Rapid determination of fibronectin by laser nephelometry. J Clin Chem Clin Biochem 18: 893, 1980

12. Mosher DF, and Williams EM: Fibronectin concentration decreased in plasma of severely ill patients with disseminated intravascular coagulation. J Lab Clin Med 91: 729, 1978

13. Goldman AS, Rudloff HB, McNamee R, Loose LD, and Diluzio NR: Deficiency of plasma humeral recognition factor activity following burn injury. J Reticuloendothelial Soc 15: 193, 1978

14. Eriksen HO, Clemmensen I, Hansen MS, and Ibsen KK: Plasma fibronectin concentration in normal subjects. Scand J Clin Lab Invest 42: 291, 1982

V.M.A. Yewdall, D.N. Bennett-Jones, J.S. Cameron,
C.S. Ogg, and D.G. Williams

109

Opsonically-Active Proteins in CAPD Fluid

SUMMARY

Concentrations of albumin, transferrin, IgG, C_3 and α_2 macroglobulin were measured by radial immunodiffusion in serum and dialysate of patients treated by CAPD. Fibronectin and CH_{50} were also measured by nephelometry and dialysate opsonic activity was determined. Transport of proteins into peritoneal dialysate was low, varied considerably from patient to patient, and showed little discrimination according to protein size. The dialysate protein level correlated with *in vitro* opsonic activity.

INTRODUCTION

It has been suggested that peritoneal host defenses may play a role in the prevention of peritonitis in certain CAPD patients.[1] The purpose of this study has been to investigate the level of certain opsonically-active proteins (IgG, C_3, and fibronectin) and selected "marker" proteins (albumin, transferrin, and α_2 macroglobulin) in the overnight dialysis effluent of patients from our CAPD program. In addition, the opsonic activity against *S. epidermidis* of the dialysate has been measured and related to the level of protein in the fluid.

From the Renal Unit, Guy's Hospital, London, United Kingdom.

METHODS

Patients were instructed to come to the clinic at the time of routine line-changes in the morning, with the overnight fluid still in their abdomen. The fluid was drained in the clinic and a sample taken. This, together with a serum sample, was stored in aliquots at $-70°$C. In occasional patients samples were taken in the 2 weeks following an intraperitoneal surgical procedure.

Serum and dialysate were analysed for albumin, transferrin, IgG, C_3, and α_2 macroblobulin by radial immunodiffusion. All measurements, except for C_3, were carried out on commercially available plates (partigen plates, Behring and Immuno-plate 111, Hyland Diagnostics) (Table 1).

Fibronectin was measured by laser nephelometer and CH_{50} by a modified tube method.[2] Opsonic activity in the dialysate was measured as the uptake, by normal polymorphs, of pre-opsonized, tritium-labeled bacteria using the method of Peterson et al.[3] In brief, a suspension of *S. epidermidis*, grown overnight in Muller-Hinton broth with tritiated adenine, was opsonized in the test PD fluid for 15 minutes at 37°C. The bacteria were washed and then incubated with normal polymorphs for 30 minutes at 37°C. Cell-associated (ingested) bacteria were separated from non-cell-associated bacteria by a process of differential centrifugation, and the percentage of bacteria ingested was calculated from the cell-associated radioactivity.

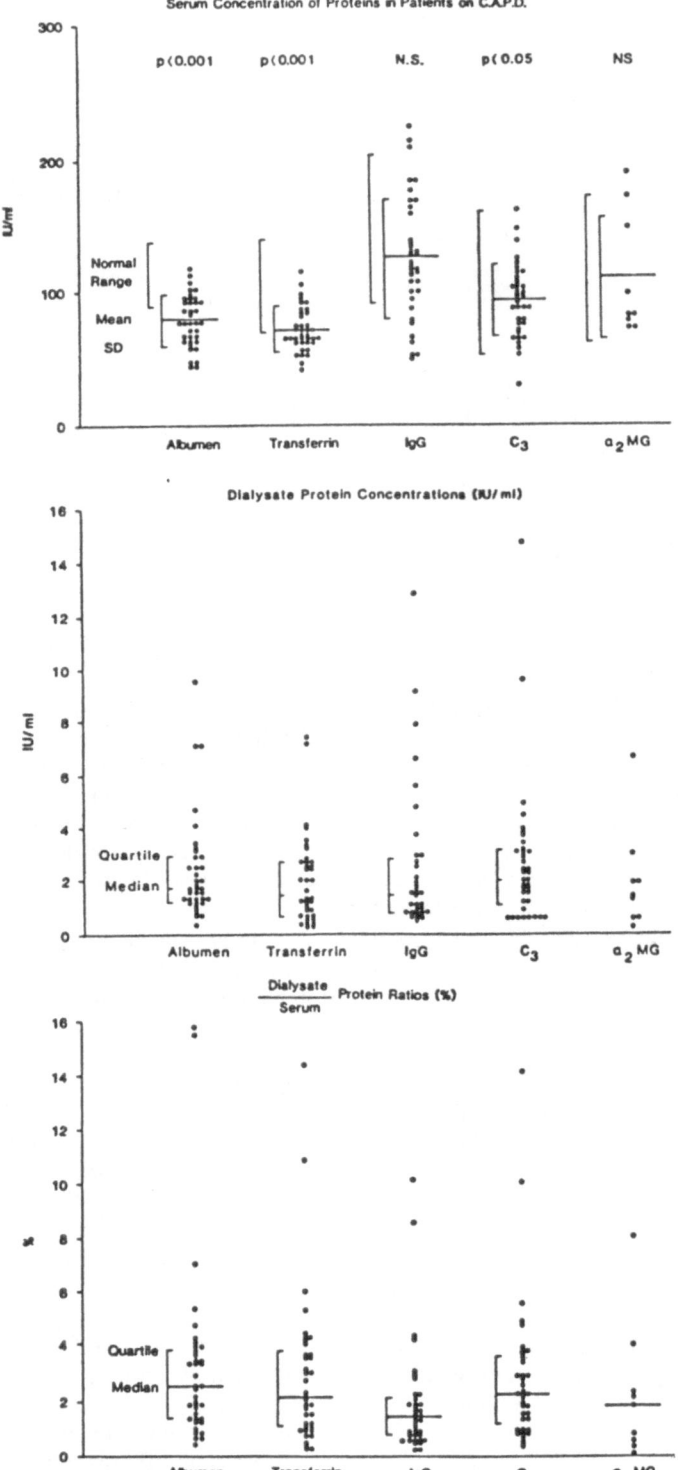

Fig. 1.   Serum and dialysis protein levels, dialysate/serum protein ratios.

Table 1. Diagnostic Tests.

	IgG	Transferrin	Albumin	α_2MG
Serum	Immuno-plate	Nor-partigen	Nor-partigen	Nor-partigen
Fluid	Immuno-plate (Low-level)	LC-partigen	M-partigen	LC-partigen

RESULTS

Serum and Dialysate Protein Levels

The levels of albumin, transferrin, C_3, IgG, and α_2 macroglobulin in serum and dialysate are shown graphically (Fig. 1). The serum levels of albumin, transferrin, and C_3 were significantly lower than in normal non-uremics, whereas there was no significant difference for IgG and α_2 macroglobulin. The dialysate levels showed a wide variation of more than 10-fold, although the highest levels occurred in patients who had undergone an intra-peritoneal procedure in the previous 2 weeks. There was a very weak correlation between the serum level of some proteins and the dialysate level—e.g., for IgG, r = 0.296, (0.05 < p < 0.1). The dialysate:serum ratio for each protein was also calculated and is shown in Figure 1.

Dialysate/Serum Protein Ratios

The correlation between the D/S ratio for IgG, C_3, and α_2 macroglobulin compared with albumin is shown in Figure 2. There is a remarkably close correlation between the concentration of all proteins measured in the dialysate when expressed in this way. It may be noted that the slope of the line as

calculated from the linear regression analysis is a measure of the mean selectivity of the peritoneal membrane for each pair of proteins—i.e., $D/S_{IgG}/D/S_{alb} = 0.60$.

The derived selectivity for each protein against albumin is as shown in Table 2. This shows a very low degree of selectivity even for proteins up to a MW 850,000 daltons. It is of interest that the passage of IgG into the peritoneal cavity is more restricted than that of C_3, which has a higher molecular weight. This phenomenon may be related to the ionic charge of the 2 molecules.

Opsonization

The opsonization of *S. epidermidis* (an isolate from a patient with peritonitis) by samples of dialysate, using the phagocytosis of radio-labeled bacteria as the assay, against the dialysate concentration of IgG is shown in Figure 3. It can be seen that there is a close correlation (r = 0.824, p < 0.001) between IgG and opsonization.

Dialysate Fibronectin Levels

We have successfully developed a nephelometric assay that detects fibronectin in the dialysate, even when there is no history of recent peritonitis.

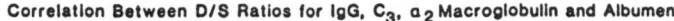

Correlation Between D/S Ratios for IgG, C₃, α₂ Macroglobulin and Albumen

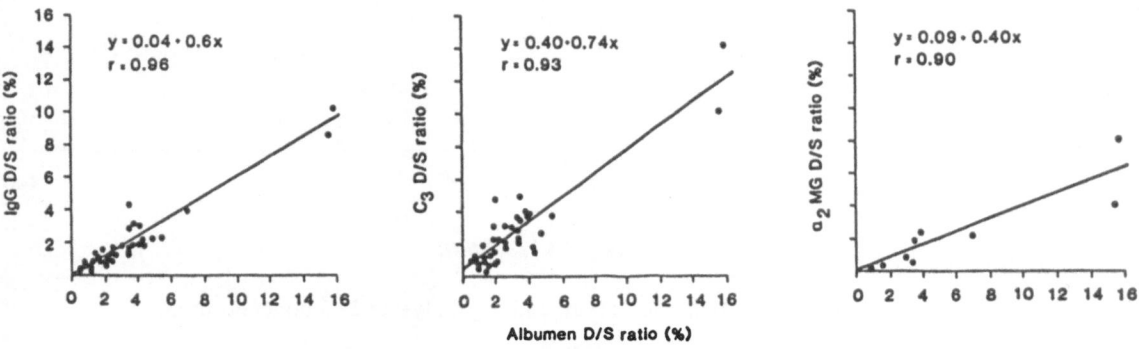

Fig. 2. Dialysate/serum protein ratios plotted against D/S ratio for albumin.

576   Yewdall, et al.

Table 2. Peritoneal Protein Selectivity.

Protein	Molecular Wt	Selectivity
IgG	150,000 daltons	0.60
C₃	185,000 daltons	0.74
α₂MG	850,000 daltons	0.40

Figure 4 shows the distribution of dialysate fibronectin levels. Unfortunately we do not have suitable samples for measuring the plasma fibronectin level in these patients and are therefore unable to give the D/P ratio. However, when plotted as a ratio to normal plasma fibronectin levels, the dialysate concentration can be seen from Figure 5 to fall on the

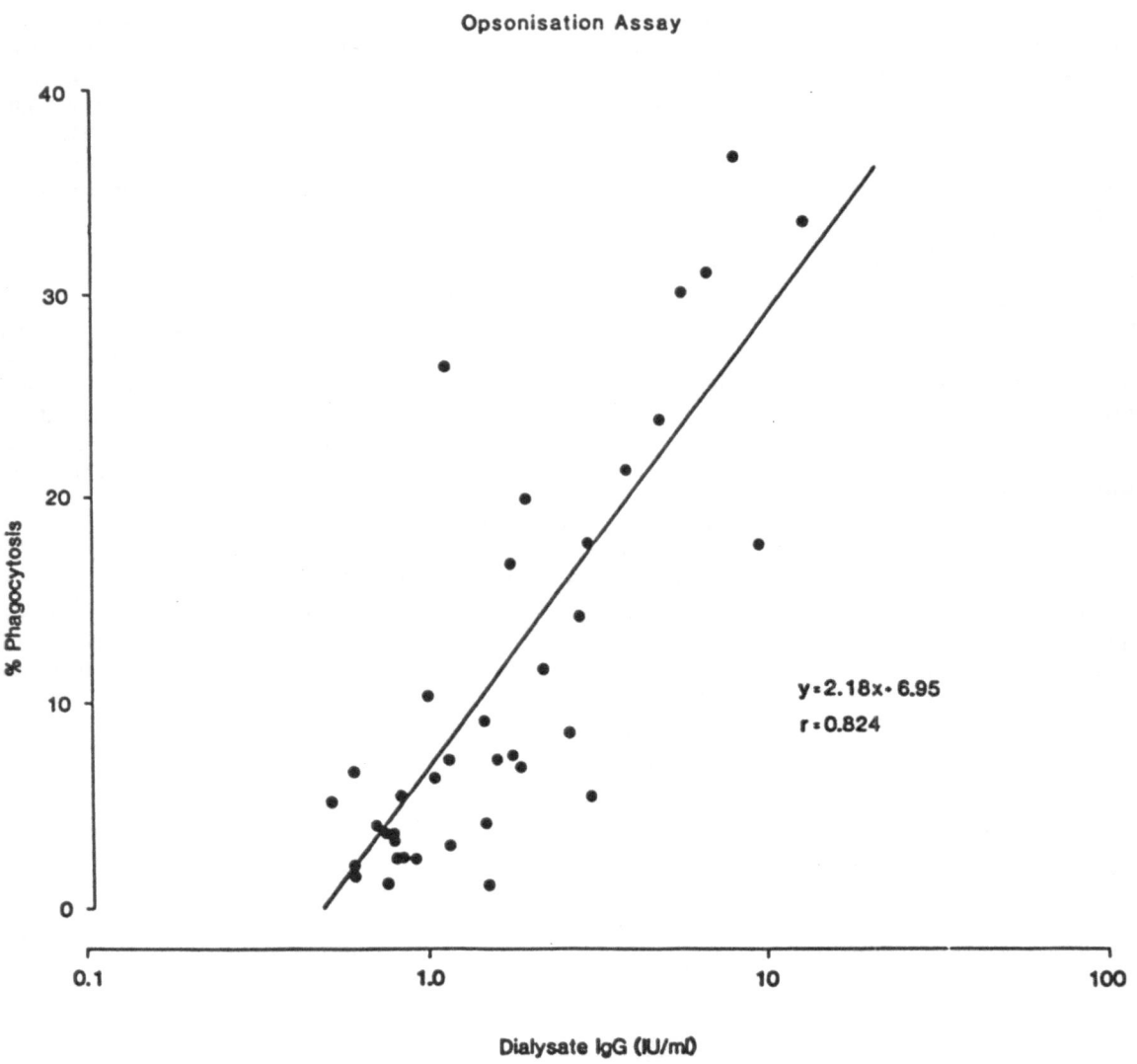

Fig. 3. Graph of opsonization assay and log dialysate IgG concentration.

Dialysate Fibronectin Levels

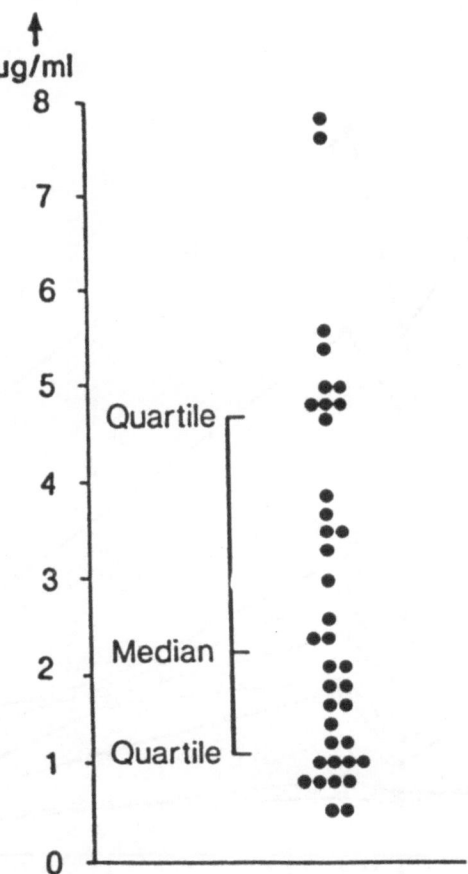

Fig. 4. Dialysate fibronectin concentration.

expected line of D/S ratio against molecular mass for each patient.

DISCUSSION

As a result of our study we can draw the following conclusions. The entry of proteins of a wide range of molecular weights (65,000–850,000 daltons) into the peritoneal cavity is highly variable from patient to patient and is increased by such surgical interventions, as catheter re-positioning. There is a very low degree of protein selectivity across the whole range of molecular weights, and patients who have a high level of one protein also have high levels of the others. The level of protein in the dialysate corresponds well with *in vitro* opsonic activity. We have no information as to which substance or substances in the dialysate is important in this process.

ACKNOWLEDGMENT

Supported by a grant from Travenol, United Kingdom.

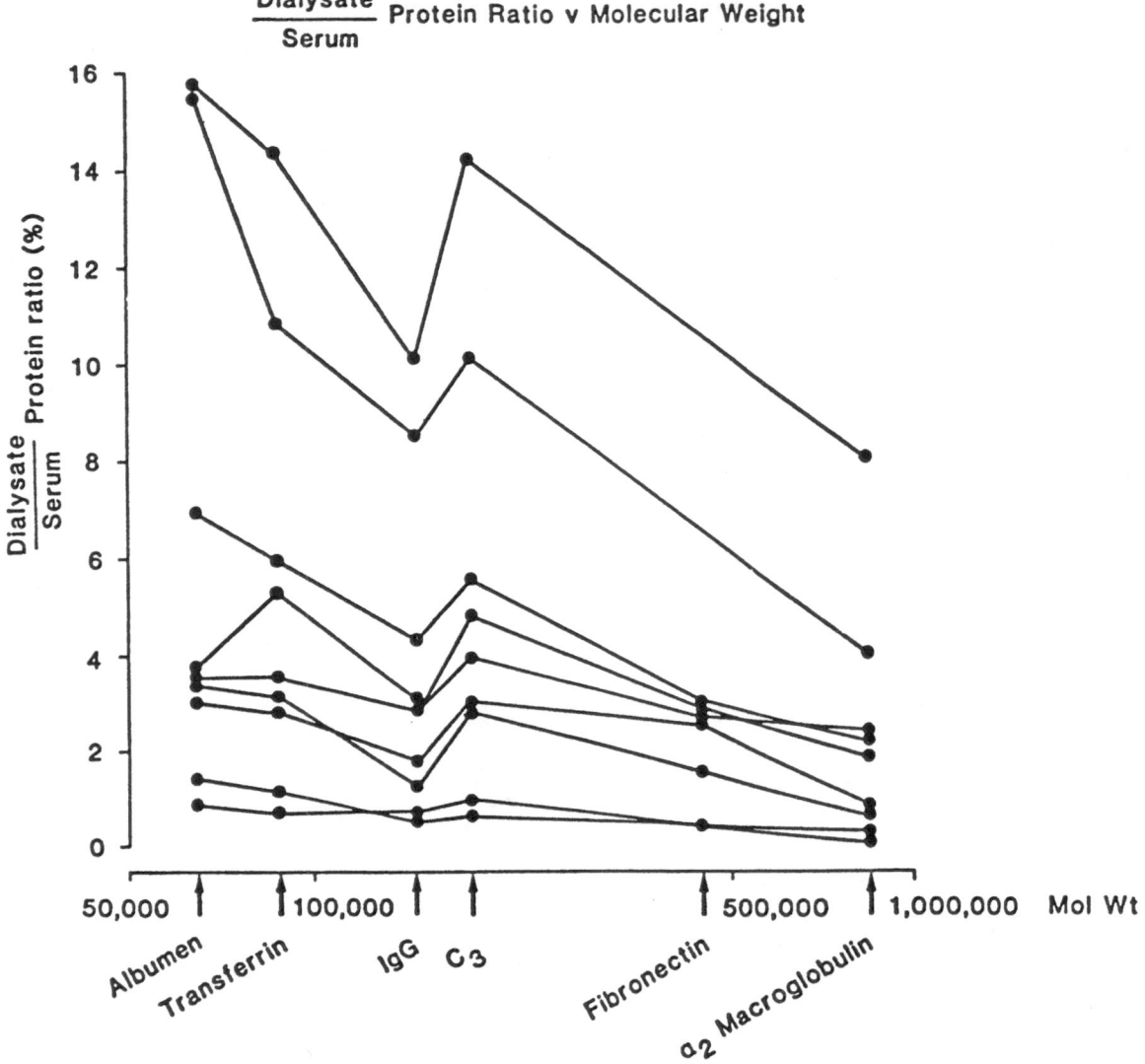

N.B. Fibronectin results expressed as Dialysate/Normal Plasma Ratio

Fig. 5.   Dialysate/serum protein ratio versus MW.

REFERENCES

1. Verbrugh HA, Keane WF, Hoidal JR, Freiberg MR, Elliott GR, and Peterson PK: Peritoneal macrophages and opsonins: Antibacterial defense in patients undergoing chronic peritoneal dialysis. J Infect Dis 147: 1018, 1983

2. Weir DM: Handbook of experimental immunology, Vol 1. Oxford: Blackwell Scientific Publications, 1973, p 5.10

3. Peterson PK, Verhoef J, Schmelling D, and Quie PG: Kinetics of phagocytosis and bacterial killing by human polymorphonuclear leukocytes and monocytes. J Infect Dis 136: 502, 1977

E. Cecchin, S. DeMarchi, P. DePaoli,
G. Santini, and F. Tesio

110

Defective Peritoneal Polymorphonuclear Leukocyte Function in Patients on Intermittent Peritoneal Dialysis: Effects of Some Divalent Ions and Fibronectin

SUMMARY

Gram-positive bacteria are the most common causative agents of peritonitis complicating peritoneal dialysis. Blood and peritoneal polymorphonuclear leukocyte (PML) function was investigated with chemiluminescence, phagocytosis and killing in ten patients with end-stage kidney disease undergoing intermittent peritoneal dialysis (IPD). Calcium (Ca), magnesium (Mg), inorganic phosphorus (P), urea, creatinine, fibronectin (Fn) concentration and pH were measured in the peritoneal dialysate. Chemiluminescence curves, phagocytosis and killing in peritoneal fluid PML were markedly depressed especially in the case of gram-positive bacteria. Phagocytosis and killing strongly correlated to Ca and Mg concentrations in the peritoneal effluent, but to the contrary there was no relationship to pH, P, urea and creatinine levels. We could not detect any significant concentration of Fn in the repeated specimens of peritoneal dialysate drainage. These findings suggest that the depletion of some divalent ions i.e. Ca and Mg, as well as the lack of Fn might play a role in impairing peritoneal fluid PML function. This study seems to provide evidence of another predisposing factor for gram-positive peritonitis in patients undergoing IPD.

From the Unit of Nephrology and Dialysis, Department of Immunology, U.S.L. 11 "Pordenonese," Stabilimento Ospedaliero di Pordenone, and the Department of Internal Medicine, U.S.L. 7 "Udinese," Stabilimento Ospedaliero di Codroipo (UD), Italy.

INTRODUCTION

Chronic peritoneal dialysis is a feasible alternative to hemodialysis for a rapidly expanding group of patients with end-stage kidney disease.[1] Despite the increasing need for peritoneal dialysis and the technological advances, peritonitis remains a major limiting complication of this form of therapy. Microorganisms isolated from patients on peritoneal dialysis with peritonitis in approximately two-thirds of cases are gram-positive.[2] *Staphylococcus epidermidis, Staphylococcus aureus*, and *Streptococcus* species are the most common agents.[3] Patients with renal failure have a heightened susceptibility to infection, secondary to both cellular immune suppression and decreased reticuloendothelial function.[4,5] Some changes in the peritoneal defense mechanisms have been reported in patients undergoing peritoneal dialysis.[6,7] The peritoneal cavity of these patients contains, instead of the normal few ml of fluid, 2 L of dialysis fluid. Further, the pH of normal peritoneal fluid is 7.4 and it is isoosmolar, whereas dialysate has a low pH (5.5) and a high osmolality because an osmotic agent (usually dextrose) is added to produce high rates of ultrafiltration. After entering the peritoneal cavity dialysate equilibrates with blood and the pH of the fluid increases toward that of the blood over 20 to 45 minutes. The decrease in osmolality is slower, usually taking about 3 hours. During the initial interval, the peritoneal phagocytic cells operate under nonphysiologic conditions. Both the low pH and the hyperosmolality are reported to depress phagocytic activity and bactericidal ability

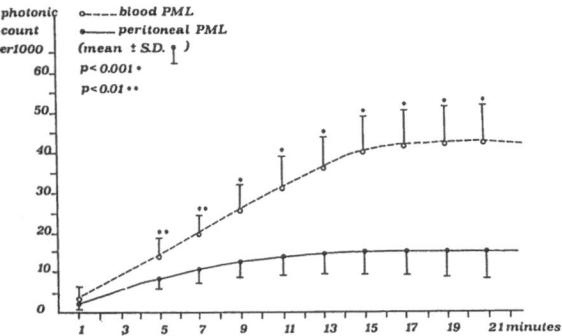

Fig. 1. Chemiluminescence curves of blood and peritoneal polymorphonuclear leukocytes (PML) of uremic patients on IPD.

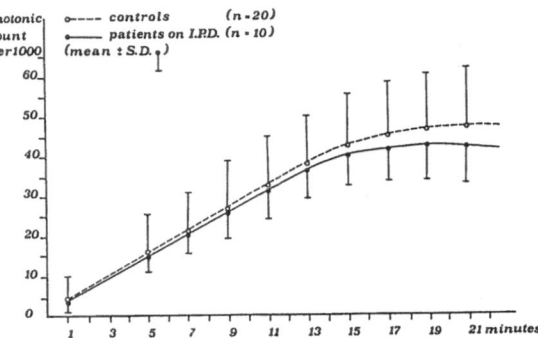

Fig. 3. Chemiluminescence curves of blood polymorphonuclear leukocytes in uremic patients on IPD and controls.

of peritoneal cells.[8,9] In addition urea, creatinine, electrolytes and other low-molecular-weight substances diffuse into the peritoneal fluid and might affect phagocytosis and bactericidal action of peritoneal phagocytic cells.

The aims of this study were to evaluate blood and peritoneal polymorphonuclear leukocyte function (PML) and to investigate the causes of the impairment of peritoneal PML which might represent another predisposing factor for peritonitis in patients with end-stage kidney disease receiving intermittent peritoneal dialysis (IPD).

MATERIALS AND METHODS

Blood and peritoneal PML function was investigated with chemiluminescence, phagocytosis and killing in ten patients with end-stage kidney disease

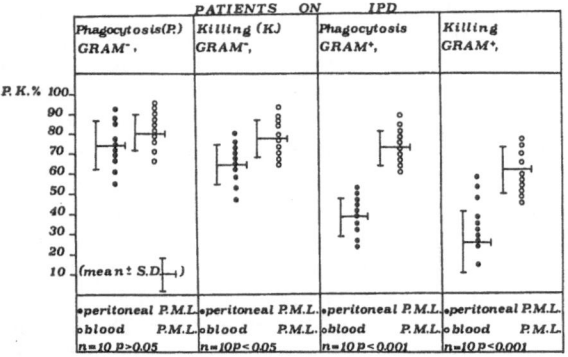

Fig. 2. Phagocytosis and killing of gram-positive and gram-negative bacteria in blood and peritoneal polymorphonuclear leukocytes (PML) of uremic patients on IPD.

receiving IPD. The patients ranged in age from 40 to 76 years (mean 58 years). Five patients were women and five were men. Before study the patients had been in the IPD program for 8 to 28 months (mean 17 months). At testing none of the patients had evidence of intraperitoneal inflammation. A control group consisted of 20 subjects (ten women and ten men; mean age 58 years, range 38–68 years) with normal renal function in which only blood PML function was investigated. We collected 20 ml of heparinized blood and peritoneal effluent from each patient. The PML were separated by dextran sedimentation, followed by density centrifugation on Ficoll-Hypaque by standard methods.[10] PML collected were 95% pure and 98% viable by trypan blue dye exlusion assay. Cells to be used for PML chemiluminescence were washed three times with Hank's balanced salt solution and then aliquoted to a final cell concentration of 1×10^6 PML/ml. PML chemiluminescence was determined by the method described by DeChatelet et al.[11] Phagocytosis and killing assay were measured by the method of Quie et al.[12] Calcium, magnesium, inorganic phosphorus, urea, creatinine, fibronectin in concentrations, and pH were measured in blood and peritoneal effluent. Urea, creatinine and inorganic phosphorus were measured by the autoanalyzer technique (Technicon). Blood pH was determined by a calibrated blood gas analyzer (Radiometer, Copenhagen, Denmark). Calcium and magnesium concentrations were measured by atomic absorption spectroscopy. Fibronectin was quantitated by Laurell's electroimmunoassay.[13] Protein standard plasma manufactured by Behring Institute served as a standard for the quantitative determination. The specific rabbit plasma fibronectin antiserum was obtained from

Behring Institute. The primary standard and unknown plasma were diluted in sodium barbital buffer. Electroimmunoassay was performed in 1% agarose containing 2% rabbit anti-human PF. Electrophoresis was performed in barbital buffer pH 8.6 for 16 hours on a cooled plate at 3 V/cm. Plates were dried, washed in 0.1 M NaCl and distilled water, dried 10 minutes at 37° C and stained with Coomassie brilliant blue. Fibronectin concentration in unknown plasma was estimated by comparing the peak area to a standard curve of four two-fold dilutions of standard plasma. Linear regression analysis and Student's t test for unpaired data were used for statistical analysis.

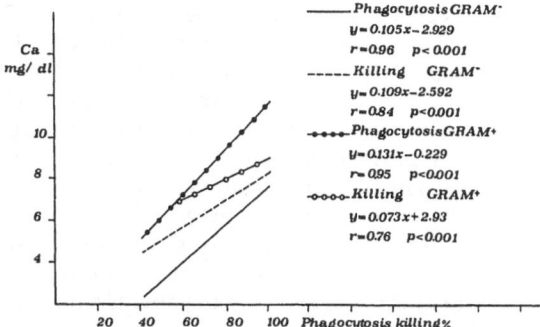

Fig. 4. Relationships between calcium concentration in peritoneal effluent (Ca) and phagocytosis and killing of gram-positive and gram-negative bacteria in peritoneal polymorphonuclear leukocytes.

RESULTS

In patients on IPD, chemiluminescence curves, phagocytosis, and killing of peritoneal effluent PML were significantly depressed as compared with those of blood PML (Figs. 1 & 2). On the other hand there was no significant difference in these parameters between blood PML of patients and those of controls (Fig. 3). The peritoneal PML function of uremic patients was markedly depressed especially in the case of gram-positive bacteria as shown in Figure 2. Phagocytosis and killing of peritoneal PML closely correlated with the peritoneal effluent concentrations of Ca and Mg (Figs. 4 & 5) whereas there was no relationship between these parameters of PML function and inorganic phosphorus, urea and creatinine concentrations. Plasma levels of fibronectin in patients on IPD did not differ significantly from those of controls (262 ± 50 mg/L vs 200 ± 40 mg/L) but we could not detect any significant concentration of fibronectin in repeated samples of peritoneal effluent.

DISCUSSION

The most important function of PML is the phagocytosis of microorganisms and particles such as immunocomplexes recognized as foreign.[14] The effective engulfment of many bacterial strains requires previous opsonization, i.e. the binding to specific IgG antibodies. Then the Fc portion of immunoglobulin can bind to the specific receptor present on the PML membrane surface and initiate the ingestion.[15] Fibronectin is a major glycoprotein that is found in a soluble form in blood and other body fluids including the peritoneal fluid.[16] Fibronectin has been shown to be a major factor influencing the

phagocytic behavior of reticuloendothelial cells.[17] Proctor et al.[18] suggested that a noncomplement, nonimmunoglobulin opsonin might play a very important role in limiting acute infection prior to the development of specific immunity and they proposed that fibronectin might be one such opsonin. It has been known that divalent ions such as calcium and magnesium have a major role in regulating PML function.[19] Our findings provide evidence of another predisposing factor for bacterial peritonitis in uremic patients receiving IPD. The peritoneal PML function in these patients is markedly depressed especially in the case of gram-positive bacteria; accordingly there is an elevated incidence of peritonitis caused by such microorganisms in our patients receiving peritoneal dialysis.[20] The positive relation-

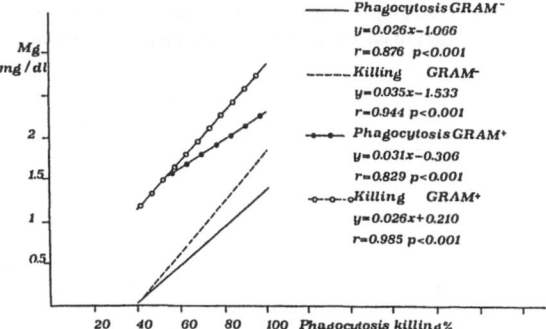

Fig. 5. Relationships between magnesium concentration in peritoneal effluent (Mg) and phagocytosis and killing of gram-positive and gram-negative bacteria in peritoneal polymorphonuclear leukocytes.

ship between calcium and magnesium concentrations and phagocytosis and killing of peritoneal PML suggest that the peritoneal fluid depletion of these divalent ions as well as the lack of a significant level of fibronectin might play a role in impairing PML function. A positive calcium and magnesium balance and a suitable concentration of these electrolytes in the dialysis solution may be important to warrant better PML function. In conclusion these data provide evidence for another predisposing factor for gram-positive peritonitis in-patients with end-stage kidney disease receiving IPD.

REFERENCES

1. Oreopoulos DG: Continuous ambulatory peritoneal dialysis in Canada. Canad Med Assoc J 120: 16, 1979
2. Rubin J, Rogers WA, and Taylor HM: Peritonitis during continuous ambulatory peritoneal dialysis. Ann Intern Med 92: 7, 1980
3. Vas SI: Microbiologic aspects of chronic ambulatory peritoneal dialysis. Kidney Int 23: 83, 1983
4. Dobbelstein H: Immune system in uremia. Nephron 17: 409, 1976
5. Goldblum SE, and Reed WP: Host defenses and immunologic alterations associated with chronic hemodialysis. Ann Intern Med 93: 597, 1980
6. Vas SI, Duwe A, and Weatherhead J: Natural defense mechanisms of the peritoneum: The effect of peritoneal dialysis fluid on polymorphonuclear cells. In Atkins RC, Thomas NM, and Farrell PC (Eds), Peritoneal dialysis. Edinburgh: Churchill Livingstone, 1981, p 41
7. Duwe AK, Vas SI, and Weatherhead JW: Effect of the composition of peritoneal dialysis fluid on chemiluminescence, phagocytosis and bactericidal activity in vitro. Infect Immunol 33: 130, 1981
8. Guckian JC, Karrh LR, Copeland JL, and McCoy J: Phagocytosis by polymorphonuclear leukocytes in patients with renal failure on chronic hemodialysis. Tex Rep Biol Med 29: 193, 1971
9. Drivas G, Rethymmiotakis N, Kalos A, and Melissinos K: Reticuloendothelial phagocytosis in patients with chronic renal failure. Invest Urol 17: 241, 1979
10. Boyum A: Isolation of leukocytes and macrophages. Scand J Immunol 5: 9, 1976
11. DeChatelet LR, Long GD, Shirley PS, Bass DA, Thomas MJ, Henderson FW, and Cohen MS: Mechanism of the luminol development chemiluminescence of human neutrophils. J Immunol 129: 1589, 1982
12. Quie P, White J, Good RA, and Holmes B: In vitro bactericidal capacity of human PMN leukocytes diminished activity in CGD of childhood. J Clin Invest 46: 4, 1967
13. Laurell CB: Electroimmunoassay of fibronectin. Scand J Clin Lab Invest 29(Suppl 124): 21, 1977
14. Stossel TP: Phagocytosis. N Engl J Med 290: 717, 1974
15. Allison F, Lancaster MG, and Crostwaite JL: Studies on the pathogenesis of acute inflammation. Am J Pathol 43: 775, 1963
16. Oh E, Pierschbacher M, and Ruoslahti E: Deposition of plasma fibronectin in tissues. Proc Natl Acad Sci U.S.A. 78: 3218, 1981
17. Saba TM, Blumenstock FA, Weber P, and Kaplan JE: Physiologic role for cold-insoluble globulin in systemic host defense: Implications of its characterization as the opsonic alpha-2-SB glycoprotein. Ann NY Acad Sci 321: 43, 1978
18. Proctor RA, Prendergast E, and Mosher DF: Fibronectin mediates attachment of Staphylococcus aureus to human neutrophils. Blood 59: 681, 1982
19. Bryant RE: Effect of divalent cation depletion on phagocytosis of staphylococci. Yale J Biol Med 41: 303, 1969
20. Cecchin E, DeMarchi S, Panarello G, Franceschin A, Chiaradia V, Santini G, and Tesio F: Torulòpsis glabrata peritonitis complicating CAPD: Successful management with oral 5-fluorocytosine. Am J Kidney Dis (in press)

B. Chandrasekaran, E.F. Schultz, V.A. DeBari,
C.T. Ronquillo, and M.A. Needle

111

Surface Marker Characterization of Peritoneal Dialysis Patients' Intraperitoneal Leukocytes by Monoclonal Antibodies

SUMMARY

The nature and quantity of leukocytes in peritoneal dialysate of uninfected patients was studied by antibody testing for the presence of various cell surface markers. About 77% of the cells were T and B lymphocytes in contrast to the predominance of macrophages harvested by saline lavage of the peritoneum. It is suggested that lymphocyte depletion may ensue from prolonged peritoneal dialysis contributing to an immunodeficiency state.

INTRODUCTION

Peritoneal dialysis (PD) for the treatment of chronic renal failure has become an important therapeutic modality. However, just as the external arterio-venous shunt used in the initial era of hemodialysis frequently led to systemic infections,[1,2] PD in its various forms is associated with a high rate of peritonitis resulting in significant morbidity and mortality.[3,4]

Patients with chronic renal failure also have immune dysfunction which further aggravates the infection problem.[5] There is, for example, a metabolic defect in the polymorphonuclear neutrophil of these patients,[6-9] which may be progressive and the

cause of which is largely unknown. As the initial phase of an investigation into immune cell function in PD, the nature and quantity of leukocytes in PD fluid from uninfected patients was studied.

MATERIALS AND METHODS

Patient Population

Patients from the PD facility at St. Joseph's Hospital and Medical Center were randomly selected for the study. The presence of an infection was the sole criterion for exclusion from the study. Signed, informed consent, as approved by the Institutional Research Committee, was obtained from each subject.

Harvesting of Peritoneal Cells

An overnight collection of 1 to 2 L peritoneal dialysate (Dianeal®, with dextrose monohydrate concentration of 1.5 to 4.25 g/dL, Travenol Laboratories, Inc., Deerfield, IL) was obtained by the nursing staff and transported to the laboratory. Aliquots of the dialysate were centrifuged at 800 x g for 10 minutes and the combined pellets were washed with Basal Medium, Eagle (minimum essential medium, MEM), buffered with Hanks salts, to which 10% heat-inactivated fetal calf serum (FCS) had been added. Both MEM and FCS were obtained from Gibco (Grand Island, NY). After washing, the cells were resuspended in MEM with 10% FCS and studied the same day.

From the Renal Laboratory and Service, and Hematology-Oncology Research Laboratory, Department of Medicine, St. Joseph's Hospital and Medical Center, Paterson; and the University of Medicine and Dentistry of New Jersey—New Jersey Medical School, Newark, New Jersey.

Table 1. Distribution of Markers on Cells from PD Fluid (Mean ± 1 SD).

Marker	Studies (No.)	Positive Cells (%)
% Monomyeloid (OKM-1) of Total	6	22.7 ± 4.8
T cells (RFC), % Total	9	64.8 ± 16.1
T 4	5	41.2 ± 19.2
T 8	5	19.2 ± 6.7
T 9	4	0.38 ± 0.75
T 11	8	54.0 ± 16.0
B cells (F(ab')$_2$), % Total	10	12.0 ± 7.0
B 1	3	18.0 ± 8.0
B 1	3	18.0 ± 8.0
B 2	3	0.23 ± 0.40
Light Chains:		
Kappa	3	9.0 ± 8.2
Lambda	4	6.9 ± 3.6

Protocol for Staining

Cell counts were adjusted to 1–2 × 10^6 cells in 0.2 ml RPMI—1640 medium (M.A. Bioproducts, Walkersville, MD) buffered with tris (hydroxymethyl) aminomethane, pH 7.2, (Fischer Scientific Corporation, Fair Lawn, NJ) containing penicillin (50 U/mL) and streptomycin (50 μg/mL) (Gibco). To the cell suspension was added 20 μl of the primary antibody (OKT4, OKT9, OKT9, OKT11, OKM1, (Ortho Diagnostic Systems, Inc., Raritan, NJ); anti-F (ab')$_2$ (Kallestad Laboratories, Chaska, MN), and anti-B1, Kappa and Lambda (Coulter Diagnostics, Hialeah, FL). These were incubated for 30 minutes at 2 to 4°C and washed thrice with cold RPMI-1640. Fifty μl of the secondary antibody (goat anti-mouse IgG, fluorescein conjugate, Hybritech, Inc., San Diego, CA) were added to the suspension, incubated at 2 to 4°C for 30 minutes, washed thrice with RPMI-1640, resuspended in buffered glycerol and counted in a Leitz transilluminated fluorescent microscope.

Table 2. Distribution of Markers on Cells from PD Patients, Using Saline Lavage Technique (n = 3) (Mean ± 1 SD).

Marker	Positive Cells (%)
M 1	61.8 ± 17.64
T 4	12.9 ± 9.4
T 8	6.4 ± 4.1
T 11	15.6 ± 10.4
F(ab')$_2$	10.0 ± 7.8

Miscellaneous Materials and Methods

Viability was determined using Erythrosin B (0.5% in phosphate-buffered saline, Sigma Chemical Corporation, St. Louis, MO), and exceeded 75%. The E-rosetting method[10] was carried out using sheep red blood cells (SRBC) from M.A. Bioproducts (40% SRBC in Alsever's solutions).

RESULTS AND DISCUSSION

In pilot studies, ordinary differential cell counts were found to be of little use, in that cell morphology appeared to be altered. Thus, the characterization of the cells from the PD exudate required the use of surface markers. The data obtained on a group of PD patients is given in Table 1.

These data indicate that most of the cells harvested are lymphocytes; T and B cells comprise roughly 77% of the total cell population. The data are in sharp contrast to those of Ganguly et al.[11] who found that the peritoneal lavage technique performed on PD patients yielded, primarily, macrophages. One important difference between their study and ours is that they used normal saline for lavage rather than PD fluid. In fact, in several cases, we performed the technique using normal saline and obtained the data in Table 2.

These data more closely resemble those reported[11] from saline lavage and suggest that the exudate cells normally appearing in PD patients are different than expected, i.e., they are, for the most part, of lymphoid origin. Because these cells are so long-lived, their depletion may lead, ultimately, to an immunodeficiency state.

REFERENCES

1. Kaslow RA, and Zellner SR: Infections in patients on maintenance haemodialysis. Lancet 1: 117, 1982
2. Montgomerie JZ, Kalmanson GM, and Guze LB: Renal failure and infection. Medicine 47: 1, 1968
3. Popovich RP, Moncreif JW, Nolph KD, Ghods AJ, Twardowski ZJ, and Pyle WK: Continuous ambulatory peritoneal dialysis. Ann Intern Med 88: 449, 1978
4. Nolph KD, Boen FST, Farrell PC, and Pyle WK: Continuous ambulatory peritoneal dialysis in Australia, Europe and the United States. Kidney Int 23: 9, 1983
5. Goldblum SE, and Reed WP: Host defenses and immunologic alterations associated with chronic hemodialysis. Ann Intern Med 93: 597, 1980
6. DeBari VA, Fingerhut MA, Keil LB, and Needle MA: Progressive peripheral phagocyte deficiency in chronic hemodialysis patients. In Condrelli L, Teodori U, Berretta A, and San Giorgi M (Eds), Internal medicine. Amsterdam: Excerpta Medica, 1980, p 773
7. Ritchey EE, Wallin JD, and Shah SV: Chemiluminescence and superoxide anion production by leukoctyes from chronic hemodialysis patients. Kidney Int 19: 349, 1980
8. Charpentier B, Lang P, Martin B, Noury J, Mathieu D, and Fries D: Depressed polymorphonuclear leukocyte functions associated with normal cytotoxic T and natural killer cells during chronic hemodialysis. Clin Nephrol 19: 288, 1983
9. DeBari VA, and Needle MA: Polymorphonuclear leukocyte defects in chronic hemodialysis patients. Clin Nephrol (in press)
10. Jondal M, Holm G, and Wigzell H: Surface markers on human B and T lymphocytes. I. A large population of lymphocytes forming non-immune rosettes with sheep red blood cells. J Exp Med 136: 207, 1972
11. Ganguly R, Milutinovitch J, Lazzell V, and Waldman RH: Studies of human peritoneal cells: A normal saline lavage technique for the isolation and characterization of cells from peritoneal dialysis patients. J Reticuloendothel Soc 27: 303, 1980

F. Giacchino, M. Formica, M. Pozzato, F. Quarello,
G. Quattrocchio, M.G. Guerra, F. Peyretti, and G. Piccoli

112

HLA Markers and Peritonitis in CAPD Patients

SUMMARY

Peripheral T and B cell subpopulations in 41 CAPD patients and 30 healthy controls were identified using monoclonal anti-T cell antibodies and immunofluorescent staining. HLA typing was also studied. OKT8 reactive cells were significantly higher in patients who had had two or more episodes of peritonitis on follow-up, with no changes from normal in those who did not develop peritonitis. The HLA-B8, DR3 haptotype was more frequent in those who did not develop peritonitis, and since HLA-B8, DR3 is known to be associated with reduced suppressor T cells, such a haplotype may confer resistance to peritonitis.

INTRODUCTION

The mechanism governing cellular immunodeficiency in uremic patients is still not well understood. *In vitro* tests have shown that lymphocytes from uremic patients proliferate less than normal with exposure to mitogens[1] or alloantigens,[2] and an imbalance of the immunoregulatory subpopulations (helper and suppressor T cells) has been found both in animals and in man with chronic renal insufficiency.[3,4] The clinical relevance of this has been observed in the high frequency of infection,[5] in an increased rate of malignancy,[6,7] and in cutaneous anergy[8,9] found in such patients.

From the Medical Nephrology Institute of the University of Turin, and the Nephrology and Dialysis Departments and Blood Bank, San Giovanni Hospital, Turin, Italy.

Peritoneal dialysis has been found to improve some aspects of cellular immunodeficiency (E-rosette count, delayed hypersensitivity skin reactions),[10,11] but not other aspects, such as T suppressor activity and T cell proliferation to mitogens.[12,13] On the other hand no correlation has been found between improved cell-mediated immunity and frequency of peritonitis.[10]

Considerable attention has been paid to the role played by blood transfusion in the immunologic alteration of patients with chronic renal insufficiency, especially in those awaiting renal allografts,[14-16] even though protein and vitamin deficiencies have also been observed to be associated with quantitative and functional abnormalities of T cell subsets.[17] This study was undertaken to evaluate more fully the immunologic patterns in CAPD patients by investigating both peripheral and peritoneal lymphocytes with specific monoclonal anti-T cell antibodies and heterologous anti-immunoglobulin antisera to B cells. Patients were studied at the onset of dialysis treatment and during peritonitis episodes.

Correlations were also sought between these results and the HLA antigen distribution, the number of blood transfusions or the state of nutrition.

MATERIALS AND METHODS

Patients

Forty-one patients on CAPD (3 to 5 exchanges a day using Dianeal® bags) were studied. Fifteen were males and 26 were females, aged between 35 and 80 years (average age 55 years.), and had been on

Table 1. Peripheral Lymphocytes in CAPD Patients and in Controls.

	CAPD	Controls
OKT3 (/mm³)	820 ± 50*	1284 ± 123
OKT3 (%)	56 ± 3.5	61 ± 6
OKT4 (%)	47 ± 4	44 ± 5
OKT8 (%)	31 ± 4	25 ± 4
S-Ig (%)	14 ± 3	16 ± 2

* $p < 0.02$ vs controls.

Table 2. Peripheral Lymphocytes in CAPD Patients during peritonitis.

	Before Peritonitis	During Peritonitis
OKT3 (%)	56 ± 3.5	59 ± 4.6
OKT4 (%)	47 ± 4	49 ± 2.7
OKT8 (%)	31 ± 3	41 ± 1.8*
S-Ig (%)	14 ± 3	16 ± 2.5

* $p < 0.05$ vs values before peritonitis.

dialysis for 5 to 39 months (average 18 months). Peripheral blood was collected before the first exchange of the morning, in a plastic tube containing 20 IU heparin (Roche)/ml of blood. Dialysate without heparin was also collected from patients at the same time as the blood samples. Thirty healthy controls (19 males and 11 females, average age 32 years) donated blood for peripheral lymphocyte subsets.

Lymphocyte Separation

Lymphocytes were obtained from 10 ml heparinized blood by separation in a Ficoll-Hypaque density gradient (Nyegaard Corporation).[18] The lymphocyte band was collected, and washed three times in 10 ml Hanks' buffered salt solution (HBSS) (pH = 7.2). Viability, as determined by eosin, was greater than 98%.

Monoclonal Antibodies to T Cell Subsets

We used the indirect immunofluorescence technique with fluorescein-conjugated goat anti-mouse IgG antibody (Bionetics Laboratories) and light microscope examination.[19] Five million cells/ml were treated with 5 μl of monoclonal antibodies (OKT3—peripheral mature T lymphocytes; OKT4—helper/inducer T lymphocytes; OKT8—suppressor/cytotoxic T lymphocytes—Orthoclone Pharmaceutical Corporation), at a dilution of 1:20, incubated at 4°C for 30 minutes and washed twice. The cells were than mixed with 5 μl of a 1:40 dilution of goat anti-mouse IgG antibody for 30 minutes, centrifuged and washed twice. The cell pellet was resuspended in one drop of mounting medium (glycerol 30% and phosphate-buffered saline)..At least 200 cells were counted under a Leitz Orthoplan microscope; monocytes were identified by phase microscopy and excluded from the counts.

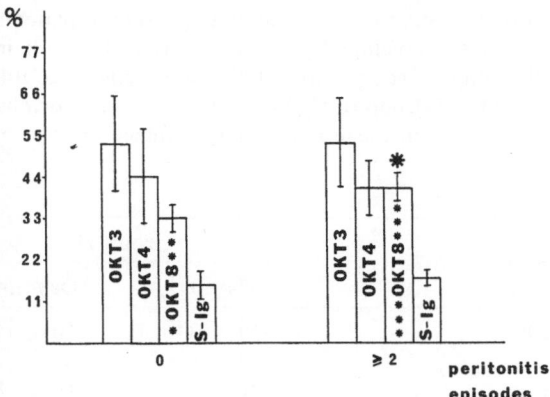

Fig. 1. Peripheral lymphocytes in CAPD patients. OKT8 reactive cells increased significantly (p < 0.05) in patients who had had two or more episodes of peritonitis compared to patients who had not had peritonitis.

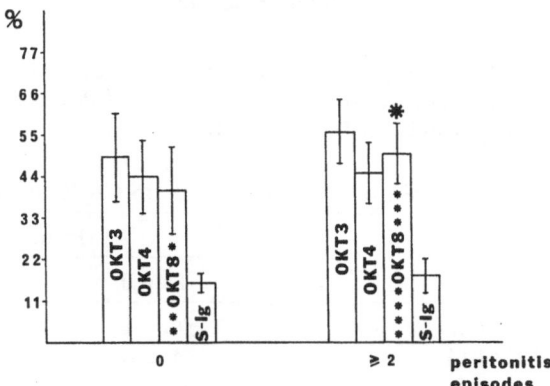

Fig. 2. Peritoneal lymphocytes in CAPD patients. OKT8 reactive cells increased significantly (p < 0.05) in patients who had had peritonitis twice or more, compared to patients who had not had peritonitis.

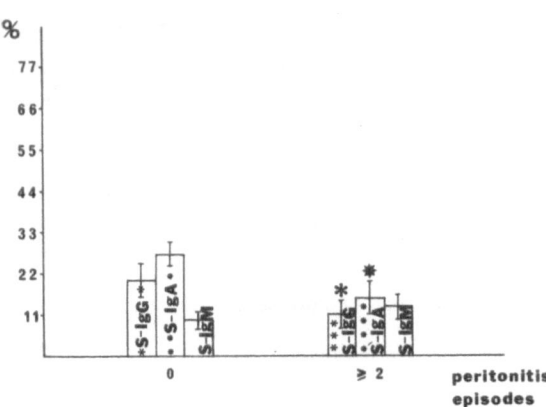

Fig. 3. Peritoneal B lymphocytes. S-IgA were significantly lower (p < 0.02) in patients who had had two or more episodes of peritonitis, compared to patients who had not had peritonitis, (S-IgG were also lower but not significantly (p < 0.5)).

Immunofluorescent Staining of B Cells

B lymphocytes were quantified by membrane immunofluorescence for surface immunoglobulins (S-Ig).[20] A lymphocyte suspension of $200\,\mu l$ (5×10^6 cells/ml) was incubated with $10\,\mu l$ of heterologous fluorescein-labeled anti-immunoglobulin antiserum (goat anti-human IgG, IgA, IgM—Behringwerke), diluted with HBSS to 1:5, at 4°C for 45 minutes. The percentage of cells was calculated with the aid of an epi-illuminated fluorescence and phase microscope. Two hundred cells per sample were counted.

Typing for HLA and D-Locus-Related Antigens

Tissue typing was performed on peripheral blood leukocytes from the laboratories of Professor E.S. Curtoni and Dr F. Peyretti.

Statistics

The data were stored in a Packard computer and statistical analyses were made by Student's and Fisher's tests and the chi square test. All values are reported as mean ± SEM.

RESULTS

CAPD patients had a significant absolute lymphopenia both in terms of total peripheral blood lymphocytes and of T cells measured by the monoclonal antibody OKT3 (p < 0.02). When these results were expressed as a percentage of OKT3 reactive cells, no difference from the control group was observed (Table 1). During peritonitis OKT8 reactive cells increased significantly (p < 0.05 vs values before peritonitis). Peripheral B lymphocytes were normal (Table 2). During the follow-up study OKT8 reactive cells were high in patients who had had two or more episodes of peritonitis, while no change was observed in the other patients (Fig. 1).

Figures 2 and 3 show details of peritoneal lymphocyte subsets. OKT8 reactive cells were higher in patients who had had two or more peritonitis episodes as compared with patients who had not had peritonitis (p < 0.05). As regards B lymphocytes, S-IgA were significantly fewer (p < 0.02) in patients who had had peritonitis twice or more as compared to the others; S-IgG were also reduced, but not significantly, in those patients.

When we compared data obtained at the beginning of the CAPD treatment, we found that an increase in OKT8 reactive cells with a reduction in S-IgG positive cells was already present in patients who later developed peritonitis (Group I), while in the other cases peritoneal T and B cells were unmodified (Group II) (Table 3). There was no correlation between these results and primary disease or

Table 3. Peritoneal Lymphocytes in CAPD Patients.

	Group I		Group II	
	Day 0	Day 150	Day 0	Day 150
OKT3 %	56 ± 4	57 ± 8	57 ± 3	50 ± 11
OKT4 %	44 ± 6	45 ± 8	45 ± 6	44 ± 10
OKT8 %	53 ± 2*	51 ± 4*	40 ± 3	40 ± 8
S-IgG %	12 ± 2	11 ± 3	17 ± 4	19 ± 4
S-IgA %	12 ± 3†	13 ± 2	25 ± 3	27 ± 3
S-IgM %	15 ± 3	13 ± 3	10 ± 2	8 ± 3

* p < 0.05 vs Group II.
† p < 0.02 vs Group II.

the number of blood transfusions received by the patients

Eight of nine patients (89%) positive for HLA-B8 (4/5 positive for HLA-DR3; 80%) did not develop peritonitis (p < 0.005 versus HLA-B8 negative patients wherein 20/30 developed peritonitis) (Table 4).

Table 4. HLA Markers and Peritonitis.

	B8+	B8−	Total	DR3+	DR3−	Total
Peritonitis	1	20	21	1	13	14
No peritonitis	8	10	18	4	5	9
Total	9	30	39	5	18	23

$\chi^2 = 8.59$; $p < 0.005$.
$\chi^2 = 4.48$; $p < 0.05$.

DISCUSSION

In this study we analyzed T and B cell subpopulations in CAPD patients, using monoclonal anti-T cell antibodies and immunofluorescent staining for B cells. Correlations were also sought for the number of blood transfusions, the state of nutrition and HLA antigen distribution.

In the follow-up study OKT8 reactive cells were significantly higher in patients who had had two or more episodes of peritonitis, while no change was observed in patients who had had no episodes of peritonitis.

Examination of peritoneal lymphocytes from the first dialysate bag of the morning showed a significant reduction in B cells bearing IgA receptors at the initiation of CAPD in patients who later developed several episodes of peritonitis; an increase in OKT8 reactive cells was also found.

An imbalance between helper and suppressor subsets has been described in malnourished patients with a decrease in helper cells.[17] In our study no correlation was found between peripheral T cell subpopulations and the nutritional state of our CAPD patients.

An increased frequency of HLA-B8, DR3 phenotype in those who did not develop peritonitis was observed in our patients. The association between HLA antigens and diseases with immunologic dysfunction has been known for several years.[21,22] HLA-B8, DR3 antigens have been associated with defective reticuloendothelial system Fc-receptor function in one study,[22] but not confirmed by others,[23,24] suggesting that this abnormality may be due to the presence of blocking factors rather than to an intrinsic monocyte defect. A decrease in T suppressor cells has also been reported in HLA-B8, DR3 positive patients.[22] That peritoneal OKT8 reactive cells were found to be normal in patients with the HLA-B8, DR3 haplotype in our study could be explained by an increase in peritoneal cytotoxic T cells, which might be responsible for the resistance to infection in such patients.

ACKNOWLEDGMENTS

The authors wish to thank the nurses of the San Giovanni Hospital home-peritoneal dialysis unit, for their excellent assistance, and Dr A. Amoroso for HLA typing.

REFERENCES

1. Quadracci LJ, Ringden O, and Krzymanski M: The effect of uremia and transplantation on lymphocyte subpopulations. Kidney Int 10: 179, 1976
2. Nakhla LS, and Coggin MJ: Lymphocyte transformation in chronic renal failure. Immunology 24: 229, 1973
3. Raskova J, and Morrison AB: A decrease in cell mediated immunity in uremia associated with an increase in activity of suppressor cells. Am J Pathol 84: 1, 1976
4. Guillou PJ, Woodhouse LF, Davison AM, and Giles GR: Suppressor cell activity of peripheral mononuclear cells from patients undergoing chronic hemodialysis. Biomedicine 32: 11, 1980
5. Siddiqui JY, Fitz AE, Lawton RL, and Kirkendall WM: Causes of death in patients receiving long-term hemodialysis. JAMA 212: 1350, 1970
6. Penn I, and Starzl TE: Malignant tumours arising de novo in immunosuppressed organ transplant recipients. Transplantation 14: 407, 1972
7. Giacchino F, Quarello F, Giachino G, Bossi P, Alloatti S, and Piccoli G: Does uremia increase malignancy? Abstracts of the 2nd Meeting of French, Italian, and Spanish Society of Nephrology, 1982, p 52
8. Wilson WEC, Kirkpatrick CH, and Talmage DW: Suppression of immunologic responsiveness in uremia. Ann Intern Med 62: 1, 1965
9. Giacchino F, Alloatti S, Quarello F, Bosticardo GM, Giraudo G, and Piccoli G: The immunological state in chronic renal insufficiency. Int J Artif Organs 5: 237, 1982
10. Giacchino F, Alloatti S, Belardi P, Quarello F, Bosticardo GM, Possato M, Aprato A, Segoloni G, and Piccoli G: Continuous ambulatory peritoneal

dialysis and cellular immunity. In Gahl GM, Kessel M, and Nolph KD (Eds), Advances in peritoneal dialysis: Proceedings of the 2nd international symposium on peritoneal dialysis. Amsterdam: Excerpta Medica, 1981, p 214

11. Giacchino F, Alloatti S, Belardi P, Coppo R, Giraudo G, Bosticardo GM, Pozzato M, and Piccoli G: The inhibitory influence of dialysis treatment on E-rosette formation. Trans Am Soc Artif Intern Organs 28: 594, 1982

12. Collart F, Tielemans C, Dratwa M, Schandene L, Wybran J, and Dupont E: Haemodialysis, continuous ambulatory peritoneal dialysis and cellular immunity. Proc Eur Dial Transplant Assoc 20: 190, 1983

13. Singh S, Hurtubise P, Michael G, Pesce A, and Pollak V: Preliminary observations on the laboratory markers of cell-mediated immunity in patients transferring from hemodialysis to continuous ambulatory peritoneal dialysis. Contrib Nephrol 36: 73, 1983

14. Fischer E, Lenhard V, Seifert P, Kluge A, and Johansen R: Blood transfusion-induced suppression of cellular immunity in man. Human Immunol 3: 187, 1980

15. Smith MD, Williams JD, Coles GA, and Salaman JR: The effect of blood transfusion on T-suppressor cells in renal dialysis patients. Transplant Proc 13: 181, 1981

16. Smith MD, Hardy G, Williams JD, and Coles GA: Suppressor cell numbers and activity in non-transfused renal dialysis patients. Clin Nephrol 20: 130, 1983

17. Chandra RK: Numerical and functional deficiency in T helper cells in protein energy malnutrition. Clin Exp Immunol 51: 126, 1983

18. Boyum A: Isolation of mononuclear cells and granulocytes from human blood. Scand J Clin Lab Invest 97(Suppl): 77, 1968

19. Reinherz EL, Kung PC, Goldstein G, and Schlossman SF: Separation of functional subsets of human T cells by a monoclonal antibody. Proc Natl Acad Sci USA 76: 4061, 1979

20. Papamichail M, Brown JC, and Holborow EJ: Immunoglobulins on the surface of human lymphocytes. Lancet 2: 850, 1971

21. Sasazuki T, McDevitt HO, and Grumet FC: The association between genes in the major histocompatibility complex and disease susceptibility. Annu Rev Med 28: 425, 1977

22. Lawley TJ, Hall RP, Fauci AS, Katz SI, Hamburger MI, and Frank MM: Defective Fc-receptor functions associated with the HLA-B8/DRw3 haplotype. N Engl J Med 304: 190, 1981

23. Fries LF, Hall RP, Lawley TJ, Crabtree GR, and Frank MM: Monocyte receptors for the Fc portion of IgG studied with monomeric IgG1: Normal in vitro expression of Fc receptors in HLA B8/DRw3 subjects with defective Fc-mediated in vivo clearance. J Immunol 129: 1041, 1982

24. Kimberly RP, Gibofsky A, Salmon JE, and Fotino M: Impaired Fc-mediated mononuclear phagocyte system clearance in HLA-DR2 and MT1-positive healthy young adults. J Exp Med 157: 1698, 1983

S. Singh, P. Hurtubise, G. Michael, A. Pesce, and V. Pollak

113

Comparison of Lymphocyte Markers and Lymphoblastic Transformation Studies of Patients Converted from Hemodialysis to CAPD

SUMMARY

Sequential studies of lymphcyte markers and *in vitro* lymphoblast transformation were performed in 15 patients who transferred voluntarily from hemodialysis to CAPD. Absolute lymphopenia was observed during hemodialysis therapy. However, there was no significant difference between lymphocyte subpopulations during hemodialysis and CAPD therapies. Mitogen induced *in vitro* lymphoblast transformation was subnormal during both therapies for all situations except 3-day pokeweed mitogen responses but there was no significant difference between the responses on the two therapies. Our results suggest that a combination of an intrinsic defect in uremic lymphocyte and an inhibitory influence of uremic serum are responsible for this hyporesponsive state.

INTRODUCTION

Chronic renal failure is often accompanied by the evidence of impaired cell mediated immunity, manifested *in vivo* by cutaneous anergy,[1] prolonged skin graft survival,[2] and altered tumor surveillance.[3] Treatment with maintenance hemodialysis does not improve this impairment. Studies to explain this phenomenon have produced controversial results.

From the University of Cincinnati Medical Center and Veterans Administration Medical Center, Cincinnati, Ohio.

Lymphopenia with decreased numbers of T and B lymphocytes have often been reported.[1,4–6] *In vitro* studies have shown that the uremic patients' lymphoblastic response to nonspecific mitogens is variable and have been reported to be diminished,[7–9] normal,[1,7,10] or increased.[11] Some have speculated that uremic serum may be the major cause for impaired lymphoblastic transformation but the results of studies measuring mitogen induced transformation of normal lymphocytes in the presence of uremic sera have been variable.[6–10,12,13] Hemodialysis is reported to cause improvement,[13] deterioration,[7,9] or no change.[1,8] The data on patients on peritoneal dialysis is scant but similar.[10,14]

The dialytic modality could possibly alter the reponsiveness of uremic lymphocytes and the ability of uremic sera to improve lymphoblastic transformation, as well as improve the uremic lymphopenia. We previously reported sequential *in vitro* studies on nine patients transferred from hemodialysis to continuous ambulatory peritoneal dialysis (CAPD) showing no change in the laboratory markers of cell-mediated immunity.[15] The scant comparative data in the literature are limited to the study of different populations on a given dialytic modality.[6,10,14] Since end stage renal disease is characterized by tremendous variability, such comparisons are of limited value. In this report we have had the opportunity to extend on our initial observations on 9 patients to 15 patients studied sequentially on hemodialysis and CAPD. These logitudinal observations eliminate group variability and allow the data to be analyzed as a function of treatment modality.

MATERIAL AND METHODS

Fifteen patients on long-term maintenance hemodialysis who wished to transfer voluntarily to CAPD were studied. Informed consent was obtained from all the participants. The patients were studied first on hemodialysis and then 3 to 4 months following transfer to CAPD. The studies during the hemodialysis phase were conducted immediately before dialysis. The hemodialysis schedule consisted of 12 to 15 hours of dialysis/week on a negative pressure delivery system and TRI-EX-1® dialyzer (Extracorporeal, King of Prussia, PA). Blood flows generally averaged 225 ml/min. The CAPD schedule consisted of 4 daily exchanges (mostly three with 1.5% and one with 4.25% dextrose dialysis solution). The patients were clinically stable and free of intercurrent illness at the time of the study.

Residual renal function, dialysis therapy, and nutritional status were carefully quantitated during the study period. Residual glomerular filtration rate was obtained by the means of urea and creatinine clearances. Total urea clearance (KT_{urea}) was obtained from the sum of dialyzer and renal clearance. Nutritional status was quantified by measuring percent ideal body weight, mid-arm muscle circumference, triceps skinfold thickness and protein catabolic rate (PCR). Drug therapy during the study was carefully recorded.

Membrane marker analysis of peripheral blood lymphocytes from patients and normal individuals was performed on mononuclear cell isolates obtained using Ficoll-Hypaque density gradient separation techniques previously described.[16] Absolute lymphocyte count was obtained from white blood cell and differential counts. The lymphocyte subpopulations were characterized by determining percentage and absolute numbers of B lymphocytes, T lymphocytes, T helper/inducer cells, and T suppressor/cytotoxic cells. B lymphocytes were identified by surface membrane immunoglobulin,[16] and T lymphocytes by sheep red blood cell rosette formation.[17] In addition, helper (OKT 4), suppressor (OKT 8) and total T lymphocytes (OKT 3) were identified by indirect immunofluorescence employing monoclonal OKT antibodies (Ortho Pharmaceutical, Raritan, NJ) as described by Hoffman et al.[18]

In vitro lymphoblast transformation was employed to evaluate lymphocyte function. The response of peripheral blood lymphocytes to stimulation by mitogens was determined by measuring the uptake of ^{3}H thymidine in 3- and 5-day cultures of stimulated lymphocytes as previously described.[19]

Doses of mitogens were-phytohemoagglutinin-M (PHA-M, General Biochemicals, Chagrin Falls, Ohio) 25 μl/10^6 cells, pokeweed mitogen (PWM, Grand Island Biological Co., Grand Island, New York) 10 μl/10^6 cells, and concanavalin A (Con-A, Pharmacia Laboratories, Piscataway, New Jersey) 25 μg/10^6 cells. PHA and Con-A are believed to be T cell mitogens. PWM stimulates B cells with additional effect on helper cells. The stimulation of patient lymphocytes to various mitogens was compared separately in cultures supplemented with 5% autologous or pooled normal human sera. Appropriate controls (without mitogen) were set up for each set of the cultures. Each culture was set up in triplicate and means were obtained.

The paired t test was used to test the difference on two therapies; log transformation on lymphoblast transformation data was required to achieve normal distribution. The data were expressed as mean ± SEM.

RESULTS

A total of 15 patients were studied, all males between 48 and 65 years of age, with a mean of 57 years. The mean duration of hemodialysis was 52 months. Primary renal disease was glomerulonephritis in 6, nephrosclerosis in 5, and polycystic kidney disease, atheroembolic renal disease, obstructive nephropathy, and diabetic glomerulosclerosis each in one. Two patients have had longstanding hepatitis B surface antigenemia without laboratory and clinical evidence of liver disease. The indices of nutritional status on the two therapies were not different. The mean body weight, serum creatinine levels, residual renal function, and urea generation rate (G_u) on the two therapies were not different. BUN levels, total urea clearance (KT_u) and KT_u/G_u on hemodialysis were significantly higher than on CAPD (Table 1).

All patients were on usual medications, which include ferrous sulfate, folic acid, multivitamins, and phosphate binders. Five patients were on metoprolol during hemodialysis, which was discontinued on CAPD in all except one.

Lymphocyte Subpopulations

Lymphocyte subpopulation data expressed as absolute number/mm^3 is summarized in Table 2. Total lymphocyte count was decreased significantly during hemodialysis therapy as compared to normal; consequently, absolute numbers of all lymphocyte

Table 1. Clinical Data (mean ± SEM).

	HD	CAPD	p Value
Weight (Kg)	74.9 ± 3.1	73.5 ± 3.2	0.179
BUN (mg/dl)	82 ± 4.7	68 ± 5.2	0.040
Creatinine (mg/dl)	16.2 ± 1.0	17.0 ± 1.2	0.323
Residual GFR (ml/min)	0.2 ± 0.1	0.05 ± 0.04	0.053
G_u (mg/min)	6.2 ± 0.5	4.8 ± 0.3	0.077
KT_u (L/wk)	3170 ± 143	1623 ± 87	0.000006
KT_u/G_u	563 ± 60	344 ± 19	0.012
PCR (g/kg/day)	0.94 ± 0.06	0.78 ± 0.05	0.068

G_u = Urea Generation, KT = Total clearance, PCR = Protein catabolic rate.

subpopulations were also depressed even though their proportions (percentages) were not different from normal. Upon transfer to CAPD, there was no significant difference from normal except for decreased number of OKT 3 positive lymphocytes. When compared with normal, these data imply that CAPD has improved the lymphocyte numbers in these patients; however, no significant difference was observed when numbers and proportions of total lymphocytes and their subpopulations during hemodialysis therapy were compared with those on CAPD.

Lymphoblastic Transformation: Intrinsic Reactivity of Uremic Lymphocytes

The responsiveness of uremic lymphocytes in both autologous (uremic) and pooled normal human sera in 3- and 5-day cultures on both hemodialysis and CAPD therapies was not different from normal (normal lymphocytes in pooled normal human sera) when PWM was used to stimulate the transformation. The response was significantly below normal for both therapies when PHA or Con-A were used in

3- or 5-day cultures enriched with either autologous (uremic) or pooled normal human sera (Figs. 1 & 2). While several patients showed impressive changes in lymphoblastic transformation upon switching to CAPD, the group means on two therapies were not different from each other. Our results suggest that institution of CAPD in previously hemodialyzed patients fails to normalize intrinsic hyporesponsiveness of patient's lymphocytes to mitogen induced *in vitro* lymphoblast transformation.

Effect of Source of Sera on Lymphoblast Transformation

The lymphocytes from these patients while on hemodialysis responded better in pooled normal human sera than in uremic (autologous) sera in both 3- and 5-day cultures except for 3-day Con-A transformation (Table 3). The uremic lymphocytes from these patients upon transfer to CAPD also responded significantly better in pooled normal human sera than in uremic (autologous) sera in all situations except for the 5-day PHA and Con-A responses. To check on the validity of these differences further, a

Table 2. Lymphocyte Subpopulations (number/mm³, mean ± SEM).

Cell Type	Normal	HD (±*)	CAPD
WBC	6525 ± 477	5160 ± 384	6940 ± 863
Total lymphocyte	2412 ± 307	1308 ± 180	1755 ± 177
T lymphocyte	1717 ± 245	964 ± 151	1300 ± 135
B lymphocyte	302 ± 59	120 ± 16	183 ± 28
OKT 3 (total T)	1910 ± 249	1034 ± 166	1231 ± 118*
OKT 4 (helper)	1108 ± 121	686 ± 79	888 ± 93
OKT 8 (suppressor)	820 ± 137	397 ± 96	660 ± 137
OKT 4/OKT 8 Ratio	1.51 ± 0.18	2.45 ± 0.30	1.93 ± 0.27

* Significantly different from normal.

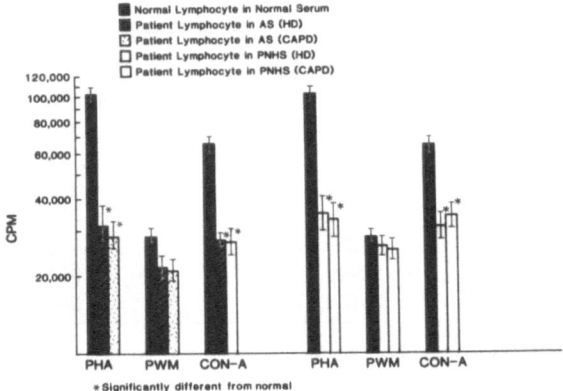

Fig. 1. Lymphoblast Transformation in 3-day cultures (mean ± SEM). PHA = Phytohemagglutinin, PWM = Pokeweed Mitogen, Con-A = Concanavalin A, AS = Autologous Sera, PNHS = Pooled Normal Human Sera, HD = Hemodialysis, CAPD = Continuous Ambulatory Peritoneal Dialysis.

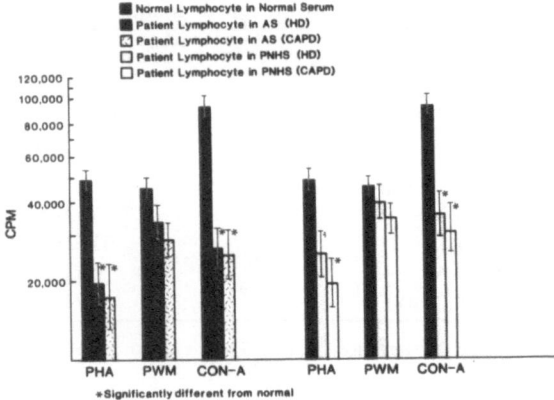

Fig. 2. Lymphoblast Transformation in 5-day cultures (mean ± SEM). PHA = Phytohemoagglutinin, PWM = Pokeweed Mitogen, Con-A = Concanavalin A, AS = Autologous Sera, PNHS = Pooled Normal Human Sera, HD = Hemodialysis, CAPD = Continuous Ambulatory Peritoneal Dialysis.

stimulation index was calculated by dividing the results of thymidine incorporation in presence of the given mitogen by those obtained in absence of any mitogen (i.e., control—see Methods). The differences reported above for normal and uremic sera were reproduced when data were transformed in this manner. However, when the ability of hemodialysis and CAPD sera to support lymphoblastic transformation of uremic lymphocytes was compared to each other, no significant difference was observed. To further elucidate the difference between hemodialysis and CAPD sera, the ratio of response in autologous (uremic) serum to that in pooled normal human serum was obtained for all patients during both therapies. Nevertheless, no significant difference was observed between sera obtained on hemodialysis and CAPD therapies. These results suggest that uremic sera, irrespective of the dialytic modality, are less supportive of mitogen induced *in vitro* lymphoblast transformation as compared to normal sera.

The results of lymphoblast transformation of uremic lymphocytes in autologous or pooled normal human sera during either therapy had no correlation

Table 3. Lymphoblast Transformation of Uremic Lymphocytes.*

Mitogen	Hemodialysis Patient Lymphocyte in			CAPD Patient Lymphocyte in		
	AS	PNHS	p	AS	PNHS	p
3-day culture						
PHA	31,300 $\overset{\times}{\div}$ 1.18	35,000 $\overset{\times}{\div}$ 1.16	.009	28,500 $\overset{\times}{\div}$ 1.15	33,100 $\overset{\times}{\div}$ 1.16	.032
PWM	21,700 $\overset{\times}{\div}$ 1.10	26,200 $\overset{\times}{\div}$ 1.09	.002	21,000 $\overset{\times}{\div}$ 1.10	25,400 $\overset{\times}{\div}$ 1.10	.002
Con-A	27,700 $\overset{\times}{\div}$ 1.06	31,300 $\overset{\times}{\div}$ 1.12	.251	27,200 $\overset{\times}{\div}$ 1.12	34,600 $\overset{\times}{\div}$ 1.12	.019
5-day culture						
PHA	19,700 $\overset{\times}{\div}$ 1.20	25,100 $\overset{\times}{\div}$ 1.22	.016	17,500 $\overset{\times}{\div}$ 1.33	19,500 $\overset{\times}{\div}$ 1.24	.303
PWM	33,700 $\overset{\times}{\div}$ 1.16	39,800 $\overset{\times}{\div}$ 1.16	.052	28,700 $\overset{\times}{\div}$ 1.16	34,600 $\overset{\times}{\div}$ 1.15	.009
Con-A	26,600 $\overset{\times}{\div}$ 1.20	35,600 $\overset{\times}{\div}$ 1.22	.004	25,300 $\overset{\times}{\div}$ 1.24	31,500 $\overset{\times}{\div}$ 1.24	.143

* Counts per minute, geometric mean ($\overline{X}g$) $\times/\div$ = antilog SEM. $\overline{X}g \times$ antilog SEM = mean + SEM; $\overline{X}g \div$ antilog SEM = mean − SEM. AS = autologous sera; PNHS = pooled normal human sera. PHA = phytohemoaggultinin; PWM = pokeweed mitogen; Con-A = Concanavalin A.

with the number of lymphocytes in various subpopulations, the ratio of helper to suppressor cells or with the ratio of lymphocytes to monocytes.

DISCUSSION

Our results show that absolute number of lymphocytes and all lymphocyte subpopulations was decreased significantly in patients during hemodialysis therapy when compared to normal controls. We believe that decrease in lymphocyte subpopulations was a consequence of absolute lymphopenia. This contention is supported by the fact that proportions of lymphocyte subpopulation during hemodialysis were not different from normal. This is similar to the findings in other studies.[1,4,6] The cell count on CAPD therapy were not significantly different from normal. While this might suggest an improvement in lymphopenia upon transfer to CAPD, there was no significant difference in cell counts on CAPD when compared to those on hemodialysis.

Intrinsic reactivity of patient lymphocytes to mitogen-induced *in vitro* lymphoblast transformation in autologous or pooled normal human sera was diminished during hemodialysis therapy. This is similar to the findings of Kauffman et al.,[8] Quadracci et al.,[6] Miller and Stewart,[20] and Holdsworth et al.[7] However, several authors have found it to be normal[1,7,10] or even increased.[11] The response was impaired to PHA and Con-A in both 3- and 5-day cultures. However, the response to PWM was not impaired. Lymphocyte reactivity remained unaltered upon institution of CAPD.

The ability of hemodialysis serum to support lymphoblast transformation of patient lymphocytes was significantly reduced as compared to pooled normal human sera except in 3-day Con-A transformation. This is similar to the findings of Newberry and Sanford[13] who found uremic sera to be inhibitory, but different from those of Touraine et al.[1] who found no difference between normal and uremic sera. Similarly, uremic sera obtained from the same patients upon transfer to CAPD was also significantly less supportive of lymphoblast transformation of patient lymphocytes in all situations except for 5-day PHA and Con-A responses. Our preliminary observations reported earlier[15] suggested this trend, but any difference between normal and uremic (both hemodialysis and CAPD) sera failed to reach statistical significance in most situations. Our extended observations reported here establish clearly that uremic sera from both hemodialysis and CAPD therapies is significantly less supportive of mitogen induced lymphoblast transformation as compared to normal sera. It may be pointed out that uremic lymphocytes were used to evaluate the ability of different sera to support blastogenesis. Since our results suggest that uremic lymphocytes often respond subnormally, cultures employing normal lymphocytes would be more appropriate to evaluate the ability of different sera to support lymphoblastic transformation. We have studied the mitogen induced transformation of normal lymphocytes in presence of uremic sera from four of these patients during hemodialysis and CAPD therapies. The response was lower in presence of uremic sera as compared to normal sera for all situations except 5-day Con-A transformation. However, the difference did not reach statistical significance, probably due to small numbers. Extension of these observations is likely to yield more conclusive information.

Intrinsic responsiveness of uremic lymphocytes as well as the ability of uremic sera to support cell transformation was depressed significantly during both hemodialysis and CAPD therapies. Moreover, no difference was observed between two therapies. This is different from the results of Kunori et al.[14] who found PHA response of patients on intermittent peritoneal dialysis to be significantly lower than that of a different group of patients on hemodialysis. However, they attributed these differences to the higher age and poorer nutrition of peritoneal dialysis patients rather than to the treatment modality. Our study design minimized various group differences and therefore would be optimal to detect true differences between dialytic modalities.

Permeability of peritoneal membrane is much higher than that of the membranes used in the dialyzers. Significantly higher clearances of substances with higher molecular weights (i.e., inulin 5200 daltons) and losses of substantial amounts of albumin (69,000 daltons) in patients on CAPD are well documented. However, the clearance of substance of lower molecular weights (i.e., urea and creatinine) are significantly higher on hemodialysis. Therefore, the composition of sera of patients on CAPD could possibly be quite different from that of patients on hemodialysis. If the suppressor factor(s) in uremic serum had a high molecular weight, CAPD would be much more suited than hemodialysis to remove such inhibitor(s). If the inhibitory effect happened to be due to the deficiency of an essential factor(s), CAPD would be more prone to produce it than hemodialysis. The converse would be true if the inhibitory (or essential) factor(s) had a lower molecular weight. However, our results suggest that the ability of hemodialysis and CAPD sera to support lymphoblast transformation of uremic lymphocytes is not different. Since the studies were conducted only 3 to 4 months after institution of CAPD, it is possible that differences may manifest later during the course of CAPD.

We conclude that intrinsic responsiveness of lymphocytes and the ability of uremic sera to support lymphoblast transformation of uremic lymphocytes are often subnormal on hemodialysis and remain so when patients are transferred to CAPD. Moreover, mitogen-induced responses had no correlation with the lymphocyte subpopulations, the ratio of helper to suppressor cells or with the ratio of lymphocytes to monocytes.

ACKNOWLEDGMENT

This work was supported by NIH grant RR-0068 and DRR CLINFO grant RR-00068-21-52, General Clinical Research Center.

REFERENCES

1. Touraine JL, Touraine F, Revillard JP, Brochier J, and Traeger J: T-lymphocytes and serum inhibitors of cell-mediated immunity in renal insufficiency. Nephron 14: 195, 1975
2. Dammin GJ, Couch NP, and Murray JE: Prolonged survival of skin homografts in uremic patients. Ann NY Acad Sci 64: 967, 1956–1957
3. Slifkin RF, Goldberg J, Neff MS, Baez A, Mattoo N, and Gupta S: Malignancy in end-stage renal disease. Trans Am Soc Artif Intern Organs 23: 34, 1977
4. Hoy WE, Cestero RVM, and Freeman RB: Deficiency of T and B lymphocytes in uremic subjects and partial improvement with maintenance hemodialysis. Nephron 20: 182, 1978
5. Jensson O: Observation on the leucocyte blood picture in acute uraemia. Br J Haematol 4: 422, 1958
6. Quadracci LJ, Ringden O, and Krzymanski M: The effect of uremia and transplantation on lymphocyte subpopulations. Kidney Int 10: 179, 1976
7. Holdsworth SR, Atkins RC, Fitzgerald MG, and Hosking CS: The effect of maintenance dialysis on lymphocyte function. Clin Exp Immunol 33: 95, 1978
8. Kauffman CA, Manzler AD, and Phair JP: Cell-mediated immunity in patients on long-term hemodialysis. Clin Exp Immunol 22: 54, 1975
9. Nelson DS, and Penrose JM: Effect of hemodialysis and transplantation on inhibition of lymphocyte transformation by sera from uremic patients. Clin Immunol Immunopathol 4: 143, 1975
10. Atkins RC, Holdsworth SR, Fitzgerald MG, and Hosking CS: The effect of maintenance dialysis on lymphocyte function. Clin Exp Immunol 33: 102, 1978
11. Slavin RG, Kelly JF, and Garrett JJ: Lymphocyte response in acute experimental renal failure. J Immunol 104: 1424, 1970
12. Kasakura S, and Lowenstein L: The effect of uremic blood on mixed leukocyte reactions and on cultures of leukocytes with phytohemagglutinin. Transplantation 5: 283, 1967
13. Newberry WM, and Sanford JP: Defective cellular immunity in renal failure: Depression of reactivity of lymphocytes to phytohemagglutinin by renal failure serum. J Clin Invest 50: 1262, 1971
14. Kunori T, Fehrman I, Ringden O, and Moller E: In vitro characterization of immunological responsiveness of uremic patients. Nephron 26: 234, 1980
15. Singh S, Hurtubise PE, Micheal G, Pesce A, and Pollak V: Preliminary observations on the laboratory markers of cell-mediated immunity in patients transferring from hemodialysis to continuous ambulatory peritoneal dialysis. Contrib Nephrol 36: 73, 1983
16. King GW, Hurtubise PE, Sagone AL, Lobuglio AF, and Metz FN: Leukemic reticuloendotheliosis. A study of the origin of the malignant cell. Am J Med 59: 411, 1975
17. Jondal M, Holm G, and Wigzel H: Surface markers on human T and B lymphocytes. I. A large population of immune lymphocytes forming nonimmune rosette with sheep red blood cells. J Exp Med 136: 207, 1972
18. Hoffman RA, Kung PC, Hansen WP, and Goldstein G: Simple and rapid measurement of human T lymphocytes and their subclasses in peripheral blood. Proc Natl Acad Sci USA 77: 4914, 1980
19. King GW, Yanes B, Hurtubise PE, Balcerzak SP, and Lobuglio AF: Immune function of successfully treated lymphoma patients. J Clin Invest 57: 1451, 1976
20. Miller TE, and Stewart E: Host immune status in uremia. I. Cell-mediated immune mechanisms. Clin Exp Immunol 41: 115, 1980

F. Collart, C. Tielemans, R. Wens, L. Schandene,
J. Wybran, E. Dupont, and M. Dratwa

114

T Lymphocytes Subsets in CAPD and Hemodialysis (HD) Patients: A Prospective Study

SUMMARY

T lymphocyte subsets were enumerated and suppressor cell activity was assessed in 17 CAPD patients. The lymphocyte population and function were comparable to values obtained in patients treated by hemodialysis. The poor lymphocyte function did not correlate with parameters implicated in cellular immunity alterations or with plasma concentrations of immune globulins.

INTRODUCTION

The abnormalities of cellular immunity of uremic patients have been studied for years and are well known. They include increased skin graft survival, decreased or abolished reactivity to hypersensitivity skin tests, and increased incidence of viral infections. Many factors have been implicated in these alterations, among which is the accumulation of middle molecules. As these middle molecules are better cleared by CAPD than by hemodialysis it was suggested that CAPD could more easily restore normal cellular immunity in such patients.[1,2] We have shown in a previous retrospective study that CAPD and HD patients displayed similar alterations in their T cells subsets and of their suppressive T cell activity.[3] For the latter we demonstrated a negative correlation with time on dialysis (Fig. 1), suggesting the

_____

From the Brugmann and Erasmus University Hospitals, Brussels, Belgium.

same negative evolution of this parameter in both groups of patients. To confirm this hypothesis we started the present prospective study with regards to T cells subsets and T cell suppressive function in CAPD and HD patients.

PATIENTS AND METHODS

Seventeen HD patients (mean age, 50.3 ± 2.9 years) were studied twice at 1 year intervals, and fourteen CAPD patients (mean age 65.7 ± 2.8 years) at a mean interval of 10 months (ranging from 7–13 months). The nephropathies these patients suffered are listed in Table 1. T lymphocyte subsets were enumerated by an indirect immunofluorescence assay with monoclonal antibodies produced by mouse hydridomas. Three monoclonal antibodies were used: OKT3, reacting with all peripheral T cells, OKT4 identifying only T cells with helper or inducer function, and OKT8 directed against a T cell subset with suppressor-cytotoxic function.

The suppressor activity was generated by incubation of the patient's lymphocytes with concanavalin-A (Con-A) for 24 hours and then assayed by measuring their inhibitory potency on the proliferative response of autologous monocytes to Con-A. We measured the proliferative response by the amount of ^{3}H-thymidine incorporated into cellular DNA in the presence and absence of the suppressor cells. The inhibition of the proliferative response was expressed as a percentage of suppression by the formula:

$$\% \text{ suppression } = 1 - \frac{\text{CPM in the presence of suppressor cells}}{\text{CPM in the absence of suppressor cells}} \times 100$$

RESULTS

Similar patterns of T lymphocytes subsets were seen in both CAPD and HD patients. There was a normal proportion of total T cells and of helper T cells, a low proportion of suppressor cytotoxic T cells, and an increased ratio of helper to suppressor cells.

At time 2, both groups showed an identical evolution of their T cells subsets. There was an increased percentage of helper T cells (statistically significant in HD patients), a lower percentage of suppressor cells (significant in CAPD patients) and an increased T4/T8 ratio (significant in both groups).

At second examination one year later, there also was a slight but not significant decrease in T cell suppressor function in HD patients but no change in CAPD patients.

Table 1. Patient Diseases Responsible for ESRD.

	HD	CAPD
Chronic pyelonephritis	7	9
Nephroangiosclerosis	4	3
Chronic glomerulonephritis	2	—
Diabetes mellitus	2	—
Polycystic kidney disease	2	2

DISCUSSION

The changes observed in T cell subsets although tenuous were the same in both CAPD and HD patients. These changes are in agreement with those reported by Singh et al.[5] who studied the changes of

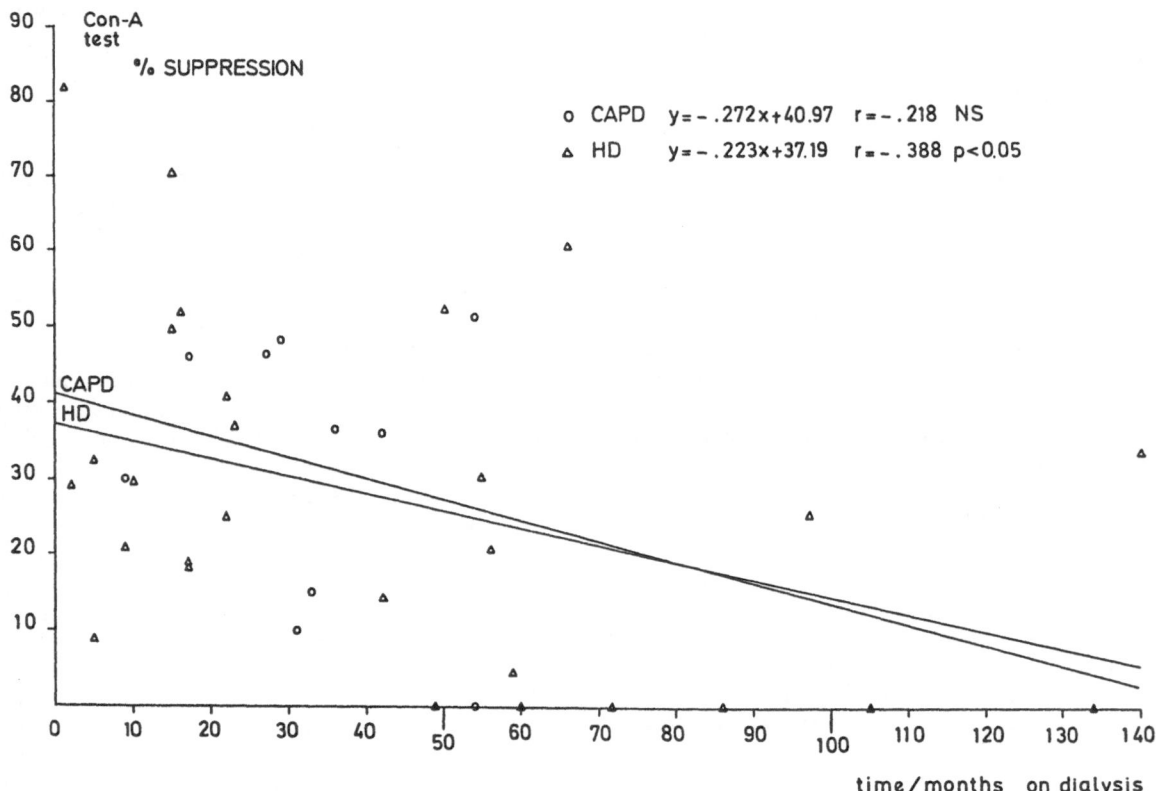

Fig. 1. Correlation between suppressor T lymphocyte function and time on dialysis in CAPD and HD patients.

Table 2. Percentage of T Cell Subsets and Con-A Stimulation at Timed Intervals in HD and CAPD Patients.

CAPD	Normals	Time 1	P	Time 2	P+
OKT3+ cells	68 ± 2	65.9 ± 2	NS	64.8 ± 1.8	NS
OKT4+ cells	41 ± 2	45.9 ± 1.7	NS	48.7 ± 2.5	NS
OKT8+ cells	27 ± 2	21.1 ± 1.1	<0.01	16.6 ± 1.4	<0.05
T4+/T8+ cells	1.6 ± 0.1	2.2 ± 0.1	<0.02	3.5 ± 0.5	<0.05
Con-A test %	45 ± 10	32.1 ± 6.3	<0.02	32.0 ± 4.2	NS

HD		Time 1	P	Time 2	P+
OKT3+ cells		61.4 ± 7.3	NS	65.1 ± 8.9	NS
OKT4+ cells		40.9 ± 7.9	NS	45.7 ± 7.8	<0.02
OKT8+ cells		20.5 ± 5.7	<0.001	18.8 ± 7.9	NS
T4+/T8+ cells		2.2 ± 0.9	<0.02	3.1 ± 1.9	<0.05
Con-A test %		30.1 ± 6.1	<0.02	26.6 ± 5.7	NS

P vs normals, P+ time 2 vs time 1.

T lymphocyte subsets of patients transferred from HD to CAPD in whom they found the same alterations as we did and no improvement with CAPD.

It has been shown that different kidney diseases (mainly extramembranous glomerulonephritis and IgA disease), even in the absence of renal failure are associated with abnormal T cell subsets.[4] Our study confirms that uremia *per se* is responsible for a change in the ratio between helper and suppressor cells.

The change in suppressor T cell activity in HD patients although not reaching the level of statistical significance is of an amplitude consistent with that predicted by the regression line between time on dialysis and suppressor function. It confirms that HD is unable to restore this parameter of cellular immunity. As no more change was found in CAPD patients we cannot find any evidence of a better evolution on this mode of treatment.

One could ask if the described changes correlate with any finding of exaggerated immune responses. However, there was no correlation between the changes observed and the plasma concentrations of IgA, IgG, IgE and IgM in our patients.

The precise reason for this poor suppressor function is unknown as it did not correlate with other parameters commonly implicated in the alterations of cellular immunity of uremic patients (plasma albumin, plasma zinc, vitamin deficiency). Nor did the low suppressor function correlate with the number of transfusions received. We then can only propose that the progressive alteration of this parameter is due to the accumulation of one or more poorly or non-dialyzable substances.

Other groups have shown with CAPD an improvement of the results of *in vitro* E-rosette tests and of the tuberculin hypersensitivity skin test, even after 6 months treatment. It should be pointed out that the tests used in those studies and ours are different: the tuberculin hypersensitivity skin test reflects the activity of different immunocompetent cells among which are mainly helper T cells, while we looked at the T cells suppressor function only. This apparent opposition between these results and ours are due to the fact that we examined different parameters of cellular immunity, whose evolution during dialysis treatment may be different.

REFERENCES

1. Giacchino F, Alloatti S, Quarello F, Coppo R, Pellerey M, and Piccoli G: The influence of peritoneal dialysis on cellular immunity. Peritoneal Dial Bull 2: 165, 1982
2. Giangrande A, Conti P, Limido A, DeFrancesco D, and Malacrida V: CAPD and cellular immunity. Proc Eur Dial Transplant Assoc 19: 372, 1982
3. Collart F, Tielemans C, Schandene L, Wybran J, Dupont E, and Dratwa M: HD, CAPD and cellular immunity. Proc Eur Dial Transplant Assoc 20: 190, 1983
4. Chatenoud L, and Boch MA: Abnormalities of T-cell subsets in glomerulonephritis and systemic lupus erythematosus. Kidney Int 20: 267, 1981
5. Singh S, Hurtubise P, Michael G, Pesce A, and Pollak V: Preliminary observations on the laboratory markers of cell-mediated immunity in patients transferring from hemodialysis to continuous ambulatory peritoneal dialysis. Contrib Nephrol 36: 73, 1983

T.H.J. Goodship, S.M. McLachlan, T.F.H. Poon, S. Lloyd, M.K. Ward, and D.N.S. Kerr

115

Immunoglobulins in CAPD

SUMMARY

Serum and peritoneal dialysate immunoglobulins were measured by immunofluoronephelometry, solid phase radioimmunoassay, or ELISA technique in CAPD patients. No sequential changes in serum immunoglobulins occurred up to 36 months after starting CAPD in 72 patients, all values being within the normal range. In addition, no correlation was found between the peritonitis rate and serum immunoglobulin at start of CAPD, nor at time of study, nor peritoneal dialysis IgG or IgM concentrations. We conclude that routine measurement of immunoglobulins has no value in clinical management of CAPD patients.

INTRODUCTION

The measurement of serum immunoglobulins is frequently used in the routine assessment of patients prior to and after starting CAPD. It is possible that these values could be useful in predicting which patients will be particularly susceptible to peritonitis and later in reflecting those patients with protein-calorie malnutrition associated with recurrent episodes of peritonitis.

It is well known that there is a variable obligatory loss of immunoglobulins in the peritoneal dialysate,[1] but it is uncertain whether this is related to levels of serum immunoglobulins or to previous peritonitis.

Interest has recently been shown in the inherent antimicrobial activity of peritoneal dialysate[2] and it is possible that immunoglobulins in the dialysate may have an opsonizing action. We have therefore studied the sequential effect of CAPD on serum immunoglobulin concentrations, the loss of IgG and IgM in peritoneal dialysate, and the possibility of an association between peritonitis and serum and peritoneal dialysate immunoglobulin concentrations.

METHODS

Sequential Study of Serum Immunoglobulins

Serum IgG, IgA, and IgM were measured by immunofluoronephelometry in 72 patients at 0, 3, 6, 12, 18, 24, 30, and 36 months after starting CAPD.

Cross Sectional Study of Serum and Peritoneal Immunoglobulins

In 38 patients with a mean time on CAPD of 19.5 ± 2 months, serum levels of IgG, IgA, and IgM were measured by immunofluoronephelometry. IgG and IgM were measured in aliquots of pooled 24 hour dialysate by solid phase radioimmunoassay[3] and IgM by an ELISA technique,[4] respectively. These methods were used in preference to immunofluoronephelometry because of the greater sensitivity of the techniques. Immunofluoronephelometric meas-

From the Department of Medicine, University of Newcastle upon Tyne, England.

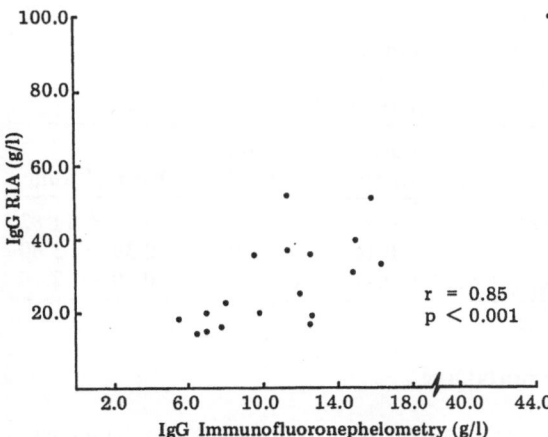

Fig. 1. IgG measured by RIA compared with IgG measured by immunofluoronephelometry.

Table 1.	Mean (±SEM) Serum Immunoglobulins (g/L) at the Start of CAPD (n = 72).	
	CAPD	Normal Range
IgG	9.17 ± 0.35	6.82 ± 14.82
IgA	2.34 ± 0.16	0.39 ± 3.80
IgM	0.84 ± 0.08	0.20 ± 2.70

urement of IgG and IgM was compared with solid phase radioimmunoassay for IgG and ELISA method for IgM by measurement of serum immunoglobulins from 20 patients using both techniques; a dilution of 1:1000 was necessary to bring the values into the range for measurement. Correlations of $r = 0.85$ and 0.87 were observed respectively for the im-

munofluoronephelometric method compared with radioimmunoassay for IgG and the ELISA technique for IgM (Figs. 1 & 2).

The peritonitis rate was calculated in three ways for the 38 patients; time to first episode in days, rate in months on CAPD per number of episodes, rate in days on CAPD per days of treatment. For the group as a whole the rate was calculated as episodes per total patient months on CAPD.

RESULTS

Sequential Study

Serum IgG, IgA, and IgM levels at the start of CAPD were all within the normal range (Table 1) and there was no significant change with time on CAPD (Figs. 3, 4, & 5).

Cross-Sectional Study

Serum IgG, IgA, and IgM levels were within the normal range at the time of study. Furthermore, in 28 of the 39 patients no significant difference was

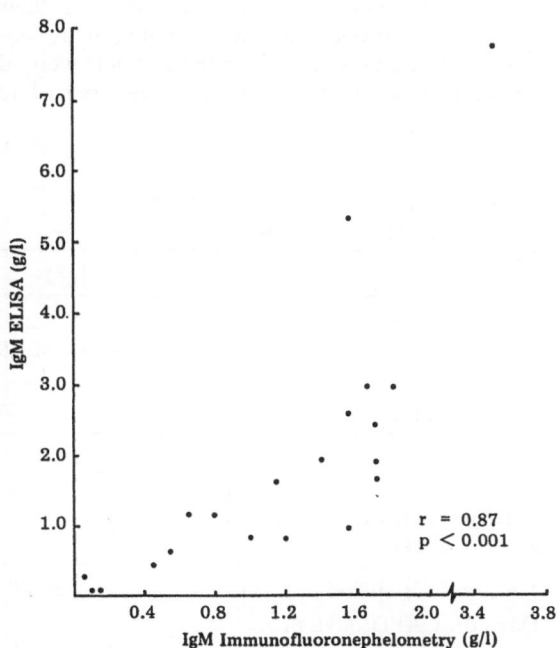

Fig. 2. IgM measured by the ELISA method compared with IgM measured by immunofluoronephelometry.

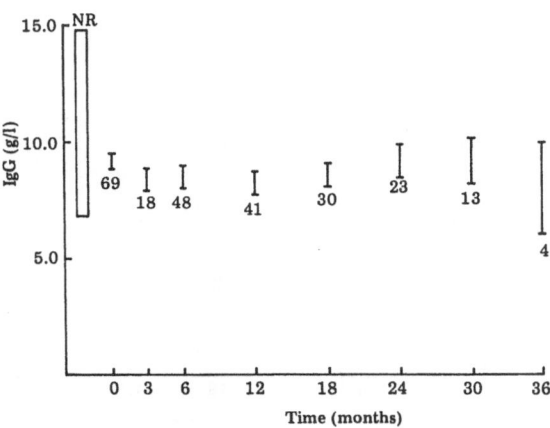

Fig. 3. Serum IgG concentrations with time on CAPD.

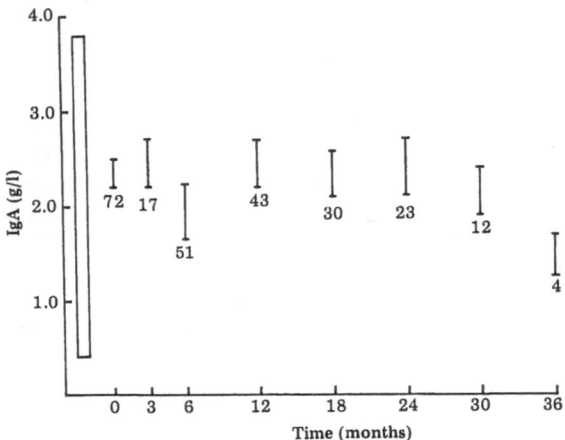

Fig. 4. Serum IgA concentrations with time on CAPD.

Table 2. Mean (±SEM) Serum Immunoglobulins (g/L) at the Start of CAPD (n = 28) and at the Time of Study (n = 38).

	At Start of CAPD	At Time of Study	Normal Range
IgG	9.74 ± 0.91	9.75 ± 0.67	6.82 ± 14.82
IgA	1.81 ± 0.14	1.90 ± 0.14	0.39 ± 3.80
IgM	0.99 ± 0.17	1.07 ± 0.17	0.20 ± 2.70

DISCUSSION

The finding that serum immunoglobulins were within the normal range and did not change with time on CAPD is in agreement with other studies.[5] Losses of IgG and IgM in the peritoneal dialysate are in a similar range to published data although previously concentration of the dialysis fluid was necessary prior to assay by radioimmunodiffusion.[1] It was perhaps not surprising that there was little or no correlation between serum and peritoneal dialysate IgG and IgM since both have high molecular weights (IgG approximately 150,000 daltons, IgM approximately 950,000 daltons) and therefore do not easily cross the peritoneal membrane. To what extent active secretion of immunoglobulins accounts for their presence in peritoneal dialysate is not certain. Neither serum nor peritoneal immunoglobulins were of any predictive or reflective value with regard to peritonitis.

observed between serum immunoglobulins assayed prior to starting CAPD and at the time of the study. (Table 2). The results for peritoneal effluent immunoglobulins are shown in Table 3. There was no correlation between serum and peritoneal dialysate IgG, but there was a weak correlation between serum and peritoneal dialysate IgM (Figs. 6 & 7). The peritonitis rate for the 38 patients at the time of study is shown in Table 4. The peritonitis rate for the group as a whole was one episode per 6.6 patient months. There was no correlation between the following parameters (all r values < 0.3). Serum immunoglobulins at the start of CAPD and peritonitis rate expressed in any of the three ways. Serum immunoglobulins at time of study and peritonitis rate. Peritoneal dialysate IgG and IgM and peritonitis rate.

Table 3. Mean (±SEM) Peritoneal Dialysate Immunoglobulins.

	IgG	IgM
Concentration (mg/L)	175.1 ± 3.6	1.08 ± 0.19
Daily Loss (mg/24 hours)	1593 ± 372	10.32 ± 1.97

Table 4. Mean (±SEM) Peritonitis Rate (n = 34, Four Patients Having No Episodes).

Time to first episode (days)	111 ± 17
Days on CAPD/days of treatment (days)	19.8 ± 3.0
Months on CAPD/episodes of peritonitis (mo)	7.2 ± 0.8

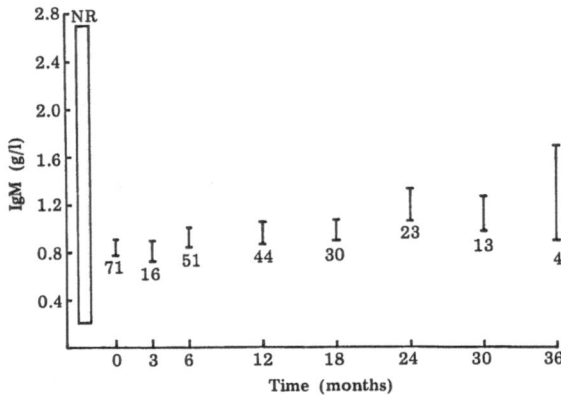

Fig. 5. Serum IgM concentrations with time on CAPD.

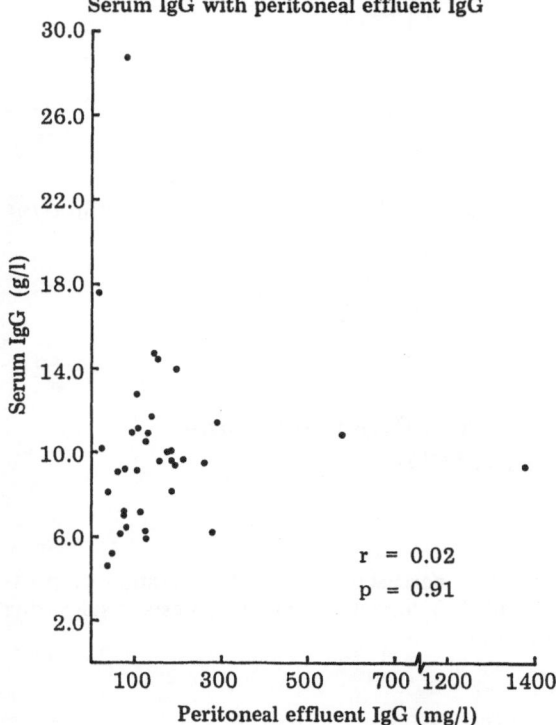

Fig. 6. Relationship between serum and peritoneal dialysate IgG concentrations.

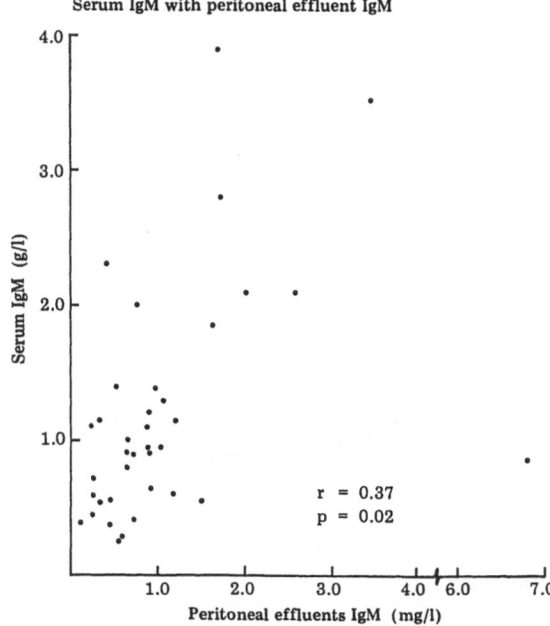

Fig. 7. Relationship between serum and peritoneal dialysate IgM concentrations.

In conclusion, this study suggests that the routine measurement of immunoglobulins in either serum or peritoneal effluent has little role in the clinical management of CAPD patients. However, we feel that further studies into the opsonizing action of immunoglobulins and peritoneal dialysate would be valuable.

ACKNOWLEDGMENT

Some of this research supported by an MRC Project Grant, No. G8115291SB and some by an MRC Project Grant, No. G8316697SB.

REFERENCES

1. Blumenkrantz MJ, Gahl GM, Kopple JD, Kamdar AV, Jones NR, Kessel M, and Coburn JW: Protein losses during peritoneal dialysis. Kidney Int 19: 593, 1981
2. Diskin CJ, Coplon N, Feldman C, and Vosti K: Antimicrobial activity in continuous ambulatory peritoneal dialysis. Peritoneal Dial Bull 3: 150, 1983
3. McLachlan SM, Rees Smith B, and Hall R: Kinetics of immunoglobulin production by cultured human peripheral blood lymphocytes. Immunol Methods 21: 211, 1978
4. Atherton MC, McLachlan SM, Pegg CAS, Dickinson A, Baylis P, Proctor SJ, and Rees Smith B: Thyroid autoantibody synthesis by blood and lymph node lymphocytes: Fractionation of B cells on density gradients. Immunology (in press)
5. Heide B, Pierratos A, Khanna R, Pettit J, Ogilvie R, Harrison J, McNeil K, and Oreopoulos DG: Nutritional status of patients undergoing CAPD. Peritoneal Dial Bull 3: 138, 1983

H.B. Steinhauer, B. Günter, and P. Schollmeyer

116

Enhanced Peritoneal Generation of Vasoactive Prostaglandins during Peritonitis in Patients Undergoing CAPD

SUMMARY

The effect of peritonitis on the peritoneal generation of prostanoids was studied during 14 episodes of bacterial peritonitis in 12 patients with end-stage renal failure undergoing CAPD. The prostaglandins; PGE_2, $PGF_{2\alpha}$, 6-keto-$PGF_{1\alpha}$, 13,14-dihydro-15-keto-$PGF_{2\alpha}$ and thromboxane (TXB_2) were determined in dialysis solution by radioimmunoassay.

The prostacyclin metabolite 6-keto-$PGF_{1\alpha}$ was found to be the major prostanoid in human peritoneal dialysate during infection-free periods and during peritonitis (420 ± 44 and 2056 ± 291 pg/ml respectively) followed by lesser amounts of PGE_2, $PGF_{2\alpha}$, TXB_2, and 13,14-dihydro-15-keto-$PGF_{2\alpha}$. The ratio of the vasodilatory prostaglandins and their metabolites respectively (PGE_2 and 6-keto-$PGF_{1\alpha}$) to the vasoconstrictors and their metabolites respectively ($PGF_{2\alpha}$ and TXB_2) increased from 6.0:1 to 12.6:1 during peritoneal inflammation. Effective therapy of peritonitis as well as the intraperitoneal administration of the cyclo-oxygenase inhibitor, indomethacin (12.5 mg/L dialysate) reduced the concentrations of all prostanoids to basal levels.

Since the peritoneal blood flow is a major determinant of solute transport across the peritoneum, vasodilator prostaglandins may play an important part in changes of the peritoneal transport properties during peritonitis. Furthermore, there is evidence that the increased peritoneal generation of prostanoids is involved in the pathogenesis of sclerosing peritonitis.

INTRODUCTION

Peritonitis continues to be a major complication of continuous ambulatory peritoneal dialysis (CAPD). Previous work has described increased peritoneal clearances and losses of protein during peritonitis.[1-5] Enhanced glucose absorption from the dialysate during inflammation results in decreased ultrafiltration rates.[5] Since local blood flow is a major determinant of solute transport across the peritoneal membrane, vasodilatation and increased vascular permeability observed during peritonitis might explain changes in the peritoneal transport properties.[5-7] The importance of endogenously generated prostaglandins on the biologic and physical qualities of the peritoneum is unknown. Intraperitoneal administration of vasodilating prostaglandins as well as drugs that result in vasodilatation enhance peritoneal mass transport.[7-9] Furthermore prostanoids are known to contribute to the genesis of the signs and symptoms of inflammatory processes and take part in control of the immunologic response.[10,11]

The present study was undertaken to investigate the effect of CAPD-associated peritonitis on the peritoneal generation of prostaglandins. Our results indicate that changes in the physical qualities and the morphological structure of the peritoneum during peritonitis are probably effected by increased generation of vasoactive prostaglandins.

From the Department of Internal Medicine, Division of Nephrology, University of Freiburg, Federal Republic of Germany.

Table 1. Clinical Data of 12 Patients with Peritonitis on CAPD.

Patient	Sex	Age (yrs)	Original Disease	Time on CAPD (mos)	Organism Isolated
A	M	65	GN	10	*Staph. epidermidis*
B	F	51	GN	10	*Acinetobacter*
C	F	36	GN	18	aerobic spore producer
				20	*Neisseria perflava*
D	M	41	AS	23	*Pseudomonas* sp.
E	M	56	DN	11	*Staph. epidermidis*
F	M	36	GN	19	*Nocardia*
				21	*Corynebacterium*
G	F	43	PN	25	*Strep. viridans*
H	M	53	GN	30	*Staph. epidermidis*
J	F	45	GN	11	no organism isolated
K	M	33	PN	7	*Staph. aureus*
L	M	39	GN	5	*Staph. epidermidis*
M	M	24	GN	26	*Staph. epidermidis*

M: male, F: female; GN: glomerulonephritis, PN: pyelonephritis.
AS: Alport's Syndrome, DN: diabetic nephropathy.

PATIENTS AND METHODS

Twelve patients (4 females, 8 males, mean age 43.5 ± 3.3 years) undergoing CAPD for end-stage renal failure were studied during 14 episodes of bacterial peritonitis and when they were doing well on CAPD (Table 1). Informed consent was obtained from all patients.

CAPD was performed with dialysis solutions containing 1.36 to 4.25% dextrose concentration (Travenol, Deerfield, IL, Fresenius, Bad Homburg, FRG), four exchanges of 1.5 to 2.0 L dialysis solution per day. Peritonitis was diagnosed by the clinical sign of abdominal tenderness accompanied by either an elevated dialysate white blood cell count (WBC) above 300/mm³ and/or a peritoneal culture yielding organism.

The therapy for bacterial peritonitis consisted of three rapid in-and-out exchanges of 2 L dialysis fluid (1.36 or 1.5% glucose concentration) without additives, followed by the administration of heparin and antibiotics to the regular dialysis solutions with a constant dwell time of 6 hours. Venous blood samples were obtained in the morning before the first dialysate exchange. Samples of dialysate were collected rapidly after the efflux and centrifuged to remove cellular blood components.

RADIOIMMUNOASSAYS

The concentrations of prostaglandins and TXB₂ were determined directly in unextracted dialysate by specific and sensitive radio-immunoassays. The RIAs for PGE_2, $PGF_{2\alpha}$, and TXB_2 were performed

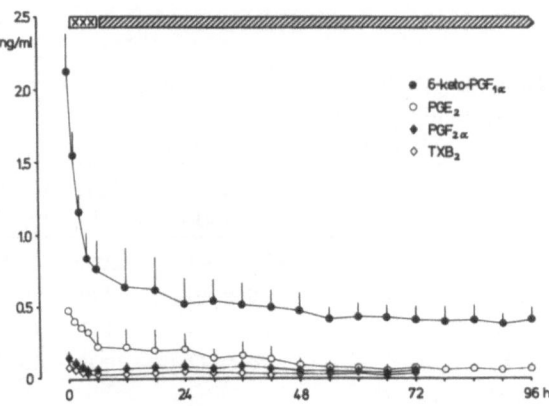

Fig. 1. Concentrations of prostanoids in peritoneal dialysate at peritonitis, $\overline{X} \pm SEM$, n = 14; ▨ : Rapid dialysate exchange, ▨ Peritoneal administration of antibiotics.

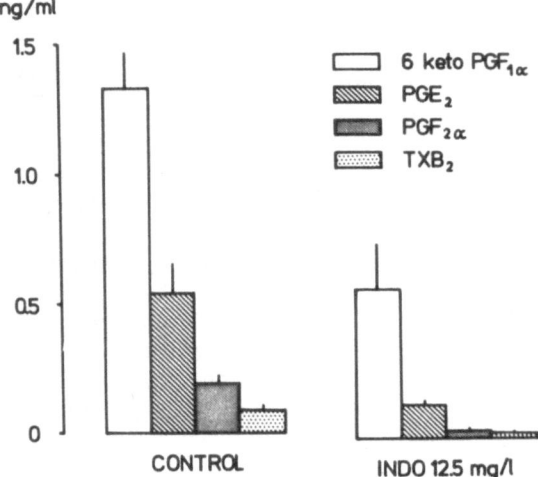

Fig. 2. Effect of indomethacin (12.5 mg/l dialysis solution) on the concentrations of prostanoids in patient F during nocardia-induced peritonitis; each column represents the mean ± SEM of four dialysates during 24 h.

as described previously[12, 13]; 6-keto-PGF$_{1\alpha}$ was determined using the double antibody method.[14] Preparation of immunogen and immunization were carried out according to the method of Peskar et al.[15] Titrated 5-keto-PGF$_{1\alpha}$ (4000 cpm/tube specific activity 120 to 180 Ci/mmol; NEN, Dreieich, FRG) in 0.1 ml phosphate buffered saline (PBS) (0.1 mol/L PBS, pH 7.4, containing 1 mg/ml gelatin) was incubated with aliquots of dialysis fluid, diluted with PBS (final volume 0.1 ml), 0.1 ml anti-6-keto-

Table 2. Dialysate Concentrations of Prostanoids during Infection-Free Periods and during Peritonitis.

	Basal* (pg/ml)	Peritonitis† (pg/ml)
6-keto-PGF$_{1\alpha}$	420 ± 44	2056 ± 291
PGE$_2$	68 ± 10	470 ± 56
PGF$_{2\alpha}$	55 ± 14	137 ± 17
TXB$_2$	26 ± 12	64 ± 13
13, 14-dihydro-15-keto-PGF$_{2\alpha}$	10 ± 2	23 ± 4

* Infection free period (four measurements per patient).
† Values represent maximal dialysate concentrations; n = 14.

PGF$_{1\alpha}$-antibody (final dilution 1/20,000) and 0.1 ml normal-rabbit-plasma (diluted 1/50 with PBS). After incubation (2 hours, at 4°C) 0.1 ml of goat antirabbit-globulin (Calbiochem, München, FRG) diluted 1 : 8 with PBS was added and incubation continued for at least 12 hours at 4°C. The precipitate was separated by centrifugation (3000 × g, for 60 minutes at 4°C), washed twice with NaCl 0.9% and dissolved in 0.5 ml of 0.1 mol/l NaOH. The radioactivity was measured in a liquid scintillation spectrometer (Packard Prias). The antibody in the final dilution of 1/20,000 bound 40% of the tracer added. Sensitivity (IC$_{50}$) and lower limit of detection (IC$_{10}$) were 180 pg and 17 pg respectively.

The 13,14-dihydro-15-keto-PGF$_{2\alpha}$-RIA was performed in detail as described previously for the radioimmunological determination of TXB$_2$[13]; 82 pg of 13,14-dihydro-15-keto-PGF$_{2\alpha}$ inhibited the binding of label to the antibody by 50%. Ten percent inhibition of binding was caused by 18 pg of 13,14-dihydro-15-keto-PGF$_{2\alpha}$. The cross-reactivity of all compounds tested was below 0.5%. The concentrations of all prostanoids determined in the dialysate decreased after intraperitoneal administration of the cyclo-oxygenase inhibitor indomethacin. None of the antibiotics used interfered with any of the radioimmunoassays. The results were expressed as means ± SEM, and compared using the Student's t test for paired observations.

RESULTS

The primary prostaglandins PGE$_2$ and PGF$_{2\alpha}$ as well as the biological inactive metabolites 6-keto-PGF$_{1\alpha}$, TXB$_2$, and 13,14-dihydro-15-keto-PGF$_{2\alpha}$ could be determined by radioimmunoassay in all samples of peritoneal dialysate during peritonitis, as well as during infection-free periods.

The concentration of prostanoids during 14 episodes of bacterial peritonitis in 12 patients are shown in Figure 1. Therapy for peritonitis reduced the concentrations of all prostaglandins to basal values within 48 hours. This decrease paralleled the normalization of the dialysate cell-count and the clinical symptoms of peritonitis.

Intraperitoneal administration of the cyclo-oxygenase inhibitor indomethacin (12.5 mg/L) reduced the dialysate concentrations of all immunoreactive prostanoids below 50% of control values (Fig. 2). The concentration of 6-keto-PGF$_{1\alpha}$ and PGE$_2$ in dialysis solution determined at the admission to the hospital during peritonitis exceeded the levels found during infection free periods for 4.9 and 6.9 times respectively (Table 2).

The dialysate concentrations of $PGF_{2\alpha}$ and its metabolite 13,14-dihydro-15-keto-$PGF_{2\alpha}$ increased 2.5 and 2.3 times respectively.

The concentration of TXB_2, the stable metabolite of the biologically active TXA_2 increased 2.5 times in comparison to infection-free periods. The ratio of PGE_2 plus 6-keto-$PGF_{1\alpha}$ to $PGF_{2\alpha}$ plus TXA_2 increased from 6.0:1 to 12.6:1. The species of microorganisms causing peritonitis, as well as the initial WBC were without significant effect on the dialysate concentrations of the various prostaglandins (Fig. 3). In one patient the development of peritonitis was observed during his stay in hospital because of non-CAPD-associated reasons. Within 12 hours (two dialysis exchanges) the concentrations of all prostaglandins and TXB_2 in dialysis fluid increased to maximal values (Fig. 4).

Two patients with repeated episodes of bacterial peritonitis (one every 3.0 and 3.3 patient-months respectively) developed histological verified sclerosing peritonitis 24 and 27 months after the onset of CAPD. Both patients never were exposed to practolol, metoprolol or acetate-containing dialysis solutions, which are believed to be involved in the pathogenesis of sclerosing peritonitis.[16-18] The ratio of dialysate prostanoids in these patients was the same as found during episodes of bacterial peritonitis in the other CAPD-patients without clinical signs of sclerosing peritonitis (data not shown). The only detectable difference between patients with and without sclerosing peritonitis was the frequency and total time of peritoneal inflammation and corresponding with this, the duration of exposure to endogenous generated prostaglandins.

DISCUSSION

Prostanoids are known to be involved in inflammatory processes as well as in the modulation of blood flow and vascular permeability.[7,9,10] Prostaglandins of the E-series and prostacyclin are potent vasodilators whereas $PGF_{2\alpha}$ and to a greater extent TXA_2 are vasoconstricting agents.[19-22] Since solute transport across the peritoneal membrane is affected by changes in local blood flow, it is reasonable to suppose that vasodilator prostaglandins modify peritoneal mass transport. Intraperitoneal administration of PGE_2 augmented the peritoneal clearances of creatinine and urea, whereas the vasoconstrictor $PGF_{2\alpha}$ significantly decreased such clearances.[7] Similar results were obtained after intraperi-

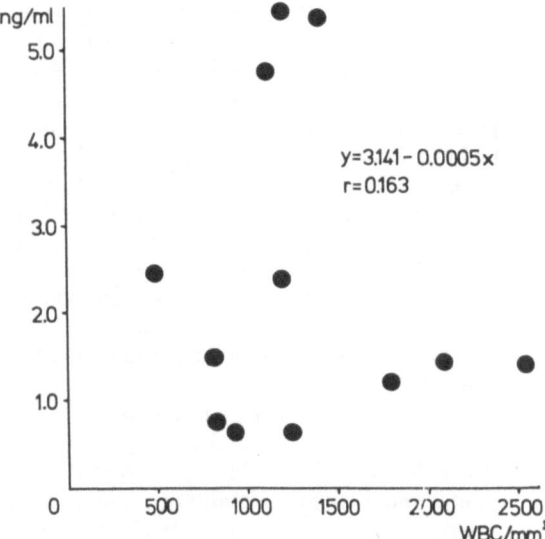

Fig. 3. Correlation between WBC/mm³ and the concentrations of 6-keto-$PGF_{1\alpha}$ in dialysis solution during peritonitis in 12 patients; values before the onset of therapy.

toneal administration of drugs that result in vasodilatation.[8,9,23]

The present results demonstrate that peritoneal generation of vasoactive prostaglandins, in patients undergoing CAPD, occurs during peritonitis as well as during infection free periods. The pros-

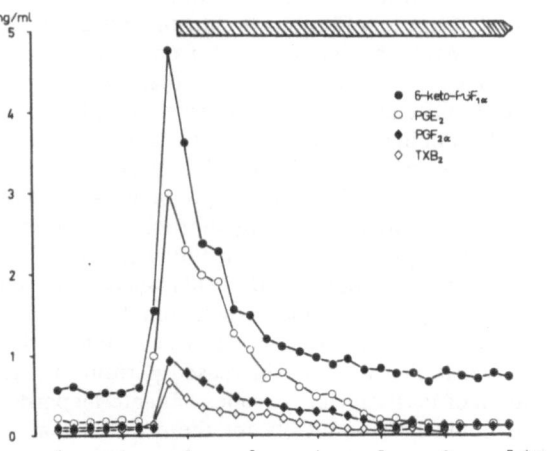

Fig. 4. Concentrations of prostanoids in peritoneal dialysate in patient H, developing peritonitis under clinical observation, [//////] : Peritoneal administration of antibiotics.

tacyclin metabolite 6-keto-$PGF_{1\alpha}$ was found to be the main dialysate prostanoid, followed by lesser amounts of immunoreactive PGE_2, $PGF_{2\alpha}$, TXB_2, and 13,14-dihydro-15-keto-$PGF_{2\alpha}$. The origin of these prostanoids is supposed to be the peritoneal mesothelium. Recent *in vitro* studies have demonstrated the generation of prostaglandins in different tissues that have mesothelial derived cells.[24] White blood cells which are known to possess the capacity for synthesizing prostaglandins, seem not to participate significantly in the generation of prostanoids, as no correlation existed between the white blood cell count and the main dialysate prostaglandin metabolite 6-keto-$PGF_{1\alpha}$.

During peritonitis the generation of all prostanoids increased. The maximal dialysate concentrations can develop within 12 hours, as observed in one patient under clinical conditions. Since local blood vessel tone is probably mediated by the vasodilators PGI_2 and PGE_2 and the antagonistic action of TXA_2, the predominance of PGI_2, determined as its biologically inactive metabolite 6-keto-$PGF_{1\alpha}$ and of PGE_2 may be responsible for the increased peritoneal blood flow during peritonitis. The augmented peritoneal clearances as well as the increased losses of proteins during peritonitis may, therefore, result from change in the physiological ratio of vasoactive prostanoids.

Since prostaglandins of the E-series were found to induce specific morphological changes in connective tissue,[25, 26] we suppose that prostanoids are involved in the pathogenesis of sclerosing peritonitis. PGE_2 can extrude enzyme-containing "matrix lysosomes" from myofibroblasts into the extracellular space.[2] After having escaped from cells, these lysosomes are no longer under direct cytoplasmic control and enzymes such as lysosomal proteases and phospholipases are set free into the extracellular area of the peritoneum. This leads to the degradation of fibrinogen and fibrin to split products, which are known to stimulate the myofibroblast proliferation.[25] This process will be maintained by an increased supply of arachidonic acid from catabolized membrane phospholipids, which stimulate the further generation of prostanoids. According to this hypothesis the observed increased peritoneal generation of PGE_2 during episodes of bacterial peritonitis could be responsible for the development of sclerosing peritonitis. Electron microscopic investigations in both patients with sclerosing peritonitis revealed the existance of extracellular "matrix lysosomes" released from proliferated peritoneal myofibroblasts.

Intraperitoneal administration of the cyclooxygenase inhibitor indomethacin was effective in reducing the generation of all prostanoids during peritonitis. The dialysate concentrations of vasodilator and vasoconstrictor prostaglandins under treatment with indomethacin were similar to those found during peritonitis free periods. Cyclooxygenase inhibitors such as indomethacin may be useful in restoring the physiologic function of the peritoneum during inflammation. Since prostaglandins seem to be mediators of inflammation-induced morphologic changes of the peritoneal membrane, inhibition of prostanoid generation may protect against the development of sclerosing peritonitis.

REFERENCES

1. Rubin J, Ray R, Barnes T, and Bower J: Peritoneal abnormalities during infectious episodes of continuous ambulatory peritoneal dialysis. Nephron 29: 124, 1981

2. Blumenkrantz MJ, Gahl G, Kopple JD, Kamdar AV, Jones MR, Kessel M, and Coburn JW: Protein losses during peritoneal dialysis. Kidney Int 19: 593, 1981

3. Verger C, Brunschvicg O, LeCharpentier Y, Lavergne A, and Vantelon J: Structural and ultrastructural peritoneal membrane changes and permeability alterations during continuous ambulatory peritoneal dialysis. Proc Eur Dial Transplant Assoc 18: 199, 1981

4. Rubin J, McFarland S, Hellems EW, and Bower JD: Peritoneal dialysis during peritonitis. Kidney Int 19; 460 1981

5. Verger C, Luger A, Moore HL, and Nolph KD: Acute changes in peritoneal morphology and transport properties with infectious peritonitis and mechanical injury. Kidney Int 23: 823, 1983

6. Nolph KD, Popovich RP, Ghods AJ, and Twardowski Z: Determinants of low clearance of small solutes during peritoneal dialysis. Kidney Int 13: 117, 1978

7. Maher JF: Pharmacological manipulation of peritoneal transport. In Nolph KD (Ed), Peritoneal dialysis. The Hague: Martinus Nijhoff 1981, p 213

8. Rubin J, Nolph KD, Arfania D, Brown P, and Prowant B: Follow up of peritoneal clearances in patients undergoing continuous ambulatory peritoneal dialysis. Kidney Int 16: 619, 1979

9. Maher JF, Hirszel P, and Lasrich M: Modulation of peritoneal transport rates by prostaglandins. In Samuelsson B, Ramwell PW, Paoletti R (Eds), Advances in prostaglandin and thromboxane research. New York: Raven Press, 1980, p 695

10. Ferreira SH, Moncàda S, and Vane JR: Prostaglandins and signs and symptoms of inflammation. In Robinson HJ, and Vane JR (Eds), Prostaglandin

synthetase inhibitors. New York: Raven Press, 1974, p 175

11. Bourne HR: Immunology. In Ramwell PW (Ed), The prostaglandins. New York: Plenum Press, 1974, p 277

12. Steinhauer HB, Anhut H, and Hertting G: The synthesis of prostaglandins and thromboxane in the mouse brain in vivo. Influence of drug induced convulsions, hypoxemia and the anticonvulsants trimethadone and diazepam. Naunyn-Schmiedeberg's Arch Pharmacol 310: 53, 1979

13. Steinhauer HB, Lubrich I, and Schollmeyer P: Response of human platelets to inhibition of thromboxane synthesis. Clin Hemorheol 3: 1, 1983

14. Morgan C, and Lazarow A: Immunoassay of insulin using a two-antibody system. Proc Soc Exp Biol Med 110: 29, 1962

15. Peskar BA, Anhut H, Kröner EE, and Peskar BM: Development, specificity and some applications of radioimmunoassays for prostaglandins and related compounds, in Advances in Pharmacologic Therapy (7). Oxford, New York: Pergamon Press, 1979, p 275

16. Brown P, Baddeley H, Read AE, Davies JD, and McGarry J: Sclerosing peritonitis, an unusual reaction to a β-adrenergic-blocking drug (practolol). Lancet 2: 1477, 1974

17. Clark CV, and Terris R: Sclerosing peritonitis associated with metoprolol. Lancet 2: 937, 1983

18. Rottembourg J, Gahl GM, Poignet JL, Mertani E, Strippoli P, Langlois P, Tanbaloc P, and Legrain M: Severe abdominal complications in patients undergoing continuous ambulatory peritoneal dialysis. Proc Eur Dial Transplant Assoc 20: 236, 1983

19. Robinson BF, Collier JG, Karim SMM, and Somers K: Effect of prostaglandins A_1, A_2, B_1, E_2 and F_2 on the forearm arterial bed and superficial hand veins in man. Clin Sci 44: 367, 1973

20. Samuelsson, Goldyne M, Granstrom E, Hamberg M, Hammarstrom S, and Malmsten C: Prostaglandins and thromboxanes. Ann Rev Biochem 47: 997, 1978

21. Moncada S, and Vane JR: Prostacyclin (PGI_2), the vascular wall and vasodilation, In Vanhoutte PM, and Leusen I (Eds), Mechanisms of vasodilation. Basel S. Karger, 1978, p 107

22. Dusting GJ, Moncada S, and Vane JR: Vascular actions of arachidonic acid and its metabolites in the perfused mesenteric and femoral beds of the dog. Eur J Phamacol 49: 65, 1978

23. Nolph KD, Ghods AJ, Van Stone J, and Brown PA: The effect of intraperitoneal vasodilators on peritoneal clearances. Trans Am Soc Artif Intern Organs 22: 586, 1976

24. Herman AG, Claeys M, Moncada S, and Vane JR: Biosynthesis of prostacyclin (PGI_2) and 121-hydroxy-5, 8, 10, 14-eicosatetranoic acid (HETE) by pericardium, pleura, peritoneum and aorta of the rabbit. Prostaglandins 18: 439, 1979

25. Riede UN: Pathogenesis of shock-induced fibrosis in man as a model of proliferative inflammation. In Deicher H, and Schulz LC (Eds), Models and mechanisms. Berlin, Heidelberg, New York: Springer, 1981, p 88

26. Joh K, Riede UN, Zahradnick HP: The effect of prostaglandins on the lysosomal function in the cervix uteri. Arch Gynecol 234: 1, 1983

M.L. Foegh, Y.T. Maddox, J.F. Winchester,
G.E. Schreiner, and P.W. Ramwell

117

Thromboxane and Prostaglandin Synthesis in Human Peritoneal Eosinophils

SUMMARY

CAPD patients occasionally exhibit peritoneal eosinophilia. Using the technique developed for routine harvesting of macrophages from waste dialysate, we harvested, isolated and purified large numbers of eosinophils over periods of several weeks in two patients on seven occasions. The number of eosinophils obtained from each bag varied from 40 to 2880 million, whereas the number of macrophages was $<1 \times 10^6$. The eosinophils were incubated in duplicate in RPMI-1640 (5×10^6 cells/ml) for 1 hour at $37°C$. Selected cyclooxygenase products, namely thromboxane A_2 (TXA_2), prostacyclin (PGI_2) and prostaglandin E_2 (PGE_2) were determined by RIA by measuring the stable metabolites thromboxane B_2 (TXB_2) and 6-keto-prostaglandin $F_{1\alpha}$ (6-keto-$PGF_{1\alpha}$) of TXA_2 and PGI_2, respectively, as well as PGE_2. The release of these products was stimulated with a calcium ionophore A23178 (5, 50, and 500 ng/ml), and zymozan (40 μg/ml) and inhibited by indomethacin (2 μg/ml). The major cyclooxygenase product measured was TXB_2: 1.56 ± 0.04 ng/ml. Only a small amount of 6-keto-$PGF_{1\alpha}$ was found (0.50 ± 0.01 ng/ml). Release was increased by A23187 and zymozan, with TXA_2 being the major metabolite. Indomethacin suppressed the release of all products to nearly nondetectable levels.

From the Division of Nephrology, Department of Medicine and Department of Physiology and Biophysics, Georgetown University Medical Center, Washington, D.C.

INTRODUCTION

Arachidonic acid metabolism through the cyclooxygenase pathway has been studied in human macrophages and the different leukocytes with the exception of eosinophils. Macrophages,[1] monocytes,[2] and polymorphonuclear leukocytes[3] synthesize prostaglandins and thromboxane while lymphocytes have not been convincingly shown to possess cyclooxygenase activity.[4] For this reason, we investigated prostaglandin and thromboxane synthesis by eosinophils prepared from dialysate of CAPD patients with the relatively rare condition of peritoneal eosinophilia.

MATERIALS AND METHODS

In our population of 150 CAPD patients, two developed intraperitoneal eosinophilia without increase in eosinophils in the peripheral blood. From these two patients, we harvested cells on seven occasions over a period of several weeks using our technique for routine harvest of macrophages from waste dialysate bags.[5] The eosinophils were isolated and purified on Percoll.[6] The purified cells were incubated in duplication in RPMI-1640 (5×10^6 cells/ml) for 1 hour at $37°C$ in the presence of either the calcium ionophore A23187 (final concentration 10^6–10^8 M), zymozan (40 μg/ml), or indomethacin (5.6×10^6 M). The arachidonate cyclooxygenase products TXA_2 and PGE_2 were determined by radioimmunoassay as TXB_2, 6-keto-$PGF_{1\alpha}$ and PGE_2,

Table 1. Mean ± SEM Concentrations (ng/ml/5 × 10⁶ cells/hour) of Arachidonic Acid Metabolites in Two CAPD Patients with Dialysate Eosinophilia, and Effects of Zymosan Incubation with the Eosinophils.

	TBX$_2$	PGE$_2$	6-keto-PGF$_{1\alpha}$
Basal	1.556 ± 0.268	0.310 ± 0.036	0.050 ± 0.010
Zymosan (40 μg/ml)	2.993 ± 0.222	0.430 ± 0.087	0.094 ± 0.008

respectively, as previously described.[1] The viability of the cells was determined by trypan blue.

RESULTS

The number of eosinophils obtained from each bag varied from 30 million to 2880 million, whereas the number of macrophages was less than one million. The major arachidonic acid metabolite measured was TXB$_2$ followed by PGE$_2$ and 6-keto-PGF$_{1\alpha}$ as seen in Table 1. The arachidonic metabolite production was stimulated by zymozan (Table 1). The calcium ionophore A23187 stimulated the release of all three products in a dose dependent manner with TXB$_2$ remaining the major product (Table 2). Indomethacin suppressed the release of all products to nearly nondetectable levels.

DISCUSSION

We have found that human peritoneal eosinophils synthesize cyclooxygenase products. Eosinophils purified on Percoll generate TXB$_2$ as the major product of the three measured: 6-keto-PGF$_{1\alpha}$ was measured in only small amounts from both unstimulated and stimulated cells. This is the first report on thromboxane synthesis by eosinophils. The amount of TXA$_2$, PGE$_2$, and PGI$_2$ synthesized from both stimulated and nonstimulated peritoneal eosinophils

were similar to that seen in both monocytes[2] and peritoneal macrophages.[1] Prostaglandin and thromboxane synthesis by human polymorphonuclear leukocytes have been reported by others.[3] However, the quantities released by these cells even on stimulation with a calcium ionophore are very small, and might be due to release from contaminating platelets. The human peripheral lymphocyte does not possess cyclooxygenase activity, but releases arachidonic acid upon stimulation.[4] Previous reports showing cyclooxygenase products being synthesized from lymphocytes, can probably be explained on the basis of impurity of the cell preparation by monocytes and platelets. One of the advantages of using human peritoneal eosinophils, rather than eosinophils from peripheral blood is that platelets are absent and macrophages/monocytes are scanty at the time of harvesting. Thus it is certain that the cyclooxygenase products found in our study are synthesized by the eosinophils.

A possible role for these arachidonic acid metabolites in the function of the eosinophils is at this stage speculative. However, in other cells of the immune system, these metabolites have been characterized as regulatory agents in the control of intracellular metabolism. These metabolites have also been proposed as intercellular humoral mediators in the immune response and they have been shown to modify many components of the immune response.

Table 2. Mean ± SEM Concentrations (ng/ml/5 × 10⁶ cells/hour) of Arachidonic Acid Metabolites after Incubation of Eosinophils with Different Concentrations (ng/ml) of Calcium Ionophore A23187.

	TXB$_2$	PGE$_2$	6-keto-PGF$_{1\alpha}$
0	1.556 ± 0.268	0.310 ± 0.036	0.050 ± 0.010
5 ng/ml	3.000 ± 0.197	0.530 ± 0.129	0.087 ± 0.030
50 ng/ml	4.197 ± 0.420	1.655 ± 0.514	0.185 ± 0.034
500 ng/ml	9.786 ± 0.620	3.258 ± 0.538	0.399 ± 0.032

For example, PGE_2, and PGI_2 inhibit and TXA_2 promotes lymphocyte proliferation.

It is also of interest to speculate about the source of the peritoneal eosinophils. The number of eosinophils are, in some instances, extremely high, with billions of cells in each dialysate bag four times a day for weeks. The half-life in the blood circulation of eosinophils is about 2 hours.[8] However, these patients had a normal eosinophil count, thus the source of these peritoneal eosinophils cannot be the peripheral blood. Bone marrow derived eosinophils are also unlikely since the mean eosinophil generation time is about 34 hours in normal individuals.[8] A possible source might be tissue-dwelling cells in that the number of eosinophils resident in tissue exceeds that in the blood by approximately 100-fold.[9]

In conclusion, we have obtained human peritoneal eosinophils from the waste dialysate of two patients with dialysate eosinophilia on CAPD. The number of eosinophils has varied, but billions of eosinophils could be obtained from each bag. We have shown for the first time that human peritoneal eosinophils produce cyclooxygenase products, with TXA_2 being the major compound in both unstimulated and stimulated cells.

REFERENCES

1. Foegh M, Maddox Y, Winchester J, Rakowski T, Schreiner G, and Ramwell PW: Prostacyclin and thromboxane release from human peritoneal macrophages. Adv Prostaglandins, Thromboxane Leukotriene Res 12: 45, 1983

2. Goldyne ME, and Stobo JD: Immunoregulatory role of prostaglandins and related lipids. CRC Crit Rev Immunol 2: 1989, 1981

3. Ramwell P, Karania J, Maggi F, Myers A, Penhos J, Watkins W, and Ramey E: Gonadal steroid regulation of vascular arachidonate metabolites. Adv Prostaglandins, Thromboxane Leukotriene Res 12:39, 1983

4. Goldyne ME, and Stobo JD: T-lymphocytes as a source of arachidonic acid and for the synthesis of eicosanoids by human monocytes/macrophages. Adv Prostaglandin, Thromboxane, Leukotriene Res 12: 39, 1983

5. Maddox Y, Foegh M, Zeligs B, Zmudka M, Bellanti J, and Ramwell P: Routine source of peritoneal macrophages. Scand J Immunol 19: 23, 1984

6. Gartner I: Separation of human eosinophils in density gradients of polyvinylpyrolidone-coated silica gel (Percoll). Immunology 40: 133, 1980

7. Leung KH, and Mihich E: Prostaglandin modulation of development of cell-mediated immunity in culture. Nature 288: 597, 1980

8. Parwaresch MR, Walle AJ, and Arndt D: The peripheral kinetics of human radiolabelled eosinophils. Virchows Arch (Cell Pathol) 21: 57, 1976

9. Stryckmans PA, Cronkite EP, Greenberg ML, and Schiffer LM: Kinetics of eosinophils leukocyte proliferation in man. Proc 12th Congr Int Soc Hematol. New York, 1963, p F19

M.W.J.A. Fieren, M.J.P. Adolfs, and I.L. Bonta

118

A Comparison of the Stimulatory Effects of Prostaglandins on Human and Rat Peritoneal Macrophage cAMP Synthesis

SUMMARY

Adenyl cyclase linked prostaglandin receptors of rat peritoneal macrophages whether resident or elicited are more sensitive to PGE_2 than to DC-PGI_2. By light microscopy macrophages isolated from patients on uncomplicated CAPD resemble elicited cells more than resident cells of the rat. Human macrophages harvested from CAPD patients are more sensitive to PGI_2 than to PGE_2, however.

INTRODUCTION

Several prostaglandins (PGs) elevated the intracellular levels of cyclic AMP (cAMP) of various cells. The PG-induced macrophage cAMP rise is associated with a down-regulation of several functions of these cells, e.g., locomotion, chemiluminescence, and phagocytosis.[1] Most experiments have been carried out in cells isolated from rodents. It is suggested that PGE_2 elevates rat peritoneal macrophage cAMP through affinity for receptors for both PGE_2 and PGI_2, whereas PGI_2 exerts its effect only through affinity to its own receptor.[2] Until now no reports have been published on cAMP synthesis following stimulation with PGs in human peritoneal macrophages. Dialysis bags of patients on continuous ambulatory peritoneal dialysis (CAPD) appear to be a practical source of human peritoneal macro-

phages.[3] Therefore we examined the sensitivity, in terms of cAMP elevation to stimulation with both PGs, of macrophages isolated from humans on CAPD and rats.

METHODS

The rat peritoneal macrophages were harvested from male Wistar rats (200 to 250 g). The macrophages were isolated using the density gradient centrifugation procedure. The macrophage population obtained was more than 90% pure and at least 95% viable as examined by trypan blue exclusion. Resident macrophages were obtained using untreated animals. Starch and carrageenin elicited cells were harvested 24 hours after an IP injection of 5 ml 1% solution of starch or 2 ml 1% solution of carrageenin. The peritoneal cavity was flushed with Gey's balanced salt solution (GBBS). Dilutions of 5×10^6 macrophages/ml GBSS were prepared for incubation. The human macrophages were harvested, using a procedure described elsewhere,[3] directly from dialysis bags of eight patients with end-stage renal disease, 4 males and 4 females, who had been treated with CAPD for several weeks or months. During the collection of the macrophages, there was no peritonitis. The dialysate contained 134 mEq/L Na, 3.5 mEq/L Ca, 1mEq/L Mg, 103.5 mEq/L Cl, 35 mEq/L lactate and 1.5, 2.3, and 4.25% dextrose. The macrophages were isolated as described in the rat experiments. The population was at least 90% pure and 95% viable. Dilutions of 5×10^5 macrophages/ml GBSS were prepared for incubations.

From the Department of Medicine I, and the Department of Pharmacology, Faculty of Medicine, Erasmus University, Rotterdam, The Netherlands.

Table 1. Effects of PGs on cAMP Levels, Expressed in % cAMP Rise.

PG Added	Resident Macrophages (%)	Starch Elicited Macrophages (%)	Carrageenin Elicited Macrophages (%)
2.8×10^{-6}M PGE$_2$	91	244	138
2.8×10^{-6}M DC-PGI$_2$	0	61	86

The samples were incubated for 10 minutes at 37°C with saline or PGs in absence or presence of 200 μM of the phosphodiesterase inhibitor isobutyl-methylxanthine (IBMX). The cAMP levels were determined using a protein binding method[4] and expressed as pmol/5×10^5 cells. The rat macrophages, resident or elicited, were stimulated with 2.8×10^{-6} M PGE$_2$ or DC-PGI$_2$, a stable analogue of PGI$_2$, in absence of IBMX. Human CAPD and starch elicited rat peritoneal macrophages were stimulated with graded concentrations of PGE$_2$ or DC-PGI$_2$, in presence of IBMX.

RESULTS

As shown in Table 1, rat peritoneal macrophages either resident or elicited, are more sensitive to stimulation with 2.8×10^{-6} M PGE$_2$ than with DC-PGI$_2$.

The results of the rat experiments carried out with graded concentrations of PGs are shown in Figure 1. The values of each concentration of DC-PGI$_2$ were significantly lower ($p < 0.05$) than those at a corresponding concentration of PGE$_2$. The results of the human CAPD experiments are shown in Figure 2. Here, the values at each concentration except 2.8×10^{-8}M DC-PGI$_2$, were significantly higher ($p < 0.05$) than those at a corresponding concentration of PGE$_2$.

DISCUSSION

Our results reported here show that adenyl cyclase linked PG receptors of rat peritoneal macro-

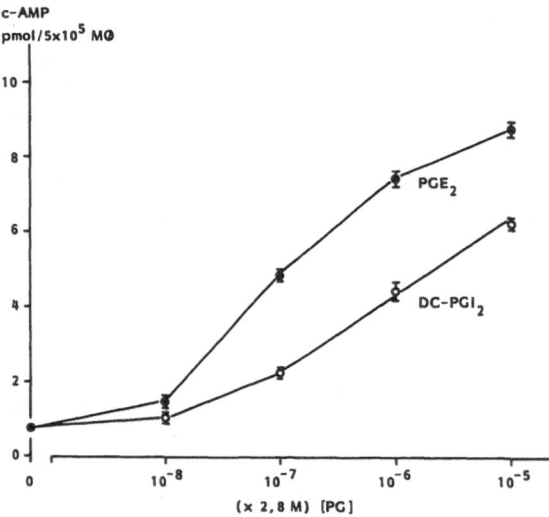

Fig. 1. Each value represents mean ± SEM of five observations (duplicate measurements) on samples from a hemogenous cell suspension of macrophages (Mo), which was pooled from ten rats.

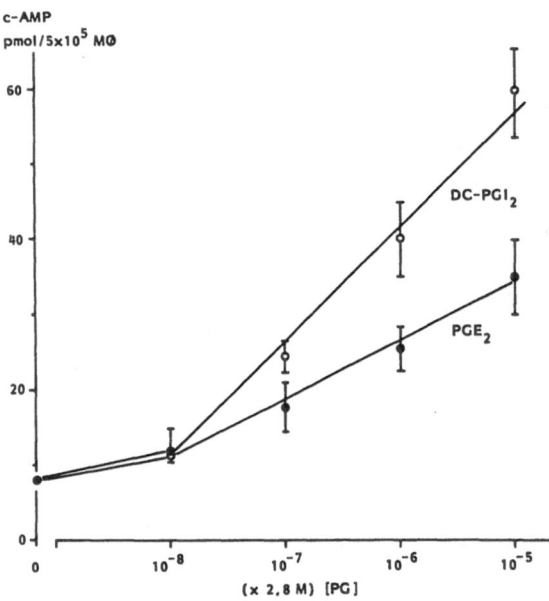

Fig. 2. The values represent the means ± SEM of individual observations (duplicate measurements) in macrophage (Mo) sampler.

phages, either resident or elicited, are more sensitive to PGE_2 than to $DC-PGI_2$ (2.8×10^{-6} M). The macrophages isolated from humans on CAPD appeared under the microscope to be more similar to elicited than to resident rat cells, i.e., the macrophages were large and contained vacuoles. In fact, these cells were almost certainly not resident cells, because there was apparently a renewed migration of macrophages after every change of dialysis bags. Therefore we compared the stimulatory effects of graded concentrations of PGE_2 and $DC-PGI_2$ on human CAPD macrophages with those on starch elicited rat peritoneal macrophages. The greater responsiveness of rat cells to PGE_2, as shown here, was also observed if experiments were carried out in absence of IBMX.[5] A similar distinction between the effects of PGE_2 and genuine PGI_2 was earlier reported in rat macrophages isolated from granuloma tissue.[6] This different sensitivity appears to be compatible with a recently reported distinction in distribution of an affinity for the binding sites of these PGs.[2] In contrast to the rat the adenyl cyclase linked PG receptors of human CAPD macrophages are more sensitive to PGI_2 than to PGE_2, although it is not known to what extent this distinction is also valid for human macrophages obtained from other sources. It is also conceivable that uremia influenced the results obtained. The data presented here indicate that macrophages obtained from CAPD dialysate could be useful in examining the effects of PGs on cAMP synthesis of macrophages of human origin. In this way the immunomodulatory functions of various PGs in man can be better defined.

ACKNOWLEDGMENTS

PGE_2 was a gift from Dr. A.J. Vergroesen, Unilever Research Laboratories, Vlaardingen, The Netherlands. $DC-PGI_2$ was obtained through courtesy of Professor C.A. Gandolfi, Farmitalia Carlo Erba, Milan, Italy.

REFERENCES

1. Bonta IL, and Parnham MJ: Immunomodulatory-anti-inflammatory functions of E-type prostaglandins. Mini review with emphasis on macrophage-mediated effects. Int J Immunopharmacol 4: 103, 1982
2. Opmeer FA, Adolfs MJP, and Bonta IL: Prostaglandin E_2 competes for adenyl cyclase coupled binding sites of (^{3}H) prostacyclin in rat peritoneal macrophages. Prostaglandins 26: 467, 1983
3. Foegh M, Maddox YT, Winchester J, Rakowski T, Schreiner G, and Ramwell PW: Prostacyclin and thromboxane release from human peritoneal macrophages. In Samuelsson B, Paoletti R and Ramwell PW (Eds), Advances in prostaglandin, thromboxane and leukotriene research Vol 12. New York: Raven Press, 1983, p 45
4. Gilman AG: Protein binding assay for adenosine-3', 5'-cyclic monophosphate. Proc Natl Acad Sci (USA) 67: 305, 1970
5. Bonta IL, Adolfs MJP, and Fieren MWJA: Cyclic AMP levels and their regulation by prostaglandins in peritoneal macrophages of rats and humans. Int J Immunopharmacol (in press)
6. Bonta IL, Adolfs MJP, and Parnham MJ: Distinction between responsiveness of macrophages to cyclic AMP elevation by prostaglandin E_2 and prostacyclin. Scand J Rheumatol 40(Suppl): 58, 1981

J. Passlick, A. Frank, M. Berger, and B. Grabensee

119

Alteration in Glucose Absorption During Peritonitis and Its Effects in Diabetic and Nondiabetic Patients Undergoing CAPD

SUMMARY

The effect of peritonitis on glucose uptake from peritoneal dialysis fluid was studied in 14 patients undergoing CAPD. No difference was noted between diabetic and nondiabetic patients. Glucose absorption increased significantly with peritonitis, however, causing a sustained elevation in plasma glucose concentration and a more rapid dissipation of the osmotic gradient.

INTRODUCTION

Patients undergoing CAPD show a loss of ultra-filtration during peritonitis, which may lead to significant fluid overload. Since there is little information, we investigated the effect of peritonitis on glucose uptake, drainage volume, serum glucose and serum insulin in nondiabetics compared to diabetics.

PATIENTS AND METHODS

Fourteen patients with end-stage renal failure undergoing CAPD, six nondiabetics, eight type I diabetics with a mean age of 46 years, age range 34–75 years were studied. Mean time on CAPD was 9

From the Medizinische Klinik, University of Düsseldorf, West Germany.

months, range 1 week–22 months. Mean duration of diabetes was 21 years, range 13–32 years. Insulin was given subcutaneously. After a standard breakfast and a 4 hour dialysis with 1.36% anhydrous dextrose dialysis fluid, the patients performed an exchange with either 1.36% or 3.86% solutions. Venous blood samples were taken at 0, 15, 30, minutes and then half-hourly. Drainage volume was measured and samples taken. Patients remained in a fasting state during the test. Dwell time was 4 hours. Statistical analysis was performed using the patient as his own control.

RESULTS

The effect of peritonitis on glucose uptake and drainage volume in nondiabetics and diabetics using 1.36% and 3.86% dextrose solution is given in Figures 1 and 2. Since the patients used 1.5 L or 2 L dialysate volume per exchange, all results are expressed as per liter instilled dialysate. Peritonitis induces a significant increase of glucose absorption and a significant decrease of drainage volume compared to uncomplicated exchanges. No significant difference in diabetic and nondiabetic patients could be demonstrated (Figs. 1 & 2). As shown in Figure 3 there is a close correlation between decrease in drainage volume and increase in glucose uptake during peritonitis using 3.86% dextrose dialysis fluid even though it is much less for the 1.36% dextrose solution. Using 1.36% dialysis fluid in diabetic pa-

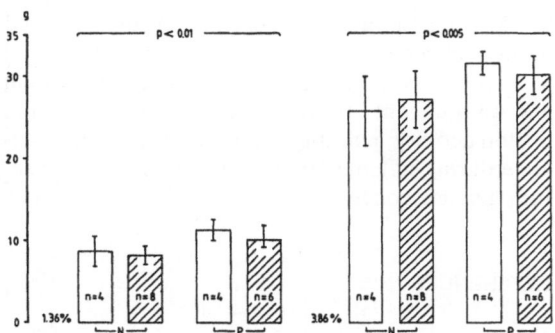

Fig. 1. Glucose uptake in diabetic and nondiabetic patients (related to 1 L infused solution) for 1.36% and 3.86% dextrose dialysis solution without (N) and with peritonitis (P).

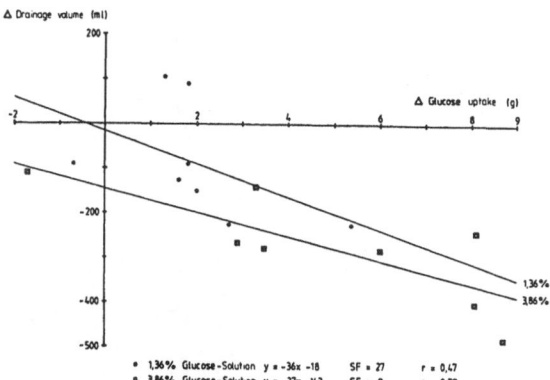

Fig. 3. Correlation of drainage volume and glucose uptake in patients on CAPD with and without peritonitis.

tients, no significant rise of serum glucose levels occurred with and without peritonitis (with peritonitis: 259 ± 117 mg/dl, without peritonitis: 239 ± 176 mg/dl). With the more concentrated solution serum glucose levels reached 251 ± 102 mg/dl without peritonitis and rose sharply in the first hour after exchange with peak levels of 396 ± 156 mg/dl in patients with peritonitis. When the 1.36% solution was employed in nondiabetic patients peak serum glucose remained below 130 mg/dl with and without peritonitis (with peritonitis: 120 ± 17 mg/dl, without peritonitis: 129 ± 23 mg/dl. Insulin remained in the normal range. An appreciable increase of glucose and insulin levels occurred while using a 3.86% dextrose dialysis solution. The maximum concentrations of serum glucose were observed in the first 1 to 2 hours subsequent to the exchange (without perito-

nitis: 160 ± 69 mg/dl and with peritonitis: 202 ± 45 mg/dl). Insulin levels reflected those of glucose, i.e., a marked increase in insulin secretion could be seen in response to the 3.86% solution especially during peritonitis with a peak level of 180 μU/ml (Figs. 4 & 5).

CONCLUSIONS

As previously shown, our study confirms that glucose absorption increases significantly during peritonitis, probably based on acute alterations of the peritoneal membrane. This results in an early dissipation of the osmotic gradient followed by a decrease of the ultrafiltration rate.[1-3] Decreased ultrafiltration secondary to increased glucose uptake

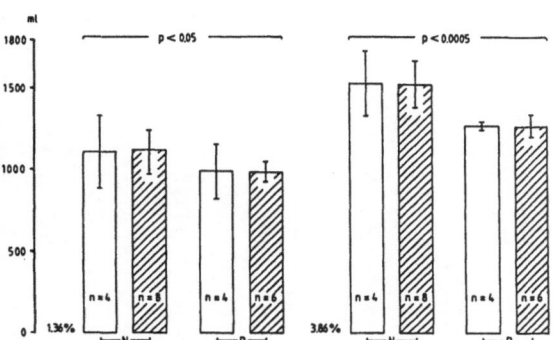

Fig. 2. Drainage volume in diabetic and nondiabetic patients (related to 1 L infused solution) for 1.36% and 3.86% dextrose dialysis solution without (N) and with peritonitis (P).

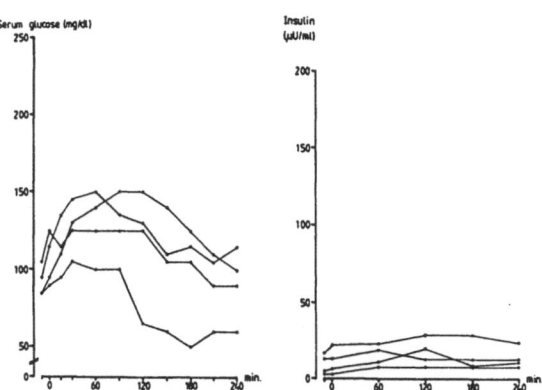

Fig. 4. CAPD with 3.86% anhydrous dextrose dialysis fluid: serum concentrations of glucose and insulin in nondiabetic patients without peritonitis.

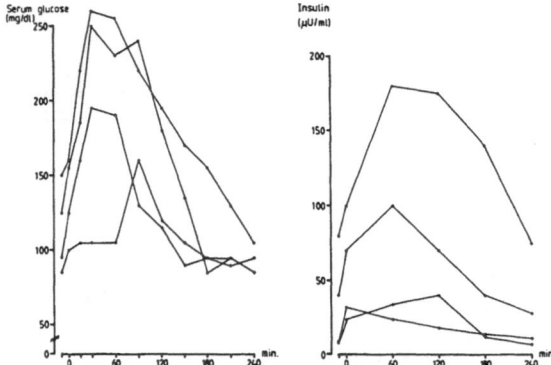

Fig. 5. CAPD with 3.86% anhydrous dextrose dialysis fluid: serum concentrations of glucose and insulin in nondiabetic patients with peritonitis.

shows no difference in diabetics or nondiabetics patients suggesting that transport of glucose depends not only on the vascular qualities of the peritoneum, but also on the altered properties of the inflamed peritoneal membrane. Even nondiabetics show a sustained elevation of serum glucose concentration and a significant but insufficient increase in serum insulin activity, pointing to peripheral insulin resistance during inflammation. Close monitoring of serum glucose concentration is therefore necessary.

REFERENCES

1. Nolph KD: Overview of the anatomy and physiology of peritoneal transport. III CAPD-Symposium Murnau (in press)
2. Raja RM, Kramer MS, Rosenbaum JL, Bolisay C, and Krug M: Contrasting changes in solute transport and ultrafiltration with peritonitis in CAPD—patients. Trans Am Soc Artif Intern Organs 28: 68, 1981
3. Rubin J, McFarland S, Hellems EW, and Bower JD: Peritoneal dialysis during peritonitis. Kidney Int 19: 460, 1981

K.I. Furman, R.O. Doehring, G.T.F. Galasko,
M.S. Kleiman, and J. Rudnick

120

Suitability of Povidone-Iodine Formulations for CAPD

SUMMARY

Views on the efficacy of povidone-iodine (PVP-I) for CAPD often vary because of failure to appreciate the difference between "available-iodine" and "free-iodine" (I_2), also the factors which control the release of I_2 from the reservoir of available iodine in PVP-I complexes, and the conversion of I_3^-, HOI and other iodine containing molecules to active I_2. Studies on the effects of diluting 10% PVP-I aqueous solutions revealed that 1:10 dilution reduces the available iodine proportionately but increases free I_2 with a parallel increase of *in vitro* antimicrobial activity. Solutions of 10% PVP-I formulated in glycol expressed from PVP-I antiseptic gauze pads (Betadine®) was found to contain less free I_2 than noted in aqueous solutions. The *in vitro* antibacterial activity was similar to that of undiluted 10% PVP-I aqueous solution against *S. aureus*, *Ps. aeruginosa* and *B. subtilis* spores, but very much less effective against *C. albicans*.

INTRODUCTION

The ideal antiseptic-disinfectant for use in CAPD should have broad-spectrum antimicrobial activity, rapid onset of action, persistent activity between applications, good surfactant action on plastic, metal, silastic, and skin surfaces, be non-

---

From the Departments of Pharmacology and Microbiology, University of the Witwatersrand, Johannesburg, South Africa.

allergenic, nonirritant to skin and catheter exit sites, easy to apply, and nonstaining. At the present time no such ideal antiseptic is available.

Elemental iodine is a powerful antimicrobial agent, which with adequate concentration and duration of exposure, can destroy all known bacteria, fungi, yeasts, viruses, and protozoa.[1] Absolute bacterial resistance to iodine is unknown. To retain the antimicrobial efficacy of iodine and avoid harmful tissue burns and staining associated with the use of the tincture or strong aqueous solutions, most treatment centers favor the use of iodine in a milder slow-release form of the iodophore polyvinylpyr-rolidine-iodine better known by its generic name povidone-iodine (PVP-I). PVP-I is now available in a variety of formulations and packings for degerming of transfer set connections with dialysate bags and catheter adaptors, and also to prevent and treat exit-site infections.

Conflicting reports appear in the literature concerning the antimicrobial efficacy of PVP-I, the most disconcerting of which relate to organisms being cultured from PVP-I solutions.[2-5] One of the most enlightening reports in this regard has been that of Berkelman et al. who investigated an alleged outbreak of *Pseudomonas cepacia* bacteremia and traced it to a batch of 10% PVP-I used to sterilize skin before venepuncture and the tops of culture bottles before injecting blood.[5] In an attempt to explain these findings Berkelman and colleagues performed an elegant series of experiments that clearly demonstrated the beneficial effects of diluting standard PVP-I solutions in increasing antibacterial efficacy.[6] Much of the misunderstanding and confusion relating to contradictory reports on PVP-I efficacy stem from a failure to appreciate the difference between the terms "available iodine" and "free-iodine".[7] Understanding the difference and the conditions under which available-iodine might become free-iodine is vital to the correct use of PVP-I in CAPD and elsewhere. In order to help explain how PVP-I can be a powerful antiseptic on the one hand, and act as a culture medium for organisms on the other, the physico-chemical characteristics of iodine and PVP-I are reviewed below, together with *in vitro* studies made in an attempt to determine how PVP-I might best be used for the purposes of CAPD.

Available-iodine in a solution is that iodine that can be titrated with sodium thiosulfate. It includes not only free-iodine (I_2), but also reservoir species of iodine such as triiodide and hypoiodous acid that lack antimicrobial activity. *Free-iodine* refers to nonionic elemental iodine as "I_2" in solution.

ELEMENTAL IODINE IN SOLUTION

I_2 is poorly soluble in water or alcohol and saturates at about 300 mg/L i.e., 300 ppm. This is therefore the strongest possible solution of iodine obtainable.

USP 2% tincture of iodine is made up with 2 g I_2/100 ml of 44–50% alcohol, an apparent 20,000 ppm. Of this, it is not possible for more than 300 ppm to be in solution without precipitation. Sodium iodide is added to the solution to provide iodide ions. These ions combine with I_2 to form triiodide which remains as a reservoir species in solution capable of reverting to I_2 when the concentration of I_2 falls below the saturation level:

$$I_2 + NaI \rightleftharpoons Na^+ + I_3^-$$

Thus USP 2% tincture of iodine has 20,000 ppm available iodine but only 300 ppm free I_2. Similarly USP 2% iodine solution has 20,000 ppm available iodine and 300 ppm free I_2.

Alkalis markedly decrease the I_2 content and consequently the antimicrobial activity of iodine solutions by converting the I_2 to hypoiodous acid. The I_2 can be restored by acidifying the solution:

$$I_2 + H_2O \rightleftharpoons HOI + H^+ + I^-$$
$$\text{(low pH} \sim 5) \qquad \text{(high pH} \sim 8).$$

The hypoiodous acid formed may react further with the oxygen in water to form iodic acid (HIO_3) and iodates.

I_2 is an avid collector of electrons to form iodide:

$$I_2 + 2e \rightleftharpoons 2I^-.$$

Electrons are collected from many organic molecules including sugars, starches, glycols, amino acids, and proteins, and is the basis of the antimicrobial action. Electrons are removed from surface molecules of bacteria etc. This is akin to an oxidation reaction. As I_2 is converted to iodide the antimicrobial potential is lost. I_2 cannot penetrate body tissues without undergoing conversion to iodide, which means that for practical purposes I_2 only has surface antimicrobial activity. Glucose also converts I_2 to iodide, so that I_2 lacks significant antibacterial action in glucose containing dialysate.[8]

POVIDONE—IODINE

The structure of the PVP-I complex is not fully understood. It has been postulated that PVP-I exists as loose spirals of varying length with hydrophilic pyrrolidine groups orientated towards the exterior and to which I^- and I_3^- bond ionically. The inner aspects of the spirals contain non-polar cavities in which the relatively insoluble I_2 molecules are held in micellar-like structures. In dry or powder form the PVP-I complexes are relatively stable and devoid of antimicrobial activity. The iodine species can only be released when the PVP-I is in solution. Besides the ions dissociating in water, the polymers separate and the shape of the spirals alter, permitting release of I_2 from the interior; i.e., adding water increases the release of I_2.[7]

USP and commercial brands of 10% PVP-I aqueous solutions are formulated to contain ± 1% or 10,000 ppm available-iodine. However these solutions have only 1 to 2 ppm free I_2 due to the very slow release of this element. Such low concentrations of I_2 have considerable antibacterial activity provided there is adequate contact time, which varies with different organisms and which for some may be quite prolonged.[1]

The PVP-I present in individually foil-wrapped antiseptic gauze pads (Betadine®) and in the disposable connection shields with PVP-I solution impregnated sponges (Travenol®) the so-called "clam shells" are formulated with 45 to 50% propylene glycol (propandiol) which imparts increased surfactant activity to the solution and prevents rapid drying on exposure. These properties are advantageous for CAPD. However the glycol appears to have an inhibitory effect on the release of free I_2 (see below). A similar inhibitory effect on I_2 has been noted when detergents are added to PVP-I in surgical scrub solutions.[5]

EXPERIMENTAL STUDIES

Free-Iodine in PVP-I Solutions

There are considerable technical difficulties associated with accurate measurement of I_2 in solution. A practical, though not entirely accurate method is to layer the solution with heptane and determine spectrophotometrically the I_2 that diffuses into the heptane.[9] However this is not valid for PVP-I solutions. The reason being that with diffusion of I_2 into the heptane layer, the equilibrium that exists between I_2 in the PVP-I and the aqueous phase is disturbed, resulting in further release of I_2 to replace that which continuously passes into the heptane. Consequently the I_2 concentration increases progressively in the heptane without reaching a steady state. Nevertheless we have been able to use this method to demonstrate relative differences of I_2 in various PVP-I solutions by determining the I_2 absorbance at a fixed time interval after layering with heptane without translating the readings to absolute mass or ppm.

METHODS

Serial dilutions of stock 10% PVP-I aqueous solution (Betadine®, Mundipharma) were made with distilled water. Similarly the glycol containing 10% PVP-I solution expressed from Betadine® (Purdue Frederick) antiseptic gauze pads was diluted serially with propandiol (Merck) and separately with distilled water. The pH was determined in all dilutions to ensure that a pH below 5 was maintained. 1.0 ml aliquots from each of the undiluted and diluted solutions were placed in a series of test-tubes. To each test-tube 10 ml analytic grade n-heptane (Merck) was added and stirred very gently for 5 minutes at 25°C, taking care to avoid emulsion formation. The tubes were allowed to stand for a further 5 minutes before aliquots of heptane were removed for determination of I_2 absorbance at 520 nm.

The available-iodine of the undiluted aqueous and glycol based PVP-I solutions was confirmed by sodium thiosulfate titration.

RESULTS

The UV absorbance in the heptane supernatant of the undiluted 10% PVP-I aqueous solution was 0.050. This increased to a maximum of 0.228 in the

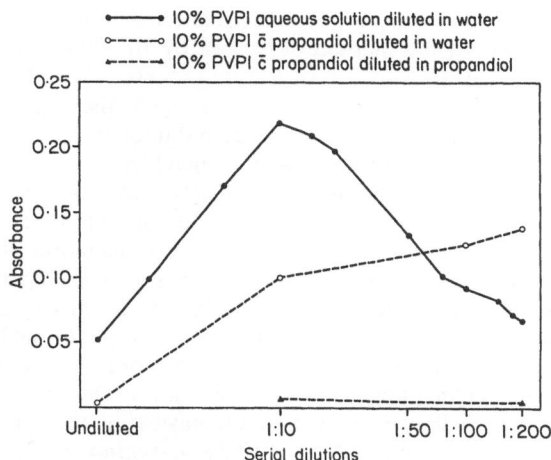

Fig. 1. Relative free-I_2 in 10% PVP-I aqueous solution undiluted and diluted with water, and in 10% PVP-I formulated with propandiol undiluted and diluted with propandiol and with water—determined by absorbance at 520 nm in supernatant heptane.

supernatant of the 1:10 dilution, indicating maximum free I_2 concentration at this dilution. The absorbance decreased to 0.091 for 1:100, and 0.068 for 1:200 dilution. (Fig. 1)

Absorbance by I_2 in the heptane supernatant of the undiluted glycol containing solution was negligible at 0.010, and remained so for the serial dilutions with propanediol. However diluting this solution with water resulted in I_2 absorbance reading of 0.102, 0.128 and 0.140 respectively, for the 1:10, 1:100, and 1:200 dilutions (Fig 1).

The available-iodine contents of the undiluted aqueous and glycol based PVP-I solutions were determined to be 1.11% and 0.95% respectively.

Antimicrobial Efficacy

METHODS

The test solutions used for this study were Betadine® (Mundipharma) 10% PVP-I aqueous solution undiluted and diluted 1:10, 1:100, and 1:200 in sterile distilled water. Also 10% PVP-I formulated in glycol expressed from Betadine® (Purdue Frederick) antiseptic gauze pads. The pH of all solutions was ascertained as being less than 5.

Challenge organisms included *Staphylococcus aureus* (ATCC 25923), *Pseudomonas aeruginosa* (ATCC 27853), *Bacillus subtilis* spores (local laboratory strain) and *Candida albicans* (clinical isolate). Following the method described by Berkelman et al.,[7] all organisms except *B. subtilis* were cultured in brain-heart infusion broth; centrifuged, the organism pellet washed, suspended, and diluted in phosphate-buffered water before being added to each of the PVP-I test solutions; I_2 was neutralized by 0.5% sodium thiosulfate at fixed time intervals of 5, 10, 15, 30, 60, and 120 seconds; and final inoculation of surviving organisms on trypticase soy blood agar plates for incubation and counting. *B. subtilis* was rendered sporing on manganese agar plates and scraping emulsified before centrifugation and suspension in phosphate-buffered water. The calculated challenge inocula in organisms/ml were as follows: *S. aureus* 1.3×10^7; *Ps. aeruginosa* $2.3 \times$ 10^6, *B. subtilis* spores 1.6×10^5; *C. albicans* 1.6×10^5. All challenge experiments were performed in duplicate and the results expressed as the mean value of surviving organisms for each pair of tests.

RESULTS

The undiluted stock and the three dilutions of the 10% PVP-I aqueous solution demonstrated rapid kill of *S. aureus*, *Ps. aeruginosa*, and *C. albicans*. Apart from a single *Pseudomonas* organism persisting in the 1:200 dilution, there were no survivors after 2 minutes contact time. The most rapid kill of both *S. aureus* and *Ps. aeruginosa* was noted in the 1:10 dilution, there being no survivors after 10 and

Table 1. Effect of Dilution of 10% Povidone-Iodine Aqueous Solution and Length of Exposure on Survival of Test Organisms.

Test Organism	Contact Time (seconds)	10% Povidone-Iodine in Aqueous Solution*			
		Undiluted	Diluted		
			1:10	1:100	1:200
Staph. aureus	5	352	4	$>10^3$	$>10^3$
(Inoculum 1.31×10^7/ml)	10	248	2	110	432
	15	10	0	21	77
	30	8	0	16	36
	60	0	0	3	4
	120	0	0	0	0
Ps. aeruginosa	5	$>10^3$	46	$>10^3$	$>10^3$
(Inoculum 2.35×10^6/ml)	10	14	1	29	$>10^3$
	15	0	1	2	30
	30	0	0	7	21
	60	0	0	1	1
	120	0	0	0	1
B. subtilis spores	5	$>10^3$	$>10^3$	$>10^3$	$>10^3$
(Inoculum 1.60×10^5/ml)	10	$>10^3$	$>10^3$	$>10^3$	840
	15	504	$>10^3$	$>10^3$	840
	30	438	558	$>10^3$	744
	60	360	732	$>10^3$	750
	120	330	768	$>10^3$	546
Candida albicans	5	$>10^3$	21	2	4
(Inoculum 1.65×10^6/ml)	10	$>10^3$	0	0	0
	15	53	0	0	0
	30	0	0	0	0
	60	0	0	0	0
	120	0	0	0	0

* Surviving Organisms (colony counts on blood agar plates).

15 seconds respectively. *C. albicans* was completely inactivated in the three diluted solutions after the first 5-second interval as compared to numerous surviving organisms being present up to 15 seconds in the undiluted PVP-I. There was poor kill of *B. subtilis* spores in all the aqueous solutions (Table 1).

The effect of the glycol containing PVP-I solution was not significantly different from that of the undiluted aqueous PVP-I solution against *S. aureus*, *Ps. aeruginosa*, and *B. subtilis* spores. However, *C. albicans* appeared to be very resistant to the antimicrobial action of this solution in that the number of surviving organisms was greater than 10^3 beyond 120 seconds contact time (Table 2).

DISCUSSION

From our studies it is evident that the commonly used 10% PVP-I aqueous solution is an effective antimicrobial agent when used in its undiluted form, and understandably has a slow action against spores. However diluting this solution 1:10 with water increases free I_2 release and the speed of antimicrobial action. The rate of kill noted in our study was more rapid than that reported by Berkelman et al.,[6] however the qualitative effect of increased bactericidal activity with dilution described by these authors was confirmed. Encouraged by our investigations we now routinely dilute stock 10% PVP-I aqueous solutions 1:10 with sterile water for use with transfer set and dialysate bag changes. Despite this, we hesitate to shorten the customary 10 minute PVP-I soak before attaching new transfer sets or changing adaptors. This because of the slow kill of spores and the possible presence of small amounts of glucose containing dialysate capable of converting I_2 to iodide. Because of the known instability of free I_2, the dilutions are freshly prepared at the beginning of each week. Unused solutions remaining from the previous week are discarded. Regular microbiologic

Table 2. Effect of 10% Povidone-Iodine Formulated with Glycol and Length of Exposure on Survival of Test Organisms.

Test Organism	Contact Time (seconds)	10% Povidone-Iodine Formulated with Glycol*
Staph. aureus (Inoculum 1.31×10^7/ml)	5	$>10^3$
	10	780
	15	532
	30	67
	60	1
	120	0
Ps. aeruginosa (Inoculum 2.35×10^6/ml)	5	246
	10	11
	15	3
	30	1
	60	0
	120	0
B. subtilis spores (Inoculum 1.60×10^5/ml)	5	$>10^3$
	10	$>10^3$
	15	$>10^3$
	30	564
	60	552
	120	648
Candida albicans (Inoculum 1.65×10^6/ml)	5	$>10^3$
	10	$>10^3$
	15	$>10^3$
	30	$>10^3$
	60	$>10^3$
	120	$>10^3$

* Surviving Organisms (colony counts on blood agar plates).

checks have not revealed any contamination or loss of efficacy in the diluted solutions kept for this period of time.

The efficacy of the glycol containing PVP-I solution appeared to be similar to that of the undiluted aqueous solution against the bacterial strains tested. How much of this antibacterial action was due to the minimal I_2 present, the glycol alone or to a combination of the two is difficult to assess. However what is significant is the fact that there was no noticeable kill of *C. albicans* after 2 minutes contact with this formulation. The commercial presentation of glycol containing PVP-I products as single sterile packed disposable units (antiseptic gauze pads and "clam shells") is certainly convenient for CAPD but does not allow for dilution. It was interesting to note in our free-I_2 study that dilution of the PVP-I solution expressed from the gauze pads with propandiol did not increase the relative free-I_2 concentration, whereas there was a prompt increase in I_2 following dilution with water (Fig. 1).

It is doubtful whether the practice of applying clam shells or taping PVP-I gauze pads around dialysate bag to transfer set connections serves anything more than a placebo effect. Use of dry sterile gauze or no dressing at all is unlikely to affect the infection rate. Thorough cleaning with a PVP-I solution immediately prior to disconnection would seem to be more important.

In the absence of an ideal antiseptic the use of PVP-I solutions is not without justification. However there are times when there is unwarrented overconfidence in the efficacy of PVP-I coupled with a failure to appreciate the numerous factors capable of reducing the concentration of free-I_2 either by inhibiting its release or facilitating conversion to inactive iodide. Important among these are evaporation, alkalinity, presence of blood or serum, glucose, glycols, detergents, and other organic matter that may either necessitate a much longer contact time to kill organisms, or permit survival of contaminants in PVP-I solutions.

A rigid "non-touch" aseptic technique is at present of much greater importance than any chemical degerming agent, and no doubt will continue to be the paramount method of combating infection and reducing the incidence of peritonitis in CAPD.

REFERENCES

1. Harvey SC: Antiseptics and disinfectants; fungicides; ectoparasiticides, In Gilman AG, Goodman LS, and Gilman A, (Eds), Goodman and Gilman's the pharmacological basis of therapeutics (6th ed). New York: Macmillan Publishing, 1980, p 973
2. Allawala NA, and Riegelman S. The properties of iodine in solutions of surface-active agents. J Am Pharm Assoc 42: 396, 1953
3. Parrott PL, Terry PM, Whitworth EN, Frawley LW, and Colbe RS: Pseudomonas aeruginosa peritonitis associated with contaminated poloxamer-iodine solution. Lancet 2: 683, 1982
4. Rodeheaver G, Bellamy W, Kody M, Spatafora G, Fitton L, Leyden K, and Edlich R: Bactericidal activity and toxicity of iodine-containing solutions in wounds. Arch Surg 117: 181, 1982
5. Berkelman RL, Lewin S, Allen JR, Anderson RL, Budnick LD, Shapiro S, Friedman SM, Nicholas P, Holzman RS, and Haley RW: Pseudobacteremia attributed to contamination of povidone-iodine with Pseudomonas cepacia. Ann Intern Med 95: 32, 1982
6. Berkelman RL, Holland BW, and Anderson RL: Increased bactericidal activity of dilute preparations of povidone-iodine solutions. J Clin Microbil 15: 635, 1982
7. Favero MS: Iodine—champagne in a tin cup. Infect Control 3: 30, 1982
8. Furman KI, Kündig H, Ninan DT, and Block JD: Reason for failure of saline-iodine flushes, In Gahl GM, Kessel M, and Nolph KD (Eds), Advances in peritoneal dialysis: Proceedings of the 2nd international symposium on peritoneal dialysis. Amsterdam: Excerpta Medica, 1981, p 281
9. Schmidt W, and Winicov M: Detergent/iodine systems. Soap Chem Specialties 43: 61, 1967

E.W. Boeschoten, P.J. Rietra, R.T. Krediet,
M.J. Visser, and L. Arisz

121

No Difference Between Oral and Intraperitoneal Treatment of CAPD Peritonitis with Cephradine

SUMMARY

After randomization 33 episodes of peritonitis in 18 patients were treated with cephradine orally and 51 episodes in 21 patients intraperitoneally. Both treatment regimens had comparably high cure rates (70 and 68%) and achieved inhibitory drug concentrations in both plasma and peritoneal dialysate of indistinguishable magnitude. Cephradine was replaced by another antibiotic when the causative organism was resistant *in vitro*. Of all episodes of peritonitis 70% were managed on an outpatient basis, and 89% were cured by drugs alone, 11% requiring catheter removal. Fourteen episodes caused by gram-positive organisms resistant to cephradine and to methicillin relapsed after an initial response.

INTRODUCTION

In the treatment of CAPD peritonitis still no consensus of opinion exists about the best therapeutic approach. Some centers start treatment with a combination of antibiotics, usually including aminoglycosides,[1,2] others use only one antimicrobial agent as drug of first choice.[3-5] In CAPD patients it is desirable to avoid aminoglycosides because the risk of ototoxicity is high, especially when treatment must be prolonged or repeated. Narrow spectrum

---

From the Departments of Medicine and Microbiology, University of Amsterdam, Academic Medical Centre, Amsterdam, The Netherlands.

antibiotics are to be preferred, but this is only possible when cure rate is good, catheter loss rare and mortality low.

Usually treatment is given intraperitoneally, but oral treatment may also succeed.[5] In most centers CAPD is continued during treatment, if possible on an outpatient basis. Since many patients are unable to inject antibiotics into the dialysate themselves the possibility of oral treatment is very important and fits better with the principle of self-care in CAPD. We questioned whether oral treatment of peritonitis would be as effective as intraperitoneal treatment. As a first-line antibiotic, cephradine was used because of its efficacy against some gram-negative and most gram-positive bacteria. Cephradine has very few adverse effects and its tendency for selection of microorganisms with antibiotic resistance is low. Cephradine can be administered orally and intraperitoneally.

PATIENTS AND METHODS

In a randomized clinical trial between January 1980 and January 1983 all peritonitis episodes in 39 adult patients (20 male, 19 female; mean age 47 years, range 21–66 years) were treated either orally (o) or intraperitoneally (IP). Peritonitis was diagnosed when the peritoneal fluid was cloudy due to a raised white cell count (more than $100/\mu l$) with or without abdominal complaints. Uncentrifugated dialysate was used for total cell count and differential cell count. The sediment of 200 ml dialysate was

Table 1. Microorganisms Isolated in 84 Peritonitis Episodes Treated According to the Protocol.

	n	%
Organisms	95	
S. epidermidis*	50	60
S. aureus	6	7
Streptococci	8	10
Enterococci	1	
Corynebacterium species	4	
P. acnes	2	
Nocardia species	1	
E. Coli	3	
Pseudomonas species	5	
Proteus species	2	
Acinetobacter species	5	
Enterobacter agglomerans	1	
Bacteroides species	2	
Candida species	1	
Ulocladium	1	
Malassezia furfur	1	
Rhodotorula rubra	1	
M. tuberculosis	1	

* 11 *S. epidermidis* strains were resistant to methicillin. In 9 episodes mixed cultures were obtained.

used for gram stain and was extensively cultured. Cephradine concentrations in serum and dialysate (overnight bags) were determined with agar diffusion technique using *B. subtilis* as the assay organism.[6]

Treatment was started before culture results were available. In all patients CAPD was continued. Lavages were not performed. The patients were randomized according to the date of catheter implantation. Implantation on an odd day: all peritonitis

episodes were treated orally (250 mg at each exchange; 500 mg first loading dose); implantation on an even day: in all episodes cephradine was given intraperitoneally (250 mg in each bag; 500 mg first loading dose). Cephradine was not used when the gram stain revealed gram-negative rods or yeasts. Cephradine was replaced by another antibiotic when the causative microorganism was found to be resistant *in vitro*. Response to treatment was judged good when peritonitis symptoms disappeared within 48 hours of treatment and cultures after the start of treatment remained negative. In cases of treatment failure peritonitis persisted despite cephradine therapy. A relapse was seen when after an initial improvement peritonitis recurred, with the same microorganism either during treatment or within two weeks after stopping the antibiotic.

RESULTS

In the 39 patients, 95 culture positive peritonitis episodes occurred, of which 84 were treated according to the protocol; 33 orally (in 18 patients) and 51 intraperitoneally (in 21 patients). The causative microorganisms of these episodes are listed in Table 1. In 11 episodes the protocol was not carried out for several reasons (Gram stain indicated the need for another antibiotic, the patients were vomiting, insufficient patient compliance, peritonitis during holiday).

The results of oral and intraperitoneal treatment were compared in peritonitis episodes caused by gram-positive bacteria (Table 2). We could not demonstrate any difference between the two forms of cephradine administration. A good response was seen in 70% (14/20) in the oral and 68% (28/41) in the intraperitoneal group. Also the time needed for the peritoneal white cell count to drop below $100/\mu l$ did

Table 2. 84 Peritonitis Episodes in 39 Patients Treated with Cephradine as Drug of First Choice.

	Peritonitis Episodes Treated	
Episode	Orally (n = 33)	Intraperitoneally (n = 51)
Gram-positive	20	41
Gram-negative	6	4
Miscellaneous	3	2
Culture negative	4	4

Episodes caused by mixed cultures or gram-positive and gram-negative bacteria are listed as gram-negative.

Table 3. Cephradine Concentrations in Serum (μg/ml) after Oral (C_o) and Intraperitoneal (C_{Ip}) Cephradine Administration.

	One Hour after First Dose	Trough <48 hours	Peak <48 hours	Trough >48 hours	Peak >48 hours
C_o mean	18.2	46.6	49.6	59.3	62.2
(range)	(<1–47.5)	(21.0–100.0)	(26.5–115.0)	(44.0–77.0)	(42.0–80.0)
n	18	15	15	13	13
C_{Ip} mean	10.3	36.9	41.3	36.0	50.7
(range)	(5.4–17.0)	(18.0–60.0)	(20.0–56.0)	(22.0–66.0)	(19.0–122.0)
n	16	15	15	14	16
p	NS	NS	NS	NS	NS

n = number of determinations.
Wilcoxon Rank Sum test ($2\alpha = 0.05$), NS = not significant.

Table 4. Cephradine Concentrations in Dialysate (μg/ml) at Various Intervals after Oral (C_o) or Intraperitoneal (C_{Ip}) Cephradine Administration (mean dwell time 8 hours).

	ca. 24 hours	2 days	4 days	7 days
C_o mean	30.1	43.1	51.0	49.0
(range)	(19.0–53.0)	(25.5–80.0)	(28.0–80.0)	(15.0–70.0)
n	22	6	21	16
C_{Ip} mean	35.7	39.2	44.9	52.7
(range)	(16.0–66.0)	(22.0–66.0)	(31.0–60.0)	(29.0–80.0)
n	22	20	19	16
p	NS	NS	NS	NS

n = number of determinations.
Wilcoxon Rank Sum test ($2\alpha = 0.05$), NS = not significant.

not differ: 3.2 days with oral and 3.6 days with intraperitoneal treatment. Relapses occurred in 14 gram-positive peritonitis episodes. Ten of them were caused by methicillin resistant *S. epidermidis*. Failures to treatment were seen in five gram-positive episodes. They were caused by *S. aureus* (2), *Nocardia*, enterococci, and *Corynebacterium* species.

Cephradine concentrations did not differ significantly in the two groups either in serum (Table 3) or in dialysate (Table 4). Dialysate cephradine concentrations at each exchange during the first 24 hours of oral treatment are shown in Figure 1. In all six patients concentrations of cephradine were well above the minimal inhibitory concentration (MIC of cephradine for susceptible gram-positive microorganisms: 1.0 to 8.0 μg/ml) even at the first exchange.

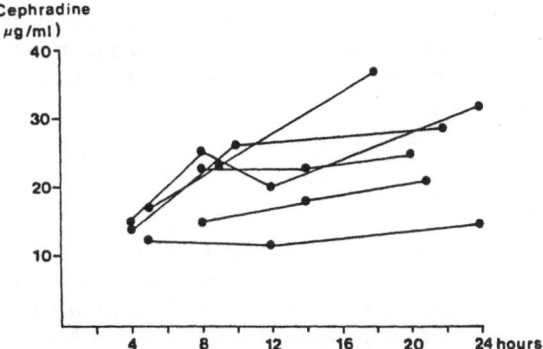

Fig. 1. Dialysate cephradine concentrations during the first 24 h with oral treatment of 6 peritonitis episodes in 6 patients.

Table 5. Treatment Outcome in 95 Culture-Positive
Peritonitis Episodes.

| | Treatment Outcome | | | | | |
| | Cure (84) | | | Catheter Removed (11) | | |
Episodes	Only C	C Replaced by Other Antibiotic	Only Other Antibiotic Used	Only C	C Replaced by Other Antibiotic	Only Other Antibiotic Used
Gram-positive (n = 71)	50	19*	—	—	2	—
Gram-negative (n = 18)	2	8	4	—	2	2
Miscellaneous (n = 6)	—	1	—	—	4	1
Total (n = 95)	52	28	4	0	8	3

* Included 14 episodes with methicillin resistant *S. epidermidis*, which relapsed after a good initial response.
C = cephradine.

Because there was no difference in treatment outcome between oral and intraperitoneal cephradine administration we could evaluate the effectiveness of cephradine as first line antibiotic by analyzing all 95 culture positive peritonitis episodes. On the basis of the gram stain seven were treated primarily with another antibiotic. Of the remaining 88 episodes 52 were cured with cephradine only (Table 5). In 14 episodes caused by methicillin resistant *S. epidermidis* a change to another antibiotic was necessary due to a relapse after a good initial response. In the other 22 episodes cephradine had to be replaced by another antibiotic because culture results required this. Finally 84 episodes (89%) were cured while CAPD was continued. Aminoglycoside antibiotics were used in only 13 of the 95 episodes. In 11 cases (11%) the catheter had to be removed because antibiotic treatment was not successful. No patient died from peritonitis. Seventy-one percent of all peritonitis episodes were treated on an outpatient basis.

DISCUSSION

In this study no difference in clinical outcome could be demonstrated between oral and intraperitoneal cephradine administration. The similarity of serum and dialysate cephradine concentrations in both treatment groups is in agreement with this result. After oral administration cephradine concentrations far above the MIC were obtained in the

dialysate within 6 hours of treatment. Cephradine proved to be a very useful first line antibiotic. It is a safe nontoxic drug that can be given orally and might select less bacterial resistance than other antibiotics. Fifty-five percent of the episodes were cured by cephradine alone. In these cases potentially toxic drugs like aminoglycosides could be avoided. In episodes where cephradine was replaced by another antibiotic the delay was not associated with a deterioration in the condition of the patients.

Of all peritonitis episodes 89% were cured by drugs and more than 70% were treated on an outpatient basis. Catheter removal was necessary in 11% which is comparable to a removal rate of 6 to 20% mentioned in other series.[3,4,7] We did not encounter *Clostridium difficile* colitis as was reported by Gokal et al.[3] None of the patients died from peritonitis.

We conclude that cephradine either orally or intraperitoneally, is a satisfactory and safe antibiotic of first choice in the treatment of CAPD peritonitis. The effectiveness of oral administration enhances the possibilities for self-care in CAPD patients.

REFERENCES

1. Vas SI: Microbiological aspects of chronic ambulatory peritoneal dialysis. Kidney Int 23: 83, 1983
2. Chan MK, Baillod RA, Chuah P, Sweny P, Raftery MJ, Varghese Z, and Moorhead JF. Three years expe-

rience of continuous ambulatory peritoneal dialysis. Lancet 1: 1409, 1981

3. Gokal R, Ramos JH, Francis DMA, Ferner RE, Goodship THJ, Proud G, Bint AJ, Ward MK, and Kerr DNS: Peritonitis in continuous ambulatory peritoneal dialysis. Lancet 2: 1388, 1982

4. Rubin J, Rogers WA, Taylor HM, Everett ED, Prowant BF, Fruto LV, and Nolph KD: Peritonitis during continuous ambulatory peritoneal dialysis. Ann Intern Med 92: 7, 1980

5. Knight KR, Polak A, Crump J, and Maskell R: Labora-

tory diagnosis and oral treatment of CAPD peritonitis. Lancet 2: 1301, 1981

6. O'Callaghan CH, and Kirby SM: Cephalosporins. In Reeves DS, et al. (Eds), Laboratory methods in antimicrobial chemotherapy. Edinburgh: Churchill Livingstone, 1978, p 181

7. Vas SI, Low DE, Layne S, et al: Microbiological diagnostic approach to peritonitis in CAPD patients. In Atkins RC, Thompson N, and Farrell PC (Eds), Peritoneal dialysis. Edinburgh: Churchill Livingstone, 1981 p 264

S. Shaldon, K.M. Koch, E. Quellhorst, and C.A. Dinarello

122

Hazards of CAPD: Interleukin-1 Production

SUMMARY

Evidence has been presented to suggest that the peritoneal macrophage is continuously stimulated during CAPD. Stimulants include pyrogen capable of making the macrophage produce interleukin-1 which in its turn will stimulate prostaglandin and fibroblast formation. Other stimulants exist and remain to be defined. The consequences of this stimulation may well be loss of ultrafiltration followed by sclerosing peritonitis in some cases.

INTRODUCTION

Loss of ultrafiltration capacity in CAPD[1] has become one of the major obstacles to the long-term viability of the treatment. It has been suggested that this complication is a precursor of sclerosing peritonitis.[2,3] Forty cases have been reported in Europe in the past year, with an 80% mortality in patients whose mean age was under 45 years. The disease may present months or years after cessation of peritoneal dialysis. The pathogenesis is unknown. The clinical features include wasting, intractable ascites,

loss of peritoneal transport function (with consequence of under dialysis if the patient is on peritoneal dialysis), and bowel obstruction. Post mortem studies reveal obliteration of the peritoneal cavity by fibrous adhesions, sacs with high protein fluid, and extreme thickening of the peritoneal membrane, which comes to resemble a fibrous band rather than an ultrathin membrane. The disease is not restricted to CAPD as it was also previously described in patients on intermittent peritoneal dialysis.[4] The pathology resembles practolol peritonitis.[5] Analysis of the risk factors in CAPD indicate a mean exposure of treatment of at least 2 years of CAPD in patients under age 60 years, often with a history of recurrent bacterial peritonitis. The incidence has been higher in patients dialysed with acetate in the fluid rather than lactate. One group[2] have a 10% incidence in their under 60 year old CAPD population with the lowest incidence of bacterial peritonitis reported in the world,[6] attributed to the use of an in-line bacterial filter, which remains in place for 14 to 28 days without being changed.

This paradox stimulated the proposition of the following explanatory hypothesis[7]: while the bacterial filter prevents bacteria arriving in the peritoneal cavity, it permits bacteria to multiply on the upstream side of the filter,[8] and allows bacterial pyrogen to traverse the filter; the pyrogen is rapidly bound to protein in the peritoneal cavity and stimulates peritoneal macrophages to produce interleukin-1 (IL-1)[9] after a suitable period of incubation, such as an overnight dwell. One of the consequences of IL-1 synthesis is the stimulation of fibroblast for-

From the Department of Nephrology, University Hospital, Nimes, France; Department of Nephrology, University Hospital, Hannover, FRG; Nephrology Center of Niedersachsen, Hann. Munden, FRG, and Department of Medicine, Tufts University School of Medicine, Boston, Massachusetts.

mation. Thus the pathogenesis of sclerosing peritonitis is induced. Of even more significance is the barrier of the peritoneum to permit transport of endogenous pyrogen (LAL) into the systemic circulation and cause fever[10]; thus the warning signs of inflammatory response to pyrogen introduction into the peritoneal cavity may be reduced or absent, leaving the patient and clinician in a state of ill advised complacency. To test this hypothesis, a series of preliminary experiments have been performed.

Table 1. LAL Content in CAPD Infusion and Drainage Fluids (n = 4).

Before filter (Sample 1)
30 pg/ml (range 0 to 45 pg/ml.)
After filter (Sample 2)
75 pg/ml (range 15 to 120 pg/ml.)
CAPD drainage fluid
Contained less than 20 pg/ml.

MATERIAL AND METHODS

In 15 patients on CAPD without clinical evidence of infection, using lactate containing fluid and no bacterial filters sterile samples were collected after an overnight dwell. In four other patients using bacterial filters, samples were collected in a sterile manner from above the filter (Sample 1); from below the filter (Sample 2); and from the drain fluid after overnight dwell (Sample 3) (Fig. 1). The samples were collected by piercing the PVC tubing with a sterile needle just prior to the tubing and filter change (which in these patients was after 4 weeks of continuous usage). The samples were stored at −70° C until they were analyzed. The following measurements were performed. An LAL estimation was performed by spectrophotometry. Interleukin-1 was measured by lymphocyte activating factor method (LAF), which measures ^{3}H uptake in murine thymocytes as an indication of DNA synthesis.[10] In samples that had not been in contact with monocytes (peritoneal macrophages), one demonstrated the presence of exogenous pyrogen by incubating the samples with human monocytes in a cell culture well at 37° C for 18 hours and then testing the supernatant fluid for its capacity to stimulate ^{3}H-thymidine uptake in murine thymocytes. In addition, in the presence of globulin, IL-1 is bound to the protein and its action on murine thymocytes is inhibited; thus in the CAPD overnight fluid it was necessary to separate the IL-1 from protein by gel chromatography using a Sephacryl S-200 column before measuring ^{3}H-thymidine uptake. The measurements of IL-1 were made in samples without prior incubation before and after gel filtration and also after incubation. In addition ^{3}H-thymidine uptake in human dermal fibroblasts was measured as an index of IL-1 ability to stimulate fibroblast formation. Specificity of IL-1 activity was confirmed by demonstration of blockade of IL-1 activity by anti-human IL-1 in both assays.

RESULTS

The preliminary results support the hypothesis and show an increase of LAL positivity across the bacterial filter (Table 1), suggesting that the filter is adding gram-negative pyrogen to the infusion fluid.

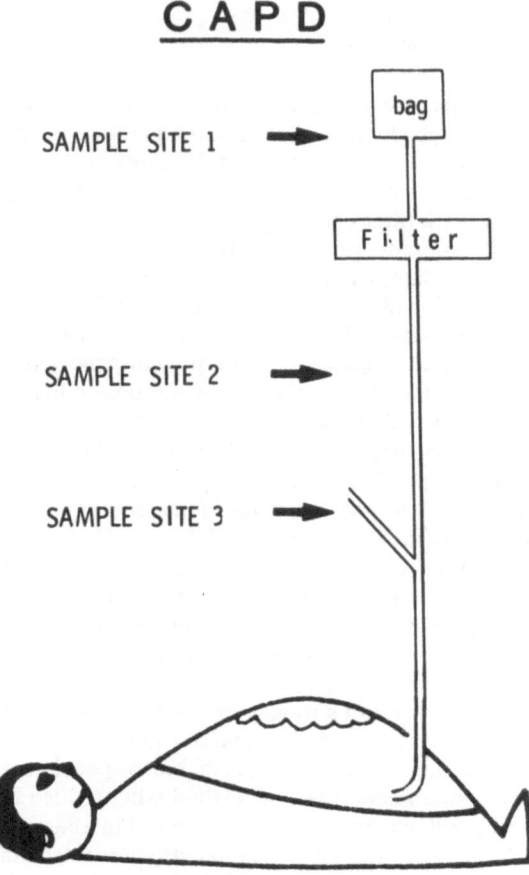

Fig. 1. The sampling sites for analysis of IL-1 and LAL activity on the samples.

In addition there was detectable pyrogen already in the dialysis fluid. The small number of samples did not permit a statistical confirmation of this trend, and it is intended to expand the experience to a larger population (Fig. 1).

Similar measurements of IL-1 in the filter group confirmed the increase in exogenous pyrogen of all varieties (including gram-positive pyrogen not detected by the LAL test) across the filter. This observation is important as LAL will be negative if all the bacterial contaminants are gram-positive which is often the case in CAPD. In addition, the highest levels of IL was seen in Sample 3, although all patients in the non filter group had IL-1 in their overnight CAPD fluid, as well, but at lower levels than in the filter population. Again, no statistical study between the two groups was undertaken, although within the non filter group the IL-1 content was significantly higher in the overnight drain fluid (Sample 3) compared to infusion fluid (Sample 1).

DISCUSSION

Thus, it would appear that CAPD is associated with the production of IL-1 in the peritoneal cavity and that the dialysate also has the capacity to stimulate fibroblast formation *in vitro*. Furthermore, patients with filters have higher levels of IL-1 in their fluid than patients without filters. From these preliminary data it is possible to speculate that at the moment it will be impossible to perform CAPD without stimulating IL-1 production. The consequence of repeated stimulation of peritoneal macrophages remains uncertain. In addition the possibility that stimulants other than exogenous pyrogen are also stimulating macrophages cannot be excluded, such as silicon particles from the catheter and plasticisers leaching from the bags and tubing sets, as well as acetate in the fluid itself. In addition to IL-1 production, it has recently been demonstrated that CAPD drainage fluid contains prostacyclin derived from peritoneal macrophages[11] and it has also been shown that IL-1 can stimulate macrophages to produce prostacyclin and thromboxane.[12] The relationship of these observations to loss of UF capability associated with an increase in glucose absorption is extremely interesting. It is reasonable to speculate that the contamination of CAPD fluid will produce IL-1 and prostaglandins and the latter will increase peritoneal blood flow if the vasodilator prostaglandins are in the majority. Increase in peritoneal blood flow will lead to a loss of UF capacity due to increased rate of glucose absorption. This mechanism being associated with IL-1 production, links loss of UF to eventual sclerosing peritonitis. Further evidence that peritoneal macrophages are under constant stimulation comes with the observation that they have a reduced phagocytic capability suggesting exhaustion from repeated stimulation.[13]

However, a fundamental question remains unanswered and is yet extremely relevant to the hypothesis: why do only 10% of patients repeatedly stimulated develop sclerosing peritonitis, if the mechanism is operative in all patients? The probability is that multiple factors are responsible, not least being the reason why fibroblast proliferation continues after the cessation of CAPD therapy. The possibility that the lesion becomes irreversible by virtue of the development of autonomous fibroblast production remains an intriguing suggestion. The true incidence of the disease remains to be evaluated.

REFERENCES

1. Nolph KD, Ryan L, Moore H, Legrain M, Mion C, and Oreopoulos DE: Factors affecting ultrafiltration in continuous ambulatory peritoneal dialysis. Peritoneal Dial Bull 4: 14, 1984
2. Slingeneyer A, Mion C, Mourad G, Canaud B, Faller B, and Beraud JJ: Progressive sclerosing peritonitis: A late and severe complication of maintenance peritoneal dialysis. Trans Am Soc Artif Intern Organs 29: 633, 1983
3. Rottembourg J, Gahl GM, Poignet JL, Mertani E, Strippoli S, Langlois P, Tranbaloc P, and Legrain M: Severe abdominal complications in patients undergoing continuous ambulatory dialysis. Proc Eur Dial Transplant Assoc 20: 236, 1983
4. Gandhi VC, Humayum H, Ing TS, Daugirdas JT, Jablokow VR, Iwatsuki S, Geis P, and Hano JE: Sclerotic thickening of the peritoneal membrane in maintenance peritoneal dialysis patients. Arch Intern Med 140: 1201, 1980
5. Marshall AJ, Baddeley H, Barritt DW, Davies JD, Lee REJ, Low-Beer TS, and Read AE: Practolol peritonitis: A study of 16 cases and a survey of small bowel functon in patients taking beta adrenergic blockers. QJ Med 46: 145, 1977
6. Mion C, Slingeneyer A, Liendo-Liendo C, Perez C, and Despaux E: Reduction in incidence of peritonitis associated with CAPD. Proc Clin Dial Transplant Forum 9: 63, 1979
7. Henderson LW, Koch KM, Dinarello CA, and Shaldon S: Hemodialysis hypotension: The interleukin hypothesis. Blood Purification 1: 3, 1983
8. Dinarello CA, and Wolff SM: Molecular basis of fever in humans. Am J Med 72: 799, 1982

9. Bennett IL: Studies on the pathogenesis of fever. V. The fever accompanying pneumococcal infection in the rabbit. Bull Johns Hopkins Hosp 98: 216, 1956

10. Dinarello CA: Interleukin-1. Rev Infect Dis 6: 51, 1984

11. Foegh M, Maddox YT, Winchester J, Rakowski T, Schreiner G, and Ramwell PW: Prostacyclin and thromboxane release from human peritoneal macrophages. In B Samuelsson, Paoletti R, and Ramwell P (Eds), Advances in prostaglandin, thromboxane, and leukotriene research. New York: Raven Press, 1983, p 45

12. Dinarello CA, Marnoy SO, and Rosenwasser LJ: Role of arachidonate metabolism in the immunoregulatory function of human leucocytic pyrogen/lymphocyte-activating factor/interleukin 1. J Immunol 130: 890, 1983

13. Keane WF, Comty CM, Verbrugh HA, and Peterson PK: Opsonic deficiency of peritoneal dialysis effluent in continuous ambulatory peritoneal dialysis. Kidney Int 25: 539, 1984

J. Manos, R.J. Postlethwaite, N.P. Mallick, and R. Gokal

123

Sclerosing Encapsulating Peritonitis and Other Complications of CAPD Peritonitis

SUMMARY

Among 97 patients treated by CAPD for a mean of 10.5 months, the peritonitis rate was 1.9 episodes/patient years and 15 patients had serious complications of peritonitis prompting a change to hemodialysis. Complications included sclerosing encapsulating peritonitis, loss of ultrafiltration capacity, loss of peritoneal surface and recurrent peritonitis. The pathogenesis of these complications of peritonitis remains unknown but these sequelae impede long-term treatment by CAPD.

INTRODUCTION

Since its introduction in 1976, CAPD has been accepted increasingly as a primary form of renal replacement therapy for patients in end-stage renal failure (ESRF).[1,2] Despite increased experience[3-5] and technical improvements, peritonitis remains a major problem, contributing to the technical failure rate sometimes reported to exceed 20 to 30% per annum,[6-8] and to an increased need for hospitalization and back up hemodialysis facilities.

Resistant or recurrent peritonitis may result in loss of ultrafiltration (UF) or loss of peritoneal space (PS). The etiology of sclerosing encapsulating peritonitis (SEP), which has recently been recognized as a serious CAPD complication[8,9] is probably multifactorial. Peritonitis seems to be the main pre-

cipitating factor; the type and strength of fluid, the material used for catheter and tubing disinfectant agents, talc, antibiotics and beta blockers have been thought to play a role.[10-17] We report here our experience regarding peritonitis related complications, in 97 patients.

PATIENTS AND METHODS

Between September 1980 and August 1983, 97 patients (mean age 40.3 years, range 16–71 years) commenced CAPD; in 87 this was the initial renal replacement therapy. Duration of CAPD ranged from 2 to 33 months (mean 10.5 months). All patients were managed on lactate containing fluids manufactured either by Travenol (T) or Fresenius (F). Most patients used four exchanges daily. The management of peritonitis consisted of continuation of CAPD (with initial lavage if the patients were very toxic), cefuroxine as the initial intra-peritoneal antibiotic, subsequently changed, if necessary, on bacteriological findings, heparin (500 U) with each exchange until the effluent became clear. A cycling machine was not used; initially, early removal of the catheter was not practiced.

RESULTS

The overall peritonitis incidence (1980-83 inclusive) was 1.9 episodes/patient year. Of the 97 patients, 18 were free of infection, 31 had one episode and eight patients each had greater than four episodes.

From the Manchester Royal Infirmary, Manchester, United Kingdom.

Table 1. Data of Patients Who Suffered Serious Abdominal Complications Following Peritonitis.

Case	Age (years)	CAPD Duration (months)	Fluid Type	β-blockers	Episodes of Peritonitis	Organism
			SEP			
1	37	16	F/T	+	2	*Pseudomonas Klebsiella*
2	8	7	F	+	2	*Staphylococcus, β. hemolytic streptococcus*
			Loss of UF			
3	27	5	F	+	2	*Staphylococcus* (×2)
4	41	2	T	+	1	fungus
			Loss of PS			
5	55	6	F	+	2	*Staphylococcus* (×2)
6	32	15	F	+	2	*E. coli, staphylococcus*
7	17	12	F	−	5	*Staphylococcus* (×4) no growth
8	20	6	F	+	3	*Staphylococcus, E. coli,* no growth
9	20	4	F	−	2	*Staphylococcus,* fungus

Complications of Peritonitis

Of the 97 patients, 15 suffered serious complications following single or multiple episodes of peritonitis such that therapy was changed to hemodialysis. Their details are shown in Tables 1 and 2; in addition, another patient (Table 1, Case 2), transferred to us for transplantation (TP), was found to have developed SEP.

SEP

Case 1 (Table 1), a 37-year-old man, previously without infection had two successive episodes of gram-negative peritonitis 14 months after starting CAPD. Following removal of the catheter and 2 weeks of hemodialysis, reinstitution of CAPD was attempted but the patient experienced severe abdominal pain and vomiting. At the time of catheter removal it was noted that his peritoneum was opaque, thickened and sclerotic, enclosing the intestine. No attempt was made to free the gut. His therapy was changed to hemodialysis and soon after he had a successful transplant. He has remained well with no intestinal problems.

Case 2 (Table 1) was a young boy who had a period of IPD for 2 months (1 episode of peritonitis) with acetate containing fluids but was then changed to hemodialysis for the next 12 months. Because of vascular access problems CAPD was started and continued for 7 months during which he had one episode of peritonitis. Following a successful TP he developed anorexia, diarrhea, vomiting, low grade fever and mild abdominal pain. He was fed intravenously but his condition progressed to intestinal obstruction. At laparotomy sclerosing encapsulating peritonitis was noted with the intestine enclosed in a

Table 2. Repeated Peritonitis Group.

Number of patients	7
Mean age (years)	39.7
Mean CAPD duration (months)	8.3
Number of peritonitis episodes	18
Rate of peritonitis (episodes/ year)	3.7
Identified organism in	15 (83%)
Staphylococcus/Streptococcus	11
Other	4
No growth	3

cocoon of thickened peritoneum. Subsequent surgical procedures led to no significant improvement and he continued to receive parenteral nutrition. Graft function remained excellent but he died 6 months later from a cerebrovascular event following intractable hypertension. Histologic appearances were typical of SEP.

Loss of Ultrafiltration

Both patients developed peritonitis early in their treatment (Table 1). Despite prompt therapy with catheter removal and apparent good initial response, recommencement of CAPD after catheter reinsertion resulted in problems of fluid overload related to loss of ultrafiltration. Both patients were managed on IPD for a period of 3 and 8 weeks until regular hemodialysis was commenced. CAPD was attempted on several occasions during the IPD phase but there was no improvement in UF. The peritoneum looked normal macroscopically at catheter removal but no histology was obtained.

Loss of Peritoneal Space

The 5 patients in this category (Table 1) had a high peritonitis rate of 3.9 episodes/patient year, which eventually resulted in reduction of the peritoneal space, which manifested as severe abdominal pain whenever peritoneal dialysis was reattempted, even with volumes as low as 500 ml. Operative findings in all cases were those of adhesions and loculus formation but there was no obvious peritoneal sclerosis.

Repeated Peritonitis

Seven patients had recurrent episodes of peritonitis (Table 2) resulting in prolonged hospitalization (mean 29 days) and were changed to hemodialysis;

partly in deference to patient preference. There was no factor that identified this group but our experience appears comparable to that of other centers.

DISCUSSION

Peritonitis still remains the major problem for patients on CAPD and is the main cause for a high technical failure rate. Even though the majority of episodes of peritonitis are treated successfully with a seemingly benign outcome, sequelae such as loss of UF, PS, or development of SEP are worrying complications.[8,9,18] Although peritonitis seems to be the main responsible factor, various other causes contributing to these complications either have been found or postulated.[10–18]

SEP is a definitive entity, with a poor prognosis, reported so far predominantly from Europe.[8,9,19] Several etiological factors have been postulated including the use of acetate solutions, beta blocking agents, disinfectant solutions used for connectors, episodes of peritonitis, plasticizers and the brand of PD fluids. We have not been able to demonstrate a single common risk factor in our two patients who developed SEP.

The loss of ultrafiltration noted in the two patients is rather surprising as it occurred very soon after commencing CAPD. One of the infections was fungal with the catheter being removed after a week. It was unfortunate that peritoneal morphology was not available in our cases. Interestingly, previous authors[21,22] have reported that patients with loss of UF are able to undergo IPD with good results as was the case in the two patients. The formation of peritoneal adhesions leading to PS loss is well documented[12] and the pathogenesis and etiology may well be similar to the aforementioned complications of SEP and UF. The mean time on CAPD of the five patients who developed this complication was only 8.6 months but their peritonitis rate was high, being 3.8 episodes/patient year. Although their peritoneum was not sclerosed it was still thickened and full of adhesions, which were very difficult to divide. There was also loss of ultrafiltration. Some of these episodes may have had too-prolonged treatment. All these cases occurred in our early experience when, because of the lack of hemodialysis facilities, CAPD was prolonged rather than removing the catheter, an important factor in treating resistant peritonitis.

The last group of our failed CAPD population comprised those seven in whom a very high peritonitis rate was recorded and resulted in a high hospitalization rate; it is not an uncommon phenomenon and one that has led to a high technique failure rate from CAPD.[3,4,6,8]

Our experience in these 15 patients, who transferred to hemodialysis, reflects the serious nature of the problem of peritonitis in CAPD patients. Although some of the serious sequelae have a small incidence, the occurrence is worrying. The etiology remains obscure and places a question mark on the long term use of CAPD for end-stage renal failure patients.

REFERENCES

1. Popovich RP, Moncrief JW, Decherd JF, Bomar JB, and Pyle WK: The definition of a novel portable/wearable equilibrium peritoneal dialysis technique. Abstr Am Soc Artif Intern Organs 5: 64, 1976
2. Oreopoulos DG, Robson M, Izatt S, Clayton S, and de Veber GA: A simple and safe technique for continuous ambulatory peritoneal dialysis (CAPD). Trans Am Soc Artif Intern Organs 24: 484, 1978
3. Gokal R, Ramos JM, Francis DMA, Ferner RE, Goodship THS, Proud G, Bint AJ, Ward MK, and Kerr DNS: Peritonitis in CAPD. Lancet 2: 1388, 1982
4. Nolph K, Boen F, Farrell P, and Pyle KW: Continuous ambulatory peritoneal dialysis in Australia, Europe and the United States. Kidney Int 23: 3, 1983
5. Wing AJ, Broyer M, Brunner FP, Challah S, Donckerwolcke RA, Gretz N, Jacobs C, Kramer P, and Selwood NH: Combined report on regular dialysis and transplantation in Europe XIII. Proc Eur Dial Transplant Assoc 20: 2, 1983
6. Prowant B, and Nolph KD: Five years' experience with peritonitis in a CAPD programme. Peritoneal Dial Bull 2: 169, 1982
7. Ramos JM, Gokal R, Siamopoulos K, Ward MK, Wilkinson R, and Kerr DNS: Continuous ambulatory peritoneal dialysis: Three years' experience. QJ Med 52: 165, 1983
8. Rottembourg J, Gahl GM, Poignet JL, Mertani E, Strippoli P, Langlois P, Tranbaloc P, and Legrain M: Severe abdominal complications in patients undergoing CAPD. Proc Eur Dial Transplant Assoc 20: 2, 1983
9. Slingeneyer A, Mion C, Mourad G, Canaud B, Faller B, and Béraud JJ: Progressive sclerosing peritonitis: a late and severe complication of maintenance peritoneal dialysis. Trans Am Soc Artif Inten Organs 29: 633, 1983
10. Tenckhoff H: Chronic peritoneal dialysis. A manual for patients, personnel and physicians. Seattle, University of Washington, School of Medicine, 1974, p 57
11. Bingswanger U, Banmatter F, Keusch G, Schiffl H, and Koller M: Chemical peritonitis during CAPD? In

Legrain M (Ed), Continuous ambulatory peritoneal dialysis. Amsterdam: Excerpta Medica, 1980, p 238
12. Mion CM, Boen ST, and Scribner P: An analysis of the factors responsible for formation of adhesions during chronic peritoneal dialysis. Am J Med Sci 250: 675, 1965
13. Schatten W: Intraperitoneal antibiotics in treatment of acute peritonitis. Surg Gynecol Obstet 102: 342, 1956
14. Lasker N, Burke JF, and Patchefsky A: Peritoneal reactions to particulate matter in peritoneal dialysis solutions. Trans Am Soc Artif Intern Organs 21: 342, 1975
15. Marshall AJ, Baddeley H, Barritt DW, Davies JD, Lee REJ, Lowbeer TS, and Read AJ: Practolol peritonitis: A study of 16 cases and a survey of small bowel function in patients taking beta adrenergic blockers. Q J Med 46: 145, 1977
16. Harty RF: Sclerosing peritonitis and propranolol. Arch Intern Med 138: 1424, 1978
17. Gandhi VS, Hymayum HM, Ing TS, Daugirdas JT, Jablokow VR, Iwatsuki S, Geis P, and Hano JE: Sclerotic thickening of the peritoneal membrane in maintenance peritoneal dialysis patients. Arch Intern Med 140: 1201, 1980
18. Slingeneyer A, Canaud B, and Mion C: Permanent loss of ultrafiltration capacity of the peritoneum in long term peritoneal dialysis: An epidemiological study. Nephron 33: 133, 1983
19. Bradley IA, Hamilton DNH, McWhinnie DL, Sternes F, MacPherson SG, Seywright M, Briggs JD, and Junor BJ: Sclerosing peritonitis after CAPD. Lancet 2: 572, 1983
20. Faller B, and Marichal JF: Evolution of ultrafiltration (UF) according to the dialysate buffer in CAPD. Abstracts of the III Int Symposium on Peritoneal Dialysis. Perit Dial Bull 4(Suppl): S22, 1984
21. Oreopoulos DG, and Khanna R: Complications of peritoneal dialysis other than peritonitis. In Nolph K (Ed), Peritoneal dialysis. The Hague, Nijhoff, 1981, p 309
22. Farrell B, and Marichal JF: Loss of ultrafiltration in CAPD: Clinical data. In Gahl GM, Kessell M, and Nolph KD (Eds), Advances in peritoneal dialysis. Proceedings of the 2nd international symposium on peritoneal dialysis. Amsterdam: Excerpta Medica, 1981, p 227
23. Backenroth-Maayan R, Longnecker R, and Kambosos D: Failure of the peritoneal membrane during chronic intermittent peritoneal dialysis. In Gahl GM, Kessell M, and Nolph KD (Eds), Advances in peritoneal dialysis. Proceedings of the 2nd international symposium on peritoneal dialysis. Amsterdam: Excerpta Medica, 1981, p 208
24. Mion C, and Slingeneyer A: Peritonitis prevention in CAPD: Long term clinical efficacy of a bacteriological filter. Proc Eur Dial Transplant Assoc 19: 388, 1982

D.L. McWhinnie, J.A. Bradley, S.P. Bramwell, D.N.H. Hamilton,
S.G. Macpherson, L.P. Cram, I.A.R. More, M.A. Forwell,
W.G.J. Smith, J.D. Briggs, and B.J.R. Junor

124

Sclerosing Peritonitis—A Further Complication of CAPD

SUMMARY

The most common complication of continuous ambulatory peritoneal dialysis (CAPD) is peritonitis which if severe or recurrent may necessitate removal of the peritoneal catheter. A further and serious complication of CAPD is sclerosing peritonitis (ScP). This condition is characterised by a partial or total encapsulation of the small bowel within a dense fibrous cocoon. Nine patients previously treated by CAPD developed ScP. The duration of CAPD ranged from 14 to 40 months and all had recurrent episodes of peritonitis often requiring catheter changes. The clinical features of ScP include recurrent abdominal pain, vomiting, malaise and weight loss preceeded by loss of ultrafiltration on CAPD. All cases required surgery for small bowel obstruction. Four patients died in the immediate post-operative period and two within 3 months from continuing small bowel obstruction. Three patients survived more than one year after operation but one subsequently died from a recurrence of ScP. The etiology of ScP is currently unclear but it represents an extremely serious potential complication of CAPD.

INTRODUCTION

The most frequent complication of continuous ambulatory peritoneal dialysis (CAPD) is peritonitis, which if severe or recurrent may necessitate

From the Departments of Surgery, Radiology, Pathology and Renal Unit, Western Infirmary Glasgow, Scotland.

catheter removal.[1] Other possible complications include exit site infection and catheter malposition.[2] Recently sclerotic thickening of the peritoneum (ScP) has been recognized as a possible late complication of both CAPD and intermittent peritoneal dialysis (IPD)[3-6] and is characterized by the deposition of a dense layer of fibrous tissue on the peritoneal surface. When severe, ScP produces partial or total encapsulation of the small bowel in a dense cocoon of fibrous tissue and this may result in small bowel obstruction.[7-10] In this report, we describe our experience of this serious complication of sclerosing peritonitis with the clinical and pathologic features.

PATIENTS, INVESTIGATIONS, AND RESULTS

Since the introduction of CAPD in the Renal Unit of the Western Infirmary, Glasgow in November 1979, we have treated over 80 patients with chronic renal failure by this method of dialysis. Our technique is that of Popovich et al.[11] as modified by Oreopoulos et al.[12] using a Tenckhoff silastic peritoneal dialysis catheter (Quinton Instrument Co, Seattle). The majority of patients carry out four 2 L exchanges of dialysis fluid each day. The dextrose concentrations of the dialysate are 1.36% and 3.86% anhydrous (Viaflex—Travenol Laboratories Limited) or 1.5% and 4.25% (Peritoflex—Fresenius) and both sources of dialysate contain lactate in a concentration of 35 mM/L.

The overall incidence of CAPD peritonitis in our unit is one episode/6.8 patient months. Peritoni-

Table 1. Patients with Sclerosing Peritonitis and Outcome.

Patient	Age/Sex	Time on CAPD (months)	Peritonitis Episodes	End CAPD to ScP (months)	Outcome
JMc	55 M	40	2	5	D
EK	30 F	24	7	11	A (transplant)
HM	60 M	14	3	13	D
DB	55 M	14	3	13	D
MG	46 F	24	6	4	D
RD	49 M	37	3	0	D
AV	45 F	24	3	1	D
JH	54 M	26	4	0	A (hemodialysis)
WC	48 M	20	5	3	D

ScP = Presentation with sclerosing peritonitis.

tis has been defined as occurring when at least two of the following criteria are met: abdominal pain with or without tenderness on palpation, cloudy peritoneal dialysate, organisms detected on Gram stain and/or culture, or a white cell count greater than 100/mm^3 dialysate. Episodes of peritonitis due to the same organism occurring within 14 days of cessation of antibiotic therapy have been classified as recurrences. Peritonitis was treated initially with intraperitoneal cefuroxime and/or gentamicin.

Nine patients of whom two were insulin-dependent diabetics developed ScP. Their age, sex, peritonitis episodes and time on and after CAPD are shown in Table 1 along with the outcome. All patients had previously demonstrated loss of ultrafiltration capacity on CAPD seen by an increasing requirement for hypertonic exchanges. This was associated with a significant fall in blood urea levels (Fig. 1) and often also in the serum creatinine.

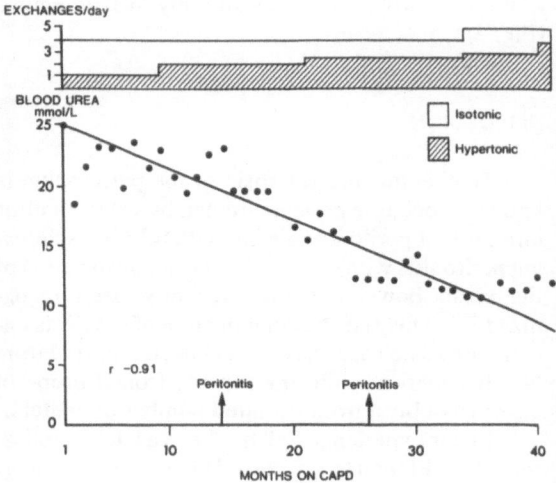

Fig. 1. Blood urea levels and use of hypertonic exchanges in patient on CAPD for 40 months with two episodes of peritonitis.

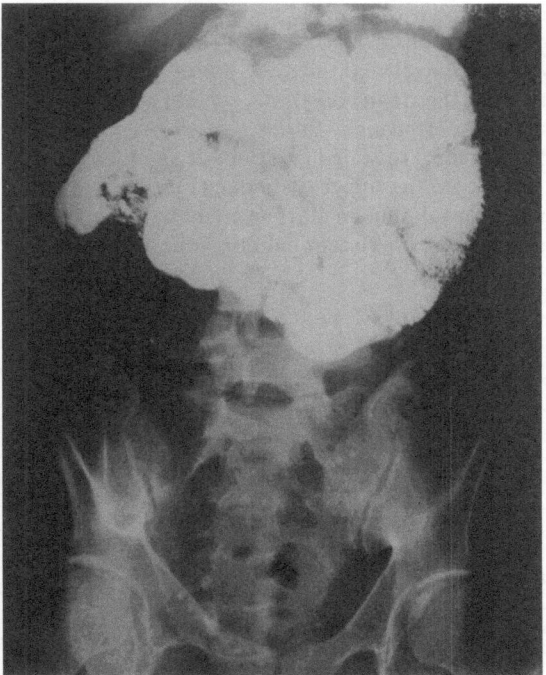

Fig. 2. Small bowel enema in ScP showing small bowel loops held in the centre of the abdomen outside the pelvis.

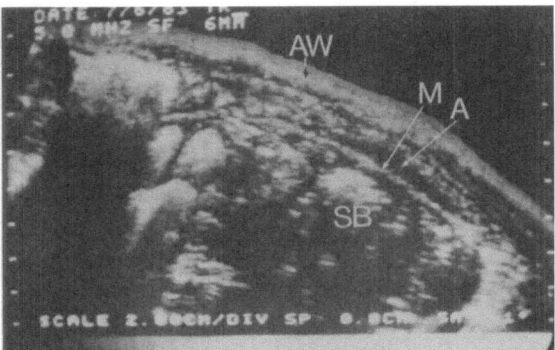

Fig. 3. Abdominal ultrasound (transverse) of abdomen showing enveloping membrane anterior to small bowel. M = membrane, A = sterile abscess cavity, SB = small bowel, AW = abdominal wall. Courtesy of Dr Patricia Morley.

In seven cases CAPD had been discontinued for recurrent or severe peritonitis, loss of ultrafiltration or transplantation before the time of presentation of ScP. The signs and symptoms were those of partial or complete small bowel obstruction with anorexia, vomiting, malaise, and weight loss. Clinical examination usually revealed a diffuse non-tender swelling in the upper abdomen. On plain abdominal x-ray there was an absence of gas shadows in the central and lower abdomen. A prolonged transit time through the small bowel was evident on barium meal and follow-through. Either a small bowel enema or barium meal revealed the loops of small bowel to be pulled into the upper abdomen (Fig. 2). In addition an encapsulating membrane could be clearly seen in some cases on abdominal ultrasound (Fig. 3).

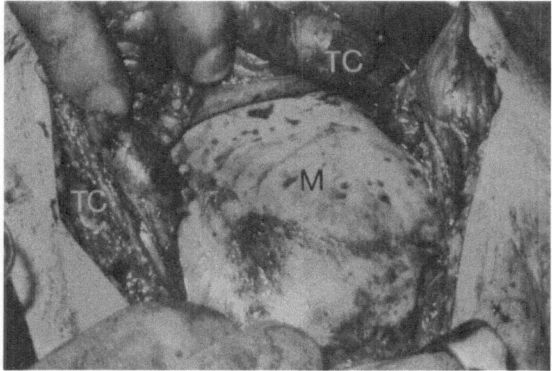

Fig. 4. Intact encapsulating membrane at laparotomy. M = membrane, TC = transverse colon.

All patients required laparotomy, in most cases as an emergency procedure for obstruction. At operation three forms of ScP were found. In some the encapsulating membrane was closely adherent to the visceral serosa of the small bowel, resulting in the bowel becoming repeatedly looped upon itself with contiguous loops adherent to each other. In others the entire small bowel was trapped behind a thickened (3 to 5 mm) flat membrane lying anterior to the small bowel while sparing the colon (Fig. 4). In these patients the small bowel was released from the thickened membrane by making multiple incisions in the membrane and excising as much of it as possible. In the third type the sclerotic process mainly affected the mesentery which was thickened and shortened resulting in small bowel obstruction.

Four patients died in the immediate post-operative period and two within 3 months of operation from persisting small bowel obstruction. Three patients survived more than one year after operation, two on hemodialysis and one following a successful cadaver transplant. One of the patients on hemodialysis however died later from a recurrence of ScP.

Biopsy of the peritoneum was performed in all cases. Microscopy showed the presence of bland fibrous tissue between and overlying loops of small bowel. There were foci of both acute and chronic inflammatory cells but no foreign material was found. While there were large areas of sclerosis there were also foci in which many small delicate blood vessels were seen. By electron microscopy the sclerotic tissue comprised scanty cells set amongst dense collagen. The cells showed features of both a fibroblastic and also a myoblastic nature (Fig. 5).

DISCUSSION

Thickening and sclerosis of the peritoneum is known to occur in patients treated by CAPD and/or intermittent peritoneal dialysis (IPD),[3,5] but sclerosing peritonitis with encapsulation and obstruction of the small bowel has only recently been recognized.[7-10] This serious complication of CAPD is uncommon as no cases have as yet been reported from North America while the reports from Europe of cases have been from a limited number of centers.

In our experience ScP has been a late complication of CAPD and has occurred up to 13 months after transfer to hemodialysis. The duration of CAPD ranged from 14 to 40 months and only one patient had symptomatic ScP within 2 years of commencing CAPD. Although the biochemical improvements we observed could be explained on the basis of a reduced protein intake this was not evident in our patients during most of the time that they were on CAPD. The association with loss of ultrafiltration suggests that there was increased permeability of the peritoneal membrane rather than a reduced peritoneal surface area.

ScP in our patients has been associated with a high mortality and four of our six patients who required emergency surgery for small bowel obstruction died in the post-operative period, as did four of the eight similar patients reported by Rottembourg et al.[7] However, if ScP can be recognized before acute bowel obstruction has occurred, it may be possible to avoid this high mortality[9, 10] but the condition may recur.

The pathogenesis of ScP resulting from CAPD is uncertain. Possible causes include exposure to constituents of the dialysis solutions of their containers. In France, the CAPD patients of Denis et al.[4] and Rottembourg et al.[7] and in North America the IPD patients described by Gandhi et al.[3] who developed ScP were all exposed to dialysis solutions containing acetate. As a consequence it has been suggested that acetate might be a possible cause.[13] However, in common with most CAPD centers in Britain and North America, the patients in this series were solely dialyzed using solutions containing lactate.

Another cause of ScP could be exposure to material in or leeching out from the catheter and it is of interest that a condition similar to ScP has been described in cirrhotic patients with ascites treated with silicone rubber LeVeen shunts.[14] The distribution of cases of ScP is not however consistent with a reaction to the catheter material being the sole causative factor and the same is true for possible reaction to the intraperitoneal use of antibiotics.

Certain beta-adrenoceptor blocking drugs, notably practolol, have been incriminated as a cause of a form of ScP.[15, 16] None of our patients had received practolol although all had previously been treated with other beta-adrenoceptor blocking drugs (propranolol, oxprenolol or atenolol). Isolated reports implying an association between ScP and propranolol and oxprenolol have appeared[17-19] but considerable doubt has been cast on these implications.[20] Although we cannot exclude with certainty a role for beta-adrenoceptor blocking drugs in causing ScP in our patients, 80% of our patients who did not develop ScP had also been on these drugs.

The peritonitis rate in patients who subsequently developed ScP was one episode/6.2 patient months, which was not significantly different from

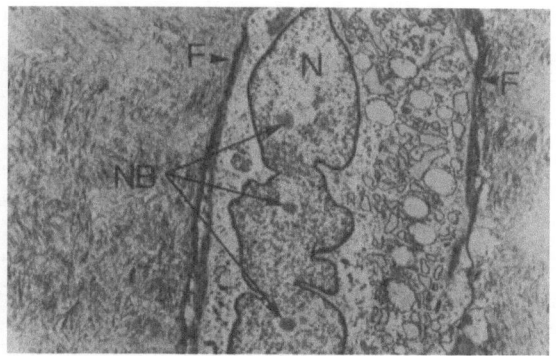

Fig. 5. Electron micrograph ($\times$ 7525) showing a myofibroblast with surrounding collagen fibres. The nucleus (N) is convoluted and contains multiple nuclear bodies (NB). The cytoplasm contains dilated cisternae of rough endoplasmic reticulum and bands of myofilament (F) with focal densities arranged parallel to the cell membrane.

the overall peritonitis rate of one episode/6.8 patient months. This is in agreement with the previous reports from France which failed to show a clear correlation between the number and severity of peritonitis episodes and the development of ScP.[7, 8] Five of our patients were transferred to hemodialysis for severe or recurrent peritonitis failing to respond to antibiotic therapy but this is no different from the practice in many CAPD centers, which have not observed cases of ScP.

There was no histologic evidence of foreign material in the abdomen or of granulomatous reaction seen to such materials as talcum powder. Currently we are investigating the role of antiseptic solution (chlorhexidine) introduced into the tubing at the time of each exchange in the development of ScP.

At present the etiology of ScP is unclear and until this is determined ScP remains an extremely dangerous potential complication of CAPD.

REFERENCES

1. Editorial: Ambulatory peritonitis. Lancet 1: 1104, 1982
2. Brown MW, Hamilton DNH, and Junor BJR: Surgical complications in patients on continuous ambulatory peritoneal dialysis. J R Coll Surg Edinburgh 28: 141, 1983
3. Gandhi VC, Humayun HM, Ing TS, Daugirdas JT, Jabolow VR, Iwatsuki S, Geis P, and Hano JE: Sclerotic thickening of the peritoneal membrane in main-

tenance peritoneal dialysis patients. Arch Intern Med 140: 1201, 1980

4. Denis J, Paineau J, Potel G, Fontenaille C, and Guenel J: Continuous ambulatory peritoneal dialysis. Ann Intern Med 93: 508, 1980

5. Gandhi VC, Ing TS, Daugirdas JT, Hagen C, Blumenkrantz MJ, and Jablokow VR: Failure of peritoneal dialysis due to peritoneal sclerosis. Int J Artif Organs 6: 97, 1983

6. Schmidt RW, and Blumenkrantz M: Peritoneal sclerosis: A "Sword of Damocles" for peritoneal dialysis? Arch Intern Med 141: 1265, 1980

7. Rottembourg J, Gahl GM, Poignet JL, Mertani E, Strippoli P, Langlois P, Tranbaloc P, and Legrain M: Severe abdominal complications in patients undergoing continuous ambulatory peritoneal dialysis. Proc Eur Dial Transplant Assoc 20: 236, 1983

8. Slingeneyer A, Canaud B, Mourad G, Bernaud JJ, Balmes M, and Mion C: Sclerosing peritonitis: Late and severe complication of long-term home peritoneal dialysis. Abst Am Soc Artif Intern Organs 12: 64, 1983

9. Bradley JA, McWhinnie DL, Hamilton DHN, Starnes F, Macpherson SG, Seywright M, Briggs JD, and Junor BJ: Sclerosing obstructive peritonitis after continuous ambulatory peritoneal dialysis. Lancet 2: 113, 1983

10. Bradley JA, Hamilton DNH, McWhinnie DL, Briggs JD, and Junor BJR: Sclerosing peritonitis after CAPD. Lancet 2: 572, 1983

11. Popovich RP, Moncrief JW, Decherd JB, Bomar JB, and Pyle WK: The definition of a portable/wearable equilibrium dialysis technique. Abst Am Soc Artif Intern Organs 5: 64, 1976

12. Oreopoulos DG, Robson M, Isatt S, Clayton S, and de Veber GA: A simple and safe technique for continuous ambulatory peritoneal dialysis. Trans Am Soc Artif Intern Organs 24: 484, 1978

13. Oreopoulos DG, Khanna R, and Wu G: Sclerosing obstructive peritonitis after CAPD. Lancet 2: 409, 1983

14. Greenlee HB, Stanley HM, Reinhardt GF, and Chejfec G: Small bowel obstruction (SBO) from compression and kinking of intestine by thickened peritoneum in cirrhosis with ascites treated with LeVeen shunt. Gastroenterology 76: 1282, 1979

15. Brown P, Baddeley H, Read AE, Davies JD, and McGarry JM: Sclerosing peritonitis, an unusual reaction of a β-adrenergic blocking drug (practolol). Lancet 2: 1477, 1974

16. Jacob H, Brandt L, Farcas P, and Frishman W: Beta-adrenergic blockade and the gastrointestinal system. Am J Med 74: 1042, 1983

17. Marshall AJ, Baddeley H, Barritt DW, Davies JD, Lee REJ, Low-Beer TS, and Read AE: Practolol peritonitis. Q J Med 46: 135, 1977

18. Harty RF: Sclerosing peritonitis and propranolol. Arch Intern Med 138: 1424, 1978

19. Ahmad S: Sclerosing peritonitis and propranolol. Chest 79: 361, 1981

20. Marigold JH, Pounder RE, Pemberton J, and Thompson RPH: Propranolol, oxprenolol and sclerosing peritonitis. Br Med J 1: 870, 1982

21. Foo KT, Ng KC, Rauff A, Foong WC, and Sinniah R: Unusual small intestinal obstruction in adolescent girls—the abdominal cocoon. Br J Surg 65: 427, 1978

22. Sieck JO, Cowgill R, and Larkworthy W: Peritoneal encapsulation and abdominal cocoon. Gastroenterology 84: 1597, 1983

J. Rottembourg, B. Issad, P. Langlois,
F. deGroc, and M. Legrain

125

Sclerosing Encapsulating Peritonitis during CAPD.
Evaluation of the Potential Risk Factors.

SUMMARY

The incidence of sclerosing encapsulating peritonitis (SEP) is one episode/16.6 patient years in a group of 163 patients treated by CAPD for a cumulative period of 237 patient years. SEP developed in 12 patients (mean age 57 ± 12 years) treated by CAPD during a mean period of 22 ± 11 months (range 7 to 42 months). Diagnosis of SEP was made in nine patients still on CAPD and in three already transferred to hemodialysis. Major clinical signs of SEP were loss of ultrafiltration, abdominal pain and intestinal obstructive episodes. Anatomical confirmation was obtained at autopsy in one patient, during an attempt to replace a catheter in five, during surgical procedures required for acute bowel obstruction in six. The outcome was severe: one patient died on CAPD, six died after surgery, five are still living on hemodialysis. The potential risk factors for SEP were analyzed comparing the 12 patients with SEP with a group without SEP. Five factors analyzed were origin of the dialysis solution, duration on CAPD, peritonitis rate and treatment, the containers and additives, and drugs.

INTRODUCTION

Since 1977 continuous ambulatory peritoneal dialysis (CAPD) was proposed as an effective maintenance therapy for patients with end-stage renal

From the Department of Nephrology, Hopital de la Pitie, Paris, France.

disease (ESRD). Large series of patients so treated have been reported with encouraging results.[1] Nevertheless recurrent peritonitis still represents a major cause of failure and a limitation to the expansion of the technique.[2] Among the severe potentially fatal abdominal complications observed in patients on CAPD, sclerosing encapsulating peritonitis (SEP) has emerged as a major problem. A recent preliminary report[3] illustrates that our observations are similar to those described earlier by Gandhi et al.[4] and Slingeneyer et al.[5] after treatment of patients with intermittent peritoneal dialysis, or as published recently in the British literature after treatment by CAPD.[6–12] Symptoms can occur weeks and even years after discontinuing peritoneal dialysis. This report deals with twelve cases, observed within a 5 year period and concentrates on analysis of the risk factors involved in the genesis of the syndrome coming from our personal data and the available literature.

PATIENTS AND METHODS

The Population at Risk

Between August 1978 and October 1983, 163 patients (104 males, 59 females) were trained to CAPD in a specialized unit in La Pitie Hospital in France. The mean age was 61.7 ± 16.6 years, with a range from 17 to 83 years. Seventy-five patients (46%) were older than 65 years at the start of treatment by CAPD.

The primary renal diseases were glomerulone-phritis in 41, insulin-dependent diabetic nephrop-athy in 47, chronic interstitial nephritis in 26, polycystic kidneys in six, nephroangiosclerosis in 16, nephropathy of various or unknown origin in 27.

The cumulative duration of treatment was 237 patient years with a mean period on CAPD of 1.5 years (range 1 to 56 months). In October 1983, 59 patients were still on CAPD, 39 were transferred to hemodialysis (HD), three received a kidney trans-plant, three recovered renal function, and 59 died while on CAPD or within 3 months after transfer to HD.

The CAPD Technique

CAPD was conducted through a double cuff Tenckhoff catheter, preferentially the curled type[13]; most patients performed four exchanges per day using routinely three 2 L bags with 1.5% dextrose concentration during the day and one 2 L bag with 4% to 4.5% dextrose concentration overnight. Ten patients were treated exclusively or temporarily by continuous cyclic peritoneal dialysis (CCPD). For various reasons including a decreasing ultrafiltration rate, 63 patients closed the catheter before sleeping and remained with an empty peritoneal cavity over-night for a period between 3 to 38 months. Most patients used chlorhexidine as an antiseptic for connections.

The peritoneal catheter was put into the perito-neal cavity in the operating room in most cases under local anesthesia. Following this procedure pa-tients were dialyzed for 2 to 3 days by continuous lavage using a cycler with 24 and 36 L/day of an acetate buffered dialysis fluid prepared by Assist-ance Publique and stored in 10 L rigid container made of polycarbonate plastic.

Diabetic patients usually used intraperitoneal injection of insulin into the catheter four times per day while changing the bag. Most patients injected once-a-day a single dose of 2500 U of heparin into the peritoneal cavity to prevent fibrin clotting formation.

Dialysis solutions from four different sources were used. Exclusive use of dialysis fluids from a single source was made in 145 patients, 65 used dialysis fluids from Assistance Publique (Paris), dur-ing 1430 patient months, 36 used Aguettant Lab, Lyon France, fluids during 450 patient months, 38 used Dianeal from Travenol, Deerfield, IL, U.S.A., during 650 patient months and 8 patients used Fresenius, W. Germany fluids during 120 patient

months. Sixteen patients have been successively dialyzed with fluids from different manufacturers; 12 initially dialyzed with fluids from Assistance Publique were transferred to Travenol Dianeal in nine cases and to Aguettant in three cases. Two initially dialyzed with fluids from Aguettant were transferred to Travenol Dianeal, and two patients dialyzed with Dianeal were transferred to Fresenius solutions.

Polyvinyl chloride (PVC) used to prepare the bags by Assistance Publique and Fresenius was manufactured by the same company, PVC used by Travenol and Aguettant Laboratories were from a different origin. The composition of dialysis fluid from different firms was almost similar. The high dextrose concentration of dialysis fluid from Travenol Aguettant, Fresenius, and Assistance Pub-lique were respectively 215, 222, 235, and 250 mmol/L. If one excludes minor differences in the potassium and magnesium concentration, the only major difference between the different solutions used was the buffer composition: sodium acetate in fluids from Assistance Publique Paris and Aguettant and sodium lactate in fluids from Travenol and Fresenius. The buffer concentration was in all cases 35 mmol ml/L.

All *peritonitis episodes* were treated by in-traperitoneal administration of antibiotics. From August 1978 until May 1981 cotrimoxazole was routinely administered as a first choice in associ-ation with continuous peritoneal lavage using a cycler.[2] Since October 1981, peritonitis episodes were treated without lavage with administration as a first choice of a combination of cephalothin and tobramycin.

RESULTS

Frequency, Symptoms, and Modalities of Diagnosis of SEP

Twelve patients (6 males, 6 females) developed the complication. The incidence being of one case of SEP for 16.6 patient years. The mean age at start of CAPD was 57 ± 12 years, ranging for 32 to 74 years. Primary renal disease was glomerulonephritis in seven, diabetic nephropathy in two, interstitial ne-phropathy, polycystic kidney, and nephropathy of unknown origin in one case respectively.

The diagnosis of SEP was made in nine pa-tients, while they were still treated by CAPD and in three cases, at 9, 12, and 15 months after transfer to HD because of recurrent peritonitis and malnutrition (cases 4, 7, and 10). The clinical symptoms observed before anatomical confirmation of the disease were decreasing ultrafiltration in seven patients and recurrent abdominal pain with anorexia nausea and vomiting in nine, leading to severe malnutrition in seven. Intermittent subocclusive intestinal episodes were observed in eight patients. Delay between the first clinical symptom and anatomical confirmation of the lesions varied from 1 to 15 months. Symptoms appeared after transfer to HD in two (Cases 4 and 10). A barium meal was given to four patients; findings were similar in all, with major signs being loss of haustration of the ileum, fixed and rigid bowel loops with ineffective peristaltic contractions seen during radioscopic examination, clear-cut separation between the loops involved in the sclerotic process, and the loops still in a free zone.

Diagnosis was anatomically confirmed in all cases. In six cases the lesions were observed during an attempt to replace a catheter. Space for cleavage was not found and the catheter was not replaced. In five cases (Cases 4, 5, 7, 10, and 11) the diagnosis was confirmed during a surgical procedure required because of acute bowel obstruction. In one case (Case 9), the diagnosis was made at autopsy. Death related mainly to acute bowel obstruction.

The lesions can extend within a very short period, for example in few weeks as observed in Case 11. At the first laparotomy for occlusion caused by ileal loop torsion, few adhesions were observed, but 6 weeks later at a second laparotomy, performed because of bowel obstruction, there was diffuse thickening of the visceral and parietal peritoneum. No peritonitis occurred and no lavage was performed between the two laparotomies.

Anatomical Lesions

Macroscopic findings observed at laparotomy were similar in all cases: the peritoneum was opaque, thickened, and sclerotic. The small bowel as a whole or partly was enclosed in a bag of thickened peritoneum. In three cases the colon was free but the root of the mesentery was sclerotic and retracted. In five cases numerous fibrous adhesions were encountered. Histological examination available in five cases showed similar lesions in all patients. Marked, diffuse thickening of the peritoneal membrane was observed due to proliferation of the connective tissue and an infiltration with inflammatory cells, mostly mononuclear. The mesothelial layer was disrupted or absent in all cases. Increased vascularity and dilated lymphatics were common

findings. Foreign body or giant cells were not observed.

Clinical Evolution after Diagnosis

All patients, except Case 9 who died while on CAPD, were transferred to HD (Table 1). The outcome was severe. Six died, 1 to 17 months after transfer. All deaths related to the sclerosing peritonitis, with persistent abdominal symptoms and malnutrition. Four patients required recurrent laparotomy for bowel obstruction. Five patients are still alive 5 to 33 months on hemodialysis, three without clinical symptoms, two with minor abdominal symptoms.

Potential Risk Factors

Treatment by CAPD including dialysis fluid composition, intraperitoneal drug administration, and any treatment delivered to the patient were analyzed. A summary of the findings is given in Table 2.

Origin of Dialysate

Patients with SEP were exclusively dialyzed with Assistance Publique dialysis fluid and three with Aguettant dialysis solution. One patient was first dialyzed with Assistance Publique solutions for 24 months and transferred to Travenol Dianeal for 13 months (Case 3). One patient (Case 7) was first dialyzed for 10 months with Travenol fluids and transferred to Assistance Publique solutions for 2 months. During this last period one severe bacterial peritonitis episode, was treated by lavage with an acetate fluid and a cycler for 40 days with a short interruption of 3 days. Until now, in this series, SEP has never been observed in patients exclusively dialyzed either with Travenol fluid during 650 patient months, nor with Fresenius fluid for 120 patient months.

Duration of Treatment by Dialysis and Relation to Dialysis Fluid Used

The mean duration of treatment by CAPD in the 12 patients with SEP was 22.6 ± 11.6 months (range from 7 to 36 months). Five patients have been dialyzed more than 2 years, including three more than 3 years, and only two patients were dialyzed for less than 1 year (Table 1). The incidence of SEP seems to increase with time and reaches 20% if one considers the three cases out of the 15 patients dialyzed at least 3 years.

Table 1. Patient Characteristics and Evolution.

Case	Sex	Age (Years)	Renal Disease*	Duration of CAPD (months)	Diagnosis of SEP Made at		Outcome after Diagnosis of SEP		
					Catheter Replacement	Bowel Surgery	On HD (months)	Still Alive	Dead
1	F	32	PN	22	+		36	+	
2	F	64	GN	42	+		1		+
3	M	49	DN	37	+		15	+	
4	F	58	GN	16		+	15		+
5	F	70	PKD	7		+	6		+
6	M	44	GN	14	+		12	+	
7	M	72	GN	13		+	1		+
8	M	60	DN	31	+		11	+	
9	F	50	unknown	10	Autopsy		—		on PD
10	M	74	GN	17		+	17	0	+
11	F	57	GN	36		+	3		+
12	M	54	GN	27	+		4	+	
mean		57 ± 12		22.6 ± 11.6					

* GN: Glomerulonephritis; PN: Pyelonephritis; PKD: Polycystic kidney disease; DN: Diabetic nephropathy.

Peritonitis Episodes. Rate and Cause

Forty-six episodes were observed in the twelve cases during the period of observation. The rate was more frequent in the group with SEP, one every 6 patient months than in the entire population (one every 9.7 patient months). Nevertheless SEP was observed in some patients with a mean rate of peritonitis below the average; e.g., one in 14 months (Case 6) and 3 in 36 months (Case 11). The organisms grown from the peritoneal fluid were Gram-positive in 34 episodes, gram-negative in eight, fungus in one, and culture negative in three episodes. Fungal infection following gram-positive infection was observed four times (Cases 3, 5, and 8).

Peritonitis Episodes. Modalities of Treatment: Lavage or Not

Twenty-six episodes occurred in eight patients and were treated by using intraperitoneal cotrimoxazole for an average of 9 days. Twelve episodes since October 1981 were treated by intraperitoneal administration of a combination of cephalothin tobramycin as a first choice. Intraperitoneal administration of other antibiotics were required in eight cases (Cases 2, 3, 4, 7, 8, 10, and 12). Twenty-one episodes in ten patients were treated by lavage with 24 to 36 L acetate buffered dialysis fluid (Assistance Publique) using a cycler. The mean duration of lavage was 3.8

± 1.2 days. A prolonged lavage was performed in three cases lasting 14 days in Case 3, 20 days in Case 8, and 40 days in Case 7 with a short interruption of 3 days. Lavage of long duration was used for fungal infection (Cases 3 and 8) and recurrent peritonitis (Case 7).

Eighteen peritonitis episodes in seven cases were never treated by lavage. Seven were "washed" for a few hours only in the outpatient clinic and two patients with SEP (Cases 5 and 12) have never been treated by peritoneal lavage.

Besides antibiotics the only drugs administered intraperitoneally were heparin and in diabetics insulin. Treatments were identical in patients without SEP.

Various Drugs Administered

Routine treatment in patients with SEP included the prolonged intake of various drugs including furosemide, clonidine, alpha-methyldopa, dihydralazine, prazosin, various sedatives, digitalis, thyroxine, calcium salts, vitamin D derivatives, and aluminum containing phosphate binders.

Eight patients with SEP received prolonged treatment with acebutolol and some of them had propranolol for a short period. Four have never received any beta-blockers. In the control group 122 out of 151 patients (81%) were treated by beta-blockers.

DISCUSSION

The peritoneal membrane, a delicate structure composed of capillaries, interstitial tissue and a simple layer of mesothelial cells,[15-17] was not designed for peritoneal dialysis. Formation of adhesions and peritoneal thickening were soon recognized as complications of chronic dialysis.[18]

Sclerosing encapsulating peritonitis is a distressing abdominal complication that can occur after either intermittent peritoneal dialysis[5] or CAPD.[6,7,9,12] The disease can progress slowly and remain asymptomatic for a long period. The first symptoms can occur several months and even a few years after transfer of the patient to either HD or transplantation.[5] However, rapid extension of the thickening of the peritoneum can be observed even in the absence of infection, as in Case 11.

Clinical symptoms are directly related to modification of gastrointestinal transit. The most common complaints are abdominal pain, nausea, vomiting and partial and intermittent bowel obstruction. Acute episodes of more or less complete intestinal occlusion can require emergency surgery. Abdominal disorders induce severe malnutrition and a life threatening situation especially if infection such as peritonitis occurs. The modification of the peritoneal membrane can induce partial loss of the ultrafiltration (UF) rate while peritoneal clearances remain unchanged. A decreased UF rate was present in seven of our 12 cases. The severity of sclerosing encapsulating peritonitis should be emphasized. Out of the 34 cases reported already in the literature[6,12] 17 have died rapidly, mostly from sepsis and malnutrition after a surgical procedure required for relief of bowel obstruction.

The factors involved in the genesis of sclerosing peritonitis are still not clearly defined. Infection should be considered as a major risk factor and the thickening of the peritoneum can be favored by recurrent inflammation of the peritoneum.[19,20,21] A history of recurrent peritonitis is encountered in many observations and in our series the rate of peritonitis, in patients with SEP, was higher than in the entire population (one every 6 patient months and one every 9.8 patient months respectively). Nevertheless SEP can occur even with a very low rate of peritoneal infection, and indeed most patients with severe recurrent peritonitis have never developed SEP. Peritonitis could be a contributing factor to SEP without being the real cause.

The origin and the composition of the dialysis fluid used may play a major role. All patients with

Table 2. Risk Factors Possibly Involved in the Genesis of Sclerosing Peritonitis.

| | Dialysis Solutions Source | | | | Peritonitis Episodes (n/patient months) | Peritoneal Lavage (n/patient months) | Drugs | |
	Aguettant	Assistance Publique	Fresenius	Travenol			Cotri-moxazole	Beta-blockers
SEP 12 cases in 22 patient years	3	8 → 1 Travenol	—	1 → 2 months AP	46 1 per 6 patient months	21 in 10 patients during a mean period of 3.8 ± 1.2 days (45% of the episodes)	8	8
Control group 151 cases in 215 patient years	35	69	8	39	255 episodes 1 per 10 patient months	68 in 43 patients (26% of the episodes)	76	122

SEP have been treated either exclusively or for a period with dialysis fluid containing acetate buffer prepared either by Assistance Publique in Paris, or Aguettant Laboratories in Lyon. No similar complications were observed when solutions from Travenol and Fresenius Laboratories were used despite similar treatment of peritonitis episodes. The major difference in the composition of the dialysis fluid between the two groups is the nature of the buffer, acetate, and lactate respectively. Dialysate containing acetate were also used to treat the patients with SEP initially reported by Gandhi et al.[4] and Slingeneyer et al.[5] However, all the cases with SEP recently reported in the English literature[6,7,9] were dialyzed using a lactate solution prepared by Fresenius.

Besides the chemical composition of the dialysate, other factors can be involved in the genesis of peritoneal inflammation; e.g., frequent use of "hypertonic" solutions[22] because of loss of ultrafiltration, presence of various particles including plasticizers coming from the bags or the containers.[19] Other factors such as the presence of formaldehyde used when reverse osmosis machines were used,[20] contamination of dialysis fluid with endotoxin[21] and very recently chlorhexidine[23] have been suspected. All our patients with SEP used chlorhexidine as an antiseptic for connection. Further research should look for factors in the dialysis fluid and the containers.

Loss of ultrafiltration has been reported as a complication occurring among patients on CAPD and increasing with time[22,24]; this early report was confirmed by other groups in patients treated by CAPD and also by IPD. A recent cooperative study clearly emphasized an increased glucose absorption through the peritoneum and a decreased UF rate, in patients dialyzed with acetate solution.[25] This complication can occur in the absence of other symptoms suggesting sclerosing peritonitis. Is loss of UF one of the preliminary manifestations of SEP or are the two diseases the consequence of a different process? Further evaluation is required to answer this question.

If one considers the different modalities of treatment for peritonitis, we were unable to detect any difference as far as intraperitoneal administration of antibiotics, including cotrimoxazole, was concerned. Peritoneal lavage to treat infection, using a cycler and a dialysate with an acetate buffer, was performed in 10 of 12 cases with SEP. But once again this mode of therapy with intraperitoneal administration of cotrimoxazole was used in all our cases until October 1981.[14] Previously no difference

in peritoneal clearances was found in patients using acetate versus lactate buffered dialysis fluid.[26,27]

Sclerosing peritonitis has been reported among patients receiving various beta-blockers including practolol,[28] propranolol,[29-31] oxprenolol,[31] atenolol, and metropolol. Treatment with beta-blockers as antihypertensive agents was routinely prescribed in our patients treated by CAPD. This treatment was mainly during the early phase of dialysis treatment but the proportion of patients treated was similar in patients with or without SEP; four of our cases with SEP had never received beta-blockers. None of the other drugs administered including antihypertensive agents, calcium salts, aluminum gels, vitamin D supplements to our knowledge induce sclerosing of the peritoneal membrane.

Sclerosing encapsulating peritonitis is a dramatic complication which jeopardizes the long term results of maintenance dialysis by peritoneal irrigation. Large discrepancies existing between the number of cases observed, the centers, countries, and the dialysis solutions used, suggest that various risk factors are involved in the genesis of the sclerosing process. Careful retrospective and prospective analysis of cases should permit detection of one or many causes of the disease and allow preventive measures. From our own experience and data from the literature, a multifactorial process seems the most likely. Presently we consider it reasonable to avoid acetate solutions, and to reduce as much as possible the indications for peritoneal lavage. Replacement of beta-blockers by other drugs when antihypertensive agents are required seems justified. Such measures are already in operation in our unit. Between October 1983 and June 1984 no new cases among the 60 patients treated in our unit and no case among our 20 new patients was observed.

REFERENCES

1. Williams CC and the University of Toronto Collaborative Dialysis Group: CAPD: An overview. Peritoneal Dial Bull 3(Suppl): S6, 1983
2. Rottembourg J, Jacq D, Singlas E, and N'Guyen J: Medical management of peritonitis. In Legrain M (Ed), Continuous ambulatory peritoneal dialysis. Amsterdam: Excerpta Medica, 1980, p 248
3. Rottembourg J, Gahl GM, Poignet JL, Mertani E, Strippoli P, Langlois P, Tranbaloc P, and Legrain M: Severe abdominal complications in patients undergoing continuous ambulatory peritoneal dialysis. Proc Eur Dial Transplant Assoc 20: 236, 1983
4. Gandhi VC, Humayun HM, Ng TS, Daugirdas JT, Jablokow VR, Iwatsuki S, Geis WP, and Hano JE:

Sclerotic thickening of the peritoneal membrane in maintenance peritoneal dialysis patients. Arch Intern Med 140: 1201, 1980

5. Slingeneyer A, Canaud B, Mourad G, Beraud JJ, Balmes M, Faller B, and Mion C: Progressive sclerosing peritonitis: A late and severe complication of maintenance peritoneal dialysis. Trans Am Soc Artif Intern Organs 12: 633, 1983

6. Bradley JA, Hamilton DNH, MacWhinnie DL, Briggs JD, and Junor BJR: Sclerosing peritonitis after CAPD. Lancet 2: 572, 1983

7. Bradley JA, MacWhinnie DL, Hamilton DHH, Starnes F, MacPherson SG, Seywright M, Briggs JD, and Junor BJR: Sclerosing obstructive peritonitis after continuous ambulatory peritoneal dialysis. Lancet 2: 113, 1983

8. Grefberg N, Nilsson P, and Andreen T: Sclerosing obstructive peritonitis; beta-blockers and continuous ambulatory peritoneal dialysis. Lancet 2: 733, 1983

9. Hauglustaine D, Monballuy J, vanMeerbeek J, Godderis P, Lauwerijns J, and Michielsen P: Sclerosing obstructive peritonitis beta-blockers and continuous ambulatory peritoneal dialysis. Lancet 2: 734, 1983

10. Oreopoulos DG, Khanna R, and Wu G: Sclerosing obstructive peritonitis after CAPD. Lancet 2: 409, 1983

11. Thomson NM, Atkins RC, Hooke D, Maydom B, and Scott DF: Long term clinical experience with continuous ambulatory peritoneal dialysis in Australia. In Atkins RC, Thomson NM, Farrell PC (Eds), Peritoneal dialysis. Edinburgh: Churchill Livingstone, 1981, p 93

12. Denis J, Paineau J, Potel G, Fontenaille C, and Guenel J: Continuous ambulatory peritoneal dialysis. Ann Intern Med 93: 508, 1980

13. Rottembourg J, Jacq D, Vonlanthen M, Issad B, and El Shahat Y: Straight or curled Tenckhoff peritoneal catheter for continuous ambulatory peritoneal dialysis. Peritoneal Dial Bull 1: 123, 1981

14. deGroc F, Rottembourg J, Jacq D, Jarlier V, N'Guyen J, and Legrain M: Les péritonites au cours de la dialyse péritonéale continue ambulatoire. Traitement par lavage ou non. Etude prospective. Nephrologie 4: 24, 1983

15. Oreopoulos DG: Peritoneal membrane handle with care. Peritoneal Dial Bull 3: 111, 1983

16. Verger C, Brunschvig O, LeCharpentier Y, Lavergne A, and Vantelon J: Structural and ultrastructural peritoneal membrane changes and permeability alterations during CAPD. Proc Eur Dial Transplant Assoc 18: 199, 1981

17. Verger C, Luger A, Moore H, and Nolph KD: Acute changes in peritoneal morphology and transport properties with infectious peritonitis and mechanical injury. Kidney Int 23: 823, 1983

18. Singer H, Rapoport A, and Crassweller PO: A case of terminal renal disease maintened for 134 days by intermittent peritoneal dialysis. Canad Med Assoc J 90: 1318, 1964

19. Lasker N, Burke JF, Patchefsky A: Peritoneal reactions to particulate matter in peritoneal dialysis solutions. Trans Am Soc Artif Intern Organs 21: 342, 1975

20. Karanicolas S, Oreopoulos DG, Izatt SH: Epidemic of aseptic peritonitis caused by endotoxin during chronic peritoneal dialysis. N Engl J Med 296: 1336, 1977

21. Binswanger U, Banmatter F, Keush G, Schiffl H, and Koller M: Chemical peritonitis during CAPD. In Legrain M (Ed), Continuous ambulatory peritoneal dialysis. Amsterdam: Excerpta Medica, 1980, p 238

22. Faller B, and Marichal JF: Loss of ultrafiltration in CAPD: Clinical data. In Gahl GM, Kessel M, Nolph KD (Eds), Advances in peritoneal dialysis. Proceedings of the 2nd international symposium on peritoneal dialysis. Amsterdam: Excerpta Medica, 1981, p 227

23. Junor BJR, Personal communication, 1984

24. Slingeneyer A, Canaud B, and Mion C: Permanent loss of ultrafiltration capacity of the peritoneum in long-term peritoneal dialysis: An epidemiological study. Nephron 33: 133, 1983

25. Factors effecting ultrafiltration in continuous ambulatory peritoneal dialysis: An international cooperative study. Peritoneal Dial Bull 4: 14, 1984

26. Rubin J, Nolph KD, and Arfania D: Comparison of the effects of lactate and acetate on clinical peritoneal clearances. Clin Nephrol 12: 145, 1979

27. LaGreca G, Basioli S, Chiaramonte S, Fabris A, Feriani M, Pisani E, and Ronco C: Acetate, lactate and bicarbonate kinetics in peritoneal dialysis. In Atkins RC, Thomson NM, Farrell PC (Eds), Peritoneal dialysis. Edinburgh, Churchill Livingstone, 1981, p 217

28. Marshall AJ, Baddeley H, Barritt OW, Davies JD, Lee REJ, Low-Beer TS, and Read AE: Practolol peritonitis: A study of 16 cases and a survey of small bowel function in patients taking beta adrenergic blockers. Q J Med New Series 46: 145, 1977

29. Harty R: Sclerosing peritonitis and propranolol. Arch Intern Med 138: 1424, 1978

30. Ahmad S: Sclerozing peritonitis and propranolol. Chest 79: 361, 1981

31. Marigold JH, Pounder RE, Pemberton J, Thompson RPH: Propranolol, oxprenolol and sclerosing peritonitis. Br Med J 284: 870, 1982

Index